handbook

S0-EAZ-826

Clinical
Drug Data

ninth edition

handbook of
Clinical Drug Data

ninth edition

EDITORS

Philip O. Anderson, PharmD, FASHP, FCSHP
Director, Drug Information Service, Department of Pharmacy
University of California Medical Center, San Diego, California
Clinical Professor of Pharmacy
University of California, San Francisco, California
San Diego Program

James E. Knoben, PharmD, MPH
Office of Clinical Standards and Quality
Health Care Financing Administration
Baltimore, Maryland

William G. Troutman, PharmD, FASHP
Regents' Professor of Pharmacy, College of Pharmacy
University of New Mexico, Albuquerque, New Mexico

APPLETON & LANGE
Stamford, Connecticut

Copyright © 1999 by Appleton & Lange
A Simon & Schuster Company
Copyright © 1997 by Appleton & Lange
Copyright © 1993 by Drug Intelligence Publications, Inc., Hamilton, Illinois

www.appletonlange.com

99 00 01 02 / 10 9 8 7 6 5 4 3 2 1

Prentice Hall International (UK) Limited, *London*
Prentice Hall of Australia Pty. Limited, *Sydney*
Prentice Hall Canada, Inc., *Toronto*
Prentice Hall Hispanoamericana, S.A., *Mexico*
Prentice Hall of India Private Limited, *New Delhi*
Prentice Hall of Japan, Inc., *Tokyo*
Simon & Schuster Asia Pte. Ltd., *Singapore*
Editora Prentice Hall do Brasil Ltda., *Rio de Janeiro*
Prentice Hall, *Upper Saddle River, New Jersey*

ISSN 1090–7971

Editor-in-Chief: Cheryl L. Mehalik
Production Editor: Mary Ellen McCourt
Designer: Janice Bielawa

ISBN 0-8385-3563-1

9 780838 535639

90000

Contributors

Brian K. Alldredge, PharmD
Professor of Clinical Pharmacy and Clinical Professor of Neurology, Departments of Clinical Pharmacy and Neurology, University of California, San Francisco, California

Andrea J. Anderson, PharmD
Clinical Program Head, Respiratory and Zyban, Clinical Applications Research, U.S. Medical Affairs Division, Glaxo Wellcome Inc., Research Triangle Park, North Carolina

Philip O. Anderson, PharmD, FASHP, FCSHP
Director, Drug Information Service, Department of Pharmacy, University of California Medical Center, San Diego, California; Clinical Professor of Pharmacy, University of California, San Francisco, California, San Diego Program

Lisa W. Ashton, PharmD
Business Manager, Advanced Healthcare Services, a division of Bristol-Myers Squibb, Princeton, New Jersey

Arasb Ateshkadi, PharmD
Assistant Professor, Western University of Health Sciences, College of Pharmacy, Pomona, California

Craig R. Ballard, PharmD, FCSHP
Antiviral and Cytokine Program Coordinator, Owen Clinic, University of California Medical Center, San Diego, California; Assistant Clinical Professor of Pharmacy, University of California, San Francisco, San Diego Program

Jerry L. Bauman, PharmD, FACC, FCCP
Professor of Pharmacy Practice, Sections of Cardiovascular Pharmacotherapy and Cardiology, University of Illinois at Chicago, Chicago, Illinois

Rosemary R. Berardi, PharmD, FASHP
Professor of Pharmacy, College of Pharmacy, University of Michigan, Ann Arbor, Michigan; Clinical Pharmacist, Gastroenterology, Department of Pharmacy Services, University of Michigan Health System, Ann Arbor, Michigan

Lawrence R. Borgsdorf, PharmD, FCSHP
Pharmacist Specialist—Ambulatory Care, Kaiser Permanente Medical Care Program, Bakersfield, California; Adjunct Professor of Clinical Pharmacy, School of Pharmacy, University of the Pacific, Stockton, California

R. Keith Campbell, BPharm, MBA
Associate Dean and Professor of Pharmacy Practice, College of Pharmacy, Washington State University, Pullman, Washington

Larry Jay Davis, PharmD
Manager, Medical Information, Gilead Sciences Inc., Foster City, California; Associate Clinical Professor of Pharmacy, University of California, San Francisco, California

Ernest J. Dole, PharmD, FASHP, BCPS
Associate Professor of Pharmacy, College of Pharmacy, The University of New Mexico, Albuquerque, New Mexico

Betty J. Dong, PharmD
Professor of Clinical Pharmacy, Department of Clinical Pharmacy; Clinical Professor of Family and Community Medicine, Division of Family and Community Medicine, University of California, San Francisco, California

Robert T. Dorr, PhD
Professor of Pharmacology, Pharmacology Department, College of Medicine, Arizona Cancer Center, University of Arizona, Tucson, Arizona

David G. Dunlop, PharmD, MPA
Chief, Inpatient Pharmacy Services, Wilford Hall Medical Center, Lackland AFB, San Antonio, Texas

John F. Flaherty, Jr., PharmD, FCCP, BCPS
Professor of Clinical Pharmacy, Department of Clinical Pharmacy, University of California, San Francisco

John G. Gambertoglio, Pharm D
Professor of Pharmacy and Biopharmaceutical Sciences, Department of Clinical Pharmacy, School of Pharmacy, University of California at San Francisco, San Francisco, California

Mildred D. Gottwald, PharmD
Assistant Clinical Professor of Pharmacy, Department of Clinical Pharmacy, University of California, San Francisco, California

Amy J. Guenette, PharmD, BCPS
Clinical Coordinator, Department of Pharmacy, Wausau Hospital, Wausau, Wisconsin

Philip D. Hansten, PharmD
Professor of Pharmacy, University of Washington, Seattle, Washington

Mark T. Holdsworth, PharmD, BCPS
Associate Professor of Pharmacy, College of Pharmacy, The University of New Mexico, Albuquerque, New Mexico

Brian P. Kearney, PharmD
Clinical Pharmacology Fellow, Drug Research Unit, Department of Clinical Pharmacy, University of California, San Francisco, California

Polly E. Kintzel, PharmD, BCPS
Clinical Pharmacy Specialist, Bone Marrow Transplantation, Harper Hospital, Department of Pharmacy, Detroit, Michigan

James E. Knoben, PharmD, MPH
Office of Clinical Standards and Quality, Health Care Financing Administration, Baltimore, Maryland

James R. Lane, Jr., PharmD
Pharmacist Specialist, Coordinator of Applied Pharmacokinetics, Department of Pharmacy, University of California Medical Center, San Diego, California, Assistant Clinical Professor of Pharmacy, University of California, San Francisco, San Diego Program

William E. Murray, PharmD
Pharmacokinetics Service Coordinator, Pharmacy Department, Children's Hospital, San Diego, California; Assistant Clinical Professor of Pharmacy, University of California, San Francisco, San Diego Program

James J. Nawarskas, PharmD
Assistant Professor of Pharmacy, College of Pharmacy, The University of New Mexico, Albuquerque, New Mexico

Robert E. Pachorek, PharmD, BCPS
Clinical Pharmacist, Mercy Hospital, San Diego, California; Adjunct Assistant Professor of Pharmacy Practice, University of Southern California, Los Angeles, California; Assistant Clinical Professor of Pharmacy, University of California, San Francisco, San Diego Program

Stephen M. Setter, PharmD
Assistant Professor of Pharmacy Practice, College of Pharmacy, Washington State University, Pullman, Washington

Fred Shatsky, BSPharm, BCNSP
Nutrition Support Pharmacist, Department of Pharmacy, University of California Medical Center, San Diego, California; Assistant Clinical Professor of Pharmacy, University of California, San Francisco, California, San Diego Program

Glen L. Stimmel, PharmD, FCCP
Professor of Clinical Pharmacy and Psychiatry, Schools of Pharmacy and Medicine, University of Southern California, Los Angeles, California

Dianne E. Tobias, PharmD
President, Tobias Consulting Services, Davis, California; Assistant Clinical Professor of Pharmacy, University of California, San Francisco

William G. Troutman, PharmD, FASHP
Regents' Professor of Pharmacy, College of Pharmacy, University of New Mexico, Albuquerque, New Mexico

John R. White, Jr., PharmD
Associate Professor, Pharmacy Practice, Washington State University, Spokane, Washington; Director, Washington State University/Sacred Heart Medical Center Drug Studies Unit, Spokane, Washington

James M. Wooten, PharmD
Assistant Professor, School of Medicine, Section of Clinical Pharmacology, Adjunct Assistant Professor, School of Pharmacy, University of Missouri, Kansas City, Missouri

Robin Swett Wooten, PharmD
Clinical Pharmacy Consultant, Lenexa, Kansas

Carolyn R. Zaleon, BSPharm
Ambulatory Care Pharmacist, Department of Pharmacy Services, University of Michigan Health-System, Ann Arbor, Michigan; Clinical Assistant Professor of Pharmacy, College of Pharmacy, University of Michigan, Ann Arbor, Michigan

Contents

Preface

The Ninth Edition of the *Handbook of Clinical Drug Data* marks the first time that a new edition is being published just two years after the previous edition. This more rapid publication schedule is in response to the rapid changes in drug therapy and record number of new drug approvals. We are pleased with the positive feedback we have received on the new format and organization of the *Handbook* introduced in the Eighth Edition. This edition contains further enhancements in organization and content.

Drug Monographs in **Part I** have many improvements. A new subheading, "Missed Doses," has been added to the Patient Instructions section of the monographs. This change makes patient counseling information required by OBRA '90 readily available to the user. Headings have been added to the Minimonograph format to assist in locating the desired data. Entire new sections have been added on monoclonal antibodies for cancer treatment and on neurodegenerative diseases, which includes drugs for Parkinson's disease, amylotropic lateral sclerosis, and Alzheimer's disease. The respiratory drugs section has been reorganized and expanded to better reflect new asthma treatment guidelines and to cover several new drugs. Important expansions have also occurred in the sections on antifungals, antiparasitics, immunosuppressants, and corticosteroids. Finally, many new individual drugs have been added and information on older drugs has been updated.

Clinical Drug Information in **Part II** has a redesigned table format to improve readability and new chapters on drug-induced pancreatitis and on ethnic and pharmacogenetic factors in drug therapy. Information in the chapters on pregnancy and lactation has been reorganized to match the section names and sequence of the drug monographs. In **Part III,** a new **Appendix** on the most useful pharmacokinetic equations has been added.

This edition also marks a turning point for the editorial staff of the *Handbook*. Bill Troutman assumed the major role in co-ordinating and editing Parts II and III and is now listed as an Editor. Larry Davis, whose career path has taken him into the drug industry, no longer serves as an assistant editor. We thank Larry for his many years of hard work and ideas for improving the *Handbook*. We would also like to thank Cheryl Mehalik of Appleton & Lange for her encouragement, and to Mary Ellen McCourt for her responsiveness to the production needs of the *Handbook*. Finally, the *Handbook* would, of course, not be what it is without the skills and knowledge of the many expert clinician–authors. Both their contributions and their forbearance with the editorial process are greatly appreciated.

Philip O. Anderson
James E. Knoben
William G. Troutman
December 1998

How to Use This Book

Part I of this book is organized around 10 major drug categories, which have been subdivided into common therapeutic groups. Within these therapeutic groups, drug information is alphabetically presented in three formats: *Monographs, Minimonographs,* and *Comparison Charts*. Monographs and Comparison Charts are *grouped together* to ensure that related drugs are easy to *compare* and *contrast*. Charts are located after the monographs to which they relate. Drug antagonists are grouped together with agonists to help simplify organization and accessibility.

Monographs are used for drugs of major importance and prototype agents.

Minimonographs are used for drugs similar to prototype drugs, those of lesser importance within a therapeutic class, and promising investigational agents. Minimonographs contain only selected subheadings of information rather than all subheadings contained in the full monographs.

Comparison Charts are used to present clinically useful information on members of the same pharmacologic class and different drugs with a similar therapeutic use, as well as to present clinically relevant information on certain other topics.

The preferred method to gain access to complete information on a *particular brand* or *generic drug* is to use the index at the end of the book. The index may also direct the user to *other pertinent* information on the drug.

MONOGRAPH FORMAT

CLASS INSTRUCTIONS

This is an optional heading at the beginning of each drug class. It consists of patient instructions that apply to more than one of the drug monographs in this subcategory. If all drugs are not identical in their instructions, only the common information is found here. The Patient Instructions section of each monograph that is affected states, *"See Class Instructions"* as the opening phrase.

GENERIC DRUG NAME   Brand Name(s)

The *nonproprietary (generic)* name is listed on the left, followed by common brand names listed on the right. Brand-name products listed are not necessarily superior or preferable to other brand-name or generic products; *"Various"* indicates the availability of additional brand and/or generic products.

Pharmacology. A description of the chemistry, major mechanisms of action, and human pharmacology of the drug in clinical application.

Administration and Adult Dosage. Route of administration, indications, and usual adult dosage range are given for the most common labeled uses. Dosages correspond to those in the product labeling or in standard reference sources. "Dose" refers to a single administration and "dosage" to a cumulative amount (eg, daily dosage).

Special Populations. Dosages in patient populations other than the typical adult are listed:

Pediatric Dosage (given by age or weight range)

Geriatric Dosage (given by age range)

Other Conditions (renal failure, hepatic disease, obesity, etc.)

Dosage Forms. The most commonly used dosage forms and available strengths are listed, as well as popular combination product dosage forms. Prediluted IV piggyback or large-volume parenteral containers are not listed unless this is the only commercially available product.

Patient Instructions. Key information that should be provided to the patient when prescribing or dispensing medication is presented. When introductions apply to an entire drug category, see "Class Instructions" at the beginning of that subcategory.

Missed Doses. What the patient should do if one or more doses are missed.

Pharmacokinetics. Data are presented as the mean $\pm$ the standard deviation. Occasionally the standard error of the mean (SE) is the only information available on variability, and it is identified as such.

Onset and Duration (time course of the pharmacologic or therapeutic effect)

Serum Levels (therapeutic and toxic plasma concentrations are given)

Fate (The course of the drug in the body is traced. Pharmacokinetic parameters are generally provided as total body weight normalized values. The volume of distribution is either a V_d in a one-compartment system or V_c and $V_{d\beta}$ in a two-compartment system.)

$t_{1/2}$ (terminal half-life is presented)

Adverse Reactions. Reactions known to be dose related are usually given first, then other reactions in decreasing order of frequency. Reaction frequency is classified into three ranges. However, percentages of reactions are provided for reactions that occur more frequently than 1%.

frequent	*(>1/100 patients)*
occasional	*(1/100 to 1/10,000 patients)*
rare	*(<1/10,000 patients)*

Contraindications. Those listed in product labeling are given. "Hypersensitivity" is not listed as a contraindication because it is understood that patients should not be given a drug to which they are allergic or hypersensitive.

Precautions. Warnings for use of the drug in certain disease states and/or patient populations, together with any cross-sensitivity with other drugs. Part II, Chapter 3, "Drug Use in Special Populations," should be consulted for more information particularly regarding pregnancy and breastfeeding.

Drug Interactions. The most important drug interactions are listed.

Parameters to Monitor. Important clinical signs and/or laboratory tests to monitor to ensure safe and effective use are presented. The frequency of monitoring may also be given; however, for many drugs the optimal frequency has not been determined.

Notes. Distinguishing characteristics, therapeutic usefulness, or relative efficacy of the drug are presented, as well as unique or noteworthy physicochemical properties, handling, storage, or relative cost.

Part

I

DRUG MONOGRAPHS

- ANALGESIC AND ANTI-INFLAMMATORY DRUGS
- ANTIMICROBIALS
- ANTINEOPLASTICS, CHEMOPROTECTANTS AND IMMUNOSUPPRESSANTS
- CARDIOVASCULAR DRUGS
- CENTRAL NERVOUS SYSTEM DRUGS
- GASTROINTESTINAL DRUGS
- HEMATOLOGIC DRUGS
- HORMONAL DRUGS
- RENAL AND ELECTROLYTES
- RESPIRATORY DRUGS

Analgesic and Anti-inflammatory Drugs ℞

Antimigraine Drugs

DIHYDROERGOTAMINE MESYLATE

D.H.E. 45, Migranal

Pharmacology. Dihydroergotamine (DHE) is a semisynthetic ergot alkaloid that is hypothesized to exert its antimigraine effect via its agonist activity at the serotonin 5-HT_{1D} receptor, resulting in vasoconstriction of intracranial blood vessels and inhibition of inflammatory neuropeptide release.[1,2] The drug also binds with high affinity to adrenergic and dopamine receptors; however, the antimigraine effect of these events is unknown. Compared to ergotamine, dihydroergotamine is a weaker vasoconstrictor, is less active as an emetic, and is less oxytocic.

Administration and Adult Dosage. **IM** 1 mg initially, then 1 mg q 1 hr prn, to a maximum of 3 mg/day or 6 mg/week. **IV** (for rapid effect) 0.5 mg, may repeat in 1 hr to a maximum of 2 mg/day or 6 mg/week. **Intranasal** one spray (0.5 mg) into each nostril; may repeat in 15 min to a maximum of 2 mg over a 24-hr period.

Special Populations. *Pediatric Dosage.* Safety and efficacy not established.

Geriatric Dosage. Same as adult dosage.

Dosage Forms. **Inj** 1 mg/mL; **Nasal Spray** 4 mg/mL.

Patient Instructions. This drug may cause numbness and tingling in fingers, toes, or face. Notify your physician if you are pregnant or have heart disease or high blood pressure. Do not exceed the maximum dosage. The nasal spray may cause local irritation. Do not reuse the applicator; use the solution right after opening. Review training materials with your health care provider and report the use of all cold or allergy medications and all over-the-counter medications.

Pharmacokinetics. *Onset and Duration.* Onset under 5 min IV, within 15–30 min after IM or intranasal spray; duration 3–4 hr. Intranasal 50–70% of patients respond in 4 hr.

Fate. The drug is absorbed directly into the systemic circulation when administered intranasally, but it undergoes extensive first-pass metabolism if given orally. Bioavailability of the nasal spray is $38 \pm 16\%$, variable depending on self-administration technique.[3] Protein binding is 93%. After administration of 1 mg, peak levels are 1 ± 0.4 μg/L (intranasal) and 4.4 μg/L (IM), occurring at 0.9 ± 0.6 hr (intranasal) and 0.4 ± 0.3 hr (IM).[3] After IM administration, V_c is 12 ± 4 L/kg, and Vd_β is 33 ± 0.2 L/kg, suggesting distribution into deep tissue compartments. Cl is 1.6 ± 0.17 L/hr/kg. The drug is metabolized to at least five metabolites, three of which are active. The major route of excretion for DHE and its metabolites is in the feces via the bile.[2,3]

3

$t_{1/2}$. α phase (intranasal) 1 ± 0.5 hr, (IM) 0.9 ± 0.3 hr; β phase (intranasal) 7.9 ± 4 hr, (IM) 7.2 ± 2.2 hr.[3]

Adverse Reactions. The most frequently reported adverse events with intranasal administration are rhinitis, pharyngitis, altered sense of taste, application site reactions, nausea, vomiting, and dizziness. With all routes of administration, nausea, vomiting, diarrhea, and localized edema occur frequently.[4,5] Occasional numbness and tingling of fingers and toes, muscle pain in extremities, weakness in legs, pruritus, rash, and infection occur. Rarely pleural and retroperitoneal fibrosis occur with prolonged use.

Contraindications. Pregnancy and lactation; peripheral vascular disease; coronary artery disease; ischemic heart disease; hemiplegic or basilar migraine; sepsis; recent history of vascular surgery; severely impaired hepatic or renal function; hypersensitivity to ergot alkaloids.

Precautions. Use caution to avoid overuse by patients with chronic vascular headaches. Patients with risk factors for coronary artery disease should undergo periodic cardiovascular evaluation.

Drug Interactions. (*See* Ergotamine Tartrate.) Dihydroergotamine may antagonize the antianginal effects of nitrates. The risk of bleeding with warfarin (eg, wound hematoma, anemia, hematuria) is worsened with co-administration of dihydroergotamine. Macrolides including erythromycin and troleandomycin may increase the risk of ergot toxicity. Sumatriptan may exacerbate coronary artery vasospasm and should not be taken within 24 hr of DHE. SSRIs may cause weakness, hyperreflexia, or incoordination.

Notes. IV dihydroergotamine is used when oral agents have failed to abort migraine and for terminating cluster or migraine headache in an emergency setting. It is not intended for prophylaxis or for the management of hemiplegic or basilar migraine. The intranasal preparation is a noninvasive option for outpatients. Intranasal administration also results in improved bioavailability over the oral form since it does not undergo a first-pass effect in the liver. Dihydroergotamine does not cause physical dependence and is associated with a more favorable side effect profile than ergotamine, especially with regard to GI and peripheral vascular effects. In one study, subcutaneously administered **sumatriptan** appeared to be more effective than DHE nasal spray; however, DHE was better tolerated.[6]

ERGOTAMINE TARTRATE   Ergomar, Ergostat, Various

Pharmacology. Ergotamine is an ergot alkaloid that is hypothesized to exert its antimigraine effects via its agonist activity at the serotonin 5-HT$_{1D}$ receptor, resulting in vasoconstriction of intracranial blood vessels and inhibition of inflammatory neuropeptide release. The drug also binds with high affinity to adrenergic receptors; however, the antimigraine effect of this binding is unknown. The mechanism in migraine is thought to be vasoconstriction of cranial blood vessels, with a concomitant decrease in the amplitude of pulsations as well as depression of serotonergic neurons that mediate pain.

Administration and Adult Dosage. *PO for migraine* 2 mg initially, then 1 mg each ½ hr prn, to a maximum of 6 mg/day or 10 mg/week; **PR** 2 mg initially, may repeat in 1 hr prn, to a maximum of 4 mg/attack or 10 mg/week; **SL** 2 mg initially, then 2 mg q 30 min as needed, to a maximum of 6 mg/day or 10 mg/week.[7] Titrate the dosage during several attacks gradually, then administer the minimum effective dosage with subsequent attacks. Patients who routinely require over 2 mg/headache can be given the total effective dosage at the onset of the headache.

Special Populations. *Pediatric Dosage.* Safety and efficacy not established. (Over 12 yr) 1 mg initially, then 1 mg q 30 min prn, to a maximum of 3 mg/attack.

Geriatric Dosage. No specific data are available.

Other Conditions. Decrease dosage by 50% in patients receiving methysergide as prophylaxis.

Dosage Forms. **SL Tab** 2 mg; **Tab** 1 mg with caffeine 100 mg (Cafergot, Ercaf, various); **Supp** 2 mg with caffeine 100 mg (Cafergot, Wigraine).

Patient Instructions. Initiate therapy at the first signs of an attack. Take only as directed and do not exceed recommended dosages. Report tingling or pain in extremities immediately.

Pharmacokinetics. *Onset and Duration.* Onset (oral) 5 hr; (rectal) 1–3 hr.[7]

Serum Levels. 200 ng/L (176 pmol/L) or greater may be therapeutic; a high frequency of adverse reactions has been associated with levels above 1.8 µg/L (1.5 nmol/L).[7]

Fate. Bioavailability 1–2% orally, 5% rectally; relative bioavailability decreases in the following order: PR > PO > SL.[7,8] Peak serum level after 2 mg rectally is 454 ± 407 ng/L (390 ± 350 pmol/L), 50 ± 43 min after the dose. Peak serum level after 2 mg with caffeine 100 mg orally is 21 ± 12 ng/L (18 ± 11 pmol/L), 69 ± 191 min after the dose.[8] V_d is 1.9 ± 0.8 L/kg; Cl is 0.68 ± 0.24 L/hr/kg.[9] The drug is extensively metabolized in the liver, with 90% of metabolites excreted in the bile.

$t_{1/2}$. 1.9 ± 0.3 hr; apparent half-life is 3.4 ± 1.9 hr after rectal administration because of slow absorption.[7,8]

Adverse Reactions. Nausea and vomiting occur frequently. Signs and symptoms of ergotamine intoxication include weakness in legs, coldness and muscle pain in extremities, numbness or tingling of fingers and toes, precordial pain, transient tachycardia or bradycardia, and localized edema; these rarely develop with recommended dosages. Frequent or worsening headaches can occur with frequent, long-term, or excessive dosages. Ergotamine dependence may result in withdrawal symptoms occurring within 24–48 hr following drug discontinuation.[7,10] Rectal or anal ulceration may occur with suppository use.

Contraindications. Pregnancy; peripheral vascular disease; coronary artery disease; hypertension; hepatic or renal impairment; sepsis; severe pruritus.

Precautions. Lactation; avoid excessive dosage or prolonged administration because of the potential for ergotism and gangrene.

Drug Interactions. β-Blockers, dopamine, and epinephrine can cause increased vasoconstriction and increased risk of peripheral ischemia or hypertension. The macrolides (especially erythromycin and troleandomycin) may inhibit the metabolism of ergot alkaloids.

Notes. The stimulant action of preparations containing **caffeine** may keep patients from the beneficial effects of sleep. Caffeine, however, may improve dissolution of the oral formulation. Ergotamine is commonly used for abortive therapy of migraine and provides relief in 50–90% of patients.[7] **Aspirin** (650 mg) or **naproxen** (750–1250 mg/day) may be effective in aborting migraine headache in mild cases or in patients who cannot take ergotamine. **Sumatriptan** appears to be more effective than ergotamine/caffeine in aborting migraine.[11] For migraine prophylaxis, **propranolol** with an initial dose of 80 mg, to a maximum of 320 mg/day, calcium-channel blocking drugs (**verapamil** or **nimodipine**), and **valproate** have been used successfully.[12]

METHYSERGIDE MALEATE   Sansert

Pharmacology. Methysergide is a semisynthetic ergot alkaloid, thought to act centrally as a serotonin agonist and to inhibit blood vessel permeability to humoral factors that affect pain threshold. Unlike other ergots, methysergide does not inhibit reuptake of norepinephrine and has minimal oxytocic, vasoconstrictor, and α-adrenergic blocking effects. Because of its toxicity, methysergide is usually used only after other prophylactic measures fail.

Adult Dosage. PO for migraine or cluster headache prophylaxis 4–8 mg/day with food. A drug-free interval of 3–4 weeks must follow each 6-month course; however, reduce the dosage gradually to avoid rebound headache.

Dosage Forms. Tab 2 mg.

Pharmacokinetics. Methysergide undergoes extensive liver metabolism to **methylergonovine**, a compound with greater activity and a longer elimination half-life than the parent drug (3.5 hr vs 1 hr). About 56% of an oral dose is eliminated in the urine as unchanged drug and metabolites.

Adverse Reactions. Insomnia, postural hypotension, nausea, vomiting, diarrhea, and peripheral ischemia occur frequently. Occasionally, heartburn, peripheral edema, rash, or arrhythmias occur. Rarely, mental depression occurs. Long-term (>6 months) therapy may cause retroperitoneal and pleuropulmonary fibrosis, and thickening of cardiac valves. The drug is contraindicated in peripheral vascular, cardiovascular, or pulmonary disease; phlebitis; pregnancy; and impaired liver or kidney function. Precautions and drug interactions are similar to ergotamine.[13]

NARATRIPTAN HYDROCHLORIDE   Amerge

Pharmacology. Naratriptan is a selective serotonin agonist at 5-HT$_{1B/1D}$ receptors that has relatively low affinity at other receptor subtypes (5-HT$_{2-5}$, 5-HT$_7$). This leads to vasoconstriction of intracranial blood vessels and inhibition of the release of inflammatory neuropeptides in the trigeminal system. Headache relief after 4 hr is similar to **sumatriptan;** however, at 24 hr, a greater percentage of patients have relief with naratriptan (53% vs 44%). Fewer patients receiving naratriptan have migraine recurrence than with sumatriptan (29% vs 44%).[14,15]

Adult Dosage. PO for migraine 2.5 mg once, to a maximum of 5 mg/24 hr. The benefits of a second dose to prevent recurrence are unknown, and it is recommended to re-evaluate the diagnosis of migraine prior to administration of a second dose.

Dosage Forms. **Tab** 2.5 mg.

Pharmacokinetics. PO 60–66% of patients respond in 4 hr. Naratriptan is rapidly and well absorbed with a bioavailability of 68% and peak plasma levels 3–4 hr after administration of a 2.5 mg oral dose during a migraine attack. Naratriptan is about 30% bound to plasma proteins. Approximately 80% of orally administered naratriptan is excreted in urine, 50% as unchanged drug and 30% as hepatic metabolites. The mean elimination half-life is 6 hr.[16]

Adverse Reactions. Adverse effects are similar to **sumatriptan** and include nausea, dizziness, drowsiness, malaise/fatigue, and pain and pressure sensations in the throat and neck. Smoking increases the clearance of the drug, whereas oral contraceptives reduce the clearance by about 32%. Contraindications are similar to those of sumatriptan; in addition, the drug is contraindicated in patients with severe renal or hepatic impairment.

Contraindications. (*See* Sumatriptan.)

RIZATRIPTAN BENZOATE   Maxalt

Pharmacology. Rizatriptan is a selective serotonin agonist at $5\text{-HT}_{1B/1D}$ receptors that has relatively low affinity at other receptor subtypes (5-HT_{1A}, $5\text{-HT}_{1E,1F}$). This leads to vasoconstriction of intracranial blood vessels and inhibition of the release of inflammatory neuropeptides in the trigeminal system. A 10 mg dose is the most efficacious, 5 mg is the best tolerated. The percentage of patients achieving headache response 2 hr after a dose are 60–62% for the 5 mg tablet and 67–77% for the 10 mg dose.

Adult Dosage. **PO for migraine** 5–10 mg; subsequent doses should be separated by at least 2 hr with no more than 30 mg taken in 24 hr. The rapidly dissolving tablet packet should be opened immediately prior to use and placed on the tongue with dry hands where it will dissolve and be swallowed with saliva.

Dosage Forms. **Tab** (conventional and rapidly dissolving [Maxalt-MLT]) 5, 10 mg.

Pharmacokinetics. Rizatriptan is rapidly and well absorbed with a bioavailability of 45%. It undergoes marked first-pass metabolism in the liver and undergoes oxidative deamination via monoamine oxidase A and demethylation to form a minor metabolite with activity similar to the parent compound. The conventional tablet has peak serum level at 1–1.5 hr after oral administration; the rapidly dissolving tablet taken without water is slightly slower in onset with a peak at 1.6–2.5 hr. Plasma concentrations are increased by 30% with hepatic impaired subjects and the AUC was increased by 44% in renally impaired subjects. About 14% of rizatriptan is bound to plasma proteins and the V_d is about 2 L/kg. The plasma elimination half-life averages 2–3 hr.

Adverse Reactions. Nausea, dizziness, dry mouth, headache, insomnia, and fatigue occur occasionally. Like other "triptan" agents it may cause pain and pressure in the chest and neck. Although the drug is a competitive inhibitor of CYP2D6, the reaction is unimportant at usual doses.

Contraindications. (*See* Sumatriptan.)

SUMATRIPTAN SUCCINATE   Imitrex

Pharmacology. Sumatriptan is a serotonin (5-HT) analogue and a selective agonist at $5-HT_{1D}$ receptors in cerebral vascular smooth muscle. Receptor activation results in migraine relief by both vasoconstriction of intracranial blood vessels and attenuation of the release of vasoactive peptides responsible for inflammation of sensory nerves.[17–19]

Administration and Adult Dosage. **PO for migraine** 25–100 mg; a second dose of up to 100 mg may be administered in 2 hr if response is unsatisfactory. If headache returns, additional doses may be given q 2 hr, up to 300 mg in a 24-hr period.[20] **SC for migraine** 6 mg; a second 6 mg injection may be administered 1 hr after the initial dose, but limited to no more than 2 injections within a 24-hr period. Controlled studies have not verified a beneficial effect of a second dose. **Intranasal** 5–20 mg in one nostril or 5 mg in each nostril; may repeat in 2 hr to a maximum of 40 mg/day.

Special Populations. *Pediatric Dosage.* (<18 yr) safety and efficacy not established.

Geriatric Dosage. Same as adult dosage.

Dosage Forms. **Tab** 25, 50 mg; **Inj** 6 mg/0.5 mL; **Nasal Spray** 5, 20 mg.

Patient Instructions. Sumatriptan is used for relief of migraine and not for the prevention of a migraine attack. Do not take this drug if you are pregnant or breastfeeding without consulting with your physician. Inform your physician if you have high blood pressure, diabetes, seizures, or heart, liver, or kidney disease. Report pain or tightness in chest, shortness of breath, wheezing, or rash immediately. **Oral.** Do not take more than 300 mg within 24 hours, and allow at least 2 hours after the first tablet. **SC Injection.** Do not take more than 2 injections within 24 hours, and allow at least 1 hour between injections. Pain or redness at injection site lasts less than 1 hour. **Nasal Spray.** If one dose does not give adequate relief, you may take another dose after 2 hours. Do not take more than 40 mg in one day.

Pharmacokinetics. *Onset and Duration.* PO 50% of patients respond in 2 hr; peak 1.5 hr. SC 70% of patients respond within 1 hr and 90% within 2 hr;[21] peak 10–15 min.[22] **Intranasal** 50–60% of patients respond in 2 hr.

Fate. Oral bioavailability is 14 ± 3% owing to presystemic metabolism and erratic absorption. Absorption is delayed by about 0.5 hr if taken with food. After a 100 mg oral dose, a peak of 54 ng/mL (0.13 μmol/L) occurs in about 1.5 hr. SC bioavailability is 97 ± 16%; a peak of 74 ng/mL (0.18 μmol/L) occurs in 12 min. After a 20 mg intranasal dose, the mean peak is 16 ng/L (6 μmol/L). Plasma protein binding is 14–21%. V_d is 2.7 L/kg; Cl is 0.96 ± 0.12 L/hr/kg. Hepatic metabolism is by monoamine oxidase A to an indole acetic acid, followed by glucuronidation and renal elimination. About 40% is found in the feces and 60% is excreted renally, 22% unchanged, and 40% as the active indole acetic acid metabolite.[23–25]

$t_{1/2}$. 1.9 ± 0.3 hr.[25]

Adverse Reactions. Frequent side effects include pain and redness at SC injection site, tingling, hot flushes, dizziness, and chest tightness or heaviness. With the nasal spray, throat discomfort and unusual taste occur frequently. With all routes of administration, occasional weakness, myalgia, burning sensation, tightness in chest, transient hypertension, drowsiness, headache, numbness, neck pain, abdominal discomfort, mouth/jaw discomfort, and sweating occur. Rarely, cardiac arrhythmias, myocardial ischemia, polydipsia, dehydration, dyspnea, skin rashes, dysuria, and dysmenorrhea occur. The drug may accumulate in melanin-rich tissues such as the eye with long-term use.

Contraindications. IV administration; ischemic heart disease; Prinzmetal's angina; uncontrolled hypertension; concurrent administration of MAO inhibitors or within 2 weeks of discontinuation; within 24 hr of an ergotamine-containing drug or ergot derivative such as methysergide or dihydroergotamine; hemiplegic or basilar migraine.

Precautions. Pregnancy. Use with caution in those with impaired hepatic function, seizure disorder, neurologic lesion, or cardiovascular disease; postmenopausal women; or men over 40 yr.

Drug Interactions. Nonselective MAO inhibitors or MAO-A inhibitors can increase the systemic availability of sumatriptan (especially after oral administration). Theoretically, ergot alkaloids and sumatriptan may cause prolonged vasospastic reactions if used together. (*See* Contraindications.)

Parameters to Monitor. Renal, hepatic, and cardiovascular status initially and q 6 months.

Notes. Sumatriptan is much more expensive than alternatives. It is effective in the treatment of cluster headache and appears to be more effective than ergotamine/caffeine in aborting migraine.[11]

ZOLMITRIPTAN   Zomig

Pharmacology. Zolmitriptan is a highly selective serotonin agonist at 5-HT$_{1B/1D}$ receptors. Activation of these receptors results in the reduction of neurogenic inflammation by inhibition of peptide release, vasoconstriction, and inhibition of neuronal depolarization at sites within the trigemino-vascular system.[26] The drug has relatively low affinity for 5-HT$_{1A}$ or 5-HT$_{1F}$ receptors. In addition to its peripheral effects, zolmitriptan is also active centrally at the brain stem level; however, the clinical relevance of this additional action is unknown. Due to its subtype selectivity, zolmitriptan may prove to be an important antimigraine agent in the setting of multiple attacks. One preliminary study showed **sumatriptan** and zolmitriptan to be equally effective and well tolerated; however, a large placebo effect occurred.[27] Larger-scale studies are needed to determine which agent should be the first-line therapy for aborting acute migrainous attacks and preventing their recurrence.

Adult Dosage. PO 2.5–5 mg. In one study a second 5 mg dose was used to treat recurrence (32% of patients); a good headache response occurred in 90% of these attacks.[28]

Dosage Forms. Tab 2.5, 5 mg.

Pharmacokinetics. Peak effect occurs in 1 hr; about 62–67% of patients respond in 2 hr.[26,28] Oral bioavailability is approximately 40%.[27] Zolmitriptan is metabolized in the liver to two inactive metabolites and one active metabolite that is up to 6 times more potent than the parent compound. Although the drug has an elimination half-life of 2.5–3 hr, its duration may be longer because elevated plasma concentrations are maintained up to 6 hr.

Adverse Reactions. Asthenia, nausea, somnolence, dizziness, and paresthesia occur. No drug interactions have been demonstrated with acetaminophen, metoclopramide, dihydroergotamine, ergotamine, or propranolol.[26]

Contraindications. (*See* Sumatriptan.)

Nonsteroidal Anti-inflammatory Drugs

ACETAMINOPHEN   Various

Pharmacology. Acetaminophen is an analgesic and antipyretic with weak anti-inflammatory action. It has the same potency as aspirin in inhibiting brain prostaglandin synthetase, but very little activity as an inhibitor of cyclo-oxygenase. Unlike other NSAIDs, it does not inhibit neutrophil activation. These differences may explain its relative lack of anti-inflammatory activity. Acetaminophen does not cause the GI erosion and bleeding associated with aspirin and has no effect on platelet function.[29]

Administration and Adult Dosage. **PO for pain or fever** (non-SR) 650–1000 mg q 4–6 hr, to a maximum of 4 g/day; (SR Tab) 1300 mg q 8 hr. **PR for pain or fever** 650 mg q 4–6 hr, to a maximum of 4 g/day.

Special Populations. *Pediatric Dosage.* **PO for pain or fever** 10–15 mg/kg q 4–8 hr, to a maximum of 5 doses/day; or (up to 3 months) 40 mg/dose, (4–11 months) 80 mg/dose, (12–23 months) 120 mg/dose, (2–3 yr) 160 mg/dose, (4–5 yr) 240 mg/dose, (6–8 yr) 320 mg/dose, (9–10 yr) 400 mg/dose, (11 yr) 480 mg/dose, to a maximum of 5 doses/day. **PR for pain or fever** (3–6 yr) 120 mg q 4–6 hr, to a maximum of 720 mg/day; (6–12 yr) 325 mg q 4–6 hr, to a maximum of 2.6 g/day; (over 12 yr) same as adult dosage.

Geriatric Dosage. Same as adult dosage.

Dosage Forms. **Cap** 325, 500 mg; **Chew Tab** 80 mg; **SR Tab** 650 mg; **Tab** 160, 325, 500, 650 mg; **Gran** 80, 325 mg; **Drp** 48, 100 mg/mL; **Elxr** 16, 24, 26, 32, 65 mg/mL; **Syrup** 32 mg/mL; **Supp** 80, 120, 125, 300, 325, 650 mg.

Patient Instructions. Do not exceed the maximum recommended daily dosage of 4 grams.

Missed Doses. If you take this drug on a regular schedule and you miss a dose, take it as soon as you remember. If it is about time for the next dose, take that dose only. Do not double the dose or take extra.

Pharmacokinetics. *Serum Levels.* (Analgesia, antipyresis) 10–20 mg/L (66–132 μmol/L). Serum concentrations over 300 mg/L (2 mmol/L) at 4 hr or 45 mg/L (300 μmol/L) at 12 hr following acute overdosage are associated with severe hepatic damage, whereas toxicity is unlikely if levels are under 120 mg/L (800 μmol/L) at 4 hr or 30 mg/L (200 μmol/L) at 12 hr.[25] (*See* Notes.)

Fate. Rapidly absorbed from GI tract, with 88 ± 15% bioavailability. Essentially unbound to plasma proteins at therapeutic doses; 20–50% bound in overdose. Extensively metabolized in the liver to inactive conjugates of glucuronic and sulfuric acids (saturable), and to a hepatotoxic intermediate metabolite (first-order) by CYP1A2 and CYP2E1. The intermediate is detoxified by glutathione (saturable). V_d is 0.95 ± 0.12 L/kg; Cl is 0.3 ± 0.084 L/hr/kg, decreased in hepatitis and increased in hyperthyroidism, pregnancy, and obesity; 3% excreted unchanged in urine.[25]

$t_{1/2}$. 2 ± 0.5 hr, decreased in hyperthyroidism and pregnancy, and increased in hepatitis and neonates.[25]

Adverse Reactions. In acute overdose, potentially fatal hepatic necrosis and possible renal tubular necrosis can occur, but clinical and laboratory evidence of hepatotoxicity may be delayed for several days. (*See* Serum Levels.) Toxic hepatitis has also been associated with long-term ingestion of 5–8 g/day for several weeks or 3–4 g/day for a year. Occasionally, erythematous or urticarial skin reactions occur; methemoglobinemia is reported rarely. Analgesic nephropathy has been associated with the consumption of 1–15.3 kg of acetaminophen over periods of 3–23 yr.[30]

Precautions. Use with caution in chronic alcoholics and in patients with G-6-PD deficiency.

Drug Interactions. Chronic alcoholics may be at increased risk for hepatic toxicity.[31] The risk of hepatotoxicity may also be increased by long-term use of other enzyme inducers (eg, barbiturates, carbamazepine, phenytoin, rifampin); acetaminophen's efficacy may also be decreased by these agents.

Notes. For the short-term treatment of osteoarthritis of the knee, acetaminophen 2.6 and 4 g/day are comparable to **naproxen** 750 mg/day and **ibuprofen** 1.2–2.4 g/day, respectively.[32] Management of acute overdosage includes emesis or gastric lavage, if no more than a few hours have elapsed since ingestion. Administration of activated charcoal is not recommended, because it may interfere with the absorption of acetylcysteine, which is used in the treatment of severe acute overdosage. Potentially dangerous acetaminophen levels (*see* Serum Levels) can be managed by the administration of 140 mg/kg acetylcysteine diluted 1:3 in a soft drink or plain water; follow with 70 mg/kg q 4 hr for 17 doses. If administered within 8–16 hr of ingestion, this therapy has been shown to minimize the expected hepatotoxicity, but treatment is still indicated as late as 24 hr after ingestion. This 72-hr oral regimen appears to be as effective as the 20-hr IV regimen, and may be superior when treatment is delayed.[29]

ASPIRIN   Various

Pharmacology. Aspirin is an analgesic, antipyretic, and anti-inflammatory agent. Anti-inflammatory properties are related to impairment of prostaglandin biosynthesis. Aspirin nonselectively inhibits both cyclo-oxygenase-1 (COX-1), which is associated with GI and renal effects and inhibition of platelet aggregation, and cyclo-oxygenase-2 (COX-2), which is associated with the inflammatory response. Unlike other NSAIDs, its antiplatelet effect is irreversible (because of transacetylation of platelet cyclo-oxygenase) for the life of the platelet (8–11 days). Salicylates without acetyl groups (eg, **sodium salicylate**) have essentially no antiplatelet effect but retain analgesic, antipyretic, and anti-inflammatory activity. Low dosages (1–2 g/day) decrease urate excretion; high dosages (>5 g/day) induce uricosuria.[29,33]

Administration and Adult Dosage. **PO or PR for fever or minor pain** 325–1000 mg q 4 hr, to a maximum of 4 g/day. **PO for arthritis and rheumatic conditions** 3.6–5.4 g/day in divided doses. **PO for acute rheumatic fever** 5–8 g/day in divided doses. **PO for prevention of transient ischemic attacks or stroke** 325–1300 mg/day in divided doses. Although higher dosages (975–1300 mg/day) are associated with slightly higher risk of GI hemorrhage, there is some evidence that they are also more effective.[34] **PO for myocardial infarction risk reduction** (primary prevention in healthy men over 50 yr with cardiovascular risk factors) 160–325 mg/day; (secondary prevention) 160–325 mg/day.[35] **PO for unstable angina** 160–325 mg/day with full dose IV heparin therapy.[35] **PO for prevention of coronary artery bypass graft occlusion** 325 mg/day started 6 hr postoperatively and continued indefinitely.[36] **PO for nonrheumatic atrial fibrillation** (patients who are poor candidates for, or decline, oral anticoagulants only) 325 mg/day; (patients under 65 yr with no stroke risk factors) 325 mg/day, although some experts recommend no antithrombotic therapy in this situation.[37]

Special Populations. *Pediatric Dosage.* **PO for juvenile rheumatoid arthritis** 60–110 mg/kg/day in divided doses. **PO for acute rheumatic fever** 100 mg/kg/day in divided doses initially for 2 weeks, then 75 mg/kg/day in divided doses for 4–6 weeks. **PO for Kawasaki disease** 80–120 mg/kg/day; decrease to 10 mg/kg/day after fever resolves. (*See* Precautions.) **PO as an analgesic/antipyretic** 10–15 mg/kg/dose q 4 hr, to a maximum of 60–80 mg/kg/day. Alternatively, (2–3 yr) 162 mg q 4 hr; (4–5 yr) 243 mg q 4 hr; (6–8 yr) 325 mg q 4 hr; (9–10 yr) 405 mg q 4 hr; (11 yr) 486 mg q 4 hr; (12 yr and over) 650 mg q 4 hr. (*See* Precautions.)

Geriatric Dosage. Use minimal effective dosages because the elderly are more susceptible to GI bleeding and acute renal insufficiency. **PO for myocardial infarction risk reduction** (healthy men over 50 yr for primary prevention with cardiovascular risk factors) 160–325 mg/day.[35]

Other Conditions. Uremia or reduced albumin levels are likely to produce higher unbound drug levels, which may increase pharmacologic or toxic effects. Dosage reduction may be required in these patients.

Dosage Forms. **Chew Tab** 81 mg; **EC Tab** 81, 165, 325, 500, 650, 975 mg; **SR Tab** 650, 800 mg; **Tab** 81, 325, 500 mg; **Supp** 120, 200, 300, 600 mg.

Patient Instructions. Children and teenagers should not use this medication for chickenpox or flu symptoms before a physician or pharmacist is consulted about Reye syndrome, a rare but serious illness. Take this drug with food, milk, or a full glass of water to minimize stomach upset; report any symptoms of GI ulceration or bleeding. Do not crush or chew enteric-coated or sustained-release preparations.

Missed Doses. If you take this drug on a regular schedule and you miss a dose, take it as soon as you remember. If it is about time for the next dose, take that dose only. Do not double the dose or take extra.

Pharmacokinetics. ***Onset and Duration.*** PO onset of analgesia 30 min.[25]

Serum Levels. (Salicylate) 150–300 mg/L (1.1–2.2 mmol/L) for rheumatic diseases, often accompanied by mild toxic symptoms. Tinnitus occurs at 200–400 mg/L (1.5–2.9 mmol/L), hyperventilation at greater than 350 mg/L (2.6 mmol/L), acidosis at greater than 450 mg/L (3.3 mmol/L), and severe or fatal toxicity at levels greater than 900 mg/L (6.6 mmol/L) 6 hr after acute ingestion.[38,39]

Fate. Rapidly absorbed from the GI tract; oral bioavailability of aspirin is 68 ± 3%. Enteric coating does not adversely affect absorption.[40] A single analgesic/antipyretic dose produces peak salicylate levels of 30–60 mg/L (0.22–0.44 mmol/L). Aspirin is 49% plasma protein bound, decreased in uremia; V_d is 0.15 ± 0.03 L/kg; Cl is 0.56 ± 0.07 L/hr/kg; 1.4% excreted unchanged in the urine. Aspirin is rapidly hydrolyzed to salicylic acid (salicylate), which is also pharmacologically active. Salicylate is metabolized primarily in the liver to four metabolites (salicyluric acid, phenolic and acyl glucuronides, and gentisic acid). Salicylate plasma protein binding is dose dependent, 95% at 15 mg/L and 80% at 300 mg/L, and decreased in uremia, hypoalbuminemia, neonates, and pregnancy; V_d is 0.17 ± 0.03 L/kg; Cl is dose dependent, 0.012 L/hr/kg at 134–157 mg/L, and decreased in hepatitis and neonates. From 2 to 30% is excreted unchanged in the urine, depending on dose and urine pH.[25]

$t_{1/2}$. (Aspirin) 0.25 ± 0.03 hr.[25] (Salicylate) dose dependent: 2.4 hr with 0.25 g, 5 hr with 1 g, 6.1 hr with 1.3 g, 19 hr with 10–20 g.[41]

Adverse Reactions. Hearing impairment, GI upset, and occult bleeding are frequent, with rare acute hemorrhage from gastric erosion. Enteric coating reduces GI bleeding.[40] As with other NSAIDs, aspirin may cause renal dysfunction, particularly in those with pre-existing renal disease or CHF.[29] Rare hepatotoxicity occurs, primarily in children with rheumatic fever or rheumatoid arthritis and adults with SLE or pre-existing liver disease[42,43]; the syndrome of asthma, angioedema, and nasal polyps may be provoked in susceptible patients.[44] A single analgesic dose may suppress platelet aggregation and prolong bleeding time for up to 1 week; large dosages may prolong PT.[45]

Precautions. Use with caution in patients with renal disease, gastric ulcer, bleeding tendencies, hypoprothrombinemia, or history of asthma, or during anticoagulant therapy. Because of the association with Reye's syndrome, the use of salicylates in children and teenagers with flu-like symptoms or chickenpox is not recommended.[46,47] Those developing bronchospasm with aspirin may develop a similar reaction to other NSAIDs.[44] Sodium salicylate and other nonacetylated salicylates (except diflunisal) are usually well tolerated in these patients.[46,48]

Drug Interactions. Alkalinizing agents (eg, acetazolamide, antacids) can reduce salicylate levels; acetazolamide may also enhance CNS penetration of salicylate. Corticosteroids can reduce serum salicylate levels. Large doses of salicylates can increase oral anticoagulant effect; even small doses can increase risk of bleeding with oral anticoagulants or heparin because of the antiplatelet effect of aspirin. Alcohol and salicylate may cause an enhanced risk of GI blood loss. Salicylates may cause an increased response to sulfonylureas, especially chlorpropamide. Salicylate decreases the uricosuric effect of uricosuric agents. Salicylate, especially in large doses, may decrease renal elimination of methotrexate and displace it from plasma protein binding sites.

Parameters to Monitor. Monitor for occult GI blood loss (periodic hematocrit, stool guaiac) in patients who ingest salicylates regularly. Serum salicylate level determinations are recommended with higher dosage regimens because of the wide variation among patients in serum levels produced. Using tinnitus as an index of maximum salicylate tolerance is *not* recommended.[38]

COX-2 INHIBITORS

CELECOXIB (Investigational–Searle)	Celebrex
MELOXICAM (Investigational–Boehringer Ingelheim)	Mobic
MK-966 (Investigational–Merck)	Vioxx

Pharmacology. Inhibition of the cyclo-oxygenase-2 (COX-2) enzyme isoform is thought to be responsible for NSAID anti-inflammatory efficacy, whereas inhibition of the cyclo-oxygenase-1 (COX-1) results in gastric and renal side effects. A relatively selective COX-2 inhibitor should combine anti-inflammatory efficacy equivalent to older, nonselective NSAIDs with improved safety. Many compounds are being studied, each with different relative selectivity for COX-1 and COX-2. In vitro tests indicate that celecoxib and MK-966 are the most selective of drugs in late stage trials, with COX-2/COX-1 activity ratios >1000. COX-2 inhibitors are being studied in rheumatoid arthritis and osteoarthritis, and as analgesics.[55-57]

Adult Dosage. PO (celecoxib) 100–400 mg bid investigationally; (meloxicam) 7.5–15 mg/day investigationally. Dosages over 15 mg/day appear to lose COX-2 selectivity; (MK-966) 12.5–25 mg/day investigationally.

Pharmacokinetics. (Meloxicam) Oral bioavailability is 89% with peak levels at steady-state occurring 5–6 hr after administration. It is 99.5% plasma protein bound. Meloxicam is metabolized extensively (up to 99%) in the liver with a half-life of 20 hr.[56]

Adverse Reactions. Safety analysis of various clinical trials suggests that COX-2 inhibitors cause GI toxicity, dyspepsia, abdominal pain, nausea, vomiting, and diarrhea at a rate similar to placebo and less than conventional NSAIDs. Whether these differences will prove to be clinically useful is still unclear. Renal and liver effects are equivalent to other NSAIDs.[55-57]

IBUPROFEN   Advil, Motrin, Nuprin, Various

Pharmacology. Ibuprofen is a nonsteroidal anti-inflammatory agent with analgesic and antipyretic properties. It is a nonselective inhibitor of cyclo-oxygenase-1 (COX-1) and cyclo-oxygenase-2 (COX-2), and it reversibly alters platelet function and prolongs bleeding time.

Administration and Adult Dosage. **PO for mild to moderate pain** 400 mg q 4–6 hr prn. **PO for primary dysmenorrhea** 400 mg q 4 hr prn. **PO for rheumatoid arthritis and osteoarthritis** 400–800 mg tid or qid, to a maximum of 3.2 g/day.

Special Populations. *Pediatric Dosage.* **PO for fever** (over 12 months) 5–10 mg/kg q 6–8 hr, to a maximum of 40 mg/kg/day. **PO for juvenile arthritis** 30–70 mg/kg/day in 3 or 4 divided doses; 20 mg/kg/day in milder disease.

Geriatric Dosage. Use minimal effective dosages because the elderly are more susceptible to GI bleeding and acute renal insufficiency.

Dosage Forms. **Cap** 400 mg; **Chew Tab** 50, 100 mg; **Tab** 100, 200, 300, 400, 600, 800 mg; **Drp** 40 mg/mL; **Susp** 20 mg/mL.

Patient Instructions. This drug may be taken with a small amount of food, milk, or antacid to minimize stomach upset. Report any symptoms of GI ulceration or bleeding, skin rash, weight gain, or edema. Dizziness may occur; until the extent of this effect is known, use appropriate caution.

Missed Doses. If you take this drug on a regular schedule and you miss a dose, take it as soon as you remember. If it is about time for the next dose, take that dose only. Do not double the dose or take extra.

Pharmacokinetics. *Serum Levels.* 10 mg/L (48 μmol/L) for antipyretic effect.[25] Serum concentrations over 200 mg/L (971 μmol/L) 1 hr after acute overdosage may be associated with severe toxicity (apnea, metabolic acidosis, and coma).[49]

Fate. Rapidly absorbed from the GI tract with bioavailability over 80%.[25] Peak serum levels in children of 17–42 mg/L (82–204 μmol/L) following a dose of 5 mg/kg and 25–53 mg/L (121–257 μmol/L) following a dose of 10 mg/kg are achieved in 1.1 ± 0.3 hr.[50] Greater than 99% plasma protein bound; metabolized to at least two inactive metabolites; V_d is 0.15 ± 0.02 L/kg, increased in cystic fibrosis; Cl is 0.045 ± 0.012 L/hr/kg, increased in cystic fibrosis. Less than 1% is excreted unchanged in the urine.[25]

$t_{1/2}$. 2 ± 0.5 hr.[25]

Adverse Reactions. Gastric distress, occult blood loss, diarrhea, vomiting, dizziness, and skin rash occur occasionally; GI ulceration (for all NSAIDs there is a greater risk in the elderly and with higher dosages) and fluid retention have been reported.[51] May occasionally cause renal dysfunction, particularly in those with pre-existing renal disease, CHF, or cirrhosis.[52] Rarely, a slight rise in the Ivy bleeding time, elevation of liver enzymes, lymphopenia, agranulocytosis, aplastic anemia, and aseptic meningitis have been reported.[53,54]

Contraindications. Syndrome of nasal polyps; angioedema; bronchospastic reactivity to aspirin or other NSAIDs.

Precautions. Avoid during pregnancy. Use with caution in patients with pre-existing renal disease, CHF, or cirrhosis[52]; a history of ulcer disease or bleeding; or risk factors associated with peptic ulcer disease (alcohol and smoking).

Drug Interactions. NSAIDs may inhibit the antihypertensive response to ACE inhibitors, ß-blockers, diuretics, and hydralazine, and also inhibit the natriuretic effect of diuretics. Possible GI bleeding and the antiplatelet effect of NSAIDs may increase the risk of serious bleeding during anticoagulant therapy. NSAIDs may decrease renal lithium clearance. Some NSAIDs (especially indomethacin and ketoprofen) reduce methotrexate clearance. Indomethacin (and probably other NSAIDs) may reduce renal function when combined with triamterene.

Parameters to Monitor. Monitor for occult blood loss, weight gain, and renal function during long-term use.

Notes. **Misoprostol** is the most effective therapy in preventing NSAID-associated GI ulceration; H_2-receptor antagonists, however, prevent duodenal, but not gastric, ulcerations. The role of **omeprazole** and **sucralfate** for prevention of GI ulceration is not firmly established.[51]

INDOMETHACIN   Indocin, Various

Pharmacology. Indomethacin is an indoleacetic acid NSAID that is one of the most potent nonselective inhibitors of cyclo-oxygenase available. In addition to its anti-inflammatory effects, indomethacin has prominent analgesic and antipyretic properties. Indomethacin is approved for treatment of rheumatoid arthritis, ankylosing spondylitis, osteoarthritis, acute gouty arthritis, acute painful shoulder, and pharmacologic closure of persistent patent ductus arteriosus in premature infants. It has also been used to suppress uterine activity and prevent premature labor.

Adult Dosage. PO for rheumatoid arthritis, rheumatoid (ankylosing) spondylitis, and osteoarthritis of the hip 25 mg bid or tid initially. Increase in 25 mg/day increments at weekly intervals until satisfactory response or to a maximum of 150–200 mg/day. Alternatively, up to 100 mg of the daily dosage may be given hs for persistent night or morning stiffness. **PO for acute gouty arthritis** 100 mg, followed by 50 mg tid until resolved. **SR Cap** 75 mg 1–2 times/day can be substituted for all uses except gouty arthritis, based on the non-SR dosage.

Pediatric Dosage. IV for pharmacologic closure of persistent patent ductus arteriosus in premature infants 0.2 mg/kg, followed by 2 additional **IV** doses of 0.1–0.25 mg/kg (depending on age) at 12- to 24-hr intervals. Alternatively, give 0.3 mg/kg as a single dose, or 1 or more doses of 0.1 mg/kg as a retention enema or via orogastric tube.[25,29,45]

Dosage Forms. Cap 25, 50 mg; **SR Cap** 75 mg; **Supp** 50 mg; **Susp** 5 mg/mL; **Inj** 1 mg.

Pharmacokinetics. Indomethacin is rapidly and well absorbed from the GI tract, with a bioavailability of 98%. Peak serum levels are reached within 2 hr with effective concentrations in the range of 0.3–3 mg/L (0.8–8 μmol/L). It is 90% plasma protein bound and has extensive O-demethylation and N-deacylation to inactive metabolites; V_d is 0.29 ± 0.04 L/kg; Cl is 0.084 ± 0.012 L/hr/kg, lower in premature infants, neonates, and the aged; $15 \pm 8\%$ is excreted unchanged in the urine. The half-life of the drug is 2.4 ± 0.4 hr, higher in premature infants, neonates, and the aged.

Adverse Reactions. Adverse effects are frequent, with about 20% of patients unable to tolerate the drug. Frontal lobe headache, drowsiness, dizziness, mental confusion, and GI distress are frequent, especially with dosages greater than 100 mg/day; occasional peripheral neuropathy, occult bleeding, and peptic ulcer occur. Rarely, pancreatitis, corneal opacities, hepatotoxicity, aplastic anemia, agranulocytosis, thrombocytopenia, aggravation of psychiatric disorders, and allergic reactions are reported. The syndrome of asthma, angioedema, and nasal polyps may be provoked in susceptible patients. Precautions, drug interactions, and monitoring are similar to other NSAIDs. (*See* Ibuprofen.)

| **NAPROXEN** | Naprosyn |
| **NAPROXEN SODIUM** | Anaprox |

Pharmacology. (*See* Ibuprofen.)

Administration and Adult Dosage. PO for mild to moderate pain, dysmenorrhea, or acute tendinitis or bursitis (naproxen) 500 mg, followed by 250 mg q 6–8 hr, to a maximum of 1250 mg/day; (naproxen sodium) 550 mg, followed by 275 mg q 6–8 hr, to a maximum of 1375 mg/day. PO for rheumatoid arthritis, osteoarthritis, and ankylosing spondylitis (naproxen) 250–500 mg bid initially, to a maximum of 1500 mg/day for limited periods; (naproxen sodium) 275–550 mg bid or 275 mg q morning and 550 mg q evening initially, to a maximum of 1650 mg/day for limited periods. If no improvement has occurred after 4 weeks of therapy, consider other drug therapy. PO for acute gout (naproxen) 750 mg, followed by 250 mg q 8 hr until resolved; (naproxen sodium) 825 mg, followed by 275 mg q 8 hr until resolved.

Special Populations. *Pediatric Dosage.* PO for juvenile arthritis 10 mg/kg/day in 2 divided doses.

Geriatric Dosage. Use minimal effective dosages because the elderly are more susceptible to GI bleeding and acute renal insufficiency.

Dosage Forms. Tab (naproxen) 250, 375, 500 mg; (naproxen sodium) 220, 275, 550 mg; EC Tab (naproxen) 375, 500 mg; SR Tab (naproxen sodium) 375, 500, 750 mg; Susp (naproxen) 25 mg/mL.

Patient Instructions. (*See* Ibuprofen.)

Pharmacokinetics. *Serum Levels.* Trough concentrations >50 mg/L (>217 μmol/L) are associated with response in rheumatoid arthritis.[25]

Fate. Rapidly absorbed from the GI tract with a bioavailability of about 99%. Greater than 99.7% plasma protein bound, saturable with increasing dosage, increased with uremia, cirrhosis, and in the elderly, and decreased in rheumatoid arthritis and hypoalbuminemia; V_d is 0.16 ± 0.02 L/kg, increased in uremia, cirrhosis, and rheumatoid arthritis. Cl is 0.0078 ± 0.0012 L/hr/kg, increased in rheumatoid arthritis and decreased in uremia; less than 1% is excreted unchanged in urine.[25]

$t_{1/2}$. 14 ± 1 hr, increased in the elderly.[25]

Adverse Reactions. May occasionally cause renal dysfunction, particularly in those with pre-existing renal disease, CHF, or cirrhosis. Interstitial nephritis and nephrotic syndrome have been reported.[58,59] (*See* Ibuprofen.)

Contraindications. (*See* Ibuprofen.)

Precautions. (*See* Ibuprofen.)

Drug Interactions. (*See* Ibuprofen.)

Parameters to Monitor. (*See* Ibuprofen.)

Notes. (*See* Ibuprofen and Nonsteroidal Anti-inflammatory Drugs Comparison Chart.)

NONSTEROIDAL ANTI-INFLAMMATORY DRUGS COMPARISON CHART

CLASS AND DRUG	DOSAGE FORMS	ADULT DOSAGE	HALF-LIFE (HR)	COX SELECTIVITY[a]		COMMENTS
				COX-1	COX-2	
ACETIC ACIDS						
Diclofenac Cataflam Voltaren Various	Tab (diclofenac) 25, 50, 75 mg Tab (diclofenac potassium) 50 mg SR Tab (diclofenac sodium) 75, 100 mg Tab (diclofenac sodium) 50, 75 mg plus misoprostol 200 μg (Arthrotec).	PO (pain, dysmenorrhea) (Cataflam) 50 mg tid; PO (arthritis) 100–200 mg/day in 2 doses. PO SR 100 mg once or twice daily (dosages expressed as diclofenac).	1.1 ± 0.2	++	++	Although it is unclear whether the risk of hepatotoxicity is any greater than with other NSAIDs, careful monitoring of symptoms and liver function tests is recommended.
Etodolac Lodine Various	Cap 200, 300, 400, 500 mg.	PO (pain) 200–400 mg q 6–8 hr; PO (arthritis) 600–1200 mg/day in 2–3 divided doses.	7.3 ± 4	++	++	Recommended for treatment of osteoarthritis; not as effective as other NSAIDs for rheumatoid arthritis.
Indomethacin Indocin Various	Cap 25, 50 mg SR Cap 75 mg Susp 5 mg/mL Supp 50 mg Inj 1 mg.	PO (gouty arthritis) 100 mg, then 50 mg tid; PO or PR (arthritis) 50–200 mg/day in 3 divided doses. SR in 1–2 doses, may substitute for equal daily dosage of non-SR.	2.4 ± 0.4	+++	+	*See* monograph. Associated with a high frequency of CNS effects such as drowsiness, dizziness, mental confusion, and frontal lobe headache.

(continued)

NONSTEROIDAL ANTI-INFLAMMATORY DRUGS COMPARISON CHART (continued)

CLASS AND DRUG	DOSAGE FORMS	ADULT DOSAGE	HALF-LIFE (HR)	COX SELECTIVITY[a] COX-1	COX-2	COMMENTS
Ketorolac Toradol Various	Tab 10 mg Inj 15, 30, 60 mg.	PO (pain, short term) 10 mg q 4–6 hr prn, to a maximum of 40 mg/day for 5 days (including IM/IV). IM or IV (short-term management of pain) 30 or 60 (IM only) mg once, then 15–30 mg q 6 hr.	4.5	—	—	For short-term (up to 5 days) use only. Do not exceed 60 mg/day parenterally in patients 65 yr or over, under 50 kg, or with elevated Cr$_s$.
Sulindac Clinoril	Tab 150, 200 mg.	PO (arthritis) 300–400 mg/day in 2 divided doses.	15 ± 4 (active sulfide metabolite)	—	—	Purported "renal-sparing" effect has been questioned. Because the active sulfide metabolite has a relatively long half-life, renal effects may not be observed for several days.
Tolmetin Tolectin Various	Cap 400 mg Tab 200, 600 mg.	PO (arthritis) 0.6– 1.8 g/day in 3–4 divided doses.	4.9 ± 0.3	—	—	Higher frequency of anaphylactoid reactions than other NSAIDs.

(continued)

NONSTEROIDAL ANTI-INFLAMMATORY DRUGS COMPARISON CHART (continued)

CLASS AND DRUG	DOSAGE FORMS	ADULT DOSAGE	HALF-LIFE (HR)	COX SELECTIVITY[a] COX-1	COX SELECTIVITY[a] COX-2	COMMENTS
ANTHRANILIC ACIDS (FENAMATES)						
Meclofenamate Meclomen Various	Cap 50, 100 mg.	PO (pain) 50 mg q 4–6 hr; PO (arthritis) 200–400 mg/day in 3–4 divided doses.	3	—	—	The fenamates as a group are more toxic than other NSAIDs and associated with headache, dizziness, and hemolytic anemia.
Mefenamic Acid Ponstel	Cap 250 mg.	PO (pain, dysmenorrhea) 250 mg q 6 hr for up to 1 week.	3	—	—	Not recommended; *see* Meclofenamate Comments.
NONACIDIC COMPOUNDS						
Nabumetone Relafen	Tab 500, 750 mg Chew Tab 1 g.	PO (arthritis) 1–2 g/day in 1–2 doses.	23 ± 4 (active 6-MNA metabolite)	++	++	Some cyclo-oxygenase-2 selectivity. Reported to have less GI toxicity than other NSAIDs; however, additional well-controlled, double-blind studies are needed.
OXICAMS						
Meloxicam Mobic (Investigational–Boehringer-Ingeheim)	—	PO (arthritis) 7.5–15 mg once daily.	20	+	+++	Greater cyclo-oxygenase-2 selectivity than nabumetone. Less mucosal damage than piroxicam.

(*continued*)

CLASS AND DRUG	DOSAGE FORMS	ADULT DOSAGE	HALF-LIFE (HR)	COX SELECTIVITY[a] COX-1	COX SELECTIVITY[a] COX-2	COMMENTS
Piroxicam Feldene Various	Cap 10, 20 mg.	PO (arthritis) 20 mg/day in 1–2 doses.	48 ± 8	++	++	Based on postmarketing surveillance data, reported to cause about 12 times more GI adverse effects than ibuprofen. High frequency of phototoxic cutaneous eruptions.
PROPIONIC ACIDS						
Fenoprofen Nalfon	Cap 200, 300 mg Tab 600 mg.	PO (pain) 200 mg q 4–6 hr; PO (arthritis) 1.2–2.4 g/day in 3–4 divided doses.	2.5 ± 0.5	—	—	Similar to ibuprofen.
Flurbiprofen Ansaid	Tab 50, 100 mg.	PO (arthritis) 200–300 mg/day in 2–4 divided doses.	3.8 ± 1.2	—	—	Similar to ibuprofen.
Ibuprofen Advil Motrin Nuprin Various	Cap 400, Chew Tab 50, 100 mg Tab 100, 200, 300, 400, 600, 800 mg Drp 40 mg/mL Susp 20 mg/mL	PO (pain, dysmenorrhea) 400 mg q 4–6 hr; PO (arthritis) 1.2–3.2 g/day in 3–4 divided doses.	2 ± 0.5	++	+	*See* monograph.
Ketoprofen Orudis Oruvail Various	Cap 25, 50, 75 mg Tab 12.5 mg SR Cap 100, 150, 200 mg.	PO (pain) 25–50 mg q 6–8 hr; PO (arthritis) 150–300 mg/day in 3 divided doses. PO SR 200 mg/day in 1 dose.	1.8 ± 0.3	—	—	Similar to ibuprofen.

(continued)

21

NONSTEROIDAL ANTI-INFLAMMATORY DRUGS COMPARISON CHART (continued)

CLASS AND DRUG	DOSAGE FORMS	ADULT DOSAGE	HALF-LIFE (HR)	COX SELECTIVITY[a] COX-1	COX SELECTIVITY[a] COX-2	COMMENTS
Naproxen Aleve Anaprox Naprelan Naprosyn Various	Tab (naproxen sodium) 220, 275, 550 mg Tab (naproxen) 250, 375, 500 mg EC Tab (naproxen) 375, 500 mg SR Tab (naproxen) 375, 500, 750 mg Susp (naproxen) 25 mg/mL.	PO (pain) 500 mg, then 250 mg q 6–8 hr; PO (arthritis) 0.5–1.25 g/day in 2 divided doses. PO (acute gout) 750 mg, then 250 mg q 8 hr. (Doses expressed as naproxen.)	14 ± 1	+++	+	*See* monograph.
Oxaprozin Daypro	Tab 600 mg.	PO (arthritis) 1.2 g/day in 1 dose.	50–60	—	—	Similar to other NSAIDs.
SALICYLATES						
Aspirin Various	*See* monograph.	PO (pain) 325–650 mg q 4 hr; PO (arthritis) 3.6–5.4 g/day in 3–4 divided doses.[b]	0.25 ± 0.03 (aspirin) 2–19 (salicylate, dose dependent)	+++	+	*See* monograph.
Choline Magnesium Trisalicylate Trilisate	Tab 500, 750 mg, 1g Liquid 100 mg/mL.	PO (pain, arthritis) 1.5–3 g/day in 1–2 divided doses.[b]	2–19 (salicylate, dose dependent)	—	—	Salicylate is only a weak inhibitor of cyclo-oxygenase. It therefore has no antiplatelet effect and can usually be administered safely to individuals with aspirin sensitivity. *See* also Aspirin monograph.

(continued)

NONSTEROIDAL ANTI-INFLAMMATORY DRUGS COMPARISON CHART (continued)

CLASS AND DRUG	DOSAGE FORMS	ADULT DOSAGE	HALF-LIFE (HR)	COX SELECTIVITY[a] COX-1	COX SELECTIVITY[a] COX-2	COMMENTS
Diflunisal Dolobid Various	Tab 250, 500 mg.	PO (arthritis) 250–500 mg bid.	11 ± 2 (dose dependent)	—	—	Not converted to salicylate; similar to other NSAIDs.
Magnesium Salicylate Doan's Various	Tab 325, 500, 545, 600 mg.	PO (pain, arthritis) 3.6–4.8 g/day in 3–4 divided doses.[b]	2–19 (salicylate, dose dependent)	—	—	*See* Choline Magnesium Trisalicylate comments and Aspirin monograph.
Salsalate Disalcid Various	Cap 500 mg Tab 500, 750 mg.	PO (arthritis) 3 g/day in 2–3 divided doses.[b]	2–19 (salicylate, dose dependent)	—	—	*See* Choline Magnesium Trisalicylate comments and Aspirin monograph.

+++ = very high; +++ = high; ++ = moderate; + = low; — = unknown.

[a]Relative cyclo-oxygenase-1 (COX-1) and cyclo-oxygenase-2 (COX-2) inhibitory selectivity. Inhibition of COX-1 causes gastric and renal side effects; inhibition of COX-2 correlates with anti-inflammatory efficacy. Not all drugs have been studied for relative COX inhibition.

[b]Long-term dosage for arthritis should be guided by serum salicylate levels; *see* Aspirin monograph.

Adapted from references 25, 29, 45, 55–65, and product information.

Opioids

Class Instructions. This drug may cause drowsiness. Until the extent of this effect is known, use caution when driving, operating machinery, or performing other tasks requiring mental alertness. Avoid excessive concurrent use of alcohol and other drugs that cause drowsiness. Prolonged use of this drug may cause constipation, and concurrent use of a stool-softening or stimulant laxative may be helpful.

For moderate to severe pain (pain rating >5 on a 0–10 scale), you must take doses at regular intervals around the clock to anticipate and prevent pain. When the drug is taken at the correct time interval and pain relief does not last for this period of time, additional "rescue" doses of a short-acting drug should be used to maintain pain relief. When more than 4 rescue doses are used in a day, contact the prescriber for a dosage increase. Addiction does not occur when these drugs are used for legitimate painful conditions. Dependence, a condition in which the body may go through withdrawal when the drug is stopped rapidly, may occur with prolonged usage but can be managed by slowly tapering the dose when the drug is no longer necessary.

Missed Doses. If you miss a dose, take it as soon as you remember. If it is about time for the next dose, take that dose only. Do not double the dose or take extra. Take subsequent doses at the same time interval previously established for pain relief.

CODEINE SALTS   Various

Pharmacology. Codeine is 3 methoxymorphine, a phenanthrene opioid with very low affinity for opioid receptors. Its analgesic activity appears to result from conversion to morphine. Poor metabolizers of debrisoquine/sparteine (approximately 7% of the Caucasian population) are unable to convert appreciable amounts of codeine to morphine and obtain no analgesia from codeine.[66–68] (*See* Morphine Sulfate.)

Administration and Adult Dosage. **PO, SC, or IM for analgesia** 15–60 mg q 4–6 hr. **PO or SC for antitussive action** 10–20 mg q 4–6 hr, to a maximum of 120 mg/day. **IV** not recommended. (*See* Precautions.)

Special Populations. *Pediatric Dosage.* **PO, SC, or IM for analgesia** (1 yr and older) 0.5 mg/kg q 4–6 hr. **PO for antitussive action** (2–6 yr) 2.5–5 mg q 4–6 hr, to a maximum of 30 mg/day; (7–12 yr) 5–10 mg q 4–6 hr, to a maximum of 60 mg/day; (over 12 yr) same as adult dosage. (*See* Notes.)

Geriatric Dosage. Same as adult dosage.[78]

Other Conditions. Reduce initial dosage in debilitated patients or those with hypoxia or hypercapnia.

Dosage Forms. **Tab** 15, 30, 60 mg; **Hyp Tab** 15, 30, 60 mg; **Inj** 30, 60 mg/mL; **Oral Liquid** 2, 2.4 mg/mL in various combinations. Formulated as phosphate or sulfate salt.

Patient Instructions. (*See* Opioids Class Instructions.)

Pharmacokinetics. *Onset and Duration.* PO, SC onset 15–30 min; IM peak analgesia 0.5–1 hr; duration (all routes) 4–6 hr.[69]

Fate. Systemic availability averages 40%, but with a wide range (12–84%), reflecting large variability in hepatic enzyme activity.[70] A single PO 15 mg dose produces serum levels of 26–33 μg/L (82–104 nmol/L) in 2 hr and 13–22 μg/L (41–69 nmol/L) in 5 hr.[71] The drug is 7% plasma protein bound. V_d is 2.6 ± 0.3 L/kg; Cl is 0.66 ± 0.12 L/hr/kg.[25] Metabolized in the liver to codeine-6-glucuronide, N-demethylated to norcodeine and O-demethylated to morphine by genetic polymorphic CYP2D6. Codeine-6-glucuronide is the major metabolite, and norcodeine and morphine are minor metabolites, each accounting for approximately 10% of the dose.[68] Accumulation of morphine occurs with repeated administration, resulting in a morphine/codeine AUC ratio of 0.29:1.[72] Variation in the reported rates of codeine conversion to morphine may be related to the assays used, with much higher concentrations of morphine reported with radioimmunoassays than with HPLC or GC-MS.[70] Primarily urinary excretion of inactive forms; 3–16% is excreted unchanged in urine.[73]

$t_{1/2}$. 2.9 ± 0.7 hr.[25]

Adverse Reactions. Sedation, dizziness, nausea, vomiting, constipation, and respiratory depression occur frequently. Dose-related signs of intoxication include miosis, drowsiness, decreased rate and depth of respiration, bradycardia, and hypotension. Dose-related adverse reactions in children include somnolence, ataxia, miosis, and vomiting at 3–5 mg/kg/day and respiratory depression at >5 mg/kg/day. Because hepatic glucuronidation is incomplete in infants, they may be at particular risk for dose-related adverse effects.[74]

Precautions. Because it can cause severe hypotension, codeine phosphate should not be administered IV.[75,76]

Drug Interactions. Potent CYP2D6 inhibitors (eg, quinidine, fluoxetine) can abolish the conversion to morphine and the pharmacologic effects of codeine.[77,78]

Notes. Codeine is no more effective than placebo in suppressing nighttime cough in children. The American Academy of Pediatrics recommends that parents be educated about the lack of proven antitussive effects and the potential risks of codeine-containing products, because overdosage has been reported.[74]

FENTANYL Duragesic, Fentanyl Oralet, Sublimaze, Various

Pharmacology. Fentanyl is a phenylpiperidine opioid agonist with predominant effects on the mu opioid receptor and is about 50–100 times more potent as an analgesic than morphine. Other related compounds include **sufentanil** (Sufenta), which is 5–7 times more potent than fentanyl; **alfentanil** (Alfenta), which is less potent than fentanyl but acts more rapidly and has a shorter duration of action; and **remifentanil** (Ultiva), which has 5–10 times the potency of fentanyl and is extremely short acting because of its rapid ester hydrolysis.[66,67] (*See* Morphine Sulfate.)

Administration and Adult Dosage. IV **patient-controlled analgesia (PCA)** 20–100 µg per activation with 3–10 min lockout period, both titrated to patient response. (*See* Patient-Controlled Analgesia Guidelines Chart, page 37.) **Epidurally for analgesia** 25–150 µg as an intermittent bolus dose or 25–150 µg/hr as a continuous infusion, titrated to patient response.[69] (*See* Notes and Intraspinal Narcotic Administration Guidelines Chart, page 37.) **Transdermal for analgesia** calculate the previous 24-hr analgesic requirement and convert this amount to the equal analgesic oral morphine dosage from the Opioid Analgesics Comparison Chart. A short-acting opioid must be used for control of breakthrough pain until sufficient transdermal fentanyl is absorbed to achieve adequate analgesia. Use the following table to determine the fentanyl transdermal dosage from the daily equivalent oral morphine dosage:

TRANSDERMAL FENTANYL COMPARISON CHART

24-HOUR ORAL MORPHINE DOSAGE[a] (MG/DAY)	FENTANYL TRANSDERMAL DOSAGE (µG/HR)
45–134	25
135–224	50
225–314	75
315–404	100
405–494	125
495–584	150
585–674	175
675–764	200
765–854	225
855–944	250
945–1034	275
1035–1124	300

[a]Assumes morphine 10 mg IM is equivalent to morphine 60 mg orally; however, because of individual variability, equivalent dosages may vary among patients. The above conversion dosages are conservative, and approximately 50% of patients are likely to require a dosage increase following initial application. (*See* Opioid Analgesics Comparison Chart.)

Initiate treatment using the recommended transdermal fentanyl dosage and increase based on response no more frequently than q 3–6 days. Multiple transdermal patches may be used to achieve appropriate dosage (do not cut patches for a partial dosage). To change treatment to another opioid, discontinue the transdermal patch for 12–18 hr and start treatment with the new opioid at about one-half the equianalgesic dosage. **IV for induction and maintenance anesthesia** (loading) 4–20 µg/kg, (maintenance) 2–10 µg/kg/hr, (additional bolus) 25–100 µg.[79] **IV for postoperative (recovery room) pain control** 50–100 µg q 1–2 hr as needed; **Lozenge for anesthesia premedication or induction of conscious sedation** 5 µg/kg (provides effects similar to 0.75–1.25 µg/kg given IM), to a maximum of 400 µg.

Special Populations. *Pediatric Dosage.* IV for sedation in neonates 9–20 µg/kg/hr; tolerance limits its usefulness for prolonged sedation.[80] **IV for induction and maintenance anesthesia** (2–12 yr) 2–3 µg/kg initially, followed by 1–5 µg/kg/hr.[79] **Lozenge for anesthesia premedication or induction of conscious sedation** (<15 kg) contraindicated; (≥15 kg) 5–15 µg/kg, to a maximum of 400 µg.

Geriatric Dosage. **Lozenge for anesthesia premedication or induction of conscious sedation** (over 65 yr) 2.5–5 µg/kg, to a maximum of 400 µg. Altered pharmacodynamics rather than pharmacokinetics appear to be responsible for increased sensitivity in elderly patients.[81]

Other Conditions. In patients with head injury, cardiovascular, pulmonary, or hepatic disease, consider a lower dosage of 2.5–5 µg/kg, to a maximum of 400 µg.

Dosage Forms. **Inj** 50 µg/mL; **SR Patch** 25, 50, 75, 100 µg/hr; **Lozenge** 100, 200, 300, 400 µg.

Patient Instructions. (*See* Opioids Class Instructions.)

Pharmacokinetics. *Onset and Duration.* IM onset 7–15 min; duration 1–2 hr. Epidural onset 5 min; duration 4–6 hr.[69] Transdermal onset 6–8 hr; peak 24–72 hr; duration after a single application 72 hr.[82,83] Greater than 17 hr required for serum levels to fall by one-half after patch removal.

Serum Levels. (Analgesia) 1–3 µg/L (3–9 nmol/L)[82,83]; (balanced anesthesia) 6–20 µg/L (18–60 nmol/L).[79]

Fate. Bioavailability is 52% with lozenge. Of the fentanyl released by the transdermal system, 92% is absorbed, but overall systemic bioavailability of the transdermal preparation is approximately 30%. The drug is 84 ± 2% plasma protein bound; it is metabolized rapidly primarily by the liver to norfentanyl and other inactive metabolites; V_d is 4 ± 0.4 L/kg; Cl is 0.78 ± 0.12 L/hr/kg, decreased in the elderly and increased in neonates and children. Pharmacokinetics are not altered in renal insufficiency or compensated hepatic cirrhosis. Less than 10% is excreted unchanged in the urine.[66,81–84]

$t_{1/2}$. 6.1 ± 2 hr[84]; 7.1–11 hr during cardiopulmonary bypass surgery.[79]

Adverse Reactions. (*See* Morphine Sulfate.) Unlike other opioids, fentanyl, alfentanil, remifentanil, and sufentanil are not associated with histamine release and may be preferable when cardiovascular stability is an issue.[79] The frequency of pruritus is lower than that of morphine but not as low as that of meperidine.[85,86] PCA fentanyl produces less depression of postoperative cognitive function in elderly patients than does PCA morphine.[87] Development of withdrawal reactions following use for sedation in neonates and infants is likely with a total dosage >2.5 mg/kg or duration of infusion >9 days.[88]

Contraindications. (*See* Morphine Sulfate.) Fentanyl SR patch is contraindicated in acute or postoperative pain, including outpatient surgery; patients <12 yr or <50 kg; pain that can be managed by conventional analgesics; and doses over 25 µg/hr at the initiation of opioid therapy. Fentanyl lozenge is contraindicated in the management of both acute and chronic pain.

Precautions. (*See* Morphine Sulfate.) Analyses of fentanyl transdermal systems after 3 days of continuous application demonstrate a considerable amount of remaining drug (28–84%), which is a potentially lethal dose (1036 μg) for a 70-kg individual.[89] Cutting the membrane-controlled fentanyl transdermal system to achieve a different dosage is not recommended, because it may damage the integrity of the semipermeable membrane. Placing a piece of impermeable material (eg, adhesive bandage) on the skin proportionate in surface area to the intended reduction in dosage may be effective.[90]

Drug Interactions. (*See* Morphine Sulfate.) The effects of fentanyl may be potentiated by other CNS depressant drugs (eg, barbiturates, general anesthetics, narcotics, and tranquilizers). Carbamazepine may decrease fentanyl's effect during anesthesia for craniotomy.

Parameters to Monitor. Monitor vital signs and pain-control ratings routinely.

Notes. Epidural administration has not been shown to be more advantageous than IV administration during surgery.[91] Lack of rapid titratability precludes the usefulness of the transdermal fentanyl system for pain control in patients with rapidly changing analgesic requirements. Transdermal fentanyl for cancer pain causes a lower frequency of constipation than SR morphine.[92] IV is the parenteral route of choice after major surgery. This route is suitable for titrated bolus or continuous administration but requires close monitoring because there is a great risk of respiratory depression with inappropriate dosage.[93]

MEPERIDINE HYDROCHLORIDE　　　　　　　　　　　Demerol, Various

Pharmacology. Meperidine is a phenylpiperidine opioid agonist with important antimuscarinic activity and negative inotropic effects on the heart. Its major metabolite, normeperidine, has excitant effects that may precipitate tremors, myoclonus, or seizures. Meperidine's antimuscarinic activity may negate the miosis that occurs with other opioids.[67] (*See* Morphine Sulfate.)

Administration and Adult Dosage. PO, IV, or SC for analgesia 50–150 mg q 3–4 hr. (*See* Notes.) Oral doses are about one-half as effective as a parenteral dose. Reduce dosage when given concomitantly with a phenothiazine or other drugs that potentiate the depressant effects of meperidine. **IV for shaking caused by general anesthesia or amphotericin B** 25–50 mg. (*See* Notes.) **IM** not recommended.[93]

Special Populations. *Pediatric Dosage.* **PO, IV, or SC for analgesia** 1–1.8 mg/kg q 3–4 hr, to a maximum of 100 mg/dose. **IM** painful and should not be used in children.[94] (*See* Notes.)

Geriatric Dosage. Same as adult dosage.

Dosage Forms. Syrup 10 mg/mL; **Tab** 50, 100 mg; **Inj** 10, 25, 50, 75, 100 mg/mL.

Patient Instructions. (*See* Opioids Class Instructions.)

Pharmacokinetics. *Onset and Duration.* PO onset about 15 min; duration 2–3 hr. SC or IM onset about 10 min; peak analgesia 0.5–1 hr; duration 2–3 hr.[25,69]

Serum Levels. From 500 to 700 μg/L (2–2.8 μmol/L) appear to be required for analgesia.[82]

Fate. Oral bioavailability is about 52 ± 3%, increasing to 80–90% in cirrhosis caused by decreased first-pass metabolism.[25,95] After a single 100 mg IM dose, mean serum levels of 670 μg/L (2.7 μmol/L) and 650 μg/L (2.6 μmol/L) are attained in 1 and 2 hr, respectively[96,97]; 58 ± 9% plasma protein bound, largely to α_1-acid glycoprotein; decreased in the elderly and in uremia.[25,98] V_d is 4.4 ± 0.9 L/kg, increased in the elderly and premature infants; Cl is 1.02 ± 0.3 L/hr/kg, reduced by 25% in surgical patients and by 50% in cirrhosis, and reduced in acute viral hepatitis.[25] Hydrolyzed and also metabolized in the liver to normeperidine (an active metabolite), which is also hydrolyzed. An average of 2% unchanged drug and 1–21% (average 6) normeperidine is excreted in urine.[98]

$t_{1/2}$. (Meperidine) α phase 12 min, β phase 3.2 hr, increasing to 7 hr in patients with cirrhosis or acute liver disease and to 14–21 hr in patients with moderate to severe renal dysfunction.[97,99,100] (Normeperidine) 14–21 hr in normals, increasing to 35 hr in renal failure.[101]

Adverse Reactions. (*See* Morphine Sulfate.) Factors that may predispose to normeperidine-induced seizures include dosage >400–600 mg/day, renal failure, history of seizures, long-term administration to cancer patients, or co-administration of agents that increase N-demethylation to normeperidine.[102] Local irritation and induration occur with repeated SC injection.

Contraindications. MAO inhibitors within the past 14–21 days; chronic pain.

Precautions. (*See* Morphine Sulfate.) Avoid in patients with reduced renal function, and avoid continuous administration for greater than a few days. The combination of meperidine with promethazine and chlorpromazine (DPT) for painful procedures is not recommended, because it has poor efficacy compared with alternative approaches and is associated with a high frequency of adverse effects.[93]

Drug Interactions. (*See* Morphine Sulfate.) Concurrent use with an MAO inhibitor may cause marked blood pressure alterations, sweating, excitation, and rigidity. Barbiturates, chlorpromazine, and phenytoin may decrease meperidine serum concentrations and increase normeperidine, reducing analgesia and increasing the risk of stimulation and seizures.[103]

Parameters to Monitor. Monitor vital signs and pain scores at regular intervals. Jerking and twitching movements may be signs of normeperidine accumulation and impending toxicity.[104]

Notes. All opioids including meperidine and morphine increase biliary tract pressure. Sphincter of Oddi spasm may be less with meperidine than with morphine, but there is little evidence that this has clinical relevance. Unlike other opioids, meperidine is useful in treating the shaking and shivering associated with general anesthesia or amphotericin B administration.[102] Because of its low therapeutic index, meperidine should be reserved for very brief courses in otherwise healthy patients who have demonstrated untoward effects during treatment with other opioids such as morphine or hydromorphone.[93] Because of its unreliable absorption and breakthrough pain when meperidine is administered IM, more rapid and predictable routes (eg, IV) are recommended.[94,105,106] Oral meperidine is not recommended for cancer pain, because the high dosage required to relieve severe pain increases the risk of CNS toxicity.[94]

METHADONE HYDROCHLORIDE
Dolophine, Various

Pharmacology. Methadone is a phenylheptylamine opioid agonist qualitatively similar to morphine but with a chemical structure unrelated to the alkaloid-type structures of the opium derivatives. Analgesic activity of (R)-methadone is 8–50 times that of (S)-methadone, and (R)-methadone has a 10-fold higher affinity for opioid receptors. Methadone is lipophilic and has considerable tissue distribution; plasma concentrations during long-term treatment are sustained by this peripheral reservoir. It does not share cross-tolerance with other opioids, and the dosage required to achieve analgesia in opioid-tolerant patients is much lower than predicted by opioid conversion tables and single-dose studies. Unlike other opioids, methadone does not have active or toxic metabolites that are associated with CNS toxicity (eg, myoclonus, seizures).[107,108] Because methadone is a long-acting narcotic agent, it can be substituted for short-acting narcotic agents for analgesia maintenance and detoxification. Methadone abstinence syndrome is similar to morphine; however, onset is slower and duration is longer. (*See also* Morphine Sulfate.)

Administration and Adult Dosage. **PO, IV, or SC for pain** 5–80 mg/day in 1–3 divided doses. Dosage escalation is slower than with other opioids and averages approximately 2%/day.[107] **PO for maintenance and detoxification treatment** the minimum effective dosage for reducing illicit heroin use is approximately 60 mg/day, with the optimum dosage ranging between 80–120 mg/day. Premature termination of treatment and use of suboptimal dosages remain common problems. If tapering is attempted, it should occur gradually over a 4–12 month period or longer.[109] **To convert from another opioid** decrease the previous opioid dosage by one-third over 24 hr and replace it with methadone using a dosage ratio of 1 mg oral methadone = 10 mg oral morphine. During day 2, attempt a further one-third decrease in the dosage of the previous opioid, and on day 3, the final one-third of the dosage of the previous opioid may be discontinued. Maintain the patient on an q-8-hr schedule with approximately 10% of the daily methadone dosage as an extra dose for breakthrough pain.[107]

Special Populations. *Pediatric Dosage.* **IV for pain** 0.1 mg/kg q 6–8 hr; **PO for pain** 0.2 mg/kg q 6–8 hr.[94]

Geriatric Dosage. Same as adult dosage.

Dosage Forms. **Tab** 5, 10 mg; **Dispersible Tab** 40 mg; **Soln** 1, 2, 10 mg/mL; **Inj** 10 mg/mL.

Patient Instructions. (*See* Opioids Class Instructions.) Dosage increases should be made cautiously and should be managed by the clinician.

Pharmacokinetics. *Onset and Duration.* (Analgesia) onset SC 10–20 min, PO 30–60 min; peak SC 0.5–1 hr; duration PO, SC, or IV 4–5 hr after a single dose, 8–48 hr with multiple doses.[82,107,108]

Serum Levels. Best rehabilitation in methadone maintenance patients has been associated with serum levels >211 μg/L (682 nmol/L).[108] There is no good correlation between serum levels and analgesia.[110]

Fate. Oral bioavailability is 92 ± 21%; 89% plasma protein bound. Pharmacokinetics are best described by a two-compartment model. $V_{d\beta}$ is 3.8 ± 0.6 L/kg; Cl is 0.084 ± 0.03 L/hr/kg. Both $V_{d\beta}$ and Cl are greater for (*R*)-methadone.[108] Extent of metabolism may increase with long-term therapy, resulting in a 15–25% decline in serum levels, although this has also been attributed to poor compliance. Metabolized in the liver to inactive metabolites via N-demethylation; metabolites are excreted in urine and bile.[107] The drug is 24 ± 10% excreted unchanged in the urine, increased by urine acidification.[25,110,111]

$t_{1/2}$. (β Phase) 35 ± 12 hr[25]; (*R*)-methadone has a longer half-life (37.5 hr) than (*S*)-methadone (28.6 hr).[108]

Adverse Reactions. (*See* Morphine Sulfate.) Because of its long half-life and lack of cross-tolerance, patients receiving methadone are at greater risk for toxicity when inappropriate dosage increases are made.

Precautions. (*See* Morphine Sulfate.) The process of switching from another opioid to methadone is complex and should only be attempted by an experienced clinician in an inpatient setting over 3–6 days. (*See* Administration and Adult Dosage.)[107]

Drug Interactions. (*See* Morphine Sulfate.) Carbamazepine, phenytoin, rifampin, and other drugs that induce CYP enzymes may decrease methadone serum levels and result in withdrawal symptoms in patients on methadone maintenance programs. Diazepam, erythromycin, fluvoxamine, and possibly other enzyme inhibitors may increase methadone levels and effects.[103]

Parameters to Monitor. During analgesia, monitor vital signs and pain ratings routinely. During methadone maintenance, monitor for signs of withdrawal, which include lacrimation, rhinorrhea, diaphoresis, yawning, restlessness, insomnia, dilated pupils, and piloerection.[109]

Notes. For treatment of narcotic addiction in detoxification or maintenance programs, methadone may be dispensed only by approved pharmacies. Maintenance therapy (treatment for longer than 3 weeks) may be undertaken only by approved methadone programs; this does not apply to addicts hospitalized for other medical conditions.

MORPHINE SULFATE
Various

Pharmacology. Morphine and other opioids interact with stereospecific opiate receptors in the CNS and other tissues. (*See* Opioid Receptor Specificity Comparison Chart.) Opioid analgesia is caused by actions at several CNS sites. Morphine and other muopioid agonists inhibit nociceptive reflexes through inhibition of neurotransmitter release, have inhibitory actions on neurons conveying nociceptive information to higher brain centers, and enhance activity in descending pathways that exert inhibitory effects on the processing of nociceptive information in the spinal cord. Mu receptors are responsible for analgesia, respiratory depression, miosis, decreased GI motility, and euphoria. Stimulation of kappa receptors results in analgesia, less intense miosis and respiratory depression, dysphoria, and psychotomimetic effects. It is unclear what the consequences of delta receptor stimulation are in humans.[66] The relief of pain is fairly specific, other sensory modalities are essentially unaffected, and mental processes are not impaired (unlike anesthetics), except when given in large doses or to opiate-naive individuals. These drugs also have antitussive effects, usually at dosages less than those required for analgesia.

Administration and Adult Dosage. With the exception of transdermal fentanyl, there is no ceiling or maximum dosage for morphine or other opioid agonists, and very large doses may be required for severe pain.[94] **PO for analgesia** 8–20 mg q 4 hr; **SR Tab, 12-hr** (narcotic-naive patients) 30 mg q 8–12 hr initially; (narcotic-tolerant patients) total daily oral morphine dosage equivalent in 2 divided doses q 12 hr; **SR Cap, 24-hr** (narcotic-naive patients) 20 mg q 24 hr initially; (narcotic-tolerant patients) total daily oral morphine dosage equivalent q 24 hr; **SC for analgesia** 5–15 mg q 4 hr (10 mg/70 kg is the optimal initial dose); **PR for analgesia** 10–20 mg q 4 hr. **IV for analgesia** 4–10 mg, dilute and inject slowly over a 2–3-min period. **IV infusion** 1–10 mg/hr[112]; some patients with chronic pain may require a dosage as high as 95 mg/hr or more.[113] **IV patient-controlled analgesia (PCA)** 1 mg per activation initially with 5–20 min lockout period, both titrated to patient response.[114,115] Continuous infusion combined with PCA is effective in chronic cancer pain.[116] **Epidural for analgesia (unpreserved solution)** (intermittent) 5 mg initially, may repeat with 1–2 mg after 1 hr; (continuous infusion) 0.05–0.1 mg/kg loading dose, then 0.005–0.01 mg/kg/hr.[117] **IT for cancer pain (unpreserved solution)** 0.4–8.3 mg/day (average 1–23 mg/day);[118] **IT for cesarean section (unpreserved solution)** 0.1 mg.[119] **Intraventricular (unpreserved solution)** 0.1–2 mg, repeated approximately q 24 hr.[120] **Inhal for dyspnea** 5–15 mg in 2 mL sterile water or NS via nebulizer q 4 hr.[121] **IM** is painful and is not recommended.[94]

Special Populations. *Pediatric Dosage.* **PO** 0.3 mg/kg q 3–4 hr. **IV** 0.05–0.2 mg/kg q 4 hr. **IV infusion** 0.01–0.04 mg/kg/hr. **Epidural** 0.05–0.08 mg/kg. **IT** 0.01–0.03 mg/kg.[94,122,123]

Geriatric Dosage. Reduce initial dosage in elderly patients, and make smaller percentage incremental increases in total daily dosage (eg, 25%) than in younger patients.

Other Conditions. Reduce initial dosage in debilitated patients.

Dosage Forms. **Soln** 2, 4, 20 mg/mL; **Supp** 5, 10, 20, 30 mg; **Tab** 10, 15, 30 mg; **SR Tab** (8, 12 hr) 15, 30, 60, 100, 200 mg; **SR Cap (24 hr)** 20, 50, 100 mg; **Inj** (unpreserved solution) 0.5, 1, 10, 25, 50 mg/mL; (preserved solution) 2, 3, 4, 5, 8, 10, 15, 25, 50 mg/mL.

Patient Instructions. (*See* Opioids Class Instructions.)

Pharmacokinetics. *Onset and Duration.* (Analgesia) onset IM 10–30 min; peak 0.5–1 hr; duration 3–5 hr.[82]

Serum Levels. It is speculated that moderate analgesia requires serum levels of at least 50 µg/L (88 nmol/L).

Fate. Well absorbed from GI tract, but first-pass conjugation is extensive, reducing oral bioavailability to $24 \pm 12\%$.[25,124] Nebulized morphine by inhalation has a low bioavailability, $5 \pm 3\%$, but a rapid peak at 10 min.[124] After an IM dose of 10 mg, peak morphine levels of about 56 µg/L (98 nmol/L) are reached within 20 min. The drug is $35 \pm 2\%$ plasma protein bound, decreased in acute viral hepatitis, cirrhosis, and hypoalbuminemia[25]; V_d is 2.12 L/kg in young normals and 1.16 L/kg in elderly patients; Cl is 2.02 L/hr/kg in young normals and 1.66 L/hr/kg in elderly patients.[112] Morphine clearance reaches adult level by age 6 months–2.5 yr.[125] Inactivated in the liver, primarily by conjugation to morphine-6-glucuronide (active) and morphine-3-glucuronide (inactive or antagonistic).[25,126] Decreased clearance of glucuronide metabolites has been demonstrated in patients with renal insufficiency.[127] Greater plasma concentrations of morphine-6-glucuronide are present with oral than with parenteral administration.[128] Mostly excreted in urine; $14 \pm 7\%$ as the active morphine-6-glucuronide and 3.4% (oral) to 9% (parenteral) of a dose is excreted unchanged.[25,126,129]

$t_{1/2}$. 1.9 ± 0.5 hr, increased in neonates and premature infants.[25]

Adverse Reactions. Respiratory and circulatory depression and constipation are major adverse effects. Patients with renal failure are more prone to develop adverse reactions.[130] Dose-related signs of intoxication include miosis, drowsiness, decreased rate and depth of respiration, bradycardia, and hypotension. Sedation, dizziness, nausea, vomiting, sweating, and constipation occur frequently. Euphoria, dysphoria, dry mouth, biliary tract spasm, postural hypotension, syncope, tachy- or bradycardia, urinary retention, and myoclonus occur occasionally. Myoclonus appears to be somewhat dose related and has been described after large doses via either IV or intraspinal routes. Myoclonus may be managed by changing to another opioid, or with either a **benzodiazepine** or **dantrolene.**[131,132] Frequent adverse effects from epidural administration include urinary retention and pruritus; the latter can be managed with **naloxone** or **butorphanol.**[117] Possible allergic-type reactions are reported occasionally. Most allergic-type reactions consist of skin rash and wheal and flare over a vein, which may occur with IV injection; these are caused by direct stimulation of histamine release, are not allergic, and are not a sign of a more serious reaction. True allergy is rare. Confusion and disorientation have been linked to phenol and formaldehyde preservatives in epidural infusions, and seizures have been associated with high-dose IV infusions containing sodium bisulfite.[133,134]

Precautions. Use with caution and in reduced dosage when giving concurrently with other CNS depressant drugs. Use with caution in pregnancy; the presence of head injury, other intracranial lesions or pre-existing increase in intracranial pressure; patients having an acute asthmatic attack; COPD or cor pulmonale; decreased respiratory reserve; pre-existing respiratory depression, hypoxia, or hypercapnia; patients whose ability to maintain blood pressure is already compromised; patients with atrial flutter or other supraventricular tachycardias; patients with prostatic hypertrophy or urethral stricture; elderly or debilitated patients; and patients with acute abdominal pain, when administration of the drug might obscure the diagnosis or clinical course. Use with caution in the elderly and neonates, and patients with renal dysfunction or elevated bilirubin or LDH levels.[125,127,128,130] Infants >1 month eliminate morphine efficiently and are unlikely to be unusually sensitive to the respiratory depressant effects but may require a longer dosage interval.[125] Do not administer IV, IT, or epidurally to opiate-naive patients unless a narcotic antagonist and facilities for assisted or controlled respiration are immediately available.

Drug Interactions. Concurrent use of opioids with other CNS depressants (eg, alcohol, antipsychotics, general anesthetics, heterocyclic antidepressants, and sedative-hypnotics) may cause respiratory depression. Cimetidine may increase serum concentration and duration of effect of the opioids.[103]

Parameters to Monitor. Monitor for pain control and signs of respiratory or cardiovascular depression.

NALOXONE HYDROCHLORIDE   Narcan, Various

Pharmacology. Naloxone, an N-allyl derivative of oxymorphone, is a narcotic antagonist that competitively binds at opiate receptors. Naloxone is essentially free of narcotic agonist properties and is used to reverse the effects of narcotic agonists and drugs with partial agonist properties.[135]

Administration and Adult Dosage. **IV (preferred) or SC for known or suspected narcotic overdose** 0.1–0.2 mg as a first dose, then progressively double the dose q 2–3 min or 0.4 mg diluted in 9 mL saline and injected in 1-mL increments q 30–60 seconds, until respiration and consciousness have become normal or until 10 mg has been given. If response occurs, to prevent recurrent toxicity due to short naloxone half-life, IV infusion at an hourly rate equal to initial dose required for arousal, with a possible repeat bolus of 50% required 20–30 minutes after start of infusion.[136,137] If a total of 10 mg has been given and there is no response, the diagnosis of narcotic overdose should be questioned. The frequency of repeat doses is based on clinical evaluation of the patient. **IV for postoperative narcotic depression** 0.1–0.2 mg initially, may repeat q 2–3 min until desired level of reversal is reached. Subsequent doses may be needed if the effect of the narcotic outlasts the action of naloxone. (*See* Notes.) **IV for epidural opioid-induced pruritus** 0.005–0.01 mg/kg either in incremental doses or as an hourly infusion.[117] **PO for opioid-induced constipation** 4–12 mg not more often than q 6 hr; more frequent administration may precipitate withdrawal.[138]

Special Populations. *Pediatric Dosage.* **IV for known or suspected narcotic overdose** 0.1–0.2 mg/kg, may repeat as needed. **IV for postoperative narcotic depression** 0.005–0.01 mg initially, may repeat q 2–3 min until desired level of reversal is reached. **IV (preferred) or SC for narcotic depression** (neonates) 0.01 mg/kg initially, may repeat q 2–3 min until desired level of reversal is reached.

Geriatric Dosage. Same as adult dosage.

Dosage Forms. **Inj** 0.02, 0.4 mg/mL.

Pharmacokinetics. *Onset and Duration.* Onset IV within 2–3 min, up to 15 min when given IM or SC; duration variable, but usually 1 hr or less.[139,140]

Fate. From 59–67% metabolized by hepatic conjugation and renal elimination of the conjugated compound.[141] V_d is approximately 2–3 L/kg;[25,142] Cl is about 1.3 L/hr/kg.[25]

$t_{1/2}$. 64 ± 12 min in adults;[143] 71 ± 36 min in neonates.[144]

Adverse Reactions. Naloxone administration has been occasionally associated with life-threatening complications, including pulmonary edema, seizures, hypertension, arrhythmias, and violent behavior within 10 min of parenteral administration.[136,137]

Contraindications. None known.

Precautions. Administration to narcotic-dependent persons (including neonates of dependent mothers) may precipitate acute withdrawal symptoms.

Drug Interactions. None known except for opioid antagonism.

Parameters to Monitor. Respiratory rate, pupil size (may not be useful in mixed drug or narcotic partial agonist overdoses), heart rate, blood pressure, and symptoms of acute narcotic withdrawal syndrome.

Notes. Naloxone is effective when administered endotracheally to patients with difficult venous access.[145] It is routinely used in the initial treatment of patients with coma of unknown origin. Its use in **clonidine** overdose has produced mixed results; use in septic and hemorrhagic shock has been disappointing.[135]

OPIOID PARTIAL AGONISTS

Pharmacology. These agents can be classified based on their effects on the opioid receptors. Opioid partial agonists have analgesic effects but are characterized by an analgesic ceiling, such that beyond a certain point, further increases in dosage do not result in additional analgesia but may produce adverse effects.[66,94] **Tramadol** is partially metabolized by CYP2D6, producing an active metabolite (M1) that binds to mu opioid receptors. Patients who are poor metabolizers of debrisoquine/sparteine have negligible M1 production and reduced analgesia, although some pain relief remains because of activation of monoaminergic antinociceptive pathways from tramadol enantiomers.[66,146]

Administration, Dosage, and Dosage Forms. (*See* Opioid Analgesics Comparison Chart.)

Patient Instructions. (*See* Opioids Class Instructions.)

Pharmacokinetics. (*See* Opioid Analgesics Comparison Chart.)

Adverse Reactions. Sedation, sweating, dizziness, nausea, vomiting, euphoria, dysphoria (agents with delta receptor activity), and hallucinations are most frequent. Occasionally, insomnia, anxiety, anorexia, constipation, dry mouth, syncope, visual blurring, flushing, decreased blood pressure, and tachycardia are reported. After parenteral use, diaphoresis, sting on injection, respiratory depression, transient apnea in newborn from use in mother during labor, shock, urinary retention, and alterations in uterine contractions during labor occur rarely. Other rarely reported effects include muscle tremor and toxic epidermal necrolysis. Local skin reactions and ulceration and fibrous myopathy at the injection site have been reported with long-term parenteral use of pentazocine.[66] **Tramadol** adverse reactions include seizures (some after the first dose) with recommended and excessive dosages. Seizure risk is increased in patients taking concomitant medications that may reduce the seizure threshold (eg, heterocyclic antidepressants, selective serotonin reuptake inhibitors, MAO inhibitors, neuroleptics) and with certain medical conditions (eg, epilepsy, head trauma, metabolic disorders, alcohol and drug withdrawal, or CNS infection). In addition, **naloxone** administration for tramadol overdose may increase the risk of seizure. Anaphylactoid reactions have also been described in tramadol postmarketing surveillance.[147–149] Dependence/addiction and major psychological disturbances have been reported with **butorphanol** nasal spray.[150]

Contraindications. (Tramadol) prior allergy to any opiate; acute intoxication with alcohol, hypnotics, centrally acting analgesics, opioids, or psychotropic drugs. (*See* Notes.)

Precautions. (*See* Morphine Sulfate.) Also, use cautiously in patients with myocardial infarction because **pentazocine** and **butorphanol** increase cardiac workload. All of these agents may produce dependence and withdrawal symptoms following extended use.

Drug Interactions. (*See* Morphine Sulfate.) With the possible exception of tramadol, these agents can precipitate acute withdrawal in narcotic-dependent individuals.[151]

Notes. Because of their ceiling effect, risk of precipitating opiate withdrawal, and marked adverse effects, these agents are not recommended for the management of cancer pain.[94] Effects of pentazocine are antagonized by naloxone only (ie, not by nalorphine or levallorphan). Naloxone in the pentazocine tablet is not absorbed orally but theoretically prevents parenteral abuse of the oral dosage form; however, IV abuse of Talwin Nx plus tripelennamine has been reported.[152]

OPIOID RECEPTOR SPECIFICITY COMPARISON CHART

	RECEPTOR TYPE		
DRUG	*Mu*	*Kappa*	*Delta*
Buprenorphine	Partial agonist-antagonist	Unknown	Minimal activity
Butorphanol	Partial agonist-antagonist	Agonist	Unknown
Dezocine	Partial agonist-antagonist	Agonist	Minimal agonist activity
Morphine	Agonist	Minimal agonist activity	Unknown
Nalbuphine	Antagonist	Agonist	Agonist
Pentazocine	Partial agonist-antagonist	Agonist	Unknown
Tramadol[a]	Partial or pure agonist[b]	Minimal activity	Unknown

[a]Also blocks norepinephrine and serotonin reuptake.
[b]Not a classic agonist-antagonist; has little or no antagonist properties but appears to have partial mu receptor agonist activity.

PATIENT-CONTROLLED ANALGESIA (PCA) GUIDELINES CHART[a]

DRUG	IV BOLUS DOSE (MG)	LOCKOUT INTERVAL (MIN)
Buprenorphine	0.03–0.2	10–20
Fentanyl	0.02–0.1	3–10
Hydromorphone	0.1–0.5	3–15
Meperidine[b]	5–30	5–15
Methadone	0.5–3	10–20
Morphine[a]	0.5–3	5–20
Nalbuphine	1–5	5–15
Oxymorphone	0.2–0.8	5–15
Pentazocine	5–30	5–15
Sufentanil	0.003–0.015	3–10

[a]Some clinicians recommend combining PCA with a basal continuous infusion of the narcotic. The hourly dosage is determined by the patient's previous narcotic dose requirements and adjusted q 8–24 hr based on the dose of PCA bolus administered, basal continuous infusion, and pain response. A typical starting hourly basal continuous infusion rate for morphine in a 70-kg adult is 0.5–3 mg/hr.
[b]Use with caution (preferably avoid) for PCA and consider factors that may predispose to seizures which include dosage over 100 mg q 2 hr for longer than 24 hr, renal failure, and history of seizure disorder.
From references 69, 114, and 116.

INTRASPINAL NARCOTIC ADMINISTRATION GUIDELINES CHART[a]

ROUTE AND DRUG	INTRASPINAL BOLUS DOSE (MG)	ONSET (MIN)	DURATION (HR)
EPIDURAL			
Alfentanil	0.7–2[b]	Rapid	1.5–1.7[c]
Fentanyl	0.025–0.15	5	2–4
Hydromorphone	1–2	15	10–16
Methadone	1–10	10	6–10
Morphine	1–10	30	6–24
Sufentanil	0.015–0.05	15	4–6
INTRATHECAL (SUBARACHNOID)			
Morphine	0.1–0.5	15	8–24

[a]Use only preservative-free preparations for intraspinal narcotic administration.
[b]Based on a 70-kg adult body weight (ie, 10–30 µg/kg).
[c]Very short duration of action; requires epidural infusion to obtain prolonged analgesia. Like fentanyl, prolonged epidural infusions produce high systemic concentrations and appear to have little advantage over IV infusion.
From references 69 and 79.

OPIOID ANALGESICS COMPARISON CHART

DRUG AND SCHEDULE[a]	DOSAGE FORMS	EQUIVALENT PARENTERAL DOSAGE[b] (MG)	EQUIVALENT ORAL DOSAGE[c] (MG)	PARENTERAL/ ORAL EFFI-CACY RATIO	DURATION OF ANALGESIA (HR)	PARTIAL ANTAGONIST ACTIVITY
Buprenorphine (C-V) Buprenex	Inj 0.324 mg/mL.	0.3–0.6 [0.4–0.8][d]	—	—	6–8	yes
Butorphanol Stadol (NC) Stadol NS (C-IV)	Inj 1, 2 mg/mL Nasal Spray 10 mg/mL (1 mg/spray).[e]	2	—	1/16	3–4	yes
Codeine (C-II) Various	Inj 30, 60 mg/mL Hyp Tab 15, 30, 60 mg Tab 15, 30, 60 mg.	120	30	1/2–2/3	4–6	no
Dezocine (NC) Dalgan	Inj 5, 10, 15 mg/mL.	10–15	—	—	3–4	yes
Fentanyl (C-II) Various	Inj 50 µg/mL SR Patch 25, 50, 75, 100 µg/hr Lozenge 100, 200, 300, 400 µg.	0.05–0.1	—	—	1–2 (patch, 72)	no
Hydrocodone and Acetaminophen (C-III) Vicodin Various	Tab 2.5, 5, 7.5 mg with aceta-minophen 500 mg, 7.5 mg with acetaminophen 750 mg, 10 mg with acetaminophen 650 mg Cap 5 mg with acetaminophen 500 mg Soln 0.5 mg/mL with aceta-minophen 33 mg/mL.	—	5	—	4–6	no

(continued)

DRUG AND SCHEDULE[a]	DOSAGE FORMS	EQUIVALENT PARENTERAL DOSAGE[b] (MG)	EQUIVALENT ORAL DOSAGE[c] (MG)	PARENTERAL/ ORAL EFFI- CACY RATIO	DURATION OF ANALGESIA (HR)	PARTIAL ANTAGONIST ACTIVITY
Hydromorphone *(C-II)* Dilaudid Various	Inj 1, 2, 3, 4, 10 mg/mL Tab 1, 2, 3, 4, 8 mg/mL Soln 1 mg/mL Supp 3 mg.	1.5	1	1/5–1/2	3–5	no
Levorphanol *(C-II)* Levo-Dromoran	Inj 2 mg/mL Tab 2 mg.	2	—	1/2	4–6	no
Meperidine *(C-II)* Demerol Various	Inj 10, 25, 50, 75, 100 mg/mL Tab 50, 100 mg Syrup 10 mg/mL.	75–100	50	1/3–1/2	2–4	no
Methadone *(C-II)* Dolophine Various	Inj 10 mg/mL Tab 5, 10 mg Dispersible Tab 40 mg Soln 1, 2, 10 mg/mL.	f	f	1/2	8–48	no
Morphine *(C-II)* Various	Inj 0.5, 1, 2, 3, 4, 5, 8, 10, 15, 25, 50 mg/mL Tab 10, 15, 30 mg Soln 2, 4, 20 mg/mL SR Cap 20, 50, 100 mg SR Tab 15, 30, 60, 100, 200 mg Supp 5, 10, 20, 30 mg.	10	5	1/3	3–5	no
Nalbuphine *(NC)* Nubain Various	Inj 10, 20 mg/mL.	10	—	1/6	3–6	yes

(continued)

39

OPIOID ANALGESICS COMPARISON CHART (continued)

DRUG AND SCHEDULE[a]	DOSAGE FORMS	EQUIVALENT PARENTERAL DOSAGE[b] (MG)	EQUIVALENT ORAL DOSAGE[c] (MG)	PARENTERAL/ ORAL EFFI- CACY RATIO	DURATION OF ANALGESIA (HR)	PARTIAL ANTAGONIST ACTIVITY
Oxycodone (C-II) Oxycontin Roxicodone	Tab 5 mg Soln 1, 20 mg/mL SR Tab 10, 20, 40, 80 mg.	—	5	—	3–4	no
Oxymorphone (C-II) Numorphan	Inj 1, 1.5 mg/mL Supp 5 mg.	1–1.5	—	1/6	4–5	no
Pentazocine (C-IV) Talwin Talwin Nx Various	Inj 30 mg/mL Tab 50 mg with naloxone 0.5 mg.	30–60	25	1/3	2–3	yes
Propoxyphene (C-IV) Darvon Various	Cap (HCl) 32, 65 mg Tab (Napsylate) 100 mg Susp (Napsylate) 10 mg/mL.	—	65 HCl 100 Napsylate	—	4–6	no
Sufentanil (C-II) Sufenta	Inj 50 μg/mL.	0.02	—	—	2.5–3.5	no
Tramadol (NC) Ultram	Tab 50 mg.	—	25	—	4–6	—

[a]Controlled Substance Schedule designated after each drug (in parentheses); NC = Not Controlled.
[b]Parenteral dose equivalent to 10 mg morphine.
[c]Oral dose equivalent to 30 mg codeine. Not for SR products.
[d]Equivalent sublingual dose.
[e]Recommended dosage is one spray in one nostril, repeated prn in 60–90 min; this cycle may then be repeated q 3–4 hr prn pain.
See Pharmacology and Notes under Methadone.
From references 66, 69, 79, 82, 83, 95, 153–156 and product information.

■ REFERENCES

1. Wyss A et al. Pharmacokinetic investigation of oral and IV dihydroergotamine in healthy subjects. *J Clin Pharmacol* 1991;41:597–602.
2. Scott AK. Dihydroergotamine: a review of its use in the treatment of migraine and other headaches. *Clin Neuropharmacol* 1992;15:289–96.
3. Humbert H et al. Human pharmacokinetics of dihydroergotamine administered by nasal spray. *Clin Pharmacol Ther* 1996;60:265–75.
4. Dihydroergotamine Nasal Spray Multicenter Investigators. Efficacy, safety, and tolerability of dihydroergotamine nasal spray as monotherapy in the treatment of acute migraine. *Headache* 1995;35:177–84.
5. Gallagher RM. Acute treatment of migraine with dihydroergotamine nasal spray. *Arch Neurol* 1996;53:1285–91.
6. Touchon J et al. A comparison of subcutaneous sumatriptan and dihydroergotamine nasal spray in the acute treatment of migraine. *Neurology* 1996;47:361–5.
7. Perrin VL. Clinical pharmacokinetics of ergotamine in migraine and cluster headache. *Clin Pharmacokinet* 1985;10:334–52.
8. Sanders SM et al. Pharmacokinetics of ergotamine in healthy volunteers following oral and rectal dosing. *Eur J Clin Pharmacol* 1986;30:331–4.
9. Ibraheem JJ et al. Kinetics of ergotamine after intravenous and intramuscular administration to migraine sufferers. *Eur J Clin Pharmacol* 1982;23:235–40.
10. Saper JR. Ergotamine dependency a review. *Headache* 1987;27:435–8.
11. The Multinational Oral Sumatriptan and Cafergot Comparative Study Group. A randomized, double-blind comparison of sumatriptan and Cafergot in the acute treatment of migraine. *Eur Neurol* 1991;31:314–22.
12. Hering R, Kuritzky A. Sodium valproate in the prophylactic treatment of migraine: a double-blind study versus placebo. *Cephalalgia* 1992;12:81–4.
13. Bredberg U et al. Pharmacokinetics of methysergide and its metabolite methylergometrine in man. *Eur J Clin Pharmacol* 1986;30:75–7.
14. Dahlof C. The ideal 5-HT1D agonist. In, Olesen J, Tfelt-Hansen P, eds. *Headache treatment: trial methodology and new drugs.* Philadelphia: Lippincott-Raven; 1997;243–51.
15. Connor HE et al. Naratriptan: biological profile in animal models relevant to migraine. *Cephalalgia* 1997;17:145–52.
16. Fuseau E et al. Absolute bioavailability of oral naratriptan. Poster presentation at the American Academy of Neurology meeting, Boston, April 13–19, 1997.
17. Dechant KL, Clissold SP. Sumatriptan. A review of its pharmacodynamic and pharmacokinetic properties, and therapeutic efficacy in the acute treatment of migraine and cluster headache. *Drugs* 1992;43:776–98.
18. Plosker GL, McTavish D. Sumatriptan. A reappraisal of its pharmacology and therapeutic efficacy in the acute treatment of migraine and cluster headache. *Drugs* 1994;47:622–51.
19. Cady RK et al. Treatment of acute migraine with subcutaneous sumatriptan. *JAMA* 1991;265:2831–5.
20. Ferrari MD et al. Oral sumatriptan: effect of a second dose, and incidence and treatment of headache recurrences. *Cephalalgia* 1994;14:330–8.
21. The Subcutaneous Sumatriptan International Study Group. Treatment of migraine attacks with sumatriptan. *N Engl J Med* 1991;325:316–21.
22. Lacey LF et al. Single dose pharmacokinetics of sumatriptan in healthy volunteers. *Eur J Clin Pharmacol* 1995;47:543–8.
23. Fowler PA et al. The clinical pharmacology, pharmacokinetics and metabolism of sumatriptan. *Eur Neurol* 1991;31:291–4.
24. Dixon CM et al. Disposition of sumatriptan in laboratory animals and humans. *Drug Metab Dispos Biol Fate Chem* 1993;21:761–9.
25. Benet LZ et al. Design and optimization of dosage regimens: pharmacokinetic data. In, Hardman JG et al., eds. *Goodman and Gilman's the pharmacological basis of therapeutics,* 9th ed. New York: McGraw-Hill; 1996:1707–92.
26. Ferrari MD. 311C90: increasing the options for therapy with effective acute antimigraine $5HT_{1B/1D}$ receptor agonists. *Neurology* 1997;48(suppl 3):S21–4.
27. Zagami AS. 311C90: long-term efficacy and tolerability profile for the acute treatment of migraine. *Neurology* 1997;48(suppl 3):S25–8.
28. Diener HC, Klein KB. The first comparison of the efficacy and safety of 311C90 and sumatriptan in the treatment of migraine. Proc 3rd European Headache Conference 1996;10–1.
29. Insel PA. Analgesic-antipyretic and anti-inflammatory agents and drugs employed in the treatment of gout. In, Hardman JG et al., eds. *Goodman and Gilman's the pharmacological basis of therapeutics,* 9th ed. New York: McGraw-Hill; 1996: 617–57.

30. Segasothy M et al. Paracetamol: a cause for analgesic nephropathy and end-stage renal disease. *Nephron* 1988;50:50–4.
31. Zimmerman HJ, Maddrey WC. Acetaminophen (paracetamol) hepatotoxicity with regular intake of alcohol: analysis of instances of therapeutic misadventure. *Hepatology* 1995;22:767–73.
32. Towheed TE, Hochberg MC. A systematic review of randomized controlled trials of pharmacological therapy in osteoarthritis of the knee, with an emphasis on trial methodology. *Semin Arthritis Rheum* 1997;26:755–70.
33. Hirsh J et al. Aspirin and other platelet-active drugs. The relationship among dose, effectiveness, and side effects. *Chest* 1995;108:247S–57S.
34. Sherman DG et al. Antithrombotic therapy for cerebrovascular disorders. An update. *Chest* 1995;108:444S–56S.
35. Cairns JA et al. Antithrombotic agents in coronary artery disease. *Chest* 1995;108:380S–400S.
36. Stein PD et al. Antithrombotic therapy in patients with saphenous vein and internal mammary artery bypass grafts. *Chest* 1995;108:424S–30S.
37. Laupacis A et al. Antithrombotic therapy in atrial fibrillation. *Chest* 1995;108:352S–9S.
38. Mongan E et al. Tinnitus as an indication of therapeutic serum salicylate levels. *JAMA* 1973;226:142–5.
39. Done AK. Aspirin-overdosage: incidence, diagnosis, and management. *Pediatrics* 1978;62(suppl):890–7.
40. Lanza FL et al. Endoscopic evaluation of the effects of aspirin, buffered aspirin, and enteric-coated aspirin on gastric and duodenal mucosa. *N Engl J Med* 1980;303:136–8.
41. Levy G. Pharmacokinetics of salicylate elimination in man. *J Pharm Sci* 1965;54:959–67.
42. Levy G, Yaffe SJ. Clinical implications of salicylate-induced liver damage. *Am J Dis Child* 1975;129:1385–6.
43. Jusko WJ, Gretch M. Plasma and tissue protein binding of drugs in pharmacokinetics. *Drug Metab Rev* 1976;5:43–140.
44. Stevenson DD, Mathison DA. Aspirin sensitivity in asthmatics. When may this drug be safe? *Postgrad Med* 1985;78:111–9.
45. Bonica JJ, ed. *The management of pain,* 2nd ed. Philadelphia: Lea & Febiger; 1990.
46. Rahwan GL, Rahwan RG. Aspirin and Reye's syndrome: the change in prescribing habits of health professionals. *Drug Intell Clin Pharm* 1986;20:143–5.
47. Pinsky PF et al. Reye's syndrome and aspirin: evidence for a dose-response effect. *JAMA* 1988;260:657–61.
48. Housholder GT. Intolerance to aspirin and the nonsteroidal anti-inflammatory drugs. *J Oral Maxillofac Surg* 1985;43:333–7.
49. Hall AH et al. Ibuprofen overdose—a prospective study. *West J Med* 1988;148:653–6.
50. Nahata MC et al. Pharmacokinetics of ibuprofen in febrile children. *Eur J Clin Pharmacol* 1991;40:427–8.
51. Hollander D. Gastrointestinal complications of nonsteroidal anti-inflammatory drugs: prophylactic and therapeutic strategies. *Am J Med* 1994;96:274–81.
52. Whelton A et al. Renal effects of ibuprofen, piroxicam, and sulindac in patients with asymptomatic renal failure. *Ann Intern Med* 1990;112:568–76.
53. Stempel DA, Miller JJ. Lymphopenia and hepatotoxicity with ibuprofen. *J Pediatr* 1977;90:657–8.
54. Bernstein RF. Ibuprofen-related meningitis in mixed connective tissue disease. *Ann Intern Med* 1980;92:206–7.
55. Riendeau D et al. Comparison of the cyclooxygenase-1 inhibitory properties of nonsteroidal anti-inflammatory drugs (NSAIDs) and selective COX-2 inhibitors, using sensitive microsomal and platelet assays. *Can J Physiol Pharmacol* 1997;75:1088–95.
56. Furst DE. Meloxicam: selective COX-2 inhibition in clinical practice. *Semin Arthritis Rheum* 1997;26 (suppl 1):21–7.
57. Wallace JL. Nonsteroidal anti-inflammatory drugs and gastroenteropathy: the second hundred years. *Gastroenterology* 1997;112:1000–16.
58. Maniglia R et al. Non-steroidal anti-inflammatory nephrotoxicity. *Ann Clin Lab Sci* 1988;18:240–52.
59. Marsh CC et al. A review of selected investigational nonsteroidal anti-inflammatory drugs of the 1980s. *Pharmacotherapy* 1986;6:10–25.
60. Vane JR, Botting RM. Mechanism of action of aspirin-like drugs. *Semin Arthritis Rheum* 1997;26 (suppl 1):2–10.
61. Litvak KM, McEvoy GK. Ketorolac, an injectable nonnarcotic analgesic. *Clin Pharm* 1990;9:921–35.
62. Brooks PM, Day RO. Nonsteroidal anti-inflammatory drugs—differences and similarities. *N Engl J Med* 1991;324:1716–25.
63. Helfgott SM et al. Diclofenac-associated hepatotoxicity. *JAMA* 1990;264:2660–2.
64. Middleton E Jr et al., eds. *Allergy principles and practice,* 3rd ed. St. Louis: CV Mosby; 1988.
65. Quercia RA, Ruderman M. Focus on nabumetone: a new chemically distinct nonsteroidal anti-inflammatory agent. *Hosp Formul* 1991;26:25–34.
66. Reisine T, Pasternak G. Opioid analgesics and antagonists. In, Hardman JG et al., eds. *Goodman and Gilman's the pharmacological basis of therapeutics,* 9th ed. New York: McGraw-Hill; 1996:521–55.

67. Way WL. Opioid analgesics and antagonists. In, Katzung BG, ed. *Basic and clinical pharmacology*, 6th ed. Norwalk, CT: Appleton & Lange; 1995:460–75.
68. Poulsen L et al. Codeine and morphine in extensive and poor metabolizers of sparteine: pharmacokinetics, analgesic effect and side effects. *Eur J Clin Pharmacol* 1995;51:289–95.
69. Bonica JJ, ed. *The management of pain*, 2nd ed. Philadelphia: Lea & Febiger; 1990.
70. Persson K et al. The postoperative pharmacokinetics of codeine. *Eur J Clin Pharmacol* 1992;42:663–6.
71. Schmerzier E et al. Gas chromatographic determination of codeine in serum and urine. *J Pharm Sci* 1966;55:155–7.
72. Guay DRP et al. Pharmacokinetics of codeine after single- and multiple-oral-dose administration to normal volunteers. *J Clin Pharmacol* 1987;27:983–7.
73. Way EL, Adler TK. The pharmacologic implications of the fate of morphine and its surrogates. *Pharmacol Rev* 1968;12:383–446.
74. American Academy of Pediatrics Committee on Drugs. Use of codeine- and dextromethorphan-containing cough remedies in children. *Pediatrics* 1997;99:918–20.
75. Cox RG. Hypoxaemia and hypotension after intravenous codeine phosphate. *Can J Anaesth* 1994;41:1211–3.
76. Parke TJ et al. Profound hypotension following intravenous codeine phosphate. Three case reports and some recommendations. *Anaesthesia* 1992;47:852–4.
77. Caraco Y et al. Pharmacogenetic determination of the effects of codeine and prediction of drug interactions. *J Pharmacol Exp Ther* 1996;278:1165–74.
78. Özdemir V et al. Pharmacokinetic changes in the elderly. Do they contribute to drug abuse and dependence? *Clin Pharmacokinet* 1996;31:372–85.
79. Bowdle TA et al., eds. *The pharmacologic basis of anesthesiology*. New York: Churchill Livingstone; 1994.
80. Arnold JH et al. Changes in the pharmacodynamic response to fentanyl in neonates during continuous infusion. *J Pediatr* 1991;119:639–43.
81. Scholz J et al. Clinical pharmacokinetics of alfentanil, fentanyl and sufentanil. An update. *Clin Pharamacokinet* 1996;31:275–92.
82. Donnelly AJ. Pharmacology of pain management agents. *Anesthesia Today* 1989;1:6–10.
83. Gourlay GK et al. The transdermal administration of fentanyl in the treatment of postoperative pain: pharmacokinetics and pharmacodynamic effects. *Pain* 1989;37:193–202.
84. Varvel JR et al. Absorption characteristics of transdermally administered fentanyl. *Anesthesiology* 1989;70:928–34.
85. Smith AJ et al. A comparison of opioid solutions for patient-controlled epidural analgesia. *Anaesthesia* 1996;51:1013–7.
86. Woodhouse A et al. A comparison of morphine, pethidine and fentanyl in the postsurgical patient-controlled analgesia environment. *Pain* 1996;64:115–21.
87. Herrick IA et al. Postoperative cognitive impairment in the elderly. Choice of patient-controlled analgesia opioid. *Anaesthesia* 1996;51:356–60.
88. Jacqz-Aigrain E, Burtin P. Clinical pharmacokinetics of sedatives in neonates. *Clin Pharamacokinet* 1996;31:423–43.
89. Marquardt KA et al. Fentanyl remaining in a transdermal system following three days of continuous use. *Ann Pharmacother* 1995;29:969–71.
90. Lee HA, Anderson PO. Giving partial doses of transdermal patches. *Am J Health-Syst Pharm* 1997;54:1759–60.
91. Guinard J-P et al. Epidural and intravenous fentanyl produce equivalent effects during major surgery. *Anesthesiology* 1995;82:377–82.
92. Ahmedzai S, Brooks D. Transdermal fentanyl versus sustained-release oral morphine in cancer pain: preference, efficacy, and quality of life. *J Pain Symptom Manage* 1997;13:254–61.
93. Acute Pain Management Guideline Panel. Acute pain management: operative or medical procedures and trauma. Clinical practice guideline. AHCPR Pub. No. 92-0032. Rockville MD: Agency for Health Care Policy and Research, Public Health Service, Department of Health and Human Services; February 1992.
94. Jacox A et al. Management of cancer pain. Clinical practice guideline No. 9. AHCPR Publication No. 94-0592. Rockville MD: Agency for Health Care Policy and Research, Public Health Service, Department of Health and Human Services; March 1994.
95. Edwards DJ et al. Clinical pharmacokinetics of pethidine: 1982. *Clin Pharmacokinet* 1982;7:421–33.
96. Fochtman FW, Winek CL. Therapeutic serum concentrations of meperidine (Demerol). *J Forensic Sci* 1969;14:213–8.
97. Klotz U et al. The effect of cirrhosis on the disposition and elimination of meperidine in man. *Clin Pharmacol Ther* 1974;16:667–75.
98. Julius HC et al. Meperidine binding to isolated alpha$_1$-acid glycoprotein and albumin. *DICP* 1989;23:568–72.

99. McHorse TS et al. Effect of acute viral hepatitis in man on the disposition and elimination of meperidine. *Gastroenterology* 1975;68:775–80.

100. Chan K et al. Pharmacokinetics of low-dose intravenous pethidine in patients with renal dysfunction. *J Clin Pharmacol* 1987;27:516–22.

101. Tang R et al. Meperidine-induced seizures in sickle cell patients. *Hosp Formul* 1980;15:764–72.

102. Clark RF et al. Meperidine: therapeutic use and toxicity. *J Emerg Med* 1995;13:797–802.

103. Quinn DI, Day RO. Drug interactions of clinical importance. An updated guide. *Drug Saf* 1995;12:393–452.

104. Geller RJ. Meperidine in patient-controlled analgesia: a near-fatal mishap. *Anesth Analg* 1993;76:655–7.

105. Erstad BL et al. Site-specific pharmacokinetics and pharmacodynamics of intramuscular meperidine in elderly postoperative patients. *Ann Pharmacother* 1997;31:23–8.

106. Isenor L, Penny-MacGillivray T. Intravenous meperidine infusion for obstetric analgesia. *J Obstet Gynecol Neonatal Nurs* 1993;22:349–56.

107. Ripamonti C et al. An update on the clinical use of methadone for cancer pain. *Pain* 1997;70:109–15.

108. Kristensen K et al. Stereoselective pharmacokinetics of methadone in chronic pain patients. *Ther Drug Monit* 1996;18:221–7.

109. Moolchan ET, Hoffman JA. Phases of treatment: a practical approach to methadone maintenance treatment. *Int J Addict* 1994;29:135–60.

110. Holmstrand J et al. Methadone maintenance: plasma levels and therapeutic outcome. *Clin Pharmacol Ther* 1978;23:175–80.

111. Berkowitz BA. The relationship of pharmacokinetics to pharmacological activity: morphine, methadone and naloxone. *Clin Pharmacokinet* 1976;1:219–30.

112. Beauclair TR, Stoner CP. Adherence to guidelines for continuous morphine sulfate infusions. *Am J Hosp Pharm* 1986;43:671–6.

113. Holmes AH. Morphine IV infusion for chronic pain. *Drug Intell Clin Pharm* 1978;12:556–7.

114. White P. Use of patient-controlled analgesia for management of acute pain. *JAMA* 1988;259:243–7.

115. Baumann TJ et al. Patient-controlled analgesia in the terminally ill cancer patient. *Drug Intell Clin Pharm* 1986;20:297–301.

116. Kerr IG et al. Continuous narcotic infusion with patient-controlled analgesia for chronic cancer pain in outpatients. *Ann Intern Med* 1988;108:554–7.

117. Lutz LJ, Lamer TJ. Management of postoperative pain: review of current techniques and methods. *Mayo Clin Proc* 1990;65:584–96.

118. Gestin Y et al. Long-term intrathecal infusion of morphine in the home care of patients with advanced cancer. *Acta Anaesthesiol Scand* 1997;41:12–7.

119. Milner AR et al. Intrathecal administration of morphine for elective Caesarean section. A comparison between 0.1 mg and 0.2 mg. *Anaesthesia* 1996;51:871–3.

120. Lobato RD et al. Intraventricular morphine for intractable cancer pain: rationale, methods, clinical results. *Acta Anaesthesiol Scand* 1987;31(suppl 85):68–74.

121. Farncombe M, Chater S. Clinical application of nebulized opioids for treatment of dyspnoea in patients with malignant disease. *Support Care Cancer* 1994;2:184–7.

122. Dews TE et al. Intrathecal morphine for analgesia in children undergoing selective dorsal rhizotomy. *J Pain Symptom Manage* 1996;11:188–94.

123. Pounder DR, Steward DJ. Postoperative analgesia: opioid infusions in infants and children. *Can J Anaesth* 1992;39:969–74.

124. Masood AR, Thomas SHL. Systemic absorption of nebulized morphine compared with oral morphine in healthy subjects. *Br J Clin Pharmacol* 1996;41:250–2.

125. McRorie TI et al. The maturation of morphine clearance and metabolism. *Am J Dis Child* 1992;146:972–6.

126. Glare PA, Walsh TD. Clinical pharmacokinetics of morphine. *Ther Drug Monit* 1991;13:1–23.

127. Davies G et al. Pharmacokinetics of opioids in renal dysfunction. *Clin Pharmacokinet* 1996;31:410–22.

128. Tiseo PJ et al. Morphine-6-glucuronide concentrations and opioid-related side effects: a survey in cancer patients. *Pain* 1995;61:47–54.

129. Stanski DR et al. Kinetics of intravenous and intramuscular morphine. *Clin Pharmacol Ther* 1978;24:52–9.

130. Chan GLC, Matzke GR. Effects of renal insufficiency on the pharmacokinetics and pharmacodynamics of opioid analgesics. *Drug Intell Clin Pharm* 1987;21:773–83.

131. Mercadante S. Dantrolene treatment of opioid-induced myoclonus. *Anesth Analg* 1995;81:1307–8.

132. Holdsworth MT et al. Continuous midazolam infusion for the management of morphine-induced myoclonus. *Ann Pharmacother* 1995;29:25–9.

133. Du Pen SL et al. Chronic epidural morphine and preservative-induced injury. *Anesthesiology* 1987;67:987–8.

134. Meisel SB, Welford PK. Seizures associated with high-dose intravenous morphine containing sodium bisulfite preservative. *Ann Pharmacother* 1992;26:1515–7.

135. Chamberlain JM, Klein BL. A comprehensive review of naloxone for the emergency physician. *Am J Emerg Med* 1994;12:650–60.

136. Hoffman RS, Goldfrank LR. The poisoned patient with altered consciousness. Controversies in the use of a 'coma cocktail.' *JAMA* 1995;274:562–9.

137. Osterwalder JJ. Naloxone—for intoxications with intravenous heroin and heroin mixtures—harmless or hazardous? A prospective clinical study. *J Toxicol Clin Toxicol* 1996;34:409–16.

138. Culpepper-Morgan JA et al. Treatment of opioid-induced constipation with oral naloxone: a pilot study. *Clin Pharmacol Ther* 1992;52:90–5.

139. Longnecker DE et al. Naloxone for antagonism of morphine-induced respiratory depression. *Anesth Analg* 1973;52:447–53.

140. Evans JM et al. Degree and duration of reversal by naloxone of effects of morphine in conscious subjects. *Br Med J* 1974;2:589–91.

141. Fishman J et al. Disposition of naloxone-7,8-^{3}H in normal and narcotic-dependent men. *J Pharmacol Exp Ther* 1973;187:575–80.

142. Vozeh S et al. Pharmacokinetic drug data. *Clin Pharmacokinet* 1988;15:254–82.

143. Ngai SH et al. Pharmacokinetics of naloxone in rats and in man: basis for its potency and short duration of action. *Anesthesiology* 1976;44:398–401.

144. Stile IL et al. The pharmacokinetics of naloxone in the premature newborn. *Dev Pharmacol Ther* 1987;10:454–9.

145. Tandberg D, Abercrombie D. Treatment of heroin overdose with endotracheal naloxone. *Ann Emerg Med* 1982;11:443–5.

146. Poulsen L et al. The hypoalgesic effect of tramadol in relation to CYP2D6. *Clin Pharmacol Ther* 1996;60:636–44.

147. Spiller HA et al. Prospective multicenter evaluation of tramadol exposure. *J Toxicol Clin Toxicol* 1997;35:361–4.

148. Kahn LH et al. Seizures reported with tramadol. *JAMA* 1997;278:1661. Letter.

149. Nightingale SL. From the Food and Drug Administration. Important new safety information for tramadol hydrochloride. *JAMA* 1996;275:1224. News.

150. Fisher MA, Glass S. Butorphanol (Stadol): a study in problems of current drug information and control. *Neurology* 1997;48:1156–60.

151. Strain EC et al. Precipitated withdrawal by pentazocine in methadone-maintained volunteers. *J Pharmacol Exp Ther* 1993;267:624–34.

152. Reed DA, Schnoll SH. Abuse of pentazocine-naloxone combination. *JAMA* 1986;256:2562–4.

153. Gourlay GK, Cousins MJ. Strong analgesics in severe pain. *Drugs* 1984;28:79–91.

154. Miller RR. Evaluation of nalbuphine hydrochloride. *Am J Hosp Pharm* 1980;37:942–9.

155. Ameer B, Salter FJ. Drug therapy reviews: evaluation of butorphanol tartrate. *Am J Hosp Pharm* 1979; 36:1683–91.

156. Dayer P et al. The pharmacology of tramadol. *Drugs* 1994;47(suppl 1):3–7.

℞ Antimicrobial Drugs

ANTIBACTERIAL DRUGS OF CHOICE

INFECTING ORGANISM	DRUG OF FIRST CHOICE	ALTERNATIVE DRUGS
GRAM-POSITIVE COCCI		
***Enterococcus*[a,1]**		
Endocarditis or other severe infection	Penicillin G or ampicillin + gentamicin or strepto-mycin	Vancomycin + gentamicin or streptomycin; quinupristin/dalfopristin[2]
Uncomplicated urinary tract infection	Ampicillin or amoxicillin	Nitrofurantoin; a fluoro-quinolone;[3] fosfomycin
Staphylococcus aureus or epidermidis		
Nonpenicillinase producing	Penicillin G or V[4]	A cephalosporin;[5,6] vanco-mycin; imipenem or meropenem; clindamycin; a fluoroquinolone[3]
Penicillinase producing	A penicillinase-resistant penicillin[7]	A cephalosporin;[5,6] vanco-mycin; amoxicillin/clavu-lanic acid; ticarcillin/cla-vulanic acid; piperacillin/tazobactam; ampicillin/sulbactam; imipenem or meropenem; clindamycin; a fluoroquinolone[3]
Methicillin resistant[8]	Vancomycin ± gentamicin ± rifampin	Trimethoprim-sulfamethoxa-zole; a fluoroquinolone;[3] minocycline[9]
***Streptococcus pyogenes* (group A) and groups C and G[10]**	Penicillin G or V[4]	Clindamycin; erythromycin; a cephalosporin;[5,6] vancomycin; clarithromy-cin;[11] azithromycin
***Streptococcus,* group B**	Penicillin G or ampicillin	A cephalosporin;[5,6] vanco-mycin; erythromycin
***Streptococcus, viridans group*[a,1]**	Penicillin G ± gentamicin	A cephalosporin;[5,6] vanco-mycin
***Streptococcus bovis*[1]**	Penicillin G	A cephalosporin;[5,6] vanco-mycin
Streptococcus, anaerobic* or *Pepto-streptococcus	Penicillin G	Clindamycin; a cephalo-sporin;[5,6] vancomycin

(continued)

46

INFECTING ORGANISM	DRUG OF FIRST CHOICE	ALTERNATIVE DRUGS
Streptococcus pneumoniae[a,12] (pneumococcus), penicillin susceptible (MIC <0.1 µg/mL)	Penicillin G or V[4]	A cephalosporin;[5,6] erythromycin; azithromycin; clarithromycin;[11] a fluoroquinolone; meropenem; imipenem; trimethoprim-sulfamethoxazole; clindamycin; a tetracycline[9]
Penicillin-intermediate resistance (MIC 0.1–1 µg/mL)	Penicillin G IV (12 million units/day for adults) or ceftriaxone or cefotaxime	Levofloxacin, grepafloxacin or trovafloxacin; vancomycin
Penicillin high-level resistance (MIC ≥2 µg/mL)	**Meningitis:** Vancomycin + ceftriaxone or cefotaxime, ± rifampin	Meropenem; imipenem
	Other infections: Vancomycin + ceftriaxone or cefotaxime; or levofloxacin, grepafloxacin, or trovafloxacin	Quinupristin/dalfopristin[2]

GRAM-NEGATIVE COCCI

Moraxella (Branhamella) catarrhalis	Trimethoprim-sulfamethoxazole	Amoxicillin/clavulanic acid; erythromycin; a tetracycline;[9] cefuroxime;[5] cefotaxime;[5] ceftizoxime;[5] ceftriaxone;[5] cefuroxime axetil;[5] cefixime;[5] cefpodoxime;[5] a fluoroquinolone;[3] clarithromycin;[11] azithromycin
Neisseria gonorrhoeae (gonococcus)[a,13]	Ceftriaxone[5] or cefixime[5] or ciprofloxacin[3] or ofloxacin[3]	Cefotaxime;[5] spectinomycin; penicillin G
Neisseria meningitidis[14] (meningococcus)	Penicillin G	Cefotaxime;[5] ceftizoxime;[5] ceftriaxone;[5] chloramphenicol;[15] a sulfonamide;[16] a fluoroquinolone[3]

GRAM-POSITIVE BACILLI

Bacillus anthracis (anthrax)	Penicillin G	Erythromycin; a tetracycline[9]
Bacillus cereus, subtilis	Vancomycin	Imipenem or meropenem; clindamycin
Clostridium perfringens[17]	Penicillin G	Clindamycin; metronidazole; imipenem or meropenem; chloramphenicol[15]

(*continued*)

INFECTING ORGANISM	DRUG OF FIRST CHOICE	ALTERNATIVE DRUGS
Clostridium tetani[18]	Penicillin G	A tetracycline[9]
Clostridium difficile[19]	Metronidazole	Vancomycin (oral)
Corynebacterium diphtheriae[20]	Erythromycin	Penicillin G
Corynebacterium, JK group	Vancomycin	Penicillin G + gentamicin; erythromycin
Erysipelothrix rhusiopathiae[a]	Penicillin G	Erythromycin, a cephalosporin,[5,6] a fluoroquinolone[3]
Listeria monocytogenes	Ampicillin ± gentamicin	Trimethoprim-sulfamethoxazole

ENTERIC GRAM-NEGATIVE BACILLI

Bacteroides[a]	Metronidazole or clindamycin	Imipenem or meropenem; amoxicillin/clavulanic acid; ticarcillin/clavulanic acid; piperacillin/tazobactam; cefoxitin;[5] cefotetan;[5] ampicillin/sulbactam; chloramphenicol;[15] cefmetazole;[5] trovafloxacin; penicillin G
Campylobacter fetus[a]	Imipenem or meropenem	Gentamicin
Campylobacter jejuni[a]	A fluoroquinolone[3] or erythromycin	A tetracycline;[9] gentamicin
Citrobacter freundi	Imipenem or meropenem[21]	A fluoroquinolone;[3] amikacin; tetracycline;[9] trimethoprim-sulfamethoxazole; cefotaxime,[5,21] ceftizoxime,[5,21] ceftriaxone,[5,21] cefepime,[5,21] or ceftazidime[5,21]
Enterobacter	Imipenem or meropenem[21]	Gentamicin, tobramycin, or amikacin; trimethoprim-sulfamethoxazole; ciprofloxacin,[22] ticarcillin,[23] mezlocillin,[23] or piperacillin;[23] aztreonam;[21] cefotaxime,[5,21] ceftizoxime,[5,21] ceftriaxone,[5,21] cefepime,[5,21] or ceftazidime[5,21]

(*continued*)

INFECTING ORGANISM	DRUG OF FIRST CHOICE	ALTERNATIVE DRUGS
Escherichia coli[a,24]	Cefotaxime, ceftizoxime, ceftriaxone, cefepime, or ceftazidime[5,21]	Ampicillin ± gentamicin, tobramycin, or amikacin; carbenicillin,[23] ticarcillin,[23] mezlocillin,[23] or piperacillin;[23] gentamicin, tobramycin, or amikacin; amoxicillin/clavulanic acid;[21] ticarcillin/clavulanic acid;[23] piperacillin/tazobactam;[23] ampicillin/sulbactam;[21] trimethoprim-sulfamethoxazole; imipenem or meropenem;[21] aztreonam;[21] a fluoroquinolone;[3] another cephalosporin[5,6]
Helicobacter pylori[a,25]	Tetracycline HCl[9] + metronidazole + bismuth subsalicylate	Tetracycline HCl + clarithromycin[11] + bismuth subsalicylate; amoxicillin + metronidazole + bismuth subsalicylate; amoxicillin + clarithromycin[11]
Klebsiella pneumoniae[a,24]	Cefotaxime, ceftizoxime, ceftriaxone, cefepime, or ceftazidime[5,21]	Imipenem or meropenem;[21] gentamicin, tobramycin or amikacin; amoxicillin/clavulanic acid;[21] ticarcillin/clavulanic acid;[23] piperacillin/tazobactam;[23] ampicillin/sulbactam;[21] trimethoprim-sulfamethoxazole; aztreonam;[21] a fluoroquinolone;[3] mezlocillin[23] or piperacillin;[23] another cephalosporin[5,6]
Proteus mirabilis[a,24]	Ampicillin[26]	A cephalosporin;[5,6,21] ticarcillin,[23] mezlocillin,[23] or piperacillin;[23] gentamicin, tobramycin, or amikacin; trimethoprim-sulfamethoxazole; imipenem or meropenem;[21] aztreonam;[21] a fluoroquinolone;[3] chloramphenicol[15]

(*continued*)

INFECTING ORGANISM	DRUG OF FIRST CHOICE	ALTERNATIVE DRUGS
Proteus, indole positive (including **Providencia rettgeri, Morganella morganii,** and **Proteus vulgaris**)[a]	Cefotaxime, ceftizoxime, ceftriaxone, cefepime, or ceftazidime[5,21]	Imipenem or meropenem;[21] gentamicin, tobramycin, or amikacin; carbenicillin,[23] ticarcillin,[23] mezlocillin,[23] or piperacillin;[23] amoxicillin/clavulanic acid;[21] ticarcillin/clavulanic acid;[23] piperacillin/tazobactam;[23] ampicillin/sulbactam;[21] aztreonam;[21] trimethoprim-sulfamethoxazole; a fluoroquinolone[3]
Providencia stuartii[a]	Cefotaxime, ceftizoxime, ceftriaxone, cefepime, or ceftazidime[5,21]	Imipenem or meropenem;[21] ticarcillin/clavulanic acid;[23] piperacillin/tazobactam;[23] gentamicin, tobramycin, or amikacin; carbenicillin;[23] ticarcillin,[23] mezlocillin,[23] or piper-acillin;[23] aztreonam;[21] trimethoprim-sulfamethoxazole; a fluoroquinolone[3]
Salmonella typhi[a,27]	A fluoroquinolone[3] or ceftriaxone[5]	Chloramphenicol;[15] trimethoprim-sulfamethoxazole; ampicillin; amoxicillin
Other Salmonella[a,28]	Cefotaxime[5] or ceftriaxone[5] or a fluoroquinolone[3]	Ampicillin or amoxicillin; trimethoprim-sulfamethoxazole; chloramphenicol[15]
Serratia[a]	Cefotaxime, ceftizoxime, ceftriaxone, cefepime, or ceftazidime[5,29]	Gentamicin or amikacin; imipenem or meropenem;[29] aztreonam;[29] trimethoprim-sulfamethoxazole; carbenicillin,[30] ticarcillin,[30] mezlocillin,[30] or piperacillin;[30] a fluoroquinolone[3]
Shigella[a]	A fluoroquinolone[3]	Azithromycin; trimethoprim-sulfamethoxazole; ampicillin; ceftriaxone[5]

OTHER GRAM-NEGATIVE BACILLI

Yersinia enterocolitica[a]	Trimethoprim-sulfamethoxazole	A fluoroquinolone;[3] gentamicin, tobramycin, or amikacin; cefotaxime or ceftizoxime[5]

(continued)

INFECTING ORGANISM	DRUG OF FIRST CHOICE	ALTERNATIVE DRUGS
Acinetobacter[a]	Imipenem or meropenem[21]	Amikacin, tobramycin, or gentamicin; ciprofloxacin;[22] trimethoprim-sulfamethoxazole; ticarcillin,[23] mezlocillin,[23] or piperacillin;[23] ceftazidime;[21] minocy-cline;[9] doxycycline[9]
Aeromonas[a]	Trimethoprim-sulfamethoxazole	Gentamicin or tobramycin; imipenem; a fluoroquinolone[3]
Bartonella		
Agent of bacillary angiomatosis (*Bartonella henselae* or *quintana*)[31]	Erythromycin	Doxycycline;[9] azithromycin
Cat scratch bacillus (*Bartonella henselae*)[31,32]	Ciprofloxacin[22]	Trimethoprim-sulfamethoxazole; gentamicin; rifampin; azithromycin
Bordetella pertussis (whooping cough)	Erythromycin	Trimethoprim-sulfamethoxazole
Brucella[a]	A tetracycline[9] + streptomycin or gentamicin	A tetracycline[9] + rifampin; chloramphenicol[15] ± streptomycin; trimethoprim-sulfamethoxazole ± gentamicin; rifampin + a tetracycline[9]
Burkholderia cepacia[a]	Trimethoprim-sulfamethoxazole	Ceftazidime;[5] chloramphenicol[15]
Calymmatobacterium granulomatis (granuloma inguinale)	Trimethoprim-sulfamethoxazole	Doxycycline[9] or ciprofloxacin ± gentamicin
Capnocytophaga canimorsus (DF-2)[33]	Penicillin G	Cefotaxime;[5] ceftizoxime;[5] ceftriaxone;[5] imipenem or meropenem; vancomycin; a fluoroquinolone;[3] clindamycin
Eikenella corrodens[a]	Ampicillin	An erythromycin; a tetracycline;[9] amoxicillin/clavulanic acid; ampicillin/sulbactam; ceftriaxone[5]
Francisella tularensis (tularemia)[a]	Streptomycin	Gentamicin; a tetracycline;[9] chloramphenicol[15]
Fusobacterium[a]	Penicillin G	Metronidazole; clindamycin; cefoxitin;[5] chloramphenicol[15]

(continued)

INFECTING ORGANISM	DRUG OF FIRST CHOICE	ALTERNATIVE DRUGS
Gardnerella vaginalis (bacterial vaginosis)	Oral metronidazole[34]	Topical clindamycin or metronidazole; oral clindamycin
Haemophilus ducreyi (chancroid)	Azithromycin or ceftriaxone	Ciprofloxacin[22] or erythromycin
Haemophilus influenzae		
Meningitis, epiglottitis, arthritis, and other serious infections	Cefotaxime or ceftriaxone[5]	Cefuroxime[5] (but not for meningitis); chloramphenicol;[15] meropenem
Upper respiratory infections and bronchitis	Trimethoprim-sulfamethoxazole	Cefuroxime;[5] amoxicillin/clavulanic acid; cefuroxime axetil;[5] cefpodoxime;[5] cefaclor;[5] cefotaxime;[5] ceftizoxime;[5] ceftriaxone;[5] cefixime;[5] a tetracycline;[9] clarithromycin;[11] azithromycin; a fluoroquinolone;[3] ampicillin or amoxicillin
***Legionella* species**[35]	Erythromycin or clarithromycin[11] or azithromycin[11] or a fluoroquinolone,[3] ± rifampin	Doxycycline[9] ± rifampin; trimethoprim-sulfamethoxazole
Leptotrichia buccalis	Penicillin G	A tetracycline;[9] clindamycin; erythromycin
Pasteurella multocida	Penicillin G	A tetracycline;[9] a cephalosporin;[5,6] amoxicillin/clavulanic acid; ampicillin/sulbactam
Pseudomonas aeruginosa[a]		
Urinary tract infection	Ciprofloxacin[22]	Carbenicillin, ticarcillin, piperacillin, or mezlocillin; ceftazidime;[5] cefepime;[5] imipenem or meropenem; aztreonam; tobramycin; gentamicin; amikacin
Other infections	Ticarcillin, mezlocillin, or piperacillin + tobramycin, gentamicin, or amikacin[36]	Ceftazidime,[5] imipenem, meropenem, aztreonam, cefepime[5] + tobramycin, gentamicin, or amikacin; ciprofloxacin;[22] trovafloxacin[22]
Pseudomonas mallei (glanders)	Streptomycin + a tetracycline[9]	Streptomycin + chloramphenicol[15]

(continued)

INFECTING ORGANISM	DRUG OF FIRST CHOICE	ALTERNATIVE DRUGS
Pseudomonas pseudomallei (melioidosis)[a]	Ceftazidime[5]	Chloramphenicol[15] + doxycycline[9] + trimethoprim-sulfamethoxazole; amoxicillin/clavulanic acid; imipenem or meropenem
Spirillum minus (rat bite fever)	Penicillin G	A tetracycline;[9] streptomycin
Stenotrophomonas maltophilia (Pseudomonas maltophilia)[a]	Trimethoprim-sulfamethoxazole	Minocycline;[9] ceftazidime;[5] a fluoroquinolone[3]
Streptobacillus moniliformis (rat bite fever; Haverhill fever)	Penicillin G	A tetracycline;[9] streptomycin
Vibrio cholerae (cholera)[37]	A tetracycline[9]	A fluoroquinolone;[3] trimethoprim-sulfamethoxazole
Vibrio vulnificus	A tetracycline[9]	Cefotaxime[5]
Yersinia pestis (plague)	Streptomycin ± a tetracycline[9]	Chloramphenicol;[15] gentamicin; trimethoprim-sulfamethoxazole
ACID-FAST BACILLI		
Mycobacterium tuberculosis[a]	Isoniazid + rifampin + pyrazinamide ± ethambutol or streptomycin[15]	Ciprofloxacin, ofloxacin, or levofloxacin;[22] cycloserine;[15] capreomycin[15] or kanamycin[15] or amikacin;[15] ethionamide;[15] clofazimine;[15] aminosalicylic acid[15]
Mycobacterium kansasii[a]	Isoniazid + rifampin ± ethambutol or streptomycin[15]	Clarithromycin;[11] ethionamide;[15] cycloserine[15]
Mycobacterium avium complex[a]	Clarithromycin[11] or azithromycin + one or more of the following: ethambutol; rifabutin; ciprofloxacin[22]	Rifampin; amikacin[15]
Prophylaxis	Clarithromycin[11]	Rifabutin
Mycobacterium fortuitum complex[a]	Amikacin + doxycycline[9]	Cefoxitin;[5] rifampin; a sulfonamide
Mycobacterium marinum (balnei)[38]	Minocycline[9]	Trimethoprim-sulfamethoxazole; rifampin; clarithromycin;[11] doxycycline[9]
Mycobacterium leprae (leprosy)	Dapsone + rifampin ± clofazimine	Minocycline;[9] ofloxacin;[22,39] sparfloxacin; clarithromycin[11,40]

(*continued*)

INFECTING ORGANISM	DRUG OF FIRST CHOICE	ALTERNATIVE DRUGS
ACTINOMYCETES		
Actinomyces israelii (actinomycosis)	Penicillin G	A tetracycline;[9] erythromycin; clindamycin
Nocardia	Trimethoprim-sulfamethoxazole	Sulfisoxazole; amikacin;[15] a tetracycline;[9] imipenem or meropenem; cycloserine[15]
Rhodococcus equi[a]	Vancomycin ± a fluoroquinolone,[3] rifampin, imipenem, or meropenem or amikacin	Erythromycin
Tropheryma whippelii[a,41] (agent of Whipple's disease)	Trimethoprim-sulfamethoxazole	Penicillin G; a tetracycline[9]
CHLAMYDIAE		
Chlamydia psittaci (psittacosis; ornithosis)	A tetracycline[9]	Chloramphenicol[15]
Chlamydia trachomatis		
(trachoma)	Azithromycin	A tetracycline[9] (topical plus oral); a sulfonamide (topical plus oral)
(inclusion conjunctivitis)	Erythromycin (oral or IV)	A sulfonamide
(pneumonia)	Erythromycin	A sulfonamide
(urethritis, cervicitis)	Azithromycin or doxycycline[9]	Erythromycin; ofloxacin;[22] amoxicillin
(lymphogranuloma venereum)	A tetracycline[9]	Erythromycin
Chlamydia pneumoniae (TWAR strain)	A tetracycline[9]	Erythromycin; clarithromycin;[11] azithromycin; a fluoroquinolone[22]
EHRLICHIA		
Ehrlichia chaffeensis	A tetracycline[9]	Chloramphenicol[15]
Agent of human granulocytic ehrlichiosis[42]	A tetracycline[9]	
MYCOPLASMA		
Mycoplasma pneumoniae	Erythromycin or a tetracycline[9] or clarithromycin[11] or azithromycin	A fluoroquinolone[3]
Ureaplasma urealyticum	Erythromycin	A tetracycline;[9] clarithromycin;[11] azithromycin; ofloxacin[22]

(*continued*)

INFECTING ORGANISM	DRUG OF FIRST CHOICE	ALTERNATIVE DRUGS
RICKETTSIA–Rocky Mountain Spotted Fever, endemic typhus (murine), epidemic typhus (louse borne), scrub typhus, trench fever, Q fever	A tetracycline[9]	Chloramphenicol;[15] a fluoroquinolone[3]
SPIROCHETES		
Borrelia burgdorferi (Lyme disease)[43]	Doxycycline[9] or amoxicillin or cefuroxime axetil[5]	Ceftriaxone;[5] cefotaxime;[5] penicillin G; azithromycin; clarithromycin[11]
Borrelia recurrentis (relapsing fever)	A tetracycline[9]	Penicillin G
Leptospira	Penicillin G	A tetracycline[9]
Treponema pallidum (syphilis)	Penicillin G[4]	A tetracycline;[9] ceftriaxone[5]
Treponema pertenue (yaws)	Penicillin G	A tetracycline[9]

[a]Resistance may be a problem; susceptibility tests should be performed.

1. Disk sensitivity testing may not provide adequate information; β-lactamase assays, "E" tests, and dilution tests for susceptibility should be used in serious infections.

2. An investigational drug in the United States (*Synercid*) available through Rhône-Poulenc Rorer (610-454-3071).

3. Among the fluoroquinolones, levofloxacin, sparfloxacin, grepafloxacin, and trovafloxacin have the greatest in vitro activity against *Streptococcus pneumoniae,* including penicillin- and cephalosporin-resistant strains. Levofloxacin, sparfloxacin, grepafloxacin, and trovafloxacin also have good activity against many strains of *Staphylococcus aureus,* but resistance has become frequent among methicillin-resistant strains. Ciprofloxacin and trovafloxacin have the greatest activity against *Pseudomonas aeruginosa.* Trovafloxacin is the most active against anaerobes. Sparfloxacin has a substantial incidence of photosensitivity reactions. For urinary tract infections, norfloxacin, lomefloxacin, or enoxacin can be used. Ciprofloxacin, ofloxacin, levofloxacin, and trovafloxacin are available for intravenous use. None of these agents are recommended for children or pregnant women.

4. Penicillin V (or amoxicillin) is preferred for oral treatment of infections caused by nonpenicillinase-producing staphylococci and other gram-positive cocci. For initial therapy of severe infections, penicillin G, administered parenterally, is first choice. For somewhat longer action in less severe infections due to group A streptococci, pneumococci, or *Treponema pallidum,* procaine penicillin G, an intramuscular formulation, is given once or twice daily. Benzathine penicillin G, a slowly absorbed preparation, is usually given in a single monthly injection for prophylaxis of rheumatic fever, once for treatment of group A streptococcal pharyngitis, and once or more for treatment of syphilis.

5. The cephalosporins have been used as alternatives to penicillins in patients allergic to penicillins, but such patients may also have allergic reactions to cephalosporins.

6. For parenteral treatment of staphylococcal or nonenterococcal streptococcal infections, a first-generation cephalosporin such as cephalothin or cefazolin can be used. For oral therapy, cephalexin or cephradine can be used. The second-generation cephalosporins cefamandole, cefprozil, cefuroxime, cefuroxime axetil, cefonicid, cef-

otetan, cefmetazole, cefoxitin, and loracarbef are more active than the first-generation drugs against gram-negative bacteria. Cefuroxime is active against ampicillin-resistant strains of *Haemophilus influenzae*. Cefoxitin, cefotetan, and cefmetazole are the most active of the cephalosporins against *Bacteroides fragilis*, but cefotetan and cefmetazole have been associated with prothrombin deficiency. The third-generation cephalosporins cefotaxime, cefoperazone, ceftizoxime, ceftriaxone, and ceftazidime and the fourth-generation cefepime have greater activity than the second-generation drugs against enteric gram-negative bacilli. Ceftazidime has poor activity against many gram-positive cocci and anaerobes, and ceftizoxime has poor activity against penicillin-resistant *S. pneumoniae* (DW Haas and T Bonczar, *J Antimicrob Chemother*, 38:293, 1996). Cefepime has in vitro activity against gram-positive cocci similar to cefotaxime and ceftriaxone and somewhat greater activity against enteric gram-negative bacilli. The activity of cefepime against *P. aeruginosa* is similar to that of ceftazidime. Cefixime, cefpodoxime, and ceftibuten are oral cephalosporins with more activity than second-generation cephalosporins against facultative gram-negative bacilli; they have no useful activity against anaerobes or *P. aeruginosa*, and cefixime and ceftibuten have no useful activity against staphylococci. With the exception of cefoperazone (which, like cefamandole, can cause bleeding), ceftazidime, and cefepime, the activity of all currently available cephalosporins against *P. aeruginosa* is poor or inconsistent.

7. For oral use against penicillinase-producing staphylococci, cloxacillin or dicloxacillin is preferred; for severe infections, a parenteral formulation of nafcillin or oxacillin should be used. Ampicillin, amoxicillin, bacampicillin, carbenicillin, ticarcillin, mezlocillin, and piperacillin are not effective against penicillinase-producing staphylococci. The combinations of clavulanic acid with amoxicillin or ticarcillin, sulbactam with ampicillin, and tazobactam with piperacillin may be active against these organisms.

8. Many strains of coagulase-positive staphylococci and coagulase-negative staphylococci are resistant to penicillinase-resistant penicillins; these strains are also resistant to cephalosporins, imipenem, and meropenem.

9. Tetracyclines are generally not recommended for pregnant women or children less than 8 years old.

10. For serious soft-tissue infection due to group A streptococci, clindamycin may be more effective than penicillin. Group A streptococci may, however, be resistant to clindamycin; therefore, some *Medical Letter* consultants suggest using both clindamycin and penicillin to treat serious soft-tissue infections. Group A streptococci may also be resistant to erythromycin, azithromycin, and clarithromycin.

11. Not recommended for use in pregnancy.

12. Some strains of *S. pneumoniae* are resistant to erythromycin, clindamycin, trimethoprim-sulfamethoxazole, clarithromycin, azithromycin, and chloramphenicol. Nearly all strains tested so far are susceptible to some of the newer fluoroquinolones (levofloxacin, sparfloxacin, grepafloxacin, and trovafloxacin) and quinupristin/dalfopristin.

13. Patients with gonorrhea should be treated presumptively for co-infection with *Chlamydia trachomatis* with azithromycin or doxycycline.

14. Rare strains of *Neisseria meningitidis* are resistant or relatively resistant to penicillin. Rifampin or a fluoroquinolone is recommended for prophylaxis after close contact with infected patients.

15. Because of the possibility of serious adverse effects, this drug should be used only for severe infections when less hazardous drugs are ineffective.

16. Sulfonamide-resistant strains are frequent in the United States; sulfonamides should be used only when susceptibility is established by susceptibility tests.

17. Debridement is primary. Large doses of penicillin G are required. Hyperbaric oxygen therapy may be a useful adjunct to surgical debridement in management of the spreading, necrotic type.

18. For prophylaxis, a tetanus toxoid booster and, for some patients, tetanus immune globulin (human) are required.

19. In order to decrease the emergence of vancomycin-resistant enterococci in hospitals, many clinicians now recommend use of metronidazole first in treatment of most patients with *Clostridium difficile* colitis, with oral vancomycin used only for seriously ill patients or those who do not respond to metronidazole (C Wenisch, *Clin Infect Dis,* 22:813, 1996).
20. Antitoxin is primary; antimicrobials are used only to halt further toxin production and to prevent the carrier state.
21. In severely ill patients, most *Medical Letter* consultants would add gentamicin, tobramycin, or amikacin.
22. Usually not recommended for use in children or pregnant women.
23. In severely ill patients, most *Medical Letter* consultants would add gentamicin, tobramycin, or amikacin (but *see* footnote 36).
24. For an acute, uncomplicated urinary tract infection, before the infecting organism is known, the drug of first choice is trimethoprim-sulfamethoxazole.
25. Eradication of *Helicobacter pylori* with various antibacterial combinations, given concurrently with an H$_2$-receptor blocker or proton pump inhibitor has led to rapid healing of active peptic ulcers and low recurrence rates (*Med Lett Drugs Ther,* 39:1, 1997).
26. Large doses (6 g or more daily) are usually necessary for systemic infections. In severely ill patients, some *Medical Letter* consultants would add gentamicin, tobramycin, or amikacin.
27. A fluoroquinolone or amoxicillin is the drug of choice for *Salmonella typhi* carriers.
28. Most cases of *Salmonella* gastroenteritis subside spontaneously without antimicrobial therapy.
29. In severely ill patients, most *Medical Letter* consultants would add gentamicin or amikacin.
30. In severely ill patients, most *Medical Letter* consultants would add gentamicin or amikacin (but *see* footnote 36).
31. W Schwartzman, *Ann Rev Med,* 47:355, 1996.
32. Role of antibiotics is not clear (JKS Chia et al., *Clin Infect Dis,* 26:193, 1998).
33. C Pers et al., *Clin Infect Dis,* 23:71, 1996.
34. Metronidazole is effective for bacterial vaginosis even though it is not usually active against *Gardnerella* in vitro.
35. JE Stout, VL Yu, *N Engl J Med,* 337:682, 1997.
36. Neither gentamicin, tobramycin, netilmicin, nor amikacin should be mixed in the same bottle with carbenicillin, ticarcillin, mezlocillin, or piperacillin for intravenous administration. When used in high doses or in patients with renal impairment, these penicillins may inactivate the aminoglycosides.
37. Antibiotic therapy is an adjunct to and not a substitute for prompt fluid and electrolyte replacement.
38. Most infections are self-limited without drug treatment (American Thoracic Society, *Am J Respir Crit Care Med,* 156:S17, 1997).
39. B Ji et al., *Antimicrob Agents Chemother,* 41:1953, 1997.
40. RH Gelber et al., *Antimicrob Agents Chemother,* 41:1618, 1997.
41. DV Durand et al., *Medicine,* 76:170, 1997.
42. RF Jacobs, GE Schatze, *J Pediatr,* 131:184, 1997.
43. For treatment of erythema migrans, facial nerve palsy, mild cardiac disease, and some cases of arthritis, oral therapy is satisfactory; for more serious neurologic or cardiac disease or arthritis, parenteral therapy with ceftriaxone, cefotaxime, or penicillin G is recommended (*Med Lett Drugs Ther,* 39:47, 1997).

From Anon. The choice of antibacterial drugs. Med Lett Drugs Ther 1998;40:33–42. Reproduced with permission.

Aminoglycosides

AMINOGLYCOSIDES

Pharmacology. Aminoglycosides are aminocyclitol derivatives that have concentration-dependent bactericidal activity against Gram-negative aerobic bacteria via binding to the interface between the 30S and 50S ribosomal subunits; anaerobic bacteria are universally resistant because aminoglycoside transport into cells is oxygen dependent. Dibasic cations (eg, magnesium, calcium) and acidic conditions decrease their in vitro action. Streptomycin and kanamycin have poor activity against some Gram-negative bacteria, especially *Pseudomonas aeruginosa.* Some Gram-positive organisms (eg, streptococci) are relatively resistant to all aminoglycosides; however, in combination with some penicillins or vancomycin, these organisms are often synergistically inhibited or killed. Aminoglycosides have a postantibiotic effect against Gram-negative bacteria, which can be exploited by using less frequent dosage intervals. Resistance is due to transferable plasmid-mediated enzymatic modification or decreased drug uptake.[1,2] (*See* Notes.)

Administration and Adult Dosage. **IM or IV by slow intermittent infusion over 30–60 min,** although 15-min infusions are safe. Newer dosage regimens combine the usual daily dosage into a **single IV infusion administered over 60 min.**[3,4] This method takes advantage of the concentration-related bactericidal effects and postantibiotic effect of aminoglycosides, and may result in less toxicity.[2–4] **IT or intraventricular administration** is usually necessary to achieve therapeutic CSF levels. (*See* Aminoglycosides Comparison Chart.)

Special Populations. *Pediatric Dosage.* (*See* Aminoglycosides Comparison Chart.)

Geriatric Dosage. Same as adult dosage, but adjust for age-related reduction in renal function.

Other Conditions. Use of IBW for determining the mg/kg dosage appears to be more accurate than dosage based on TBW. In morbid obesity, dosage requirement may best be estimated using a dosing weight of IBW + 0.4 (TBW – IBW).[1,2] With conventional dosage methods, serum drug levels should be targeted for high peaks (>6 mg/L with gentamicin and tobramycin) because these may be associated with better outcome in bacteremia, pneumonia, and other systemic infections.[1,2] Critically ill patients with serious infections or in disease states known to markedly alter aminoglycoside pharmacokinetics (eg, cystic fibrosis, burns, or major surgery)[1,2] often have variable distribution and excretion of the drugs. Serum level monitoring is unnecessary in patients with less serious infections without appreciable renal impairment. (*See* Aminoglycosides Comparison Chart.)

When the drug is administered once daily, very high peak concentrations (>16 mg/L with gentamicin and tobramycin) are achieved; given the lack of association between specific concentrations and therapeutic and/or toxic outcomes, the exact role of serum level monitoring is unclear.[3–5] (*See* Aminoglycosides Comparison Chart.)

Adjust dosage based on renal function. Individualization is critical because these agents have a low therapeutic index. In renal impairment, the following guidelines may be used to determine initial dosage (modified from reference 6):

1. Select loading dose in mg/kg (LBW or dosing weight as above) to provide peak serum levels in the range listed below for the desired aminoglycoside.

AMINOGLYCOSIDE	USUAL LOADING DOSE	EXPECTED PEAK SERUM LEVEL
Tobramycin Gentamicin	1.5–2 mg/kg	4–10 mg/L
Amikacin	5–7.5 mg/kg	15–30 mg/L

2. Select maintenance dose (as percentage of chosen loading dose) to continue peak serum levels indicated above, according to desired dosage interval and the patient's corrected Cl_{cr}.

PERCENTAGE OF LOADING DOSE REQUIRED FOR DOSAGE INTERVAL SELECTED

CL_{CR} (ML/MIN)	HALF-LIFE[a] (HR)	8 HR	12 HR	24 HR
90	3.1	84%	—	—
80	3.4	80	91%	—
70	3.9	76	88	—
60	4.5	71	84	—
50	5.3	65	79	—
40	6.5	57	72	92%
30	8.4	48	63	86
25	9.9	43	57	81
20	11.9	37	50	75
17	13.6	33	46	70
15	15.1	31	42	67
12	17.9	27	37	61
10[b]	20.4	24	34	56
7[b]	25.9	19	28	47
5[b]	31.5	16	23	41
2[b]	46.8	11	16	30
0[b]	69.3	8	11	21

[a]Alternatively, 50% of the chosen loading dose may be given at an interval approximately equal to the estimated half-life.
[b]Dosage adjustment for patients with Cl_{cr} <10 mL/min should be assisted by measured serum levels. Give supplemental doses of 50–75% of the loading dose after each hemodialysis period.

These guidelines are based on population data; serum levels in individual patients may deviate from guideline estimates. No guidelines have been developed for netilmicin or streptomycin.

Dosage Forms. (*See* Aminoglycosides Comparison Chart.)

Patient Instructions. Report any dizziness or sensations of ringing or fullness in the ears.

Pharmacokinetics. *Serum Levels.* (*See* Aminoglycosides Comparison Chart.)

Fate. Absorption after oral or rectal administration is about 0.2–2%; absorption across denuded skin may reach 5%. Irrigation of vascularized areas (eg, peritoneal cavity) results in absorption approximating IM use.[7] IM administration is followed by rapid and complete absorption, with peak serum levels occurring after 0.5–1.5 hr. IV infusions over 0.5–1 hr produce serum levels similar to equal IM doses. Binding of aminoglycosides to plasma proteins is low. These agents distribute rapidly into the extracellular fluid compartment with a V_d of about 0.3 ± 0.08 L/kg, which is increased by fever, edema, ascites, and fluid overload, and in neonates.[8] Aminoglycosides accumulate markedly in some tissues, especially the renal cortex, to levels many times those found in the serum,[2,8] particularly with frequent dosage intervals compared with the same dosage given at less frequent intervals.[2,3] Levels in the CSF of patients with meningitis generally do not exceed 25% of serum levels, except in neonates;[2,8] penetration into the eye is inadequate for treatment of intraocular infections. Penetration into lung tissues and sputum is low, and large doses may be necessary to optimally treat pneumonias with relatively insensitive organisms (eg, *Pseudomonas aeruginosa*). Distribution of aminoglycosides into the peritoneal cavity of patients with peritonitis is therapeutically adequate.[7,8] Elimination is via glomerular filtration of unchanged drug;[1,2] Cl is about 80% of Cl_{cr}. After discontinuation, low levels of aminoglycoside can be detected in the urine for several days caused by excretion of drug that had accumulated in deep tissue compartments.[2,8]

$t_{1/2}$. α Phase 5–15 min; β phase (adults) about 2 ± 0.4 hr with normal renal function (1.5–9 hr in neonates <1 week and 3 hr in older infants); may be more variable in certain groups (eg, obstetric and burn patients) despite normal renal function; 50–70 hr in anuria. A prolonged γ elimination phase is observed when concentrations fall to the lower range of detectability, representing egress from deep tissue compartments and subsequent renal elimination; the half-life of this phase ranges from 60–350 hr (usually 150–200).[2–8] β Phase half-life is most important for use in calculating individualized dosage, but the γ phase may account for the gradual rise of serum levels and apparent increase in half-life with continued therapy, despite stable renal function.[2,8]

Adverse Reactions. Aminoglycoside-induced nephrotoxicity is usually mild and reversible; progression to severe renal disease and dependence on dialysis is rare. Nephrotoxicity is manifested by elevations in Cr_s, BUN, and aminoglycoside concentrations and appearance of renal tubular casts, enzymes, and β_2-microglobulin and occurs in 5–30% of patients, depending on the criteria used and the population risk factors present.[1,2,9] Duration of therapy, prior aminoglycoside therapy, advanced age, pre-existing renal disease, liver disease, volume depletion, and female sex have been identified as risk factors for nephrotoxicity.[1,2] Concomitant use of nephrotoxic drugs also increases the risk of nephrotoxicity. Elevated trough levels are *not* a risk factor but often a result of nephrotoxicity.[2,10] There is no evidence that there are clinically important differences in nephrotoxicity between gentamicin, tobramycin, netilmicin, and amikacin.[9] Depletion of magnesium and other minerals caused by increased renal excretion occurs. Occasional, but often permanent, vestibular toxicity is reported, usually in association with streptomycin. Subclinical vestibular disturbances can be detected in 40% or more of patients receiving aminoglycosides.[1,2,9] Early cochlear damage can be detected only by sequential audiometric examination, because hearing loss in conversational frequencies is a sign of advanced auditory impairment. Furthermore, early auditory damage is not as apparent in the elderly or others with pre-existing high-tone deficits. Risk factors for ototoxicity include duration of therapy, bacteremia, hypovolemia, peak temperature, and liver disease.[1,2] Elevated serum concentrations are apparently not associated with increased ototoxicity risk,[10] nor do there appear to be any clinically important differences between gentamicin, tobramycin, netilmicin, and amikacin.[9] Oral aminoglycosides, primarily neomycin, have been associated with a spruelike malabsorption syndrome.[1,2] Neuromuscular blockade with respiratory failure is rare, except in predisposed patients. (*See* Precautions.)

Precautions. Pregnancy; pre-existing renal impairment; vestibular or cochlear impairment; myasthenia gravis; hypocalcemia; postoperative or other conditions that depress neuromuscular transmission.

Drug Interactions. Concurrent or sequential use of other nephro- or ototoxic agents may increase the risk of aminoglycoside toxicities. Concurrent use of aminoglycosides with neuromuscular blocking agents may potentiate neuromuscular blockade and cause respiratory paralysis.[2] The action of oral anticoagulants may be potentiated by oral neomycin, presumably via reduced absorption or synthesis of vitamin K. Ticarcillin and acylampicillins may degrade aminoglycosides in vitro, resulting in artificially low levels; the extent of degradation is dependent on time, temperature, and β-lactam concentration.[8,11] Degradation can occur in vivo in patients with renal insufficiency.[12] Amikacin is the aminoglycoside least susceptible to β-lactam inactivation.[8,11]

Parameters to Monitor. Renal function tests before and q 2–3 days during therapy. Audiometry and electronystagmography may be performed in patients able to cooperate. Peak and trough serum aminoglycoside levels are useful for individualizing dosage and assuring the presence of effective serum levels. In neonates or other patients with rapidly changing renal function, obtain serum drug concentrations initially and q 2–3 days until stable. However, with once- or twice-daily dosage and in pediatric patients, trough serum levels may be undetectable and other sampling strategies are necessary.[3–5,13] Routine monitoring may not be cost effective in patients without underlying disease between 3 and 18 yr of age.[14] (*See also* Special Populations, Other Conditions.)

Notes. Of the available aminoglycosides, gentamicin, tobramycin, netilmicin, and amikacin are the most clinically useful. **Streptomycin** use is largely restricted to the treatment of enterococcal endocarditis (in combination with ampicillin), tuberculosis, brucellosis, plague, and tularemia; however, it is currently available only for compassionate use from the manufacturer. Amikacin is often used as part of a combination regimen for treatment of *Mycobacterium avium* complex infection. **Neomycin** is much more toxic than the other aminoglycosides when given parenterally; it is restricted to oral use for gut sterilization and topical use for minor infections. Resistance among Gram-negative organisms, especially *P. aeruginosa,* has virtually eliminated the systemic use of **kanamycin. Tobramycin** is roughly equivalent to gentamicin therapeutically, although it is about 2–4 times more active against *P. aeruginosa* than is gentamicin, is often active against gentamicin-resistant *P. aeruginosa,* and may be preferred because of a superior peak-to-MIC ratio.[15] Resistance of Gram-negative bacilli is lowest with amikacin; amikacin use does not appear to result in increased resistance to the drug.[1,2]

AMINOGLYCOSIDES COMPARISON CHART

DRUG	DOSAGE FORMS	ADULT DOSAGE[a]	PEDIATRIC DOSAGE[a]	USUAL THERAPEUTIC SERUM LEVELS (MG/L)[b]	
				Peak[c]	*Trough*
Amikacin Sulfate Amikin	Inj 50, 250 mg/mL.	IM or IV 15–20 mg/kg/day in 2 equally divided doses; IT 5–20 mg/day.	IM or IV (<1 week) 12–15 mg/kg q 36–48 hr; IM or IV (infants >1 week) 12 mg/kg q 24 hr; IM or IV (children) same as adult mg/kg dosage.	20–35	≤10
Gentamicin Sulfate Garamycin Various	Inj 10, 40 mg/mL IT Inj 2, 10 mg/mL Ophth Oint 3 mg/g Ophth Soln 3 mg/mL Top Crm 1% Top Oint 1%.	IM or IV 5–6 mg/kg/day in 3 equally divided doses q 8 hr or in a single-dose IV q 24 hr; IM or IV for less serious infections[d] 3–5 mg/kg/day in 3 equally divided doses q 8 hr or in a single-dose IV q 24 hr; IT 4–8 mg q 24 hr.	IM or IV (<1 week) 4–5 mg/kg q 36–48 hr; IM or IV (infants >1 week) 4 mg/kg q 24 hr; IM or IV (children) 6–7.5 mg/kg/day (7–10 mg/kg/day in cystic fibrosis) in 3–4 equally divided doses q 6–8 hr; IT 1–2 mg q 24 hr.	6–12	≤2
Netilmicin Sulfate Netromycin	Inj 100 mg/mL.	IM or IV 3[d]–6.5 mg/kg/day in 1–3 equally divided doses q 8–24 hr,	Same as gentamicin.	6–12	≤2

(continued)

AMINOGLYCOSIDES COMPARISON CHART (continued)

DRUG	DOSAGE FORMS	ADULT DOSAGE[a]	PEDIATRIC DOSAGE[a]	USUAL THERAPEUTIC SERUM LEVELS (MG/L)[b] Peak[c]	Trough
Streptomycin Sulfate Various	Inj 400 mg/mL.	IM 15–25 mg/kg/day (usually 1–2 g/day) in 2 equally divided doses q 12 hr; IM for TB 12–15 mg/kg/day to a maximum of 1 g or 22–25 mg/kg to a maximum of 1.5 g 2–3 times/week.	IM (neonates) 20–30 mg/kg/day in 2 equally divided doses q 12 hr; IM (children) 20–40 mg/kg/ day in 2 equally divided doses q 12 hr; IM for TB 20–40 mg/kg/ day or 25–30 mg/kg 2–3 times/week.	15–30	≤5
Tobramycin Sulfate Nebcin Tobi	Inj 10, 40 mg/mL Ophth Oint 3 mg/g Ophth Soln 3 mg/g.	IM or IV 5–6 mg/kg/day in 3 equally divided doses q 8 hr or in a single-dose IV q 24 hr; IM or IV for less serious infections[d] 3–5 mg/kg/day in 3 equally divided doses q 8 hr or IV q 24 hr; IV for cystic fibrosis 10 mg/kg/day; Inhal for cystic fibrosis 300 mg q 12 hr for 28 days. IT 4–8 mg q 24 hr.	IM or IV same as gentamicin; IV for cystic fibrosis 10 mg/kg/day; Inhal for cystic fibrosis 300 mg q 12 hr for 28 days.	6–12	≤2

[a]For systemic infections; UTIs are adequately treated with lower dosages.

[b]Based on divided doses given q 8–12 hr; higher peaks and lower (or undetectable) troughs are seen when less frequent dosage intervals are used.

[c]As seen 30 min after a 30-min IV infusion or approximately 1 hr after IM administration of a usual adult dose. Uncomplicated UTIs may be treated with smaller doses that produce much lower serum levels; however, serious infections, such as Gram-negative bacteremia, pneumonia, or endocarditis may require doses resulting in serum levels in the higher part of the range. Clinical efficacy appears to increase as the ratio of the peak serum level to the MIC of the pathogen increases.[15]

[d]These doses conform to those used in published clinical trials, but higher dosages may be necessary in certain patient populations.

Antifungal Drugs

AMPHOTERICIN B	Fungizone
AMPHOTERICIN B CHOLESTERYL SULFATE	Amphotec
AMPHOTERICIN B LIPID COMPLEX	Abelcet
LIPOSOMAL AMPHOTERICIN B	AmBisome

Pharmacology. Amphotericin B is a polyene macrolide antifungal drug isolated from the bacteria *Streptomyces nodosus*. It acts by binding to ergosterol constituents within the cytoplasmic membrane of fungi, with subsequent disruption of membrane integrity and function. Innate or acquired resistance to amphotericin B is rare. Sensitivity of fungi to amphotericin B is related to the concentration of ergosterol present in the fungal cytoplasmic membrane.[16]

Drug binding to cholesterol in cell membranes contributes to amphotericin B–induced nephrotoxicity. Lipid-based formulations provide a carrier for amphotericin B that effectively sequesters the drug to reduce cholesterol interactions, thereby reducing drug-induced nephrotoxicity.

Administration and Adult Dosage. (*See* Amphotericin B Products Comparison Chart.) **IV test dose given before the first amphotericin B dose** (conventional amphotericin B) 1 mg in 20 mL D5W, or (any amphotericin B formulation) 2–5% of the initial dose mixed with an adequate admixture volume to infuse over 10–20 min. Give no premedication and closely monitor the patient for 30–60 min following the test dose.[16] A test dose is used to identify patients particularly sensitive to infusion-related adverse effects or with hypersensitivity to an alternative amphotericin B formulation. However, the utility of the test dose has been questioned, and therapy of a serious fungal infection should not be delayed to administer a test dose.[17] The manufacturer of amphotericin B lipid complex recommends against a test dose. **IV for fungal infections,** initiate with the full treatment dose for patients with life-threatening disease. Initiation at a fraction of the therapeutic dose with daily incremental increases has been advocated to improve patient tolerance of infusion-related adverse effects but has not been evaluated in a controlled manner.[16,18] **Duration of therapy** not well defined; patients with life-threatening mycotic disease must receive amphotericin B until resolution of clinical and microbiologic evidence of fungal infection, or until unacceptable drug-induced toxicity occurs. Cumulative dosages of amphotericin B are generally 10–20 mg/kg.[16,18] **IV for maintenance therapy** (conventional amphotericin B and amphotericin B lipid complex) full daily dosage, given every other day (eg, q M, W, F).[16,19] **IV prophylaxis after bone marrow transplantation** (conventional amphotericin B) 0.1 mg/kg/day or 5–10 mg/day has been used.[20] **PO for oral candidiasis** (amphotericin B suspension) 1 mL qid. Swish and hold in mouth for 1 min, or as long as possible, then swallow. Continue for at least 2 weeks. **Top for candidiasis** (Crm, Lot, or Oint) apply to affected area 2–4 times/day for 1–4 weeks. (*See* Topical Antifungals Comparison Chart.)

Alternative Routes. Amphotericin B is given by various alternative routes occasionally to facilitate drug availability to a sanctuary site or to minimize systemic toxicity. Administration by these routes is based primarily on case reports. Therefore, administration of amphotericin B by an alternative route should *never* replace standard therapy. **IT** (conventional amphotericin B) 0.025–0.05 mg, increased in 0.025–0.05 mg/day increments to the desired therapeutic or maximum tolerated dosage. Doses of 0.5–1 mg 2–3 times/week or 0.3 mg/day have been reported. Administration is usually via an Ommaya reservoir. Although an Ommaya reservoir is not mandatory for IT administration, the device facilitates repeated drug administration with more precise drug delivery, improved patient tolerance, and clarified CSF diagnostic quality. **Lumbar puncture and intracisternal injection** have been reported.[16] **Intra-articular for fungal arthritis** 5–50 mg q 2–7 days; the dose is determined by the size of the infected joint.[21] **Intracavitary for pulmonary aspergillomas** 5–50 mg in D5W daily or 2–3 times/week has been used in patients unable to undergo surgical resection.[22] **Inhal for prophylaxis against *Aspergillus* spp. following bone marrow transplantation** 0.15% in D5W nebulized to deliver 10 mg/day in 2 divided doses.[23] **Intranasal for prophylaxis in bone marrow transplant recipients** 0.5% in sterile water 10 mg/day in divided doses.[24] **IP for the treatment of fungal peritonitis** 1–2 mg/L dialysate for 7–14 days has been used in patients receiving peritoneal dialysis; instillation is problematic because amphotericin B is physically incompatible with ionic solutions (eg, dialysate).[16] **Bladder irrigation for uncomplicated fungal cystitis** 50 mg/L in sterile water q 24 hr.[16] **Ocular for keratomycosis** 0.15% (0.1–0.25%) in preservative-free sterile water q 30–60 min for the initial 48–72 hr concurrently with atropine. Subsequent to subjective improvement and ocular re-epithelization, the dosage interval may be prolonged to qid and therapy continued for at least 1 month.[16,25] **Intravitreal for fungal keratomycosis** 5 μg/0.1 mL preservative-free sterile water as a one-time dose.[26] **Ocular by subtenonian injection for postoperative fungal endophthalmitis** 500–750 μg/day for 8 doses.[16] **IM or PO administration of injectable amphotericin B** is not recommended.

Special Populations. *Pediatric Dosage.* **IV** (all products) same as adult dosage. **PO** same as adult dosage. **Top** same as adult dosage.

Geriatric Dosage. Same as adult dosage, but long-term IV administration is more likely to be limited by renal impairment. Co-morbid conditions may reduce patient tolerance of ancillary medications used for management of infusion-related adverse effects (eg, corticosteroid-induced sodium retention).

Other Conditions. In pre-existing chronic renal dysfunction, no dosage adjustment is necessary. The duration of the IV infusion with conventional amphotericin B must be 4–6 hr to prevent drug-related hyperkalemia. In acute renal dysfunction, interrupt treatment, extend the dosage interval, or decrease the dosage as the patient's clinical condition allows to reduce exacerbation of renal impairment.[18] In obesity, for patients ≥1.3 times IBW, calculate dosage based on IBW or adjusted body weight (IBW + 0.4 × [adjusted body weight − IBW]).[27]

Dosage Forms. **Inj** (*See* Amphotericin B Products Comparison Chart.) **Oral Susp** 100 mg/mL; **Top Crm** 30 mg/g; **Top Lot** 30 mg/mL; **Top Oint** 30 mg/g.

Patient Instructions. Injection. Infusion reactions, including shaking, chills, increased temperature, nausea, and other symptoms may occur when this medication is being given. Although uncomfortable, these effects are transient. Certain medications reduce infusion reactions for most people. Amphotericin B may affect your kidneys. If this occurs, you may need to take supplemental minerals by mouth (eg, potassium, magnesium). **Oral Suspension.** Shake well before using. Swish and hold in mouth for 1 minute, or as long as possible, then swallow. Discontinue if mouth irritation occurs. **Topical.** This preparation may stain clothing.

Missed Doses. (Oral, topical) If you take this drug on a regular schedule and you miss a dose, take it as soon as you remember. If it is about time for the next dose, take that dose only. Do not double the dose or take extra.

Pharmacokinetics. Preclinical and phase I testing of conventional amphotericin B preceded development of HPLC and refinement of pharmacokinetic methodology. Pharmacokinetic parameters quoted in tertiary literature may actually reflect drug concentration analysis using microbiologic bioassays.

Serum Levels. A correlation between serum concentrations and therapeutic or toxic drug effects has not been identified or defined for any commercially available amphotericin B formulation.

Fate. (Conventional amphotericin B) poor PO and IM absorption.[16] End of infusion serum concentration is 0.984 ± 0.056 mg/L following administration of conventional amphotericin B 0.25 mg/kg. Extensively bound (>90%) to plasma lipoproteins.[16] Accumulation in hepatic, splenic, pulmonary, and renal tissue.[27] The pharmacokinetics of lipid-based formulations are influenced by the lipid carrier. (*See* Amphotericin B Products Comparison Chart.) The liposome carrier of liposomal amphotericin B is sufficiently small to evade elimination by macrophages of the reticuloendothelial system. Subsequently, the systemic bioavailability of this formulation exceeds that of amphotericin B cholesteryl sulfate and amphotericin B lipid complex. In contrast, the larger lipid carriers of amphotericin B cholesteryl sulfate and amphotericin B lipid complex are recognizable by phagocytic cells and readily distribute to tissues rich in macrophages. Metabolites of amphotericin B have not been identified.[16] Urinary elimination is 3–8%.[16,28] For pharmacokinetic parameters, *see* Amphotericin B Products Comparison Chart.

$t_{1/2}$. (*See* Amphotericin B Products Comparison Chart.)

Adverse Reactions. Frequent adverse effects include infusion-related reactions, nephrotoxicity, normochromic normocytic anemia, and phlebitis. Infusion reactions ordinarily include rigors, chills, and fever. Less common infusion-related reactions include nausea, tachycardia, tachypnea, hypotension, hypertension, bradycardia, myalgia, and arthralgia. Symptoms generally occur during or within 60–90 min following completion of the infusion and decrease with ancillary medications and repeated administration. **Meperidine** 25–50 mg IV reduces the duration and intensity of rigors and chills. **Acetaminophen** 325–650 mg PO reduces fever and is often administered as premedication. **Diphenhydramine** 25–50 mg PO/IV is often included as a premedication. **Hydrocortisone,** which reduces fever, chills, and nausea, is reserved for patients with infusion reactions refractory to other ancillary medications. Case reports describe the use of **dantrolene** for refractory rigors and chills. Although premedication with **ibuprofen** reduces the rigors and chills, most patients receiving amphotericin B are at risk for adverse effects from the nephrotoxic and antiplatelet effects of NSAIDs.[16,19] The prevalence of infusion reactions is greater with conventional amphotericin B or amphotericin B cholesteryl sulfate, relative to amphotericin B lipid complex or liposomal amphotericin. The frequency and intensity of infusion-related reactions is similar with administration of conventional amphotericin B over 1–2 hr and 4–6 hr; however, rapid IV infusion (<60 min) of amphotericin B can cause hyperkalemia and cardiovascular collapse in anephric or hyperkalemic patients. To prevent drug-induced hyperkalemia, infuse amphotericin B over 4–6 hr in patients with renal failure, pre-existing hyperkalemia, or markedly reduced potassium clearance.[19] Amphotericin B cholesteryl sulfate, amphotericin B lipid complex, and liposomal amphotericin are each less nephtrotoxic than conventional amphotericin B. However, these formulations are not devoid of nephrotoxicity. Nephrotoxicity is generally reversible. Permanent renal impairment may occur, particularly in patients receiving conventional amphotericin B >1 mg/kg/day, or with pre-existing renal impairment, prolonged therapy with amphotericin B, sodium depletion, or concurrent nephrotoxic drugs. Signs of nephrotoxicity include increased Cr_s and BUN, hypomagnesemia, hypokalemia, isosthenuria, and renal tubular acidosis. Nephrotoxicity may be reduced with IV infusion of 0.9% NaCl 250–500 mL over 30–45 min immediately before amphotericin B. The patient's body size and cardiovascular status must be considered when selecting the volume and rate of 0.9% NaCl infusion. The saline infusion may be repeated immediately after amphotericin B administration. Normochromic normocytic anemia, which is secondary to amphotericin B–induced nephrotoxicity, is mild and transient and rarely requires intervention. Phlebitis is secondary to chronic peripheral administration of conventional amphotericin B. Some advocate use of **heparin** 1 IU/mL admixture to minimize phlebitis.[16,18]

Rare adverse effects reported with conventional amphotericin B include premature ventricular contraction, dilated cardiomyopathy, hypertension, and diffuse alveolar hemorrhage.[16,18,29,30] Infusion-related respiratory difficulty has been reported with amphotericin B cholesteryl sulfate and amphotericin B lipid complex. Rarely, allergic reactions may occur with liposomal amphotericin B.

IT administration of amphotericin B causes headache, nausea, vomiting, abdominal pain, urinary retention, tinnitus, visual changes, ventriculitis, parethesias, numbness, mono- or paraparesis, arachnoiditis, focal neurologic defects, and chemical or bacterial meningitis. Life-threatening brain puncture and hemorrhage may occur with intracisternal injection.[16]

Precautions. Pregnancy. Impaired renal function. Avoid rapid infusions (<4 hr) in patients with Cl_{cr} <20 mL/min, hyperkalemia, or reduced ability to excrete potassium.[31] Separate from neutrophil infusions by at least 6 hr.[31]

Drug Interactions. Additive nephrotoxicity may occur with cyclosporine, tacrolimus, aminoglycosides, loop diuretics, and other nephrotoxic agents. Toxicity of flucytosine may be increased. Corticosteroids may enhance potassium loss.

Parameters to Monitor. Monitor Cr_s, BUN, magnesium, and potassium before therapy and at least twice weekly during therapy. Monitor patients at risk for acute or worsening renal dysfunction daily. Monitor hemoglobin at least weekly. Monitor microbiologic, radiographic, and clinical signs of fungal infection. Ancillary use of hydrocortisone, acetaminophen, or aspirin may mask fevers.

Notes. To ensure even lipid complex distribution, invert admixtures of amphotericin B lipid complex several times immediately before start of infusion and q 2 hr thereafter. Because amphotericin B has a propensity to precipitate, avoid direct admixture or Y-site mixture of all amphotericin B formulations with IV fluids (except dextrose solution), other IV drugs, or blood products. Admixture expiration of conventional amphotericin B and amphotericin B cholesteryl sulfate is determined by sterility more than chemical stability or physical incompatibility. Avoid admixture of conventional amphotericin B with lipid emulsion (eg, Intralipid). Physical incompatibility of this admixture results in particles >10 μM and phase separation.[32]

Prospective, comparative clinical trials support equivalent efficacy of lipid-based amphotericin B and conventional amphotericin B (amphotericin B cholesteryl sulfate) for the treatment of invasive aspergillosis, (amphotericin B lipid complex) treatment of invasive candidiasis, and (amphotericin B cholesteryl sulfate, liposomal amphotericin B) the management of persistent neutropenic fevers. Relative to historical controls, amphotericin B lipid complex is as effective as conventional amphotericin B for the treatment of invasive aspergillosis. Case reports or small clinical series describe successful treatment of mucormycosis, fusariosis, cryptococcoses using lipid-based amphotericin B. Prospective comparative trials evaluating the relative efficacy of lipid-based amphotericin B formulations have not been conducted.

AMPHOTERICIN B PRODUCTS COMPARISON CHART

	CONVENTIONAL AMPHOTERICIN B	AMPHOTERICIN B CHOLESTERYL SULFATE	AMPHOTERICIN B LIPID COMPLEX	LIPOSOMAL AMPHOTERICIN B
	Fungizone	*Amphotec*	*Abelcet*	*AmBisome*
LIPID CHEMISTRY				
Lipid component	Deoxycholate	Cholesteryl Sulfate	DMPG, DMPC	HSPC, DSPC
Diameter (nm)	50	120–140	1600–11,000	80
Configuration	Micelle	Discoid	Ribbon-like	Spherical liposome
PHARMACEUTICAL CHARACTERISTICS				
Vial size (mg)	50	50, 100	100	50
Storage conditions	2–8°C	15–30°C	2–8°C	2–8°C
Compatible IV fluids	D5W	D5W	D5W	D5W
ADMINISTRATION AND DOSAGE				
Daily dosage (mg/kg)				
Sensitive fungi	0.5–1	3–4	5	1–3
Less-sensitive fungi	1–1.5	6	5	3–5
Infusion duration (hr)	1–6	2–6	2	1
In-line filter	Not recommended.	Do not filter.	Do not filter.	May use if pore size ≥1 micron.

(continued)

AMPHOTERICIN B PRODUCTS COMPARISON CHART (continued)

	CONVENTIONAL AMPHOTERICIN B *Fungizone*	AMPHOTERICIN B CHOLESTERYL SULFATE *Amphotec*	AMPHOTERICIN B LIPID COMPLEX *Abelcet*	LIPOSOMAL AMPHOTERICIN B *AmBisome*
PHARMACOKINETICS				
V_{dss} (L/kg)	0.74–3.99	(Adult) 4.2 ± 1.4 (Child) 4.6 ± 1.7	3.9 ± 0.3	0.37
Clearance (L/hr/kg)	0.01 ± 0.001	(Adult) 0.11 ± 0.03 (Child) 0.14 ± 0.02	0.08 ± 0.02	0.023
AUC (mg/L/hr)[a]	—	(Adult) 9.6 ± 2.6 (Child) 7.1 ± 2.6	2.8 ± 0.25	423
Half-life (hr)	25–50	32 ± 5.6	45 ± 6.3	α phase 1.7 β phase 23.6

DMPC = dimyristoylphosphatidyl choline; DMPG = dimyristoylphosphatidyl glycerol; DSPC = distearoylphosphatidyl choline; HSPC = hydrogenated soy phosphatidyl choline.

[a]AUC values normalized to a dosage of 1 mg/kg/day.

From references 16, 27, 28, 33, 34 and product information.

71

CLOTRIMAZOLE
Gyne-Lotrimin, Lotrimin, Mycelex

Pharmacology. Clotrimazole is an imidazole used for local therapy of fungal infections. The topical formulations are equivalent to other topical antifungals in the treatment of *Candida* spp. or dermatophyte skin infections.[35] (*See* Topical Antifungals Comparison Chart.)

Adult Dosage. **Top for tinea infections** apply to affected area bid. **Vag Tab for vulvovaginal candidiasis** 100 mg/day at bedtime for 7 days; or, 2 100 mg tablets once daily at bedtime for 3 days; or 1 500 mg tablet once at bedtime. **Vag Crm for vulvovaginal candidiasis** 1 applicatorful (50 mg) at bedtime for 6–14 days. **PO to treat oropharyngeal candidiasis** dissolve 10 mg troche in the mouth 5 times/day; **PO for prophylaxis of oral candidiasis in patients receiving immunosuppressive drugs** dissolve 10 mg troche in the mouth tid.

Pediatric Dosage. **Top** same as adult dosage. **Troche** (<3 yr) safety and efficacy not established; (≥3 yr) same as adult dosage. **Vag Crm, Tab** (<12 yr) safety and efficacy not established; (≥12 yr) same as adult dosage.

Dosage Forms. **Top Crm, Top Lot, Top Soln, Vag Crm** 1%; **Troche** 10 mg; **Vag Tab** 100, 500 mg.

Adverse Reactions. Nausea, vomiting, bad taste, and mildly abnormal liver function tests have occurred with oral troche. Vulvovaginal burning, itching, and irritation have been reported with vaginal products. Skin rash occurs occasionally with vaginal or topical use.

FLUCONAZOLE
Diflucan

Pharmacology. Fluconazole is a triazole antifungal agent that is highly water soluble and is active in vivo against many fungal species (especially *Cryptococcus* spp.). The drug is active against *Candida* spp., *Blastomyces dermatitidis, Coccidioides immitis,* and *Histoplasma capsulatum.* Antifungal effects are caused by inhibition of fungal cytochrome P450–dependent enzymes that prevent conversion of lanosterol to ergosterol.[36–38]

Administration and Adult Dosage. **PO or IV for oropharyngeal or esophageal candidiasis** 200 mg on day 1, then 100 mg/day for 10–14 days. Severe esophageal candidiasis may require up to 400 mg/day.[36,39] **PO or IV for cryptococcal meningitis: short-term therapy** 400 mg/day for 6–10 weeks; **maintenance therapy in patients with AIDS** 200 mg/day indefinitely. Dosages up to 1 g/day have been used for cryptococcal meningitis. **PO for uncomplicated vaginal candidiasis** 150 mg as a single dose.[38] **PO or IV for coccidioidal meningitis** 400 mg/day indefinitely[40]; dosages up to 800 mg/day have been used. **PO or IV for prophylaxis of candidiasis in bone marrow transplantation** 400 mg/day and continued for 7 days after granulocyte count exceeds 1000/μL. Initiate therapy several days prior to onset of neutropenia.[39]

Special Populations. *Pediatric Dosage.* **PO or IV for candidiasis** 6 mg/kg once, then 3 mg/kg/day for at least 2 weeks for oropharyngeal candidiasis and for at least 3 weeks (or 2 weeks after symptom resolution) for esophageal candidiasis; dosages up to 12 mg/kg/day have been used. **PO or IV for systemic candidiasis**

6–12 mg/kg/day. **PO or IV for treatment or prophylaxis of cryptococcal meningitis** 12 mg/kg once, then 6 mg/kg/day; continue treatment for at least 10–12 weeks after CSF cultures become negative. Prophylaxis in HIV-infected children continues indefinitely.

Geriatric Dosage. (>65 yr) although half-life is prolonged, dosage adjustment appears unnecessary, unless renal impairment is severe.[37] (*See* Other Conditions.)

Other Conditions. Reduce dosage in impaired renal function: for Cl_{cr} of 20–50 mL/min, give the usual dose q 48 hr; Cl_{cr} of 10–19 mL/min, 50–200 mg q 48 hr; Cl_{cr} <10 mL/min, 50–100 mg q 48 hr. Give a full dose after hemodialysis. Patients on chronic ambulatory peritoneal dialysis may receive 50–200 mg/day.

Dosage Forms. **Tab** 50, 100, 150, 200 mg; **Susp** 10, 40 mg/mL; **Inj** 2 mg/mL.

Patient Instructions. Take with a meal if stomach upset occurs. Report changes in appetite, dark urine, or light stools.

Missed Doses. Take this drug at regular intervals. If you miss a dose of this medicine, take it as soon as you remember. If it is almost time for your next dose, take that dose only and go back to your regular dosage schedule. Leave a minimum of 12 hours between doses. Do not double the dose or take extra.

Pharmacokinetics. *Fate.* Rapidly and well absorbed (90%) orally, unaffected by gastric pH. Peak concentrations of 1.8–2.8 mg/L (5.9–9 μmol/L) achieved 2–4 hr after administration of 100–150 mg orally. Plasma protein binding is 11–12%; penetrates well into CSF (over 60% of simultaneous serum levels). V_d is 0.65 ± 0.2 L/kg; Cl is 0.015 ± 0.006 L/hr/kg. About 64–90% of a dose is excreted unchanged in urine.[37]

$t_{1/2}$. 22 ± 4 hr; 37 hr in patients over 65 yr; up to 125 hr in patients with renal impairment.[37]

Adverse Reactions. Occasional nausea, vomiting, diarrhea, abdominal pain, or elevations of liver transaminases occur. Severe hepatitis or exfoliative skin reactions occur rarely.[36,39]

Precautions. Observe patients who develop rash for worsening of the lesions and discontinue the drug if necessary.

Drug Interactions. Rifampin induces the metabolism of fluconazole and may lead to clinical failure. Fluconazole inhibits metabolism of phenytoin, warfarin, and, to a minor extent, cyclosporine. Low dosages have been shown to increase the serum levels of tolbutamide, glipizide, glyburide, and possibly other sulfonylureas. This could lead to a greater hypoglycemic effect, and dosage reduction may be necessary.[39]

Parameters to Monitor. Liver function tests weekly initially, then monthly. Monitor renal function tests weekly if abnormal at outset of therapy. (*See* Precautions.) Monitor patients with elevated transaminases more carefully for hepatitis.

Notes. Combination therapy with fluconazole and **flucytosine** for treatment of cryptococcal meningitis appears to be superior to single-agent therapy;[36] further studies of this combination, as well as fluconazole plus **amphotericin B** are needed. Fluconazole-resistant *Candida albicans* has been clinically demonstrated;

increased use of prophylactic fluconazole may increase the likelihood of the emergence of resistant strains such as *Candidia krusei.*[39]

FLUCYTOSINE   Ancobon

Pharmacology. Flucytosine (5-FC) is a fluorinated cytosine analogue that appears to be deaminated to the cytotoxic antimetabolite fluorouracil by cytosine deaminase, an enzyme present in fungal but not human cells. It has a narrow spectrum of activity and is used with other antifungals because resistance develops rapidly when used alone in *Candida* and *Cryptococcus* spp. infections.[35]

Administration and Adult Dosage. PO 50–150 mg/kg/day in 4 divided doses; the use of higher dosages has been suggested to prevent the emergence of resistance. Duration of therapy must be guided by severity of the infection and response to therapy.

Special Populations. *Pediatric Dosage.* PO same as adult dosage in mg/kg.

Geriatric Dosage. Same as adult dosage, but adjust for age-related reduction in renal function.

Other Conditions. Reduce dosage in impaired renal function. An approximate dosage reduction can be determined by administering doses at intervals in hours equal to four times the Cr_s in mg/dL. Alternative regimens such as reduced doses at 6-hr intervals have been recommended. In patients on maintenance hemodialysis q 48–72 hr, give 20–50 mg/kg after each dialysis.[35,41] Use normal dosage in liver disease.

Dosage Forms. Cap 250, 500 mg.

Patient Instructions. Take the capsules required for a single dose over a 15 min period with food to minimize stomach upset.

Missed Doses. Take this drug at regular intervals. If you miss a dose of this medicine, take it as soon as you remember. If it is almost time for your next dose, take that dose only and go back to your regular dosage schedule. Leave a minimum of 4 hours between doses. Do not double the dose or take extra.

Pharmacokinetics. *Serum Levels.* Toxicity most likely over 100 mg/L (780 μmol/L). (*See also* Precautions.)

Fate. Rapidly and well absorbed (about 90%), with peak about 1–2 hr after administration of a 500 mg dose to adults averaging 8–12 mg/L (62–93 μmol/L) in patients with normal renal function. Negligible binding to plasma proteins; V_d is 0.7 L/kg. Widely distributed throughout the body, including the CSF and eye. Eliminated almost entirely (average 90%) in the urine by glomerular filtration unchanged, with urine levels many times greater than serum levels. Low serum concentrations of **fluorouracil** have been found in patients taking flucytosine and may be responsible for hematologic toxicity.[35,41]

$t_{1/2}$ 6 ± 0.6 hr; up to 100 hr or greater with renal impairment.[35,41]

Adverse Reactions. Occasional nausea, vomiting, diarrhea, bone marrow suppression (often dose limiting in HIV-infected patients), and elevated liver function tests (usually asymptomatic and rapidly reversible). Diarrhea occurs occasionally; ulcerating enteritis occurs rarely.[35,41]

Precautions. Pregnancy; severe renal impairment (elimination is highly variable and monitoring of serum levels is recommended, keeping peak concentrations under 100 mg/L); impaired hepatic function; hematologic disorders; or history of therapy with myelosuppressive drugs (eg, zidovudine, ganciclovir, cancer chemotherapy) or radiation.[35,41]

Drug Interactions. Amphotericin B can increase the toxicity of flucytosine by increasing its cellular penetration and impairing its elimination secondary to nephrotoxicity.

Parameters to Monitor. Before, and frequently during therapy, monitor BUN, Cr_s, Cl_{cr}, full hematology, and liver function tests. (*See also* Precautions.)

Notes. Flucytosine may be synergistic with **amphotericin B,** depending on the organism involved; the combination is useful in treating cryptococcal meningitis in AIDS and non-AIDS patients,[42] although the superiority of the combination in AIDS patients has not been established. Flucytosine may be additive or synergistic with **fluconazole** for the treatment of cryptococcal meningitis; however, further experience in clinical trials is needed before this combination can be recommended.[43]

GRISEOFULVIN   Fulvicin, Grifulvin V, Grisactin

Pharmacology. Griseofulvin is a fungistatic agent that appears to affect mitosis in fungal cells. It is active against dermatophytes and is not useful in the treatment of yeast or other fungal infections.[35]

Adult Dosage. PO (microsize) 0.5–1 g/day in a single or 2–4 divided doses; (ultramicrosize) 330–660 mg/day in 1–2 divided doses. Therapy usually must be continued for at least 3 weeks; infections of the palms or soles require 4–8 weeks of therapy; nail infections usually require 6–12 months of therapy. Instruct patients to take the drug with meals to enhance absorption, avoid prolonged sun exposure, and avoid alcohol.

Pediatric Dosage. (microsize) 11 mg/kg/day; (ultramicrosize) 7.3 mg/kg/day, given as for adults.

Dosage Forms. (microsize) **Cap** 125, 250 mg; **Tab** 250, 500 mg; **Susp** 25 mg/mL; (ultramicrosize) **Tab** 125, 165, 250, 330 mg.

Adverse Reactions. Adverse reactions include occasional nausea and vomiting. Photosensitivity reactions, peripheral neuritis, and leukopenia are rare. The drug may exacerbate acute intermittent porphyria.

ITRACONAZOLE   Sporanox

Pharmacology. Itraconazole is a synthetic triazole antifungal agent that is more active than ketoconazole or fluconazole against certain fungi, notably *Aspergillus* spp. It also has activity against *Coccidioides, Cryptococcus, Candida, Histoplasma, Blastomyces,* and *Sporotrichosis* spp. Itraconazole inhibits fungal cytochrome P450–dependent enzymes. This inhibition blocks ergosterol biosynthesis, creating disturbances in membrane function and membrane-bound enzymes and affecting fungal cell growth and viability.[39,44]

Administration and Adult Dosage. **PO for systemic fungal infections** 200–600 mg/day, depending on site and severity of infection. Give dosages over 200 mg/day in 2–3 divided doses. **PO for vulvovaginal candidiasis** 200 mg bid for 1 day or 200 mg/day for 7 days. **PO for dermatomycoses** 100 mg/day for 15 days or 200 mg/day for 7 days. **PO for pityriasis versicolor** 200 mg/day for 7 days. **PO for plantar tinea pedis and palmar tinea manum** 100 mg/day for 30 days or 200 mg bid for 7 days. **PO for onychomycosis** 200 once daily for 3 months.[45]

Special Populations. *Pediatric Dosage.* Safety and efficacy not established.

Geriatric Dosage. Same as adult dosage.

Other Conditions. Dosage reduction in patients with hepatic impairment may be necessary, but guidelines are not established. No dosage adjustment is necessary in renal impairment.

Dosage Forms. **Cap** 100 mg; **Soln** 10 mg/mL.

Patient Instructions. Take this drug with food to ensure maximal absorption. Do not take with medications that decrease stomach acid (eg, antacids, H_2-blockers, omeprazole). Report symptoms of fatigue, loss of appetite, nausea, vomiting, yellowing of the skin, dark urine, or pale stools.

Missed Doses. Take this drug at regular intervals. If you miss a dose of this medicine, take it as soon as you remember. If it is almost time for your next dose, take that dose only and go back to your regular dosage schedule. Leave a minimum of 12 hours between doses. Do not double the dose or take extra.

Pharmacokinetics. *Serum Levels.* Levels <5 mg/L (<7 µmol/L) are associated with treatment failure in *Aspergillus* infections.[46]

Fate. Relative oral bioavailability of the capsules compared to an oral solution is over 70%[39]; the solubility of itraconazole is aided by an acidic environment, and food increases absorption. Peak serum concentration occurs in 4–5 hr; peak concentration is 20 µg/L (28 nmol/L) after a single 100 mg oral dose during fasting, increasing to 180 µg/L (0.26 µmol/L) when taken with food.[44] The drug is over 99% protein bound, primarily to albumin, with only 0.2% available as free drug.[44] It is highly lipid soluble, and concentrations are much higher in tissues than in serum. Itraconazole is metabolized in the liver and exhibits dose-dependent elimination.[39] One metabolite, hydroxyitraconazole, has antifungal activity, and serum concentrations are double those of itraconazole at steady state.

$t_{½}$ 24–42 hr; possibly longer with large daily dosages.[39]

Adverse Reactions. Itraconazole is well tolerated with long-term use. Occasional rash, pruritus, nausea, vomiting, abdominal discomfort, headache, dizziness, decreased libido, and hypertension occur. Mild transient elevations of transaminases occur frequently, but hepatotoxicity is rare. There are no apparent adverse effects on testicular or adrenal steroidogenesis.[39,44]

Contraindications. Co-administration with astemizole or cisapride.

Precautions. Pregnancy; lactation.

Drug Interactions. Itraconazole inhibits CYP3A3/4 and inhibits metabolism of certain drugs such as astemizole, cisapride, cyclosporine, terfenadine, and warfarin. (*See* Contraindications.) Warfarin dosage reduction may be necessary during concurrent use. Cyclosporine dosage may need to be reduced by 50% with itraconazole dosages over 100 mg/day. Avoid concurrent carbamazepine, phenytoin, or rifampin because they may dramatically reduce the serum itraconazole concentration.[46,47]

Parameters to Monitor. Closely monitor prothrombin time in patients on concurrent warfarin and cyclosporine levels in patients taking these drugs. Monitor liver function tests in patients with pre-existing hepatic impairment. Serum drug concentrations may be monitored if poor absorption or increased metabolism of itraconazole is suspected.

KETOCONAZOLE   Nizoral

Pharmacology. Ketoconazole is an imidazole antifungal agent that exerts its antifungal effects through inhibition of the synthesis of ergosterol (a fungal cell wall component) by inhibiting fungal cytochrome P450. It is primarily used for mucocutaneous fungal infections, including candidiasis, and in tinea versicolor unresponsive to topical therapy. It is used to treat blastomycosis, histoplasmosis, and paracoccidioidiomycosis in immunocompetent patients. It appears to suppress rather than eliminate coccidiomycosis. Because of its poor CSF penetration, ketoconazole is not recommended for fungal infections of the CNS.[41,44] Because of its effects on steroid synthesis (*see* Adverse Reactions) the drug has been used in prostatic cancer and Cushing syndrome.

Administration and Adult Dosage. PO 200–400 mg daily or bid, depending on site and severity of infection. **Top** apply once daily or bid for dermatophytoses, superficial mycoses, or seborrheic dermatitis. **Top for dandruff** apply shampoo twice weekly for 4 weeks.

Special Populations. *Pediatric Dosage.* PO (<2 yr) not established; (>2 yr) 3.3–6.6 mg/kg/day in 1 or 2 divided doses. The drug is bioavailable when tablets are crushed and mixed in applesauce or juice. **Top** apply once daily.

Geriatric Dosage. Same as adult dosage.

Other Conditions. Limited data suggest that dosage adjustment is unnecessary in patients with hepatic impairment; however, definitive studies are needed. No adjustment is necessary in renal dysfunction.

Dosage Forms. **Tab** 200 mg; **Crm** 2%; **Shampoo** 1, 2%.

Patient Instructions. This drug may be taken with meals if stomach upset occurs, but do not take with medications that decrease stomach acid (eg, antacids, H₂-blockers, omeprazole). Report symptoms of fatigue, loss of appetite, yellowing of the skin, dark urine, or pale stools. Taking this drug with an acidic beverage (eg, a cola drink) can increase the absorption substantially. In patients receiving the drug in 0.1 N HCl to promote absorption, the solution should be sipped through a straw to avoid damaging the teeth.

Missed Doses. Take this drug at regular intervals. If you miss a dose of this medicine, take it as soon as you remember. If it is almost time for your next dose, take that dose only and go back to your regular dosage schedule. Leave a minimum of 12 hours between doses. Do not double the dose or take extra.

Pharmacokinetics. *Fate.* Bioavailability is about 75% and is dose dependent. An acidic environment is necessary for dissolution and absorption. Bioavailability appears to be decreased by 20–40% when the drug is administered with food and is even more markedly reduced if gastric pH is elevated. Poor absorption may occur in AIDS patients because of achlorhydria and other pathologic changes in the GI track. Peak serum levels of 3.4 ± 0.3 mg/L (6.4 ± 0.6 μmol/L) are attained following a 200 mg dose taken with a meal. The drug is 93–96% plasma protein bound. V_d is estimated to be 0.36 ± 0.1 L/kg with a single dose, increasing to 2.4 ± 1.6 L/kg during long-term therapy; Cl is estimated to be 0.5 ± 0.25 L/hr/kg during long-term therapy. Ketoconazole is extensively metabolized by the liver to inactive metabolites, with only 2–4% of a dose excreted unchanged in urine.[35,48,49]

$t_{1/2}$. 8.7 ± 0.2 hr after a single dose, decreasing to 3.3 ± 1 hr during long-term therapy.[35,48]

Adverse Reactions. Generally well tolerated, with the most frequent side effects being nausea, vomiting, pruritus, and abdominal discomfort. Hepatotoxicity, including massive hepatic necrosis, occurs occasionally, but mild elevations of transaminases occur frequently. Gynecomastia occurs, probably caused by ketoconazole-induced suppression of testosterone synthesis. Ketoconazole also blocks cortisol production; however, clinically apparent hypoadrenalism occurs rarely. Irritation, pruritus, and stinging may occur with topical use.

Contraindications. Co-administration with astemizole or cisapride.

Precautions. Pregnancy; lactation.

Drug Interactions. Ketoconazole inhibits human CYP3A4 and inhibits metabolism of certain drugs such as astemizole, cyclosporine, methylprednisolone, terfenadine, and warfarin. (*See* Contraindications.) Warfarin dosage reduction may be necessary during concurrent use. H_2-receptor antagonists, antacids, and probably omeprazole and lansoprazole may reduce ketoconazole oral absorption.

Parameters to Monitor. Monitor liver function tests before starting therapy and often during therapy. Closely monitor prothrombin time in patients on concurrent warfarin and cyclosporine levels in patients taking this drug.

Notes. Achlorhydric patients may be given the drug with glutamic acid hydrochloride or 0.1 N HCl (using a drinking straw) to increase absorption.[49] An acidic drink (eg, a cola) may also be used to increase ketoconazole absorption by about 65% in achlorhydria.[50]

MICONAZOLE	Monistat IV
MICONAZOLE NITRATE	Monistat, Micatin, Various

Pharmacology. Miconazole is an imidazole antifungal agent available in topical preparations and as a solubilized IV preparation in a polyethoxylated castor oil (Cremophor EL).[35] (*See* Topical Antifungals Comparison Chart.)

Adult Dosage. **IV** 1.2–3.6 g/day in 3 divided doses, diluted in at least 200 mL of D5W or NS and infused over 30–60 min. **Top for tinea infections** apply bid. **Vag**

Tab for vulvovaginal candidiasis 100 mg at bedtime for 7 days, or 200 mg hs for 3 days. **Vag Crm for vulvovaginal candidiasis** 5 g hs for 7 days.

Pediatric Dosage. IV (<1 yr) 15–30 mg/kg/day; (1–12 yr) 20–40 mg/kg/day. Do not exceed 15 mg/kg/dose. **Top** same as adult dosage; **Vag Crm, Tab** (<12 yr) safety and efficacy not established; (≥12 yr) same as adult dosage.

Dosage Forms. **Inj** 10 mg/mL; **Top Crm, Top Spray, Top Pwdr, Vag Crm,** 2%; **Vag Supp** 100, 200 mg.

Adverse Reactions. Phlebitis, pruritus, nausea, vomiting, fever, chills, and rash are frequent side effects of IV miconazole.

Notes. Because of the serious toxicity (eg, cardiorespiratory arrest, hyponatremia) of the parenteral preparation (most likely caused by the vehicle) and data challenging the clinical effectiveness of this agent, restrict parenteral use to treating fungal infections known to be resistant to amphotericin B (eg, *Scadosporium apiospermum*). Vaginal and topical effects are similar to those of clotrimazole.

NYSTATIN   Mycostatin, Nilstat, Various

Pharmacology. Nystatin is a polyene antifungal agent very similar to amphotericin B but too toxic for parenteral use. Oral absorption is negligible, and there is no absorption through intact skin or mucous membranes.[35] (*See* Topical Antifungals Comparison Chart.)

Adult Dosage. **PO for oral candidiasis** (Susp) 400,000–600,000 units qid (as a "swish and swallow"); (troches) 200,000–400,000 units 4–5 times/day. Treat for at least 48 hr after oral symptoms have cleared and cultures have returned to normal. Immunocompromised patients require a longer duration of therapy (eg, 10–14 days). The vaginal tablet has been successfully used orally in place of the oral suspension; its slow dissolution allows prolonged contact time. **PO for GI candidiasis** 500,000–1,000,000 units tid. **Vag for candidiasis** 100,000 units daily or bid for 2 weeks.

Pediatric Dosage. **PO for candidiasis** (newborns) 100,000 units qid; (older infants and children) 200,000–400,000 units qid. **Top** same as adult dosage.

Dosage Forms. **PO Tab** 500,000 units; **PO Troche** 200,000 units; **Susp** 100,000 units/mL; **Top Crm, Oint, Pwdr** 100,000 units/g; **Vag Tab** 100,000 units.

Adverse Reactions. Nontoxic by oral, topical, and vaginal routes. Allergic sensitization occurs rarely.

TERBINAFINE   Lamisil

Pharmacology. Terbinafine is a synthetic allylamine antifungal agent that exerts its activity by inhibiting fungal ergosterol synthesis through inhibition of squalene epoxidase. Terbinafine is active orally and topically. It has demonstrated activity against dermatophyte infections but is less active than azole antifungal against yeast species.[35,51] (*See* Topical Antifungals Comparison Chart.)

Adult Dosage. **PO** 250 mg once daily for 6 weeks for onychomycosis of fingernails or for 12 weeks for onychomycosis of the toenails. Reduce dosage in severe hepatic or renal dysfunction. **Top for tinea corporis or cruris, or cutaneous**

candidiasis apply cream bid for 1 week; **Top for tinea pedis** apply solution or spray bid for 1 week, cream may require therapy up to 4 weeks, especially for plantar infections; **Top for tinea versicolor** apply solution or spray bid for 1 week.

Pediatric Dosage. Safety and efficacy not established <12 yr.

Dosage Forms. Crm 1%; **Top Spray** 1%; **Top Soln** 1%; **Tab** 250 mg.

Pharmacokinetics. Terbinafine is 70–80% orally absorbed regardless of the presence of food. Peak concentrations after 250 and 500 mg oral doses are 0.9 mg/L (3.1 μmol/L) and 2 mg/L (6.9 μmol/L), respectively, within 2 hr. Terbinafine is highly lipophilic and is widely distributed with a V_d of 13.5 L/kg. It is extensively metabolized to inactive metabolites, and its elimination half-life ranges from 11 to 16 hr; however, an additional elimination phase of 200–400 hr may reflect the gradual release of terbinafine from adipose tissue.

Adverse Reactions. Frequent adverse reactions during oral therapy are dyspepsia, abdominal pain, diarrhea, skin reactions, malaise, lethargy, and taste disturbance.

Drug Interactions. Terbinafine does not appear to affect cytochrome P450 isozymes markedly, but its clearance is increased 100% by rifampin and decreased 33% by cimetidine.

TOPICAL ANTIFUNGALS COMPARISON CHART

CLASS AND DRUG	DOSAGE FORMS	ADULT DOSAGE[a]	COMMENTS
ALLYLAMINES AND BENZYLAMINES			
Butenafine Hydrochloride Mentax	Top Crm 1%.	Top (tinea pedis) apply daily for 1–4 weeks.	A benzylamine similar to the allylamines.
Naftifine Hydrochloride Naftin	Top Crm 1% Top Gel 1%.	Top (tinea) apply bid for 4 weeks.	First agent of allylamine class; response is faster than with imidazoles.
Terbinafine Hydrochloride Lamisil	Top Crm 1% Top Soln 1% Top Spray 1%.	Top (tinea cruris or corporis) apply daily–bid for 1–4 weeks; (tinea pedis) apply bid for up to 4 weeks.	Allylamine; 10–100 times more potent than naftifine. Response is more rapid than imidazoles, and it has excellent penetration in tinea pedis.
IMIDAZOLES			
Butoconazole Nitrate Femstat	Vag Crm 2%.	Vag (nonpregnant) 2% crm hs for 3–6 days; (pregnant, 2nd or 3rd trimester) 2% crm hs for 6 days.	Spectrum similar to other imidazoles.
Clotrimazole Lotrimin Mycelex	Top Crm 1% Top Lot 1% Top Soln 1% Vag Tab 100, 500 mg Vag Crm 1%.	Vag 100 mg supp or 1% crm hs for 7 days; 500 mg supp hs once; Top (*Candida*, tinea) apply bid.	Useful for 1st trimester *Trichomonas* vaginitis, but less effective than metronidazole.
Econazole Nitrate Spectazole	Top Crm 1%.	Top (*Candida*) apply bid; (tinea) apply once daily.	Activity similar to other imidazoles.

(continued)

81

TOPICAL ANTIFUNGALS COMPARISON CHART (continued)

CLASS AND DRUG	DOSAGE FORMS	ADULT DOSAGE[a]	COMMENTS
Ketoconazole Nizoral	Top Crm 2%. Shampoo 1, 2%.	Top (*Candida*, tinea) apply daily for 2–6 weeks; (seborrhea) apply bid for 4 weeks; (shampoo) twice weekly for 4 weeks, then prn.	Possibly less effective than some newer topical imidazoles.
Miconazole Nitrate Micatin, Monistat	Top Crm 2%. Vag Supp 100, 200 mg. Vag Crm 2%.	Vag 100 mg supp or 2% crm hs for 7 days or 200 mg supp hs for 3 days. Top apply bid.	Similar to other imidazoles; superior to tolnaftate in dermatomycoses.
Oxiconazole Nitrate Oxistat	Top Crm 1%. Top Lot 1%.	Top (tinea) apply daily–bid for 2–4 weeks.	Similar to other imidazoles, but superior to miconazole in dermatomycoses.
Sulconazole Nitrate Exelderm	Top Crm 1%. Top Soln 1%.	Top (tinea) apply daily–bid for 3–4 weeks.	Similar to other imidazoles, but superior to miconazole in vaginal candidiasis.
Terconazole Terazol	Vag Crm 0.4, 0.8%. Vag Supp 80 mg.	Vag 0.4% crm hs for 7 days; 0.8% crm or supp hs for 3 days.	Possibly more effective than older imidazoles; appears effective in vaginal trichomoniasis.
Tioconazole Vagistat-1	Vag Oint 6.5%.	Vag hs once.	
POLYENES			
Amphotericin B Fungizone	Top Crm 3% Top Lot 3% Top Oint 3%.	Top (*Candida*) apply bid–qid for 1–4 weeks.	Inconvenient application schedule.

(continued)

TOPICAL ANTIFUNGALS COMPARISON CHART (continued)

CLASS AND DRUG	DOSAGE FORMS	ADULT DOSAGE[a]	COMMENTS
Nystatin Mycostatin Nilstat	Top Crm 100,000 units/g Top Oint 100,000 units/g Top Pwdr 100,000 units/g Vag Tab 100,000 units.	Top (*Candida*) apply bid-tid. Vag 1 tab hs for 14 days.	Similar to amphotericin B.
MISCELLANEOUS			
Ciclopirox Olamine Loprox	Top Crm 1% Top Lot 1%.	Top (*Candida,* tinea) apply bid.	A hydroxypyridone. More effective than clotrimazole for tinea versicolor.
Haloprogin Halotex	Top Crm 1% Soln 1%.	Top (tinea) apply bid for 2–4 weeks.	Equivalent to tolnaftate.
Tolnaftate Tinactin Ting	Top Crm 1% Top Soln 1% Top Gel 1% Pwdr 1% Spray Liquid 1% Spray Pwdr 1%.	Top (tinea) apply bid for 2–6 weeks.	A thiocarbamate. Possibly slightly less effective than imidazoles in dermatomycoses.

[a]The dosage for vaginal creams for candidal infections is one applicatorful at the interval shown. Tinea pedis should be treated at the maximum dosage (usually bid) for the longest time mentioned, usually 4 weeks.
From reference 35 and product information.

83

Antimycobacterial Drugs

CLOFAZIMINE
Lamprene

Pharmacology. Clofazimine is a lipophilic rhimophenazine dye approved for treating leprosy and used in atypical *Mycobacterium* infections, discoid lupus erythematosus, and pyoderma gangrenosum.[52,53]

Adult Dosage. **PO for leprosy, *Mycobacterium avium* complex infections, and for discoid lupus erythematosus** 100 mg/day with food; dosages up to 200 mg/day are used for erythema nodosum leprosum. **PO for pyoderma gangrenosum** 300–400 mg/day have induced remission, but the manufacturer states that dosages greater than 200 mg/day are not recommended.

Pediatric Dosage. **PO for leprosy** 1 mg/kg/day; **PO for *M. avium* complex** 1–2 mg/kg/day.

Dosage Forms. Cap 50, 100 mg.

Pharmacokinetics. The drug is about 50% bioavailable. A peak serum concentration of 0.5–2 mg/L (1–4 μmol/L) 2 hr after an oral 100 to 200 mg dose is proposed as evidence of adequate absorption. Clofazimine accumulates in fatty tissues and the reticuloendothelial system, and is eliminated with a half-life of about 70 days.

Adverse Reactions. Bodily secretions, skin, conjunctivae, cornea, urine, and feces may turn red to brownish black; an orange–pink skin discoloration is common and may take months to years to disappear after stopping the drug. Dose-related GI pain, nausea, vomiting, and diarrhea may occur because of crystalline deposits in GI tissue. Eosinophilic enteritis and splenic infarction occur rarely at dosages greater than 100 mg/day. (*See also* Second-Line Antituberculosis Agents Comparison Chart.)

ETHAMBUTOL
Myambutol

Pharmacology. Ethambutol is a tuberculostatic agent that is only active against mycobacteria, including *Mycobacterium avium* complex. It does not directly enhance short course (6–9 months) regimens of isoniazid, rifampin, and pyrazinamide. Ethambutol is recommended to be included as part of a 4-drug initial regimen if there is a possibility of drug resistance and should be continued for 12 months if isoniazid resistance is demonstrated. Ethambutol is also used in combination with clarithromycin to treat disseminated *M. avium intracellulare* (MAI) infection in patients with AIDS.[53–57]

Adult Dosage. **PO for tuberculosis** 15–25 mg/kg/day as a single dose given in combination with isoniazid and/or rifampin and/or pyrazinamide. **PO for MAI** 15 mg/kg/day, to a maximum of 1 g/day as a single dose in combination with clarithromycin or azithromycin.

Pediatric Dosage. Same as adult dosage.

Dosage Forms. Tab 100, 400 mg.

Pharmacokinetics. Ethambutol is about 80% absorbed from the GI tract with complex disposition characteristics. A peak serum concentration of 2–6 mg/L (8–25 μmol/L) 2 hr after an oral 15–25 mg/kg dose is proposed as evidence of adequate absorption. Its half-life is 4–6 hr, increasing to 32 hr in severe renal impairment. Approximately 80% is excreted unchanged in urine.

Adverse Reactions. Adverse reactions are rare with the recommended dosage of 15–25 mg/kg/day. Optic neuritis (manifested as blurred vision, color blindness, and restricted visual fields) occurs rarely with dosages of 15 mg/kg/day, and is usually reversible with prompt drug discontinuation. Hyperuricemia may occur because of impairment of uric acid excretion.

ISONIAZID   Various

Pharmacology. Isoniazid (INH) is a synthetic hydrazine derivative of isonicotinic acid that inhibits the synthesis of mycolic acid, a component of the mycobacterial cell wall; it probably has other actions. Its activity is limited to mycobacteria; it is tuberculostatic or tuberculocidal depending on concentration and reproductive rate of the organism. Resistance is uncommon in preventive therapy, but can develop rapidly if used alone in active tuberculosis. Primary resistance is becoming increasingly common in certain communities, and has occurred in a variety of institutional settings (eg, hospitals, prisons). These settings are characterized by a high prevalence of HIV infection.[53,54,56,58]

Administration and Adult Dosage. PO for prophylaxis of tuberculosis 5 mg/kg/day (usually 300 mg) as a single daily dose, to a maximum of 300 mg/day, given as a single agent for 1 yr.[57,58] (*See* Notes.) **PO for treatment of tuberculosis** same dosage as above combined with rifampin 600 mg/day and pyrazinamide 15–30 mg/kg/day for 8 weeks, followed by 16 weeks of INH and rifampin. Alternatively, give the doses of INH, rifampin, ethambutol, and pyrazinamide for 2 weeks, followed by INH 15 mg/kg (to a maximum of 900 mg), rifampin 600 mg, ethambutol 50 mg/kg (to a maximum of 2.5 g), and pyrazinamide 50–70 mg/kg (to a maximum of 4 g) in 2 or 3 divided doses twice weekly for a total of 6 weeks by directly observed therapy (DOT), then continue INH and rifampin twice weekly for 16 weeks by DOT.[55,56] In 3-times-a-week regimens, ethambutol dosage is 25–30 mg/kg/day (to a maximum of 2.5g), with INH, rifampin, and pyrazinamide at the same doses as in the twice-weekly regimen, but continued for 6 months by DOT. If pyrazinamide cannot be taken, a 9-month course may be administered in which INH in the above dosage is combined with rifampin 600 mg/day. **IM or IV** (rarely used) same as oral dosage.

Special Populations. *Pediatric Dosage.* **PO for prophylaxis of tuberculosis** 10–15 mg/kg/day as a single dose, to a maximum of 300 mg/day, given as a single agent for a minimum of 6 months.[55] **PO for treatment of pulmonary tuberculosis** same dosage as above, but combine with rifampin 10–20 mg/kg (to a maximum of 600 mg), and pyrazinamide 15–30 mg/kg/day (to a maximum of 2 g) in 2 or 3 divided doses for 8 weeks followed by 16 weeks of INH and rifampin. Alternatively, give the daily doses of INH, rifampin, ethambutol, and pyrazinamide for 2 weeks, followed by INH 20–40 mg/kg (to a maximum of 900 mg), rifampin 10–20 mg/kg (to a maximum of 600 mg), ethambutol 50 mg/kg (to a maximum of 2.5 g), and pyrazinamide 50–70 mg/kg (to a maximum of 4 g) in 2 or 3 divided doses twice weekly for a total of 6 weeks by DOT, then continue INH and rifampin twice weekly for 16 weeks by DOT. In 3-times-a-week regimens, pyrazinamide dosage is 50–70 mg/kg/day (to a maximum of 3 g) in 2–3 divided doses. If pyrazinamide cannot be taken, a 9-month course may be administered in which INH in the above dosage is combined with rifampin 10–20 mg/kg (to a maximum of 600 mg).[55,56] **IM or IV** (rarely used) same as oral dosage.

Geriatric Dosage. Same as adult dosage.

Other Conditions. Acetylator phenotype has not been evaluated as a parameter for dosage individualization; however, some sources recommend a dosage of 150–200 mg/day in slow acetylators with renal impairment.[59] In individuals with HIV infection being treated for tuberculosis, treatment regimens are not altered, but should continue for a total of 9 months and at least 6 months beyond culture conversion.

Dosage Forms. **Tab** 50, 100, 300 mg; **Cap** 150 mg with rifampin 300 mg (Rifamate); **Tab** 50 mg with rifampin 120 mg and pyrazinamide 300 mg (Rifater); **Inj** 100 mg/mL.

Patient Instructions. Report any burning, tingling, or numbness in the extremities; unusual malaise; fever; dark urine; or yellowing of the skin or eyes.

Missed Doses. Take this drug at regular intervals. If you miss a dose of this medicine, take it as soon as you remember. If it is almost time for your next dose, take that dose only and go back to your regular dosage schedule. Leave a minimum of 12 hours between doses. Do not double the dose or take extra.

Pharmacokinetics. *Serum Levels.* A peak serum level of 3–5 mg/L (22–36 μmol/L) 2 hr postdose is proposed as evidence of adequate absorption.[53]

Fate. Rapid and nearly complete oral absorption with peak serum concentrations of 1–5 mg/L (7–36 μmol/L) 1 hr after a 5 mg/kg dose.[58] Widely distributed in body tissues including the CSF of normal patients and those with meningitis. V_d is 0.67 ± 0.15 L/kg; Cl is 0.22 ± 0.07 L/hr/kg in slow acetylators and 0.44 ± 0.12 L/hr/kg in rapid acetylators.[48] Eliminated primarily by acetylation in the liver to inactive metabolites which are excreted in the urine. Specific pattern of elimination depends on acetylator phenotype of the individual.[59]

$t_{1/2}$. (Rapid acetylators) 1.1 ± 0.1 hr, (slow acetylators) 2.1 ± 1.1 hr. Increased to 4 hr with renal impairment, and 6.7 hr with liver disease.

Adverse Reactions. Pyridoxine-responsive peripheral neuropathy can occur, especially in alcoholics, diabetics, patients with renal failure, malnourished patients, and slow acetylators, and with dosages >5 mg/kg/day.[59] Subclinical hepatitis is frequent (10–20%) and characterized by usually asymptomatic elevation of AST and ALT, which may return to normal despite continued therapy; it may be more frequent with combined INH–rifampin therapy.[60] Clinical hepatitis is rare in those <20 yr, but is strikingly related to age (rising to 2–3% in 50–65-yr-old patients). Rare cases of massive liver atrophy resulting in death usually appear in association with alcoholism or pre-existing liver disease; most severe cases occur within the first 6 months.[60] With acute overdosage (usually 6–10 g), INH may produce severe CNS toxicity including coma and seizures as well as hypotension, acidosis, and occasionally death.[59]

Contraindications. Acute or chronic liver disease; previous INH-associated hepatitis.

Precautions. Pregnancy; lactation. Use with caution in daily users of alcohol, elderly patients, and those with a slow acetylator phenotype.

Drug Interactions. INH may inhibit the metabolism of carbamazepine and phenytoin, increasing the risk of toxicity, particularly of phenytoin in slow acetylators. Mental changes may result from effects of INH and disulfiram on metabolism of adrenergic neurotransmitters; avoid the use of disulfiram in patients who must take INH. Aluminum-containing antacids may interfere with INH absorption. Rifampin may increase the metabolism of INH to hepatotoxic metabolites.

Parameters to Monitor. Question for prodromal signs of hepatitis (eg, fever, malaise) and signs of peripheral neuropathy (eg, burning, tingling, numbness) monthly during therapy. Baseline and monthly AST and ALT are recommended only in high-risk groups (those >35 yr, daily alcohol users, and those with a history of liver dysfunction),[60] although they are not predictive of clinical hepatitis.

Notes. It is generally recommended that all patients receive INH for prophylaxis of tuberculosis who have had a positive reaction to intermediate-strength Purified Protein Derivative (PPD, 5 Tuberculin Units) and who (1) are household contacts of patients with active tuberculosis; (2) converted their PPD to positive within the past 12–24 months; (3) have radiologic evidence of inactive tuberculosis or a history of inadequately treated active tuberculosis; (4) are foreign-born persons (and their families) from high-prevalence areas who have entered the United States within the past 2 years; (5) are persons with known or suspected HIV infection; (6) are persons with medical or iatrogenic conditions that increase the risk of tuberculosis—silicosis, gastrectomy, jejunoileal bypass, weight of 10% or more below ideal, chronic renal failure, diabetes mellitus, corticosteroid or other immunosuppressive therapy, hematopoietic malignancy, other malignancy, and other conditions in which immunosuppression results from the disease or its treatment. Most sources suggest that the use of INH prophylaxis in patients >35 yr should be further restricted because of the increased risk of fatal hepatotoxicity, although this is controversial. Limiting the duration of prophylaxis to 6 months appears to be cost effective compared to 9- or 12-month regimens, and may improve compliance, although HIV-infected patients should receive 12 months of therapy.[58]

To prevent peripheral neuropathy, give **pyridoxine** in a dosage of 50 mg/day to adults receiving large dosages of INH (10 mg/kg/day or more) and those who are predisposed to peripheral neuritis (eg, diabetics, HIV-infected, alcoholics). Pyridoxine IV in a dosage equal to the estimated amount of INH ingested is recommended for acute INH overdose.[61]

Add **ethambutol** or **streptomycin** to the initial treatment regimen until drug susceptibility studies are available, or unless there is little possibility of drug resistance (ie, there is <4% primary resistance to INH in the patient's community, and the patient has had no previous treatment with antituberculosis medications, is not from a country with a high prevalence of drug resistance, and has no known exposure to a drug-resistant case.)[55,62]

PYRAZINAMIDE   Various

Pharmacology. Pyrazinamide is a synthetic analogue of niacinamide that is only active against mycobacteria. The mode of action is unknown. The drug is most active at acid pH, and is active against intracellular organisms. Resistance develops rapidly when used alone, but no cross-resistance with isoniazid is observed.[55-58]

Adult Dosage. (*See* Isoniazid Dosage.)

Dosage Forms. **Tab** 500 mg; **Tab** 300 mg with isoniazid 50 mg and rifampin 120 mg (Rifater).

Pharmacokinetics. The drug is well absorbed from the GI tract with serum concentrations of 40–50 mg/L (0.3–0.4 mmol/L) achieved about 2 hr after a 1 g dose. A peak serum concentration of 20–60 mg/L (163–488 μmol/L) 2 hr after an oral 1–2 g dose is proposed as evidence of adequate absorption. The parent compound and several metabolites are excreted in urine.

Adverse Reactions. Frequent hyperuricemia, probably caused by prevention of uric acid excretion by one of the metabolites, and occasional dose-dependent hepatotoxicity occur. As many as 1–5% of patients taking regimens including isoniazid, rifampin, and pyrazinamide develop laboratory evidence of hepatic damage.

RIFABUTIN   Mycobutin

Pharmacology. Rifabutin is a rifamycin similar to rifampin chemically and in antibacterial spectrum. Rifabutin is more active against mycobacteria than rifampin, including some rifampin-resistant strains of *Mycobacterium tuberculosis* and atypical mycobacteria, and is particularly active against *Mycobacterium avium intracellulare* (MAI).[63-66]

Adult Dosage. PO for prophylaxis of MAI infections in patients with advanced HIV infection 300 mg/day.

Dosage Forms. **Cap** 150 mg.

Pharmacokinetics. Well absorbed orally, but rifabutin has a low bioavailability of 12–20% because of first-pass metabolism. Rifabutin is widely distributed in the body and is concentrated intracellularly to a greater extent than rifampin. It is 71 ± 2% plasma protein bound and has an estimated V_d of 45 ± 17 L/kg and Cl of 0.69 ± 0.32 L/hr/kg. The drug is hepatically metabolized to a number of compounds, with about 10% excreted unchanged in urine. It induces its own metabolism; its terminal half-life after long-term use is 45 ± 16 hr.

Adverse Reactions. The most frequent adverse reactions include rash, taste alterations, anorexia, nausea, insomnia, nervous system disorders (facial paralysis, twitching, and peripheral neuritis), leukopenia, and bilirubinemia. Uveitis has occurred with dosages >300 mg/day.

Drug Interactions. Rifabutin induces the metabolism of drugs metabolized via CYP3A4; although the clinical importance of this effect is not clear, it appears to be less than that of rifampin.

RIFAMPIN	Rimactane, Rifadin, Various

Pharmacology. Rifampin is a synthetic rifamycin B derivative that inhibits the action of DNA-dependent RNA polymerase. It is highly active against mycobacteria, most Gram-positive bacteria, and some Gram-negative bacteria, most notably, *Neisseria meningitidis*. It is also used to enhance bactericidal activity of other antistaphylococcal agents in refractory or chronic infections. Antagonism with vancomycin is observed in vitro, but is probably not clinically relevant. Primary resistance is uncommon, but resistance can develop rapidly if used alone.[67]

Administration and Adult Dosage. PO or IV (rarely used) for treatment of tuberculosis 600 mg/day as a single daily dose in combination with at least one other antitubercular agent. (*See* Isoniazid.)[55,56] **PO for prophylaxis of meningococcal meningitis** 600 mg/day for 4 days or 600 mg bid for 2 days. **PO for staphylococcal infection** 600 mg/day as a single dose in combination with another antistaphylococcal agent.

Special Populations. *Pediatric Dosage.* **PO for treatment of tuberculosis** (>5 yr) 10–20 mg/kg/day as a single daily dose, to a maximum of 600 mg/day, in combination with at least one other antitubercular agent.[55,56] **PO for prophylaxis of meningococcal meningitis** (<1 month) 5 mg/kg bid for 2 days; (1 month–12 yr) 10 mg/kg/day, to a maximum of 600 mg/day for 4 days, or 10 mg/kg bid, to a maximum of 600 mg bid for 2 days.

Geriatric Dosage. Same as adult dosage.

Other Conditions. Accumulation is expected in patients with hepatic dysfunction or biliary obstruction, but dosage guidelines are not available. No dosage adjustment is necessary in patients with impaired renal function.

Dosage Forms. Cap 150, 300 mg; **Cap** 300 mg with isoniazid 150 mg (Rifamate); **Tab** 120 mg with isoniazid 50 mg and pyrazinamide 300 mg (Rifater); **Inj** 600 mg.

Patient Instructions. Take this medication with a full glass of water on an empty stomach (1 hour before or 2 hours after meals) for best absorption. It is important to take this medication regularly as directed, because inconsistent use may increase its toxicity. This drug may cause harmless red–orange discoloration of sweat, tears (it may permanently discolor soft contact lenses), saliva, feces, and urine.

Missed Doses. Take this drug at regular intervals. If you miss a dose of this medicine, take it as soon as you remember. If it is almost time for your next dose, take that dose only and go back to your regular dosage schedule. Leave a minimum of 12 hours between doses. Do not double the dose or take extra.

Pharmacokinetics. *Serum Levels.* A peak serum level of 8–24 mg/L (10–29 μmol/L) 2 hr after a 600–750 mg oral dose is proposed as evidence of adequate absorption.[53]

Fate. 100% absorbed orally, with a 600 mg dose producing a peak serum concentration of approximately 10 mg/L (12 µmol/L) 1–3 hr after administration. Food delays absorption but does not affect overall bioavailability. First-pass hepatic extraction is substantial but saturated with doses >300–450 mg; thus, larger doses produce disproportionate increases in serum levels. Widely distributed throughout the body; however, useful amounts appear in the CSF only in the presence of inflamed meninges. About 80% plasma protein bound; V_d is 0.97 ± 0.36 L/kg; Cl is 0.21 ± 0.1 L/hr/kg. Eliminated primarily by deacetylation in the liver to a partially active metabolite that is extensively enterohepatically recirculated, producing very high biliary concentrations. About 50–60% of a dose is eventually excreted in the feces. Urinary excretion is variable and appears to increase with the dose. At usual dosages, 12–15% is excreted unchanged in the urine.[66]

t½. 3.5 ± 0.8 hr. Half-life increases with higher doses, but may become shorter over the first few weeks of treatment. It is not changed by renal impairment, but is increased unpredictably by liver disease or biliary obstruction.[66]

Adverse Reactions. Adverse reactions are more frequent and severe with intermittent, high-dose administration. GI symptoms are frequent. Acute, reversible renal failure, characterized as tubular damage with interstitial nephritis, sometimes appearing with concomitant hepatic failure has been reported rarely, especially in association with intermittent administration.[58,59] Asymptomatic elevation of liver enzymes occurs frequently, whereas clinical hepatitis is rare, but more common with pre-existing liver disease or alcoholism; the effect of **isoniazid** co-administration on the frequency of hepatitis is unclear.[60] Competition with bile for biliary excretion may produce jaundice, especially with pre-existing liver disease. Intermittent therapy is also associated with thrombocytopenia and a flu-like syndrome (ie, fever, joint pain, muscle cramps).

Contraindications. Hypersensitivity to any rifamycin derivative.

Precautions. Pregnancy; lactation. Use with caution in daily users of alcohol, those with pre-existing liver disease, and those with a history of drug-associated hepatic damage (especially from antituberculars).

Drug Interactions. Rifampin accelerates the metabolism of many drugs such as oral contraceptives, corticosteroids, cyclosporine, digitoxin, enalapril, HIV protease inhibitors, propranolol, methadone, metoprolol, mexiletine, phenytoin, quinidine, theophylline, tolbutamide, oral verapamil, warfarin, and zidovudine because of potent inducing effects on CYP3A.[68] The dosage of these drugs may need to be increased during concurrent use. Rifampin may increase the metabolism of isoniazid to hepatotoxic metabolites.

Parameters to Monitor. Question for prodromal signs of hepatitis (eg, fever, malaise). Baseline and monthly AST and ALT have been recommended, especially for patients with factors predisposing to hepatotoxicity (eg, alcoholism, pre-existing liver disease), although they are not predictive of clinical hepatitis in the absence of symptoms.

Notes. Rifampin is a useful drug for tuberculosis, but should be used only in combination regimens because of rapid emergence of resistant mutants of *Mycobac-*

terium tuberculosis when it is used alone. The recent emergence of multiple drug resistance among strains of *M. tuberculosis* in patients with AIDS includes high-level rifampin resistance. The routine use of rifampin in methicillin-resistant *Staphylococcus aureus* (MRSA) endocarditis is not recommended except after failure of conventional therapy and possibly with renal, myocardial, splenic, or cerebral abscess. If rifampin is added to vancomycin for treatment of MRSA, add a third drug (eg, gentamicin) to reduce the likelihood of resistance development. In nonendocarditis infections caused by MRSA, do not use rifampin unless there is inadequate response to vancomycin alone.

RIFAPENTINE   Priftin

Pharmacology. Rifapentine is a rifamycin, similar to rifampin and rifabutin. It is used in the treatment of pulmonary tuberculosis and is similar in efficacy to daily rifampin, although relapse rates may be greater with rifapentine.

Adult Dosage. PO for tuberculosis 600 mg twice weekly for 2 months with at least 72 hr between doses, then once weekly for 4 months. It should be used in conjunction with other antitubercular drugs in both phases. The drug may be taken with food to decrease nausea, vomiting, or GI upset.

Dosage Forms. Tab 150 mg.

Pharmacokinetics. Peak serum levels occur 5–6 hr after an oral dose. Food increases the bioavailability and peak serum level. Rifapentine is 93% bound to serum albumin. V_d is estimated to be 70 ± 1 L/kg. Cl is 2.5 ± 0.14 L/hr/kg in males and 1.7 ± 0.41 L/hr/kg in females. The drug is hydrolyzed by an esterase to the active metabolite 25-desacetyl rifapentine. Half-lives of the drug and metabolite are each about 13 hr.

Adverse Reactions. The most frequent side effects in combination regimens were neutropenia, leukopenia, increased liver enzymes, dyspepsia, and anorexia, although these appeared to be less frequent than equivalent rifampin-containing regimens. Pyuria and hematuria occurred more frequently with rifapentine than with rifampin. Patients should have baseline liver enzymes, bilirubin, CBC, and platelet count before starting therapy. Routine laboratory monitoring during therapy is not necessary unless clinically indicated.

Contraindications. Hypersensitivity to any rifamycin.

Drug Interactions. Rifapentine induces CYP2C8/9 and 3A4. It may increase the metabolism of drugs metabolized by these isozymes. Rifapentine decreases indinavir peak by 55% and AUC by 70%. It is should be used with great caution in conjunction with protease inhibitors and other drugs metabolized by CYP2C8/9 or 3A4.

SECOND-LINE ANTITUBERCULOSIS AGENTS COMPARISON CHART[a]

DRUG	DOSAGE FORMS	ADULT DOSAGE	PEDIATRIC DOSAGE	SERUM LEVELS[b] (MG/L)	HALF-LIFE		MAJOR ADVERSE EFFECTS
					Normal	Renal Impairment	
Aminosalicylic Acid Salts[c] Various	Tab 500 mg.	PO 8–12 g/day in 2–4 divided doses (as the acid).	150–300 mg/kg/day in 3–4 divided doses, to a maximum of 12 g/day.	20–60[d] (4 g)	1 hr	—	GI intolerance; hepatitis; lupuslike syndrome. Rarely used.
Capreomycin Sulfate Capastat	Inj 1 g.	Same as streptomycin.	Same as streptomycin.	Same as streptomycin.	2.5 hr	↑	Nephrotoxicity; ototoxicity.
Clofazimine Lamprene	Cap 50, 100 mg.	PO 100–200 mg/day.	Not well established.	0.5–2 (100–200 mg)	70 days	—	Brown–black discoloration of skin and bodily secretions; nausea; vomiting; GI pain because of deposition in GI tissues.
Cycloserine Seromycin	Cap 250 mg.	PO 15–20 mg/kg/day (usually 500 mg) in 2 divided doses, to a maximum of 1 g/day.	PO 10–15 mg/kg/day to a maximum of 1 g/day.	20–35 (250–500 mg)	10 hr	↑	CNS (drowsiness, dizziness, headache, depression, rare seizures, and psychosis).
Ethionamide Trecator-SC	Tab 250 mg.	PO 15–20 mg/kg/day (usually 500–750 mg) as a single daily dose, to a maximum of 1 g/day.	PO 15–20 mg/kg/day to a maximum of 1 g/day.	1–5 (250–500 mg)	3 hr	—	GI intolerance; hepatitis; CNS (drowsiness, dizziness, headache, depression, rare seizures).

(continued)

DRUG	DOSAGE FORMS	ADULT DOSAGE	PEDIATRIC DOSAGE	SERUM LEVELS[b] (MG/L)	HALF-LIFE Normal	HALF-LIFE Renal Impairment	MAJOR ADVERSE EFFECTS
Kanamycin Sulfate Kantrex	Inj 37.5, 250, 333 mg/mL.	Same as streptomycin.	Same as streptomycin.	Same as streptomycin.	2–3 hr	80–90 hr	Nephrotoxicity; ototoxicity.
Rifabutin Mycobutin	Cap 150 mg.	PO 300 mg/day as a single dose.	Not well established. (1 yr) 15–25 mg/kg/day; (2–10 yr) 4–19 mg/kg/day; (14–16 yr) 2.8–5.4 mg/kg/day.	—	45 ± 16 hr	—	See monograph.
Streptomycin Sulfate Various	Inj 400 mg/mL.	IM 12–15 mg/kg/day to a maximum of 1 g, or 22–25 mg/kg to a maximum of 1.5 g 2–3 times/ week.	IM 20–40 mg/kg/ day to a maximum of 1 g, or 25–30 mg/kg to a maximum of 1.5 g 2–3 times/week.	35–40 (12–15 mg/kg) 65–80 (22–25mg/kg)	2–3 hr	↑	Vestibular ototoxicity.

[a]Use only in combination with other effective antituberculars.
[b]Peak serum level 1 hr (parenteral) or 2 hr (oral) after the adult dose in parentheses that is evidence of adequate absorption.
[c]Sodium salt contains 73% aminosalicylic acid; increase dosage accordingly. Sodium content is 4.7 mEq/g.
[d]Peak serum level 6 hr after a dose of Paser granules (investigational).
Adapted from references 53, 55, 58, and 59.

Antiparasitic Drugs

Class Instructions: Pinworms. Purgation, enemas, or special dietary restrictions are unnecessary with this drug, which may be taken with food or beverages. To avoid reinfestation with pinworms, wash the perianal area thoroughly each morning. Change and wash nightclothes, undergarments, and bedclothes daily. Wash hands and under fingernails thoroughly after bowel movements and before eating. Treat all family members simultaneously and clean bedroom and bathroom floors thoroughly at the end of the course of treatment. In order to demonstrate a cure, no eggs must be found in the anal area at least 5 weeks after the end of treatment.

ALBENDAZOLE   Albenza

Pharmacology. Albendazole is a benzimidazole drug related to mebendazole and has a similar mechanism of action; however, it has a broader range of activity than mebendazole.

Administration and Adult Dosage. **PO for hydatid cyst** 400 mg bid for 28 days, followed by a 2-week drug-free interval; repeat to a total of three cycles. **PO for cysticercosis** 400 mg bid for 8–30 days; repeat courses of therapy may be needed. **PO for** *Clonorchis sinensis* 10 mg/kg/day for 7 days; **PO for toxocariasis** 400 mg bid for 3–5 days.[69]

Special Populations. *Pediatric Dosage.* Safety and efficacy not established. **PO for hydatid cyst** 15 mg/kg/day for 28 days; repeat course of therapy prn. **PO for cysticercosis** 15 mg/kg/day in 2–3 divided doses for 8–28 days; repeat course of therapy prn. **PO for toxocariasis** 400 mg bid for 3–5 days.[69]

Geriatric Dosage. Same as adult dosage.

Dosage Forms. **Tab** 200 mg.

Patient Instructions. Take this drug with a fatty meal to increase absorption and improve effectiveness.

Missed Doses. Take this drug at regular intervals. If you miss a dose of this medicine, take it as soon as you remember. If it is almost time for your next dose, take that dose only and go back to your regular dosage schedule. Do not double the dose or take extra.

Pharmacokinetics. *Fate.* Absorption is poor, but is enhanced by fat. Oral bioavailability of unchanged albendazole is negligible because of first-pass metabolism to albendazole sulfoxide, the active form of the drug. The sulfoxide has a peak serum level 2–3 hr after a dose. CNS concentrations are 40% of serum levels; concentration in echinococcal cysts is about 25% of serum levels. The absorbed drug is primarily excreted in urine as metabolites.[70]

$t_{1/2}$. (Albendazole sulfoxide) 10–15 hr.[70]

Adverse Reactions. Occasionally, diarrhea, abdominal pain, and migration of roundworms through the mouth and nose occur. Rarely, leukopenia, alopecia, or increased transaminases occur.[69]

Precautions. Pregnancy; liver dysfunction.

Drug Interactions. Concurrent dexamethasone increases serum levels by 50%.[70]

Parameters to Monitor. Monitor hepatic transaminases and WBC count during prolonged therapy.

Notes. Albendazole is also an alternative in ascariasis, capillariasis, cutaneous larva migrans, eosinophilic enterocolitis, gnathostomiasis, hookworm, microsporidiosis (in AIDS), pinworms, strongyloidiasis, trichostrongyloidiasis, and whipworm.[69,71]

MEBENDAZOLE   Vermox, Various

Pharmacology. Mebendazole is active against many intestinal roundworms. It binds to helminth tubulin, and inhibits glucose uptake in the parasite with no effect on blood glucose concentrations in the host.[70]

Administration and Adult Dosage. **PO for pinworms** 100 mg in a single dose; repeat in 2 weeks. **PO for roundworms, whipworms, and hookworms** 100 mg bid for 3 days.[69]

Special Populations. *Pediatric Dosage.* (<2 yr) Safety and efficacy not established. **PO for pinworms, roundworms, whipworms, and hookworms** same as adult dosage.[69]

Geriatric Dosage. Same as adult dosage.

Dosage Forms. **Chew Tab** 100 mg.

Patient Instructions. (*See* Pinworms Class Instructions.) Chew tablets before swallowing.

Pharmacokinetics. *Fate.* Poorly absorbed orally. Almost all eliminated unchanged in the feces, but up to 10% may be recovered in the urine 48 hr after a dose, primarily as the decarboxylated metabolite.[70]

Adverse Reactions. Occasional abdominal pain and diarrhea in cases of massive infestation and expulsion of worms. Occasionally, migration of roundworms through the mouth and nose occurs. Rarely, leukopenia, agranulocytosis, and hypospermia have been reported.[69]

Precautions. Pregnancy.

Drug Interactions. Carbamazepine and hydantoins may reduce mebendazole serum levels.

Parameters to Monitor. When treating whipworm, take a stool sample for egg count 3 weeks after treatment to detect frequent (about 30%) persistent infestation requiring retreatment.

Notes. Mebendazole is the agent of choice for whipworm, producing about a 70% cure rate with a single treatment; the cure rate is 90–100% with roundworms, hookworms, and pinworms. Particularly useful in mixed infestations. It is also used in several other infestations, such as trichinosis, eosinophilic enterocolitis, capillariasis, angiostrongyliasis, and visceral larva migrans.[69,70]

PERMETHRIN   Acticin, Elimite, Nix

Pharmacology. Permethrin is a pyrethroid that acts on arthropod nerve cell membranes to cause delayed polarization and paralysis. It is active against lice (including unhatched eggs) and mites (eg, scabies).

Administration and Adult Dosage. Top for head lice apply 1% cream rinse to hair one time after washing hair. Leave on for no longer than 10 min and rinse with water. If live lice are seen after 7 or more days, reapply as above. Alternatively, 5% cream left on the hair overnight under a shower cap has been suggested.[69] **Top for pubic lice** although not FDA-approved, application as for head lice has been used; repeat application at 10 days has been recommended.[72,73] **Top for scabies** thoroughly massage 5% cream into the skin from the head to the soles of the feet. Remove by showering or bathing after 8–14 hr.

Special Populations. *Pediatric Dosage.* **Top for lice** (<2 months) safety and efficacy not established; (>2 months) same as adult dosage. **Top for scabies** (<2 months) safety and efficacy not established. Neonates have been treated, but cream should be removed after 6 hr;[74] (>2 months) same as adult dosage.

Geriatric Dosage. Same as adult dosage.

Dosage Forms. Liquid (creme rinse) 1% (Nix); **Crm** 5% (Acticin, Elimite).

Patient Instructions. Lice. Wash hair and towel dry. Apply enough creme rinse to saturate hair and scalp, especially behind the ears and on the nape of the neck. Use the comb provided with the product to remove nits. Wash all headgear in hot, soapy water and dry using the hot cycle of a dryer for at least 20 minutes. Clothing and bedding that cannot be washed should be sealed in a plastic bag for 2 weeks or dry cleaned. Soak combs in hot water for 5–10 minutes. Thoroughly vacuum the room(s) inhabited by the affected person(s). If infestation of the eyebrows or eyelashes occurs, consult your health care provider. **Scabies.** Itching, mild burning, or stinging may occur after application. Itching usually resolves by 4 weeks. If irritation persists, consult your health care provider.

Pharmacokinetics. *Fate.* Usually <2% absorbed after topical application. Permethrin is rapidly metabolized by ester hydrolysis to inactive metabolites which are excreted in urine.[75]

Adverse Reactions. Adverse reactions are mild and occur only occasionally with the treatment of lice. With the 5% cream for treatment of scabies, mild, transient burning, stinging, or tingling occurs in about 10% of patients. Itching, edema, and erythema are often symptoms of scabies and may be exacerbated temporarily by treatment with permethrin. Intolerable burning and stinging may occur in patients with AIDS and scabies.[75] Itching and skin irritation may persist after successful treatment because of local allergic reactions to the dead mites. Allergic reactions are rare and may be caused by the formaldehyde preservative.

Contraindications. Documented allergy to any pyrethroid or vehicle component.

Precautions. Pregnancy, although animal studies indicate no teratogenicity. During lactation, discontinue nursing temporarily during treatment with 5% cream;

use of 1% creme rinse poses little risk during breastfeeding. Avoid contact with eyes and mucous membranes.

Drug Interactions. None known.

Paramenters to Monitor. Observe for parasites 7–10 days after treatment of lice infestation or 14 days after treatment of scabies.

Notes. Permethrin is the drug of choice for pediculosis and scabies. **Malathion** 0.5% lotion (Ovide) is an alternative for pediculosis. **Synergized pyrethrins** (pyrethrins and piperonyl butoxide) have efficacy similar to permethrin for head lice, but they are not as persistent as permethrin and require a repeat treatment after 1 week. A single dose of **ivermectin** 200 μg/kg PO is effective for scabies and head lice.[69] In scabies, permethrin is safer and slightly more effective than **lindane** and more effective and easier to use than **crotamiton**.[73,75] Lindane is not recommended because resistance occurs frequently and lindane is a persistent environmental contaminant.[73]

PRAZIQUANTEL   Biltricide

Pharmacology. Praziquantel causes a loss of intracellular calcium, resulting in paralysis and dislodgement of worms from sites of attachment. In higher dosages, it damages the parasite's surface membrane, allowing the host's immune response to destroy the worm.[71]

Administration and Adult Dosage. PO for schistosomiasis (*Schistosoma haematobium, Schistosoma mansoni*) 40 mg/kg in 2 divided doses the same day, but heavy infestations require 60 mg/kg in 3 divided doses at 4–6-hr intervals,[69,71] (*Schistosoma japonicum, Schistosoma mekongi*) 60 mg/kg in 3 doses at 4–6-hr intervals. PO for flukes (eg, fascioliasis, clonorchiasis, opisthorchiasis) 25 mg/kg tid for 1 day; (paragonimiasis) 25 mg/kg tid for 2 days.[69,71] **PO for tapeworms** (beef, dog, fish, pork) 5–10 mg/kg as a single dose; (dwarf tapeworm) 25 mg/kg as a single dose. **PO for neurocysticercosis** 50 mg/kg/day in 3 doses for 15 days.[69] (*See* Notes.)

Special Populations. *Pediatric Dosage.* (<4 yr) safety and efficacy not established. **PO** same as adult dosage.

Geriatric Dosage. Same as adult dosage.

Dosage Forms. **Tab** 600 mg.

Patient Instructions. Take with liquid during meals, but do not chew tablets. This drug may cause dizziness or drowsiness. Use caution when driving, operating machinery, or performing other tasks requiring mental alertness.

Pharmacokinetics. *Fate.* The drug is 80% absorbed orally, but undergoes extensive first-pass metabolism. CSF concentrations are 14–20% of serum levels. The drug is metabolized and metabolites are excreted primarily in urine.

$t_{1/2}$. 1.1 ± 0.3 hr.

Adverse Reactions. Side effects are usually mild. Dizziness, headache, and malaise occur frequently after large doses. Occasionally, abdominal discomfort, fever, sweating, and eosinophilia occur. Drowsiness or fatigue may occur because of a structural similarity to benzodiazepines. Pruritus and rash occur rarely.[69] In patients treated for cysticercosis, an inflammatory response, presumably caused by dead and dying organisms, occurs that is manifested by headache, seizures, and increased intracranial pressure.

Contraindications. Ocular cysticercosis.

Precautions. Pregnancy; liver disease; avoid breastfeeding for 72 hr after the last dose.

Drug Interactions. Drugs that induce CYP3A3/4 (eg, dexamethasone, carbamazepine, phenobarbital, phenytoin) can increase clearance, decrease bioavailability, and cause treatment failure; drugs that inhibit CYP3A3/4 (eg, cimetidine, ketoconazole, erythromycin) decrease clearance, increase serum levels, and lengthen half-life.[70,71]

Parameters to Monitor. Observe for CNS toxicity when treating cysticercosis.

Notes. Concomitant corticosteroid therapy is recommended for patients treated for neurocysticercosis.

PYRANTEL PAMOATE   Antiminth, Various

Pharmacology. Pyrantel is a depolarizing neuromuscular blocker that produces spastic paralysis of the parasite with no similar effects on the host after oral use. It also inhibits acetylcholinesterases.[70]

Administration and Adult Dosage. PO for roundworms and pinworms 11 mg/kg, to a maximum of 1 g in a single dose; for pinworms repeat after a 2-week interval. PO for hookworms and eosinophilic enterocolitis 11 mg/kg/day, to a maximum of 1 g for 3 days.[69] Doses are expressed as base equivalent.

Special Populations. *Pediatric Dosages.* Safety and efficacy not established <2 yr. PO same as adult dosage.

Geriatric Dosage. Same as adult dosage.

Dosage Forms. Susp 50 mg/mL (strength expressed as base equivalent).

Patient Instructions. (*See* Pinworms Class Instructions.)

Pharmacokinetics. *Fate.* Slight oral absorption. Over 50% is excreted unchanged in feces, and less than 15% of the dose is excreted as parent drug and metabolites in the urine.[70]

Adverse Reactions. Occasional nausea, vomiting, headaches, dizziness, rash, and transient AST elevations.[69]

Contraindications. Liver disease.

Precautions. Avoid during pregnancy.

Drug Interactions. Piperazine and pyrantel may be mutually antagonistic in ascariasis.

Notes. Virtually 100% effective for pinworms and roundworms; ineffective for whipworm and *Strongyloides* spp.

THIABENDAZOLE

Pharmacology. Although the exact mechanism is unknown, thiabendazole inhibits the helminth-specific enzyme, fumarate reductase, and may interfere with microtubule assembly and inhibit glucose uptake in the parasite.[70]

Administration and Adult Dosage. PO for strongyloidiasis 25 mg/kg bid for 2 days; continue therapy of disseminated strongyloidiasis for at least 5 days. **PO for cutaneous larva migrans** 25 mg/kg bid for 2–5 days; concomitantly apply thiabendazole oral suspension topically qid directly over the end of the larval tunnel in the skin. **PO for visceral larva migrans** 25 mg/kg bid for 7 days. Do not exceed a dosage of 3 g/day for any indication.[69] (*See* Notes.)

Special Populations. *Pediatric Dosage.* (<13.6 kg) safety and efficacy not established. **PO** same as adult dosage.

Geriatric Dosage. Same as adult dosage.

Dosage Forms. Susp 100 mg/mL; **Chew Tab** 500 mg.

Pharmacokinetics. *Fate.* Well absorbed after oral administration. Most of the drug is metabolized to inactive glucuronide or sulfate compounds and excreted in urine within 24 hr.

Adverse Reactions. CNS effects such as dizziness, drowsiness, and giddiness occur frequently; nausea and vomiting are also common. Diarrhea, epigastric pain, fever, chills, flushing, and headache occur occasionally, as do allergic manifestations (eg, pruritus, rash, angioedema). Seizures, leukopenia, lymphadenopathy, and liver damage occur rarely.[69]

Precautions. Pregnancy.

Drug Interactions. Thiabendazole may inhibit hepatic metabolism of xanthines (eg, theophylline).

Notes. A systemic corticosteroid may be indicated to reduce inflammation caused by dying larvae when the drug is used to treat visceral larva migrans of the eye.

Antiviral Drugs

Class Instructions: HIV Drugs. Underdosage, noncompliance, or partial compliance with drug regimens for these drugs may result in development of a resistant strain(s) of HIV that will not be susceptible to treatment. Do not stop taking this medication unless told to do so by your health care provider. This drug should be used in combination with other anti-HIV medications. Protease inhibitors do not cure or prevent HIV infection. It is still possible for a person taking this medication to transmit the virus to another person. Opportunistic infections and other complications associated with HIV infection may continue to develop while you take this medication. Protease inhibitors have a potential for serious interactions with a large number of commonly prescribed drug products. Always check with your health care provider before starting any new medication.

Missed Doses. Missing doses may result in the development of resistance which may lead to treatment failure. If you forget a dose, take it as soon as you remember. If it is almost time for your next scheduled dose (within 4 hr), skip the missed dose. Do not double your dose.

| **ACYCLOVIR** | Zovirax, Various |
| **VALACYCLOVIR** | Valtrex |

Pharmacology. Acyclovir is an acyclic nucleoside analogue of deoxyguanosine that is selectively phosphorylated by the virus-encoded thymidine kinase to its monophosphate form. Cellular enzymes then convert the monophosphate to the active antiviral acyclovir triphosphate, which inhibits viral DNA synthesis by incorporation into viral DNA, resulting in chain termination. Acyclovir has potent activity against herpes simplex virus I and II (HSV), and also herpes zoster virus (varicella-zoster virus [VZV]). Activity against cytomegalovirus, which lacks a specific virus-encoded thymidine kinase, is limited, but resistance can be overcome with high serum concentrations in some patient populations. Acyclovir inhibits Epstein-Barr virus, but it has not been found clinically useful. Human herpesvirus 6 is resistant.[76–78] Valacyclovir is the L-valyl ester of acyclovir, which undergoes extensive first-pass hydrolysis to yield high serum acyclovir concentrations.

Administration and Adult Dosage. **IV for severe localized HSV infection** (acyclovir) 5 mg/kg q 8 hr for 5 days for nonimmunocompromised patients or 7–10 days for immunocompromised patients; **IV for VZV infection in immunocompromised patients** 10 mg/kg q 8 hr for 7–10 days; **IV for HSV encephalitis** 10 mg/kg q 8 hr for 10–14 days. Dilute to 50–250 mL and infuse over 60 min. Maintain minimum urine output of 500 mL/24 hr for each gram of acyclovir administered. **PO for primary or recurrent genital HSV infection** (acyclovir) 200 mg 5 times/day for 10 days; (valacyclovir, immunocompetent patients) 500 mg bid for 5 days. **PO for prevention of recurrent genital HSV infection** (acyclovir) 400 mg bid or 200 mg 3–5 times/day; **PO for active VZV (chickenpox) or herpes zoster** (acyclovir) 800 mg q 4 hr 5 times/day for 5 days (chickenpox) or 7–10 days (zoster). **PO for herpes zoster in immunocompetent patients** (valacyclovir) 1 g q 8 hr for 7 days. **Top for initial genital HSV infection and limited non–life-threatening mucocutaneous HSV infections in immunocompromised patients** (acyclovir) 0.5-inch ribbon to cover 4-square-inch affected skin area q 3 hr 6 times/day for 7 days.

Special Populations. *Pediatric Dosage.* (All dosages apply to acyclovir.) **IV for HSV infection** (neonates) 10 mg/kg q 8 hr for 10–14 days[77]; (13 months–11 yr) 750 mg/m^2/day in 3 divided doses for 7 days. **IV for VZV (chickenpox) in immunocompromised children** (13 months–11 yr) 1500 mg/m^2/day in 3 divided doses. **IV for HSV encephalitis** (6 months–11 yr) 1500 mg/m^2/day in 3 divided doses for 10 days. **PO for VZV (chickenpox)** (acyclovir) (>2 yr and <40 kg) 20 mg/kg/dose, to a maximum of 800 mg q 6 hr for 5 days; (>40 kg) same as adult dosage; (valacyclovir) safety and efficacy not established.

Geriatric Dosage. Same as adult dosage, but adjust for age-related reduction in renal function.

Other Conditions. (Acyclovir) in obesity, base dosage on IBW. In renal insufficiency, reduce parenteral and oral dosage as follows: Cl_{cr} 25–50 mL/min, give the usual dose q 12 hr; Cl_{cr} 10–25 mL/min, give the usual dose q 24 hr; Cl_{cr} 0–10 mL/min, give 50% of the usual dose q 24 hr. For patients on hemodialysis, give the usual daily dosage after dialysis. (Valacyclovir) in renal insufficiency, reduce the dosage as follows: Cl_{cr} 30–49 mL/min, 1 g q 12 hr; Cl_{cr} 10–29 mL/min, 1 g q 24 hr; Cl_{cr} <10 mL/min, 500 mg q 24 hr.

Dosage Forms. (Acyclovir) **Cap** 200; **Tab** 400, 800 mg; **Inj** 500 mg, 1 g; **Oint** 5%; **Susp** 40 mg/mL. (Valacyclovir) **Tab** 500 mg.

Patient Instructions. Use a finger cot or latex glove when applying acyclovir ointment to avoid autoinoculation. The ointment may cause transient burning or stinging.

Missed Doses. Take this (oral) drug at regular intervals. If you miss a dose of this medicine, take it as soon as you remember. If it is almost time for your next dose, take that dose only and go back to your regular dosage schedule. Leave a minimum of 4 hours between doses. Do not double the dose or take extra.

Pharmacokinetics. ***Fate.*** Oral bioavailability of acyclovir is estimated to be 15–30%; valacyclovir is well absorbed, with a bioavailability of 54%.[79] Valacyclovir is extensively converted to acyclovir after oral administration. After 200–600 mg of acyclovir orally, mean peak steady-state levels are 0.56–1.3 mg/L (2.5–5.9 μmol/L); levels after IV doses of 2.5–15 mg/kg are 5–24 mg/L (23–105 μmol/L). After an oral dose of 1 g of valacyclovir, mean peak steady-state acyclovir level is 5–6 mg/L (22–27 μmol/L).[80] CSF acyclovir concentrations are 25–70% of simultaneous serum level. Decay is biphasic, with $V_{d\beta}$ of 0.69 ± 0.19 L/kg; Cl is 0.21 ± 0.03 L/hr/kg with normal renal function[79]; 86–92% is excreted unchanged in urine; the remainder is metabolized to 9-carboxymethoxymethylguanine. Renal clearance is 75–80% of total clearance and is markedly reduced by concomitant probenecid.[81]

$t_{1/2}$. (Acyclovir) α phase 0.34 hr, β phase 2.9 ± 0.8 hr in adult patients, increasing to nearly 20 hr in end-stage renal disease; 5.7 hr on dialysis; about 4 hr in neonates.[81]

Adverse Reactions. (Acyclovir) nephrotoxicity, thought to be caused by precipitation of acyclovir crystals in the nephron, occurs in about 10% of patients if the drug is given by bolus (<10 min) injection. Phlebitis at injection site occurs frequently with IV infusion because of the high pH (9–11) of the product. Other side effects reported are CNS toxicity (eg, headache, lethargy, tremulousness, delirium, seizures), nausea, vomiting, and skin rash. CNS toxicity occurs primarily in patients with underlying neurologic disease or end-stage renal disease, or with cancer chemotherapy and irradiation to the CNS, and may not be primarily caused by the drug. Topical application to herpes lesions may be painful.[76–77] (Valacyclovir) adverse reactions appear comparable to acyclovir. Nausea, vomiting, diarrhea, abdominal pain, and headache have been reported frequently with valacyclovir use. Thrombotic thrombocytopenic purpura/hemolytic-uremic syndrome has been reported in patients with advanced HIV disease and in bone marrow and renal transplant patients. This phenomenon has not been reported in immunocompetent patients.[80]

Contraindications. (Valacyclovir) allergy to any component of the drug or to acyclovir.

Precautions. Use with caution in renal impairment, dehydration, and pre-existing neurologic disorders. Valacyclovir is not indicated in immunocompromised patients.

Drug Interactions. Zidovudine and acyclovir may result in drowsiness and lethargy. Probenecid may increase oral bioavailability and half-life of acyclovir.

Parameters to Monitor. Monitor renal function and injection site for signs of phlebitis daily. Carefully monitor patients with underlying neurologic diseases for evidence of neurotoxicity. (*See* Adverse Reactions.)

Notes. Acyclovir-resistant strains of virus that are deficient in thymidine kinase have been isolated from patients after treatment. Although thought to be less virulent than sensitive strains, HSV strains resistant to acyclovir have been described in AIDS patients.[77]

CIDOFOVIR   Vistide

Pharmacology. Cidofovir (HPMPC) is a nucleotide analogue with potent in vitro and in vivo activity against cytomegalovirus (CMV) and other herpesviruses. Cidofovir contains a phosphonate group that enables it to bypass initial virus-dependent phosphorylation. Cellular enzymes convert cidofovir to cidofovir diphosphate, the active intracellular metabolite.[82–84]

Adult Dosage. **IV induction for CMV retinitis** 5 mg/kg infused over 1 hr once weekly for 2 weeks, then **IV maintenance** 5 mg/kg once every other week. Reduce dosage to 3 mg/kg if Cr_s increases by 0.3–0.4 mg/dL above baseline or if $\geq$2+ proteinuria occurs. It is essential to give the following with cidofovir: PO 2 g **probenecid** 3 hr before administration and IV 1 L of NS over 1 hr just prior to administration. If tolerated, give another liter of NS with or after cidofovir administration; finally, give PO 1 g probenecid 2 hr and 8 hr after the end of cidofovir infusion. Cidofovir is also being investigated as an intravitreal injection for CMV retinitis.

Dosage Forms. **Inj** 75 mg/mL.

Pharmacokinetics. Peak serum cidofovir concentration averages 26.1 $\pm$ 3.2 mg/L (83 $\pm$ 10 μmol/L) after a 5 mg/kg IV infusion with concomitant probenecid and hydration. Cidofovir is not appreciably bound to plasma proteins; V_d averages 0.5 L/kg. Cidofovir is excreted almost entirely unchanged in the urine. The elimination half-life of cidofovir is 3–6 hr when administered with probenecid. Cidofovir diphosphate has a prolonged intracellular half-life, ranging from 17–65 hr, which allows infrequent administration schedules of once weekly to once every other week.

Adverse Reactions. Nephrotoxicity is the most frequent adverse reaction, and high-dose probenecid (*see* Adult Dosage) must be used with administration of cidofovir. Probenecid decreases uptake of cidofovir in proximal renal tubular cells, decreasing the risk of nephrotoxicity. Other frequent adverse reactions are proteinuria, elevated Cr_s, nausea, vomiting, fever, asthenia, neutropenia, rash, headache, diarrhea, alopecia, anemia, and abdominal pain. Ocular hypotony and decreased intraocular pressure have been reported occasionally. Nausea, vomiting, fever, rash, and chills are frequent reactions reported with probenecid.

DIDANOSINE   Videx

Pharmacology. Didanosine (dideoxyinosine; ddI) is a purine nucleoside that undergoes complex metabolism in vivo to dideoxyadenosine (ddA), which ultimately undergoes metabolism to an active triphosphorylated form (ddATP). Incorporation of ddATP into viral DNA leads to chain termination, and ddATP is a competitive inhibitor of HIV reverse transcriptase, which further contributes to the interference of HIV replication.[85]

Administration and Adult Dosage. PO for HIV infection ($\geq$60 kg) 200 mg (as 2 tablets) q 12 hr, or 250 mg (as powder) q 12 hr; (<60 kg) 125 mg (as 2 tablets) q 12 hr, or 167 mg (as powder) q 12 hr. Take each dose as 2 whole (not partial) tablets to provide adequate buffering.

Special Populations. *Pediatric Dosage.* PO for HIV infection (BSA 1.1–1.4 m^2) 100 mg (as 2 tablets) q 12 hr, or 125 mg (as pediatric powder) q 12 hr; (BSA 0.8–1 m^2) 75 mg (as 2 tablets) q 12 hr, or 94 mg (as pediatric powder) q 12 hr; (BSA 0.5–0.7 m^2) 50 mg (as 2 tablets) q 12 hr, or 62 mg (as pediatric powder) q 12 hr; (BSA $\leq$0.4 m^2) 25 mg (as 1 tablet) q 12 hr, or 31 mg (as pediatric powder) q 12 hr.[86,87]

Geriatric Dosage. Same as adult dosage, but not studied in this population.

Other Conditions. Consider dosage reduction in patients with renal or hepatic impairment. Some clinicians suggest reduction of didanosine dosage by 75% in patients with severe renal impairment. Didanosine is removed by hemodialysis, but the quantity removed is low and supplemental doses are not recommended.[88]

Dosage Forms. **Chew/Dispersible Tab** 25, 50, 100, 150 mg; **Pwdr for Oral Soln** 100, 167, 250, 375 mg; **Pwdr for Oral Soln (pediatric)** 2, 4 g.

Patient Instructions. *(See* HIV Drugs Class Instructions.) Didanosine is not a cure for HIV infection, and opportunistic infections and other complications associated with HIV infection may continue to occur. Didanosine must be taken on an empty stomach 1 hour before or 2 hours after a meal. It is essential that the 2-tablet dose be taken each time to avoid destruction of the drug by stomach acid. For children >1 year, use the 2-tablet dose; for those <1 year of age, use the 1-tablet dose. Tablets may be chewed and swallowed, or dissolved in at least 30 mL of water and swallowed immediately. Do *not* swallow the tablets whole. Reconstituted solution may be stored for up to 30 days when refrigerated. Shake solution thoroughly before administering each dose.

Missed Doses. Take this drug at regular intervals. If you miss a dose of this medicine, take it as soon as you remember. If it is almost time for your next dose, take that dose only and go back to your regular dosage schedule. Leave a minimum of 12 hours between doses. Do not double the dose or take extra.

Pharmacokinetics. *Fate.* Didanosine is rapidly degraded at acidic pH. Appreciable interpatient variability and dose-dependent characteristics affect didanosine absorption. Oral bioavailability of the buffered powder for oral solution is 33 ± 11%.[89,90] The chewable/dispersible buffered tablets are 20–25% more bioavailable than the buffered powder for solution. The peak serum concentration is 1.1 ± 0.7 mg/L (4.7 ± 2.9 μmol/L) after a 375 mg oral dose of buffered powder for solution. Protein binding is less than 5%. CSF concentration 1 hr after infusion of didanosine averages 21% of the concurrent serum concentration. $V_{d\beta}$ is 1 ± 0.7 L/kg; Cl is 1 ± 0.08 L/hr/kg.[88] Up to 60% of dose is excreted unchanged in the urine; the remainder is extensively metabolized to ddATP, hypoxanthine, and uric acid.[85,88]

$t_{1/2}$. 1.75 ± 0.99 hr;[88] in vitro intracellular half-life of ddATP is 8–43 hr.[91]

Adverse Reactions. Pancreatitis has occurred at a frequency of 5–9% in clinical trials at or below current recommended dosages and can be fatal. Peripheral neuropathy is frequent and occurs in 16–34% of patients, with 12% requiring dosage reduction. Diarrhea has been reported with the buffered powder for oral solution at a frequency of 34%. In children, pancreatitis and peripheral retinal depigmentation have occurred frequently, although the latter has not been associated with visual impairment.[92] Peripheral neuropathy has not occurred in children.

Precautions. Avoid didanosine tablets in patients with phenylketonuria because these contain phenylalanine. Didanosine has been associated with hyperuricemia; use caution in patients with a history of gout or baseline hyperuricemia; avoid in individuals with a history of pancreatitis.

Drug Interactions. Administration with fluroquinolones may reduce fluoroquinolone serum levels because of buffers in formulation. Avoid concurrent administration with dapsone, indinavir, itraconazole, ketoconazole, or other medications requiring an acidic environment for absorption because of buffers in didanosine formulation. Both ganciclovir and trimethoprim-sulfamethoxazole appear to increase didanosine's bioavailability, but the clinical importance is unknown. Use with alcohol, high-dose trimethoprim-sulfamethoxazole, or other pancreatitis-associated drugs may increase the risk of pancreatitis.[93,94]

Parameters to Monitor. Obtain serum amylase, lipase, and triglycerides monthly. Symptoms of abdominal pain, nausea, and vomiting may indicate pancreatitis. Symptoms of distal numbness, tingling, or pain in the feet or hands may indicate neuropathy and may necessitate dosage modification. Monitor clinical signs, symptoms, and laboratory markers for progression of HIV disease to help decide regimen changes in antiretroviral therapy. Baseline CD4 and HIV-1 RNA polymerase chain reaction viral load tests are useful to measure clinical benefit of therapy. Repeat tests after 1 month and q 3–4 months thereafter have been suggested to monitor benefit of antiretroviral therapy.

Notes. At present there are no results from clinical trials regarding the effect of didanosine on the clinical progression of HIV infection, such as frequency of opportunistic infections and improvement of survival. Combination therapy with **zidovudine** has been used by some clinicians to decrease viral resistance and improve clinical benefit. As with other nucleoside reverse transcriptase inhibitors, drug-resistant HIV-1 isolates emerge with long-term didanosine therapy ($\geq$12 months).[87] (*See* Antiviral Drugs for HIV Infection Comparison Chart.)

FAMCICLOVIR	Famvir
PENCICLOVIR	Denavir

Pharmacology. Famciclovir is the diacetyl, 6-deoxy ester of the antiviral guanosine analogue penciclovir. Famciclovir is absorbed rapidly and converted to penciclovir in the intestinal wall and liver. Viral thymidine kinase converts penciclovir to its monophosphate form. Cellular enzymes then convert the monophosphate to the active antiviral penciclovir triphosphate. The triphosphate inhibits viral DNA synthesis by incorporation into viral DNA, resulting in termination of the chain. Penciclovir has potent activity against herpes simplex virus I and II (HSV) and herpes zoster virus (varicella-zoster). Penciclovir also has some activity against Epstein-Barr virus and cytomegalovirus, but has not demonstrated clinical usefulness against infections with these agents.[94–96]

Adult Dosage. PO for herpes zoster (famciclovir) 500 mg q 8 hr for 7 days. In renal insufficiency, reduce the dosage as follows: Cl_{cr} 40–59 mL/min, 500 mg q 12 hr; Cl_{cr} 20–39 mL/min, 500 mg q 24 hr; Cl_{cr} <20 mL/min, 250 mg q 48 hr; with hemodialysis, 250 mg after each dialysis. **PO for recurrent genital HSV infection** (famciclovir) 125 mg bid for 5 days. In renal insufficiency, reduce the dosage as follows: Cl_{cr} 20–39 mL/min, 125 mg q 24 hr; Cl_{cr} <20 mL/min, 125 mg q 48 hr; with hemodialysis, 125 mg after each dialysis. **Top for herpes labialis** (penciclovir) apply to lesions q 2 hr while awake for 4 days, starting as early as possible at the beginning of an outbreak.

Dosage Forms. **Crm** (penciclovir) 1%; **Tab** (famciclovir) 125, 250, 500 mg.

Pharmacokinetics. Topical penciclovir is virtually unabsorbed. The absolute bioavailability of penciclovir is 77% after a 500 mg oral dose of famciclovir. Peak serum concentrations are 0.84 ± 0.22 (3.3 ± 0.9 µmol/L) and 3.34 ± 0.58 mg/L (13 ± 2.3 µmol/L) 45 min after 125- and 500 mg oral doses of famciclovir, respectively. Penciclovir is <20% protein bound, and the V_d is approximately 1 L/kg. Penciclovir is eliminated primarily by renal excretion. The elimination half-life is approximately 2 hr with normal renal function, increasing to over 13 hr in patients with severely impaired renal function.

Adverse Reactions. Nausea, vomiting, diarrhea, and headache occur frequently with famciclovir. Pruritus, paresthesias, and fatigue occur occasionally. Penciclovir may cause mild erythema occasionally.

Drug Interactions. Cimetidine may enhance the bioavailability of famciclovir and its conversion to penciclovir somewhat.

FOSCARNET SODIUM	Foscavir

Pharmacology. Foscarnet sodium (phosphonoformic acid; PFA) is a pyrophosphate analogue. Foscarnet actively inhibits viral DNA polymerases in its parent form and does not require phosphorylation for optimal antiviral activity. It has antiviral activity against herpes simplex virus I and II, human cytomegalovirus (CMV), Epstein-Barr virus, hepatitis B virus, varicella-zoster virus, and some retroviruses including HIV. Foscarnet sodium inhibits DNA synthesis in CMV and other herpesviruses by inhibiting viral DNA polymerase.[97]

Administration and Adult Dosage. **IV induction for CMV retinitis in AIDS patients** 60 mg/kg q 8 hr or 90 mg/kg q 12 hr for 14–21 days.[98] **IV maintenance for CMV retinitis in AIDS patients** 90–120 mg/kg/day in 1 dose. **IV for acyclovir-resistant herpesvirus infections** 40 mg/kg q 8 hr or 60 mg/kg q 12 hr until clinical resolution.[98] **IV for acyclovir-resistant varicella-zoster infections in immunocompromised patients** 40 mg/kg q 8 hr or 60 mg/kg q 12 hr for 10–21 days or until clinical resolution.[78,99]

Special Populations. *Pediatric Dosage.* Safety and efficacy not established.

Geriatric Dosage. Same as adult dosage, but adjust for age-related reduction in renal function.

Other Conditions. Reduce dosage in renal function impairment. (*See* product information.)

Dosage Forms. **Inj** 24 mg/mL.

Patient Instructions. Foscarnet is not a cure for cytomegalovirus retinitis, and progression of disease may continue during or following treatment. Regular eye examinations are important to monitor for disease progression. Report symptoms of tingling around the mouth or numbness in extremities, which may indicate a need for temporary discontinuation of foscarnet.

Missed Doses. Take this drug at regular intervals. If you miss a dose of this medicine, take it as soon as you remember. If it is almost time for your next dose, take that dose only and go back to your regular dosage schedule. Leave a minimum of 12 hours between doses. Do not double the dose or take extra.

Pharmacokinetics. *Fate.* After twice-daily infusion of 90 mg/kg over 2 hr, peak serum levels are 98 ± 27 mg/L (577 ± 161 μmol/L) and troughs are 6.4 ± 8.3 mg/L (38 ± 49 μmol/L).[98] Plasma protein binding is 14–17%. CSF concentrations range from 35–103% of simultaneous serum levels. V_{dss} is 0.3–0.7 L/kg; Cl is 0.13 ± 0.05 L/hr/kg. Foscarnet is not metabolized and is 70–90% excreted unchanged in the urine.[98]

$t_{1/2}$. α phase 1.4 ± 0.6 hr, β phase 6.8 ± 5 hr in patients receiving continuous or intermittent infusions. A terminal half-life of 36–196 hr may represent release of the drug from binding sites in bone.[98]

Adverse Reactions. Abnormal renal function, including decreased Cl_{cr} and acute renal failure, occurs in about one-third of patients. Electrolyte abnormalities including hypocalcemia, hypophosphatemia, hyperphosphatemia, hypokalemia, and hypomagnesemia occur in 6–16% of patients. Seizures have been reported in 10% of patients and may be related to electrolyte abnormalities or underlying disease. Other adverse reactions frequently reported are fever 65%, nausea 47%, anemia 33%, diarrhea 30%, vomiting 26%, headache 26%, and granulocytopenia 14%. Local irritation, inflammation, and pain may occur at the injection site with peripheral administration at a frequency of 1–5%.[98,100,101]

Precautions. Use with extreme caution in patients with renal impairment of nephrotoxic drugs, pre-existing cytopenias, pre-existing electrolyte abnormalities, or underlying neurologic disorders.

Drug Interactions. Concurrent use of nephrotoxic drugs such as aminoglycosides or radiologic contrast media may increase risk and severity of nephrotoxicity. IV pentamidine may increase the risk of hypocalcemia; avoid this combination, if possible, although inhaled pentamidine does not seem to be a risk factor.[94]

Parameters to Monitor. Monitor Cr_s 2 or 3 times/week during induction therapy and weekly during maintenance therapy. Monitor serum calcium, magnesium, potassium, and phosphorus at the same frequency as Cr_s. Symptoms of perioral tingling, numbness in extremities, or other paresthesias may indicate electrolyte abnormalities and may require more frequent monitoring and a need to obtain ionized calcium levels.

GANCICLOVIR   Cytovene, Vitrasept

Pharmacology. Ganciclovir (DHPG) is a synthetic acyclic nucleoside analogue of guanine structurally related to acyclovir. The antiviral activity of ganciclovir appears to be a result of its conversion to the triphosphate form, which functions as both an inhibitor of and faulty substrate for viral DNA polymerase. Ganciclovir has antiviral activity both in vitro and in vivo against herpes simplex virus I and II, human cytomegalovirus (CMV), Epstein-Barr virus, and varicella-zoster virus.[75,101]

Administration and Adult Dosage. **IV for treatment of CMV retinitis (induction)** 5 mg/kg q 12 hr for 14–21 days, then (**maintenance**) 5 mg/kg once daily for 7 days each week or 6 mg/kg once daily for 5 days each week. Induction treatment may be repeated for patients who experience disease progression. **IV for prevention of CMV disease in transplant recipients** 5 mg/kg q 12 hr for 7–14 days, followed by 5 mg/kg once daily for 7 days each week or 6 mg/kg once daily for 5 days each week. Duration of treatment depends on the duration and degree of immunosuppression. Dilute each IV dose in 100 mL NS or D5W and infuse over 60 min. **PO for CMV retinitis (maintenance after IV induction)** 1 g q 8 hr with food. **PO for prophylaxis of CMV disease** 1 g q 8 hr with food indefinitely.

Special Populations. *Pediatric Dosage.* Safety and efficacy not established. The adult dosage in mg/kg has been used.

Geriatric Dosage. Same as adult dosage, but adjust for age-related reduction in renal function.

Other Conditions. In renal insufficiency, reduce *parenteral induction* dosage as follows: Cl_{cr} 50–69 mL/min, give 2.5 mg/kg q 12 hr; Cl_{cr} 25–49 mL/min, 2.5 mg/kg q 24 hr; Cl_{cr} <25 mL/min, give 1.25 mg/kg q 24 hr; for patients on hemodialysis, 1.25 mg/kg 3 times/week. On hemodialysis days, give the dose after hemodialysis because dialysis reduces serum levels by approximately 50%. Reduce *parenteral maintenance* dosage in renal insufficiency as follows: Cl_{cr} 50–69 mL/min, give 2.5 mg/kg q 24 hr; Cl_{cr} 25–49 mL/min, 1.25 mg/kg q 24 hr; Cl_{cr} 10–24 mL/min, 0.625 mg/kg q 24 hr; for patients on hemodialysis, 0.625 mg/kg 3 times/week following hemodialysis. Reduce *oral maintenance* dosage in renal insufficiency as follows: Cl_{cr} 50–69 mL/min, give 1.5 g once daily or 500 mg tid; Cl_{cr} 25–49 mL/min, 1 g/day in 1 or 2 doses; Cl_{cr} 10–24 mL/min, 500 mg/day; Cl_{cr} <10 mL/min, 500 mg 3 times/week following hemodialysis.

Dosage Forms. **Cap** 250, 500 mg; **Inj** 500 mg; **Ocular Implant** 4.5 mg (nominal release).

Patient Instructions. Ganciclovir is not a cure for cytomegalovirus retinitis, and progression of disease may continue during or following treatment. Concurrent use with zidovudine may result in severe reduction in white blood cell count; therefore, report any signs or symptoms of infection, such as fever, chills, or sweats. Take oral ganciclovir with food.

Missed Doses. Take this drug at regular intervals. If you miss a dose of this medicine, take it as soon as you remember. If it is almost time for your next dose, take that dose only and go back to your regular dosage schedule. Leave a minimum of 4 hours between doses. Do not double the dose or take extra.

Pharmacokinetics. *Fate.* Ganciclovir is absorbed poorly from the GI tract; oral bioavailability is 6% when taken with food (about 20% greater than when taken on an empty stomach). Average peak serum concentration of 0.34 ± 0.13 mg/L (1.3 ± 0.5 μmol/L) occurs 1–2 hr after a single 1 g oral dose. Mean peak and trough steady-state levels after IV doses of 5 mg/kg q 12 hr in patients with normal renal function are 5.3 ± 2.8 mg/L (21 ± 11 μmol/L) and 1.1 ± 0.4 mg/L (4.3 ± 1.5 μmol/L), respectively. Ganciclovir is 1–2% plasma protein bound; CSF concentration is 24–67% of simultaneous serum level. V_c is 0.26 ± 0.08 L/kg; $V_{dβ}$ is 1.17 ± 0.54 L/kg; Cl is 0.25 ± 0.13 L/hr/kg with normal renal function. The drug is 90–99% excreted unchanged in the urine. Hemodialysis reduces serum levels by 53 ± 12%. Renal excretion occurs principally via glomerular filtration, although limited renal tubular secretion may also occur.[101,102]

$t_{1/2}$. α phase 0.76 ± 0.67 hr; β phase 3.6 ± 1.4 hr in adult patients, increasing to 11.5 ± 3.9 hr in renal insufficiency.[101,102]

Adverse Reactions. Granulocytopenia (ANC <1000/μL) occurs in 13–67% of patients and is the most frequent dose-limiting adverse effect.[101] Thrombocytopenia (platelets <50,000/μL) occurs in 20% of patients. CNS toxicity (headache, lethargy, dizziness, confusion, seizure, coma) has been reported at a frequency of 5–17%. Phlebitis, inflammation, and pain at the site of IV infusion occur frequently because of the high pH of the solution. Anemia, fever, rash, and abnormal liver function tests occur in about 2% of patients.[101,103]

Contraindications. Hypersensitivity to acyclovir or ganciclovir.

Precautions. Use with caution in renal impairment, pre-existing cytopenias, or concurrent myelosuppressive drug therapy.

Drug Interactions. Didanosine AUC may be increased when given within 2 hr of ganciclovir. Probenecid may decrease the renal excretion of ganciclovir. Use extreme caution in combination with zidovudine because of additive myelosuppression. Concurrent nephrotoxic drugs (eg, cyclosporine, zidovudine) may increase the nephrotoxicity of ganciclovir. Concurrent cytotoxic drugs may increase the toxicity of ganciclovir. Seizures have been reported with concurrent use of ganciclovir and imipenem-cilastatin.

Parameters to Monitor. Monitor CBC and platelet count twice weekly during induction treatment and at least weekly during maintenance treatment. Monitor renal function at least q 2 weeks. Check injection site for phlebitis and infection daily.

Notes. Ganciclovir-resistant CMV strains have been isolated from patients during treatment.[104] Disease progression caused by these strains has been observed and may require changing therapy to an alternative antiviral (eg, foscarnet).

INDINAVIR   Crixivan

Pharmacology. Indinavir is an HIV protease inhibitor with a mechanism of action similar to saquinavir.[105] (*See* Antiviral Drugs for HIV Infection Comparison Chart.)

Adult Dosage. PO for HIV infection 800 mg q 8 hr. Each dose should be taken on an empty stomach with water or other fat-free liquid or with light, fat-free foods (eg, toast, jelly, corn flakes, skim milk, sugar, coffee). In patients with mild to moderate hepatic insufficiency caused by cirrhosis, the dosage is 600 mg q 8 hr.

Dosage Forms. Cap 200, 400 mg.

Pharmacokinetics. Indinavir is rapidly absorbed in the fasting state. Administration of indinavir with a meal high in calories, fat, or protein decreases oral absorption by about 75%. The absolute bioavailability has not been determined in humans, but the fasting bioavailability ranges from 14–70% in animals. Indinavir is 60% bound to human plasma proteins. It is primarily metabolized by CYP3A4, and less than 20% is excreted unchanged in the urine; half-life is 1.8 ± 0.4 hr.

Adverse Reactions. Frequent adverse reactions include nausea, vomiting, abdominal pain, diarrhea, headache, asthenia, insomnia, taste perversion, transient elevations of hepatic transaminases, asymptomatic hyperbilirubinemia, and nephrolithiasis. Dizziness, somnolence, anorexia, malaise, and dry mouth occur occasionally. Nephrolithiasis occurred in 4% of patients in clinical trials and can be managed with hydration and temporary drug discontinuation. Patients should drink at least 1.5 L/day of liquids to ensure adequate hydration while taking indinavir.

LAMIVUDINE   Epivir

Pharmacology. Lamivudine (3TC) is a synthetic pyrimidine nucleoside that has activity against HIV-1, HIV-2, and hepatitis B virus. Lamivudine is metabolized intracellularly to lamivudine triphosphate and acts as a chain terminator of viral DNA. It also acts as a competitive inhibitor of HIV reverse transcriptase. Use of lamivudine alone to treat HIV infection leads to rapid emergence of high-level resistance; therefore, it is used in combination with zidovudine. Resistance to zidovudine is markedly delayed when the drug is used with lamivudine, and the combination results in greater and more sustained elevations in CD4 cell counts than zidovudine monotherapy.[88,92,106–108] (*See* Antiviral Drugs for HIV Infection Comparison Chart.)

Adult Dosage. PO with zidovudine for HIV 150 mg bid with zidovudine 200 mg PO tid. Reduce dosage in renal impairment.

Pediatric Dosage. PO (3 months–12 yr) 4 mg/kg, to a maximum of 150 mg bid with zidovudine.

Dosage Forms. Tab 150 mg; **Soln** 10 mg/mL.

Pharmacokinetics. Oral bioavailability is 82%. V_d is 1.3 L/kg; elimination half-life is 2.5 hr. Excretion is primarily by the renal route, with 68–71% of drug excreted unchanged in urine.

Adverse Reactions. The most frequently reported adverse effects have been headache, fatigue, nausea, insomnia, neuropathy, and musculoskeletal pain.

NELFINAVIR MESYLATE   Viracept

Pharmacology. Nelfinavir mesylate is an antiviral that inhibits HIV-1 and HIV-2 proteases by binding to the active enzymatic site, preventing cleavage of polyprotein precursors. This cleavage is essential for maturation of infectious virus, and its inhibition results in the formation of immature, noninfectious HIV particles. (*See* Antiviral Drugs for HIV Infection Comparison Chart.)

Administration and Adult Dosage. PO for HIV disease in combination with nucleoside analogues 750 mg tid or 1250 mg bid.[109]

Special Populations. *Pediatric Dosage.* **PO for HIV disease in combination with nucleoside analogues** (<2 yr) safety and efficacy not established; (2–13 yr) 20–30 mg/kg tid.

Geriatric Dosage. Not studied, but expected to be the same as adult dosage.

Dosage Forms. Tab 250 mg; **Pwdr** 50 mg nelfinavir base/level scoopful (1 g).

Patient Instructions. (*See* HIV Drugs Class Instructions.) Each dose must be taken orally with a light snack or meal to increase the amount of the drug absorbed. If you are taking an oral contraceptive, you should use an alternate or additional contraceptive measure. Store nelfinavir in a dry place at room temperature. New onset diabetes mellitus, exacerbation of pre-existing diabetes mellitus, and hyperglycemia have been reported in HIV-infected patients receiving protease inhibitors. Some patients require either initiation or dosage adjustments of insulin or oral hypoglycemic agents. Diabetic ketoacidosis has also occurred. Hyperglycemia persisted in some cases after drug discontinuation.

Pharmacokinetics. *Fate.* Bioavailability is unknown in humans, but animal data suggest an oral bioavailability of 20–80%. Nelfinavir absorption is increased 2- to 3-fold when administered with food. Peak serum concentrations occur 2–4 hr after a dose. After multiple oral doses of 750 mg tid, peak serum concentrations average 3–4 mg/L (5.3–7 μmol/L) and trough concentrations average 1–3 mg/L (1.8–5.3 μmol/L). Plasma protein binding is >98%. Nelfinavir is metabolized by cytochrome P450 enzymes, primarily CYP3A4 and to a minor extent by CYP2C9, 2C19, and 2D6. The major oxidative metabolite has in vitro antiviral activity comparable to the parent drug. Less than 2% of nelfinavir is excreted unchanged in urine.

$t_{1/2}$. 3.5–5 hr.

Adverse Reactions. Diarrhea, abdominal pain or discomfort, flatulence, nausea, rash, and difficulty swallowing tablets are frequent. Diarrhea often resolves spontaneously 1–2 weeks after initiation of therapy. Antidiarrheal medications are often beneficial in alleviating or minimizing symptoms. Occasional reactions include asthenia, headache, and fatigue.

Contraindications. (*See* Drug Interactions.)

Precautions. Do not use nelfinavir as monotherapy. Appropriate use is with other antiretroviral therapy to reduce potential for developing drug resistance. Nelfinavir powder for oral solution contains 11.2 mg phenylalanine/g of powder and should be used cautiously in patients with phenylketonuria.

Drug Interactions. Nelfinavir is an inhibitor of CYP3A and it may cause increased serum concentrations of drugs primarily metabolized by CYP3A. It is also a substrate for CYP3A and nelfinavir concentrations may be affected by the induction or inhibition of CYP3A by other drugs. Do not co-administer nelfinavir with rifampin because it decreases nelfinavir's steady-state AUC by 82%. Co-administration with rifabutin reduces nelfinavir's AUC by 32% and increases rifabutin's AUC by 207%. If administered together, the manufacturer recommends reducing the rifabutin dosage by 50%, although alternatives should be considered. Avoid other drugs (eg, carbamazepine, phenobarbital, phenytoin) that strongly induce CYP3A4 because they may substantially reduce nelfinavir serum concentrations. Avoid co-administration with astemizole or cisapride because of possible prolonged QT intervals and serious cardiovascular adverse events. Co-administration with ethinyl estradiol/norethindrone resulted in a 47% decrease in ethinyl estradiol serum concentration and an 18% decrease in norethindrone serum concentration. Alternative contraceptives need to be used while receiving nelfinavir therapy. Co-administration with indinavir results in an 83% increase in nelfinavir AUC and a 51% increase in indinavir AUC. Co-administration with ritonavir results in a 152% increase in nelfinavir AUC and minimal change in ritonavir AUC. Various protease inhibitor combinations are under study, but safety and efficacy of these combinations have not been established.

Parameters to Monitor. Monitor clinical signs, symptoms, and laboratory markers for progression of HIV disease to help decide regimen changes in antiretroviral therapy. Baseline CD4+ and HIV-1 RNA polymerase chain reaction viral load tests are standard of practice markers to measure clinical benefit of therapy. Adherence to the drug regimen should be assessed throughout treatment course to help in assessment of effectiveness. Repeat tests after 1 month and q 3–4 months to monitor benefit of antiretroviral therapy.

NEVIRAPINE   Viramune

Pharmacology. Nevirapine is a dipyridodiazepinone nonnucleoside HIV-1 reverse transcriptase inhibitor. Nevirapine and other nonnucleoside reverse transcriptase inhibitors are not active against HIV-2 reverse transcriptase. The inhibition by nevirapine is noncompetitive, and the binding site is located near but not directly at the catalytic amino acid residues, which may provide nevirapine activity against HIV-1 mutants that are resistant to nucleoside reverse transcriptase inhibitors. Nevirapine provides added benefit (eg, increased CD4 count, decreased viral load) in combination with zidovudine and didanosine.[110-113] (*See* Antiviral Drugs for HIV Infection Comparison Chart.)

Adult Dosage. PO for HIV 200 mg/day for 2 weeks, followed by 200 mg bid or 400 mg once daily.

Pediatric Dosage. PO (<13 yr) 120 mg/m^2/day for 2 weeks, then bid.

Dosage Forms. Tab 200 mg; Susp 10 mg/mL.

Pharmacokinetics. Oral absorption is not affected by food or antacids; bioavailability is 90%. The median time to peak concentration is 4 hr after a 400 mg dose with average peak concentrations after the first dose of 3.4 ± 1 mg/L. Peak and trough concentrations average 7.2 ± 1.4 mg/L (27 ± 5 μmol/L) and 4 ± 1.2 mg/L (15 ± 4 μmol/L), respectively, after 14 days of therapy. The average elimination half-life is 45 hr in the initial 2-week period and decreases to 25–30 hr thereafter because of metabolic autoinduction mediated by the cytochrome P450 system. Less than 3% of the dose is excreted renally.

Adverse Reactions. A mild to moderate rash occurs in up to 48% of patients. Rash may be associated with liver function test elevations and a low frequency of clinical hepatitis. The risk of developing rash is highest within 2 weeks of drug initiation or dosage escalation to 400 mg/day and is reduced by following the recommended dosage escalation schedule. Other occasional adverse reactions include arthralgia, fatigue, fever, myalgia, and somnolence.

RITONAVIR   Norvir

Pharmacology. Ritonavir is an HIV protease inhibitor with a mechanism of action similar to saquinavir.[114,115] (*See* Antiviral Drugs for HIV Infection Comparison Chart.)

Adult Dosage. PO for treatment of HIV 600 mg q 12 hr with food in combination with nucleoside analogues. Ritonavir may be better tolerated initially if the dosage is initiated at 300 mg q 12 hr and increased to 600 mg q 12 hr over 10–14 days. If the 600 mg q 12-hr dosage is not reached after 2 weeks of therapy, discontinue therapy, because the risk of developing viral resistance to ritonavir or cross-resistance to other protease inhibitors is increased with lower dosages.

Dosage Forms. Cap 100 mg; Soln 80 mg/mL. Capsules must be refrigerated.

Pharmacokinetics. Ritonavir is rapidly absorbed, and is increased by approximately 15% with food. Absolute bioavailability has not been determined in humans, but bioavailability ranges from 30–70% in animals. Ritonavir is 98–99% protein bound, primarily to albumin and α$_1$-acid glycoprotein. After a 600 mg oral dose taken with food, a peak serum concentration of 11.2 ± 3.6 mg/L (15.5 ± 5 μmol/L) occurs at 3.3 ± 2.2 hr and the trough is 3 ± 2.1 mg/L (4.2 ± 2.9 μmol/L). Serum concentrations may decrease over time because of autoinduction of the CYP3A and CYP2D isoenzymes responsible for metabolism of ritonavir.

Adverse Reactions. Nausea, vomiting, diarrhea, asthenia, anorexia, abdominal pain, taste perversion, perioral paresthesia, peripheral paresthesia, headache, insomnia, and elevated serum triglyceride concentrations occur frequently. Occasionally, elevations of hepatic transaminases and CPK occur.

Drug Interactions. Ritonavir is a potent inhibitor of several cytochrome P450 enzymes (CYP2C9, 2C19, 2D6, and 3A3/4) and can produce large increases in serum concentrations of highly metabolized drugs. Consult the product information for contraindicated drugs and carefully review patient's medication list for interactions before starting this therapy.

SAQUINAVIR	Fortovase
SAQUINAVIR MESYLATE	Invirase

Pharmacology. Saquinavir is a synthetic peptidelike substrate analogue that inhibits HIV protease. Inhibition of HIV protease prevents the cleavage of polyprotein precursors which is essential for maturation of infectious virus.[116,117] Saquinavir mesylate is formulated in a hard gelatin capsule. Saquinavir has been reformulated into a soft gelatin capsule that combines saquinavir base in an oil-like substance allowing microdispersion upon contact with gastric fluids enhancing oral bioavailability. (*See* Antiviral Drugs for HIV Infection Comparison Chart.)

Administration and Adult Dosage. PO for advanced HIV disease in combination with other nucleoside analogues (saquinavir mesylate) 600 mg q 8 hr; (saquinavir) 1200 mg q 8 hr.

Special Populations. *Pediatric Dosage.* (<16 yr) safety and efficacy not established.

Geriatric Dosage. Not studied, but expected to be same as adult dosage.

Dosage Forms. (Saquinavir mesylate) **Cap** 200 mg; (saquinavir) **Cap** 200 mg.

Patient Instructions. (*See* HIV Drugs Class Instructions.) Saquinavir mesylate must be taken within 2 hours after a full meal to achieve adequate concentrations of drug to inhibit viral replication. Saquinavir (Fortovase) is better absorbed and requires a snack or some food to help increase the amount of medication getting into the blood. Saquinavir should be kept in the refrigerator. New onset diabetes mellitus, worsening of pre-existing diabetes mellitus, and hyperglycemia have been reported in HIV-infected patients receiving protease inhibitors. Some patients require either initiation or dosage adjustments of insulin or oral hypoglycemic agents. Diabetic ketoacidosis has also occurred. Hyperglycemia persists in some cases after drug discontinuation.

Pharmacokinetics. *Fate.* Oral absorption of saquinavir mesylate is erratic and the drug undergoes extensive first-pass metabolism. Approximately 30% of a 600 mg dose is absorbed when given within 2 hr after food; absolute bioavailability averages 4%. Saquinavir bioavailability relative to saquinavir mesylate is 331%. Saquinavir is 98% plasma protein bound; concentrations in the CSF are negligible. Saquinavir undergoes metabolism primarily by CYP3A4; Cl is 1.14 L/hr/kg.[111]

$t_{1/2}$. 12 hr.

Adverse Reactions. Abdominal discomfort or pain, diarrhea, anorexia, and nausea occur frequently. Occasional adverse reactions include asthenia, rash, elevations of transaminases, and headache. Rare reactions include ataxia, confusion, hemolytic anemia, thrombophlebitis, attempted suicide, seizures, and exacerbation of chronic liver disease.

Contraindications. (*See* Drug Interactions.)

Precautions. Do not use saquinavir as monotherapy because of the greater potential for developing resistance.

Drug Interactions. Do not administer saquinavir with rifampin because steady-state AUC of saquinavir decreases by 80%. Administration with rifabutin reduces saquinavir plasma concentrations by 40% and alternatives to this combination should be considered. Avoid other drugs that strongly induce CYP3A4, because they may substantially decrease saquinavir serum concentrations. Avoid co-administration with astemizole or cisapride because of possible prolonged QT intervals and serious cardiovascular adverse events. Concurrent ketoconazole, and possibly other inhibitors of CYP3A4, may increase the bioavailability and half-life of saquinavir. (*See* Cytochrome P450 Enzyme Interactions.) Ingesting grapefruit juice with saquinavir has been suggested to increase the bioavailability of saquinavir by inhibition of CYP3A4. However, the grapefruit juice must be concentrated, taken with every dose of saquinavir, and contain flavinoids to have any benefit. This method is not likely to be palatable to most patients because of gastric irritation and appears unnecessary with the soft gelatin capsule formulation of saquinavir.

Parameters to Monitor. (*See* Nelfinavir.)

Notes. Saquinavir (Fortovase) should be refrigerated; once brought to room temperature (≤25°C), it should be used within 3 months. Fortovase has a dosage of 1200 mg tid to achieve saquinavir plasma concentrations sufficient to inhibit the replication of HIV. The hard gelatin capsule formulation dosage of 600 mg tid does not consistently achieve adequate saquinavir plasma concentrations. The use of **ritonavir** 400 mg bid and saquinavir 400 mg bid in combination has been used to improve concentrations of saquinavir and tolerance of ritonavir.

STAVUDINE	Zerit

Pharmacology. Stavudine (d4T) is a synthetic pyrimidine nucleoside reverse transcriptase inhibitor that is structurally similar to zidovudine and has been shown to inhibit HIV replication in vitro. Stavudine is phosphorylated by cellular enzymes to stavudine triphosphate, which acts both as a competitive inhibitor of HIV reverse transcriptase and as an alternative nucleoside substrate, which leads to premature elongation of viral DNA.[118,119] (*See* Antiviral Drugs for HIV Infection Comparison Chart.)

Adult Dosage. PO for HIV (<60 kg) 30 mg bid; (≥60 kg) 40 mg bid. Dosage can be reduced to 15 mg q 12 hr for patients <60 kg or 20 mg q 12 hr for patients ≥60 kg if they are at risk for peripheral neuropathy. Reduce dosage in renal impairment.

Dosage Forms. Cap 15, 20, 30, 40 mg.

Pharmacokinetics. Stavudine is well absorbed with or without food and oral bioavailability is 82%. Average time to peak concentration is 1 hr with serum concentrations of about 1.2 mg/L after a single 0.67 mg/kg dose. V_d is 0.53 L/kg. Limited data suggest that stavudine distributes into the CSF, with concentrations approximately 40% of serum concentration. Renal clearance is about 40% of total clearance, with the remaining drug metabolized to thymine and eventually to β-aminoisobutyric acid.

Adverse Reactions. The most frequent adverse effect is peripheral neuropathy; occasionally, elevated hepatic transaminases occur.

ZIDOVUDINE	Retrovir

Pharmacology. Zidovudine (azidothymidine; AZT) is a thymidine analogue that inhibits HIV replication. It is converted to the active monophosphate form by thymidine kinase and ultimately to zidovudine triphosphate by intracellular enzymes. This form exerts its activity at viral DNA polymerase (reverse transcriptase) by competing with other cellular deoxynucleosides and by acting as a chain terminator of DNA synthesis.[85] (*See* Antiviral Drugs for HIV Infection Comparison Chart.)

Administration and Adult Dosage. The optimal dosage is not established; large interpatient pharmacokinetic variability necessitates individualization of dosage. **PO for HIV infection with** 300 mg bid or 200 mg tid. **PO for maternal-fetal HIV transmission (maternal)** 300 mg bid, begun after the 14th week of pregnancy and continued throughout the pregnancy, then **IV during labor** 2 mg/kg over 1 hr, followed by a continuous infusion of 1 mg/kg/hr until delivery. (*See also* Pediatric Dosage.) **PO for combination therapy with zalcitabine** 200 mg q 8 hr with zalcitabine 0.75 mg q 8 hr. **PO for postexposure prophylaxis** 1–1.5 g/day in 4 or 5 divided doses has been used[120]; however, the effectiveness of this regimen is not confirmed in humans and informed consent should be obtained. **IV for patients unable to take oral medication** 1–2 mg/kg q 4 hr infused over 1 hr, only until oral therapy can be initiated.

Special Populations. *Pediatric Dosage.* **PO for prevention of maternal HIV transmission** 2 mg/kg/dose q 6 hr for first 6 weeks of life, beginning 8–12 hr after birth.[121] **IV for prevention of maternal HIV transmission if unable to receive PO** 1.5 mg/kg/dose q 6 hr until oral therapy can be initiated. **PO for HIV infection** (0–2 weeks) 2 mg/kg/dose q 6 hr; (2–4 weeks) 3 mg/kg/dose q 6 hr; (4 weeks–13 yr) 180 mg/m²/dose (to a maximum of 200 mg) q 6 hr; (over 13 yr) 100 mg q 4 hr 5 times/day.[87]

Geriatric Dosage. Same as adult dosage, but adjust for age-related reduction in renal function.

Other Conditions. Reduce dosage by 50% in patients with Cl_{cr} <25 mL/min,[88] and decrease by 75% in cirrhosis.[122]

Dosage Forms. **Cap** 100 mg; **Tab** 300 mg; **Syrup** 10 mg/mL; **Inj** 10 mg/mL.

Patient Instructions. (*See* HIV Drugs Class Instructions.) This drug is not a cure for HIV disease. Opportunistic infections and other complications associated with HIV infection may continue to develop. This drug may be taken with food to decrease abdominal discomfort or nausea. It is important to have blood counts followed closely during therapy to monitor for decreases in blood cell counts.

Pharmacokinetics. *Serum Levels.* Not established; intracellular concentrations of zidovudine triphosphate may correlate with therapeutic benefit, but in vivo data are not available.

Fate. Zidovudine undergoes marked presystemic metabolism. Oral bioavailability is 60–70%, possibly reduced with high-fat meals. Peak serum levels are approximately 1.2 mg/L (4.5 μmol/L) after a 250 mg oral dose. Protein binding is less than 25%. CSF concentrations are 24% of serum in children receiving a continuous infusion of the drug. V_{dss} is 1.6 ± 0.6 L/kg; Cl is 1.3 ± 0.3 L/hr/kg in adults and 36.4 ± 11.5 L/hr/m^2 in children. Zidovudine (ZDV) is rapidly metabolized to the inactive ether glucuronide (GZDV). GZDV formation is reduced, and zidovudine AUC and half-life are increased in patients with cirrhosis. About 60% of an oral dose is excreted as GZDV in urine. GZDV excretion is reduced in patients with renal dysfunction; hemodialysis removes GZDV but not ZDV.[88,122,123]

$t_{1/2}$. (Adults) 1.1 ± 0.2 hr; 2.1 hr in uremia; 2.4 hr in cirrhosis.[88] (Children) 1.5 ± 0.6 hr.

Adverse Reactions. Severe anemia and granulocytopenia occur frequently and may necessitate blood transfusions; epoetin may help alleviate anemia in patients with low serum erythropoietin levels. Other frequent adverse reactions associated with zidovudine in placebo-controlled trials include abdominal discomfort, nausea, vomiting, isomnia, myalgias, and headaches. Adverse reactions that occasionally occur with long-term use (>12 weeks) include myopathy and nail pigmentation.[85]

Contraindications. Life-threatening allergy to the drug or its components.

Precautions. Pregnancy; lactation. Use with caution in liver disease or hepatomegaly, especially obese women.

Drug Interactions. Several drugs decrease the glucuronidation of zidovudine, including atovaquone, methadone, probenecid, valproic acid, and possibly fluconazole; rifampin increases zidovudine glucuronidation; however, the clinical importance of these interactions is not established.[94] Initial studies showed that prolonged administration of acetaminophen was associated with increased hematologic toxicity from zidovudine, but further study does not support this finding.[124]

Parameters to Monitor. Hemoglobin, hematocrit, MCV, and WBC for hematologic toxicity. Monitor clinical signs, symptoms, and laboratory markers for progression of HIV disease to help decide regimen changes in antiretroviral therapy. Baseline CD4 and HIV-1 RNA polymerase chain reaction viral load tests are useful to measure clinical benefit of therapy. Repeat tests after 1 month and q 3–4 months thereafter have been suggested to monitor benefit of antiretroviral therapy.

Notes. Viral resistance to zidovudine has occurred in vitro with isolates recovered from patients and is associated with prolonged zidovudine use and more advanced disease; correlation between viral resistance in vitro and progression of disease has not been established. Studies with **lamivudine** (3TC) suggest that the combination can delay or prevent HIV-1 viral resistance to zidovudine.

ANTIRETROVIRAL THERAPY FOR HIV

The use of protease inhibitors in combination with reverse transcriptase inhibitors has dramatically changed the treatment of HIV infection. Regimens containing a protease inhibitor have enhanced the ability to inhibit replication of HIV, impacting immunologic and viral markers, delaying progression of disease, and improving survival. Many formidable hurdles stand in the way of effective treatment, including patient adherence to dosage regimens, adverse effects, and drug–drug interactions. These hurdles interfere with quality of life and control of the viral burden and also contribute to the emergence of resistance. It is essential for health care providers and patients to appreciate the complexity of antiretroviral medication regimens in order to achieve harmony between goals of antiretroviral therapy and optimal patient care. General principals of treatment that guide contemporary treatment decisions are outlined below:

- Viral load monitoring is essential to guide decision making.
- Attaining and maintaining an undetectable HIV RNA in blood (which may indirectly reflect lymph concentrations) is the goal of therapy.
- Effective antiretroviral therapy should be introduced *before* extensive immune system damage has occurred.
- Three-drug combination therapy, preferably including a potent protease inhibitor, is the regimen most likely to achieve the goal of an undetectable HIV RNA level and provide a durable response.
- Compliance with the treatment regimen is critical to success and must be considered in initiating and choosing regimens.
- Most or all drugs in a failing regimen should be changed simultaneously.

For further information and clarification on appropriate use of antiretroviral therapy, refer to U.S. Public Health Service guidelines for the use of antiretroviral agents in pediatric HIV infection and HIV-infected adults and adolescents (references 125 and 126).

ANTIVIRAL DRUGS FOR HIV INFECTION COMPARISON CHART

DRUG	DOSAGE FORMS	ADULT DOSAGE	PEDIATRIC DOSAGE	EFFECT ON CYP450 ISOZYMES	ADVERSE REACTIONS	COMMENTS
HIV NUCLEOSIDE REVERSE TRANSCRIPTASE INHIBITORS						
Abacavir Ziagen	Tab 300 mg Soln 20 mg/mL.	PO 300 mg bid.	PO 8 mg/kg bid.	No effect.	Rash, asthenia, hypersensitivity reaction.	Patients who have a hypersensitivity reaction must not take the drug; it could be fatal.
Didanosine Videx	Chew Tab 25, 50, 100, 150 mg Pwdr for Oral Soln (adult) 100, 167, 250, 375 mg Pwdr for Oral Soln (pediatric) 2, 4 g.	PO (<60 kg) 125 mg q 12 hr or 167 mg q 12 hr (as powder); (≥60 kg) 200 mg q 12 hr or 250 mg q 12 hr (as powder). Once daily administration is being investigated.	(*See* monograph.)	No effect.	Neuropathy, pancreatitis, nausea, dysgeusia, diarrhea, hyperuricemia, headache, asthenia, seizures, pruritus.	$Cl_{cr} \leq 60$ mL/min, consider dosage reduction, but no specific recommendations are available.

(*continued*)

DRUG	DOSAGE FORMS	ADULT DOSAGE	PEDIATRIC DOSAGE	EFFECT ON CYP450 ISOZYMES	ADVERSE REACTIONS	COMMENTS
Lamivudine Epivir	Tab 150 mg Soln 10 mg/mL.	PO 150 mg bid.	PO (3 mo–12 yr) 4 mg/kg q 12 hr, to a maximum of 150 mg q 12 hr.	No effect.	Nausea, headache, rash, fatigue, anorexia; generally well tolerated, but pancreatitis is a risk in pediatric population, but not in adults.	Reduce dosage in renal impairment: Cl_{cr} 30–49 mL/min, 150 mg/day; Cl_{cr} 15–29 mL/min, 150 mg once, then 100 mg/day; Cl_{cr} 5–14 mL/min, 150 mg once, then 50 mg/day; Cl_{cr} <5 mL/min, 50 mg once, then 25 mg/day.
Stavudine Zerit	Cap 15, 20, 30, 40 mg Soln 1 mg/mL.	PO (≤60 kg) 30 mg bid; PO (>60 kg) 40 mg bid. Reduce dosage for mild to moderate peripheral neuropathy.	PO (≤30 kg) 1 mg/kg q 12 hr.	No effect.	Neuropathy, headache, nausea, asthenia, insomnia, elevated hepatic enzymes.	Reduce dosage in renal impairment: Cl_{cr} 26–50 mL/min, reduce dosage by 50% and give q 12 hr; Cl_{cr} 10–25 mL/min, reduce dosage by 50% and give q 24 hr.
Zalcitabine Hivid	Tab 0.375, 0.75 mg.	PO 0.75 mg tid. Reduce dosage for symptoms of peripheral neuropathy.	Not established.	No effect.	Neuropathy, oral and esophageal ulceration, elevated hepatic enzymes, pancreatitis, rash, pruritus.	Reduce dosage in renal impairment: Cl_{cr} 10–40 mL/min, same dose q 12 hr; Cl_{cr} <10 mL/min, same dose q 24 hr.

(continued)

ANTIVIRAL DRUGS FOR HIV INFECTION COMPARISON CHART (continued)

DRUG	DOSAGE FORMS	ADULT DOSAGE	PEDIATRIC DOSAGE	EFFECT ON CYP450 ISOZYMES	ADVERSE REACTIONS	COMMENTS
Zidovudine Retrovir	Cap 100 mg Tab 300 mg Syrup 10 mg/mL Inj 10 mg/ML.	PO 200 mg tid or 300 mg bid. (*See* monograph for other indications.)	PO (neonates) 2 mg/kg q 6 hr; IV (neonates) 1.5 mg/kg q 6 hr (infants and children) 80 mg/m² q 6 hr.	No effect.	Bone marrow suppression (anemia, neutropenia), nausea, abdominal pain, elevated hepatic enzymes, headache, malaise, elevated CPK, myopathy, nail discoloration.	Reduce dosage in renal impairment: Cl$_{cr}$ ≤25 mL/min, reduce recommended dosage by 50%.
Zidovudine and Lamivudine Combivir	Tab 300 mg zidovudine plus 150 mg lamivudine.	PO 1 tablet bid.	Not recommended.	No effect.	(*See* lamivudine and zidovudine.)	Contraindicated in renal impairment.
HIV NUCLEOTIDE REVERSE TRANSCRIPTASE INHIBITORS						
Adefovir Preveon (Investigational, Gilead)	Tab 60, 120 mg.	PO 60–120 mg/day with L-carnitine. (*See* comments.)	Not established.	No effect.	Nausea, vomiting, diarrhea, neutropenia, thrombocytopenia, Fanconi syndrome (↑Cr$_s$, proteinuria) ↑LFTs, ↓serum free carnitine.	Must take carnitine 500 mg/day during therapy. Nephrotoxicity is frequent.

(*continued*)

ANTIVIRAL DRUGS FOR HIV INFECTION COMPARISON CHART (continued)

DRUG	DOSAGE FORMS	ADULT DOSAGE	PEDIATRIC DOSAGE	EFFECT ON CYP450 ISOZYMES	ADVERSE REACTIONS	COMMENTS
NONNUCLEOSIDE REVERSE TRANSCRIPTASE INHIBITORS						
Delavirdine Rescriptor	Tab 100 mg.	PO 400 mg tid.	Not established.	*Inhibits* CYP2C9 CYP2C19 CYP3A4	Rash, headache, elevated hepatic enzymes.	Tablets may be dispersed in water to allow easier administration.
Efavirenz Sustiva	Cap 50, 100, 200 mg.	PO 600 mg qd.	(10–14 kg) 200 mg/day; (15–19 kg) 250 mg/day; (20–24 kg) 300 mg/day; (25–32.5 kg) 350 mg/day; (32.5–39 kg) 400 mg/day; (≥40 kg) 600 mg/day.	*Induces* CYP3A4 *Inhibits* CYP2C9 CYP2C19 CYP3A4	CNS symptoms, dizziness, rash, dysphoria, anxiety, nausea, insomnia, inability to concentrate.	CNS symptoms frequently resolve within 2–4 weeks of initiating therapy. It may be helpful to take dose at bedtime or to take in 2–3 divided doses to help reduce symptoms. Rash frequent in first 2 weeks, but usually resolves in 2 months.
Nevirapine Viramune	Tab 200 mg Susp 10 mg/mL (investigational).	PO 200 mg/day for 14 days, then 400 mg/day in 1 or 2 doses. (*See* comments.)	PO initiate with 120 mg/m² once daily for 14 days, then increase to full dosage of 120–200 mg/m² q 12 hr.	*Induces* CYP3A4	Rash, hepatitis, fatigue, headache.	To reduce the frequency of rash, it is essential to increase the dosage over 14 days. Increase to full dosage only if no rash or other adverse effects occur.

(*continued*)

121

ANTIVIRAL DRUGS FOR HIV INFECTION COMPARISON CHART (continued)

DRUG	DOSAGE FORMS	ADULT DOSAGE	PEDIATRIC DOSAGE	EFFECT ON CYP450 ISOZYMES	ADVERSE REACTIONS	COMMENTS
PROTEASE INHIBITORS						
Amprenavir Agenerase	Cap 150 mg Liquid 15 mg/mL.	PO 1.2 g bid.	PO 20–22.5 mg/kg bid.	*Inhibits* CYP3A4 CYP2C19 CYP2E1	Rash (frequent), nausea, vomiting, diarrhea, flatulence, perioral paresthesias. Triglycerides, LFTs, and glucose.	Rash usually occurs within 9 days and resolves in 1 week after discontinuation; Stevens-Johnson syndrome has occurred.
Indinavir Mesylate Crixivan	Cap 200, 400 mg.	PO 800 mg q 8 hr.	PO 500 mg/m² q 8 hr (under study in clinical trials).	*Inhibits* CYP3A4	Nausea, headache, abdominal pain, hyperbilirubinemia, insomnia, dizziness, nephrolithiasis.	Administer on an empty stomach 1 hr before or 2 hr after a meal (or can take with a light meal). Adequate hydration is required to minimize risk of nephrolithiasis.
Nelfinavir Mesylate Viracept	Tab 250 mg Pwdr 50 mg nelfinavir free base per level scoopful (1 g).	PO 750 mg tid or 1250 mg bid.	PO 20–30 mg/kg tid.	*Inhibits* CYP3A4	Diarrhea, nausea, dysphagia, rash.	Administer with food or light snack to increase absorption 2- to 3-fold.

(continued)

ANTIVIRAL DRUGS FOR HIV INFECTION COMPARISON CHART (continued)

DRUG	DOSAGE FORMS	ADULT DOSAGE	PEDIATRIC DOSAGE	EFFECT ON CYP450 ISOZYMES	ADVERSE REACTIONS	COMMENTS
Ritonavir Norvir	Cap[a] 100 mg Soln[a] 80 mg/mL.	PO 600 mg q 12 hr.[b] *Combination:* PO 400 mg q 12 hr with saquinavir; PO 400 mg q 12 hr.	PO 400 mg/m^2 q 12 hr.[c]	*Inhibits* CYP3A4 CYP2C9 CYP2C19 CYP2D6	Nausea, vomiting, diarrhea, headache, circumoral and extremity paresthesias, asthenia, taste perversion, elevated serum triglycerides, hepatic transaminases, CPK, uric acid.	Titrate dosage from 300 mg q 12 hr to 600 mg q 12 hr over 10–14 days to reduce adverse events.
Saquinavir Fortovase	Cap 200 mg.	PO 1.2 g tid. *Combination:* PO 400 mg q 12 hr with ritonavir 400 mg PO q 12 hr.	Not established.	*Inhibits* CYP3A4	Abdominal cramping, nausea, diarrhea, headache.	Bioavailability relative to Invirase formulation is 331%. Refrigerate capsules, but may keep at room temperature for 90 days.

(continued)

ANTIVIRAL DRUGS FOR HIV INFECTION COMPARISON CHART (continued)

DRUG	DOSAGE FORMS	ADULT DOSAGE	PEDIATRIC DOSAGE	EFFECT ON CYP450 ISOZYMES	ADVERSE REACTIONS	COMMENTS
Saquinavir Mesylate Invirase	Cap 200 mg.	PO 600–1800 mg tid. *Combination:* PO 400 mg q 12 hr with ritonavir 400 mg PO q 12 hr.	Not established.	*Inhibits* CYP3A4	Nausea, headache, elevated hepatic transaminases.	Bioavailability is 4% and erratic.

[a]Ritonavir capsules must be kept refrigerated. Ritonavir solution must be stored in the original container.
[b]Adult dosage escalation for ritonavir: days 1–2, 300 mg PO bid; days 3–5, 400 mg PO bid; days 6–13, 500 mg PO bid; day 14, 600 mg PO bid.
[c]Pediatric dosage escalation for ritonavir: Initiate therapy at 250 mg/m^2 q 12 hr and increase stepwise to full dosage over 5 days as tolerated.
From references 125–127 and product information.

β-Lactams

AMOXICILLIN

Pharmology. Amoxicillin differs from ampicillin by the presence of a hydroxyl group on the amino side chain. It has activity essentially identical to ampicillin.[128,129] (*See* β-Lactams Comparison Chart.)

Adult Dosage. PO 250–500 mg q 8 hr, to a maximum of 4.5 g/day. **PO for endocarditis prophylaxis** 2 g 1 hr prior to dental or upper airway procedures.

Pediatric Dosage. PO 20–40 mg/kg/day in 3 equally divided doses q 8 hr. **PO for endocarditis prophylaxis** 50 mg/kg 1 hr prior to dental or upper airway procedures.

Dosage Forms. **Cap** 250, 500 mg; **Chew Tab** 125, 250 mg; **Drp** 50 mg/mL; **Susp** 25, 50 mg/mL.

Pharmacokinetics. Amoxicillin is completely absorbed, with about 85% bioavailability because of a small first-pass effect. Serum concentrations are greater than those after equal doses of ampicillin; postabsorptive pharmacokinetics are identical to those of ampicillin.

Adverse Reactions. Adverse effects are similar to ampicillin, although diarrhea and rashes are much less frequent with amoxicillin.

AMOXICILLIN AND POTASSIUM CLAVULANATE

Pharmacology. Clavulanic acid has weak antibacterial activity, but is a potent inhibitor of plasmid-mediated β-lactamases, including those produced by *Haemophilus influenzae, Moraxella (Branhamella) catarrhalis, Staphylococcus aureus, Neisseria gonorrhoeae,* and *Bacteroides fragilis.* Thus, when combined with certain other β-lactam antibiotics, the combination is very active against many bacteria resistant to the β-lactam alone.[130,131]

Adult Dosage. PO One "250" or "500" tablet tid or 1 "875" tablet bid. (*See* Dosage Forms.)

Pediatric Dosage. PO 20–45 mg/kg/day (of the amoxicillin component) in 2 or 3 divided doses. (*See* Dosage Forms.)

Dosage Forms. Do not substitute combinations of lower-dose tablets to make a higher dose, because diarrhea is markedly increased. **Tab** (8-hr) 250 mg amoxicillin/125 mg clavulanic acid, 500 mg amoxicillin/125 mg clavulanic acid; (12-hr) 875 mg amoxicillin/125 mg clavulanic acid; **Chew Tab** (8-hr) 125 mg amoxicillin/31.25 mg clavulanic acid, 250 mg amoxicillin/62.5 mg clavulanic acid; (12-hr) 200 mg amoxicillin/28.5 mg clavulanic acid, 400 mg amoxicillin/57 mg clavulanic acid; **Susp** (8-hr) 25 mg amoxicillin/6.25 mg clavulanic acid/mL, 50 mg amoxicillin/12.5 mg clavulanic acid/mL; (12-hr) 40 mg amoxicillin/5.7 mg clavulanic acid/mL, 80 mg amoxicillin/11.4 mg clavulanic acid/mL.

Pharmacokinetics. Peak serum clavulanate concentration is 2.6 mg/L 40–60 min following an oral dose of 250 mg amoxicillin/125 mg clavulanate. Amoxicillin pharmacokinetics are not affected by clavulanic acid. Clavulanic acid half-life is approximately 60 min.

Adverse Reactions. Adverse effects of this preparation include those of amoxicillin; however, diarrhea is more frequent with the combination and depends on the dosage of clavulanate. The 12-hr formulations reduce the frequency of diarrhea. Nausea and diarrhea may occur less frequently when this preparation is administered with food. (*See* β-Lactams Comparison Chart.)

AMPICILLIN   Various

Pharmacology. Ampicillin has a similar mechanism of action and is comparable in activity to penicillin G against Gram-positive bacteria, but is more active than penicillin G against Gram-negative bacteria.[128,129] (*See* β-Lactams Comparison Chart.)

Adult Dosage. PO 250–500 mg qid. **IM or IV** 100–200 mg/kg/day in 4–6 divided doses. Give the same dose q 12 hr with a Cl_{cr} <20 mL/min. **IV or IM for endocarditis prophylaxis** 2 g within 30 min of procedure.

Pediatric Dosage. PO (<20 kg) 50–100 mg/kg/day in 2–4 divided doses; (>20 kg) 100–400 mg/kg/day in 4–6 divided doses. **IV** (neonates) 25–100 mg/kg/dose q 6–12 hr—higher dosages for meningitis; (<20 kg) 50–100 mg/kg/day in 2–4 divided doses; (>20 kg) 400 mg/kg/day in 4–6 divided doses. **IV or IM for endocarditis prophylaxis** 50 mg/kg within 30 min of procedure.

Dosage Forms. **Cap** 250, 500 mg; **Chew Tab** 125 mg; **Drp** 100 mg/mL; **Susp** 25, 50, 100 mg/mL; **Inj** 125, 250, 500 mg, 1, 2, 10 g.

Pharmacokinetics. Oral forms are about 50% absorbed in the fasting state; food delays absorption. Plasma protein binding is low, and therapeutic concentrations are attained in most tissues and fluids including CSF (in the presence of inflammation). About 90% is excreted unchanged in urine. Half-life is 1.2 hr, 2 hr in neonates, increasing to 20 hr in anuric patients.

Adverse Reactions. Nausea and diarrhea occur frequently with oral therapy. Other reactions include frequent skin rash (more frequent in patients receiving allopurinol and very frequent in patients with Epstein-Barr virus infection [mononucleosis]). Most of these eruptions are probably not hypersensitivity reactions, but are immunologically mediated. They are generally dose related (higher frequency at higher dosages), are macular rather than urticarial, and disappear with continued administration of the drug.

ANTISTAPHYLOCOCCAL PENICILLINS

Pharmacology. Methicillin, nafcillin, oxacillin, cloxacillin, and dicloxacillin are similar to other penicillins in their mechanism of action. However, these drugs are not hydrolyzed by staphylococcal penicillinases. Therefore, nearly all isolates of *Staphylococcus aureus* and some isolates of coagulase-negative staphylococci are susceptible to these drugs. Methicillin- (actually β-lactam-) resistant staphylococci have altered penicillin-binding proteins (transpeptidases). Although these drugs are primarily used in staphylococcal infection, they retain good activity against most streptococci, except enterococci.[126,128,132]

Adult Dosage. Oral administration of nafcillin and oxacillin is not recommended because they are poorly absorbed. (*See* β-Lactams Comparison Chart.)

Pediatric Dosage. (*See* β-Lactams Comparison Chart.)

Dosage Forms. (*See* β-Lactams Comparison Chart.)

Pharmacokinetics. Only cloxacillin and dicloxacillin are adequately absorbed from the GI tract. Except for methicillin, these drugs are mostly hepatically eliminated by metabolism and biliary excretion.

Adverse Reactions. Interstitial nephritis is frequent with methicillin, but occurs only rarely with the other drugs. Hepatic damage occurs rarely with oxacillin. Nafcillin has a propensity for local irritation at the IV infusion site, and may cause neutropenia more frequently than other antistaphylococcal penicillins.

AZTREONAM   Azactam

Pharmacology. Aztreonam is a monobactam with activity similar to that of third-generation cephalosporins against most Gram-negative aerobic bacteria (including *Pseudomonas aeruginosa*), but it is inactive against Gram-positive bacteria and anaerobes.[133–135] (*See* β-Lactams Comparison Chart.)

Adult Dosage. IM or IV 500 mg–2 g q 6–12 hr, to a maximum of 8 g/day, depending on severity and site of infection. Reduce maintenance dosage by 50% with a Cl_{cr} of 10–30 mL/min and by 75% with a Cl_{cr} <10 mL/min. One-eighth of the initial dose should be given after hemodialysis.

Pediatric Dosage. IV (9 months–16 yr) 30 mg/kg q 6–8 hr. Dosages as high as 50 mg/kg q 6 hr have been used in children with serious Gram-negative infections (eg, *P. aeruginosa*).

Dosage Forms. Inj 500 mg, 1, 2 g.

Pharmacokinetics. Peak serum concentrations of 164 and 255 mg/L occur after a 30-min IV infusion of 1 and 2 g, respectively. With inflamed meninges, CSF concentrations are similar to those observed with comparable dosages of third-generation cephalosporins, but experience in treating meningitis is limited. The drug is 60% plasma protein bound and has a V_d of about 0.24 L/kg; 60–70% is excreted in urine unchanged. The half-life is 1.5–2 hr, increasing to 6 hr in renal failure and 3.2 hr in alcoholic cirrhosis.

Adverse Reactions. Adverse effects of aztreonam are minimal. Cross-allergenicity between aztreonam and other β-lactams is low, and aztreonam has been used safely in penicillin- or cephalosporin-allergic patients.

CEPHALOSPORINS

Pharmacology. Cephalosporin antibiotics have broad-spectrum activity against many Gram-positive and Gram-negative pathogens. These agents are generally considered to be bactericidal through binding to various penicillin-binding proteins in bacteria, which results in changes in cell wall structure and function. Members of this class are frequently subdivided into "generations" based on their antimicrobial activity (as well as order of introduction into clinical use).[135–139]

First-generation cephalosporins have activity against Gram-positive bacteria (eg, *Staphylococcus* spp.) as well as a limited, but important, number of species of aerobic Gram-negative bacilli (eg, *Escherichia coli, Klebsiella* spp., *Proteus mirabilis*). *Haemophilus influenzae* and most other aerobic Gram-negative bacilli often indigenous to hospitals (eg, *Enterobacter* spp., *Pseudomonas* spp.) are resistant to these drugs. Anaerobic bacteria isolated in the oropharynx are generally susceptible to these agents; however, anaerobes such as *Bacteroides fragilis* are resistant.[135,139]

The **second-generation cephalosporins** cefamandole, cefonicid, ceforanide, and cefuroxime all differ from first-generation agents in their improved activity against *H. influenzae* and some strains of *Enterobacter* spp., *Providencia* spp., and *Morganella* spp.[135,139] The oral second-generation cephalosporins cefuroxime axetil, cefprozil, cefonicid, and loracarbef (a carbacephem) have similar but less potent activity.[140-143] Cefoxitin, cefmetazole, and cefotetan (which are actually cephamycins) have increased activity against anaerobes, including *B. fragilis*[135,144,145]; the other second-generation cephalosporins have poor activity against this organism.[135]

Third-generation cephalosporins are noteworthy for their marked potency against common Gram-negative organisms (eg, *E. coli, Klebsiella pneumoniae*) as well as their activity against Gram-negative bacilli resistant to older agents (eg, *Serratia* spp., *Pseudomonas aeruginosa*). Although grouped together, some agents have better activity against certain organisms (eg, ceftazidime is better against *P. aeruginosa*), and poorer activity against others (eg, cefixime and ceftazidime are poorer against *Staphylococcus aureus*).[135,136,138,139]

Fourth-generation cephalosporins have a spectrum similar to the third-generation drugs, plus activity against some Gram-negative strains that are resistant to the third-generation agents, such as *Enterobacter* spp. Their antianaerobic activity is poor.

Resistance to cephalosporins is mediated by β-lactamase, reduction in outer cell wall membrane permeability, and alteration of the affinity of these agents for penicillin-binding proteins. Resistance among certain β-lactamase–producing organisms (eg, *Enterobacter* and *Citrobacter* spp.) to third-generation cephalosporins has increased in recent years such that these agents cannot be relied upon to provide effective therapy.[139]

Administration and Adult Dosage. (*See* β-Lactams Comparison Chart.)

Special Populations. *Pediatric Dosage.* (*See* β-Lactams Comparison Chart.)

Geriatric Dosage. Same as adult dosage, but adjust for age-related reduction in renal function.

Other Conditions. Most agents require dosage modification in renal dysfunction; exceptions are ceftriaxone and cefoperazone, which have biliary and renal or primarily biliary elimination, respectively.[138] Dosage reduction of all agents is required in patients with concomitant hepatic and renal dysfunction. (*See* β-Lactams Comparison Chart.)

Pharmacokinetics. Some of the greatest differences between agents reside in their pharmacokinetic properties. Of note is the improved CSF penetration of certain later-generation agents over the first-generation agents. Therapeutic CSF concentrations are achieved with cefotaxime, moxalactam, ceftriaxone, and ceftazidime; these agents have proven efficacy in the treatment of meningitis caused by susceptible organisms in adults and children.[135,138,139] Adequate CSF concentrations of ceftizoxime have also been observed, although its use in the treatment of meningitis is less well established. Cefuroxime penetrates adequately into CSF, but is less effective for meningitis than third-generation agents.[135,146] (*See* β-Lactams Comparison Chart.)

Adverse Reactions. Most cephalosporins are generally well tolerated, although a few agents have unique adverse reactions. Hypersensitivity reactions may occur in approximately 10% of patients known to be allergic to penicillin; do not administer these agents to patients with a history of an immediate reaction to penicillin.[147] Nausea and diarrhea occur with all agents; however, diarrhea is more common with ceftriaxone and cefoperazone because of high biliary excretion.[135,138,139] Colitis caused by *Clostridium difficile* has been reported with all the cephalosporins, but may be more common with ceftriaxone and cefoperazone. Nephrotoxicity is rare, particularly when used without other nephrotoxic agents.[139] All agents with an N-methylthiotetrazole (NMTT) moiety in the three position of the cephem nucleus (cefoperazone, cefamandole, cefotetan, and cefmetazole) may produce a disulfiram-like reaction in some patients upon ingestion of alcohol-containing beverages. In addition, these agents may be associated to varying degrees with bleeding secondary to hypoprothrombinemia, which is corrected or prevented by vitamin K administration.[135,138,139,148] Although controversial, the mechanism of this reaction appears to involve inhibition of enzymatic reactions requiring vitamin K in the activation of prothrombin precursors by NMTT. However, other factors (eg, malnutrition, liver disease) may be more important risk factors for bleeding than the NMTT-containing cephalosporins.[148] Thus, cautious use (and perhaps even avoidance) of agents with the NMTT side chain is recommended in patients with poor oral intake and critical illness. Administration of vitamin K and monitoring of the prothrombin time is indicated with these agents, particularly when therapy is prolonged. Positive direct Coombs' tests occur frequently, but hemolysis is rare.[135,139] Ceftriaxone has been associated with biliary pseudolithiasis (sludging), which may be asymptomatic or resemble acute cholecystitis.[149] This adverse effect occurs most often with dosages of ≥2 g/day, especially in patients receiving prolonged therapy or those with impaired gallbladder emptying. The mechanism is ceftriaxone-calcium complex formation, and it is usually reversible upon drug discontinuation.[150] Neonates given ceftriaxone can develop kernicterus caused by displacement of bilirubin from plasma protein binding sites; its use in this population is best avoided. Development of resistance during treatment of infections caused by *Enterobacter* spp., *Serratia* spp., and *P. aeruginosa* has occurred with all these agents.[135,138,139]

Precautions. Penicillin allergy. Use agents with NMTT side chain with caution in patients with underlying bleeding diathesis, poor oral intake, or critical illness. Use with caution in renal impairment and in those on oral anticoagulants (especially NMTT-containing drugs). Avoid use of ceftriaxone in neonates, particularly premature infants.

Drug Interactions. Avoid concomitant ingestion of alcohol or alcohol-containing products with agents containing the NMTT side chain. Probenecid reduces renal clearance and increases serum levels of most agents, except those that do not undergo renal tubular secretion (eg, ceftazidime, ceftriaxone, moxalactam).

Parameters to Monitor. Monitor prothrombin time 2–3 times/week with agents having an NMTT side chain, particularly when using large dosages; monitor bleeding time with moxalactam and with high dosages of other agents having an NMTT side chain. Obtain antimicrobial susceptibility tests for development of resistance in patients relapsing during therapy. Monitor renal function tests initially and periodically during high-dose regimens or when the drug is used concurrently with nephrotoxic agents. Monitor for diarrhea, particularly with ceftriaxone and cefoperazone; test stool specimen for *C. difficile* toxin if diarrhea persists or is associated with fever or abdominal pain.

CEFAZOLIN SODIUM   Ancef, Kefzol, Various

Pharmacology. Cefazolin is a first-generation cephalosporin with activity against most Gram-positive aerobic organisms except enterococci and some Gram-negative bacilli (eg, *Escherichia coli, Klebsiella* spp., *Proteus mirabilis*).[137,139]

Adult Dosage. IM or IV for treatment 250 mg–1 g q 6–12 hr (usually 1 g q 8 hr), to a maximum of 6 g/day. Decrease dosage in renal impairment. (See β-Lactams Comparison Chart.) **IM or IV for surgical prophylaxis** 1 g 30–60 min prior to surgery. **IM or IV for endocarditis prophylaxis** 1 g within 30 min prior to a dental or upper airway procedure.

Pediatric Dosage. IM or IV (≤ 1month) 25 mg/kg/dose given q 8–12 hr; (>1 month) 50–100 mg/kg/day in 3 divided doses given q 8 hr. **IM or IV for endocarditis prophylaxis** 25 mg/kg within 30 min prior to a dental or upper airway procedure.

Dosage Forms. Inj 250, 500 mg, 1, 5, 10, 20 g.

Pharmacokinetics. Cefazolin is 75–85% plasma protein bound, and widely distributed throughout the body with high concentrations in many tissues and cavities, but subtherapeutic concentrations in the CSF. Virtually 100% is excreted unchanged in the urine via filtration and secretion; the half-life is about 1.8 hr, increasing to 30–40 hr in renal impairment.

Adverse Reactions. (*See* Cephalosporins.)

CEFEPIME HYDROCHLORIDE   Maxipime

Pharmacology. Cefepime is a fourth-generation cephalosporin with a broader spectrum of activity than other cephalosporins. It has similar activity to ceftazidime against Gram-negative bacteria, including *Pseudomonas aeruginosa,* but is also active against some isolates resistant to third-generation cephalosporins (eg, *Enterobacter* spp.). Cefepime has greater potency against Gram-positive organisms (eg, staphylococci) than ceftazidime, and is similar in activity to ceftriaxone. Its anaerobic activity is poor, particularly against *Bacteroides fragilis.*[150–152]

Administration and Adult Dosage. IM or IV 500 mg–2 g q 12 hr; moderate to severe infections are treated with IV 1–2 g q 12 hr.

Special Populations. *Pediatric Dosage.* (<12 yr) safety and efficacy not established. **IM or IV** dosages of 150 mg/kg/day in 3 divided doses, to a maximum of 200 mg/dose, have been used in serious childhood infections such as cystic fibrosis and meningitis.

Geriatric Dosage. Same as adult dosage, adjusting for age-related renal impairment.

Other Conditions. In patients with Cl_{cr} of 30–60 mL/min, the usual dose is given q 24 hr; with a Cl_{cr} of 10–30 mL/min, 50% of the usual dose is given q 24 hr; and with a Cl_{cr} <10 mL/min, 25% of the dose (but no less than 250 mg) is given q 24 hr.

Dosage Forms. Inj 500 mg, 1, 2 g.

Pharmacokinetics. *Fate.* Following a 30-min IV infusion of 1 g, serum concentrations of 79 mg/L are achieved. It is about 20% plasma protein bound. Cefepime penetrates most tissues and fluids well; CSF concentrations are 3.3–6.7 mg/L after 50 mg/kg q 8 hr. About 85% of a dose is eliminated renally by glomerular filtration. Elderly patients have a slightly lower total clearance, which parallels Cl_{cr}.

$t_{½}$. 2.3 hr.

Adverse Reactions. The most common adverse reactions are injection-site reactions, rash, positive direct Coombs' test without hemolysis, decreased serum phosphorus, increased hepatic enzymes, eosinophilia, and abnormal PT and PTT. Encephalopathy has been reported in patients with renal impairment given unadjusted dosages. (*See* Cephalosporins monograph.)

Contraindications. Previous immediate hypersensitivity reaction to any β-lactam.

Precautions. Adjust dosage in patients with impaired renal function. Use with caution in patients with GI disease, especially colitis.

Parameters to Monitor. Obtain renal and hepatic function tests, and PT and PTT periodically.

CEFOTAXIME SODIUM   Claforan

Pharmacology. Cefotaxime is a third-generation cephalosporin with activity against Gram-negative organisms resistant to first- and second-generation cephalosporins (eg, indole-positive *Proteus* spp., *Serratia* spp.). Its desacetyl metabolite (DACM) has good activity and may be synergistic with cefotaxime against certain organisms. The activity of cefotaxime against *Pseudomonas aeruginosa* is inferior to ceftazidime, and against *Staphylococcus aureus* is inferior to cefazolin. Cefotaxime is more active than other cephalosporins (except ceftriaxone) against *Streptococcus pneumoniae* that are intermediately resistant to penicillin G.[135,136,138,139,153]

Adult Dosage. IM or IV 250 mg–2 g q 6–12 hr (usually 1–2 g q 8–12 hr), to a maximum of 12 g/day. Reduce dosage by 50% in patients with a Cl_{cr} <20 mL/min.

Pediatric Dosage. IV (newborns up to 1 week of age) 50 mg/kg q 12 hr; (newborns 1–4 weeks) 50 mg/kg q 8 hr; (older infants and children) 50–200 mg/kg/day (200 mg/kg/day for meningitis) given in 3–4 divided doses q 6–8 hr.

Dosage Forms. Inj 500 mg, 1, 2, 10 g.

Pharmacokinetics. CSF concentrations range from 0.3 to 0.44 mg/L after a 1 g dose, and in higher dosages cefotaxime is effective for treatment of meningitis. About 50% of a dose is excreted unchanged in urine and 50% metabolized to DACM. DACM is metabolized to inactive metabolites and excreted unchanged in urine.

Adverse Reactions. Cefotaxime is well tolerated, with coagulopathies only rarely reported. (*See* Cephalosporins.)

CEFOTETAN DISODIUM
Cefotan

Pharmacology. Cefotetan is a cephamycin, structurally and pharmacologically similar to the cephalosporins, particularly second-generation agents, and it contains an N-methylthiotetrazole side chain. It has greater activity against enteric Gram-negative bacteria than first- and second-generation cephalosporins and superior activity against *Bacteroides fragilis* and other anaerobic bacteria (comparable to cefoxitin and cefmetazole). Gram-positive activity is less than cefazolin.[135,144,145]

Adult Dosage. IV or IM for treatment 500 mg–2 g q 12–24 hr (usually 1–2 g q 12 hr), to a maximum of 6 g/day; **IV or IM for surgical prophylaxis** 1–2 g 30–60 min prior to surgery, then 1–2 g q 12 hr for up to 24 hr postoperatively. Reconstitute the drug with 0.5% lidocaine for IM administration because IM injection is painful. Reduce dosage by 50% with a Cl_{cr} of 10–30 mL/min, and by 75% in patients with a Cl_{cr} <10 mL/min.

Pediatric Dosage. Safety and efficacy not established. **IV** 40–60 mg/kg/day given in equally divided doses q 12 hr has been reported.

Dosage Forms. Inj 1, 2, 10 g.

Pharmacokinetics. Cefotetan is excreted primarily unchanged in urine, with an elimination half-life of 3.5 hr.

Adverse Reactions. (*See* Cephalosporins.)

CEFTAZIDIME
Ceptaz, Fortaz, Tazicef, Tazidime

Pharmacology. Ceftazidime is a third-generation cephalosporin with activity generally similar to cefotaxime, but having superior activity against *Pseudomonas aeruginosa* and inferior activity against Gram-positive (particularly against *Staphylococcus aureus* and penicillin-resistant pneumococci) and anaerobic bacteria.[135–139,153]

Adult Dosage. IM or IV 500 mg–2 g q 8–12 hr; q 12-hr administration appears to be adequate in the elderly. Reduce dosage by 50% with a Cl_{cr} of 30–50 mL/min; with a Cl_{cr} of 15–30 mL/min, the maximum dosage is 1 g q 24 hr; with a Cl_{cr} <15 mL/min, the dosage is 500 mg q 24–48 hr.

Pediatric Dosage. **IV** (newborns) 30 mg/kg q 8–12 hr; (older infants and children) **IM or IV** 30–50 mg/kg q 8 hr, to a maximum of 6 g/day (225 mg/kg/day for treatment of meningitis).

Dosage Forms. **Inj** 500 mg, 1, 2, 6 g. Conventional formulations of ceftazidime release carbon dioxide during reconstitution; the lysine formulation (eg, Ceptaz) avoids this problem.

Pharmacokinetics. Ceftazidime is less than 30% plasma protein bound and is 80–90% excreted unchanged in urine by filtration, with a half-life of 1.6 hr, increasing to 25–34 hr in renal failure.

Adverse Reactions. The drug is generally well tolerated. (*See* Cephalosporins.)

CEFUROXIME SODIUM	Kefurox, Zinacef
CEFUROXIME AXETIL	Ceftin

Pharmacology. Cefuroxime is a second-generation cephalosporin with greater activity than cefazolin, but less than cefotaxime, against *Haemophilus influenzae,* including β-lactamase–producing strains. The activity of cefuroxime against *Staphylococcus aureus* is slightly less than that of cefazolin. Its activity against anaerobes is poor, similar to the first-generation cephalosporins.[135,139,146,154]

Adult Dosage. **IM or IV for treatment** 750 mg–1.5 g q 8 hr (q 6 hr in serious infections); **IM or IV for prophylaxis** 1.5 g 1 hr prior to surgery; doses of IM or IV 750 mg may be given q 8 hr for up to 24 hr postoperatively (1.5 g q 12 hr to a total of 6 g for open heart surgery). Reduce parenteral dosage in renal impairment; with a Cl_{cr} of 10–20 mL/min, give the usual dose q 12 hr; with a Cl_{cr} <10 mL/min, give the usual dose q 24 hr. **PO** 125–500 mg q 12 hr.

Pediatric Dosage. **IM or IV** (newborns) 10–25 mg/kg q 12 hr; (older infants and children) 50–100 mg/kg/day, to a maximum of 250 mg/kg/day for meningitis in 3–4 divided doses. **PO** 15–20 mg/kg q 12 hr in children (40 mg/kg/day for otitis media); it may be given in applesauce.

Dosage Forms. **Inj** 750 mg, 1.5 g; **Susp** 25 mg/mL; **Tab** 125, 250, 500 mg. Do not interchange the tablets and suspension on a mg/kg basis. (*See* β-Lactams Comparison Chart.)

Pharmacokinetics. In adults, oral bioavailability appears to be lower with the suspension than with the tablets, and food increases the bioavailability of the tablets. After absorption of oral cefuroxime axetil, it is hydrolyzed in the bloodstream to cefuroxime. Cefuroxime's pharmacokinetics are similar to cefazolin's, but CSF concentrations are adequate for treatment of meningitis caused by certain organisms; however, the third-generation agents ceftriaxone and cefotaxime are superior in *H. influenzae* meningitis. Over 95% of the drug is excreted unchanged in the urine and the elimination half-life is 1.2 hr.

Adverse Reactions. The drug is generally well tolerated. (*See* Cephalosporins.)

EXTENDED-SPECTRUM PENICILLINS

Pharmacology. The carboxypenicillin ticarcillin and the acylureidopenicillins (mezlocillin and piperacillin) have the same mechanism of action as other penicillins, but are more active against enteric Gram-negative bacteria and *Pseudomonas aeruginosa.* Tiearcillin is not active against *Klebsiella* spp., but the acylureido derivatives do have activity and are generally more potent against susceptible isolates. The acylureidopenicillins also have activity comparable to ampicillin against enterococci. The combination of clavulanic acid plus ticarcillin is active against *Klebsiella* spp. as well as β-lactamase–producing staphylococci, *Haemophilus influenzae,* and *Bacteroides* spp. The combination of tazobactam plus piperacillin is similar to clavulanic acid plus ticarcillin. These two combination products are not appreciably more active against *P. aeruginosa* or *Enterobacter cloacae* than ticarcillin or piperacillin alone.[128,129,131,155–157]

Adult Dosage. (*See* β-Lactams Comparison Chart.)

Pediatric Dosage. (*See* β-Lactams Comparison Chart.)

Dosage Forms. (*See* β-Lactams Comparison Chart.)

Pharmacokinetics. Usual half-life is 1–1.5 hr, which is prolonged in anuria, although acylureido derivatives are partially metabolized and accumulate to a lesser extent. The acylureidopenicillins are also subject to capacity-limited elimination (ie, increasing dosage results in progressive saturation of elimination pathways, resulting in decreased clearance), which allows administration of higher doses at 6- to 8-hr intervals.

Adverse Reactions. Adverse effects are similar to other penicillins. Sodium content of the usual daily dosage of parenteral ticarcillin approaches the equivalent of 1 L of NS. The carboxylic acid function in the carboxypenicillin structure produces prolongation in bleeding time with systemic dosages as a result of binding to platelets and preventing aggregation.

IMIPENEM AND CILASTATIN SODIUM   Primaxin

Pharmacology. Imipenem is a carbapenem with an extremely broad spectrum against many aerobic and anerobic Gram-positive and Gram-negative bacterial pathogens. The commercial preparation contains an equal amount of cilastatin, a renal dehydropeptidase inhibitor that has no antimicrobial activity but prevents imipenem's metabolism by proximal tubular kidney cells, thus increasing urinary imipenem concentrations and possibly decreasing nephrotoxicity.[135,157,158] (*See* Notes.)

Administration and Adult Dosage. **IV** 1–4 g/day in 3 or 4 divided doses (usually 500 mg q 6–8 hr). For severe, life-threatening infections, a dose of 1 g q 6 hr is recommended (not to exceed 60 mg/kg/day).[157] Infuse 250 to 500 mg doses over 20–30 min and 1 g doses over 40–60 min; reduce infusion rate if nausea and/or vomiting develops. **IM** 1–2 g/day in 3 or 4 divided doses.

Special Populations. *Pediatric Dosage.* (<1 week) 25 mg/kg q 12 hr; (1–4 weeks) 25 mg/kg q 8 hr; (4 weeks–3 months) 25 mg/kg q 6 hr; (3 months–3 yr) 15–25 mg/kg q 6 hr; (>3 yr) 15 mg/kg q 6 hr.[157,159]

Geriatric Dosage. Same as adult dosage, but adjust for age-related reduction in renal function.

Other Conditions. Reduce dosage with renal insufficiency as follows: Cl_{cr} 30–70 mL/min, give 75% of the usual dosage; Cl_{cr} 20–30 mL/min, give 50% of the usual dosage; Cl_{cr} <20 mL/min, give 25% of the usual dosage. Give a supplemental dose following hemodialysis.[157]

Dosage Forms. **Inj (IV)** 250 mg imipenem/250 mg cilastatin, 500 mg imipenem/500 mg cilastatin; **Inj (Susp, IM only)** 500 mg imipenem/500 mg cilastatin, 750 mg imipenem/750 mg cilastatin. (*See* Notes.)

Pharmacokinetics. *Fate.* Peak serum imipenem concentrations are 22 and 52 mg/L after 30-min infusions of 500 mg and 1 g, respectively; levels are <1 mg/L at 6 hr. CSF levels range from 0.5 to 11 mg/L with inflamed meninges and appear to be adequate to treat meningitis, but experience in treating meningitis is limited and seizures may occur in such patients. Imipenem is 20% plasma protein bound; V_d is 0.26 L/kg. Probenecid increases imipenem serum levels and prolongs its half-life. About 70% of imipenem is excreted unchanged in urine when given with cilastatin, with the remainder excreted as metabolite; cilastatin is excreted 90% unchanged in urine.[157,158]

$t_{½}$. (Imipenem) 0.9 ± 0.1 hr; 3–4 hr in renal failure. (Cilastatin) 0.8 ± 0.1 hr; 17 hr in renal failure.[157,158]

Adverse Reactions. Nausea and vomiting occur, sometimes associated with hypotension or diaphoresis, particularly with high doses and rapid infusion.[157,158] Rashes occur occasionally, and cross-allergenicity with penicillins has been documented. Convulsions have occurred, primarily in the elderly, in those with underlying CNS disease, with overdosage in patients with renal failure, or with other predisposing factors.[157,158,160,161]

Precautions. Use with caution in elderly patients, or those with a history of seizures or who are otherwise predisposed. Adjust dosage carefully in renal impairment. Imipenem may cause immediate hypersensitivity reactions in patients with a history of anaphylaxis to penicillin.[161]

Drug Interactions. Concomitant administration with probenecid produces higher and prolonged serum concentrations of imipenem and cilastatin. Imipenem has been shown in vitro to antagonize the activity of other β-lactams (eg, acylureidopenicillins, most cephalosporins, aztreonam) presumably via β-lactamase induction; although the clinical relevance is unclear, avoid co-administration.[158] Co-administration of imipenem/cilastatin with ganciclovir has been associated with generalized seizures in a few patients; the mechanism of this interaction is unknown.

Parameters to Monitor. Obtain renal function tests periodically.

Notes. Used alone, emergence of resistance during treatment of *Pseudomonas aeruginosa* infections occurs frequently; however, cross-resistance to other classes (eg, aminoglycosides, cephalosporins) does not occur.[157,158] Addition of an aminoglycoside may prevent development of resistance, but in vitro synergism occurs only infrequently.

Vials may be reconstituted into a suspension using 10 mL of the infusion so-lution and then further diluted by transferring the suspension into the infusion container; alternatively, the powder in the 120-mL vials can be diluted initially with 100 mL of solution. The initial dilution must be shaken well to ensure sus-pension/solution. Do not inject the suspension. The resulting solution ranges from colorless to yellow. Reconstituted solutions are stable in dextrose-containing solu-tions for 4 hr at room temperature and 24 hr under refrigeration, and in normal saline for 10 hr at room temperature and 48 hr under refrigeration. With IM ad-ministration use 2 mL of lidocaine 1% injection to reconstitute a 500 mg vial and give the suspension by deep IM injection into a large muscle mass (eg, gluteal muscle).[158]

MEROPENEM
Merrem

Pharmacology. Meropenem is a carbapenem with a mechanism of action similar to imipenem. Unlike imipenem, meropenem is not appreciably degraded by renal dehydropeptidase-I, and thus does not require concomitant administration of a de-hydropeptidase inhibitor.[158,162,163] (*See* Notes.)

Administration and Adult Dosage. IV for less severe infections 500 mg–1 g q 8–12 hr; **IV for severe or life-threatening infections (eg, meningitis)** 2 g q 8 hr.

Special Populations. *Pediatric Dosage.* IV (<3 months) safety and efficacy not established, but 20 mg q 12 hr has been used; (3 months–12 yr) 10–20 mg/kg q 8 hr; in meningitis 40 mg/kg q 8 hr has been used.[162]

Geriatric Dosage. Same as adult dosage, but adjust for age-related reduction in renal function.

Other Conditions. Reduce dosage in renal impairment. With a Cl_{cr} of 26–50 mL/min, give the normal dose q 12 hr; with Cl_{cr} of 11–25 mL/min, the dosage is reduced by 50%; with Cl_{cr} <10 mL/min, give one-half the dose once daily.[162,164]

Dosage Forms. Inj 500 mg, 1 g.

Pharmacokinetics. *Fate.* The pharmacokinetics of meropenem are similar to those of imipenem, although meropenem can be given by both infusion and IV bolus.[160,162] After IV infusion of 1 g, the peak serum concentration is 55 mg/L; the drug distributes well into most tissues and fluids, including the CSF. Plasma protein binding is low and the V_{dss} is 0.32 ± 0.03 L/kg. Meropenem is primarily eliminated renally by both glomerular filtration and tubular secretion. Up to 70% of a dose is recovered unchanged in the urine, with a renal metabolite accounting for the remainder of the dose (up to 30%). Meropenem is appreciably removed by hemodialysis, and a supplemental dose is required following dialysis. Children have pharmacokinetics similar to adults; increased clearance and reduced half-life occur in cystic fibrosis.[164]

$t_{1/2}$. 0.9 ± 0.09 hr, increasing to 6.8–13.7 hr in end-stage renal disease.[164]

Adverse Reactions. Adverse effects are similar to imipenem; the most common include injection-site reactions, rash, nausea, vomiting, and diarrhea.[158,162] Ani-mal studies suggest that meropenem has a lower epileptogenic potential, which has been supported by a low frequency of seizures in clinical trials, including studies in patients with meningitis.[162]

Precautions. Use with caution in patients with hypersensitivity to penicillins, because meropenem may cause immediate hypersensitivity reactions in patients allergic to penicillins.[161] Adjust dosage in renal impairment.

Drug Interactions. Probenecid can reduce renal clearance of meropenem and increase half-life by 38% and AUC by 56%. The combination should be avoided.

Parameters to Monitor. Obtain renal function tests periodically.

Notes. Meropenem is more active than imipenem against enteric Gram-negative bacilli; the two have equivalent activity against *Pseudomonas aeruginosa* and *Bacteroides fragilis,* and meropenem is slightly less active than imipenem against Gram-positive organisms.[158,162]

PENICILLIN G SALTS   Various

Pharmacology. Penicillin G has activity against most Gram-positive organisms and some Gram-negative organisms, notably *Neisseria* spp. It acts by interfering with late stages of bacterial cell wall synthesis; resistance is primarily caused by bacterial elaboration of β-lactamases; some organisms have altered penicillin-binding protein targets (eg, enterococci and pneumococci); others have impermeable outer cell wall layers.[128,129]

Administration and Adult Dosage. **PO** 250–500 mg (400,000–800,000 units) q 6 hr for mild to moderate infections. **IV** 2–24 million units/day in 4–12 divided doses, depending on infection. **IM** not recommended (very painful); use benzathine or procaine salt form as indicated.

Special Populations. *Pediatric Dosage.* **PO** (<12 yr) 25,000–90,000 units/kg/day in 3–6 divided doses; (>12 yr) same as adult dosage. **IV (preferably) or IM** (neonates) 25,000–50,000 units/kg q 6–12 hr; up to 400,000 units/kg/day has been used in meningitis; (>1 month) 100,000–300,000 units/kg/day in 4–6 divided doses.

Geriatric Dosage. Same as adult dosage, but adjust for age-related reduction in renal function.

Other Conditions. With usual oral dosage, no dosage adjustment is required in patients with impaired renal function; however, in treating more severe infections with larger IV dosages, careful adjustment is necessary. In anuric patients, give no more than 3 million units/day.[165]

Dosage Forms. **Susp/Syrup** (as potassium salt) 40,000, 80,000 units/mL (reconstituted); **Tab** (as potassium salt) 200,000, 250,000, 400,000, 500,000, 800,000 units; **Inj** (as potassium salt) 1, 5, 10, 20 million units; **Inj** (as sodium salt) 5 million units.

Patient Instructions. Take this (oral) drug with a full glass of water on an empty stomach (1 hour before or 2 hours after meals) for best absorption; refrigerate solution.

Missed Doses. Take this drug at regular intervals. If you miss a dose, take it as soon as you remember. If it is about time for the next dose, take that dose only.

Leave a minimum of 4–6 hours between doses. Do not double the dose or take extra.

Pharmacokinetics. *Fate.* Only 15–30% orally absorbed because of its high susceptibility to gastric acid hydrolysis; peak concentrations of 1.5–2.7 mg/L occur 0.5–1 hr after administration of 500 mg. Widely distributed in body tissues, fluids, and cavities, with biliary levels up to 10 times serum levels; 30–60% plasma protein bound. Penetration into CSF is poor, even with inflamed meninges; however, large parenteral dosages (>20 million units/day) adequately treat meningitis caused by susceptible organisms. From 80 to 85% of the absorbed dose is excreted unchanged in the urine.[128,129]

$t_{1/2}$. 30–40 min; 7–10 hr in patients with renal failure; 20–30 hr in patients with hepatic and renal failure.[165]

Adverse Reactions. Occasionally, nausea or diarrhea occurs after usual oral doses. As with all penicillins, CNS toxicity may occur with massive IV dosages (60–100 million units/day) or excessive dosage in patients with impaired renal function (usually >10–20 million units/day in anuric patients); characterized by confusion, drowsiness, and myoclonus, which may progress to convulsions and result in death. Large dosages of the sodium salt form may result in hypernatremia and fluid overload with pulmonary edema, especially in patients with impaired renal function or CHF. Large dosages of the potassium salt form may result in hyperkalemia, especially in patients with impaired renal function and with rapid infusions. Occasional positive Coombs' reactions with rare hemolytic anemia have been reported after large IV doses. Interstitial nephritis has been rarely reported following large IV dosages. Hypersensitivity reactions (primarily rashes) occur in 1–10% of patients. Most serious hypersensitivity reactions follow injection rather than oral administration.[128,161]

Contraindications. History of anaphylactic, accelerated (eg, hives) or serum sickness reaction to previous penicillin administration. (*See* Notes.)

Precautions. Use caution in patients with a history of penicillin or cephalosporin hypersensitivity reactions, atopic predisposition (eg, asthma), impaired renal function (hence neonates and geriatric patients), impaired cardiac function, or preexisting seizure disorder.

Drug Interactions. Physically and/or chemically incompatible with aminoglycosides leading to drug inactivation; never mix them together in the same IV solution or syringe. Probenecid competes with penicillin for renal excretion, resulting in higher and prolonged serum concentrations.[128,129]

Parameters to Monitor. Obtain renal function tests initially when using high dosages. During prolonged high-dose therapy, monitor renal function tests and serum electrolytes periodically.

Notes. A dose of 250 mg equals 400,000 units of penicillin G. Penicillin V potassium is preferred to penicillin G potassium for oral administration because of more complete (60%) and reliable absorption. Skin testing with **penicilloylpolylysine** (PPL, Pre-Pen) and **minor determinant mixture** (MDM) can help determine the likelihood of serious reactions to penicillin in penicillin-allergic individuals.[128,166] Availability of MDM is limited; it is locally available in small amounts only at larger medical centers. Desensitization is recommended in pregnant women with syphilis and may be attempted (rarely) in patients with life-threatening infections that are likely to be responsive only to penicillin, but this is a dangerous procedure and many alternative antibiotics are available.[128] (*See* also β-Lactams Comparison Chart.)

β-LACTAMS COMPARISON CHART

DRUG CLASS AND DRUG	DOSAGE FORMS	ADULT DOSAGE	PEDIATRIC DOSAGE	ADULT DOSAGE IN RENAL IMPAIRMENT[a]	PEAK SERUM LEVELS (MG/L)[b]	PERCENTAGE PROTEIN BOUND	COMMENTS
CARBAPENEMS							
Imipenem and Cilastatin Sodium Primaxin	Inj (IV) 250 plus 250 mg, 500 plus 500 mg; (IM) 500 plus 500 mg, 750 plus 750 mg.	IV 1–4 g/day (1–2 g/ day preferred) in 3 or 4 divided doses; IM 1–2 g/day in 3 or 4 divided doses.	(<3 months) *See* monograph; IV (3 mo–3 yr) 25 mg/kg q 6 hr; (>3 yr) 15 mg/kg q 6 hr.	Cl$_{cr}$ 30–70 mL/min: 75% of usual dosage; Cl$_{cr}$ <20 mL/min: 50% of usual dosage; Cl$_{cr}$ <20 mL/min: 25% of usual dosage.	22 (IV 500 mg imipenem)	20	Very broad activity against most aerobic and anaerobic bacteria. Frequent nausea and dose-related seizure potential.
Meropenem Merrem	Inj 500 mg, 1 g.	IV 500 mg–1 g q 8–12 hr; 2 g q 8 hr in life-threatening infections.	(<3 months) *See* monograph; IV (3 mo–12 yr) 10–20 mg/kg q 8 hr; 40 mg/ kg q 8 hr in meningitis.	Cl$_{cr}$ 26–50 mL/min: usual dose q 12 hr; Cl$_{cr}$ 11–25 mL/min: 50% of usual dose q 12 hr; Cl$_{cr}$ <10 mL/min: 50% of usual dose q 24 hr.	55	Low	Less active than imipenem against Gm+ and more active against most Gm– bacteria; equivalent against *P. aeruginosa* and *B. fragilis.* Less seizure potential than imipenem.

(*continued*)

DRUG CLASS AND DRUG	DOSAGE FORMS	ADULT DOSAGE	PEDIATRIC DOSAGE	ADULT DOSAGE IN RENAL IMPAIRMENT[a]	PEAK SERUM LEVELS (MG/L)[b]	PERCENTAGE PROTEIN BOUND	COMMENTS
CEPHALOSPORINS, FIRST-GENERATION							
Cefadroxil Duricef Various	Cap 500 mg Susp 25, 50, 100 mg/mL Tab 1 g.	PO 500 mg–1 g q 12–24 hr; PO for endocarditis prophylaxis 2 g 1 hr prior to dental procedure.	PO 30 mg/kg/ day in 1 or 2 divided doses; PO for endocarditis prophylaxis 50 mg/kg 1 hr prior to dental procedure.	PO 1 g, then 500 mg at intervals below: Cl_{cr} 26–50 mL/min: 12 hr; Cl_{cr} 10–25 mL/min: 24 hr; Cl_{cr} <10 mL/min: 36 hr.	12–16	20	Spectrum similar to cefazolin.

(continued)

β-LACTAMS COMPARISON CHART (continued)

DRUG CLASS AND DRUG	DOSAGE FORMS	ADULT DOSAGE	PEDIATRIC DOSAGE	ADULT DOSAGE IN RENAL IMPAIRMENT[a]	PEAK SERUM LEVELS (MG/L)[b]	PERCENTAGE PROTEIN BOUND	COMMENTS
Cefazolin Sodium Ancef Kefzol Various	Inj 250, 500 mg, 1, 5, 10, 20 g.	IM or IV 250 mg–1 g q 6–12 hr; IM or IV for surgical prophylaxis 1 g 30–60 min prior to surgery; IM or IV for endocarditis prophylaxis 1 g within 30 min prior to upper airway procedure.	IM or IV (neonates <1 month) 25 mg/kg q 8–12 hr; (infants >1 month) 50–100 mg/kg/day in 3 divided doses. IM or IV for endocarditis prophylaxis 25 mg/kg within 30 min of procedure.	Cl_{cr} 10–35 mL/min: 50% of usual dose q 12 hr; Cl_{cr} <10 mL/min: 50% of usual dose q 18–24 hr.	80–110	75–85	Good Gm+ coverage (including *S. aureus*), plus some Gm– activity (*E. coli, Klebsiella* spp.).Sodium = 2 mEq/g.
Cephalexin Keflex Keftab Various	Cap 250, 500 mg Drp 100 mg/mL Susp 25, 50 mg/mL Tab 250, 500 mg, 1 g.	PO 250 mg–1 g q 6 hr; PO for endocarditis prophylaxis 2 g 1 hr prior to dental procedure.	PO 25–50 mg/kg/day in 4 divided doses; PO for endocarditis prophylaxis 50 mg/kg 1 hr prior to dental procedure.	Cl_{cr} 10–50 mL/min: 50% of usual dosage; Cl_{cr} <10 mL/min: 25% of usual dosage.	10–20	6	Oral absorption is almost complete; spectrum similar to cefazolin.

(continued)

β-LACTAMS COMPARISON CHART (continued)

DRUG CLASS AND DRUG	DOSAGE FORMS	ADULT DOSAGE	PEDIATRIC DOSAGE	ADULT DOSAGE IN RENAL IMPAIRMENT[a]	PEAK SERUM LEVELS (MG/L)[b]	PERCENTAGE PROTEIN BOUND	COMMENTS
Cephalothin Sodium Various	Inj 1, 2, 4, 10, 20 g.	IV 500 mg–1 g q 4–6 hr; IM not recommended.	IV (neonates <7 days) 20 mg/kg q 8–12 hr; (infants >7 days) 75–125 mg/kg/day in 4–6 divided doses.	Cl_{cr} 10–25 mL/min: 1 g q 6 hr; Cl_{cr} <10 mL/min: 500 mg q 6–8 hr.	15–30	65	Spectrum similar to cefazolin. Painful IM injection. Sodium = 2.8 mEq/g.
Cephapirin Sodium Cefadyl Various	Inj 500 mg, 1, 2, 4, 20 g.	IM or IV 500 mg–1 g q 4–6 hr.	Same as cephalothin.	Same as cephalothin.	10–20	45–50	Very similar to cephalothin. Sodium = 2.4 mEq/g.
Cephradine Anspor Velosef Various	Cap 250, 500 mg Susp 25, 50 mg/mL Tab 1 g Inj 250, 500 mg, 1, 2, 4 g.	PO 250 mg–1 g q 6 hr; IM or IV 500 mg–1 g q 4–6 hr.	IM or IV same as cephalothin; PO same as cephalexin.	IM or IV same as cephalothin; PO same as cephalexin.	10–20 (PO) 15–30 (IV)	5–20	Oral form comparable to cephalexin; spectrum similar to cefazolin. Sodium = 6 mEq/g injection.

(continued)

143

β-LACTAMS COMPARISON CHART (continued)

DRUG CLASS AND DRUG	DOSAGE FORMS	ADULT DOSAGE	PEDIATRIC DOSAGE	ADULT DOSAGE IN RENAL IMPAIRMENT[a]	PEAK SERUM LEVELS (MG/L)[b]	PERCENTAGE PROTEIN BOUND	COMMENTS
CEPHALOSPORINS, SECOND-GENERATION							
Cefaclor Ceclor Various	Cap 250, 500 mg SR Tab 375, 500 mg Susp 25, 37.5, 50, 75 mg/mL.	PO 250 mg–1 g q 6–8 hr SR Tab 375–500 mg q 12 hr.	PO 40 mg/kg/day in 3 divided doses.	Cl_{cr} 10–50 mL/min: 50% of usual dosage; Cl_{cr} <10 mL/min: 25% of usual dosage.	10–15	25	Spectrum similar to cefazolin, but includes some ampicillin-resistant *H. influenzae.*
Cefamandole Naftate Mandol	Inj 500 mg, 1, 2, 10 g.	IM or IV 500 mg–1 g q 4–8 hr.	IM or IV 50–150 mg/kg/day in 4–6 divided doses.	Cl_{cr} 10–50 mL/min: 50% of usual dose q 8 hr; Cl_{cr} <10 mL/min: 25% of usual dose q 12 hr.	80–90	56	NMTT side chain. Spectrumsimilar to cefuroxime. Sodium = 3.3 mEq/g.
Cefonicid Sodium Monocid	Inj 500 mg, 1, 10 g.	IM or IV 500 mg–2 g/day as a single dose.	Not established.	IM or IV 7.5 mg/kg, then 25–50% of usual dose given: Cl_{cr} 10–50 mL/min: q 24–48 hr; Cl_{cr} <10 mL/min; q 3–5 days.	220 (IV bolus)	83–98[c]	Poor activity against *Staphylococcus* spp. Unbound drug levels low and excreted rapidly because of saturable protein binding. Sodium = 3.7 mEq/g.

(continued)

DRUG CLASS AND DRUG	DOSAGE FORMS	ADULT DOSAGE	PEDIATRIC DOSAGE	ADULT DOSAGE IN RENAL IMPAIRMENT[a]	PEAK SERUM LEVELS (MG/L)[b]	PERCENTAGE PROTEIN BOUND	COMMENTS
Cefotetan Disodium Cefotan	Inj 1, 2 g.	IM or IV 500 mg–2 g q 12–24 hr.	Not established.	IM or IV give usual dose at intervals below: Cl_cr 10–30 mL/min: 24 hr; Cl_cr <10 mL/min: 48 hr.	140–180 (IV bolus)	78–91[c]	NMTT side chain. Spectrum similar to cefoxitin. Sodium = 3.5 mEq/g. Reconstitute IM with 0.5% lidocaine.
Cefoxitin Sodium Mefoxin	Inj 1, 2, 10 g.	IV 1–2 g q 6–8 hr.	IV 80–160 mg/kg/day in 4–6 divided doses.	Cl_cr 10–50 mL/min: 50% of usual dose q 6–8 hr; Cl_cr <10 mL/min: 25% of usual dose q 12 hr.	30–50	75	Gm+ activity less than cefazolin, but better Gm− and anaerobic activity. Sodium = 2.3 mEq/g.
Cefprozil Cefzil	Tab 250, 500 mg Susp 25, 50 mg/mL.	PO 500 mg daily–bid.	PO (6 mo–12 yr) 15 mg/kg q 12 hr.	Cl_cr ≤30 mL/min: 50% of usual dose at same interval.	10.5	36	Spectrum similar to cefaclor, but more active against *H. influenzae*.
Cefuroxime Sodium Keftrox Zinacef	Inj 750 mg, 1.5 g.	IM or IV 750 mg–1.5 g q 6–8 hr.	IM or IV (neonates) 10–25 mg/kg q 12 hr; (children) 50–100 mg/kg/day in 3–4 divided doses.	IM or IV: Cl_cr 10–20 mL/min: usual dose q 12 hr; Cl_cr <10 mL/min: usual dose q 24 hr.	140 (IV bolus)	33	Gm+ activity similar to cefazolin, but better Gm− activity, including *H. influenzae*. Sodium = 2.4mEq/g. *(continued)*

β-LACTAMS COMPARISON CHART (continued)

DRUG CLASS AND DRUG	DOSAGE FORMS	ADULT DOSAGE	PEDIATRIC DOSAGE	ADULT DOSAGE IN RENAL IMPAIRMENT[a]	PEAK SERUM LEVELS (MG/L)[b]	PERCENTAGE PROTEIN BOUND	COMMENTS
Cefuroxime Axetil Ceftin	Susp 25 mg/mL Tab 125, 250, 500 mg.	PO 125–500 mg bid.	PO 15–40 mg/kg/day in 2 divided doses.	—	3.6 (PO)	33	Do not interchange suspension and tablets.
Loracarbef Lorabid	Cap 200, 400 mg Susp 20, 40 mg/mL.	PO 200–400 mg q 12 hr.	PO (6 mo–12 yr) 7.5–15 mg q 12 hr.	Cl_{cr} 10–49 mL/min: 50% of usual dosage; Cl_{cr} <10 mL/min: usual dose q 3–5 days.	6.8 (PO 200 mg)	25	Carbacephan analogue of cefaclor with similar spectrum; must be taken on an empty stomach.
CEPHALOSPORINS, THIRD-GENERATION							
Cefdinir Omnicef	Cap 300 mg Susp 25 mg/mL.	PO 600 mg/day in 1 or 2 doses.	PO 14 mg/kg/day in 1 or 2 doses.	Cl_{cr} <30 mL/min: 300 mg/day.	2.9 (PO 600 mg)	60–70	Spectrum similar to cefpodoxime.
Cefixime Suprax	Tab 200, 400 mg Susp 20 mg/mL.	PO 200–400 mg q 12–24 hr; PO for gonorrhea 400 mg once.	PO 8 mg/kg/day in 1 or 2 divided doses.	Cl_{cr} 20–60 mL/min: 75% of usual dosage; Cl_{cr} <20 mL/min: 50% of usual dosage.	4.9	70	More active than cefuroxime or cefaclor against *H. influenzae*, but less Gm+ activity.

(*continued*)

DRUG CLASS AND DRUG	DOSAGE FORMS	ADULT DOSAGE	PEDIATRIC DOSAGE	ADULT DOSAGE IN RENAL IMPAIRMENT[a]	PEAK SERUM LEVELS (MG/L)[b]	PERCENTAGE PROTEIN BOUND	COMMENTS
Cefopera-zone Sodium Cefobid Various	Inj 1, 2 g.	IM or IV 2–8 g/day in 2–4 divided doses.	IM or IV (neonates) 50 mg/kg/dose q 12 hr; (children) 50–75 mg/kg q 8–12 hr.	No change.	125	85–95[c]	Less active than ceftazidime against *P. aeruginosa* NMTT side chain. Sodium = 1.5 mEq/g.
Cefotaxime Sodium Claforan	Inj 500 mg, 1, 2, 10 g.	IM or IV 1–2 g q 8–12 hr.	IM or IV (neonates ≤1 week) 50 mg/kg q 12 hr; (neonates 1–4 weeks) 50 mg/kg q 8 hr; (infants >4 weeks) 50–200 (200 in meningitis) mg/kg/day in 3–4 divided doses.	Cl$_{cr}$ <20 mL/min: 50% of usual dosage.	40	37	Good Gm+ and Gm− activity except for *P. aeruginosa*; modest antianaerobic activity. Sodium = 2.2mEq/g.
Desacetyl-cefota-xime					1–65	—	Active metabolite of cefotaxime.

(continued)

147

β-LACTAMS COMPARISON CHART (continued)

DRUG CLASS AND DRUG	DOSAGE FORMS	ADULT DOSAGE	PEDIATRIC DOSAGE	ADULT DOSAGE IN RENAL IMPAIRMENT[a]	PEAK SERUM LEVELS (MG/L)[b]	PERCENTAGE PROTEIN BOUND	COMMENTS
Cefpodoxime Proxetil Vantin	Tab 100, 200 mg Susp 10, 20 mg/mL.	PO 100–400 mg q 12 hr; PO for gonorrhea 200 mg once.	PO 5 mg/kg q 12 hr.	Cl_{cr} <30 mL/min: usual dose given q 24 hr.	23 (PO 200 mg)	18–30	Spectrum similar to cefixime, but better Gm+ activity.
Ceftazidime Ceptaz Fortaz Tazicef Tazidime	Inj 500 mg, 1, 2, 6 g.	IM or IV 500 mg– 2 g q 8–12 hr.	IM or IV (neonates ≤1 month) 30 mg/ kg/dose q 8–12 hr; (infants >1 month) 30–50 mg/kg/ dose q 8 hr.	Cl_{cr} 30–50 mL/min: 50% of usual dose q 12–24 hr; Cl_{cr} 15–30 mL/min: 1 g q 24 hr; Cl_{cr} <15 mL/min: 500 mg q 24– 48 hr.	80	17	Best activity against *P. aeruginosa*; poor Gm+ activity. Sodium = 2.3 mEq/g.
Ceftibuten Cedax	Cap 400 mg Susp 18, 36 mg/mL.	PO 200–400 mg q 24 hr.	PO 9 mg/kg/day in 1 or 2 divided doses.	Cl_{cr} 30–49 mL/min: 4.5 mg/kg or 200 mg q 24 hr; Cl_{cr} 5–29 mL/min: 2.25 mg/kg or 100 mg q 24 hr.	60–77	11 (PO 200 mg)	Spectrum similar to cefixime.

(continued)

β-LACTAMS COMPARISON CHART (continued)

DRUG CLASS AND DRUG	DOSAGE FORMS	ADULT DOSAGE	PEDIATRIC DOSAGE	ADULT DOSAGE IN RENAL IMPAIRMENT[a]	PEAK SERUM LEVELS (MG/L)[b]	PERCENTAGE PROTEIN BOUND	COMMENTS
Ceftizoxime Sodium Cefizox	Inj 1, 2g.	IM or IV 1–2 g q 8–12 hr.	IM or IV (>6 months) 50 mg/ kg/dose q 6–8 hr.	Cl$_{cr}$ 10–50 mL/min: 50% of usual dose q 12–24 hr; Cl$_{cr}$ <10 mL/min: 25–50% of usual dose q 24–48 hr.	75–90	31	Spectrum similar to cefotaxime except slightly more active against anaerobes. Sodium = 2.6 mEq/g.
Ceftriaxone Disodium Rocephin	Inj 250, 500 mg, 1, 2, 10 g.	IM or IV 500 mg–2 g/day as a single dose; IM for gonorrhea 250 mg once.	IM or IV 50–100 (100 in meningitis) mg/kg/ day in 2 divided doses.	No change. (see Comments.)	145	83–96[c]	Spectrum similar to cefotaxime. Reduce dose with concurrent renal and hepatic dysfunction. Sodium = 3.6 mEq/g.

(continued)

β-LACTAMS COMPARISON CHART (continued)

DRUG CLASS AND DRUG	DOSAGE FORMS	ADULT DOSAGE	PEDIATRIC DOSAGE	ADULT DOSAGE IN RENAL IMPAIRMENT[a]	PEAK SERUM LEVELS (MG/L)[b]	PERCENTAGE PROTEIN BOUND	COMMENTS
CEPHALOSPORINS, FOURTH-GENERATION							
Cefepime Maxipime	Inj 500 mg, 1, 2 g.	IM or IV 500 mg–2 g q 12 hr.	<12 yr safety and efficacy not established.	Cl$_{cr}$ 30–60 mL/min: usual dose q 24 hr; Cl$_{cr}$ 10–29 mL/min: 50% of usual dose q 24 hr; Cl$_{cr}$ <10 mL/min: 25% of usual dose q 24 hr.	79	16	Spectrum similar to ceftazidime; more active against Gm+ organisms; also active against resistant *Enterobacter* spp.
MONOBACTAM							
Aztreonam Azactam	Inj 500 mg, 1, 2 g.	IM or IV 0.5–2 g q 6–12 hr.	Safety and efficacy not established. IV 30 mg/kg q 6–8 hr (50 mg/kg q 4–6 hr in *P. aeruginosa*) has been used.	Cl$_{cr}$ 10–30 mL/min: 50% of usual dosage; Cl$_{cr}$ <10 mL/min: 25% of usual dosage.	164	60	Spectrum similar to ceftazidime against aerobic Gm– organisms only. No cross-allergenicity in penicillin-allergic patients.

(continued)

DRUG CLASS AND DRUG	DOSAGE FORMS	ADULT DOSAGE	PEDIATRIC DOSAGE	ADULT DOSAGE IN RENAL IMPAIRMENT[a]	PEAK SERUM LEVELS (MG/L)[b]	PERCENTAGE PROTEIN BOUND	COMMENTS
PENICILLIN G AND V							
Penicillin G Potassium Various	Inj 1, 5, 10, 20 million units Tab, Susp (*see* monograph.)	IV 1–5 million units q 4–6 hr.	IV (neonates) 25,000–50,000 units/kg q 6–12 hr; (>1 month) 100,000–300,000 units/kg/day in 4–6 divided doses.	Cl_{cr} <40 mL/min: IV dose (in million units/day) = 3.2 + (Cl_{cr}/7).	1.5–2.7 (IV 500 mg)	60	Gm+ (except most *Staphylococcus* strains), some Gm– (*Neisseria* spp.), and anaerobes (except *B. fragilis*). Poor oral absorption Potassium = 1.7 mEq/ million units.
Penicillin G Benzathine Various	Inj 300,000, 600,000, 1.2 million units/ mL.	IM for *Strep.* pharyngitis 1.2 million units once; IM for syphilis (early) 2.4 million units once; (late) 2.4 million units/ week for 3 weeks.	IM for *Strep.* pharyngitis (<27 kg) 300,000–600,000 units once; (>27 kg) 900,000 units once.	No change.	0.063 (IM 600,000 units)	60	Use limited to syphilis and *Strep.* pharyngitis. For IM use only.

(continued)

151

β-LACTAMS COMPARISON CHART (continued)

DRUG CLASS AND DRUG	DOSAGE FORMS	ADULT DOSAGE	PEDIATRIC DOSAGE	ADULT DOSAGE IN RENAL IMPAIRMENT[a]	PEAK SERUM LEVELS (MG/L)[b]	PERCENTAGE PROTEIN BOUND	COMMENTS
Penicillin G Procaine Various	Inj 300,000, 500,000, 600,000 units/mL.	IM 600,000–1.2 million units q 12–24 hr.	IM (neonates) 50,000 units/kg/day in 1–2 divided doses; (>27 kg) 900,000 units once.	No change.	0.9 (IM 300,000 units)	60	For IM use only.
Penicillin V Potassium Pen VK Veetids Various	Tab 125, 250, 500 mg Susp 25, 50 mg/mL.	PO 250–500 mg q 6 hr.	PO 15–50 mg/kg/day in 3–4 divided doses.	No change.	3–8	78	Spectrum similar to penicillin G. About 60% absorbed; preferred oralform of penicillin.
ANTISTAPHYLOCOCCAL PENICILLINS							
Cloxacillin Sodium Cloxapen Tegopen Various	Cap 250, 500 mg Susp 25 mg/mL.	PO 250–500 mg q 6 hr.	PO (<20 kg) 50–100 mg/kg/day in 4 divided doses; (>20 kg) same as adult dosage.	No change.	7	94	Used primarily for *S. aureus* infections. Suspension may be better tolerated than dicloxacillin.

(continued)

β-LACTAMS COMPARISON CHART (continued)

DRUG CLASS AND DRUG	DOSAGE FORMS	ADULT DOSAGE	PEDIATRIC DOSAGE	ADULT DOSAGE IN RENAL IMPAIRMENT[a]	PEAK SERUM LEVELS (MG/L)[b]	PERCENTAGE PROTEIN BOUND	COMMENTS
Dicloxacillin Sodium Dynapen Pathocill Various	Cap 125, 250, 500 mg Susp 12.5 mg/mL.	PO 125–500 mg q 6 hr.	PO 12.5–25 mg/ kg/day in 4 divided doses.	No change.	12.4	98	Comparable to cloxacillin.
Methicillin Sodium Staphcillin	Inj 1, 4, 6, 10 g.	IV 100–200 mg/kg/ day in 4–6 divided doses.	IV (neonates ≤14 days) 25 mg/kg q 8–12 hr; (neonates 15–30 days) 25 mg/kg q 6 hr; (children) same as adult dosage.	Cl$_{cr}$ <10 mL/min: decrease dosage by 50%.	60	40	Least potent of class; most likely to cause interstitial nephritis. Sodium = 2.9 mEq/g.
Nafcillin Sodium Nafcil Unipen	Cap 250 mg Tab 500 mg Inj 500 mg, 1, 2, 10 g.	IV 50–150 mg/kg/ day in 4–6 divided doses; PO 50–100 mg/ kg/day in 4 divided doses, but not recommended.	IV (neonates <7 days) 25 mg/kg q 8–12 hr; (neonates >7 days) 25 mg/ kg q 6–8 hr.	No change.	3.4 (PO) 20–40 (IV)	89	Comparable to oxacillin. Reversible neutropenia may be more common with nafcillin. Poorly absorbed orally; cloxacillin or dicloxacillin preferred. IV sodium = 2.9 mEq/g. *(continued)*

153

β-LACTAMS COMPARISON CHART (continued)

DRUG CLASS AND DRUG	DOSAGE FORMS	ADULT DOSAGE	PEDIATRIC DOSAGE	ADULT DOSAGE IN RENAL IMPAIRMENT[a]	PEAK SERUM LEVELS (MG/L)[b]	PERCENTAGE PROTEIN BOUND	COMMENTS
Oxacillin Sodium Bactocill Prostaphlin	Cap 250, 500 mg Susp 50 mg/mL Inj 250, 500 mg, 1, 2, 4, 10 g.	IV 50–200 mg/kg/day in 4–6 divided doses; PO 250–500 mg q 6 hr, but not recommended.	IV (neonates) same as methicillin; (children) same as adult dosage.	No change.	2.5 (PO) 40 (IV)	92	Poorly absorbed orally; cloxacillin or dicloxacillin preferred. Rare hepatic toxicity. IV sodium = 2.9 mEq/g.
AMPICILLIN DERIVATIVES							
Amoxicillin Amoxil Various	Cap 250, 500 mg Chew Tab 125, 250 mg Drp 50 mg/mL Susp 25, 50 mg/mL.	PO 250–500 mg tid, to a maximum of 6 g/day; PO for endocarditis prophylaxis 2 g 1 hr before procedure.	PO 20–40 mg/kg/day in 3 divided doses; PO for endocarditis prophylaxis 50 mg/kg 1 hr before procedure.	No change.	9	20	Spectrum similar to ampicillin, but better bioavailability (85%) and less diarrhea.

(continued)

DRUG CLASS AND DRUG	DOSAGE FORMS	ADULT DOSAGE	PEDIATRIC DOSAGE	ADULT DOSAGE IN RENAL IMPAIRMENT[a]	PEAK SERUM LEVELS (MG/L)[b]	PERCENTAGE PROTEIN BOUND	COMMENTS
Ampicillin Sodium Various	Cap 250, 500 mg Chew Tab 125 mg Drp 100 mg/mL Susp 25, 50, 100 mg/mL Inj 125, 250, 500 mg, 1, 2, 10 g.	PO 250–500 mg qid; IM or IV 100–200 mg/kg/day in 4–6 divided doses.	PO (<20 kg) 50–100 mg/kg/day in 2–4 divided doses; PO or IV (>20 kg) 100–400 mg/kg/day in 4–6 divided doses.	Cl_{cr} <20 mL/min: same dose q 12 hr.	4 (PO) 58 (IV)	22	About 50% oral bio-availability; GI side effects and rashes are frequent. IV sodium = 3 mEq/g.
Bacampi-cillin Spectrobid	Tab 400 mg (278 mg ampicillin) Susp 25 mg (17.5 mg ampicillin)/mL.	PO 400–800 mg bid.	PO 25–50 mg/kg/day in 2 divided doses.	No change.	12 (PO 800 mg)	22 (ampicillin)	Inactive ester of am-picillin; essentially equivalent to am-oxicillin.
EXTENDED-SPECTRUM PENICILLINS							
Mezlocillin Sodium Mezlin	Inj 1, 2, 3, 4, 20 g.	IV 200–300 mg/kg/day in 3–4 divided doses.	IV (neonates <7 days) 50–100 mg/kg q 12 hr; (neonates >7 days) 50–100 mg/kg q 6–8 hr; (children) same as adult dosage.	Cl_{cr} 10–30 mL/min: 3 g q 8 hr; Cl_{cr} <10 mL/min: 2 g q 8 hr.	263 (IV 4 g)	35	Spectrum similar to ticarcillin, but bet-ter enterococcal coverage. Sodium = 1.85 mEq/g.

(continued)

155

β-LACTAMS COMPARISON CHART (continued)

DRUG CLASS AND DRUG	DOSAGE FORMS	ADULT DOSAGE	PEDIATRIC DOSAGE	ADULT DOSAGE IN RENAL IMPAIRMENT[a]	PEAK SERUM LEVELS (MG/L)[b]	PERCENTAGE PROTEIN BOUND	COMMENTS
Piperacillin Sodium Pipracil	Inj 2, 3, 4, 40 g.	IV 200–300 mg/kg/day in 4–6 divided doses.	Not well established. IV (neonates) 50–100 mg/kg q 8–12 hr; (children) 200–300 (350–500 in cystic fibrosis) mg/kg/day in 4–6 divided doses.	Cl_{cr} 20–40 mL/min: 4 g q 8 hr; Cl_{cr} <20 mL/min: 4 g q 12 hr.	244 (IV 4 g)	35	Best activity against *P. aeruginosa.* Sodium = 1.85 mEq/g.
Ticarcillin Disodium Ticar	Inj 1, 3, 6, 20, 30 g.	IV 200–300 mg/kg/day in 4–6 divided doses.	IV (neonates ≤7 days and <2 kg) 75 mg/kg q 12 hr; (neonates >7 days and <2 kg or ≤7 days and >2 kg) 75 mg/kg q 8 hr; (neonates >7 days and >2 kg) 100 mg/kg q 8 hr.	Cl_{cr} 30–60 mL/min: 2 g q 4 hr; Cl_{cr} 10–30 mL/min: 2 g q 8 hr; Cl_{cr} <10 mL/min: 2 g q 12 hr.	324 (IV 3 g)	65	Less active than piperacillin against *P. aeruginosa;* no activity against *Klebsiella* spp. More antiplatelet effect than mezlocillin or piperacillin. Sodium = 5.2–6.5 mEq/g.

(continued)

DRUG CLASS AND DRUG	DOSAGE FORMS	ADULT DOSAGE	PEDIATRIC DOSAGE	ADULT DOSAGE IN RENAL IMPAIRMENT[a]	PEAK SERUM LEVELS (MG/L)[b]	PERCENTAGE PROTEIN BOUND	COMMENTS
PENICILLIN AND β-LACTAMASE COMBINATIONS							
Amoxicillin and Clavulanate Potassium Augmentin	Chew Tab 125 mg amoxicillin plus 31.25 mg clavulanate, 250 mg amoxicillin plus 62.5 mg clavulanate Susp 25 mg amoxicillin plus 6.25 mg clavulanate/ mL, 50 mg amoxicillin plus 12.5 mg clavulanate/mL Tab 250 mg amoxicillin plus 125 mg clavulanate, 500 mg amoxicillin plus 125 mg clavulanate, 875 mg amoxicillin plus 125 mg clavulanate.	PO "250" or "500" tablet tid, or "875" tablet bid.	PO 20–40 mg/ kg/day (of amoxicillin) in 3 divided doses.	No change.	9 (PO 500 mg amoxicillin) 2.6 (PO 125 mg clavulanate)	20 (amoxicillin) 22 (clavulanate)	Active against ampicillin-resistant *S. aureus*, *B. fragilis*, and β-lactamase-producing Enterobacteriacae. More diarrhea than with amoxicillin. Do not substitute 2 "250" tablets for 1 "500" tablet.

(continued)

β-LACTAMS COMPARISON CHART (continued)

DRUG CLASS AND DRUG	DOSAGE FORMS	ADULT DOSAGE	PEDIATRIC DOSAGE	ADULT DOSAGE IN RENAL IMPAIRMENT[a]	PEAK SERUM LEVELS (MG/L)[b]	PERCENTAGE PROTEIN BOUND	COMMENTS
Ampicillin Sodium and Sulbactam Sodium Unasyn	Inj 1 g ampicillin plus 500 mg sulbactam/vial, 2 g ampicillin plus 1 g sulbactam/vial.	IM or IV 1.5–3 g of the combination q 6–8 hr.	<12 yr safety and efficacy not established.	Cl$_{cr}$ 15–30 mL/min: same dose q 12 hr; Cl$_{cr}$ 5–14 mL/min: same dose q 24 hr.	58 (IV 1 g ampicillin) 30 (IV 500 mg sulbactam)	22 (ampicillin) 38 (sulbactam)	Spectrum similar to Augmentin. Sodium = 5 mEq/1.5 g.
Piperacillin Sodium and Tazobactam Sodium Zosyn	Inj 2.25, 3.375, 4.5 (0.5 g tazobactam/ 4 g piperacillin).	IV 3.375 g q 6 hr; 4.5 g q 6 hr for *P. aeruginosa*.	Safety and efficacy not established.	Cl$_{cr}$ 20–40 mL/min: 2.25 g q 6 hr; Cl$_{cr}$ <20 mL/min: 2.25 g q 8 hr.	224 (IV 4 g piperacillin) 34 (IV 0.5 g tazobactam)	20 (piperacillin) 1 (tazobactam)	Similar spectrum to Timentin, but better activity against *P. aeruginosa* and enterococci. Sodium = 2.35 mEq/g of piperacillin.
Ticarcillin Disodium and Clavulanate Potassium Timentin	Inj 3.1, 31 g (100 mg clavulanate/3 g ticarcillin).	IV 3.1 g q 4–6 hr.	IV (≥3 months) <60 kg: 50 mg/kg (of ticarcillin) q 4–6 hr; ≥60 kg: same as adult dosage.	Cl$_{cr}$ 30–60 mL/min: 3.1 g q 6 hr; Cl$_{cr}$ 10–30 mL/min: 3.1 g q 8 hr; Cl$_{cr}$ <10 mL/min: 3.1 g q 12 hr.[d]	324 (IV 3 g ticarcillin) 8 (IV 100 mg clavulanate)	65 (ticarcillin) 22 (clavulanate)	Improved activity over ticarcillin against *S. aureus*, *H. influenzae*, and anaerobes, but not *P. aeruginosa* or *E. cloacae*. Sodium = 4.7 mEq/g of ticarcillin.

[a]Usual *dose* means individual doses given at the specified interval; usual *dosage* means total daily dosage.
[b]Average peak serum concentrations following administration of a 500 mg oral dose or a 1 g IV infusion over 30 min, except as noted.
[c]Concentration dependent.
[d]With dosages recommended in marked renal impairment, clavulanate concentrations may provide ineffective synergism with ticarcillin.[173]
From references 155–157, 167–173 and product information.

Macrolides

AZITHROMYCIN
Zithromax

Pharmacology. Azithromycin is a macrolide with a 15-membered ring (making it an azalide) that is slightly less active than erythromycin against Gram-positive bacteria, but substantially more active against *Moraxella (Branhamella) catarrhalis, Haemophilus* spp., *Legionella* spp., *Neisseria* spp., *Bordetella* spp., *Mycoplasma* spp., and *Chlamydia trachomatis.* The drug also has activity against aerobic Gram-negative bacilli and *Mycobacterium avium,* and is comparable to erythromycin in activity against *Campylobacter* spp. It is the most active macrolide for *Toxoplasma gondii,* including activity against the cyst form.[174–176]

Administration and Adult Dosage. PO for mild to moderate acute bacterial exacerbations of chronic obstructive pulmonary disease, pneumonia, pharyngitis or tonsillitis, and uncomplicated skin and skin structure infections 500 mg as a single dose on the first day followed by 250 mg/day on days 2–5 for a total dosage of 1.5 g. PO for nongonococcal urethritis and cervicitis caused by *C. trachomatis* or for chancroid *(Haemophilus ducreyi)* 1 g as a single dose.[177] PO for treatment of *M. avium* complex in AIDS patients 500 mg/day in combination with ethambutol.[178] PO for prophylaxis of *M. avium* complex in AIDS patients 1.2 g once weekly alone or in combination with rifabutin 300 mg/day.[179] PO for endocarditis prophylaxis 500 mg 1 hr prior to procedure. IV for pelvic inflammatory disease 500 mg/day for 1–2 days, followed by PO 250 mg/day to complete 7 days of therapy. IV for community-acquired pneumonia 500 mg/day for at least 2 days followed by PO 500 mg/day to complete 7–10 days of therapy.

Special Populations. *Pediatric Dosage.* PO for otitis media (≥6 months) 10 mg/kg as a single daily dose on day 1, followed by 5 mg/kg/day as a single dose on days 2–5. PO for streptococcal pharyngitis/tonsillitis (≥2 yr) 12 mg/kg/day as a single dose for 5 days.[180–182] PO for endocarditis prophylaxis 15 mg/kg 1 hr prior to procedure. IV (<16 yr) safety and efficacy not established.

Geriatric Dosage. Same as adult dosage.

Other Conditions. Dosage reduction may be needed in severe hepatic impairment, but guidelines are not available.

Dosage Forms. Cap 250 mg; Tab 250, 600 mg; Susp 20, 40 mg/mL; Pwdr for Oral Soln 1 g; Inj 500 mg.

Patient Instructions. Take the capsules with a full glass of water on an empty stomach (1 hour before or 2 hours after meals) for best absorption. Tablets may be taken without regard to meals. Do not take aluminum- or magnesium-containing antacids with azithromycin.

Missed Doses. Take this drug at regular intervals. If you miss a dose take it as soon as you remember. If it is about time for the next dose, take that dose only. Leave a minimum of 12 hours between doses. Do not double the dose or take extra.

Pharmacokinetics. *Fate.* Oral bioavailability is 37%. After a 500 mg oral capsule, a peak serum concentration of 0.41 mg/L (0.55 μmol/L) is achieved in 2 hr. Plasma protein binding ranges from 7–50%, primarily to α_1-acid glycoprotein. Azithromycin penetrates both macrophages and polymorphonuclear leukocytes, accounting for intracellular concentrations that are 40-fold extracellular concentrations. Azithromycin is widely distributed throughout the body, and tissue concentrations (including the CNS) range from 10- to 150-fold higher than those in serum. Tissue concentrations peak 48 hr after administration, and high concentrations persist for several days after drug discontinuation. Elimination is polyphasic, reflecting rapid initial distribution into tissues, followed by slow elimination. V_d is 23–31 L/kg; Cl is 38 L/hr in adults. Azithromycin is metabolized in the liver and elimnated largely through biliary excretion; only 6% is excreted unchanged in urine.[175,183,184]

$t_{1/2}$. Terminal phase 11–68+ hr.[175,184]

Adverse Reactions. The drug is well tolerated. Frequent adverse effects are mild to moderate diarrhea, nausea, and abdominal pain. Headache and dizziness occur occasionally. Rash, angioedema, hepatomegaly, and cholestatic jaundice are reported rarely.[175]

Contraindications. Hypersensitivity to any macrolide.

Precautions. Use during pregnancy only if clearly needed. Use caution in patients with impaired hepatic function or severely impaired renal function.

Drug Interactions. Azithromycin does not interact with hepatic cytochrome P450 enzymes and, unlike erythromycin and clarithromycin, is not associated with these types of interactions.[185]

Parameters to Monitor. Baseline and periodic liver function tests during prolonged therapy.

CLARITHROMYCIN   Biaxin

Pharmacology. Clarithromycin is a semisynthetic macrolide antibiotic that is slightly more active than erythromycin against Gram-positive bacteria, *Moraxella (Branhamella) catarrhalis,* and *Legionella* spp. It is very active against *Chlamydia* spp., and is superior to other macrolides in its activity against *Mycobacterium avium* complex (MAC).[175,183]

Administration and Adult Dosage. **PO for respiratory and skin infections** 250–500 mg bid; **PO for MAC in AIDS patients** 500 mg bid. **PO for endocarditis prophylaxis** 500 mg 1 hr prior to procedure. **PO for eradication of *Helicobacter pylori*** 500 mg tid in combination with proton pump inhibitors and other drugs. (*See* Gastrointestinal Drugs, Treatment of *Helicobacter pylori* Infection in Peptic Ulcer Disease Chart.)[186]

Special Populations. *Pediatric Dosage.* **PO for community-acquired pneumonia** 15 mg/kg q 12 hr for 10 days; **PO for other indications** 7.5 mg/kg bid, to a maximum of 500 mg bid. **PO for endocarditis prophylaxis** 15 mg/kg 1 hr prior to procedure.

Geriatric Dosage. Same as adult dosage.

Other Conditions. Reduce dosage by 50% with Cl_{cr} <30 mL/min.

Dosage Forms. **Tab** 250, 500 mg; **Susp** 25, 50 mg/mL.

Pharmacokinetics. *Fate.* Clarithromycin is acid-stable and absorbed well with or without food. Bioavailability is 55%, with peak serum concentrations of about 2 mg/L attained after a 400 mg oral dose. The hydroxy metabolite is active and may be synergistic in vitro with the parent drug.[184]

$t_{1/2}$. (Clarithromycin) 4.5 hr; (hydroxy-metabolite) 4–9 hr.[184]

Adverse Reactions. Similar to erythromycin, but clarithromycin has better GI tolerance.

Contraindications. Hypersensitivity to any macrolide antibiotic; concurrent use with certain other drugs. (*See* Drug Interactions.)

Precautions. Use with caution in severe renal or hepatic function impairment; dosage reduction is advised.

Drug Interactions. Clarithromycin has a lower affinity for CYP3A4 than erythromycin and therefore has fewer clinically important drug interactions; however, its use is contraindicated with astemizole or cisapride. Serum concentrations of theophylline and carbamazepine may also be increased by clarithromycin.

ERYTHROMYCIN AND SALTS   Various

Pharmacology. Erythromycin is a bacteriostatic macrolide antibiotic with a spectrum similar to penicillin G; it is also active against *Mycoplasma pneumoniae* and *Legionella pneumophila.*[187–189] It acts by binding to the 50S ribosomal subunit, inhibiting protein synthesis. Gram-positive organisms develop resistance via R-factor mediated alteration of the binding site. Gram-negative organisms are resistant because of cell wall impermeability.

Administration and Adult Dosage. (*See* Macrolide Antibiotics Comparison Chart.) **For gastroparesis** 200 mg IV of the lactobionate salt, 250 mg PO of the ethylsuccinate salt or 500 mg PO of the base 15–120 min before meals and at bedtime appear to be effective.[190]

Special Populations. *Pediatric Dosage.* (*See* Macrolide Antibiotics Comparison Chart.)

Geriatric Dosage. Same as adult dosage.

Other Conditions. Dosage adjustment is probably unnecessary in renal impairment.[180,187]

Dosage Forms. (*See* Macrolide Antibiotics Comparison Chart.)

Patient Instructions. Take this drug with a full glass of water on an empty stomach (1 hour before or 2 hours after meals) for best absorption. Refrigerate the suspension.

Missed Doses. Take this drug at regular intervals. If you miss a dose take it as soon as you remember. If it is about time for the next dose, take that dose only. Leave a minimum of 4–6 hours between doses. Do not double the dose or take extra.

Pharmacokinetics. *Fate.* Oral absorption varies widely with the salt and dosage form (*see* Macrolide Antibiotics Comparison Chart), with peak serum concentrations occurring from 30 min (suspension) to 4 hr (coated tablet) after administration. However, enteric-coated erythromycin base tablets, stearate tablets, and estolate capsules produce equivalent erythromycin serum levels when administered to fasting subjects. Food or restricted water intake (ie, 20 mL or less) with a dose dramatically lowers the absorption of the stearate form. The drug is $83 \pm 5\%$ plasma protein bound and widely distributed into most tissues, cavities, and body fluids except the brain and CSF (even with meningeal inflammation). V_d is 0.6 ± 0.1 L/kg; Cl is 0.55 ± 0.25 L/hr/kg. Erythromycin is partially metabolized in the liver by CYP3A3/4, and is excreted primarily as unchanged erythromycin with high concentrations in the bile and feces. Only 12–15% of an IV dose is excreted unchanged in urine.[48,187]

$t_{1/2}$. 1.6 ± 0.7 hr; unchanged or slightly prolonged in anuric patients, based on minimal data; prolonged in cirrhosis.[48]

Adverse Reactions. Frequent GI distress. IM form is very painful, despite local anesthetic (butamben) in the product, and may produce sterile abscesses. IV administration frequently produces pain, venous irritation, and phlebitis. Mild elevations of serum hepatic enzymes occur frequently. Transient deafness occurs occasionally with high dosages.[187,191] Rare, but potentially serious, reversible intrahepatic cholestatic jaundice occurs primarily with the estolate and ethylsuccinate forms, usually in adults after 10–14 days of therapy, although it may occur after the first dose if there is a history of previous use. Prodrome includes malaise, nausea, vomiting, fever, and abdominal pain (which may be severe and misdiagnosed as acute surgical abdomen). Symptoms resolve in 1–2 weeks, and serum enzymes return to normal over several months.

Contraindications. Concurrent use with astemizole or cisapride; IM form in patients with hypersensitivity to local anesthetics of the para-aminobenzoic acid type (eg, procaine); hepatic dysfunction (estolate and ethylsuccinate forms).

Precautions. Pregnancy. Use with caution in patients with liver disease because of possibly impaired excretion.

Drug Interactions. Erythromycin inhibits CYP3A4 and can reduce hepatic metabolism of some drugs, including astemizole, carbamazepine, cisapride, cyclosporine, theophylline, triazolam, warfarin, and others.[192] (*See* Contraindications.)

Parameters to Monitor. Liver function tests in patients who experience prodromal symptoms (*see* Adverse Reactions) while receiving the estolate or ethylsuccinate form; check daily for vein irritation and phlebitis in patients receiving IV forms. Closely monitor the effects of other drugs which interact with erythromycin during concurrent use.

Notes. Avoid injectable forms if at all possible. Erythromycin is more active in an alkaline environment. Unrelated to its antibacterial effect, erythromycin in low doses binds to motilin receptors in the GI tract to stimulate gastric emptying. It is the most prokinetic macrolide and has been used in gastroparesis and in other GI motility disorders.[190,193–196]

MACROLIDE ANTIBIOTICS COMPARISON CHART

DRUG	DOSAGE FORMS	ADULT DOSAGE	PEDIATRIC DOSAGE	COMMENTS
Azithromycin Zithromax	Cap 250 mg. Tab 250, 600 mg Susp 20, 40 mg/mL Pwdr for Oral Soln 1 g Inj 500 mg.	PO 500 mg once, then 250 mg/day for 4 days; PO for urethritis and cervicitis 1 g; PO for MAC treatment 500 mg/day; PO for MAC prophylaxis 1.2 g once/week. IV 500 mg/day.	PO for otitis media or pneumonia, 10 mg/kg once, then 5 g/kg/day for 4 days; PO for pharyngitis/tonsilitis 12 mg/kg/day for 5 days.	Broader spectrum than erythromycin. Food interferes with absorption. Less GI intolerance than erythromycin. Little or no P450 inhibition.
Clarithromycin Biaxin	Tab 250, 500 mg Susp 25, 50 mg/mL.	PO 250–500 mg bid; PO for MAC 500 mg bid; PO for *H. pylori* 500 mg tid with other agents.	PO for pneumonia 15 mg/kg q 12 hr for 10 days; PO for other uses 7.5 mg/kg bid.	Broader spectrum than erythromycin. Food does not decrease absorption. Less GI intolerance than erythromycin. Less inhibition of CYP3A3/4 than erythromycin.
Dirithromycin Dynabac	EC Tab 250 mg.	PO 500 mg once daily for 7–14 days.	<12 yr not recommended.	Spectrum similar to erythromycin, but less GI intolerance and little or no P450 inhibition.
Erythromycin Base E-Mycin Ery-Tab ERYC Various	EC Tab 250, 333, 500 mg EC Cap Pellets 250 mg.	PO 1 g/day in 2–4 doses, to a maximum of 4 g/ day.	PO 30–50 mg/kg/day in 4 doses; may double in severe infection.[a]	Food interferes with absorption of uncoated products; EC products appear to be among the best tolerated erythromycin formulations.[b]

(continued)

163

MACROLIDE ANTIBIOTICS COMPARISON CHART (continued)

DRUG	DOSAGE FORMS	ADULT DOSAGE	PEDIATRIC DOSAGE	COMMENTS
Erythromycin Estolate Ilosone Various	Cap 250 mg Susp 25, 50 mg/mL (reconstituted) Tab 500 mg.	PO 250–500 mg q 6 hr, to a maximum of 4 g/day.	PO 30–50 mg/kg/day in 3–4 doses.[a]	PO well absorbed; unaffected by food and highly resistant to gastric acid hydrolysis; absorbed as propionate ester which predominates in serum (8:1) and may be less active; rare intrahepatic cholestatic jaundice.[b]
Erythromycin Ethylsuccinate E.E.S. EryPed Various	Drp 40 mg/mL Susp 40, 80 mg/mL Chew Tab 200 mg Tab (coated) 400 mg.	PO 400 mg q 6 hr, to a maximum of 4 g/day.	PO 30–50 mg/kg/day in 3–4 doses; may double in severe infection.	Absorbed better than base; intermediate susceptibility to gastric acid hydrolysis. Absorbed as ester, which predominates in serum (3:1) and may be less active. Rare intrahepatic cholestatic jaundice.[b]
Erythromycin Gluceptate Ilotycin	Inj (IV only) 1 g.	IV 15–20 mg/kg/day in 3–4 doses, to a maximum of 4 g/day.	IV same as adult dosage in 2–4 doses; may double in severe infection.[a]	Painful; phlebitis frequent; avoid use if possible. Infuse over 20–60 minutes.[b]

(continued)

MACROLIDE ANTIBIOTICS COMPARISON CHART (continued)

DRUG	DOSAGE FORMS	ADULT DOSAGE	PEDIATRIC DOSAGE	COMMENTS
Erythromycin Lactobionate Erythrocin Various	Inj (IV only) 500 mg, 1 g.	Same as erythromycin gluceptate.	Same as erythromycin gluceptate. [a]	Same as erythromycin gluceptate. [b]
Erythromycin Stearate Erythrocin Various	Tab (film coated) 250, 500 mg.	PO 1 g/day in 2 or 4 doses, to a maximum of 4 g/day.	PO 30–50 mg/kg/day in 4 doses; may double in severe infections.	Absorption about equal to ethylsuccinate, although food interferes markedly with absorption. Hydrolyzed to free base before absorption. [b]

[a] In newborns, data are available for erythromycin estolate only, suggesting an oral dosage of 40 mg/kg/day in 2–4 divided doses.
[b] Despite differences in oral absorption, no clinical studies have shown any salt to be clearly superior in any particular therapeutic use.
From references 197–202 and product information.

165

Quinolones

CIPROFLOXACIN Cipro

Pharmacology. Ciprofloxacin is a fluoroquinolone that inhibits bacterial DNA-gyrase, an enzyme responsible for the unwinding of DNA for transcription and subsequent supercoiling of DNA for packaging into chromosomal subunits. It is highly active against Enterobacteriaceae, with MICs often <0.1 mg/L. It is also active against some strains of *Pseudomonas aeruginosa* and *Staphylococcus* spp., with an MIC_{90} of 0.5–1 mg/L. However, recent reports indicate increasing resistance to this agent in methicillin-resistant *S. aureus*. It has poor activity against streptococci and anaerobes.[203,204]

Administration and Adult Dosage. **PO for uncomplicated urinary tract infections** 250 mg q 12 hr. **PO for moderate to severe systemic infections** 500–750 mg q 12 hr. **PO for gonorrhea** 500 mg once. **PO for chancroid** 500 mg q 12 hr for 3 days.[177] **IV** 400 mg q 12 hr.

Special Populations. *Pediatric Dosage.* (<16 yr) safety and efficacy not established. Use has been limited because of the potential for arthropathy. Ciprofloxacin has been used in children 6–16 yr old in limited situations to treat serious infections. **IV for *P. aeruginosa* infections in cystic fibrosis** 30 mg/kg/day in 3 divided doses. **PO for *P. aeruginosa* infections in cystic fibrosis** 40 mg/kg/day in two divided doses.[205]

Geriatric Dosage. Reduce dosage for age-related reduction in renal function, although dosage reduction is not necessary with only minor age-related renal function changes.[206]

Other Conditions. Reduce dosage by 50% or double the dosage interval when Cl_{cr} is <30 mL/min; special dosage adjustments in patients with cystic fibrosis are not necessary.[207]

Dosage Forms. **Inj** 200, 400 mg; **Susp** 50, 100 mg/mL; **Tab** 250, 500, 750 mg; **Ophth Drp** 0.3%; **Otic Susp** 2 mg plus hydrocortisone 10 mg/mL.

Patient Instructions. This drug may be taken with food to minimize stomach upset. Avoid antacid use during treatment; calcium, iron, or zinc supplements may also reduce absorption. Avoid excessive exposure to sunlight during ciprofloxacin treatment. Report any tendon pain or inflammation that occurs during therapy.

Missed Doses. Take this drug at regular intervals. If you miss a dose take it as soon as you remember. If it is about time for the next dose, take that dose only. Leave a minimum of 6–8 hours between doses. Do not double the dose or take extra.

Pharmacokinetics. *Serum Levels.* A peak serum level of 4–6 mg/L (12–18 μmol/L) 2 hr after an oral 750 to 1000 mg dose is proposed as evidence of absorption adequate for tuberculosis therapy.[53]

Fate. Approximately 70% absorbed orally; food decreases the rate but not the extent of absorption. Aluminum-, calcium-, or magnesium-containing antacids or sucralfate markedly decrease the extent of absorption. Peak serum concentrations are 3 ± 0.6 mg/L (9 ± 1.8 μmol/L) following a 750 mg oral dose; a 200 mg IV dose infused over 30 min results in a peak concentration of about 3.2 ± 0.6 mg/L. V_d averages 2 L/kg. Renal clearance averages 0.26 L/hr/kg. Less than 30% is plasma protein bound. Ciprofloxacin attains very high concentrations in many body fluids and tissues, most notably urine, prostate, and pulmonary mucosa. CSF concentrations are <1 mg/L; experience with the drug in the treatment of meningitis is very limited. From 45–60% of a parenteral dose is recovered unchanged in urine; the remainder is excreted as four metabolites or eliminated in feces.[184,206–210]

$t_{1/2}$. 4.2 ± 0.63 hr,[209] 6.9 ± 2.9 hr in severe renal impairment.[210]

Adverse Reactions. GI intolerance (nausea, vomiting, diarrhea, abdominal discomfort) occurs frequently. CNS effects such as headaches and restlessness have occurred in 1–2% of patients. Other CNS effects (eg, dizziness, insomnia, anxiety, irritability, and seizures) have been reported in less than 1% of patients. Skin rashes and photosensitivity occur occasionally. Anaphylaxis occurs rarely.[184]

Contraindications. Hypersensitivity to any quinolone.

Precautions. Pregnancy; lactation.

Drug Interactions. Aluminum-, calcium-, or magnesium-containing antacids markedly reduce oral absorption. Although there is some information that spacing administration by 2 hr or more may minimize these interactions, it is probably best not to use ciprofloxacin in patients taking long-term antacid therapy. Iron supplements and zinc-containing multivitamins may reduce absorption. Theophylline clearance may be reduced in some patients receiving ciprofloxacin. Patients receiving fluoroquinolones and methylxanthines such as theophylline or caffeine may be at increased risk of CNS toxicity (eg, convulsions). Warfarin metabolism may be impaired by ciprofloxacin, although studies with the fluoroquinolone enoxacin indicate that only the metabolism of the less active (R)-warfarin is affected. Use caution when adding ciprofloxacin in a patient taking warfarin. The solubility of ciprofloxacin is reduced at higher pH values; thus, avoid alkalinization of the urine.[208]

Parameters to Monitor. Monitor serum theophylline levels closely in patients receiving theophylline. Monitor prothrombin time and signs of bleeding in patients on warfarin.

OFLOXACIN	Floxin
LEVOFLOXACIN	Levaquin

Pharmacology. Ofloxacin is a systemic fluoroquinolone similar to ciprofloxacin. Levofloxacin is the active L-isomer of ofloxacin which allows higher dosages of the active form to be given with fewer side effects. Ofloxacin has greater activity against *Chlamydia trachomatis, Ureaplasma urealiticum, Mycoplasma pneumoniae,* and *Mycobacterium tuberculosis* than ciprofloxacin, but less activity against *Pseudomonas aeruginosa.*[53,184,203,204,211] (*See* Fluoroquinolones Comparison Chart.)

Adult Dosage. (Ofloxacin) **IV or PO for systemic infections** 400 mg q 12 hr; **PO for nongonococcal urethritis** 300 mg q 12 hr for 7 days; **PO for acute, uncomplicated gonorrhea** 400 mg once; **IV or PO for urinary tract infections**

200 mg q 12 hr. (Levofloxacin) **IV or PO** 250–500 mg once daily. Reduce the dosage of both drugs in renal impairment. (*See* Fluoroquinolones Comparison Chart.)

Pediatric Dosage. (<18 yr) safety and efficacy not established.

Dosage Forms. (Ofloxacin) **Inj** 200, 400 mg; **Tab** 200, 300, 400 mg. (Levofloxacin) **Inj** 25 mg/mL; **Tab** 250, 500 mg.

Pharmacokinetics. Ofloxacin is >95% bioavailable orally. A peak serum concentration of 8–12 mg/L (22–33 μmol/L) 2 hr after an oral dose of 600–800 mg is proposed as evidence of absorption adequate for tuberculosis therapy. Ofloxacin is predominantly renally excreted with a half-life of 5–7 hr.

Adverse Reactions. (*See* Ciprofloxacin.)

Drug Interactions. Ofloxacin does not alter hepatic metabolism of methylxanthine compounds (eg, caffeine, theophylline). However, like other fluoroquinolones, cations markedly reduce the absorption of this agent.

FLUOROQUINOLONES COMPARISON CHART

DRUG	DOSAGE FORMS	ADULT DOSAGE	DOSAGE IN RENAL IMPAIRMENT	ORAL BIOAVAILABILITY (PERCENT)	PEAK SERUM LEVELS (MG/L)[a]	COMMENTS[b]
Ciprofloxacin Cipro Ciloxan	Tab 250, 500, 750 mg Inj 200, 400 mg Ophth Drp 0.3% (Ciloxan) 2.5, 5 mL.	PO 250–750 mg q 12 hr; PO for gonorrhea 500 mg once; IV 200–400 mg q 12 hr; Ophth 2 drops q 15 min–4 hr.	Cl$_{cr}$ 30–50 mL/min: PO 250–500 mg q 12 hr; IV usual dosage; Cl$_{cr}$ 5–29 mL/min: PO 250–500 mg q 18 hr; IV 200–400 mg q 18–24 hr; Dialysis: PO 250–500 mg q 24 hr after dialysis.	60–80	3 ± 0.6 (PO 750 mg) 3.2 ± 0.6 (IV 200 mg)	Most active against *P. aeruginosa*.
Enoxacin Penetrex	Tab 200, 400 mg.	PO 200–400 mg q 12 hr.	Cl$_{cr}$ 5–15 mL/min: usual dose q 24 hr.	83–90	5.5 (PO 400 mg) 8.2 (IV 400 mg)	Most potent inhibitor of theophylline metabolism.
Fleroxacin Megalone (Investigational, Roche)	—	PO or IV 200–400 mg/day in 1 dose.	Cl$_{cr}$ 16–30 mL/min: 50% of usual dose q 24 hr; Cl$_{cr}$ 5–15 mL/min: 25% of usual dose q 24 hr.	>90	5.6 (PO 400 mg)	Under investigation for single daily dose administration.

(continued)

FLUOROQUINOLONES COMPARISON CHART (continued)

DRUG	DOSAGE FORMS	ADULT DOSAGE	DOSAGE IN RENAL IMPAIRMENT	ORAL BIOAVAILABILITY (PERCENT)	PEAK SERUM LEVELS (MG/L)[a]	COMMENTS[b]
Grepafloxacin Raxar	Tab 200 mg.	PO 400–600 mg/day in one dose; PO for gonorrhea 400 mg once.	No dosage changes required.	NA	1.5 (PO 400 mg)	Long half-life of 12 hr. Can be administered with or without food.
Levofloxacin Levaquin	Tab 250, 500 mg Inj 25 mg/mL.	PO or IV 250–500 mg q 24 hr.	Cl_{cr} 20–49 mL/min: Usual dose once, then 250 mg q 24 hr; Cl_{cr} 10–19 mL/min: Usual dose once, then 250 mg q 48 hr; Hemodialysis or peritoneal dialysis: 500 mg once, then 250 mg q 48 hr.	95–100	5.7 (PO 500 mg) 6.4 (IV 500 mg)	Active S–(–) isomer of ofloxacin. Levofloxacin is not appreciably removed from the body during hemodialysis or peritoneal dialysis.
Lomefloxacin Maxaquin	Tab 400 mg.	PO 400 mg once daily.	Cl_{cr} <40 mL/min: PO 400 mg once, then 200 mg/day.	95–98	25 (PO 400 mg)	No effect on theophylline metabolism. Long half-life of 8 hr. Relatively weak antibacterial. Photo-toxic.

(continued)

FLUOROQUINOLONES COMPARISON CHART (continued)

DRUG	DOSAGE FORMS	ADULT DOSAGE	DOSAGE IN RENAL IMPAIRMENT	ORAL BIOAVAILABILITY (PERCENT)	PEAK SERUM LEVELS (MG/L)[a]	COMMENTS[b]
Norfloxacin Noroxin Chibroxin	Tab 400 mg Ophth Drp 0.3% (Chibroxin) 5 mL.	PO 200–400 mg q 12 hr; PO for gonorrhea 800 mg once; Ophth 1 or 2 drops q 2 hr–qid.	Cl_{cr} <30 mL/min: PO 400 mg/day.	35–45 (estimated)	1.4–1.6 (PO 400 mg)	Used in urinary and GI tract infections only because of poor oral bioavailability.
Ofloxacin Floxin Ocuflox	Tab 200, 300, 400 mg Inj 200, 400 mg Ophth Drp 0.3% (Ocuflox).	PO or IV 200–400 mg q 12 hr. PO for gonorrhea 400 mg once. Ophth 1 or 2 drops q 2–4 hr for 2 days, then qid up to 5 days.	Cl_{cr} 10–50 mL/min: usual dose q 24 hr; Cl_{cr} <10 mL/min: 50% of usual dose q 24 hr.	95–100	3.5–5.3 (PO 400 mg)	Most active against *Chlamydia* spp.; little effect on theophylline metabolism.
Sparfloxacin Zagam	Tab 200 mg.	PO 400 mg once, then 200 mg q 24 hr.	Cl_{cr} <50 mL/min: 400 mg once, then 200 mg q 48 hr.	90	0.62–0.71 (PO 200 mg) 0.56–1.60 (PO 400 mg)	Can be taken with or without food. No effect on theophylline metabolism. Phototoxic.

(continued)

FLUOROQUINOLONES COMPARISON CHART (continued)

DRUG	DOSAGE FORMS	ADULT DOSAGE	DOSAGE IN RENAL IMPAIRMENT	ORAL BIOAVAILABILITY (PERCENT)	PEAK SERUM LEVELS (MG/L)[a]	COMMENTS[b]
Trovafloxacin Alatrofloxacin Mesylate Trovan	Tab 100, 200 mg. Inj 5 mg/mL.	PO 200 mg/day; PO for gonorrhea 100 mg once; IV 200–300 mg/day.	No adjustment needed in renal impairment or dialysis.	88	1.1 (PO 100 mg) 3.3 (PO 300 mg)	Broad spectrum of activity. Penetrates into CSF better than other quinolones. May have benefit against resistant organisms.

[a]Peak serum concentrations following administration of the dose shown in parentheses.
[b]All fluoroquinolones are associated with tendon rupture. Discontinue therapy at the first sign of tendon pain or inflammation, and patients should refrain from exercise until the diagnosis of tendinitis can be confidently excluded.[203]

From references 184, 203–217.

Sulfonamides

TRIMETHOPRIM AND SULFAMETHOXAZOLE   Bactrim, Septra, Various

Pharmacology. Sulfamethoxazole (SMZ) is a synthetic analogue of para-aminobenzoic acid (PABA) which competitively inhibits the synthesis of dihydropteric acid (an inactive folic acid precursor) from PABA in microorganisms. Trimethoprim (TMP) acts at a later step to inhibit the enzymatic reduction of dihydrofolic acid to tetrahydrofolic acid. The most important determinant of efficacy is usually the level of susceptibility to TMP; resistance to the combination is uncommon, but appears to be increasing worldwide. The combination is active against many bacteria except anaerobes, *Pseudomonas aeruginosa,* and many *Streptococcus faecalis* spp. It is also highly active and effective against the protozoan *Pneumocystis carinii*. TMP/SMZ demonstrates in vitro activity against methicillin-resistant *Staphylococcus aureus* (MRSA), but clinical success has been variable and unpredictable.[218–221]

Administration and Adult Dosage. **PO for UTI** 160 mg of TMP and 800 mg of SMZ q 12 hr for 10–14 days. **PO for prophylaxis of recurrent UTI** 40 mg TMP and 200 of SMZ at bedtime 3 times a week. **PO for shigellosis** 160 mg of TMP and 800 of SMZ q 12 hr for 5 days. **IV for severe Gram-negative infections or shigellosis** 8–10 mg/kg/day of TMP and 40–50 mg/kg/day of SMZ, in 2–4 equally divided doses, q 6–12 hr for 5 days for shigellosis and up to 14 days for severe UTI. **PO or IV for *P. carinii* pneumonia (PCP)** 12.5–20 mg/kg/day of TMP and 62.5–100 mg/kg/day of SMZ, in 2–4 equally divided doses, for up to 21 days. **PO for PCP infection prophylaxis** 160 mg of TMP and 800 mg of SMZ once daily; intermittent dosage (eg, 3 times a week) is also used. In patients with HIV infection, the drug is indicated if there was a previous episode of PCP or CD4 counts are <200/µL.[219] (*See* Notes.)

Special Populations. *Pediatric Dosage.* **PO for UTI or shigellosis** (2 months–12 yr) 8 mg/kg/day of TMP and 40 mg/kg/day of SMZ (Susp 1 mL/kg/day) in 2 equally divided doses; (over 12 yr) same as adult mg/kg dosage. **PO for otitis media** same as UTI dosage. **IV for severe Gram-negative infection or shigellosis** (2 months and over) same as adult mg/kg dosage. **PO or IV for PCP** same as adult mg/kg dosage. **PO for *P. carinii* infection prophylaxis** 150 mg/m^2/day of TMP and 750 mg/m^2/day of SMZ, in divided doses, given 3 days a week.[222]

Geriatric Dosage. Reduce dosage for age-related reduction in renal function, although dosage reduction is not necessary with only minor age-related renal function changes. (*See* Precautions.)

Other Conditions. For a Cl_{cr} <30 mL/min, give normal dosage for 1–6 doses; then, with a Cl_{cr} of 15–30 mL/min, follow with 50% of the usual dosage; with a Cl_{cr} <15 mL/min, follow with 25–50% of the usual dosage in 1 or 2 divided doses. Give patients on hemodialysis a normal dose after each dialysis procedure. For systemic infections treated with higher dosages, monitor serum levels.

Dosage Forms. **Susp** 8 mg/mL of TMP and 40 mg/mL of SMZ; **Tab** 80 mg of TMP and 400 mg of SMZ (single strength), 160 mg of TMP and 800 mg of SMZ (double strength); **Inj** 16 mg/mL of TMP and 80 mg/mL of SMZ.

Patient Instructions. Take this medication with a full 8 fl. oz. glass of water on an empty stomach (1 hour before or 2 hours after meals) for best absorption. Drink several additional glasses of water daily, unless directed otherwise.

Missed Doses. Take this drug at regular intervals. If you miss a dose take it as soon as you remember. If it is about time for the next dose, take that dose only. If you are taking the drug once a day, leave a minimum of 10–12 hours between doses. If you are taking the drug twice a day, leave a minimum of 5–6 hours between doses. Do not double the dose or take extra.

Pharmacokinetics. *Serum Levels.* Trimethoprim levels >5 mg/L (>17 μmol/L) and SMZ peak levels of about 100 mg/L (396 μmol/L) may be required in *P. carinii* pneumonia.[219,223]

Fate. TMP and SMZ are 90–100% absorbed orally. In normal adults, peak serum concentrations of 0.9–1.9 mg/L (3.1–6.5 μmol/L) of TMP and 20–50 mg/L (79–198 μmol/L) of SMZ occur about 1–4 hr after 160 mg of TMP and 800 mg of SMZ. An additional 10–20 mg/L of SMZ exists in the serum as inactive metabolites. IV infusion of 160 mg of TMP and 800 mg of SMZ over 1 hr produces peak serum levels of 3.4 mg/L (11.7 μmol/L) of TMP and 46.3 mg/L (183 μmol/L) of SMZ. TMP and SMZ are widely distributed in the body, although TMP is much more widely distributed because of its greater lipophilicity. TMP is 45% plasma protein bound and has a V_d of 1–2 L/kg; SMZ is 60% plasma protein bound and has a V_d of 0.36 L/kg. TMP concentrations in various tissues and fluids (including the prostrate, bile, and sputum) are several times greater than concomitant serum concentrations; CSF concentrations in normal adults are approximately 50% of serum concentrations. Nearly all TMP is excreted in the urine within 24–72 hr, 50–75% as unchanged drug. SMZ undergoes extensive liver metabolism, producing N^4-acetylated and N^4-glucuronidated derivatives; 85% is excreted in the urine within 24–72 hr, 10–30% as unchanged drug. The pharmacokinetics of these drugs are essentially unchanged when given in combination. The pH of the urine influences renal excretion of both drugs, but does not markedly alter overall elimination.[219,224]

$t_{1/2}$. 11 ± 2.3 hr for TMP and 8 ± 0.4 hr for SMZ in normal adults.[224] 20–30 hr or more for TMP in severe renal failure; 18–24 hr for SMZ in anuria.[221]

Adverse Reactions. Gastrointestinal irritation including nausea, vomiting, and anorexia occurs frequently, and both the frequency and severity appear to be dose related. Rashes and other hypersensitivity reactions similar to those caused by other sulfonamides occur occasionally. In patients with AIDS, allergic skin reactions, rash (usually diffuse, erythematous or maculopapular, and pruritic) are frequent and may be associated with fever, leukopenia, neutropenia, thrombocytopenia, and increased transaminase levels.[225] Desensitization has been successful, though. (*See* Notes.) In patients without underlying myelosuppression and treated with conventional dosages, the frequency of megaloblastic anemia and other hematologic disorders is rare, but may be higher in folate-deficient patients. Hepatotoxicity and nephrotoxicity are rare; renal dysfunction may occur in patients with pre-existing renal disease, but it is reversible.[221,224] Allergic skin reactions, including toxic epidermal necrolysis, exfoliative dermatitis, Stevens-Johnson syndrome, erythema multiforme, and fixed drug eruptions occur rarely. Other rare adverse effects include cholestatic jaundice, pancreatitis, pseudomembranous colitis, hyperkalemia, myalgia, headache, insomnia, fatigue, ataxia, vertigo, depression, and anaphylaxis.[221]

Contraindications. Pregnancy; infants under 2 months; history of hypersensitivity reaction to sulfonamide derivatives or trimethoprim; megaloblastic anemia caused by folate deficiency. Lactation is stated by manufacturer to be a contraindication, but risk is probably limited to nursing infants under 2 months of age.

Precautions. G-6-PD deficiency; impaired renal or hepatic function. Adverse reactions may be more frequent in the elderly, especially with impaired hepatic or renal function or in those taking thiazide diuretics.

Drug Interactions. The effects of methotrexate, sulfonylureas, and warfarin are increased when used with trimethoprim-sulfamethoxazole. Enhanced bone marrow suppression may occur with the combination of trimethoprim/sulfamethoxazole and mercaptopurine. A decreased effect of cyclosporine and an increased risk of nephrotoxicity may occur. High-dose trimethoprim-sulfamethoxazole with didanosine may increase the risk of pancreatitis. Phenytoin clearance may be decreased with concurrent use.

Parameters to Monitor. Baseline and periodic CBC for patients on long-term or high-dose treatment. Monitor SMZ serum levels in patients treated for PCP if absorption is questionable or response is poor.[219] In patients with AIDS, monitor for hypersensitivity skin reactions (rash and urticaria).

Notes. Protect all dosage forms from light. The efficacy and safety of TMP and SMZ have been demonstrated in numerous infectious conditions (eg, chronic UTI, chronic bronchitis, sepsis, enteric fever, prostatitis, endocarditis, meningitis, and gonorrhea), and the combination is considered an effective alternative to conventional therapy in most cases.[219,224] Efficacy of TMP and SMZ in the treatment of *Pneumocystis carinii* pneumonitis is equivalent to **pentamidine,** which makes the combination the therapy of choice because of its greater safety and lower cost.[223] Oral desensitization or rechallenge with TMP/SMZ has been successful in permitting continued use in patients with AIDS who experience hypersensitivity reactions.[226] Sulfamethoxazole is also available as a single agent (Gantanol **Susp** 100 mg/mL; **Tab** 500 mg).

Tetracyclines

DOXYCYCLINE AND SALTS   Vibramycin

Pharmacology. Tetracyclines are broad-spectrum bacteriostatic compounds that inhibit protein synthesis at the 30S ribosomal subunit. Activity includes Gram-positive, Gram-negative, aerobic, and anaerobic bacteria, as well as spirochetes, mycoplasmas, rickettsiae, chlamydiae, and some protozoa. Many bacteria have developed plasmid-mediated resistance. Most Enterobacteriacae and *Pseudomonas aeruginosa* are resistant. Doxycycline is somewhat more active than other tetracyclines against anerobes and facultative Gram-negative bacilli.[227,228]

Administration and Adult Dosage. **PO** 100 mg q 12 hr for 2 doses, then 50–100 mg/day in 1 or 2 doses, depending on the severity of the infection, to a maximum of 200 mg/day. **PO for uncomplicated chlamydial genital infections** 100 mg bid for at least 7 days. **PO for primary and secondary syphilis** 100 mg tid for at least 10 days. **PO for prophylaxis against travelers' diarrhea** 200 mg en route, then 100 mg/day for duration of travel (6 weeks maximum). **PO for malaria prophylaxis in short-term (<4 months) travelers** 100 mg/day beginning 1–2 days before travel to malarious areas, and for 4 weeks after leaving the area. **IV** 200 mg in 1 or 2 divided doses for 1 day, followed by 100–200 mg/day, infused at a concentration of 0.1–1 g/L over 1–4 hr; double maintenance dosage in severe infections. **Intrapleural for pleural effusions** 500 mg in 25–30 mL of NS has been used; most patients require 2–4 infusions for maximum efficacy.[229] **Not for SC or IM use.**

Special Populations. *Pediatric Dosage.* **Not recommended under 8 yr. PO** (>8 yr, <45 kg) 2.2 mg/kg q 12 hr for 2 doses, then 2.2–4.4 mg/kg/day in 1 or 2 divided doses, depending on the severity of the infection; (>45 kg) same as adult dosage. **PO for malaria prophylaxis in short-term (<4 months) travelers** (>8 yr) 2.2 mg/kg/day to a maximum of 100 mg/day beginning 1–2 days before travel to malarious areas, and for 4 weeks after leaving the area. **IV** (<45 kg) 4.4 mg/kg in 1 or 2 divided doses for 1 day followed by 2.2–4.4 mg/kg/day in 1 or 2 divided doses, infused at a concentration of 0.1–1 g/L over 1–4 hr; (>45 kg) same as adult dosage.

Geriatric Dosage. Same as adult dosage.

Other Conditions. No dosage adjustment is necessary in renal impairment.

Dosage Forms. **Cap** (as hyclate) 50, 100 mg; **Tab** (as hyclate) 50, 100 mg; **Susp** (as monohydrate) 5 mg/mL (reconstituted); **Syrup** (as calcium) 10 mg/mL; **Inj** (as hyclate) 100, 200 mg.

Patient Instructions. Take doxycycline by mouth with a full glass of water on an empty stomach, but if stomach upset occurs, the drug may be taken with food or milk, but not antacids or iron products. Avoid prolonged exposure to direct sunlight while taking this drug.

Missed Doses. Take this drug at regular intervals. If you miss a dose take it as soon as you remember. If it is about time for the next dose, take that dose only. Leave a minimum of 6–8 hours between doses. Do not double the dose or take extra.

Pharmacokinetics. *Onset and Duration.* Duration of protection against travelers' diarrhea is about 1 week after drug discontinuation.[230]

Fate. About 93% is orally absorbed, producing a peak of 3 mg/L (6.5 μmol/L) 2–4 hr after administration of a 200 mg dose; antacids and iron may markedly impair oral absorption; milk causes about a 30% decrease in bioavailability and food has little effect. Widely distributed in the body, penetrating most cavities including CSF (12–20% of serum levels). The drug is $88 \pm 5\%$ plasma protein bound. V_d is 0.75 ± 0.32 L/kg; Cl is 0.032 ± 0.01 L/hr/kg. About $41 \pm 19\%$ is excreted unchanged in the urine in normal adults; the remainder is eliminated in feces via intestinal and biliary secretion.[48,230,231]

$t_{1/2}$. 16 ± 6 hr in normal adults; slightly prolonged in severe renal impairment.[48,230]

Adverse Reactions. IV administration frequently produces phlebitis. Oral doxycycline causes less alteration of intestinal flora than other tetracyclines, but it may cause nausea and diarrhea with equal frequency. It binds to calcium in teeth and bones, which may cause discoloration of teeth in children, especially during growth; however, doxycycline has a lower potential for this effect than most other tetracyclines. In contrast to other tetracyclines, doxycycline is not very antianabolic and will not further increase azotemia in renal failure. Phototoxic skin reactions occur occasionally.[227,228,230]

Contraindications. Hypersensitivity to any tetracycline.

Precautions. Not recommended in pregnancy or in children ≤8 yr because permanent staining of the child's teeth will occur. Use with caution in severe hepatic dysfunction. The syrup contains sulfites.

Drug Interactions. Antacids containing di- or trivalent cations, bismuth salts, or zinc salts interfere with absorption of oral tetracyclines. Oral iron salts lower doxycycline serum levels, even of IV doxycycline, by interfering with absorption and enterohepatic circulation. Barbiturates, carbamazepine, and phenytoin may enhance doxycycline hepatic metabolism, possibly decreasing its effect. Tetracyclines may interfere with enterohepatic circulation of contraceptive hormones, causing menstrual irregularities and possibly unplanned pregnancies. Combined use of tetracyclines with the bactericidal agents such as penicillins may result in decreased activity in some infections.

Parameters to Monitor. Check for signs of phlebitis daily during IV use.

Notes. Doxycycline is the tetracycline of choice because it is better tolerated than other tetracyclines, although tetracyclines are the drugs of choice for very few infections.[227,228] Each vial contains 480 mg of ascorbic acid per 100 mg of doxycycline hyclate for injection. (*See* Tetracyclines Comparison Chart.)

TETRACYCLINE AND SALTS   Various

Pharmacology. Tetracycline has an antimicrobial spectrum of activity similar to doxycycline. Current uses are for treatment of infection caused by *Chlamydia* spp., *Mycoplasma* spp., and *Brucella* spp.[227,228] It is also used as a treatment for acne and in some regimens against *Helicobacter pylori*. (*See* Gastrointestinal Drugs, Treatment of *Helicobacter pylori* Infection in Peptic Ulcer Disease.)

Adult Dosage. PO 1–2 g/day in 2–4 divided doses. Reduce dosage, or preferably use another drug, in severe renal or hepatic impairment.

Pediatric Dosage. PO (<8 yr) not recommended; (>8 yr) 25–50 mg/kg/day in 2–4 divided doses.

Dosage Forms. (*See* Tetracyclines Comparison Chart.)

Pharmacokinetics. Tetracycline is well absorbed from the GI tract. Multivalent cations chelate tetracyclines and inhibit absorption; warn patients to avoid concurrent antacids, dairy products, iron, or sucralfate. The half-life of tetracycline is about 10 hr, increasing to as high as 108 hr in anuria.[48]

Adverse Reactions. GI irritation is frequent and may result in esophageal ulceration if the drug is taken at bedtime with insufficient fluid. Disruption of bowel flora occurs frequently and may result in diarrhea, candidiasis, or rarely pseudomembranous colitis. Antianabolic effects produce elevated BUN, hyperphosphatemia, and acidosis in patients with renal failure. Acute fatty infiltration of the liver with pancreatitis occurs rarely with large (>2 g) IV doses, especially in pregnancy; avoid tetracyclines in pregnancy. Tetracyclines should not be given to children <8 yr because of binding of calcium in teeth and resultant discoloration.

Drug Interactions. Oral absorption is markedly inhibited by di- and trivalent cations (eg, antacids).

TETRACYCLINES COMPARISON CHART

DRUG	DOSAGE FORMS	ADULT DOSAGE	PERCENTAGE ORAL ABSORPTION	HALF-LIFE (HOURS) Normal	HALF-LIFE (HOURS) Anuria	PERCENTAGE EXCRETED UNCHANGED IN URINE	COMMENTS
Demeclocycline Hydrochloride Declomycin	Cap 150 mg Tab 150, 300 mg.	PO 600 mg/day in 2-4 divided doses. PO for SIADH 300 mg tid-qid.	66	15	40-60	42	Most phototoxic tetracycline; causes nephrogenic diabetes insipidus rarely.
Doxycycline Calcium **Doxycycline Hyclate** **Doxycycline Monohydrate** Vibramycin Various	Cap 50, 100 mg Tab 100 mg Susp 5 mg/mL Syrup 10 mg/mL Inj 100, 200 mg.	PO 100 mg q 12 hr for 2 doses, then 50-100 mg/day in 1-2 divided doses; IV 200 mg in 1-2 divided doses on day 1, then 100-200 mg/day.	93	16 ± 6	12-22	41	Safest in renal failure because of its lack of accumulation and lack of antianabolic effects. Well tolerated when given IV.
Minocycline Hydrochloride Minocin Various	Cap 50, 100 mg Tab 50, 100 mg Susp 10 mg/mL Inj (IV only) 100 mg.	PO or IV 200 mg initially, then 100 mg q 12 hr.	95-100	16 ± 2	11-23	11	Very frequent transient vestibular toxicity.

(continued)

179

TETRACYCLINES COMPARISON CHART (continued)

DRUG	DOSAGE FORMS	ADULT DOSAGE	PERCENTAGE ORAL ABSORPTION	HALF-LIFE (HOURS) Normal	HALF-LIFE (HOURS) Anuria	PERCENTAGE EXCRETED UNCHANGED IN URINE	COMMENTS
Oxytetracycline **Oxytetracycline Hydrochloride** **Oxytetracycline Calcium** Various	Cap 250 mg Inj (IM only, contains 2% lidocaine) 50, 125 mg/mL.	PO 1–2 g/day in 2–4 divided doses; IM 250 mg once daily to 300 mg/day in 2–3 doses.	58	9	47–66	70	Seldom used. IM produces lower serum levels than oral.
Tetracycline Various	Cap 100, 250, 500 mg	PO 1–2 g/day in 2–4 divided doses.	77	10.6 ± 5	57–108	60	(*See* monograph.)
Tetracycline Hydrochloride Various	Tab 250, 500 mg Susp 25 mg/mL Top Soln 2.2 mg/mL Top Oint 3%.	Top (soln) for acne apply in the morning and evening.					

From reference 48 and product information.

Miscellaneous Antimicrobials

ATOVAQUONE   Mepron

Pharmacology. Atovaquone is a highly lipophilic hydroxynaphthoquinone with activity against *Pneumocystis carinii, Toxoplasma gondii,* and *Plasmodium* spp. It is a structural analogue of ubiquinone, a small hydrophobic respiratory chain electron carrier molecule found in mitochondria. The mechanism of antipneumocystis activity by atovaquone is unclear, but may be inhibition of the mitochondrial electron transport chain, causing inhibition of pyrimidine synthesis and leading to inhibition of nucleic acid and ATP synthesis.[232,233]

Administration and Adult Dosage. PO for *P. carinii* pneumonia 750 mg bid for 21 days.

Special Populations. *Pediatric Dosage.* Safety and efficacy not established.

Geriatric Dosage. (>65 yr) not evaluated, but dosage adjustment appears not to be necessary.

Other Conditions. Dosage alteration is not required with renal or hepatic impairment.

Dosage Forms. Susp 150 mg/mL.

Patient Instructions. It is extremely important to take this medication with food to increase absorption; failure to do so may limit response to therapy. Shake the suspension gently prior to use.

Missed Doses. Take this drug at regular intervals. If you miss a dose take it as soon as you remember. If it is about time for the next dose, take that dose only. Leave a minimum of 6–8 hours between doses. Do not double the dose or take extra.

Pharmacokinetics. *Serum Levels.* Steady-state serum levels >14 mg/L (>38 μmol/L) are correlated with survival in patients with PCP; serum levels <6 mg/L (<16 μmol/L) may be ineffective.[233]

Fate. Atovaquone exhibits slow, irregular absorption, depending on the formulation. A high-fat meal increases absorption of the suspension 2.3-fold compared with the fasting state. A peak concentration of 11.5 mg/L (31 μmol/L) is achieved with a single 750 mg dose of the suspension. Oral administration of 750 mg bid as the suspension produces a steady-state level of 24 mg/L (65 μmol/L). More than 99.9% is protein bound, and the drug does not appear to cross the blood-brain barrier well. It appears to undergo enterohepatic cycling, with >94% excreted over 21 days in the feces, with no metabolite identified, and <0.6% renally excreted.[233]

$t_{1/2}$. 67 ± 10 hr.[233]

Adverse Effects. Maculopapular rash occurs frequently, but many patients are able to continue atovaquone therapy, and in most instances, the rash resolves without sequelae. GI disturbances including abdominal pain, nausea, vomiting, and diarrhea occur frequently. Fever, headaches, and insomnia have also been reported frequently. Elevations of hepatic transaminases and hyponatremia occur frequently, but do not require cessation of therapy.

Contraindications. Severe diarrhea or malabsorption syndrome, because pre-existing diarrhea is associated with poor outcome, presumably as a result of decreased absorption and serum levels.

Precautions. Lactation. Consider alternative therapy in patients who cannot take the drug with food or with GI disorders that may decrease oral absorption.

Drug Interactions. Rifampin may decrease atovaquone serum levels.

Parameters to Monitor. Baseline and periodic liver function tests for patients on prolonged treatment.

Notes. Atovaquone has been used for prevention of *P. carinii* pneumonia in patients who are unable to tolerate or who have failed other traditional prevention medication; although clinical trials are ongoing, the safety, efficacy, and optimal dosage for this indication are not well established.

CHLORAMPHENICOL AND SALTS   Chloromycetin, Various

Pharmacology. Chloramphenicol is a broad-spectrum bacteriostatic antibiotic isolated from *Streptomyces venezuelae* and is particularly useful against ampicillin-resistant *Haemophilus influenzae, Salmonella* spp., rickettsial infections such as Rocky Mountain Spotted Fever, typhoid fever, and most anerobic organisms. It inhibits protein synthesis by binding the 50S ribosomal subunit and may be bactericidal against some bacteria including pneumococci, meningococci, and *H. influenzae.* Chloramphenicol has variable activity against vancomycin-resistant enterococcal infection. Resistance occurs because of impermeability of the cell wall or bacterial production of chloramphenicol acetyltransferase, a plasmid-mediated enzyme that acetylates chloramphenicol into a microbiologically inert form.[189,228,234,235]

Administration and Adult Dosage. **IV** 50–100 mg/kg/day depending on severity, location, and organism in 4 divided doses. **IM not recommended.**

Special Populations. *Pediatric Dosage.* **IV** (<7 days or <2 kg) 25 mg/kg once daily; (neonates >7 days and >2 kg) 25 mg/kg q 12 hr; (older infants and children) 50–100 mg/kg/day given q 6 hr. These regimens produce unpredictable levels, and serum level monitoring is recommended.[236] **IM not recommended.**

Geriatric Dosage. Same as adult dosage.

Other Conditions. Reduce dosage with impaired liver function as guided by serum levels; no alteration necessary in impaired renal function.[236]

Dosage Forms. **Inj** (as sodium succinate) 1 g (100 mg/mL when reconstituted); **Ophth Oint** 10 mg/g; **Ophth Pwdr for Soln** 25 mg/vial; **Ophth Soln** 5 mg/mL; **Otic Soln** 5 mg/mL; **Top Crm** 10 mg/g (expressed as chloramphenicol base).

Pharmacokinetics. *Serum Levels.* (*See* Adverse Reactions.)

Fate. IV 1 g produces levels of 5–12 mg/L (15–37 μmol/L) 1 hr after administration to normal adults. In infants and young children, hydrolysis of succinate to the active form may be slow and incomplete. IM administration may produce serum levels of active drugs that are 50% lower than the equivalent oral dose. The drug attains therapeutic levels in most body cavities, the eye, and CSF; it is 53%

plasma protein bound. V_d is 0.94 ± 0.06 L/kg; Cl is 0.14 ± 0.01 L/hr/kg. Most of the drug is eliminated by glucuronidation in the liver followed by excretion in the urine; the remainder is excreted in the urine unchanged. The rate of glucuronidation and renal elimination is greatly reduced in neonates; 6.5–80% of succinate may be excreted unhydrolyzed. Urine concentrations may be inadequate to treat UTIs, especially in patients with moderately to severely impaired renal function. A small amount (2–4%) of a dose appears in the bile and feces, mostly as the glucuronide.[48,228]

$t_{1/2}$. 4 ± 2 hr in healthy adults;[48] extremely prolonged and variable in neonates, infants, and young children. Unpredictable in patients with impaired liver function. Some normal patients and patients with impaired renal function exhibit impaired free drug elimination.

Adverse Reactions. Serum levels >25 mg/L (>77 μmol/L) frequently produce reversible bone marrow depression with reticulocytopenia, decreased hemoglobin, increased serum iron and iron-binding globulin saturation, thrombocytopenia, and mild leukopenia.[236] The drug inhibits iron uptake by bone marrow, and anemic patients do not respond to iron or vitamin B_{12} therapy while receiving chloramphenicol. This anemia most often follows parenteral therapy, large dosages, long duration of therapy, or impaired drug elimination. Complete recovery usually occurs within 1–2 weeks after drug discontinuation. Aplastic anemia occurs rarely (1/12,000 to 1/50,000) and may be fatal. It is not dose related and can occur long after a short course of oral or parenteral therapy;[236] its occurrence following ophthalmic or parenteral use is controversial.[237] Fatal cardiovascular-respiratory collapse (gray syndrome) may develop in neonates given excessive dosages. This syndrome is associated with serum levels of about 50–100 mg/L (155–310 μmol/L).[236] A similar syndrome has been reported in children and adults given large overdoses.

Contraindications. Trivial infections; prophylactic use; uses other than those for which it is indicated.

Precautions. Pregnancy; lactation. Use with caution in patients with liver disease (especially cirrhosis, ascites, and jaundice) or pre-existing hematologic disorders, or patients receiving other bone marrow depressants. May cause hemolytic episodes in patients with G-6-PD deficiency; observe dosage recommendations closely in neonates and infants.

Drug Interactions. Chloramphenicol increases serum concentrations of phenytoin, warfarin, and sulfonylurea oral hypoglycemic agents. Both phenytoin and phenobarbital can decrease serum levels of chloramphenicol.

Parameters to Monitor. CBC, with platelet and reticulocyte counts before and frequently during therapy; serum iron and iron-binding globulin saturation may also be useful. Liver and renal function tests before and occasionally during therapy.

CLINDAMYCIN SALTS
Cleocin, Various

Pharmacology. Clindamycin is a semisynthetic 7-chloro, 7-deoxylincomycin derivative that is active against most Gram-positive organisms except enterococci and *Clostridium difficile*. Gram-negative aerobes are resistant, but most anerobes are sensitive. It inhibits bacterial protein synthesis by binding to the 50S ribosomal subunit; it is bactericidal or bacteriostatic depending on the concentration, organism, and inoculum.[238,239]

Administration and Adult Dosage. **PO** 150–450 mg q 6 hr; **PO for prevention of endocarditis in patients at risk undergoing dental, oral, or upper respiratory tract procedures, and who are allergic to penicillin** 600 mg 1 hr before procedure.[199] **IM or IV** 600 mg–2.7 g/day in 2–4 divided doses, to a maximum of 4.8 g/day. **IV for endocarditis prophylaxis** 600 mg within 30 min prior to dental procedure. Single IM doses >600 mg are not recommended; infuse IV no faster than 30 mg/min. **Top for acne** apply bid. **Vag for bacterial vaginosis** 1 applicatorful hs for 7 days.

Dosage Individualization. *Pediatric Dosage.* **PO** (<10 kg) give no less than 37.5 mg q 8 hr; (>10 kg) 8–25 mg/kg/day in 3 or 4 divided doses; **PO for endocarditis prophylaxis** 20 mg/kg 1 hr prior to dental procedure. **IM or IV** (<1 month) 15–20 mg/kg/day in 3 or 4 divided doses; the lower dosage may be adequate for premature infants; (>1 month) 15–40 mg/kg/day in 3 or 4 divided doses (not less than 300 mg/day in severe infection, regardless of weight). **IV for endocarditis prophylaxis** 20 mg/kg within 30 min prior to dental procedure.

Geriatric Dosage. Same as adult dosage.

Other Conditions. Dosage adjustment is unnecessary in renal impairment or cirrhosis, although the effect of acute liver disease is unknown.[231,238,240]

Dosage Forms. **Cap** (as hydrochloride) 75, 150, 300 mg; **Soln** (as palmitate) 15 mg/mL (reconstituted); **Inj** (as phosphate) 150 mg/mL; **Top Soln** (as phosphate) 1%; **Top Gel** (as phosphate) 1%; **Vag Crm** 2%.

Patient Instructions. Report any severe diarrhea or blood in the stools immediately and do *not* take antidiarrheal medication. Do not refrigerate the reconstituted oral solution because it will thicken.

Missed Doses. Take this drug at regular intervals. If you miss a dose take it as soon as you remember. If it is about time for the next dose, take that dose only. Leave a minimum of 4–6 hours between doses. Do not double the dose or take extra.

Pharmacokinetics. *Fate.* Absorption is nearly 87% and is the same from the capsule or the solution; food may delay, but not decrease, absorption. The palmitate and phosphate esters are absorbed intact and rapidly hydrolyzed to the active base. Unhydrolyzed phosphate ester usually constitutes <20% of the total peak serum level after parenteral clindamycin, but may increase to 40% in patients with impaired renal function. A 500 mg oral dose produces a peak serum level of 5–6 mg/L (12–14 μmol/L) in 1 hr. A 300 mg IM dose produces a peak level of 5–6 mg/L 1–2 hr postinjection. A 600 mg IV dose infused over 30 min produces a peak serum level of 10 mg/L (23 μmol/L). The drug is widely distributed throughout the body except the CSF. It is 94% plasma protein bound; V_d is 1.1 ± 0.3 L/kg; Cl is 0.28 ± 0.08 L/hr/kg. There is hepatic metabolism and excretion of active forms in the bile. From 5–10% of the absorbed dose is recovered as unchanged drug and active metabolites in the urine within 24 hr.[48,231,238,241]

$t_{1/2}$. 2.9 ± 0.7 hr; increased in premature infants;[48] unchanged or slightly increased in severe renal disease; may be increased or unchanged in liver disease.[239]

Adverse Reactions. After oral administration anorexia, nausea, vomiting, cramps, and diarrhea occur frequently.[231,238,240] Oral and, rarely, parenteral clindamycin may cause severe, sometimes fatal, pseudomembranous colitis (PMC), which may be clinically indistinguishable at onset from non-PMC diarrhea.[238] Antibiotic-associated PMC is secondary to overgrowth of toxin-producing *Clostridium difficile.* Symptoms usually appear 2–9 days after initiation of therapy. PMC has been reported after topical administration.[240] PMC is terminated in many patients by discontinuing the antibiotic immediately; however, if diarrhea is severe or does not improve promptly after discontinuation, treat with metronidazole or vancomycin.[238,239] The value of corticosteroids, cholestyramine, and antispasmodics in the management of antibiotic-associated diarrhea and PMC has not been established.[238] Antidiarrheals such as diphenoxylate or loperamide may worsen PMC and should *not* be used.

Precautions. Pregnancy; lactation. Use with caution in neonates under 4 weeks of age, and in patients with liver disease. Discontinue *immediately* if severe diarrhea occurs. Drug accumulation may occur in patients with severe concomitant hepatic and renal dysfunction, but data are lacking.

Drug Interactions. Clindamycin may enhance the action of nondepolarizing neuromuscular blocking agents. Kaolin-pectin mixture delays but does not decrease oral absorption of clindamycin.

Parameters to Monitor. Observe for changes in bowel frequency.

Notes. Oral solution is stable for 2 weeks at room temperature following reconstitution; do not refrigerate.

METRONIDAZOLE   Flagyl, MetroGel, Various

Pharmacology. Metronidazole is a synthetic nitroimidazole active against *Trichomonas vaginalis* (trichomoniasis), *Entamoeba histolytica* (amebiasis), and *Giardia lamblia* (giardiasis); it is bactericidal against nearly all obligate anerobic bacteria including *Bacteroides fragilis.* It is inactive against aerobic bacteria and requires microbial reduction by a nitroreductase enzyme to form highly reactive intermediates that disrupt bacterial DNA and inhibit nucleic acid synthesis, leading to cell death.[236]

Administration and Adult Dosage. **PO or IV for anaerobic infections** 15 mg/kg (usually 1 g) initially, followed by 7.5 mg/kg (usually 500 mg) q 8–12 hr, to a maximum of 2 g/day. Infuse each IV dose over 1 hr. **PO for antibiotic-associated colitis** 250 mg qid for 7–10 days.[242] (*See* Notes.) **PO for trichomoniasis** 2 g as a single dose or in 2 doses on the same day, or 500 mg bid for 7 days.[177] **PO for giardiasis** 250 mg tid for 5 days. (*See* Notes.)[242] **PO for symptomatic intestinal amebiasis** (amebic dysentery) 750 mg tid for 10 days. **PO for extraintestinal**

amebiasis 750 mg tid for 10 days;[242] some practitioners include a drug effective against the intestinal cyst form, because occasional failures with metronidazole therapy have been reported. **PO for bacterial vaginosis** 500 mg bid for 7 days, or 2 g as a single dose.[177] **Vag for bacterial vaginosis** 1 applicatorful (5 g) bid for 5 days. **Top for rosacea** apply bid.

Special Populations. *Pediatric Dosage.* **IV for anaerobic infections** (preterm infants) 15 mg/kg once, then 7.5 mg/kg q 24–48 hr; (term infants) 15 mg/kg once, then 7.5 mg/kg q 12–24 hr; (infants >1 week old and children) same as adult mg/kg dosage. **PO for giardiasis** 15 mg/kg/day in 3 divided doses for 5 days, to a maximum of 750 mg/day. (*See* Notes.) **PO for amebic dysentery or extraintestinal amebias is** 35–50 mg/kg/day in 3 divided doses for 10 days, to a maximum of 2.5 g/day.

Geriatric Dosage. (>65 yr) decreased clearance may result in accumulation of the drug. Dosage reduction or changing dosage interval to once or twice daily are reasonable modifications to avoid potential adverse reactions.[243]

Other Conditions. No dosage alteration required with renal impairment. Patients with substantial liver dysfunction metabolize metronidazole slowly, with resultant accumulation of metronidazole and its metabolites in the serum. For such patients, it has been suggested that dosage intervals be increased to 12–24 hr, although specific guidelines are not available.[243]

Dosage Forms. **Tab** 250, 500 mg; **Inj** 500 mg; **Top Gel** 0.75%; **Vag Gel** 0.75%.

Patient Instructions. This drug may be taken with food to minimize stomach upset. It may cause a harmless dark discoloration of the urine and metallic taste in the mouth. Nausea, vomiting, flushing, and faintness may occur if alcohol is taken during therapy with this drug.

Missed Doses. Take this drug at regular intervals. If you miss a dose take it as soon as you remember. If it is about time for the next dose, take that dose only. Leave a minimum of 4–6 hours between doses. Do not double the dose or take extra.

Pharmacokinetics. *Serum Levels.* Not used clinically.

Fate. IV 500 mg q 12 hr over 1 hr produces steady-state peak and trough levels of 23.6 mg/L (138 μmol/L) and 6.7 mg/L (39 μmol/L), respectively. IV 500 mg q 8 hr over 1 hr produces steady-state peak and trough levels of 27.4 mg/L (160 μmol/L) and 15.5 mg/L (91 μmol/L), respectively. Well absorbed orally with levels similar to those following IV infusion; 250 and 500 mg doses produce peak concentrations of 4–6 mg/L (23–35 μmol/L) and 10–13 mg/L (58–76 μmol/L), respectively, at 1–2 hr in adults. Bioavailability of vaginal gel is 53–58%. Less than 20% plasma protein bound; wide distribution with therapeutic levels in many tissues, including abscesses, bile, bone, breast milk, CSF, and saliva. V_d is 0.85 ± 0.25 L/kg; Cl is 0.07 ± 0.02 L/hr/kg. Extensively metabolized in the liver by hydroxylation, oxidation, and glucuronide formation; 44–80% excreted in the urine in 24 hr, about 6–18% as unchanged drug.[242,243]

$t_{1/2}$. 6–10 hr in adults; not increased with impaired renal function; prolonged variably with severe hepatic impairment.[48,242,243]

Adverse Effects. Metallic taste in mouth and GI complaints occur frequently with high dosages. Occasional dizziness, vertigo, and paresthesias have been reported with very high dosages. Reversible mild neutropenia reported occasionally.[189,242] Reversible, rare, but severe peripheral neuropathy may occur with high dosages given over prolonged periods. Antibiotic-associated colitis has been reported rarely with oral metronidazole. The IV preparation is occasionally associated with phlebitis at the infusion site. Experimental production of tumors in some rodent species and mutations in bacteria have raised concern regarding potential carcinogenicity; to date, mammalian testing and human epidemiologic research have not detected an appreciable risk, although further data are needed.[242]

Contraindications. First trimester of pregnancy, although there is no direct evidence of teratogenicity in humans or animals.[189]

Precautions. Pregnancy; lactation; active CNS disease or neutropenia.

Drug Interactions. Disulfiram-like reactions are reported with concurrent alcohol use, but are uncommon. Confusion and psychotic episodes have been reported with concurrent disulfiram; avoid this combination, if possible. Metronidazole inhibits CYP3A3/4 and may affect the metabolism of many drugs; the best documented is an enhanced hypoprothrombinemic response to warfarin. Phenytoin metabolism may also be inhibited.

Parameters to Monitor. Before and after the completion of any lengthy or repeated courses of therapy, monitor WBC count. Monitor serum metronidazole levels as well as signs of toxicity in patients with severe liver disease.[243]

Notes. The treatment of *asymptomatic* trichomoniasis is controversial. Signs of endocervical inflammation or erosion on physical examination are considered an indication for treatment. Also, most practitioners treat asymptomatic male consorts, because lack of such treatment may be a cause of treatment failure or recurrent infection of the female partner.[177] Metronidazole has been used in combination regimens to treat *Helicobacter pylori* infected patients with duodenal or gastric ulcers. (*See* Gastrointestinal Drugs, Treatment of *Helicobacter pylori* in Peptic Ulcer Disease Comparison Chart.) Although it is slightly less effective than **vancomycin,** metronidazole is considered by some to be the drug of choice for antibiotic-associated pseudomembranous colitis because of its lower cost[244] and because of the emergence of vancomycin-resistant enterococci because of vancomycin overuse.

NITROFURANTOIN   Macrodantin, Macrobid, Various

Pharmacology. Nitrofurantoin is a synthetic nitrofuran that is active against most bacteria that cause UTIs except *Pseudomonas aeruginosa, Proteus* spp., many *Enterobacter* spp., and *Klebsiella* spp. The drug is used primarily to prevent recurrent UTIs, but is also effective in the treatment of uncomplicated UTIs.[245]

Adult Dosage. PO for UTI (macrocrystals) 50–100 mg qid with meals and hs for treatment; (Macrobid) 100 mg bid for 7 days. **PO for chronic suppression** 50–100 mg hs. The drug should be taken with food.

Pediatric Dosage. PO for UTI 5–7 mg/kg/day in 4 divided doses for treatment; **PO for chronic suppression** 1 mg/kg/day in 1–2 doses.

Dosage Forms. Cap (macrocrystals) 25, 50, 100 mg; **Susp** 5 mg/mL; **Cap** containing 25 mg as macrocrystals and 75 mg in an SR form (Macrobid).

Pharmacokinetics. Following oral absorption, serum and extraurinary tissue concentrations are subtherapeutic. About 25–35% is excreted in urine with a urine concentration of about 200 mg/L from an average dose.

Adverse Reactions. Adverse effects are primarily nausea, vomiting, and diarrhea, and are dose related; use of the macrocrystalline form and administration with food may minimize GI distress. Hypersensitivity reactions, such as rash, occur only rarely. Acute allergic pneumonitis is reversible with discontinuation of therapy. Chronic interstitial pulmonary fibrosis also occurs occasionally with long-term therapy and may be irreversible. Ascending polyneuropathy associated with prolonged high-dose therapy or use of the drug in renal failure is only slowly reversible. Intravascular hemolysis may occur in patients with severe G-6-PD deficiency. Although the drug is mutagenic in mammalian cells, there is no clinical evidence of carcinogenicity or teratogenicity.

PENTAMIDINE ISETHIONATE   Pentam 300, NebuPent

Pharmacology. Pentamidine is an aromatic diamidine used in the treatment of trypanosomiasis and *Pneumocystis carinii* pneumonia. Pentamidine inhibits dihydrofolate reductase, interferes with anaerobic glycolysis, inhibits oxidative phosphorylation, and limits nucleic acid and protein synthesis, but the mechanism by which pentamidine kills *P. carinii* is unclear.[246]

Administration and Adult Dosage. **IV (preferred) or IM** 3–4 mg/kg/day as a single dose for 2–3 weeks; infuse IV over 60 min. **Inhal for *P. carinii* pneumonia prophylaxis in high-risk HIV-infected patients** 300 mg q 4 weeks via special nebulizer. (*See* Notes.)

Special Populations. *Pediatric Dosage.* Same as adult dosage.

Geriatric Dosage. Same as adult dosage.

Other Conditions. Dosage adjustment does not appear necessary in renal impairment.[247]

Dosage Forms. **Inj** 300 mg; **Inhal** 300 mg.

Pharmacokinetics. *Serum Levels.* Not used clinically.

Fate. Negligible oral absorption. Peak serum levels of 0.5–3 mg/L (1.5–8.8 μmol/L) occur after 4 mg/kg IV infusion. Serum levels are very low after inhalation (<0.1 mg/L). About 70% plasma protein bound; distributed widely in tissues, with highest concentrations found in spleen, liver, kidneys, and adrenal glands. V_c is 3 L/kg; terminal V_d is 190 ± 70 L/kg; Cl is 1.08 ± 0.42 L/hr/kg. There are no data on the effects of liver impairment. Less than 20% of a dose is excreted unchanged in urine.[48,248]

$t_{1/2}$. α phase 1.2 ± 0.6 hr; terminal elimination half-life is up to 29 ± 25 days, suggesting rapid tissue uptake with slow release and subsequent urinary excretion.[247]

Adverse Reactions. With IV administration, nephrotoxicity occurs in up to 25% of patients, hypoglycemia in up to 27%, and hypotension in up to 10% of patients. Fever, rash, leukopenia, and liver damage occur occasionally. Hyperglycemia and type 1 diabetes mellitus have been reported as well as pancreatitis. Pentamidine-induced torsades de pointes has been reported rarely. IM injection frequently produces pain and abscess formation at the injection site. With aerosolized pentamidine, reversible bronchoconstriction and unpleasant taste occur frequently. Severe adverse reactions are less frequent, but reports of pancreatitis, hypoglycemia, and cutaneous eruptions have occurred rarely, suggesting some systemic absorption.[246]

Precautions. Use with caution in diabetes mellitus.

Drug Interactions. IV pentamidine may increase the risk of hypocalcemia with foscarnet; avoid this combination, if possible, although inhaled pentamidine does not seem to be a risk factor.

Parameters to Monitor. Obtain serum glucose, Cr_s, BUN, liver function tests, electrolytes, CBC, and platelet count daily. Monitor blood pressure after administration.

Notes. Concomitant therapy with both pentamidine and **trimethoprim-sulfamethoxazole** appears to offer no benefit and may be additively toxic. There is concern about occupational exposure with inhalation therapy. No studies have yet determined the health effects of exposure to pentamidine itself; however, transmission of tuberculosis to health care workers has been attributed partly to the use of aerosolized pentamidine among clinic patients coinfected with HIV and tuberculosis. Health care workers administering aerosolized pentamidine should wear masks and protective eye wear.[246]

QUINUPRISTIN AND DALFOPRISTIN　　Synercid
(Investigational, Rhone-Poulenc Rorer)

Pharmacology. Quinupristin and dalfopristin is a combination of two streptogramin antibiotics that are naturally occurring compounds isolated from *Streptomyces pristinaspiralis.* Quinupristin, a derivative of pristinamycin IA, and dalfopristin, a derivative of pristinamycin IIA, are combined in a fixed ratio of 30:70 (w/w). This combination inhibits protein synthesis by sequential binding to the 50S subunit of bacterial ribosomes; its synergistic activity may be caused by binding of dalfopristin, altering conformation of the ribosome such that its affinity for quinupristin is increased. Individually, pristinamycin I and pristinamycin II are bacteriostatic, but in combination they are bactericidal against Gram-positive bacteria, including methicillin-resistant *Staphylococcus aureus* (MRSA). Synergy has been reported with vancomycin against MRSA and multiply resistant enterococci. It also has activity against anaerobic organisms, but most Gram-negative organisms such as the Enterobacteriacae, *Acinetobacter* spp., and *Pseudomonas aeruginosa* are resistant.[249–251] Although the drug is effective for many types of infections, it should generally be reserved for treating resistant organisms.

Adult Dosage. IV 7.5 mg/kg (of the combination) q 8–12 hr infused in D5W over 60 min has been used investigationally. A dosage reduction to 5 mg/kg q 8–12 hr should be considered in patients with renal or hepatic impairment who do not tolerate the usual dosage.

Dosage Forms. Inj 500 mg (quinupristin 150 mg/dalfopristin 350 mg).

Pharmacokinetics. The pharmacokinetics are complex and not fully elucidated. Quinupristin peak concentrations are 2.4–2.8 mg/L (2.3–2.7 μmol/L) and dalfopristin's are 6.2–7.2 mg/L (9–10.4 μmol/L) after a 7.5 mg/kg dose in healthy volunteers. Quinupristin is about 90% protein bound and dalfopristin is 10–36% bound in vitro. Clearance of both drugs decreases with repeated doses and in obese patients. Dalfopristin may have an active metabolite. Both drugs are primarily eliminated in feces, with only about 15–20% excreted unchanged in urine. Half-lives are about 1 hr for quinupristin and 0.5–1 hr for dalfopristin, both possibly increased in cirrhosis.

Adverse Reactions. Mild to moderate local reactions of itching, pain, and burning at the injection site are frequent and subside with continued use. Nausea, vomiting, diarrhea, and headache have also been reported frequently. Occasionally, reversible myalgia and arthralgia occur and liver function tests are increased.

Drug Interactions. Quinupristin/dalfopristin inhibits CYP3A4 and markedly impairs cyclosporine clearance, requiring cyclosporine dosage reduction.

TRIMETHOPRIM   Proloprim, Trimpex, Various

Pharmacology. Trimethoprim is a synthetic folate-antagonist antibacterial. (*See* Trimethoprim and Sulfamethoxazole.) Trimethoprim is effective in acute UTI. It has a potential advantage over the sulfa-containing combination in patients with allergy or toxicity attributed to sulfonamides; however, the relative potential for trimethoprim alone to permit the development of resistance is undetermined. Used alone, trimethoprim is ineffective against *Pneumocystis carinii,* but in combination with **dapsone** (a sulfone), it is effective in treating mild to moderate *P. carinii* pneumonia (PCP).[224,225]

Adult Dosage. **PO for uncomplicated acute UTI** 200 mg/day in 1 or 2 doses for 10 days. **PO for the treatment of mild to moderate (PaO$_2$ >60 mm Hg) PCP** 20 mg/kg/day in 3 or 4 divided doses with dapsone 100 mg once daily.

Dosage Forms. Tab 100, 200 mg.

Pharmacokinetics. Trimethoprim is rapidly absorbed orally. A 100 mg dose yields a serum concentration of 1 mg/L (3.4 μmol/L) 1–4 hr after the dose. It is 20% plasma protein bound and 40–50% is excreted unchanged in urine. Half-life is 8–10 hr with normal renal function.

Adverse Reactions. Occasional adverse effects are mild thrombocytopenia, nausea, fever, and rash; the frequency appears to be dose related. Methemoglobinemia and dose-related hemolysis have occurred in patients with G-6-PD deficiency receiving dapsone with trimethoprim; it is important to check G-6-PD status prior to initiating combination therapy.

TRIMETREXATE   Neutrexin

Pharmacology. Trimetrexate is a lipophilic analogue of methotrexate that inhibits dihydrofolate reductase, leading to the disruption of purine biosynthesis. It has activity against *Pneumocystis carinii* and *Toxoplasma gondii* and has demonstrated modest efficacy against a number of malignancies. It is approved for the treatment of moderate to severe *P. carinii* pneumonia (PCP) in immunocompromised patients and has also been used investigationally in advanced solid tumors alone or in combination with **fluorouracil** and **leucovorin**.[252-254]

Adult Dosage. IV for moderate to severe PCP 45 mg/m^2/day infused over 60–90 min for 21 days. Give IV or PO calcium leucovorin 20 mg/m^2 q 6 hr concomitantly and continue it for 3 days after the end of trimetrexate administration. **IV for colorectal cancer** 110 mg/m^2 on day 1, followed by leucovorin 200 mg/m^2 and a fluorouracil-leucovorin regimen on day 2. **IV for advanced urogenital cancer** 8 mg/m^2/day for 5 days q 3 weeks.[255] Reduce dosage by 50% in patients with Cr_s >1.6 mg/dL.

Dosage Forms. Inj 25 mg.

Pharmacokinetics. Trimetrexate has at least two metabolites, both of which inhibit dihydrofolate reductase. It is eliminated primarily by hepatic metabolism; less than one-third is excreted unchanged in urine. The elimination half-life ranges from 4–12 hr in patients with AIDS and PCP, and from 8–26 hr in patients with cancer.

Adverse Reactions. The primary toxicity is myelosuppression (neutropenia, thrombocytopenia, and anemia); myelosuppression is minimized with concurrent administration of calcium leucovorin. Hypoalbuminemia (≤3.5 g/dL) or hypoproteinemia (≤6 g/dL) increase the risk of severe or life-threatening myelosuppression, presumably because of increased unbound drug levels.[256] Elevated liver function tests, fever, rash, peripheral neuropathy, mucositis, and nausea or vomiting occur frequently. Hypersensitivity reactions and seizures are reported rarely.

VANCOMYCIN HYDROCHLORIDE   Vancocin, Various

Pharmacology. Vancomycin binds irreversibly to the cell wall in a manner slightly different from β-lactams. Many Gram-positive cocci and bacilli, including methicillin-resistant *Staphylococcus aureus* and *Clostridium difficile* are inhibited. Most Gram-negative bacteria are resistant, and vancomycin-resistant enterococci have been reported in association with overuse of vancomycin.[221]

Administration and Adult Dosage. IV 20–30 mg/kg/day (usually 2 g/day) in 2–4 divided doses as a dilute infusion over 1–2 hr. **PO for staphylococcal enterocolitis** 2 g/day in 2–4 divided doses. **PO for antibiotic-associated colitis** 125–500 mg q 6 hr for 7–10 days; retreat with a longer course if relapse occurs. (*See* Notes.) **Not for IM use.**

Dosage Individualization. *Pediatric Dosage.* **IV** (neonates) 20 mg/kg/day; (older infants and children) 40 mg/kg/day in 2–4 divided doses. **PO** 10–50 mg/kg/day in 4 divided doses. **Not for IM use.**

Geriatric Dosage. Same as adult dosage, but adjust for age-related reduction in renal function.

Other Conditions. Adjust dosage carefully in renal impairment; Cl is directly related to Cl_{cr}. Anuric patients on hemodialysis have been given the usual dose q 7–14 days, although one source recommends 8 mg/kg given q 6–24 hr according to renal function.[257] Dosage adjustment is unnecessary in liver disease.

Dosage Forms. Cap 125, 250 mg; **Susp** 1, 10 g; **Inj** 500 mg, 1 g.

Patient Instructions. Report pain at infusion site, dizziness, or fullness or ringing in ears with IV use; nausea or vomiting with oral use.

Missed Doses. (Oral) if you miss a dose, take it as soon as you remember. If it is about time for the next dose, take that dose only.

Pharmacokinetics. *Serum Levels.* Therapeutic range is not well defined. Ototoxicity has been associated with high serum concentrations, but has also been noted at lower levels.[257,258] Peaks associated with efficacy are between 20–40 mg/L (14–28 μmol/L); troughs >15 mg/L (10 μmol/L) may be excessive.

Fate. Oral absorption is negligible, although appreciable serum levels may be observed in patients with renal dysfunction receiving oral vancomycin for *C. difficile*–induced antibiotic-associated colitis. Fecal concentrations with PO 500 mg q 6 hr reach 3 mg/g. IV 500 mg produces serum levels of 6–10 mg/L (4–7 μmol/L) in 1 hr. Plasma protein binding is 30 ± 10%. The drug is widely distributed, except into the CSF, although some success has been reported in the treatment of meningitis, particularly in children. V_c is 0.1–0.15 L/kg; $V_{d\beta}$ is 0.39 ± 0.06 L/kg; Cl is 0.084 L/hr/kg with normal renal function. In renal impairment, Cl (in mL/min) may be estimated as $[0.79 \times Cl_{cr}$ (in mL/min)] + 3.5. Metabolism and biliary excretion are negligible; 80–90% is excreted unchanged in the urine within 48 hr.[48,259]

$t_{1/2}$. β phase 5.6 ± 1.8 hr, 6–10 days with renal impairment. No change with hepatic disease.[48,256]

Adverse Reactions. Chills, fever, nausea, and phlebitis may occur frequently, especially with direct injection of undiluted drug (not recommended). Rapid infusion may cause transient systolic hypotension.[260] The "red man" or "red neck" syndrome of erythema, pruritus, and localized edema is associated with histamine release caused by rapid infusions of doses of 500 mg or greater; it often does not occur or is less severe with subsequent doses.[261] Extravasation causes local tissue necrosis. Ototoxicity (auditory and vestibular) and possibly nephrotoxicity occur, but have not been definitely linked to high serum levels.[258,262] Eosinophilia, neutropenia, and urticarial rashes have been reported frequently. Side effects of vancomycin may not be as prevalent today as in the past, perhaps because of changes in the manufacturing process that eliminated some impurities.[263]

Precautions. Pregnancy. Use with caution in patients with impaired renal function or pre-existing hearing loss, or in those receiving other ototoxic or nephrotoxic agents.

Drug Interactions. Administration with an aminoglycoside may increase the risk of nephrotoxicity.[263]

Parameters to Monitor. With IV use, obtain initial renal function tests and repeat twice weekly during therapy. Routine monitoring of serum levels in patients with normal renal function is not recommended because it has questionable value, but is often performed.[262] Check for signs of phlebitis daily.

Notes. An alternative agent for treatment or prophylaxis of staphylococcal or streptococcal infections when a less toxic agent is inappropriate (eg, penicillin or cephalosporin allergy, or resistant organisms) or has not produced an adequate therapeutic response. Use of vancomycin in antibiotic-associated colitis is becoming less desirable because of the emergence of vancomycin-resistant enterococci caused by overuse of vancomycin. Reserve vancomycin for cases refractory to metronidazole.[244]

■ REFERENCES

1. Lortholary O et al. Aminoglycosides. *Med Clin North Am* 1995;79:761–87.
2. Gilbert DN. Aminoglycosides. In, Mandell GL et al., eds. *Principles and practice of infectious diseases*, 4th ed. Churchill Livingstone: New York; 1995:279–306.
3. Preston SL, Briceland LL. Single daily dosing of aminoglycosides. *Pharmacotherapy* 1995;15:297–306.
4. Nicolau DP et al. Experience with a once-daily aminoglycoside program administered to 2184 patients. *Antimicrob Agents Chemother* 1995;39:650–5.
5. Blaser J et al. Monitoring serum concentrations for once-daily netilmicin dosing regimens. *J Antimicrob Chemother* 1994;33:341–8.
6. Sarubbi FA, Hull JH. Amikacin serum concentrations, predictions of levels and dosage guidelines. *Ann Intern Med* 1978;89:612–8.
7. Walshe JJ et al. Crossover pharmacokinetic analysis comparing intravenous and intraperitoneal administration of tobramycin. *J Infect Dis* 1986;153:796–9.
8. Zaske DE. Aminoglycosides. In, Evans WE et al., eds. *Applied pharmacokinetics. Principles of therapeutic drug monitoring.* 3rd ed. Vancouver, WA: Applied Therapeutics; 1992:14-1–47.
9. Kahlmeter G, Dahlager JI. Aminoglycoside toxicity—a review of clinical studies published between 1975 and 1982. *J Antimicrob Chemother* 1984;13(suppl A):9–22.
10. McCormack JP, Jewesson PJ. A critical reevaluation of the "therapeutic range" of aminoglycosides. *Clin Infect Dis* 1992;14:320–9.
11. Pickering LK et al. Effect of concentration and time upon inactivation of tobramycin, gentamicin, netilmicin, and amikacin by azlocillin, carbenicillin, mecillinam, mezlocillin, and piperacillin. *J Pharmacol Exp Ther* 1981;217:345–9.
12. Thompson MIB et al. Gentamicin inactivation by piperacillin or carbenicillin in patients with end-stage renal disease. *Antimicrob Agents Chemother* 1982;21:268–73.
13. Erdmay SM et al. An updated comparison of drug dosing methods. Part III. Aminoglycoside antibiotics. *Clin Pharmacokinet* 1991;20:374–88.
14. Massey KL et al. Identification of children in whom routine aminoglycoside serum concentration monitoring is not cost-effective. *J Pediatr* 1986;109:897–901.
15. Moore RD et al. Clinical response to aminoglycoside therapy: importance of the ratio of peak concentration to minimum inhibitory concentration. *J Infect Dis* 1987;155:93–9.
16. Gallis HA et al. Amphotericin B: 30 years of clinical experience. *Rev Infect Dis* 1990;12:308–9.
17. Griswold MW et al. Is amphotericin B test dose needed? *Ann Pharmacother* 1998;32:475–7.
18. Kintzel PE et al. Practical guidelines for preparing and administering amphotericin B. *Am J Hosp Pharm* 1992;49:1156–64.
19. Kline S et al. Limited toxicity of prolonged therapy with high doses of amphotericin B lipid complex. *Clin Infect Dis* 1995;21:1154–8.
20. O'Donnell MR et al. Prediction of systemic fungal infection in allogeneic marrow recipients: impact of amphotericin B prophylaxis in high-risk patients. *J Clin Oncol* 1994;12:827–34.
21. Bennett JE. Antifungal drugs. In, Mandell GL et al, eds. *Principles and practice of infectious diseases.* 3rd ed. New York: Churchill Livingstone; 1990:361–76.
22. Varkey B et al. Pulmonary aspergilloma. A rational approach to treatment. *Am J Med* 1976;61:626–31.
23. Conneally E et al. Nebulized amphotericin B as prophylaxis against invasive aspergillosis in granulocytopenic patients. *Bone Marrow Transplant* 1990;5:403–6.
24. Meunier-Carpentier F et al. Amphotericin B nasal spray as prophylaxis against aspergillosis in patients with neutropenia. *N Engl J Med* 1984;311:1056. Letter.
25. Gordon MA et al. Corneal allescheriosis. *Arch Ophthalmol* 1959;62:758–63.
26. Perraut LE et al. Successful treatment of *Candida albicans* endophthalmitis with intravitreal amphotericin B. *Arch Ophthalmol* 1981;99:1565–7.
27. Christiansen KJ et al. Distribution and activity of amphotericin B in humans. *J Infect Dis* 1985;152:1037–43.
28. Kan VL et al. Comparative safety, tolerance, and pharmacokinetics of amphotericin B lipid complex and amphotericin desoxycholate in healthy male volunteers. *J Infect Dis* 1991;164:418–21.

29. Levy M et al. Amphotericin B-induced heart rate decrease in children. *Clin Pediatr* 1995;34:358–64.

30. Le Y et al. Amphotericin B-associated hypertension. *Ann Pharmacother* 1996;30:765–7.

31. Wright DG et al. Lethal pulmonary reactions associated with the combined use of amphotericin B and leukocyte transfusions. *N Engl J Med* 1981;304:1185–9.

32. Trissel LA. Amphotericin B does not mix with fat emulsion. *Am J Health-Syst Pharm* 1995;52:1463–4. Letter.

33. Amantea MA et al. Population pharmacokinetics and renal function-sparing effects of amphotericin B colloidal dispersion in patients receiving bone marrow transplants. *Antimicrob Agent Chemother* 1995;39:2042–7.

34. Heinemann V et al. Pharmacokinetics of liposomal amphotericin B (AmBisome) versus other lipid-based formulations. *Bone Marrow Transplant* 1994;14(suppl 5):S8–9.

35. Hoy JF. Antifungal drugs. In, Kucers A et al., eds. *The use of antibiotics.* 5th ed. Oxford. Butterworth-Heinemann, 1997:1245–505.

36. Powderly WG. Fluconazole. *Infect Med* 1995;12:257, 281–82.

37. Debruyne D, Ryckelynck J-P. Clinical pharmacokinetics of fluconazole. *Clin Pharmacokinet* 1993;24:10–27.

38. Perry CM et al. Fluconazole. An update of its antimicrobial activity, pharmacokinetic properties, and therapeutic use in vaginal candidiasis. *Drugs* 1995;49:984–1006.

39. Como JA, Dismukes WE. Oral azole drugs as systemic antifungal therapy. *N Engl J Med* 1994;330:263–72.

40. Galgiani JN et al. Fluconazole therapy for coccidioidal meningitis. *Ann Intern Med* 1993;119:28–35.

41. Terrell CL, Hughes CE. Antifungal agents for deep-seated mycotic infections. *Mayo Clin Proc* 1992;67:69–91.

42. Bennett JE et al. A comparison of amphotericin B alone and combined with flucytosine in the treatment of cryptococcal meningitis. *N Engl J Med* 1979;301:126–31.

43. Allendoerfer R et al. Combined therapy with fluconazole and flucytosine in murine cryptococcal meningitis. *Antimicrob Agents Chemother* 1991;35:726–9.

44. Lyman CA, Walsh TJ. Systemically administered antifungal agents. A review of their clinical pharmacology and therapeutic applications. *Drugs* 1992;44:9–35.

45. Haria M et al. Itraconazole. A reappraisal of its pharmacological properties and therapeutic use in the management of superficial fungal infections. *Drugs* 1996;51:585–620.

46. Tucker RM et al. Interaction of azoles with rifampin, phenytoin, and carbamazepine: in vitro and clinical observations. *Clin Infect Dis* 1992;14:165–74.

47. Ducharme MP et al. Itraconazole and hydroxyitraconazole serum concentrations are reduced more than tenfold by phenytoin. *Clin Pharmacol Ther* 1995;58:617–24.

48. Benet LZ et al. Design and optimization of dosage regimens: pharmacokinetic data. In, Hardman JG et al., eds. *Goodman and Gilman's the pharmacological basis of therapeutics.* New York: McGraw-Hill; 1996: 1707–92.

49. Barriere SL. Pharmacology and pharmacokinetics of traditional antifungal agents. *Pharmacotherapy* 1990; 10(suppl):134S–40S.

50. Chin TWF et al. Effects of an acidic beverage (Coca-Cola) on absorption of ketoconazole. *Antimicrob Agents Chemother* 1995;39:1671–5.

51. Balfour JA, Faulds D. Terbinafine: a review of its pharmacodynamic and pharmacokinetic properties, and therapeutic potential in superficial mycoses. *Drugs* 1992;43:259–84.

52. Arbiser JL et al. Clofazimine: a review of its medical uses and mechanisms of action. *J Am Acad Dermatol* 1995;32:241–7.

53. Peloquin CA. Pharmacology of the antimycobacterial drugs. *Med Clin North Am* 1993;77:1253–62.

54. Brausch LM, Bass JB. The treatment of tuberculosis. *Med Clin North Am* 1993;77:1277–90.

55. Bass JB Jr et al. Treatment of tuberculosis and tuberculosis infection in adults and children. *Am J Resp Crit Care Med* 1994;149:1359–74.

56. Initial therapy for tuberculosis in the era of multidrug resistance. *MMWR* 1993;42(RR-7):1–8.

57. Heifets LB. Antimycobacterial drugs. *Semin Respir Infect* 1994;9:84–103.

58. van Scoy RE, Wilkowske CJ. Antituberculous agents. *Mayo Clin Proc* 1992;67:179–87.

59. Pratt WB, Fekety R. Drugs that act on mycobacteria. In, Pratt WB, Fekety R, eds. *The antimicrobial drugs.* New York: Oxford University Press; 1986:277–316.

60. Alexander MR et al. Isoniazid-associated hepatitis. *Clin Pharm* 1982;1:148–53.

61. Holdiness MR. Neurological manifestations and toxicities of the antituberculous drugs. *Med Toxicol Adv Drug Exp* 1987;2:33–51.

62. O'Brien RJ. Drug-resistant tuberculosis: etiology, management and prevention. *Semin Respir Infect* 1994;9:104–12.

63. Skinner MH et al. Pharmacokinetics of rifabutin. *Antimicrob Agents Chemother* 1989;33:1237–41.

64. Nightingale SD et al. Two controlled trials of rifabutin prophylaxis against *Mycobacterium avium* complex infection in AIDS. *N Engl J Med* 1993;329:828–33.

65. Masur H. Recommendations on prophylaxis and therapy for disseminated *Mycobacterium avium* complex disease in patients infected with the human immunodeficiency virus. Public Health Service Task Force on Prophylaxis and Therapy for *Mycobacterium avium* Complex. *N Engl J Med* 1993;329:898–904.

66. Blaschke TF, Skinner MH. The clinical pharmacokinetics of rifabutin. *Clin Infect Dis* 1996;(suppl 1):S15–22.

67. Thornsberry C et al. Rifampin: spectrum of antibacterial activity. *Rev Infect Dis* 1983;5(suppl 3):S412–7.

68. Venkatesan K. Pharmacokinetic drug interactions with rifampicin. *Clin Pharmacokinet* 1992;22:47–65.

69. Anon. Drugs for parasitic infections. *Med Lett Drugs Ther* 1998;40:1–12.

70. Jernigan JA, Pearson RD. Antiparasitic drugs. In, Mandell GL et al., eds. *Principles and practice of infectious diseases.* 4th ed. New York: Churchill Livingstone; 1995:458–92.

71. Liu LX, Weller PF. Antiparasitic drugs. *N Engl J Med* 1996;334:1178–84.

72. Kalter DC et al. Treatment of pediculosis pubis. *Arch Dermatol* 1987;123:1315–9.

73. Brown S et al. Treatment of ectoparasitic infections: review of the English-language literature, 1982–9. *Clin Infect Dis* 1995;20(suppl 1):S104–9.

74. Quarterman MJ, Lesher LJ Jr. Neonatal scabies treated with permethrin 5% cream. *Pediatr Dermatol* 1994;11:264–6.

75. Meinking TL, Taplin D. Safety of permethrin vs lindane for the treatment of scabies. *Arch Dermatol* 1996;132:959–62. Editorial.

76. Elion GB. Acyclovir: discovery, mechanism of action, and selectivity. *J Med Virol* 1993;(suppl 1):2–6.

77. Whitley RJ, Gnann JW. Acyclovir: a decade later. *N Engl J Med* 1992;327:782–9.

78. Nikkels AF, Pierard GE. Recognition and treatment of shingles. *Drugs* 1994;48:528–48.

79. Soul-Lawton J et al. Absolute bioavailability and metabolic disposition of valaciclovir, the L-valyl ester of acyclovir, following oral administration to humans. *Antimicrob Agents Chemother* 1995;39:2759–64.

80. Jacobson MA. Valaciclovir (BW256U87): the L-valyl ester of acyclovir. *J Med Virol* 1993;(suppl 1):150–3.

81. Laskin OL. Acyclovir, pharmacology and clinical experience. *Arch Intern Med* 1984;144:1241–6.

82. Cundy KC et al. Clinical pharmacokinetics of cidofovir in human immunodeficiency virus–infected patients. *Antimicrob Agents Chemother* 1995;39:1247–52.

83. Lalezari JP et al. (S)-1-[3-hydroxy-2-(phosphonylmethoxy)propyl]cytosine (cidofovir): results of a phase I/II study of a novel antiviral nucleotide analogue. *J Infect Dis* 1995;171:788–96.

84. Flaherty JF. Current and experimental therapeutic options for cytomegalovirus disease. *Am J Health-Syst Pharm* 1996;53(suppl 2):S4–11.

85. Neuzil KM. Pharmacologic therapy for human immunodeficiency virus infection: a review. *Am J Med Sci* 1994;307:368–73.

86. Working group on Antiretroviral Therapy: National Pediatric HIV Resource Center. Antiretroviral therapy and medical management of the human immunodeficiency virus-infected child. *Pediatr Infect Dis J* 1993;12:513–22.

87. Johnson VA. Nucleoside reverse transcriptase inhibitors and resistance of human immunodeficiency virus type 1. *J Infect Dis* 1995;17(suppl 2):S140–9.

88. Dudley MN. Clinical pharmacokinetics of nucleoside antiretroviral agents. *J Infect Dis* 1995;171(suppl 2):S99–112.

89. Knupp CA et al. Pharmacokinetics of didanosine in patients with acquired immunodeficiency syndrome or acquired immunodeficiency syndrome–related complex. *Clin Pharmacol Ther* 1991;49:523–35.

90. Hartman NR et al. Pharmacokinetics of 2′,3′-dideoxyinosine in patients with severe human immunodeficiency infection. II. The effects of different oral formulations and the presence of other medications. *Clin Pharmacol Ther* 1991;50:278–85.

91. Stretcher BN. Pharmacokinetic optimisation of antiretroviral therapy in patients with HIV infection. *Clin Pharmacokinet* 1995;29:46–65.

92. van Leeuwen R et al. The safety and pharmacokinetics of a reverse transcriptase inhibitor, 3TC, in patients with HIV infection: a phase I study. *AIDS* 1992;6:1471–5.

93. Moore KHP et al. Pharmacokinetics of lamivudine administered alone and with trimethoprim-sulfamethoxazole. *Clin Pharmacol Ther* 1996;59:550–8.

94. Taburet A-M, Singlas E. Drug interactions with antiviral drugs. *Clin Pharmacokinet* 1996;30:385–401.

95. Pue MA et al. Linear pharmacokinetics of penciclovir following administration of single oral doses of famciclovir 125, 250, 500 and 750 mg to healthy volunteers. *J Antimicrob Chemother* 1994;33:119–27.

96. Perry CM, Wagstaff AJ. Famciclovir: a review of its pharmacological properties and therapeutic efficacy in herpesvirus infections. *Drugs* 1995;50:396–415.

97. Minor JR, Baltz JK. Foscarnet sodium. *DICP* 1991;25:41–7.

98. Wagstaff AJ, Bryson HM. Foscarnet. A reappraisal of its antiviral activity, pharmacokinetic properties and therapeutic use in immunocompromised patients with viral infections. *Drugs* 1994;48:199–226.

99. Sasadeusz JJ, Sacks SL. Systemic antivirals in herpesvirus infections. *Dermatol Clin* 1993;11:171–85.

100. Jacobson MA et al. Foscarnet-induced hypocalcemia and effects of foscarnet on calcium metabolism. *J Clin Endocrinol Metab* 1991;72:1130–5.

101. Crumpacker CS. Ganciclovir. *N Engl J Med* 1996;335:721–9.

102. Sommadossi J-P et al. Clinical pharmacokinetics of ganciclovir in patients with normal and impaired renal function. *Rev Infect Dis* 1988;10(suppl 3):S507–14.

103. Morris DJ. Adverse effects and drug interactions of clinical importance with antiviral drugs. *Drug Saf* 1994;10:281–91.

104. Erice A et al. Progressive disease due to ganciclovir-resistant cytomegalovirus in immunocompromised patients. *N Engl J Med* 1989;320:289–93.

105. Moyle G, Gazzard B. Current knowledge and future prospects for the use of HIV protease inhibitors. *Drugs* 1996;51:701–12.

106. Hart GJ et al. Effects of (–)-2′-deoxy-3′-thiacytidine (3TC) 5′-triphosphate on human immunodeficiency virus reverse transcriptase and mammalian DNA polymerases alpha, beta, and gamma. *Antimicrob Agents Chemother* 1992;36:1688–94.

107. Merrill DP et al. Lamivudine or stavudine in two- and three-drug combinations against human immunodeficiency virus type I replication in vitro. *J Infect Dis* 1996;173:355–64.

108. Eron JJ et al. Treatment with lamivudine, zidovudine, or both in HIV-positive patients with 200 to 500 CD4+ cells per cubic millimeter. *N Engl J Med* 1995;333:1662–9.

109. Peterson A et al. Comparison of bid and tid dosing of nelfinavir (NFV) in combination with stavudine (d4T) and lamivudine (3TC): an interim look. Presented at the 5th Conference on Retroviruses and Opportunistic Infections. February 1–5, 1998; Chicago. Abstract 373.

110. Cheeseman S et al. Phase I/II evaluation of nevirapine alone and in combination with zidovudine for infection with human immunodeficiency virus. *J Acquir Immune Defic Syndr Hum Retrovirol* 1995;8:141–51.

111. Havlir D et al. High-dose nevirapine: safety, pharmacokinetics, and antiviral effect in patients with human immunodeficiency virus infection. *J Infect Dis* 1995;171:537–45.

112. Investigational drug brochure: Viramune (nevirapine) expanded access program. Ridgefield, CT: Boehringer Ingelheim, March 1996.

113. D'Aquila RT et al. Nevirapine, zidovudine, and didanosine compared with zidovudine and didanosine in patients with HIV-1 infection. A randomized, double-blind, placebo-controlled trial. *Ann Intern Med* 1996;124:1019–30.

114. Danner SA et al. A short-term study of the safety, pharmacokinetics, and efficacy of ritonavir, an inhibitor of HIV-1 protease. *N Engl J Med* 1995;333:1528–33.

115. Markowitz M et al. A preliminary study of ritonavir, an inhibitor of HIV-1 protease, to treat HIV-1 infection. *N Engl J Med* 1995;333:1534–9.

116. Kitchen VS et al. Safety and activity of saquinavir in HIV infection. *Lancet* 1995;345:952–5.

117. Vella S. Update on a proteinase inhibitor. *AIDS* 1994;8(suppl 3):S25–9.

118. Sommadossi J-P. Comparison of metabolism and in vitro antiviral activity of stavudine versus other 2′,3′-dideoxynucleoside analogues. *J Infect Dis* 1995;171(suppl 2):S88–92.

119. Murray HW et al. Stavudine in patients with AIDS and AIDS-related complex: AIDS clinical trials group 089. *J Infect Dis* 1995;171(suppl 2):S123–30.

120. Lange JM et al. Failure of zidovudine prophylaxis after accidental exposure to HIV-1. *N Engl J Med* 1990;322:1375–7.

121. Recommendations of the U.S. Public Health Service task force on the use of zidovudine to reduce perinatal transmission of human immunodeficiency virus. *MMWR* 1994;43(RR-11):1–20.

122. Taburet AM et al. Pharmacokinetics of zidovudine in patients with liver cirrhosis. *Clin Pharmacol Ther* 1990;47:731–9.

123. Acosta EP et al. Clinical pharmacokinetics of zidovudine: an update. *Clin Pharmacokinet* 1996;4:251–62.

124. Steffe EM et al. The effect of acetaminophen on zidovudine metabolism in HIV-infected patients. *J Acuir Immune Defic Syndr* 1990;3:691–4.

125. Panel on Clinical Practices for Treatment of HIV Infection. Guidelines for the use of antiretroviral agents in HIV-infected adults and adolescents. MMWR 1998;47(RR-5):43–82.

126. Panel on Clinical Practices for Treatment of HIV Infection. Guidelines for the use of antiretroviral agents in pediatric HIV Infection. MMWR 1998;47(RR-4):1–43.

127. Centers for Disease Control and Prevention. Public Health Service Task Force recommendations for the use of antiretroviral drugs in pregnant women infected with HIV-1 for maternal health and for reducing perinatal HIV-1 transmission in the United States. MMWR 1998;47(RR-2):1–30.

128. Chambers HF, Neu HC. Penicillins. In, Mandell GL et al., eds. *Principles and practice of infectious diseases.* 4th ed. New York: Churchill Livingstone; 1995:233–46.

129. Barza M. Antimicrobial spectrum, pharmacology and therapeutic use of antibiotics. Part 2: Penicillins. *Am J Hosp Pharm* 1977;34:57–67.

130. Weber DJ et al. Amoxicillin and potassium clavulanate: an antibiotic combination. *Pharmacotherapy* 1984;4:122–36.

131. Sutherland R. β-lactam/β-lactamase inhibitor combinations: development, antibacterial activity and clinical applications. *Infection* 1995;23:191–200.

132. Neu HC. Antistaphylococcal penicillins. *Med Clin North Am* 1982;66:51–60.

133. Johnson DH, Cunha BA. Aztreonam. *Med Clin North Am* 1995;79:733–43.

134. Brogden RN, Heel RC. Aztreonam. A review of its antibacterial activity, pharmacokinetic properties and therapeutic uses. *Drugs* 1986;31:96–130.

135. Donowitz GR, Mandell GL. Beta-lactam antibiotics (2 parts). *N Engl J Med* 1988;318:419–26, 490–500.

136. Cunha BA. Third-generation cephalosporins: a review. *Clin Ther* 1992;14:616–47.

137. Nightingale CH et al. Pharmacokinetics and clinical use of cephalosporin antibiotics. *J Pharm Sci* 1975;64:1899–927.

138. Barriere SL, Flaherty JF. Third-generation cephalosporins: a critical evaluation. *Clin Pharm* 1984;3:351–73.

139. Karchmer AW. Cephalosporins. In, Mandell GL et al., eds. *Principles and practice of infectious diseases.* 4th ed. New York: Churchill Livingstone; 1995:247–64.

140. Rodman DP et al. A critical review of the new oral cephalosporins. *Arch Fam Med* 1994;3:975–80.

141. Fassbender M et al. Pharmacokinetics of new oral cephalosporins, including a new carbacephem. *Clin Infect Dis* 1993;16:646–53.

142. Force RW, Nahata MC. Loracarbef: a new orally administered carbacephem antibiotic. *Ann Pharmacother* 1993;27:321–9.

143. Cooper RDG. The carbacephems: a new beta-lactam antibiotic class. *Am J Med* 1992;92(suppl 6A):2S–6S.

144. DiPiro JT, May JR. Use of cephalosporins with enhanced anti-anaerobic activity for treatment and prevention of anaerobic and mixed infections. *Clin Pharm* 1988;7:285–302.

145. Ward A, Richards DM. Cefotetan. A review of its antibacterial activity, pharmacokinetic properties and therapeutic use. *Drugs* 1985;30:382–426.

146. Schaad UB et al. A comparison of ceftriaxone and cefuroxime for the treatment of bacterial meningitis in children. *N Engl J Med* 1990;322:141–7.

147. Petz LD. Immunologic cross-reactivity between penicillins and cephalosporins: a review. *J Infect Dis* 1978;137(suppl):S74–9.

148. Lipsky JJ. Antibiotic-associated hypoprothrombinemia. *J Antimicrob Chemother* 1988;21:281–300.

149. Schaad UB et al. Reversible ceftriaxone-associated biliary pseudolithiasis in children. *Lancet* 1988;2:1411–3.

150. Shiffman ML et al. Pathogenesis of ceftriaxone-associated biliary sludge. *Gastroenterology* 1990;99:1772–8.

151. Cunha BA, Gill MV. Cefepime. *Med Clin North Am* 1995;79:721–32.

152. Barradell LB, Bryson HM. Cefepime. A review of its antibacterial activity, pharmacokinetic properties and therapeutic use. *Drugs* 1994;47:471–505.

153. Friedland IR, McCracken GH Jr. Management of infections caused by antibiotic-resistant *Streptococcus pneumoniae.* *N Engl J Med* 1994;331:377–82.

154. Smith BR, LeFrock JL. Cefuroxime: antibacterial activity, pharmacology, and clinical efficacy. *Ther Drug Monit* 1983;5:149–60.

155. Drusano GL et al. The acylampicillins: mezlocillin, piperacillin, and azlocillin. *Rev Infect Dis* 1984;6:13–32.

156. Holmes B et al. Piperacillin. A review of its antibacterial activity, pharmacokinetic properties and therapeutic use. *Drugs* 1984;28:375–425.

157. Clissold SP et al. Imipenem/cilastatin. A review of its antibacterial activity, pharmacokinetic properties and therapeutic efficacy. *Drugs* 1987;33:183–241.

158. Norrby SR. Carbapenems. *Med Clin North Am* 1995;79:745–59.

159. Ahonkhai VI et al. Imipenem-cilastatin in pediatric patients: an overview of safety and efficacy in studies conducted in the United States. *Pediatr Infect Dis J* 1989;8:740–7.

160. Calandra GB et al. Review of adverse experiences and tolerability in the first 2,516 patients treated with imipenem/cilastatin. *Am J Med* 1985;78(suppl 6A):73–8.

161. Saxon A. Immediate hypersensitivity reactions to beta-lactam antibiotics. *Ann Intern Med* 1987;107:204–15.

162. Wiseman LR et al. Meropenem. A review of its antibacterial activity, pharmacokinetic properties and clinical efficacy. *Drugs* 1995;50:73–101.

163. Pryka RD, Haig GM. Meropenem: a new carbapenem antimicrobial. *Ann Pharmacother* 1994;28:1045–54.

164. Mouton JW, van den Anker JN. Metropenem clinical pharmacokinetics. *Clin Pharmacokinet* 1995;28:275–86.

165. Wright AJ, Wilkowske CJ. The penicillins. *Mayo Clin Proc* 1987;62:806–20.

166. Weiss ME, Adkinson NF Jr. β-lactam allergy. In, Mandell GL et al., eds. *Principles and practice of infectious diseases.* 4th ed. New York: Churchill Livingstone; 1995:272–8.

167. Plaisance KI, Nightingale CH. Pharmacology of cephalosporins. In, Queener SF et al., eds. *Beta-latam antibiotics for clinical use.* New York: Marcel Dekker; 1986:285–347.

168. Dudley MN, Nightingale CH. Effects of protein binding on the pharmacology of cephalosporins. In, Neu HC, ed. *New beta-lactam antibiotics: a review from chemistry to clinical efficacy of the new cephalosporins.* Philadelphia: Francis Clarke Wood Institute for the History of Medicine; 1982;227–39.

169. Carver P et al. Comparative pharmacokinetic study of cefotetan and cefoxitin in healthy volunteers. *Infect Surg* 1986;(April suppl):11–4.

170. Wise R. The pharmacokinetics of the oral cephalosporins: a review. *J Antimicrob Chemother* 1990;26(suppl E):13–20.

171. Melikian DM, Flaherty JF. Antimicrobial agents. In, Schrier RW, Gambertoglio JG, eds. *Handbook of drug therapy in liver and kidney disease.* Boston: Little, Brown; 1991:14–45.

172. Klepser ME et al. Clinical pharmacokinetics of newer cephalosporins. *Clin Pharmacokinet* 1995;28:361–84.

173. Hardin TC et al. Comparison of ampicillin-sulbactam and ticarcillin-clavulanic acid in patients with chronic renal failure: effects of differential pharmacokinetics on serum bactericidal activity. *Pharmacotherapy* 1994;14:147–52.

174. Bahal N, Nahata MC. The new macrolide antibiotics: azithromycin, clarithromycin, dirithromycin, and roxithromycin. *Ann Pharmacother* 1992;26:46–55.

175. Schlossberg D. Azithromycin and clarithromycin. *Med Clin North Am* 1995;79:803–15.

176. Berry A et al. Azithromycin therapy for disseminated *Mycobacterium avium-intracellulare* in AIDS patients. First National Conference on Human Retroviruses. Washington, DC; 1993. Abstract #292.

177. 1993 Sexually Transmitted Diseases Treatment Guidelines. *MMWR* 1993;42(RR-14):1–102.

178. Centers for Disease Control and Prevention. Recommendations on prophylaxis and therapy for disseminated *Mycobacterium avium* complex for adults and adolescents infected with human immunodeficiency virus. *MMWR* 1993;42(RR-9):14–20.

179. Havlir D et al. Prophylaxis against disseminated *Mycobacterium avium* complex with weekly azithromycin, daily rifabutin, or both. *N Engl J Med* 1996;335:392–8.

180. McLinn S. Double blind and open label studies of azithromycin in the management of acute otitis media in children: a review. *Pediatr Infect Dis J* 1995;14:S62–6.

181. Hopkins SJ, Williams D. Clinical tolerability and safety of azithromycin in children. *Pediatr Infect Dis J* 1995;14:S67–71.

182. Nahata MC. Pharmacokinetics of azithromycin in pediatric patients: comparison with other agents used for treating otitis media and streptococcal pharyngitis. *Pediatr Infect Dis J* 1995;14:S39–44.

183. Piscitelli SC et al. Clarithromycin and azithromycin: new macrolide antibiotics. *Clin Pharm* 1992;11:137–52.

184. Rodvold KA, Piscitelli SC. New oral macrolide and fluoroquinolone antibiotics: an overview of pharmacokinetics, interactions, and safety. *Clin Infect Dis* 1993;17(suppl 1):S192–9.

185. Dunn CJ, Barradell LB. Azithromycin: a review of its pharmacological properties and use as 3-day therapy in respiratory tract infections. *Drugs* 1996;51:483–505.

186. Markham A, Mctavish D. Clarithromycin and omeprazole as *Helicobacter pylori* eradication therapy in patients with *H. pylori*-associated gastric disorders. *Drugs* 1996;51:161–78.

187. Brittain DC. Erythromycin. *Med Clin North Am* 1987;71:1147–54.

188. Washington JA, Wilson WR. Erythromycin: a microbial and clinical perspective after 30 years of clinical use. (2 parts). *Mayo Clin Proc* 1985;60:189–203, 271–8.

189. Smilack JD et al. Tetracyclines, chloramphenicol, erythromycin, clindamycin, and metronidazole. *Mayo Clin Proc* 1991;66:1270–80.

190. Weber FH et al. Erythromycin: a motilin agonist and gastrointestinal prokinetic agent. *Am J Gastroenterol* 1993;88:485–90.

191. Eichenwald HF. Adverse reactions to erythromycin. *Pediatr Infect Dis J* 1986;5:147–50.

192. Amsden GW. Macrolides versus azalides: a drug interaction update. *Ann Pharmacother* 1995;29:906–17.

193. Peeters TL. Erythromycin and other macrolides as prokinetic agents. *Gastroenterology* 1993;105:1886–99.

194. Lartey PA et al. New developments in macrolides: structures and antibacterial and prokinetic activities. *Adv Pharmacol* 1994;28:307–43.

195. Kreek MJ, Culpepper-Morgan JA. Constipation syndromes. In, Lewis JH, ed. *A pharmacologic approach to gastrointestinal disorders.* Baltimore: Williams & Wilkins; 1994:179–208.

196. Dive A et al. Effect of erythromycin on gastric motility in mechanically ventilated critically ill patients: a double-blind, randomized, placebo-controlled study. *Crit Care Med* 1995;23:1356–62.

197. Guay DRP. Macrolide antibiotics in paediatric infectious diseases. *Drugs* 1996;51:515–36.

198. Bloomfield G. A comparison of gastrointestinal tolerance to five different forms of erythromycin. *P&T* 1996;(April):209–14.
199. Dajani AS et al. Prevention of bacterial endocarditis. Recommendations by the American Heart Association *JAMA* 1990;264:2919–22.
200. Ginsburg CM. Pharmacology of erythromycin in infants and children. *Pediatr Infect Dis J* 1986;5:124–9.
201. Brogden RN, Peters DH. Dirithromycin. A review of its antimicrobial activity, pharmacokinetic properties and therapeutic efficacy. *Drugs* 1994;48:599–616.
202. Anon. Dirithromycin. *Med Lett Drugs Ther* 1995;37:109–10.
203. Just PM. Overview of the fluoroquinolone antibiotics. *Pharmacotherapy* 1993;13:4S–17S.
204. Suh B, Lorber B. Quinolones. *Med Clin North Am* 1995;79:869–94.
205. Schaad UB et al. Use of fluoroquinolones in pediatrics: consensus report of an international society of chemotherapy commission. *Pediatr Infect Dis J* 1995;14:1–9.
206. Schentag JJ, Gross TF. Quinolone pharmacokinetics in the elderly. *Am J Med* 1992;92(suppl 4A):33S–7S.
207. Nightingale CH. Pharmacokinetic considerations in quinolone therapy. *Pharmacotherapy* 1993;13:34S–8S.
208. Radandt JM et al. Interactions of fluoroquinolones with other drugs mechanisms, variability, clinical significance, and management. *Clin Infect Dis* 1992;14:272–84.
209. Dudley MN et al. Effect of dose on the serum pharmacokinetics of intravenous ciprofloxacin with identification and characterization of extravascular compartments using noncompartmental and compartmental pharmacokinetic models. *Antimicrob Agents Chemother* 1987;31:1782–6.
210. Forrest A et al. Relationships between renal function and disposition of oral ciprofloxacin. *Antimicrob Agents Chemother* 1988;32:1537–40.
211. Davis R. Bryson HM. Levofloxacin. *Drugs* 1994;47:677–700.
212. Balfour JA et al. Fleroxacin. A review of its pharmacology and therapeutic efficacy in various infections. *Drugs* 1995;49:794–850.
213. Wadworth AN, Goa KL. Lomefloxacin. *Drugs* 1991;42:1018–60.
214. Goa KL et al. Sparfloxacin. *Drugs* 1997;53:700–25.
215. Wagstaff AJ, Balfour JA. Grepafloxacin. *Drugs* 1997;53:817–24.
216. Fish DN, Chow AT. The clinical pharmacokinetics of levofloxacin. *Clin Pharmacokinet* 1997;32:101–19.
217. Haria M, Lamb HM. Trovafloxacin. *Drugs* 1997;54:435–45.
218. Foltzer MA, Reese RE. Trimethoprim-sulfamethoxazole and other sulfonamides. *Med Clin North Am* 1987;71:1177–94.
219. Cockerill FR, Edson RS. Trimethoprim-sulfamethoxazole. *Mayo Clin Proc* 1991;66:1260–9.
220. Markowitz N et al. Trimethoprim-sulfamethoxazole compared with vancomycin for the treatment of *Staphylococcus aureus* infection. *Ann Intern Med* 1992;117:390–8.
221. Lundstrom TS, Sobel JD. Vancomycin, trimethoprim-sulfamethoxazole, and rifampin. *Infect Dis Clin North Am* 1995;9:747–67.
222. Goodwin SD. *Pneumocystis carinii* pneumonia in human immunodeficiency virus–infected infants and children. *Pharmacotherapy* 1993;13:640–6.
223. Davey RT Jr, Masur H. Recent advances in the diagnosis, treatment, and prevention of *Pneumocystis carinii* pneumonia. *Antimicrob Agents Chemother* 1990;34:499–504.
224. Pratt WB, Fekety R. The antimetabolites. In, Pratt WB, Fekety R., eds. *The antimicrobial drugs.* New York: Oxford University Press; 1986:229–51.
225. Masur H. Prevention and treatment of pneumocystis pneumonia. *N Engl J Med* 1992;327:1853–60.
226. Absar N et al. Densensitization to trimethoprim/sulfamethoxazole in HIV-infected patients. *J Allergy Clin Immunol* 1994;93:1001–5.
227. Standiford HC. Tetracyclines and chloramphenicol. In, Mandell GL et al., eds. *Principles and practice of infectious diseases.* 4th ed. New York. Churchill Livingstone; 1995:306–17.
228. Kapusnik-Uner JE et al. Antimicrobial agents: tetracyclines, chloramphenicol, erythromycin and miscellaneous antibacterial agents. In, Hardman JG et al., eds. *Goodman and Gilman's the pharmacological basis of therapeutics.* New York: McGraw-Hill; 1996:1130–5.
229. Fingar BL. Sclerosing agents used to control malignant pleural effusions. *Hosp Pharm* 1992;27:622–8.
230. Francke EL, Neu HC. Chloramphenicol and tetracyclines. *Med Clin North Am* 1987;71:1155–68.
231. Wilson WR, Cockerill FR. Tetracyclines, chloramphenicol, erythromycin, and clindamycin. *Mayo Clin Proc* 1987;62:906–15.
232. Haile LG, Flaherty JF. Atovaquone: a review. *Ann Pharmacother* 1993;27:1488–94.
233. Spencer CM, Goa KL. Atovaquone. A review of its pharmacological properties and therapeutic efficacy in opportunistic infections. *Drugs* 1995;50:176–96.
234. Norris AH et al. Chloramphenicol for the treatment of vancomycin-resistant enterococcal infections. *Clin Infect Dis* 1995;20:1137–44.

235. Greenfield RA. Symposium on antimicrobial therapy X. Chloramphenicol, clindamycin, and metronidazole. *J Okla State Med Assoc* 1993;86:336–41.

236. Smilack JD et al. Tetracyclines, chloramphenicol, erythromycin, clindamycin and metronidazole. *Mayo Clin Proc* 1991;66:1270–80.

237. Rayner SA, Buckley RJ. Ocular chloramphenicol and aplastic anemia. Is there a link? *Drug Saf* 1996;14:273–6.

238. Pratt WB, Fekety R. Bacteriostatic inhibitors of protein synthesis. In, Pratt WB, Fekety R, eds. *The antimicrobial drugs.* New York: Oxford University Press; 1986:184–228.

239. Dhawan VK, Thadepalli H. Clindamycin: a review of 15 years of clinical experience. *Rev Infect Dis* 1982;4:1133–53.

240. Klainer AS. Clindamycin. *Med Clin North Am* 1987;71:1169–76.

241. Van Arsdel PP et al. The value of skin testing for penicillin allergy diagnosis. *West J Med* 1986;144:311–4.

242. Falagas ME, Gorbach SL. Clindamycin and metronidazole. *Med Clin North Am* 1995;79:845–67.

243. Lau AH et al. Clinical pharmacokinetics of metronidazole and other nitroimidazole anti-infectives. *Clin Pharmacokinet* 1992;23:328–64.

244. Wenisch C et al. Comparison of vancomycin, teicoplanin, metronidazole, and fusidic acid for treatment of *Clostridium difficile*-associated diarrhea. *Clin Infect Dis* 1996;22:813–8.

245. Black M et al. Antimicrobial agents: sulfonamides, trimethoprim-sulfamethoxazole, quinolones. In, Hardman JG et al., eds. *Goodman and Gilman's the pharmacological basis of therapeutics.* New York: McGraw-Hill; 1996:1069–70.

246. Wispelwey B, Pearson RD. Pentamidine: a review. *Infect Control Hosp Epidemiol* 1991;12:375–82.

247. Conte JE Jr. Pharmacokinetics of intravenous pentamidine in patients with normal renal function or receiving hemodialysis. *J Infect Dis* 1991;163:169–75.

248. Donnelly H et al. Distribution of pentamidine in patients with AIDS. *J Infect Dis* 1988;157:985–9.

249. Chant C, Rybak MJ. Quinupristin/dalfopristin (RP 59500): a new streptogramin antibiotic. *Ann Pharmacother* 1995;29:1022–7.

250. Bryson HM, Spencer CM. Quinupristin-dalfopristin. *Drugs* 1996;52:406–16.

251. Griswold MW et al. Quinupristin-dalfopristin (RP 59500): an injectable streptogramin combination. *Am J Health-syst Pharm* 1996;53:2045–53.

252. Fulton B et al. Trimetrexate. A review of its pharmacodynamic and pharmacokinetic properties and therapeutic potential in the treatment of *Pneumocystis carinii* pneumonia. *Drugs* 1995;49:563–76.

253. Marshall JL, DeLap RJ. Clinical pharmacokinetics and pharmacology of trimetrexate. *Clin Pharmacokinet* 1994;26:190–200.

254. Blanke CD et al. Phase II study of trimetrexate, fluorouracil, and leucovorin for advanced colorectal cancer. *J Clin Oncol* 1997;15:915–20.

255. Witte RS et al. An Eastern Cooperative Oncology Group phase II trial of trimetrexate in the treatment of advanced urothelial carcinoma. *Cancer* 1994;73:688–91.

256. Grem JL et al. Correlates of severe of life-threatening toxic effects from trimetrexate. *J Natl Cancer Inst* 1988;80:1313–8.

257. Lake KD, Peterson CD. A simplified method for initiating vancomycin therapy. *Pharmacotherapy* 1985;5:340–4.

258. Rybak MJ et al. Nephrotoxicity of vancomycin, alone and with an aminoglycoside. *J Antimicrob Chemother* 1990;25:679–87.

259. Matzke GR et al. Clinical pharmacokinetics of vancomycin. *Clin Pharmacokinet* 1986;11:257–82.

260. Newfield P, Roizen MF. Hazards of rapid administration of vancomycin. *Ann Intern Med* 1979;91:581.

261. Healy DP et al. Vancomycin-induced histamine release and "red man syndrome": comparison of 1- and 2-hour infusions. *Antimicrob Agents Chemother* 1990;34:550–4.

262. Edwards DJ, Pancorbo S. Routine monitoring of serum vancomycin concentrations: waiting for proof of its value. *Clin Pharm* 1987;6:652–4.

263. Farber BF, Mollering RC. Retrospective study of the toxicity of preparations of vancomycin from 1974–1981. *Antimicrob Agents Chemother* 1983;23:138–41.

Antineoplastics, Chemoprotectants, and Immunosuppressants

Antineoplastics

Antineoplastics. The agents included in this section are those having widespread use in cancer chemotherapy. Agents with therapeutic importance in small patient populations are not included.

Information on the dosage of these drugs has largely been determined empirically, and clinical investigations are continually being performed to find safer and more effective dosage regimens. Thus, dosages in this section should only be considered as guidelines based on the most widely accepted usage at the time of this writing. Because space does not permit detailed discussions of the toxicity, dosage regimens, and other aspects of these drugs, the reader should become familiar with specific agents before initiating treatment.[1] References are provided in this section for more detailed information concerning the proper and safe use of these agents. If specific investigational protocols are available, these may also provide information that is unavailable from other sources, especially with regard to dosage and regimens.

Cancer chemotherapeutic agents as a class are the most toxic drugs in use. Adverse reactions listed represent those most likely to occur with the usual doses and methods of use. Infrequent, but serious, reactions are also listed; however, the lists of adverse reactions are not comprehensive. Nausea and vomiting are important side effects of these agents that can be adequately treated by current antiemetics alone or in combination. In order to tailor antiemetic therapy better to the emetic potential of the chemotherapy, a standard rating scale is used in these monographs. Several points to remember are that emetogenicity is dose dependent, combinations of chemotherapeutic agents result in greater emetogenic potential than the drug(s) used alone, and emetogenic potentials are best defined in adults and do not necessarily apply to children. The categories of emetogenicity used are as follows:[2]

CATEGORY	PERCENTAGE OF PATIENTS AFFECTED
High	>90
Moderately high	60–90
Moderate	30–60
Moderately low	10–30
Low	<10

Class Instructions: Antineoplastics. This drug is very potent, and some side effects can be expected to occur with its use. Be sure that you understand the possible dangers as well as the possible benefits of the drug before you begin to take it.

Cytotoxic Agents. Because this drug can decrease your body's ability to fight infections, report any signs of infection such as fever, shaking chills, or sore throat immediately. Also report any unusual bruising or bleeding, shortness of breath, or painful or burning urination. Avoid the use of aspirin-containing products, and avoid alcohol or use it in moderation. Nausea, vomiting, or hair loss may sometimes occur with this drug. The severity of these effects depends on the individual, the dosage, and other drugs that may be given at the same time. This drug may cause temporary or sometimes permanent sterility in men and women. It may also cause birth defects if the father is taking the drug at the time of conception or if the mother is taking it any time during pregnancy. If you are breastfeeding, this drug may appear in the milk and cause problems in your baby; therefore, use an alternate method of feeding your baby.

Missed Doses. This drug should be taken at regular intervals exactly as prescribed. If a dose is missed, it should be taken as soon as it is remembered. If it is almost time for the next dose, only that dose should be taken and the regular dosage schedule should be resumed. The dose should never be doubled or extra doses taken.

Alkylating Agents

ALTRETAMINE   Hexalen

Pharmacology. Altretamine (formerly hexamethylmelamine) acts primarily as an alkylating agent. It is used in combination chemotherapy of ovarian cancer and is also active in cervical and lung cancers.[3–5]

Adult Dosage. PO as a single agent 260 mg/m^2/day in 4 divided doses for as long as 2–5 weeks. Lower dosages are required if altretamine is combined with other myelosuppressive agents.

Dosage Forms. Cap 50 mg.

Pharmacokinetics. Oral bioavailability is incomplete and erratic, and may be dose dependent. Altretamine is N-demethylated to pentamethylmelamine by hepatic microsomal enzymes. The serum half-life ranges from 4.7–10.2 hr, with >50% of a dose renally excreted in 24 hr and less than 1% excreted unchanged.

Adverse Reactions. Nausea, vomiting, and abdominal cramps may be dose limiting in some patients. Neurotoxic effects are frequent, including agitation, hallucinations, and confusion; these are reversible and amenable to dosage reduction. Anemia, leukopenia, and thrombocytopenia are typically mild.

BUSULFAN   Myleran

CHLORAMBUCIL   Leukeran

MELPHALAN   Alkeran

Pharmacology. These drugs are water-soluble compounds that alkylate DNA, forming a variety of covalent cross-links. The drugs are polyfunctional and may form more than one covalent bond to susceptible cell constituents (typically the N^7 position of guanine). They are cell cycle phase nonspecific and chemically stable enough for oral absorption before appreciable alkylator activation occurs.

Administration and Dosage.

	BUSULFAN	CHLORAMBUCIL	MELPHALAN
Administration	PO.	PO.	PO; IV.
Adult Dosage	Up to 8 mg/day (usually 1–3 mg/day).	0.1–0.2 mg/kg/day for 1 day; or 6–12 mg/day maintenance; or 0.4 mg/kg q 2–4 weeks.[6]	PO 7 mg/m² for 4 days; or 2–4 mg/day maintenance for multiple myeloma.[7] IV 16 mg/m² q 2 weeks for 4 doses, then q 4 weeks
Pediatric Dosage	CML 0.06–0.12 mg/kg.	Non-Hodgkin's lymphoma, CLL, nephrotic syndrome, rheumatoid arthritis (initial) 0.1–0.2 mg/kg/day.	—
Geriatric Dosage	Same as adult dosage, but adjust for age-related reduction in renal function.		

[a]CLL = chronic lymphoblastic leukemia; CML = chronic myelocytic leukemia

Special Populations. *Other Conditions.* Elimination is significantly correlated with the GFR. Studies in nephrectomized animals demonstrate markedly increased myelotoxicity with unadjusted melphalan doses. Thus, one group currently recommends a 50% decrease in the melphalan dosage for BUN >30 mg/dL or Cr_s >1.5 mg/dL.[8] Reduce IV melphalan dosage to 75% of normal for WBC counts of 3000–4000/µL or platelet counts of 75,000–100,000/µL, or to 50% for WBC counts of 2000–3000/µL or platelet counts of 50,000–75,000/µL, respectively; do not give it with WBC counts of <2000/µL or platelet counts of <50,000/µL.[9]

Dosage Forms. (Busulfan) **Tab** 2 mg. (Chlorambucil) **Tab** 2 mg. (Melphalan) **Tab** 2 mg; **Inj** 50 mg.

Patient Instructions. (*See* Antineoplastics Class Instructions.)

Pharmacokinetics.

Fate.

	BUSULFAN	CHLORAMBUCIL	MELPHALAN
Absorption	Reported by manufacturer to be well absorbed orally.	Oral bioavailability is about 87 ± 20% by radiolabeled drug studies;[10,11] reduced by 10–20% if ingested with food.[12]	Oral bioavailability erratic and incomplete, (mean of 56%, range 25–89%); some patients have no levels after standard doses.[13,14]

(*continued*)

	BUSULFAN	CHLORAMBUCIL	MELPHALAN
Distribution	Homogeneous; good ascites penetration; V_d is 0.99 ± 0.23 L/kg;[10] extensively bound to proteins.	V_d is 0.29 ± 0.21 L/kg; 99% plasma protein bound.[10]	V_d is 0.45 ± 0.15 L/kg; 90 ± 5% plasma protein bound.[10]
Metabolism	Extensively metabolized, major fraction as methanesulfonic acid. Cl is 0.27 ± 0.05 L/hr/kg.[10]	Rapid metabolism to a number of inactive metabolites. Cl is 0.16 ± 0.04 L/hr/kg.[10]	Not actively metabolized; spontaneous chemical degradation to mono- and dihydroxy products. Cl is 0.31 ± 0.17 L/hr/kg.[10]
Excretion	No unchanged drug found in urine; however, metabolites are renally excreted.	Less than 1% excreted unchanged in urine over 24 hr.	Unchanged drug 24-hr urinary excretion is 10–15% of a dose.
$t_{1/2}$	Rapid initial serum clearance: 90% of dose after 3 min. $t_{1/2\beta}$ is 2.6 ± 0.5 hr.[10]	1.3 ± 0.9 hr (unchanged drug); 2.5 hr (major metabolite, an aminophenylacetic acid derivative).[9,10]	IV: $t_{1/2\alpha}$ 8 min; $t_{1/2\beta}$ 1.4 ± 0.2 hr.[10,13,14]

Adverse Reactions. Emetic potential is low. Nausea and vomiting are rare with long-term administration, although large single doses can be strongly emetogenic. Dose-limiting toxicity for this group is typically myelosuppression, with nadirs of 14–21 days for leukopenia and thrombocytopenia after pulse dosage regimens; daily administration results in chronic low indices with cumulative effects. Not uncommonly, blood counts continue to drop after drug discontinuation; fatal pancytopenia has been reported. Therefore, hematologic assessments are important with long-term daily regimens. There may be some selectivity for different normal cell lines by these drugs; busulfan, and perhaps chlorambucil, selectively depresses granulocytes, relatively sparing platelets and lymphoid elements. The nadir for melphalan can be prolonged (4–6 weeks); continuous administration frequently leads to severe myelosuppression (especially platelets) that continues after the drug is discontinued. Pulmonary fibrosis can occasionally occur with all these drugs, especially busulfan; symptoms include cough, dyspnea, and fever; histopathologic changes include bilateral fibrosis. A high-dose glucocorticoid may help early evolving pulmonary disease caused by melphalan and chlorambucil, but "busulfan lung" is usually fatal within 6 months of diagnosis.[15–17] Busulfan frequently causes hyperpigmentation (especially of intertriginous areas) and broad suppression of testicular, ovarian, and adrenal function (occasionally leading to Addisonian crisis). Long-term daily administration of these drugs predisposes patients to drug-induced carcinogenesis, often heralded by preleukemic pancytopenia and culminating in acute myelocytic leukemia. Allergic hypersensitivity reported, especially with melphalan. With prolonged use, sterility occurs with all akylators; women appear more sensitive than men.

Contraindications. Documented hypersensitivity; inadequate marrow reserve.

Precautions. *See* Special Populations for melphalan use in renal impairment.

Drug Interactions. None known.

Parameters to Monitor. WBC and platelet counts at least monthly; reduce dosage at first sign of appreciable myelosuppression (ie, WBC <3000/µL or platelets <75,000/µL). Conversely, assess patients receiving oral melphalan for evidence of mild to moderate myelotoxicity to ensure that some absorption is occurring.

CARBOPLATIN
Paraplatin

Pharmacology. Carboplatin is a more stable cyclobutane carboxylato derivative of cisplatin that is slowly activated to expose two DNA binding sites on the platinum II coordinate complex. The drug binds to DNA by both inter- and intrastrand crosslinks in a fashion similar to, but more delayed than that with cisplatin.[18] It is more water soluble and commensurately less nephrotoxic than cisplatin. Action is cell cycle phase nonspecific.

Administration and Adult Dosage. **IV for refractory ovarian cancer** 360 mg/m^2 q 4 weeks. Administration by continuous infusion has been reported, but is not commonly used.[19–21]

Special Populations. *Pediatric Dosage.* Although not specifically labeled for pediatric use, carboplatin has been safely administered to children. **IV for recurrent brain tumors** 175 mg/m^2/week for 4 weeks.[22]

Geriatric Dosage. Same as adult dosage, but adjust for age-related reduction in renal function.

Other Conditions. Reduce dosage in patients with reduced renal function, a history of prior myelosuppressive therapy, and/or poor bone marrow reserve. Reduce dosage by about 25% if the prior nadir WBC count is <500/µL or the platelet count is <50,000/µL. When Cl$_{cr}$ is 41–59 mL/min, a dose of 250 mg/m^2 is recommended; for Cl$_{cr}$ of 16–40 mL/min, 200 mg/m^2 is recommended. Two prospectively validated formulas for dosage individualization are available. One formula seeks to achieve different target serum AUC values in untreated or pretreated patients: dose (mg) = AUC $\times$ (Cl$_{cr}$ + 25), wherein "desired" AUC ranges are 6–8 mg/mL·min for untreated patients and 4–6 mg/mL·min for previously treated patients.[23] The second does not require Cl$_{cr}$ estimates and uses a complex mathematical formula.[24]

Dosage Forms. **Inj** 50, 150, 450 mg.

Patient Instructions. (*See* Antineoplastics Class Instructions, particularly regarding infection risk.)

Pharmacokinetics. *Fate.* About 30% of carboplatin is irreversibly bound to plasma proteins; the half-life of this protein-bound fraction is >5 days.[25] V$_d$ is 16–20 L for carboplatin. Carboplatin is slowly hydrolyzed in vivo to a form with two DNA binding sites; the rate of hydrolysis is much slower than the rate of chloride loss with cisplatin. The free (unbound) fraction of carboplatin and its hydrolyzed species are excreted in urine via both glomerular filtration and tubular secretion. Urinary elimination accounts for over 65% of drug elimination in patients with normal renal function.

$t_{1/2}$. (Unbound) α phase 90 ± 50 min; β phase 180 ± 50 min.[25]

Adverse Reactions. The emetic potential is moderately high to high, but is much less severe than with cisplatin and is easily controlled with antiemetics. Myelosuppression is the primary dose-limiting effect of carboplatin, and thrombocytopenia tends to be more severe than leukopenia; about 25% of previously untreated and 35% of previously treated ovarian cancer patients experience thrombocytopenia. The thrombocytopenic nadir for carboplatin as a single agent is approximately 21 days, and patients with pre-existing renal dysfunction or poor bone marrow reserve have an increased risk for severe thrombocytopenia. Anemia of a mild degree can also occur in up to 90% of patients; in some studies over 40% of patients required transfusions and 5% of patients experienced hemorrhage. Diarrhea, abdominal pain, or constipation occur in 6–17% of patients. Nephrotoxicity occurs in 1–22% of patients. Unlike cisplatin, carboplatin does not cause cumulative damage to renal tubules. Transient decreases of 20–30% in some serum electrolytes occur, specifically magnesium, potassium, sodium, and calcium. Hepatic enzyme elevations may occur in one-third of patients, but they are not associated with serious or prolonged liver injury. Peripheral neuropathies occur in less than 10% of patients; however, the risk increases in patients over 65 yr or if large dosages of cisplatin have been administered. CNS symptoms occur in 5% or less of patients, and ototoxicity occurs in 1% of patients. Occasional reactions include allergic hypersensitivity, alopecia, and various cardiovascular events (eg, embolism, cerebrovascular accident, cardiac failure).

Contraindications. The manufacturer lists pre-existing renal impairment and myelosuppression as contraindications, but the drug has been given with appropriate dosage modification. (*See* Special Populations, Other Conditions.)

Precautions. Use with caution in patients with hearing impairment or reduced renal function, or if extensive prior chemotherapy has been administered. Patients with a history of prior cisplatin therapy are at a higher risk for nephrotoxic and neurotoxic sequelae. Vigorous hydration and diuretics are not usually required with carboplatin.

Drug Interactions. Myelotoxicity of carboplatin is additive with other myelotoxic drugs. Concurrent use of other nephrotoxic drugs (such as aminoglycosides) may delay carboplatin elimination and enhance toxicity. Although not well documented, cisplatin interactions may also occur with carboplatin, but at a lesser intensity.

Parameters to Monitor. Measure Cl_{cr} prior to dosage calculation. Monitor platelet and granulocyte counts, and Cr_s during therapy.

CISPLATIN   Platinol, Various

Pharmacology. Cisplatin is a planar coordinate dichlorodiammino compound of platinum in the +II valence state. It is aquated in vivo to a positively charged species that can alkylate nucleophilic sites in DNA such as purine and pyrimidine bases. Its action is cell cycle phase nonspecific.

Administration and Adult Dosage. IV bolus or continuous infusion (usually with aggressive hydration) single doses of up to 120 mg/m^2 have been used.[26] **IV in the Einhorn testicular cancer regimen** 20 mg/m^2/day for 5 days.[27] (*See* Notes.)

Special Populations. *Pediatric Dosage.* **IV** 10–20 mg/m^2/day for 4–5 days, repeat q 3–4 weeks. **IV** maximum single dose is 100 mg/m^2 given q 2–3 weeks.[26]

Geriatric Dosage. Same as adult dosage, but adjust for age-related reduction in renal function.

Other Conditions. Reduce dosage in renal impairment; specific dosage reduction guidelines have not been established.

Dosage Forms. Inj 10, 50 mg.

Patient Instructions. (*See* Antineoplastics Class Instructions.) Be prepared for severe nausea and vomiting following drug administration.

Pharmacokinetics. *Serum Levels.* In vitro cell culture data suggest cytotoxicity at levels of 50 mg/L for 1 hr or 5 mg/L for 8 hr.

Fate. Peak serum levels of free platinum following a 100 mg/m^2 bolus are about 3.4 mg/L when given with mannitol (12.5 g) and 2.7 mg/L without mannitol.[28] Over 90% of platinum is protein bound to RBCs, albumin, and prealbumin. It is freely distributed to most organs including kidneys, liver, skin, and lungs, and has minimal accumulation in CSF only after repeated doses. Cumulative 24-hr urinary excretion of platinum is 20% with mannitol, 40% without.

t$_{\frac{1}{2}}$. Free platinum 48 min (without mannitol); 59 min (with mannitol). Terminal half-life is 58–73 hr, probably reflecting slow release of protein-bound drug.[28,29]

Adverse Reactions. Emetic potential is high. Nausea and vomiting are severe and often prolonged (days), and may be managed with aggressive prophylaxis using a serotonin 5HT$_3$-antagonist, butyrophenone (eg, droperidol), metoclopramide, a high-dose glucocorticoid, or a combination. Primary toxicity is dose-related nephrotoxicity, especially proximal tubular impairment. Ototoxicity and elevated hepatic enzymes occur frequently; total dose-related hypomagnesemia and severe cumulative peripheral neuropathy occur. Slight leukopenia, thrombocytopenia, and frequent anemia also occur. Epoetin alfa is useful in preventing severe anemia caused by cisplatin. Rare toxicities include transient cortical dysfunction (blindness) and hypersensitivity (including anaphylaxis).

Contraindications. Renal insufficiency (Cr$_s$ >1.5–2 mg/dL or Cl$_{cr}$ <60 mL/min); myelosuppression; hearing impairment; previous anaphylaxis. However, some patients with prior anaphylaxis have been successfully retreated with cisplatin and concomitant antihistamine, epinephrine, and glucocorticoid.

Precautions. Use with caution in renal impairment and with other nephrotoxic drugs, especially aminoglycosides.[30] Assure adequate hydration prior to administration. Both furosemide and mannitol are used to decrease platinum nephrotoxicity, although each apparently retards free platinum elimination.

Drug Interactions. Cisplatin may enhance nephrotoxicity and ototoxicity of the aminoglycosides. Use with ifosfamide may increase nephrotoxicity and potassium and magnesium loss, especially in children. Furosemide ototoxicity may be increased by cisplatin. Cisplatin can increase methotrexate serum levels and its toxicity. Cisplatin can decrease absorption and serum levels of valproic acid. Phenytoin serum levels may be decreased following cisplatin-containing combination regimens.

Parameters to Monitor. Assess renal function prior to each dose (eg, serial BUN or Cr_s) and serum magnesium levels periodically.

Notes. Reconstitute with sterile water; it may then be mixed in saline-containing solutions. It is stable for 24 hr in mannitol. Do not expose solution to metals (eg, metal drippers or cannulae), because platinum may rapidly plate onto these surfaces. Hydrate the patient with at least 1 L of a saline-containing solution with 20 mEq of KCl and 3 g of $MgSO_4/L$.[31]

CYCLOPHOSPHAMIDE   Cytoxan, Various

Pharmacology. Cyclophosphamide is inactive in vitro and must be enzymatically activated in the liver to yield both active alkylating compounds and toxic metabolites.[32] Cell cycle phase nonspecific.

Administration and Adult Dosage. IV or PO alone or in combination regimens 250–500 mg/m² q 3–4 weeks. **IV (usually) or PO in high-dose intermittent regimens (including bone marrow transplant)** maximum of 40–50 mg/kg given once or over 2–5 days, repeat q 2–4 weeks—these doses are not well tolerated orally. IV doses may be given in any convenient volume of all common IV solutions or by IV push. **Continuous daily administration PO** 1–5 mg/kg/day; during continuous therapy, dosage must be individualized based on patient bone marrow response.

Special Populations. *Pediatric Dosage.* **IV, PO for malignancies** same as adult dosage. **PO for nephrotic syndrome** 2.5–3 mg/kg/day for up to 8 weeks.

Geriatric Dosage. Same as adult dosage.

Other Conditions. No dosage alteration appears necessary in renal impairment, because differences in toxicity between normals and patients with renal failure have not been reported.[33]

Dosage Forms. Tab 25, 50 mg; **Inj** 100, 200, 500 mg, 1, 2 g.

Patient Instructions. (*See* Antineoplastics Class Instructions.) Drink 2–3 quarts of fluids daily (1–2 quarts in smaller children) and urinate frequently; do *not* take oral doses at bedtime. Report any blood in the urine.

Pharmacokinetics. *Fate.* Oral absorption is 74 ± 22%.[10] Metabolized to active compounds (including the highly toxic nonalkylating aldehyde, acrolein, and the principal alkylator, phosphoramide mustard) primarily by hepatic microsomal mixed-function oxidases. Cyclophosphamide is 13% plasma protein bound; its alkylating metabolites are 50% bound. V_d is 0.78 ± 0.57 L/kg for parent drug; Cl is 0.078 ± 0.03 L/hr/kg.[10] Renal elimination accounts for 6.5 ± 4.3% of unchanged drug and 60% of metabolites,[34] with a mean renal clearance of 0.66 L/hr of unchanged drug.[33] Clearance may be reduced in obese patients. Elimination is linear over a wide range of doses.[32]

$t_{1/2}$. (Serum alkylating activity) 7.5 ± 4 hr, slightly longer in patients on allopurinol or those previously exposed to cyclophosphamide;[10,33,34] unchanged in renal dysfunction.[35]

Adverse Reactions. Emetic potential is moderate to high (>1 g). Nausea, vomiting, and alopecia are frequent and dose dependent. Dose-limiting toxicity is myelosuppression with a WBC nadir of about 10 days; platelets are also suppressed, perhaps to a lesser extent. Transient, reversible blurred vision occurs frequently. The drug is locally nonirritating. Renally eliminated active metabolites occasionally cause sterile hemorrhagic cystitis, which may resolve slowly, often leading to a fibrotic, contracted bladder. Bladder epithelial changes range from minimal to frank neoplasia. An early sign of cystitis is microscopic hematuria, which can lead to hemorrhage. Prophylactic hydration is recommended. To prevent urotoxicity with high-dose regimens, administer **mesna.** (*See* Mesna.) **Acetylcysteine** (Mucomyst) bladder irrigations may have antidotal activity. Rarely, bladder dysplasia can lead to bladder cancer after very high doses or with concurrent or prior bladder radiation. Cross-allergenicity with other alkylators (eg, mechlorethamine) may occur. Ovarian and testicular function may be permanently lost following high-dose, long-term therapy. Rare reactions include a high-dose fatal cardiomyopathy, "allergic" interstitial pneumonitis, and a transient condition similar to SIADH that is preventable with vigorous isotonic hydration.

Contraindications. Previous life-threatening hypersensitivity to cyclophosphamide; marked leukopenia and thrombocytopenia; hemorrhagic cystitis; severe pulmonary toxicity caused by prior alkylator therapy.

Precautions. Pregnancy. Consider dosage reduction or discontinuation of drug in patients who develop infections.

Drug Interactions. Cyclophosphamide may prolong the action of neuromuscular blocking agents. Allopurinol and cimetidine may enhance cyclophosphamide myelotoxicity.

Parameters to Monitor. Prior to induction therapy, assess the patient for adequate numbers of WBCs (>3500/μL) and platelets (>120,000/μL). With long-term use, assess these counts at least monthly. Monitor closely for hematuria, especially if the patient has received a large cumulative dosage.

Notes. Do not dilute with benzyl alcohol–preserved solutions. Diluted solution is stable for 24 hr at room temperature and 6 days under refrigeration. Widely used in both hematologic and solid malignancies, and as an immunosuppressant in a variety of autoimmune disorders.

DACARBAZINE   DTIC-Dome

Pharmacology. Dacarbazine is an imidazole analogue of a purine precursor that alkylates DNA via methyldiazonium in a cell cycle phase nonspecific fashion. It is used in malignant melanoma with about a 10–20% objective response rate.[36,37]

Adult Dosage. **IV as a single dose** up to 850 mg/m^2, repeated in 3–4 weeks. Alternatively, it may be given in a dosage of up to 250 mg/m^2/day for 5 days, repeated in 3–4 weeks. Reduce the dosage in renal and/or hepatic impairment.

Dosage Forms. Inj 100, 200, 500 mg.

Pharmacokinetics. Dacarbazine is extensively metabolized, some microsomally mediated (50% by N-demethylation); it is 5% plasma protein bound, with 30–45% of a dose excreted unchanged in the urine. The drug has an α half-life of 35 min and a β half-life of about 5 hr; in one patient with renal and hepatic dysfunction, the terminal half-life increased to 7.2 hr.

Adverse Reactions. Nausea and vomiting, which are occasionally severe, occur almost invariably; these may decrease in severity with successive courses of therapy. Dose- and duration-dependent sterility, mutagenicity, and teratogenicity have been reported. Pain on injection also occurs. The dose-limiting toxicity is myelosuppression, with a leukopenic nadir at 21–25 days. Occasionally, a flu-like syndrome of myalgia, fever, and malaise occurs within 1 week of drug administration. Use dacarbazine with caution in patients with pre-existing bone marrow aplasia, and avoid exposure to sunlight because of possible photosensitivity reactions. The drug is light sensitive, therefore minimize exposure to light after reconstitution. The reconstituted solution is clear to pale yellow and is stable for 8 hr after reconstitution at room temperature; pink discoloration denotes drug decomposition.

IFOSFAMIDE   Ifex

Pharmacology. Ifosfamide is a structural analogue of the alkylating agent cyclophosphamide (CTX). The rate of hepatic conversion of ifosfamide to the active metabolite 4-hydroxyifosfamide is slightly slower than with CTX, although formation of the bladder toxin acrolein is not reduced. The ultimate metabolite ifosforamide mustard crosslinks DNA to impair cell division. The drug is always given with mesna to prevent urotoxicity. Although labeled for use in refractory testicular cancer, ifosfamide also has useful activity against soft tissue sarcoma, malignant lymphoma, and small cell lung cancer.[38] Ifosfamide is cell cycle phase nonspecific.

Administration and Adult Dosage. **IV for refractory testicular cancer** 1.2 g/m^2/day over 30 min to 4 hr for 5 days, or 2 g/m^2/day for 3 consecutive days. The recommended concurrent IV **mesna** dose is 20% of the ifosfamide dose, given 15 min before ifosfamide and again at 4 and 8 hr. It can be directly admixed with ifosfamide. The latter two mesna doses can be given orally at twice the dose (ie, each at 40% of the ifosfamide dose) if patient compliance and a lack of emesis can be assured.[39] **Alternatively, IV by continuous infusion** 5–8 g/m^2 over 24 hr with mesna added at the same concentration as ifosfamide.[40] However, more severe nephrotoxicity may occur with this regimen.[41]

Special Populations. *Pediatric Dosage.* **IV for sarcomas (Ewing's and osteosarcoma)** 1.2 g/m^2/day over 30 min for 5 days, each with 3 IV mesna doses as above.[42,43]

Geriatric Dosage. Same as adult dosage, but adjust for age-related reduction in renal function.

Other Conditions. Dosage reduction is indicated in patients with reduced renal function, although specific guidelines are not available.

Dosage Forms. Inj 1, 3 g.

Patient Instructions. (*See* Antineoplastics Class Instructions.)

Pharmacokinetics. *Fate.* Ifosfamide, but not its metabolites, penetrates into the CNS; CSF levels are about 38–49% of simultaneous serum levels. Ifosfamide is metabolized to the active alkylating agent ifosforamide mustard by CYP2B6, which converts ifosfamide to 4-hydroxyifosfamide (which may act as the transport form of the molecule). The 4-hydroxy metabolite is then chemically and enzymatically broken down to active and inactive metabolites. Inactive metabolites include 4-carboxyifosfamide and several dechloroethylated species such as thiodiacetic acid. About 60–80% of a dose is excreted in the urine over 72 hr, including up to 50% of unchanged drug. In addition to 4-hydroxyifosfamide, the bladder irritant acrolein is also excreted renally and can accumulate to high concentrations in the urinary bladder.[44,45]

$t_{1/2}$. 6.9 hr.[46]

Adverse Reactions. Emetic potential is moderate; nausea and vomiting can be readily managed with antiemetics. Alopecia occurs in most patients treated with ifosfamide. The major dose-limiting effect of ifosfamide is urotoxicity manifested as hematuria. The frequency of microscopic hematuria with ifosfamide and the chemoprotectant mesna ranges from 5–18% of courses;[38] gross hematuria is less common (<5%). (*See* Mesna.) Renal tubular toxicity, manifested by elevations in BUN and Cr_s, occurs in <10% of patients. It is more frequent in patients who are poorly hydrated or have pre-existing abnormal renal function,[47] those with renal cell cancer,[48] those given high-dose 24-hr continuous ifosfamide infusions,[49] and those receiving concomitant treatment with other nephrotoxins.[47] Myelosuppression primarily involves leukopenia with a 7- to 14-day nadir. This effect is less severe than with cyclophosphamide and rarely affects platelets. However, in combination with other myelosuppressive drugs, additive leukopenia may occur that is not reduced by mesna. Leukopenia has been particularly severe in nephrectomized patients with renal cell cancer.[49] CNS toxicities occur in up to 50% of patients, but risk factors, including dosage, are unclear. The most common effect is a slight sedation or somnolence, which rarely proceeds to coma and death. These signs appear within 2 hr and typically remit 1–3 days after drug administration. Other rare CNS neurotoxicities include cerebellar toxicity (ataxia), urinary incontinence, and seizures.[50] Some of these CNS effects may be caused by the minor metabolite chloracetaldehyde, which is excreted in the urine and accumulates in renal failure.[51] Transient elevation in liver function tests is frequently reported, but is rarely clinically important. Other occasional toxic effects include allergic reactions, diarrhea, peripheral neuropathy, and stomatitis.

Contraindications. Severe pre-existing myelosuppression.

Precautions. Because of more severe nephrotoxicity and CNS toxicities, patients with reduced renal function, and particularly nephrectomized renal cell cancer patients, are poor candidates for this agent. Withhold repeat therapy until there is resolution of microscopic hematuria (<10 RBCs per high-power field). An adequate state of hydration is critical to reducing urotoxicity.

Drug Interactions. Use with cisplatin may increase nephrotoxicity and potassium and magnesium loss, especially in children. Nephrotoxicity is also enhanced when ifosfamide is combined with other nephrotoxic drugs.

Parameters to Monitor. Ensure that renal function and peripheral WBC counts are normal prior to administration. During therapy, monitor hematuria daily because dosage reduction or higher mesna dosage may prevent more serious urotoxicity.

Notes. Ifosfamide is compatible with D5W, NS, Ringer's lactate injection, and sterile water. It can also be directly mixed with mesna. Exercise caution to reduce exposure during handling and disposal.

MECHLORETHAMINE HYDROCHLORIDE   Mustargen

Pharmacology. Mechlorethamine (nitrogen mustard; HN_2) is a prototype bis-chloroethylamine, polyfunctional alkylating agent. In solution, the compound readily ionizes to an active form, which can alkylate at a number of nucleophilic protein sites, principally the N^7 position of guanine in both DNA and RNA. This action is cell cycle phase nonspecific.

Administration and Adult Dosage. **IV for Hodgkin's disease** (in the classical MOPP regimen) 6 mg/m^2 by careful push on days 1 and 8 of a monthly treatment cycle.[52] Irritation, spasm, and sclerosis occur in exposed veins; therefore, it is common to begin venipunctures low on the limb and move up serially, and to administer mechlorethamine last in a combination drug sequence. **IV as a single agent** up to 0.4 mg/kg as a single monthly dose. **Top for mycosis fungoides and psoriasis** 10 mg/60 mL of water, applied to the affected body areas 1 or 2 times a day.[53]

Special Populations. *Pediatric Dosage.* **IV** same as adult dosage.

Geriatric Dosage. Same as adult dosage.

Dosage Forms. **Inj** 10 mg.

Patient Instructions. (*See* Antineoplastics Class Instructions.)

Pharmacokinetics. *Fate.* Chemical cyclization occurs in vivo to form positively charged carbonium ions, which rapidly react with various cellular components; unchanged drug cannot be detected in the blood within minutes of administration. Less than 0.01% of unchanged drug is recovered in the urine; however, up to 50% of radioactively labeled products may be found in urine within 24 hr.[1]

Adverse Reactions. Emetic potential is high; nausea and vomiting within the first 3 hr are severe and may last over 1 day. The major dose-limiting toxicity is myelosuppression: leukopenic nadir occurs at 6–8 days, thrombocytopenic nadir at 10–16 days. Extravasation causes delayed and protracted (months) ulceration and necrosis; a 1/6 molar sodium **thiosulfate** solution (4 mL of 10% sodium thiosulfate plus 6 mL sterile water) and copious flushing with water may be used as topical antidotes to lessen serious tissue damage. Primary reproductive failure and alopecia are frequent in both males and females. IV or topical use can cause maculopapular rashes and sometimes severe sensitivity reactions (anaphylaxis and occasional cross-reactivity with other alkylating agents).

Contraindications. Prior severe hypersensitivity reactions; pre-existing profound myelosuppression; infection.

Precautions. Give patients with lymphomas (especially "bulky" lymphomas) prophylactic allopurinol 2–3 days prior to and throughout therapy to prevent hyperuricemia and urate nephropathy following massive tumor lysis. Make every effort to avoid topical contact with this highly vesicant drug by health personnel.

Drug Interactions. None known.

Parameters to Monitor. Pretreatment and at least monthly assessment of bone marrow function, particularly WBC and platelet counts.

Notes. Mechlorethamine is a powerful vesicant and should be prepared with great caution. Use mask and rubber gloves during preparation and avoid inhalation of dust and vapors, or contact with skin and mucous membranes, especially the eyes. Use the injection within 1 hr of preparation; topical solution and ointment are stable for 1 month under refrigeration.[54] Because of its extreme acute toxicity, use is limited primarily to malignant lymphomas[52] and topically in mycosis fungoides, a cutaneous non-Hodgkin's T-cell lymphoma.[55]

MITOMYCIN   Mutamycin

Pharmacology. Mitomycin (mitomycin C) is an antibiotic that contains quinone, urethane, and aziridine groups. It is activated chemically and metabolically to alkylating species; it is cell cycle phase nonspecific, but maximum efficacy is in the G_1 and S phases. Mitomycin is used primarily in GI tract tumors intravenously and in bladder cancer intravesically.[56-59]

Adult Dosage. **IV as a single agent** 10–15 mg/m^2 in a single dose and repeated q 6 weeks if hematologic toxicity has resolved. **IV in combination regimens** 5–10 mg/m^2 repeated in 4–6 weeks. **Intravesically in bladder cancer** up to 60 mg/week.

Dosage Forms. **Inj** 5, 20, 40 mg.

Pharmacokinetics. Following IV doses of 15 mg/m^2, the peak serum level is about 1 mg/L (3 μmol/L). The drug is eliminated primarily by hepatic clearance, with about 20% hepatic extraction and 10–30% recovery of unchanged drug in the urine. Cl is 0.3–0.4 L/hr/kg. The drug has an α half-life of 5–10 min after IV injection and β half-life of 46 min.

Adverse Reactions. Nausea, vomiting, diarrhea, alopecia, and nephrotoxicity occur frequently. The drug also produces sterility, mutagenicity, and teratogenicity. The dose-limiting toxicities are myelosuppression (with a long leukopenic nadir of 3–4 weeks), thrombocytopenia, and anemia, all of which may be cumulative. Monitor the patient carefully for delayed and prolonged myelosuppression. Severe ulceration may occur if the drug is extravasated (topical **DMSO** may be useful). Interstitial pneumonia, for which a glucocorticoid is helpful, occurs occasionally. Long-term therapy occasionally causes hemolytic-uremic syndrome. Mitomycin is contraindicated in patients with pre-existing severe myelosuppression or anemia.

NITROSOUREAS:

CARMUSTINE	BiCNU
LOMUSTINE	CeeNU

Pharmacology. Carmustine (BCNU) and lomustine (CCNU) are highly lipid soluble drugs which are metabolized to active alkylating and carbamoylating moieties. Several key cellular enzymatic steps are inhibited, including those involving DNA polymerase and RNA and protein synthesis. There is typically only partial cross-resistance to classical alkylators. The nitrosoureas are cell cycle phase nonspecific and even have activity on G_0 (resting phase) cells.

Administration and Dosage. (*See also* Notes.)

	CARMUSTINE	LOMUSTINE
Administration	IV in 100–200 mL D5W in glass containers only over 15–45 min.	PO only.
Adult Dosage	75–100 mg/m²/day for 1–2 days or 200 mg/m² as a single dose, or 80 mg/m²/day for 3 days. Repeat at 6- to 8-week intervals.	100–130 mg/m² as a single dose, repeat at 6- to 8-week intervals.
Pediatric Dosage	Same as adult dosage.	Same as adult dosage.
Geriatric Dosage	Reduce dosage by 25–50% and/or increase treatment interval to at least 8 weeks.	Same as adult dosage.
Other Conditions	Treat patients with heavily pretreated bone marrow with 50–75% of the recommended dosage and/or at lengthened treatment intervals (8 weeks minimum).	

Dosage Forms. (Carmustine) **Inj** 100 mg with alcohol diluent. (Lomustine) **Cap** 10, 40, 100 mg—commercial packet contains two of each strength for a total of 300 mg. (*See* Notes.)

Patient Instructions. (*See* Antineoplastics Class Instructions.) Take lomustine on an empty stomach.

Pharmacokinetics.

Fate.

	CARMUSTINE	LOMUSTINE
Absorption	—	Complete after 30 min.[60]
Distribution	Both drugs are diffusely distributed with decreasing relative concentrations in spleen, liver, and ovaries; both achieve substantial penetration into CNS with simultaneous CSF levels of >50% of serum for intact carmustine and its metabolites[61] and >30% for intact lomustine and its metabolites;[60] enterohepatic cycling of active metabolites is possible and may explain subsequent peaks in nitrosourea serum levels at 1 and 4 hr.	

(continued)

	CARMUSTINE	**LOMUSTINE**
Metabolism	Both drugs are rapidly and extensively metabolized (partially by liver microsomal enzymes) to a number of active products which have long serum half-lives compared to the parent compounds.	
Excretion	30% urinary drug recovery as metabolites after 24 hr, 65% after 96 hr.[61]	50% urinary drug recovery as metabolites after 12 hr, 60% after 48 hr; <5% fecal excretion.[60]
$t_{1/2}$	Intact drug 5 min; biologic effect 15–30 min; metabolites, slow decay over 3–4 days.[61]	Intact drug 15 min; cyclohexyl and carbonyl metabolites: α phase 4–5 hr, ß phase 30–50 hr; chloroethyl metabolite 72 hr.[60]

Adverse Reactions. Emetic potential is moderately high to high; prophylactic antiemetics are recommended. Major dose-limiting toxicity is delayed and potentially cumulative myelosuppression; nadirs are unusually prolonged, with leukopenia at approximately 35 days and thrombocytopenia at about 30 days. Thus, doses are not repeated more often than q 6 weeks.[62] Carmustine frequently causes severe pain at injection site and venospasm, which may be reduced by slow, dilute infusions. Both drugs may transiently elevate liver enzymes. Pulmonary fibrosis may occur following cumulative dosages over 1 g/m²; nephrotoxicity consistently occurs following cumulative dosages of 1.5 g/m² or more.[63] Variant carmustine-induced pulmonary fibrosis, highly responsive to early drug discontinuation and a glucocorticoid, has been reported.[64] Other occasional toxicities include CNS effects (eg, confusion, lethargy, ataxia), stomatitis, and alopecia. In animal models, the nitrosoureas are highly carcinogenic and several clinical cases of leukemia after nitrosourea therapy have been reported.

Contraindications. Demonstrated hypersensitivity; marked pre-existing myelosuppression.

Precautions. Pregnancy.

Drug Interactions. Experimentally in rats, carmustine, lomustine, and the investigational drug semustine are cleared much more rapidly (with reduced antitumor activity) by pretreatment with phenobarbital, which stimulates microsomal enzymes. Conversely, cimetidine can impair metabolism and increase nitrosourea myelotoxicity. Clinical resistance to carmustine and perhaps other nitrosoureas is reduced by concomitant amphotericin B. Digoxin and phenytoin serum levels may be decreased following carmustine-containing combination regimens.

Notes. Store carmustine under refrigeration; appearance of an oily film in the vial is evidence of decomposition, and such vials should be discarded. Carmustine is incompatible with sodium bicarbonate. Lomustine absorption is rapid; thus, vomiting 45 min or more after ingestion does not require readministration.

Carmustine implant wafers (Gliadel) contain 7.7 mg of carmustine in a biodegradable, hydrophilic polyanhydride polymer (Polifeprosam 20). They are indicated for implantation in the resection cavity of patients undergoing surgery for recurrent glioblastoma multiforme. In a multicenter, placebo-controlled trial, 6-month survival in patients with glioblastoma was 50% greater with carmustine implants than with placebo. The typical adult dosage is 8 wafers (61.6 mg of carmustine) implanted at the time of surgery. In experimental systems, the polymer releases carmustine over a 2- to 3-week period in vivo. Intracranial infections occur at a higher rate (4% vs. 1%) and seizures are more frequent with carmustine wafers than in untreated patients. Mild to moderate healing abnormalities occur in 4% of treated patients compared to 1% of untreated patients. Other systemic and CNS side effects are equivalent in treated and untreated patients.[65,66]

PROCARBAZINE HYDROCHLORIDE   Matulane

Pharmacology. Procarbazine is an N-methylhydrazine derivative that undergoes auto-oxidation and microsomal activation to form several alkylating species, including the diazonium ion as well as several oxygen free radicals such as H_2O_2, $\cdot OH$ and $\cdot O_2$ (superoxide). It is cell cycle phase nonspecific and used in brain tumors and Hodgkin's and non-Hodgkin's lymphomas.[67]

Adult Dosage. PO 50–200 mg/m^2/day for 10–25 days, repeated in 3–4 weeks. Calculate the dosage based on ideal body weight and reduce dosage for a BUN >40 mg/dL, Cr_s >2 mg/dL, or serum bilirubin >3 mg/dL.

Dosage Forms. Cap 50 mg.

Pharmacokinetics. The drug is rapidly and well absorbed after oral administration; CNS levels are equal to serum after 0.5–1.5 hr. Procarbazine is 70% recovered in the urine, primarily as an acid metabolite, with <5% excreted unchanged.

Adverse Reactions. Frequent CNS side effects include dizziness, headache, ataxia, nightmares, depression, and hallucinations (in up to 30% of patients). Paresthesias may also occur occasionally. Mild to moderate nausea and vomiting occur in 60–90% of patients, but tolerance usually develops rapidly. Dose- and duration-dependent sterility, mutagenicity, and teratogenicity are reported. The drug predisposes patients to secondary acute nonlymphocytic leukemias. The dose-limiting toxicity is myelosuppression with a pancytopenic nadir at 2–3 weeks. Occasional side effects include a flu-like syndrome, allergic pneumonitis, and rash. Procarbazine is contraindicated in patients with *severe* hypersensitivity to the drug or pre-existing bone marrow aplasia. Periodic evaluations of neurologic status and monthly CBCs may be useful.

Drug Interactions. Avoid concurrent use with MAO inhibitors, alcohol, heterocyclic antidepressants, sympathomimetics, or tyramine-containing foods. Microsomal enzyme-inducing drugs may augment procarbazine cytotoxicity. Procarbazine potentiates barbiturates, narcotics, and other hepatically metabolized drugs.

STREPTOZOCIN   Zanosar

Pharmacology. Streptozocin (streptozotocin) is a glucose-containing nitrosourea. It has some selective cytotoxic activity in insulinomas and malignant carcinoid, and is active to a lesser extent in other adenocarcinomas of the GI tract. The drug inhibits DNA synthesis via inhibition of pyrimidine biosynthesis and blockade of key enzymatic reactions in gluconeogenesis pathways. It is cell cycle phase non-specific.[68]

Adult Dosage. IV as a single agent 1–1.5 g/m^2/week for 6 weeks, followed by a 4-week observation period; **IV in combination** 0.5–1 g/m^2/day for 5 days q 4–6 weeks.

Dosage Forms. Inj 1 g.

Pharmacokinetics. Streptozocin is highly lipophilic, achieving good CNS penetration. Streptozocin and metabolites have a short distribution phase ($t_{1/2}$, 6 min) followed by possibly two elimination phases representing active metabolites ($t_{1/2\beta}$, 3.5 hr; $t_{1/2\gamma}$, 40 hr). The drug is rapidly and extensively metabolized (unchanged drug half-life is 35 min), and only 10–20% is excreted unchanged in urine.

Adverse Reactions. Frequent acute toxicities include nausea, vomiting, and phlebitis; carefully avoid extravasation. The drug is moderately myelotoxic, but extremely nephrotoxic. Signs of streptozocin nephrotoxicity include various renal tubular defects and proteinuria; adequate hydration may offer some protection. It also selectively destroys pancreatic β cells.

THIOTEPA

Pharmacology. Thiotepa (TESPA, TSPA) is a thiophosphoramide compound that is slowly hydrolyzed to release ethylenimine moieties that alkylate DNA. It is used systemically in the treatment of breast cancer, intracavitarily for bladder or pleural disease and intrathecally for CNS disease. It is also given in high doses with autologous bone marrow transplantation.[69]

Adult Dosage. IV, IM, or SC 0.5 mg/kg monthly or 6 mg/m^2/day for 4 days. Reduce the dosage by all routes in patients with pre-existing bone marrow suppression. **Intracavitary** 60 mg; **IT** 1–10 mg/m^2.

Dosage Forms. Inj 15 mg.

Pharmacokinetics. Thiotepa is slowly metabolized, primarily to TEPA. Total body Cl is 8.5 $L/hr/m^2$, with 15% recovered in the urine as TEPA in 24 hr. Thiotepa has an α half-life of 7.5 min and a β half-life of 109 min.

Adverse Reactions. Mild nausea and vomiting occur frequently. The dose-limiting toxicity is myelosuppression (both granulocytes and platelets). Myelosuppression can occur after intravesicular or intrapleural administration. Anaphylaxis occurs rarely, and mutagenicity, teratogenicity, and sterility have been reported.

Antimetabolites

CLADRIBINE
Leustatin

Pharmacology. Cladribine (2CdA) is the 20-chloro analogue of deoxyadenosine. It is a purine nucleoside that is avidly phosphorylated to toxic metabolites that accumulate intracellularly. Lymphocytes, which lack inactivating deaminase activity, are selectively destroyed by inhibition of both DNA synthesis and repair. Cladribine is highly active in hairy cell leukemia; other responsive tumors include malignant lymphoma and acute and chronic myelogenous leukemias. It is also promising in the treatment of chronic progressive multiple sclerosis.[70-73]

Adult Dosage. **IV for hairy cell leukemia** 0.09 mg/kg/day for 7 days by continuous infusion. New dosage regimens are exploring single daily SC injections because of the prolonged intracellular retention of active metabolites.

Dosage Forms. **Inj** 1 mg/mL.

Pharmacokinetics. Studies with oral administration indicate a bioavailability of 48%, implying that doubling the IV dose may allow oral administration in hairy cell leukemia. The drug has a $V_{d\beta}$ of 9.2 ± 5.4 L/kg and biphasic elimination with half-lives of 35 min and 6.7 hr. About 40% of a dose is excreted renally as parent drug and metabolites.

Adverse Reactions. Frequent adverse reactions include severe neutropenia with fever and infection (70%), anemia (37%), and thrombocytopenia (12%). A flu-like syndrome is also common. Suppression of immune system function because of helper T-lymphocyte depletion can be quite long-lived and presents a risk of systemic opportunistic infections by fungi, bacteria, and/or parasites such as *Pneumocystis carinii*.

CYTARABINE
Cytosar-U

Pharmacology. Cytarabine (cytosine arabinoside, Ara-C) is an arabinose sugar analogue of the natural pyrimidine nucleoside deoxycytidine. Cytarabine is converted to the triphosphate derivative, ara-CTP, which interferes with one or more DNA polymerases and is incorporated into DNA strands, leading to DNA fragmentation and chain termination. Once a threshold level of ara-C-mediated DNA damage is exceeded, apoptosis occurs.[74] Cytarabine is cell cycle S phase specific, with activity markedly enhanced by continuous administration over several days.

Administration and Adult Dosage. **IV for remission induction** 100–150 mg/m²/day as a continuous infusion for 5–10 days. Experimental therapy has successfully used induction doses of 2–3 g/m² q 12 hr as a 2-hr infusion for 4–12 doses in refractory AML.[75] **IV or SC for remission induction** 100 mg/m² q 12 hr for 5–10 days. **SC for remission maintenance** 70–100 mg/m²/day for 5 days in 4 divided doses. (*See* Notes.)

Special Populations. *Pediatric Dosage.* **IV or SC** same as adult dosage.

Geriatric Dosage. Same as adult dosage.

Dosage Forms. **Inj** 100, 500 mg, 1, 2 g.

Patient Instructions. (*See* Antineoplastics Class Instructions.)

Pharmacokinetics. *Serum Levels.* 50–100 mg/L (0.2–0.4 mmol/L) are required for cytotoxic effects.[76]

Fate. Not systemically available following oral absorption. After injection, there is a large interpatient variation in serum levels attained as measured by various assay techniques.[77] Serum levels of 100–400 mg/L (0.4–1.6 mmol/L) are produced by a 60-min continuous infusion of 300 mg/m².[78] Serum levels up to 240 mg/L (1 mmol/L) are achieved with high-dose regimens. It is widely distributed and deactivated by cytidine deaminase, primarily in the liver. The CSF to serum ratio is 0.1–0.14:1 with bolus doses and up to 0.4–0.5:1 with continuous infusion. There is slow elimination from the CSF caused by low CNS deaminating activity; however, to attain therapeutic CSF concentrations following standard IV doses, intrathecal administration is required. Tear fluid concentrations are detectable after high-dose therapy. The drug is about 13% plasma protein bound. V_d is 3 ± 1.9 L/kg; Cl is 0.78 ± 0.24 L/hr/kg.[10] The deamination product, uracil arabinoside (ara-U) is inactive and rapidly excreted in the urine; 24 hr after injection, 72% of the dose is recovered in the urine as Ara-U, only $11 \pm 8\%$ as unchanged drug.[10,79]

$t_{\frac{1}{2}}$. α phase 1.6–12 min; β phase 2.6 ± 0.6 hr.[10,78–80]

Adverse Reactions. Emetic potential is moderate (<250 mg) to moderately high (250 mg–1 g); prophylactic antiemetics are very effective. The principal side effect is dose-related myelosuppression with a leukopenic nadir of 3–11 days and a thrombocytopenic nadir of 12–14 days; megaloblastosis is typically noted in the recovering bone marrow and in the rare cases in which anemia develops. Ocular toxicity is frequent with high-dose therapy; typically, conjunctival injection and central punctate corneal opacities occur. Concurrent use of glucocorticoid eye drops is recommended with high-dose therapy.[81] Occasionally, mild oral ulceration and a flu-like syndrome, manifested by arthralgias, fever, and sometimes rash, occur. Irreversible cerebellar toxicity (ataxia, cognitive dysfunction) is a risk after cumulative doses of 30 g/m^2 or greater.[82] Hepatic enzyme elevation is rare, even with 3 g/m^2 doses; one instance of SIADH was reported with this large dose.[75] Cutaneous small vessel necrotizing vasculitis has occurred rarely after high-dose cytarabine, 3–5 days after initiation of therapy.[83]

Precautions. Myelosuppression is *not* a contraindication, because marrow hypoplasia with complete suppression of the leukemic clone is the desired clinical endpoint; however, extensive supportive facilities must be available during therapy, including WBC and platelet transfusion capability.

Drug Interactions. Digoxin bioavailability from tablets may be decreased following cytarabine-containing combination regimens.

Parameters to Monitor. Routine WBC and platelet counts; RBC indices.

Notes. Patients may be taught sterile technique for self-administration of SC drug for leukemia remission maintenance. The use of small reconstitution volumes (1 mL/100 mg) and rotation of injection sites should be observed. Clinical activity is limited primarily to selected hematologic malignancies (eg, AML, ALL, DHL). The combination of cytarabine and **interferon** increases the rate of response and prolongs survival in patients with the chronic phase of chronic myelogenous leukemia compared to interferon alone.[84]

Cytarabine is given by IT injection or intraventricular injection via an implanted Ommaya reservoir to prevent or treat malignant metastases from acute myeloid leukemia and other cancers. The usual adult dosage is 70 mg/m^2 (or a fixed 100 mg) per dose once or twice weekly. IT doses should not be repeated more often than q 3–5 days in adults. In children, the dose is reduced as follows: (<1 yr) reduce by one-half; (1–2 yr) reduce by one-third; (2–3 yr) reduce by one-sixth. The drug should be diluted only with nonpreserved, isotonic solutions such as NS, or preferably, Ringer's lactate (because of its buffering capacity). In these dilutions, cytarabine is physically compatible with hydrocortisone sodium succinate and methotrexate if a neutral pH is maintained. The half-life in CSF ranges from 2–11 hr (mean 3.5 hr). Typical toxicities include headache and vomiting which are dose- and frequency-related. Patients with blocked or impaired CSF outflow may experience greater toxicity. With frequent, repeated administration, seizures and paraplegia can occur.[80,81]

FLOXURIDINE   FUDR, Various

Pharmacology. Floxuridine is the deoxyribose metabolite of fluorouracil. The drug inhibits DNA synthesis by binding to thymidylate synthetase in S phase of cell division.

Administration and Adult Dosage. Intra-arterially for colon cancer metastases to the liver 0.1–0.6 mg/kg/day for 1–6 weeks by continuous hepatic artery perfusion.[85] Hospitalize patients for at least the first course of therapy.

Special Populations. *Pediatric Dosage.* Safety and efficacy not established.

Geriatric Dosage. Same as adult dosage.

Other Conditions. Reduce dosage when combined with other myelosuppressive drugs or in patients experiencing severe toxicity (usually mucositis or diarrhea) from previous doses.

Dosage Forms. Inj 500 mg.

Patient Instructions. (*See* Antineoplastics Class Instructions.)

Pharmacokinetics. *Fate.* Floxuridine has a high degree (69–92%) of hepatic extraction. A large fraction is converted to the active phosphorylated metabolite 5-fluorodeoxyuridylate monophosphate (FdUMP). Ultimately, the drug is almost completely metabolized to inactive compounds, which are eliminated by exhalation (60% of a dose) or by urinary excretion (about 10–30% of a dose).[86]

$t_{1/2}$. <15 min.

Adverse Reactions. Emetic potential with intra-arterial administration is low. Diarrhea and stomatitis occur frequently. Stomatitis can be life-threatening, as can an unusual dermatitis affecting the hands and feet; both toxicities are much more frequent with prolonged infusions. The primary dose-limiting toxicity of floxuridine is myelosuppression, principally leukopenia with some thrombocytopenia. Liver enzyme elevations occur frequently, but they rarely herald serious hepatic complications. Local complications involving the hepatic catheter include thrombosis, leakage, embolism, and infection. Some catheter placements can also result in gastric ulcers or biliary sclerosis if their respective arterioles are inadvertently perfused.[85]

Contraindications. Pregnancy; poor nutrition; pre-existing myelosuppression; serious infection.

Precautions. Biliary sclerosis may occur, requiring repositioning or removal of the catheter.

Drug Interactions. None known.

Parameters to Monitor. Monitor WBC count prior to and following each treatment. Observe for diarrhea (fluid and electrolyte status). Monitor for severe hepatic enzyme elevations, which may indicate biliary sclerosis.

Notes. Floxuridine can be administered in NS or D5W and it is compatible with heparin.

FLUDARABINE PHOSPHATE   Fludara

Pharmacology. Fludarabine is a fluorinated nucleotide analogue of vidarabine. It is rapidly converted to 2-fluoro-ara-A, which is then phosphorylated to 2-fluoro-ara-ATP, which inhibits DNA synthesis. Fludarabine has little cross-resistance with other agents used for chronic lymphocytic leukemia (CLL).

Adult Dosage. **IV for B-cell CLL that has not responded to at least one standard alkylating agent regimen** 25 mg/m²/day for 5 days given over 30 min in 100–125 mL of D5W or NS. Refrigerate the drug before reconstitution and use within 8 hr after reconstitution.

Dosage Forms. **Inj** 50 mg.

Pharmacokinetics. The metabolite 2-fluoro-ara-A has a V_d of 98 L/m², a Cl of 8.9 L/hr/m², and a half-life of about 10 hr. About 23% of a dose is excreted in the urine as unchanged 2-fluoro-ara-A, and clearance is proportional to Cl_{cr}.

Adverse Reactions. The most frequent adverse effects are myelosuppression (neutropenia, thrombocytopenia, and anemia), fever and chills, infection, rash, myalgia, nausea, vomiting, and diarrhea. Frequent pulmonary symptoms include pneumonia, cough, and dyspnea. Fludarabine produced severe CNS toxicity (ie, blindness, coma, and death) in 36% of patients treated with a dosage of 4 times the currently recommended dosage. Similar CNS toxicity occurs occasionally ($\leq 0.2\%$ of patients) with recommended dosages. Other CNS effects include weakness, visual disturbances, paresthesias, agitation, confusion, and peripheral neuropathy.

FLUOROURACIL   Various

Pharmacology. Fluorouracil (5-fluorouracil, 5-FU) is a fluorinated antimetabolite of the DNA pyrimidine precursor uracil. It inhibits thymidine formation, thereby blocking DNA synthesis. Some fluorouracil may be incorporated into RNA, inhibiting subsequent protein synthesis. It is cell cycle S phase specific.

Administration and Adult Dosage. **Rapid IV** 15 mg/kg/week for 4 weeks followed by 20 mg/kg/week until severe toxicity develops. The drug is stopped until resolution is complete, then resumed at 5 mg/kg/week.[87] **IV "loading course"** 12 mg/kg (800 mg maximum) as a single daily dose for 4 days, then 12–15 mg/kg/week is recommended by manufacturer; however, this regimen has been associated with severe, life-threatening bone marrow toxicity.[88] **IV continuous infusion** 1–2 g/day for up to 5 days has been used by special treatment centers; continuous infusion does not consistently increase antitumor efficacy, but does appear to lessen hematologic toxicity.[89] **IV for Dukes' stage C colon cancer following resection in combination with levamisole** 450 mg/m²/day for 5 days initially, then 450 mg/m² once a week beginning in 28 days and continued for 1 yr. (*See* Notes.) **PO** doses are associated with low bioavailability and short clinical response. **Intra-arterial, intraperitoneal, and intracavitary** administration have also been used, although floxuridine is preferred. **Top for neoplastic keratoses** apply daily for 1–2 weeks as a thin layer with gloved hand or nonmetal applicator. Skin response progresses sequentially through erythema, vesiculation, erosion, ulceration, necrosis, and finally regranulation. Treatment is usually stopped once erosion is evident to allow healing to occur over the next 1–2 months. **Vag for condylomata acuminata** ⅓ applicatorful (1.5 g) of 5% cream once a week hs for 10 weeks.[90]

Special Populations. *Pediatric Dosage.* Generally indicated for adult malignancies, although theoretically, equivalent mg/kg doses could be used in children.

Geriatric Dosage. Same as adult dosage.

Other Conditions. Base dosage on ideal body weight in obesity or if the patient has excessive fluid retention.

Dosage Forms. **Inj** 50 mg/mL; **Top Crm** 1.5%; **Top Soln** 1, 2, 5%.

Patient Instructions. (*See* Antineoplastics Class Instructions.) Avoid prolonged exposure to strong sunlight; report any severe sores in the mouth immediately.

Pharmacokinetics. *Fate.* Oral doses are erratically and incompletely absorbed with bioavailability of 28%, worsened by mixing with acidic fruit juices.[90] The drug is 8–12% plasma protein bound. The drug diffuses into effusions and CSF (peak CSF levels of 60–80 nmol/L after a 15 mg/kg IV bolus). V_d is about 25 ± 12 L/kg; Cl is 0.96 ± 0.42 L/hr/kg.[10] Extensively and rapidly metabolized, primarily in the liver, to a variety of inactive metabolites that are renally excreted. Up to 15% is renally excreted unchanged, 90% within 6 hr of administration. Fluoroacetate and citrate metabolites found in the CSF are believed to mediate rare CNS (cerebellar) toxicities.

$t_{1/2}$. α phase about 8 min; β phase 11 ± 4 min.[10,91]

Adverse Reactions. Emetic potential is moderately low (<1 g) to moderate (>1 g). Dose-limiting toxicity is myelosuppression (when given by bolus injection) with leukopenic and thrombocytopenic nadirs at 7–14 days. Severe stomatitis 5–8 days after therapy can herald severe impending myelosuppression; this occurs unpredictably with large bolus doses (>12 mg/kg). With continuous infusions, myelosuppression is reduced considerably, but mucositis and diarrhea may be dose limiting. Oral administration increases severity of the frequent mild diarrhea. GI ulceration is occasionally severe. Cutaneous toxicities include mild to moderate alopecia, hyperpigmentation of skin and veins, and rashes that are often worsened by sunlight. Excessive lacrimation is frequent; occasionally tear duct fibrosis develops. Rare toxicities involve CNS dysfunction manifested by ataxia, confusion, visual disturbances, and headache. Cardiotoxicity occurs rarely.

Contraindications. Pregnancy. Pre-existing severe myelosuppression (WBCs <2000/μL, platelet count <100,000/μL); poor nutritional state; serious infections.

Precautions. Use with caution in patients with pre-existing coronary artery disease.

Drug Interactions. Concurrent allopurinol appears to block one activation pathway, thereby reducing fluorouracil hematologic toxicity. Fluorouracil can inhibit the antipurine effects of methotrexate. The clinical importance of these two interactions is unclear.

Parameters to Monitor. Pretreatment and monthly assessment of bone marrow function, particularly WBC and platelet counts. In the weeks following administration, observe for severe stomatitis, which may herald life-threatening myelosuppression.

Notes. If a precipitate is noted in the ampule, gently warm in a water bath and/or vigorously shake to redissolve. Fluorouracil is physically incompatible with diazepam, doxorubicin, cytarabine, and methotrexate injections. Mild to moderate activity in GI tract tumors and in breast cancer; topical application of cream is often curative in superficial skin cancers. **Leucovorin** has been used with fluorouracil to increase fluorouracil binding to the target enzyme, thymidylate synthetase. **Levamisole** (Ergamisol) is an immunomodulator used to enhance fluorouracil efficacy in Dukes' C colon cancer. It is given orally in a dosage of 50 mg q 8 hr for 3 days, q 14 days for 1 yr.

GEMCITABINE   Gemsar

Pharmacology. Gemcitabine is a difluorinated nucleoside analogue of cytarabine that is phosphorylated by intracellular deoxycytidine kinase to the active di- and triphosphate forms. These antimetabolites inhibit ribonucleotide reductase and reduce the normal pool of deoxycytidine triphosphate, respectively. This leads to an inhibition of DNA synthesis (both replication and repair). Compared to cytarabine, gemcitabine is preferentially phosphorylated and retained intracellularly. It is approved for palliative therapy in pancreatic cancer, and is also active in breast cancer and non–small cell lung cancer.[92-94] (*See* Notes.)

Administration and Adult Dosage. IV 1 g/m^2/week infused over 30 min for 7 consecutive weeks, followed by 1 week rest, then once weekly for 3 weeks with 1 week rest thereafter.

Dosage Forms. **Inj** 100, 500 mg.

Patient Instructions. (*See* Antineoplastics Class Instructions.) Take acetaminophen prior to each dose to reduce flu-like symptoms.

Pharmacokinetics. *Fate.* A peak serum level of 14.7 mg/L (56 μmol/L) occurs following a 1 g/m^2 IV dose. The drug is metabolized to active di- and triphosphate forms and also deaminated to inactive difluorodeoxyuridine (dFdU) in liver and blood. Cl is 408 ± 121 L/hr/m^2 in men, and 31% lower in women. Renal elimination of dFdU is 77% of a dose; 5% of a dose is recovered unchanged in urine.[92]

$t_{1/2}$. (Gemcitabine) 8–14 min (dose and infusion duration dependent); (dFdU) 10–14 hr.[92]

Adverse Reactions. Emetic potential is moderately low and is well controlled by antiemetics. Thrombocytopenia is the dose-limiting toxicity; cumulative-dosage anemia is next most common. Neutropenia occurs, but is rarely dose limiting. A transient, acute flu-like syndrome consisting of fever, fatigue, chills, headache, and arthralgias occurs in most patients. Fever responds to acetaminophen and usually does not recur. Erythematous pruritic maculopapular rashes on the neck and extremities are frequent, but usually respond to a tropical glucocorticoid. Hepatic transaminases may increase in two-thirds of patients, but this is rarely serious. Diarrhea occurs rarely.

Contraindications. Severe pre-existing thrombocytopenia.

Precautions. Thrombocytopenia may lead to serious bleeding and anemia, and may require transfusion therapy. Based on a similarity to cytarabine, CNS (cerebellar) toxicities may occur after high cumulative dosages, especially with impaired renal function.

Drug Interactions. None known.

Parameters to Monitor. Monitor platelet count, RBC count, and hemoglobin levels, and serum hepatic transaminase levels monthly.

Notes. Gemcitabine is clinically active in pancreatic cancer, breast cancer, and non–small cell lung cancer, although objective increases in tumor shrinkage and survival are minimal.[91–94] Gemcitabine produces primarily palliative responses such as reduced pain and enhanced quality of life with minimal serious toxicity compared to other cytotoxic agent therapies.

METHOTREXATE
Mexate, Various

Pharmacology. Methotrexate is a folic acid analogue that binds to dihydrofolate reductase, blocking formation of the DNA nucleotide thymidine; purine synthesis is also inhibited. It is most active in S phase.

Administration and Adult Dosage. *Single Agent Therapy.* **IM, IV, or PO for choriocarcinoma** 15–30 mg/day for 5 days, repeated q 1–2 weeks for 3–5 courses; **IM for mycosis fungoides** 50 mg once weekly or 25 mg twice weekly; **IM, IV, or PO for head and neck cancer** 25–50 mg/m^2 once weekly (watch for cumulative myelosuppression with continued administration of this regimen). **IT for meningeal leukemia** 12 mg/m^2 in a preservative-free, isotonic diluent (eg, Elliott's B solution, patient's own CSF, or D5LR); **IV high-dose therapy** (1–3 g/m^2) with leucovorin rescue should be used only by experts in major research centers; **IM or PO for psoriasis or arthritis** maintenance 5–10 mg initially, then **IM, IV, or PO** 10–25 mg/week, to a maximum of 50 mg/week, depending on clinical response; long-term daily administration results in increased hepatotoxicity compared to weekly oral or parenteral doses. **IM in glucocorticoid-dependent asthma** 7.5 mg, then 15 mg 1 week later, with subsequent weekly doses adjusted to 15–50 mg depending on 24-hr serum levels.[95] **PO for glucocorticoid-dependent asthma** 15 mg/week has been used.[96] **IM for ectopic pregnancy** 50 mg/m^2; some investigators repeat dose in 1 week if β-hCG levels do not drop.[97,98] **IM for induction of abortion** 50 mg/m^2, followed in 3–7 days by misoprostol 500–800 µg vaginally; exact timing of misoprostol dosage and oral administration of methotrexate are under investigation.[99–101]

Combined Modality Therapy. **For acute lymphocytic leukemia** various schedules are reported for remission-maintenance therapy: **IM or IV** 30 mg/m^2 twice weekly, or 7.5 mg/kg/day for 5 days, or **PO** 2.5 mg/kg/day for 2 weeks; repeat at monthly intervals. **IM, IV, or PO for Burkitt's lymphoma** 0.625–2.5 mg/kg/day for 1–2 weeks, then off drug for 7–10 days; **IM or IV for breast cancer** (combined with cyclophosphamide and fluorouracil) 40 mg/m^2 on days 1 and 8, then repeat monthly.[102]

Special Populations. *Pediatric Dosage.* **IM or IV for remission maintenance** same as adult dosage for acute lymphoblastic leukemia. **IT for meningeal cancer** use age-adjusted dosage rather than mg/m^2 dose:[103]

AGE (YR)	IT DOSE (MG)
>3	12
2–3	10
1–2	8
<1	6

Geriatric Dosage. Same as adult dosage, but adjust for age-related reduction in renal function.

Other Conditions. Patients with any "third space" fluid (eg, ascites, pleural effusions) should have fluid removed before drug administration because of drug retention and slow release of drug from these compartments.[104] Reduce dosage in renal impairment as follows:[105]

CREATININE CLEARANCE (ML/MIN)	PERCENTAGE OF DOSAGE RECOMMENDED
>50	60–100 (0–40% reduction)
10–50	30–50 (50–70% reduction)
<10	15 (85% reduction)

Dosage Forms. **Tab** 2.5 mg; **Inj** (as sodium) 2.5, 25 mg/mL (preserved solution); 25 mg/mL (nonpreserved solution); 20, 25, 50, 100, 250 mg, 1 g (nonpreserved powder).

Patient Instructions. (*See* Antineoplastics Class Instructions.)

Pharmacokinetics. *Serum Levels.* Following high-dose therapy, a threshold for bone marrow and mucosal toxicity is approximately 1 μmol/L 48 hr after administration. To prevent fatal bone marrow toxicity, keep serum levels below 10 μmol/L at 24 hr, 500 nmol/L at 48 hr, and 50 nmol/L at 72 hr.[106]

Fate. PO and IM absorption are rapid, peaking at 1–2 and 0.1–1 hr, respectively. Oral bioavailability is dose related, but averages 30%.[105] Following IT administration, the drug slowly diffuses into the bloodstream. About 34% is plasma protein bound; V_d is 0.55 ± 0.19 L/kg; Cl is 0.126 ± 0.048 L/hr/kg.[10] Over 90% of a dose is excreted in the urine, 90% unchanged after IV administration of high doses. Methotrexate solubility is markedly enhanced in slightly alkaline urine and reduced in acidic urine.

$t_{\frac{1}{2}}$. α phase 0.75 min; β phase 2 hr; γ phase 7.2 ± 2.1 hr.[10,107]

Adverse Reactions. Unless otherwise indicated, these reactions apply to high-dose chemotherapy of malignancies. Emetic potential is moderate. Nearly all reactions are dose and duration related. The primary toxicity is hematologic suppression, principally leukopenia, with the nadir at 7–14 days depending upon the administration schedule (more prolonged with daily administration). Thrombocytopenia and macrocytic anemia, dose-related nephrotoxicity, and ocular irritation occur frequently. Hepatotoxicity occurs frequently. Diarrhea and mucosal ulcerations of the mouth and tongue may occasionally become severe within 1–3 weeks after administration, sometimes heralding severe myelotoxicity. Erythematous rashes have been reported. Leukoencephalopathy occurs rarely with either IV or IT use. Other toxicities following intrathecal use include nausea and vomiting, meningismus, paresthesias, and rarely convulsions. Long-term daily administration in psoriasis has led to hepatocellular damage including fibrotic liver changes and atrophy of the liver; the frequency may be lower with larger intermittent doses. A single low dose for use in medical abortion is generally well tolerated, with none of the severe reactions reported above.

Contraindications. Pregnancy; severe renal or hepatic dysfunction; psoriasis patients with pre-existing bone marrow depression.

Precautions. Renal function must be determined prior to administration. Alkalinize the urine prior to high doses to enhance methotrexate solubility.

Drug Interactions. Concomitant vinca alkaloids (vincristine or vinblastine) can impair methotrexate elimination from the CSF and may enhance methotrexate toxicity. Cisplatin, NSAIDs, omeprazole, high-dose penicillins, probenecid, and sulfonamides can increase methotrexate serum levels and toxicity. Salicylate may decrease renal elimination of methotrexate and displace it from plasma protein binding sites. Alcohol may enhance hepatotoxicity of methotrexate. Asparaginase given 1 week prior to 24 hr after methotrexate appears to reduce methotrexate hematologic toxicities. Cholesterol-binding resins may decrease oral methotrexate absorption. Broad-spectrum antibiotics may decrease methotrexate serum levels and efficacy after oral administration.

Parameters to Monitor. Monitor pretreatment and periodic hepatic, renal, and bone marrow function (including WBCs, platelets, and RBCs). Follow high doses with 24-hr and/or 48-hr serum methotrexate levels and institution of appropriate leucovorin rescue.

Notes. Reconstitute lyophilized forms with NS, D5W, or Elliott's B solution (for intrathecal use). Reconstituted solutions are chemically stable for 7 days at room temperature. Methotrexate is physically incompatible with fluorouracil, prednisolone sodium phosphate, and cytarabine. It is clinically useful in a variety of hematologic and solid tumors as well as nonmalignant hyperplastic conditions such as psoriasis. If overdosage occurs, the antidote is **calcium leucovorin** (citrovorum factor), which can be given IV or IM in methotrexate-equivalent doses up to 75 mg q 6 hr for 4 doses. A delay of greater than 36 hr lessens the chance of rescue.[106]

PENTOSTATIN   Nipent

Pharmacology. Pentostatin (formerly 2'deoxycoformycin) is an analogue of a normal purine intermediate involved in the conversion of adenosine to inosine. It is an irreversible inhibitor of the enzyme adenosine deaminase (ADA), which is primarily found in lymphoid cells. Pentostatin-induced inhibition of ADA leads to a buildup of deoxyadenosine and several phosphorylated derivatives that deplete cellular ATP. These metabolic products ultimately inhibit DNA synthesis in lymphatic tumor cells, including chronic lymphocytic leukemia, acute lymphoblastic leukemia, and especially hairy cell leukemia. There are some data to suggest that the cytotoxic effect is cell cycle phase specific for the G_1 phase.[108,109]

Adult Dosage. **IV for hairy cell leukemia refractory to interferon alfa** 4 mg/m^2 every other week.

Dosage Forms. **Inj** 10 mg.

Pharmacokinetics. Serum levels after doses of 2–10 mg/m^2 average 1.5–4.7 mmol/L. V_d is 20–23 L/m^2; Cl is 3.1 L/hr/kg. The terminal half-life of pentostatin averages 5–10 hr. Up to 90% of a dose is excreted in the urine in an active form, and dosage reduction is indicated in patients with reduced renal function.

Adverse Reactions. Renal tubular toxicity and myelosuppression are the major dose-limiting toxicities of pentostatin. Renal toxicity manifested by Cr_s elevation is much more frequent at doses over 5 mg/m^2/day. Adequate hydration and the avoidance of other nephrotoxins can reduce the frequency and severity of pentostatin-induced nephrotoxicity. Lymphocytopenia is frequent with both B- and T-lymphocytes depressed, possibly explaining the relatively frequent, severe systemic infections with organisms that include Gram-negative bacteria, *Candida albicans,* herpes zoster (varicella), and herpes simplex. Neurologic effects are frequent with pentostatin and include lethargy and fatigue; these rarely progress to coma and are more common and severe with high-dose regimens. Mild to moderate nausea and vomiting also occur frequently, but are easily controlled with standard antiemetic regimens.

PURINE ANALOGUES:

MERCAPTOPURINE   Purinethol

THIOGUANINE

Pharmacology. Mercaptopurine (6-MP) and thioguanine (6-TG) are thiolated purines that act as antimetabolites following metabolic activation to the nucleotide forms (phosphorylated ribose sugar attachment). Subsequently, de novo purine biosynthesis is interrupted at a number of enzymatic sites, including the conversion of inosinic acid to adenine- or xanthine-based ribosides. DNA and RNA synthesis is halted in a cell cycle S phase specific fashion.

Administration and Adult Dosage. (Mercaptopurine) **PO, IV** (investigational) 75–100 mg/m^2/day.[110] (*See* Drug Interactions.) (Thioguanine) **PO, IV** (investigational) 2–3 mg/kg/day.

Special Populations. *Pediatric Dosage.* Same as adult dosage.

Geriatric Dosage. Same as adult dosage.

Other Conditions. Purine antimetabolite toxicities are not consistently increased in patients with renal failure.[111,112] (*See* Precautions.)

Dosage Forms. (Mercaptopurine) **Tab** 50 mg; **Inj** (investigational) 500 mg. (Thioguanine) **Tab** 40 mg; **Inj** (investigational) 75 mg.

Patient Instructions. (*See* Antineoplastics Class Instructions.) To maximize absorption, do not take these drugs with meals. Nausea and vomiting are uncommon with usual doses.

Pharmacokinetics. *Fate.* (Mercaptopurine) $12 \pm 7\%$ oral bioavailability, increasing to 60% with concurrent allopurinol.[113] The drug is approximately 20–30% plasma protein bound and freely distributed throughout the body including placental transfer; the CSF/serum ratio is 0.19–0.27. Mercaptopurine is metabolized extensively by xanthine oxidase, also methylated to active metabolite and sulfated to inactive thiouric acid. V_d is 0.56 ± 0.38 L/kg; Cl is 0.66 ± 0.24 L/hr/kg; 22% excreted unchanged in urine.[10] (Thioguanine) oral bioavailability is unknown. The drug is approximately 20–30% plasma protein bound and freely distributed throughout the body, including placental transfer; the CSF/serum ratio is 0.16. Thioguanine is metabolized predominantly to inactive metabolites.

$t_{\frac{1}{2}}$. (Mercaptopurine) 0.9 ± 0.37 hr;[10] (thioguanine) α phase 15 min, β phase 11 hr.

Adverse Reactions. Emetic potential is low to moderate. The dose-limiting toxicity is myelosuppression (leukopenia and thrombocytopenia). Mild to moderate mucositis occurs with large doses with low daily maintenance doses. Predominantly cholestatic liver toxicities occur frequently with long-term therapy. Marked crystalluria with hematuria has occurred with large IV mercaptopurine doses.[114] A variety of rashes have also been described with these drugs. Long-term immunosuppressive therapy with any of these agents predisposes patients to carcinogenesis; CNS lymphomas and acute myeloid leukemia are the most frequent malignancies.[115]

Contraindications. Pregnancy; pre-existing severe bone marrow depression.

Precautions. Investigational use of mercaptopurine for inflammatory bowel disease may predispose to pancreatitis.

Drug Interactions. Patients taking allopurinol *must* receive substantially reduced doses of oral mercaptopurine (25–33% of the normal dose), to avoid life-threatening myelosuppression caused by blocked inactivation. Thioguanine is primarily inactivated by methylation; thus, no dosage reduction is necessary with concomitant allopurinol. Enhanced bone marrow suppression may occur with the combination of trimethoprim/sulfamethoxazole and mercaptopurine.

Parameters to Monitor. WBC and platelet counts and total bilirubin at least monthly.

Notes. There is usually complete cross-resistance between mercaptopurine and thioguanine.

UFT (Investigational—Tahio)   Orzel

Pharmacology. UFT is a combination containing the fluorouracil prodrug **tega-fur** (formerly ftorafur) and the ribonucleoside pyrimidine **uracil** in a fixed molar ratio of 1:4 (tegafur:uracil). Tegafur is gradually converted to the antimetabolite fluorouracil by metabolism in the liver. This approximates a continuous infusion of fluorouracil following oral ingestion of UFT. The uracil component slows the metabolism of fluorouracil and reduces production of the toxic metabolite, 2-fluoro-β-alanine, resulting in reduced GI and myelosuppressive toxicity with the combination.[116,117]

Administration and Adult Dosage. **PO for colorectal cancer** 800–900 mg/m^2 weekly or daily for 5 consecutive days, repeated q 28 days. Alternatively 360–400 mg/m^2/day for 28 consecutive days, repeated q 35–42 days. All daily dosages are given in 3 divided doses q 8 hr.[116]

Special Populations. *Pediatric Dosage.* Safety and efficacy not established.

Geriatric Dosage. Same as adult dosage.

Dosage Forms. **Cap** containing tegafur 100 mg and uracil 224 mg.

Patient Instructions. (*See* Antineoplastics Class Instructions.) Take this drug on an empty stomach with 4–8 fl. oz. of water.

Missed Doses. If you are taking this drug daily, take a missed dose as soon as possible if you remember within 12 hours. If it is within 2 hours of next dose, skip the missed dose and do not double the next dose. If you miss 2 or more doses, contact your physician. If you are taking this drug weekly and miss a dose, contact your physician.

Pharmacokinetics. *Serum Levels.* No correlation has been found between the peak level or AUC of any component of UFT and myelotoxicity.

Fate. Both tegafur and uracil are rapidly absorbed, but levels of tegafur are higher than uracil, despite the 4-fold higher uracil dosage. With a daily dosage of 800–900 mg/m^2, peak levels of tegafur, uracil, and 5-FU are 24.6, 13.6, and 1.4 mg/L, respectively. Tumor levels of 5-FU and its nucleotide metabolites are higher than in normal tissue. Uracil is quickly metabolized and excreted via non-biliary pathways. Some tegafur metabolites are excreted in bile.[116]

Adverse Reactions. The dose-limiting toxicity in phase I trials using daily doses was GI, including nausea, vomiting, anorexia, and diarrhea. With daily schedules, the GI effects tend to be cumulative, resulting in moderate mucositis and diarrhea. Fatigue also occurs in over one-half of patients treated using the 28-day dosage schedule. With the shorter 5-day schedules, myelosuppression, principally neutropenia, is dose-limiting.

Notes. UFT may also be combined with oral **leucovorin** in the treatment of advanced colorectal cancer.[117]

Cytokines

ALDESLEUKIN
Proleukin

Pharmacology. Aldesleukin (interleukin-2; IL-2) is a cytokine produced by activated T-lymphocytes. It binds to T-cell receptors to induce a proliferative response and differentiation into lymphokine activated killer (LAK) cells in the blood and tumor-infiltrating lymphocytes (TIL-cells) in specific tumors. The pharmaceutical product is a nonglycosylated molecule produced by recombinant DNA techniques in *Escherichia coli*.[118,119]

Administration and Adult Dosage. IV for metastatic renal cell carcinoma 600,000 IU/kg over 15 min q 8 hr for 14 doses; repeat after 9 days of rest for a total of 28 doses. **IV infusion** 3–6 million IU/m² infused over 6 hr is commonly used.

Special Populations. *Pediatric Dosage.* (<18 yr) safety and efficacy not established.

Geriatric Dosage. Same as adult dosage.

Other Conditions. Interpatient pharmacokinetic differences are not known; however, withholding dose(s) is required if severe cardiovascular collapse, or pulmonary or renal insufficiency, coma, psychosis, or GI toxicity occurs.

Dosage Forms. Inj 22 million IU (1.3 mg protein). (*See* Notes.)

Patient Instructions. (*See* Antineoplastics Class Instructions.)

Pharmacokinetics. *Fate.* Limited human data indicate that the drug undergoes biphasic elimination after IV administration. The kidney is believed to be the major organ of elimination, and the drug undergoes intrarenal metabolism to inactive fragments.[120]

$t_{1/2}$. α phase 14 ± 7.7 min; β phase 80 ± 34 min.[120]

Adverse Reactions. Emetic potential is low. Severe cardiovascular toxicities include fluid retention (over 10% of body weight) and pulmonary interstitial edema. Hypotension requiring treatment has occurred 2–4 hr after treatment with a high-dose bolus or continuous infusions as well as with low-dose SC regimens. Anemia occurs in up to 77% of high-dose bolus IV regimens. Frequently, nausea, vomiting, diarrhea, rash, pruritus, and nasal congestion occur. Abnormal laboratory findings include frequent increased Cr$_s$, oliguria, eosinophilia, and thrombocytopenia.[118] Increased serum transaminases and bilirubin occur occasionally; hepatic dysfunction occurs rarely. Myocardial ischemia may also occur and fatal MI has been reported. Capillary leak syndrome may occur and requires close monitoring of fluid balance.[118] When combined with adoptive cellular therapy (reinfused LAK cells), immediate fever and chills result; **indomethacin** 50 mg orally or **meperidine** 25–50 mg IM or IV may lessen these.

Precautions. Aldesleukin has produced severe cardiopulmonary toxicity and must be cautiously used in any patient with a history of cardiac insufficiency from any cause. Patients must also be in good general physical condition in order to tolerate the hypotension and pulmonary edema that can complicate high-dose aldesleukin therapy.

Drug Interactions. Glucocorticoids block some aldesleukin actions and are usually reserved for treating severe toxicity.

Parameters to Monitor. Monitor blood pressure, cardiac output, and fluid balance closely.

Notes. Some studies describe IL-2 activity in different units or by weight. Aldesleukin is labeled in IU (18 million IU = 1.1 mg protein), and doses for other IL-2 products should be converted to IU for proper dosage. Aldesleukin is active in metastatic renal cell carcinoma (MRCC) and metastatic malignant melanoma. In MRCC, response rates are 15% (with some complete remissions), lasting a median of 23 months. Response rates are higher in patients with good performance status and especially those with pulmonary metastases as the main site of disease.

INTERFERON ALFA:	
ALFA-2A	Roferon-A
ALFA-2B	Intron A
ALFA-N3	Alferon N

Pharmacology. Alpha interferons are single-chain proteins. The alfa-2 interferons are biosynthetic; alfa-2a has a lysine at position 23, alfa-2b an arginine. Alfa-n3 interferon is a multisubspecies form of natural interferons isolated from human leukocytes. Interferons bind to specific membrane receptors and are then taken up intracellularly to affect diverse cellular functions. These include cell membrane alterations (eg, enhanced antigen expression), cell cycle blockade at the G_1-S portion, enhanced antiviral enzyme synthesis (eg, $2',5'$-oligo-adenylate synthetase with resultant products, which destroy double and single stranded viral RNA), and immunomodulatory activity (eg, increased activity of natural killer [NK] lymphocytes and phagocytic macrophages). General cellular protein synthesis is also decreased, including cytochrome P450 enzymes.[121]

Administration and Adult Dosage. **IM or SC for hairy cell leukemia** (alfa-2a or 2b) 2 million IU/m^2 daily or 3 times a week. **IM or SC for AIDS-related Kaposi's sarcoma** (alfa-2b) slowly increase dose from 5 million IU/day up to 20–36 million IU/day.[122] **Intralesionally for condylomata acuminata** (alfa-2b) 1 million IU/wart 3 times weekly for 3 weeks, to a maximum 5 warts a day (use only the 10 million IU vial); (alfa-n3) 250,000 IU (0.05 mL)/wart twice weekly for up to 8 weeks, to a maximum 0.5 mL/day. **IM or SC for chronic hepatitis B** 5 million IU/day or 10 million IU 3 times a week for 16 weeks.[123] **IM or SC for chronic hepatitis C** 3 million IU 3 times a week for 6 months. (*See* Notes.) **IV and SC for malignant melanoma** (alfa-2b) 20 million IU/m^2 IV 5 times a week for 4 weeks, then 10 million IU/m^2 SC 3 times a week for 48 weeks. **IM or SC for chronic myeloid leukemia** (alfa-2a) 3–6 million IU/day.

Special Populations. *Pediatric Dosage.* (<18 yr) not recommended.

Geriatric Dosage. Same as adult dosage.

Dosage Forms. (Alfa-2a) **Inj** 3, 6, 10, 36 million IU. (Alfa-2b) **Inj** 3, 5, 10, 18, 25, 50 million IU. (Alfa-n3) **Inj** 5 million IU.

Patient Instructions. (Subcutaneous use) Instruct in proper method of aseptic preparation of vials and syringes, proper technique for SC administration, and proper disposal of syringes and needles. Rotate SC injection sites. Acetaminophen is recommended to reduce frequent flu-like symptoms, which usually decrease with continued therapy.

Missed Doses. Take this drug at regular intervals. If you miss a dose of this medicine, call your physician for instructions. Do not double the dose or take extra.

Pharmacokinetics. *Fate.* Alfa-2a and 2b are 100% bioavailable after IM or SC administration, with an absorption half-life of about 6 hr. IM or SC doses of 10 million IU produce peak serum levels of 100–200 IU/mL within 4 hr; the same dose IV produces peak serum levels of 500–600 IU/mL within 15–30 min. Alfa-n3 is not detectable in serum after intralesional administration, although a small amount is probably absorbed. The majority of a dose is thought to be metabolized, with none filtered or secreted by the kidney.[124,125]

$t_{\frac{1}{2}}$. α phase 0.11 hr; β phase (IV or IM) 2 hr, (SC) 3 hr.[124,125]

Adverse Reactions. Emetic potential is negligible. The most frequent reactions include fever to 38–39°C, chills, arthralgias, headache, malaise, and myalgias (flu-like syndrome). These reactions are more severe upon initiation of therapy and are ameliorated by acetaminophen or dosage reduction. Anorexia and nausea without vomiting are also frequent. With large doses (generally over 1 million IU), hematologic suppression (eg, mild thrombocytopenia, leukopenia) occurs, as does slight elevation of hepatic enzymes (AST, LDH, alkaline phosphatase), and mild hypertension, occasionally associated with tachycardia. Very high doses (≥30 million IU) are associated with somnolence, dizziness, and confusion. Mild erythema and pruritus at the injection site can also occur. Interferons are not mutagenic nor carcinogenic in standard animal or in vitro models.

Contraindications. Severe hypersensitivity; development of a neutralizing serum antibody (precludes the use of alternate recombinant product, switch to natural interferon alfa-n3). (*See* Notes.)

Precautions. Pregnancy. Use with caution in patients with cardiovascular disease, seizure disorder, or hepatic or renal impairment. Proper hydration during therapy may help lessen hypotensive reactions. Neutralizing serum antibodies can form after prolonged interferon administration. This has been associated with reduced toxicities and antitumor effects.[126]

Drug Interactions. Interferon may worsen the neutropenia of zidovudine in Kaposi's sarcoma. Interferon may increase theophylline serum levels. Combination with vidarabine may result in increased neurotoxicity.

Notes. A clear dose–response relationship is established for toxicity, but not for antitumor effectiveness (except for Kaposi's sarcoma). Alpha interferons have activity in reducing the symptomatology of hairy cell leukemia; hematologic response rates of 80–90% are possible in this disease. Other cancers responsive to interferon alfa include renal cell cancer (10–30% partial response rate); acute leukemias (15–30% response rate), and the nonblastic phase of CML (40–60% response rate). Although not a labeled use, interferon alfa-n3 can be used systemically and is specifically recommended for antibody-positive patients receiving recombinant products. Patients who fail interferon treatment for hepatitis C can be given interferon alfa-2b plus oral **ribavirin** (Rebetol). It is available in a combination package (Rebetron).

DNA Intercalating Drugs

ANTHRACYCLINES:

DAUNORUBICIN HYDROCHLORIDE	Cerubidine
DOXORUBICIN HYDROCHLORIDE	Adriamycin, Rubex
IDARUBICIN HYDROCHLORIDE	Idamycin

Pharmacology. Daunorubicin (daunomycin), doxorubicin (hydroxydaunomycin), and idarubicin (4-demethoxydaunomycin) are tetracyclic amino sugar-linked antibiotics that are actively taken up by cells and concentrated in the nucleus; intercalation or fitting between DNA base pairs occurs, which impairs DNA synthesis. Other biochemical lesions produced include quinone moiety-generated production of oxygen and hydroxyl free radicals with lipid peroxidation of cellular membranes. The anthracyclines also interfere with the activity of the G_2-specific enzyme, topoisomerase-II, which leads to the formation of cleavable complexes between enzyme and DNA, resulting in DNA double strand breaks. These agents are primarily cell cycle phase nonspecific, but with slightly greater activity in late S or G_2 phase cells.

Administration and Dosage.

	DAUNORUBICIN	DOXORUBICIN	IDARUBICIN
Administration	IV push, infusion.	IV push, infusion.	IV push, infusion.
	These compounds are extremely toxic (potent vesicants) if inadvertently extravasated; very careful IV technique is mandatory.		
Adult Dosage	IV 30–45 mg/m²/day for 1–3 days; generally not repeated more often than q 3 weeks.	IV 60–90 mg/m² for 1 dose or 20–30 mg/m²/day for 3 days; generally not repeated more often than q 3 weeks. Alternatively, 20 mg/m²/week.	IV 12 mg/m²/day for 3 days.[127]
Pediatric Dosage	Same as adult dosage.	Same as adult dosage.	Same as adult dosage.[128]

(continued)

	DAUNORUBICIN	**DOXORUBICIN**	**IDARUBICIN**
Cumulative Lifetime Dosage Limits[a]	550 mg/m^2, up to 850 mg/m^2.	550 mg/m^2. 400 mg/m^2 with prior chest irradiation or pre-existing heart disease.[b]	Unknown.

[a]Attainment of maximal cumulative dosage generally precludes continued use, despite evidence of continuing drug response; however, some patients may continue to respond without development of cardiomyopathy.[129] Use of dexrazoxane can extend dosage limits in breast cancer. (*See* Dexrazoxane.)

[b]Low weekly doses or continuous 96-hr infusion[130] appear to be less toxic and may allow attainment of greater cumulative dosages (>550 mg/m^2).[131,132]

Special Populations. *Other Conditions.* Cumulative dosages of all agents must be reduced in patients with prior irradiation of the cardiac chest region, pre-existing heart disease, or prior large cyclophosphamide dosage. Doxorubicin requires no dosage adjustment for severe renal impairment, whereas with daunorubicin 75% of the dosage is recommended in severe renal impairment. Doxorubicin dosages, however, must be substantially reduced with severe hepatic dysfunction.[133] Idarubicin dosage reductions are indicated for bilirubin of 2.6–5 mg/dL or Cr_s ≥2 mg/dL. For severe mucositis, administration is delayed until mucositis resolves, then dosage is reduced by 25%.

SERUM BILIRUBIN (MG/DL)	**PERCENTAGE OF DOSE RECOMMENDED**	
	DOXORUBICIN	**IDARUBICIN**
≤1.2	100 (no reduction)	—
1.2–3	50	—
>3	25 (75% reduction)	50 (50% reduction)

Dosage Forms. (Daunorubicin) **Inj** 20 mg. (Doxorubicin) **Inj** 10, 20, 50, 100, 150, 200 mg. (Idarubicin) **Inj** 5, 10 mg.

Patient Instructions. (*See* Antineoplastics Class Instructions.) Immediately report any change in sensation (eg, stinging) at injection site during infusion (this may be an early sign of infiltration). Red-colored urine does not indicate toxicity.

Pharmacokinetics.

	DAUNO- RUBICIN	**DOXO- RUBICIN**	**IDARUBICIN**	**IDA- RUBICINOL**
FATE				
Absorption	Extensively degraded to inactive aglycone in GI tract.		About 24% oral bioavail- ability.[134]	The primary active metabolite of idarubicin.

(*continued*)

	DAUNO-RUBICIN	DOXO-RUBICIN	IDARUBICIN	IDA-RUBICINOL
Distribution	Both drugs enter cells rapidly and concentrate in the nuclei. Tissue concentrations are highest in lung, kidney, small intestine, and liver; trivial amounts found in the CNS. Avid tissue binding is probably responsible for prolonged terminal half-lives and V_d of 500–600 L/m^2.		Peak serum level of 2 µg/L after a dose of 7–9 mg/m^2.[135] 94% plasma protein bound; V_d about 1700 L/m^2.	Peak serum level of 15 µg/L.[135] 94% plasma protein bound; V_d about 1700 L/m^2.
Metabolism	Both drugs are extensively metabolized, initially to less active alcohol metabolites; further metabolized by liver microsomes to inactive aglycones and demethylated glucuronide and sulfate conjugates.[136]		Both agents are partially metabolized and excreted as glucuronide conjugates. Idarubicin Cl is 60–77 L/hr/m^2.	

EXCRETION

	DAUNO-RUBICIN	DOXO-RUBICIN	IDARUBICIN	IDA-RUBICINOL
Biliary	20–30% of a dose.	40–60% of a dose.	Primary route of excretion.	Primary route of excretion.
Urinary	14–23% as unchanged drug and metabolites (primarily daunorubicinol).	5–10% as metabolites over 5 days.[133]	8% of a dose over 24 hr.	8% of a dose over 24 hr.
$t_{1/2}$.	α 45 min β 18.5 hr (daunorubicinol 27 hr).	α 30 min β 3 hr γ 17 hr (metabolites 32 hr).[133]	α 14 min[137] β 19–34 hr.[135,137]	65.5 hr.[137]

Adverse Reactions. Emetic potential is moderate to moderately high with all three drugs. Stomatitis, nausea, and vomiting are dose dependent and frequent; prophylactic antiemetics are often helpful. Myelosuppression, affecting both platelets and neutrophils, is the major acute dose-limiting side effect. Typical nadirs range from 9–14 days, with recovery nearly complete within 3 weeks of administration. Hemorrhage occurs in up to 10% of induction courses with idarubicin. Excessive lacrimation is reported in about 25% of patients receiving doxorubicin. Alopecia usually occurs; during low-dose adjuvant chemotherapy administration, regional scalp hypothermia may decrease hair loss.[138] Severe, protracted ulceration and necrosis can occur with inadvertent perivenous infiltration; partially effective local treatments include limb elevation, ice packing, and topical **DMSO.** (*See* Notes.) Large evolving lesions necessitate early plastic surgery consultation. Long-term anthracycline use can lead to severe and often fatal cardiomyopathy. (*See* Cumulative Dosage Limits and Notes.) Symptoms are nonspecific and indicative of advanced CHF such as shortness of breath, edema, and fatigue. The frequency is low (overall 2.2%) when total dosage limits are observed and may be lower when monthly doses are given over several days or by continuous 96-hr infusion.[139] Late cardiotoxicity is reported in children receiving total dosages of doxorubicin <500 mg/m^2.[140] During drug infusion, various non-specific ECG changes may occur; these do not imply an increased risk of cardiotoxicity. Graded endomyocardial biopsy and graded radionuclide angiography have proved most effective for assessment of the emergence of severe cardiomyopathy. Other reactions include transient erythema and phlebitis during administration and a radiation-synergy phenomenon involving heightened tissue reactions in concurrently or previously irradiated tissues, especially the esophagus (avoid by spacing weeks apart). Urine remains red for 1–2 days after administration.

Contraindications. Pre-existing bone marrow suppression (WBCs <3000/μL; platelets <120,000/μL; MI in previous 6 months; history of CHF). Marrow suppression is not a contraindication in relapsed leukemia patients.

Precautions. Careful administration technique is mandatory to avoid extravasation and tissue necrosis. Hepatocellular disease or cirrhosis may slow production of alcohol metabolites.

Drug Interactions. A number of drugs may interact with the anthracyclines: vinca alkaloids (cross-resistance), amphotericin B (increased drug uptake), and cyclosporine and streptozocin (reduced drug clearance and increased toxicity).[141] Most of these drug interactions have only been studied in vitro and require clinical confirmation.

Parameters to Monitor. Obtain pretreatment and at least biweekly nadir WBC and platelet counts. Monitor general cardiac status and serial radionuclide scans of the heart in high-risk patients. Add up prior doses to estimate cardiotoxicity dosage limit.

Notes. These drugs are compatible with usual IV solutions but incompatible with heparin, sodium bicarbonate, and fluorouracil. IV push doses are best reconstituted with NS or D5W. These solutions are stable for prolonged periods and can withstand freezing and thawing.[142] Doxorubicin is widely effective in numerous solid tumors, such as ovarian, thyroid, and gastric carcinomas, sarcomas, and cancer of the breast, as well as hematologic malignancies, such as the lymphomas and leukemias. The iron-chelating agent dexrazoxane reduces doxorubicin-induced cardiotoxicity in patients with breast cancer.[143] (*See* Dexrazoxane.) The activity of idarubicin and daunorubicin is limited primarily to AML. Topical **DMSO** (1.5 mL of a 90% w/v solution q 6 hr for 2 weeks) has been effective at preventing extravasation ulceration in one trial.[144]

DAUNORUBICIN CITRATE, LIPOSOMAL   DaunoXome

Pharmacology. Daunorubicin is encapsulated in the lipid component of this red emulsion formulation, which consists of distearoylphosphatidylcholine and cholesterol in a fixed lipid:daunorubicin ratio of 1:18.6 (in mg/mL). These liposomes are taken up into tumor and reticuloendothelial system cells, which release prolonged but low serum levels of daunorubicin over time.[145] Murine studies suggest selective (enhanced) uptake of liposomal daunorubicin into tumor tissues compared to normal organs.[146] Liposomal daunorubicin is used to treat AIDS-related Kaposi's sarcoma.

Administration and Adult Dosage. **IV for Kaposi's sarcoma** 40 mg/m^2 q 2 weeks.

Special Populations. *Pediatric Dosage.* Safety and efficacy not established.

Geriatric Dosage. Same as adult dosage.

Other Conditions. Based on studies with daunorubicin, reduce dose by 25% for a serum bilirubin of 1.2–3 mg/dL and by 50% for a serum bilirubin or Cr$_s$ >3 mg/dL. Do not administer if absolute granulocyte count is under 750/μL.

Dosage Forms. **Inj** 50 mg.

Patient Instructions. (*See* Antineoplastics Class Instructions.)

Pharmacokinetics. *Fate.* Mean peak serum levels (free plus liposomal) after doses of 20, 40, 60, and 80 mg/m^2 are 8.2, 18.2, 36.2, and 43.6 mg/L, respectively.[145] Compared to equivalent doses of the nonliposomal drug, the free drug levels are 100-fold lower, and persist for up to 2.5 days after administration. In adults, V$_d$ is 2.9–4.1 L; Cl ranges from 0.4–0.9 L/hr, about 5% of the Cl of the free drug.[145] Thus, the AUC is increased, Cl is slowed, but peak levels are low with the liposomal formulation.

t$_{1/2}$. 2.8–5.2 hr (total of liposomal plus free drug).

Adverse Reactions. Emetic potential is low to moderate. The most frequent symptoms are mild to moderate fatigue, which occurs in 56% of patients, and low-grade fever in 26% of patients. An acute triad of back pain, flushing, and chest tightness may occur in up to 14% of patients, usually upon initial administration. This liposomal-component reaction subsides with interruption of the infusion and typically does not recur upon restarting at a slower infusion rate. Neutropenia occurs in 17% of patients; mild anemia and thrombocytopenia occur in 7 and 4% of treatment courses, respectively. Diarrhea occurs in 10% of patients; mild liver enzyme elevation occurs in 4% of patients.[145] Cardiac toxicity appears to be less with this formulation than with aqueous daunorubicin.

Contraindications. Previous serious allergy to the drug or any component of the formulation. (*See* Anthracyclines, Daunorubicin.)

Precautions. Pregnancy; lactation. Do not administer if absolute granulocyte count is under 750/μL.

Drug Interactions. Not well studied with this formulation. (*See* Anthracyclines.)

Parameters to Monitor. Monitor the number of Kaposi's sarcoma lesions for response or evidence of disease progression (10 or more new lesions or an increase of 25%). Obtain WBC count prior to administration. Monitor left ventricular ejection fraction at cumulative dosages of 320 and 480 mg/m^2, and q 240 mg/m^2 thereafter.

Notes. Mix only in D5W; do not filter.

DOXORUBICIN HYDROCHLORIDE, LIPOSOMAL   Doxil

Pharmacology. Doxorubicin is encapsulated in the aqueous core of small (100-nm) liposomes composed of a phospholipid bilayer with an outer coating of polyethylene glycol (PEG). The small liposome size and PEG coating mask recognition by reticuloendothelial cells, thereby increasing the half-life of the liposomes in vivo. Once the liposomes accumulate in tissues, free doxorubicin is slowly released to exert its antitumor effect. Most toxicities are reduced by the liposomal formulation without compromising efficacy in solid tumors such as Kaposi's sarcoma. (*See* Anthracyclines.)

Administration and Adult Dosage. IV for AIDS-related Kaposi's sarcoma 20 mg/m^2 q 3 weeks.

Special Populations. *Pediatric Dosage.* Safety and efficacy not established.

Geriatric Dosage. Same as adult dosage.

Other Conditions. (Liver dysfunction) Reduce dosage 50% for serum bilirubin 1.2–3 mg/dL; reduce dosage by 75% for bilirubin over 3 mg/dL. (Stomatitis) For patients who develop stomatitis, wait 1 week, re-evaluate, and readminister at 100% for Grade II severity (painful ulcers, but able to eat), 75% for Grade III severity (painful ulcers and unable to eat), 50% for Grade IV severity (extensive, disabling stomatitis requiring nutritional support). (Hematologic toxicity) Reduce dose and/or delay administration to allow for ANC and platelet count (PC) to return to at least 1000/μL and 50,000/μL, respectively. Then readminister at 100% of dosage if nadir ANC was 1000–1500/μL and/or PC was 50,000–150,000/μL; 75% of dosage if nadir ANC was 500/μL and/or PC was 25,000–50,000/μL; or 50% of dosage if nadir ANC was under 500/μL and/or PC was under 25,000/μL, respectively. (Erythrodysesthesia) For Grade I erythrodysesthesia (mild swelling or erythema) present 4 weeks after the dose, administer 75% of standard dosage. For Grade II erythrodysesthesia (erythema or desquamation not precluding physical activity) present 3 weeks after the dose, delay the dose for 1 week; if present 4 weeks after the dose, reduce the next dose by 50%. For Grade III erythrodysesthesia (palmar–plantar [hand/foot] that is severe [diffuse blistering]) 3 weeks after drug administration, hold the next dose for 1 week; if it is still present at 4 weeks, discontinue the drug.

Dosage Forms. Inj 2 mg/mL.

Patient Instructions. (*See* Antineoplastics Class Instructions.)

Pharmacokinetics. *Fate.* Mean peak serum levels (±SE) after 10 and 20 mg/m^2 doses are 4.1 ± 0.2 and 8.3 ± 0.5 μg/mL, respectively. Most of this level is liposomally encapsulated drug; the assay does not differentiate. Liposomal doxorubicin has a smaller V$_d$ (2.2–4.4 L/m^2) than free doxorubicin; Cl is 0.034–0.108 L/hr/m^2. The AUC for the 10 and 20 mg/m^2 doses are 277 ± 33 (±SE) and 590 ± 59 (±SE) mg·L/hr. A small amount (0.8–2.6 ng/mL) of the doxorubicinol metabolite is found in serum following a dose. Cl of parent drug ranges from 24–35 L/hr/m^2. Tissue concentrations of drug may be 19 times higher in Kaposi's sarcoma lesions than in adjacent normal skin.[147]

t$_{½}$. (Liposomal and free drug) α phase 5.2 ± 1.4 hr; β phase 55 ± 4.8 hr.[147]

Adverse Reactions. Similar to free doxorubicin. Myelosuppression, principally neutropenia, occurs in 49% of patients and sepsis in 5%. Opportunistic infections also occur in AIDS patients, especially those with a high tumor burden, low CD4 count, or pre-existing infection. Palmar–plantar erythrodysesthesia is cumulative. It is manifested as painful red soles and palms, which can progress to ulceration and debilitating infection if doses are not reduced and/or delayed. Doxorubicin-induced cumulative dosage cardiomyopathy and inadvertent extravasation necrosis may be lessened, but not entirely eliminated, with the liposomal formulation. Radiation recall soft tissue toxicity has been reported.

Contraindications. (*See* Anthracyclines, Doxorubicin.)

Precautions. May sensitize soft tissues to radiation damage. To lessen frequency of irreversible cardiomyopathy, observe the cumulative anthracycline dosage limit of 500 mg/m^2. Avoid extravasation, and do not give IM or SC.

Drug Interactions. (*See* Anthracyclines.)

Parameters to Monitor. Obtain absolute neutrophil count and platelet count, serum bilirubin level, and severity of stomatitis and palmar–plantar erythrodysesthesia prior to administration.

Notes. Do not filter. Overall response rates of 40–60% are reported for patients with AIDS-related Kaposi's sarcoma;[147,148] it may also be effective in other solid tumors in HIV-negative patients.

DACTINOMYCIN   Cosmegen

Pharmacology. Dactinomycin (actinomycin D) is a tricyclic, peptide-containing antibiotic that acts as an intercalator of DNA, resulting in decreased mRNA transcription in a phase nonspecific fashion. It is used in the treatment of sarcomas and choriocarcinoma.[149,150]

Adult Dosage. IV 2 mg/week or 500 μg/day for up to 5 days, repeated at 3- to 4-week intervals. Reduce dosage in the presence of hepatobiliary dysfunction. Reconstitute dactinomycin with preservative-free diluents. It is bound by cellulose filters, so avoid in-line filtration.

Pediatric Dosage. IV 450 μg/m^2/day, to a maximum of 500 μg/day, for up to 5 days; the course is repeated in 3 weeks. (*See* Adult Dosage.)

Dosage Forms. **Inj** 0.5 mg.

Pharmacokinetics. About 30% of the drug is recovered from the feces and urine after 1 week; there is no CNS penetration, and it is probably concentrated in the bile. The terminal half-life is over 36 hr.

Adverse Reactions. Nausea, vomiting, mucositis, diarrhea, and reversible alopecia occur frequently. Dose- and duration-dependent hepatotoxicity and genotoxic effects have been reported. Severe ulceration occurs if the drug is extravasated. The dose-limiting toxicity is myelosuppression with a leukopenic nadir at 7–10 days. Rarely, radiation recall occurs.

MITOXANTRONE   Novantrone

Pharmacology. Mitoxantrone is a substituted salt of a planar anthracene. The drug binds to DNA by intercalation and inhibits topoisomerase II, producing DNA strand breaks; DNA synthesis is impaired in a cell cycle phase nonspecific fashion.[151]

Administration and Adult Dosage. **IV for solid tumors** 12 mg/m^2 q 4 weeks or 5 mg/m^2/week for 3 weeks. **IV for leukemia** 10–12 mg/m^2/day for 3 days.

Special Populations. *Pediatric Dosage.* **IV for leukemia** up to 8 mg/m^2/week for 3 weeks or up to 18 mg/m^2 q 4 weeks.[152]

Geriatric Dosage. Same as adult dosage.

Other Conditions. Reduce doses by approximately 30–50% in patients with abnormal hepatobiliary function and/or appreciable third-space fluid accumulations.[153] Reduced doses are also required in patients with poor bone marrow reserve. No dosage alteration is required with renal function impairment.

Dosage Forms. **Inj** 2 mg/mL.

Patient Instructions. (*See* Antineoplastics Class Instructions.) This drug may turn urine blue-green for 24 hr after administration because of the dark blue drug color. Discoloration of the whites of the eyes may also occur.

Pharmacokinetics. *Fate.* The drug is over 95% plasma protein bound and exhibits prolonged retention in tissues. Some liver metabolism to glucuronyl and glutathione conjugates occurs. Urinary recovery is <8% of a dose; the majority is eliminated in the bile; fecal recovery averages 18% of a dose over 5 days.[153]

$t_{\frac{1}{2}}$. α phase 14 min; β phase 1.1 hr; γ phase 38–43 hr.[153]

Adverse Reactions. Emetic potential is low. Myelosuppression, principally granulocytopenia (nadir at 10–14 days), occurs and is most severe in heavily pretreated or irradiated patients. Mucositis, which is dose limiting, occurs only with weekly regimens. CHF has been reported frequently, most often after prior anthracycline therapy. Cumulative cardiotoxicity limits are not well established, but may approach 125 mg/m^2 with prior anthracyclines and 160 mg/m^2 without.[151] Alopecia and extravasation necrosis are minimal.

Precautions. Reduce the dosage in patients with poor hepatobiliary function. Dosage reduction may also be necessary in patients previously treated with marrow suppressant or cardiotoxic agents.

Drug Interactions. None known.

Parameters to Monitor. Obtain serum bilirubin before each dose. Assess cardiac function in patients with prior anthracycline therapy or severe pre-existing cardiovascular disease. Monitor absolute granulocyte levels prior to each dose; nadir counts 7–10 days after the dose are optimal.

Notes. Mitoxantrone is not usually a vesicant, although it can rarely cause necrosis and usually tints the tissues a blue color.

PLICAMYCIN   Mithracin

Pharmacology. Plicamycin (mithramycin) is a complex, polycyclic, sugar-linked antibiotic that acts by DNA binding in a cell cycle phase nonspecific fashion; it also has a separate calcium-lowering effect. It is used in testicular cancer and to control severe hypercalcemia caused by malignancy.[154,155]

Adult Dosage. **IV for testicular tumors** 25–30 μg/kg/day for up to 5 days, repeat in 4 weeks if toxicity has resolved. **IV for hypercalcemia** 25 μg/kg/day for 3–4 days. Reduce dosage by 25–50% in moderate to severe renal impairment. *Note:* dosage is in μg/kg with no single dose over 3 mg.

Dosage Forms. Inj 2.5 mg.

Pharmacokinetics. The metabolic fate of the drug is unknown, but the drug penetrates well into the CNS and 40% of radioactivity from a radiolabled dose appears in the urine.

Adverse Reactions. Mild to moderate myelosuppression with a leukopenic nadir at 7–12 days, nausea, and vomiting occur frequently. Dose- and duration-dependent nephrotoxicity (increased Cr_s and proteinuria) and hepatotoxicity (increased LDH and AST) occur frequently. Sterility, mutagenicity, and teratogenicity have been reported. The dose-limiting toxicity is a hemorrhagic tendency characterized by decreased platelet count and responsiveness, and depressed clotting factor synthesis. Rarely, stomatitis, progressive skin thickening, and hyperpigmentation occur. The drug is an irritant, but not a vesicant if extravasated. The drug is contraindicated in patients with pre-existing bleeding diatheses, hypocalcemia, or severe renal or hepatic dysfunction. Use cautiously, if at all, with other drugs affecting platelet function (eg, aspirin).

Hormonal Drugs and Antagonists

AROMATASE INHIBITORS:

AMINOGLUTETHIMIDE	Cytadren
ANASTROZOLE	Arimidex
LETROZOLE	Femara

Pharmacology. Aminoglutethimide, anastrozole, and letrozole inhibit the metabolic conversion of androstenedione to estradiol, which is mediated by aromatase, primarily in peripheral adipose tissues. In postmenopausal women, this deprives hormonally sensitive breast cancers of estrogenic stimulation. Aminoglutethimide is less specific and also blocks the cholesterol-based biosynthesis of all corticosteroid precursors (eg, hydrocortisone, aldosterone) in the adrenal gland and at peripheral sites.[156–158] Anastrozole and letrozole are much more specific inhibitors of estrogen synthesis that do not affect synthesis of other steroids.

Administration and Adult Dosage. (Aminoglutethimide) **PO** 750 mg–1.5 g/day; (anastrozole) **PO** 1 mg/day; (letrozole) **PO** 2.5 mg/day.

Dosage Forms. (Aminoglutethimide) **Tab** 250 mg. (Anastrozole) **Tab** 1 mg. (Letrozole) **Tab** 2.5 mg.

Dosage Modification. *Pediatric Dosage.* (Aminoglutethimide) Safety and efficacy not established, but the following has been used: **PO for adrenal hyperplasia and adrenal tumors** (>2.5 yr) 0.375–1.5 g/day. (Anastrozole, letrozole) Safety and efficacy not established.

Geriatric Dosage. Same as adult dosage.

Other Conditions. (Anastrozole) No change required in hepatic or renal impairment. (Letrozole) No dosage adjustment is required with $Cl_{cr} \geq 10$ mL/min.

Patient Instructions. (Aminoglutethimide) If severe stress or trauma occurs, increased hydrocortisone dosage may be needed. Marked drowsiness may occur during therapy. Skin rashes are common, especially at the start of therapy. (Letrozole) This drug may be taken with food.

Missed Doses. This drug should be taken at regular intervals exactly as prescribed. If a dose is missed, it should be taken as soon as it is remembered. If it is almost time for the next dose, take only that dose and resume the regular dosage schedule. Do not double the dose.

Pharmacokinetics. *Fate.* (Aminoglutethimide) A 1 g oral dose yields serum levels of 9 μg/mL. Cl averages 5.5 L/hr in adults. About 50% is metabolized in liver to a less active N-acetyl derivative; this and other metabolites are excreted renally.[1,156] (Anastrozole) Extensively metabolized and excreted renally (10% as parent, 60% as metabolites).[157] (Letrozole) Well absorbed. V_d is 1.9 L/kg. The drug is metabolized to a glucuronide metabolite which is excreted in urine. Only 5% is excreted in urine unchanged.

$t_{1/2}$. (Aminoglutethimide) α phase 2.5 hr; β phase 13.3 hr. (Anastrozole) 50 hr. (Letrozole) about 2 days.[1,156–158]

Adverse Reactions. (Aminoglutethimide) Lethargy and somnolence (80%); skin rashes (50%); visual blurring, dizziness (15–30%, especially in the elderly); nausea, vomiting, and hypotension (15%); hypothyroidism (5%); hematologic suppression (eg, agranulocytosis, pancytopenia) (<1%). (Anastrozole) Asthenia (16%); nausea (15%); headache (13%); hot flashes (12%); back pain (10%); emesis (9%); dizziness, rash, constipation (<5%). (Letrozole) musculoskeletal pain, nausea, hot flashes, headache, sweating, hair thinning, and edema are frequent.

Contraindications. None known.

Precautions. (Aminoglutethimide) Supplemental **hydrocortisone** 50–100 mg/day and **fludrocortisone** 0.1 mg/day are required during therapy.

Drug Interactions. (Aminoglutethimide) Several drug interactions may occur because of the drug's enhancement of CYP3A metabolism; the effects of dexamethasone, digoxin, medroxyprogesterone, tamoxifen, theophylline, and warfarin may be reduced. Aminoglutethimide also induces its own metabolism, which decreases blood levels and half-lives during long-term therapy. (Letrozole) Letrozole inhibits CYP2A6 and CYP2C9.

Parameters to Monitor. (Aminoglutethimide) Monitor thyroid function and blood pressure periodically during therapy.

BICALUTAMIDE	Casodex
FLUTAMIDE	Eulexin
NILUTAMIDE	Nilandron

Pharmacology. These drugs are nonsteroidal antiandrogens that competitively inhibit binding of testosterone at androgen receptors in the testes and prostate gland, reducing androgen-stimulated cell growth. They are used together with a luteinizing hormone-releasing hormone (LHRH) analogue (eg, leuprolide or goserelin). Bicalutamide has a longer half-life and 4-fold higher affinity than flutamide for the androgen receptor, which allows once-daily administration.[159,160]

Administration and Adult Dosage. **PO for prostatic carcinoma** together with an LHRH analogue (Bicalutamide) 40 mg once daily; (Flutamide) 250 mg q 8 hr; (Nilutamide) 300 mg/day for 30 days, then 150 mg/day.

Special Populations. *Pediatric Dosage. Geriatric Dosage.* Same as adult dosage.

Other Conditions. If prostate specific-antigen (PSA) levels rise together with clinical disease progression, consider discontinuing the antiandrogen temporarily and continuing the LHRH antagonist to re-establish androgen receptor sensitivity. Renal or hepatic impairment does not appear to alter elimination of either drug.

Dosage Forms. (Bicalutamide) **Tab** 50 mg. (Flutamide) **Tab** 125 mg. (Nilutamide) **Tab** 50 mg.

Patient Instructions. Take therapy continuously without interruption. Start bicalutamide at the same time as the LHRH agonist. Hot flashes and some feminizing side effects (especially breast enlargement or tenderness) may occur during therapy.

Missed Doses. Take a missed dose as soon as possible. If you take the drug once daily and it is time for the next dose, take it at the regular time. Do not double the dose. If you take two or more doses daily, and it is about time for the next dose, skip the missed dose. Do not double the dose. If you miss two or more doses contact your physician.

Pharmacokinetics. *Fate.* These agents are well absorbed orally and absorption is unaffected by food, but absolute bioavailability is unknown. (Bicalutamide) With an oral dose of 50 mg/day, bicalutamide attains a peak serum level of 8.9 mg/L (21 μmol/L) 31 hr after a dose at steady state. Cl of (R)-bicalutamide is 0.32 L/hr. The active (R)-enantiomer of bicalutamide is oxidized to an inactive metabolite, which, like the inactive (S)-enantiomer, is glucuronidated and cleared rapidly by elimination in the urine and feces.[160] (Flutamide) Flutamide attains peak serum levels of 78 μg/L (283 nmol/L) 2–4 hr after a 250 mg dose at steady state, and its metabolite (α-hydroxyflutamide) achieves levels of 0.720–1.68 mg/L. Flutamide and its active metabolite α-hydroxyflutamide are bound to plasma proteins. Both drugs are extensively metabolized. The majority of a flutamide dose is excreted in the urine as 2-amino-5-nitro-4-(trifluoromethyl) phenol (inactive) with little parent and active metabolite (4.2% of a dose) excreted in the bile or feces.[161,162]

$t_{\frac{1}{2}}$. (Bicalutamide) 5.8 days; (Flutamide) 7.8 hr; (Nilutamide) 41–49 hr.[160–162]

Adverse Reactions. These agents are relatively well tolerated. When the drugs are combined with an LHRH agonist, the following side effects occur: hot flashes (50%), general pain (25%), back pain (16%), asthenia (16%), pelvic pain (12%), constipation (15%), diarrhea (10–24%, higher with flutamide, possibly because of lactose intolerance),[163] nausea (11%), nocturia (10%), liver enzyme elevation (6–10%), abdominal pain (8%), and chest pain (5%). Hepatic injury and jaundice occur rarely.

Contraindications. None known.

Precautions. Discontinue these drugs if liver function tests are consistently over twice the upper limits of normal in the absence of hepatic metastases.

Drug Interactions. Dosage adjustment of warfarin, based on INR, may be necessary when bicalutamide is administered because it can displace warfarin from protein binding sites in vitro.

Parameters to Monitor. Monitor PSA levels q 3 months as an index of disease response. Obtain serum transaminases q 3–4 months to rule out drug-induced hepatic injury.

ESTRAMUSTINE PHOSPHATE   Emcyt

Pharmacology. Estramustine is a conjugate of nor-nitrogen mustard linked by a carbamate bond to the 3 position of the steroidal nucleus of estradiol. Phosphorylation at position 17 adds water solubility. Estramustine was originally thought to act as a hormonally directed alkylating agent, but later studies suggest an alternate effect, impairment of mitotic spindle formation. Dephosphorylated estradiol and estrone metabolites produce typical estrogenic effects.[164]

Administration and Adult Dosage. **PO for prostatic carcinoma** 14 mg/kg/day in 3–4 divided doses.

Special Populations. *Geriatric Dosage.* Same as adult dosage.

Other Conditions. Diabetic and hypertensive patients may require increased doses of insulin or antihypertensives because of estrogenic effects.

Dosage Forms. **Cap** 140 mg.

Patient Instructions. Take this drug on an empty stomach; particularly avoid taking with milk, milk products, or calcium-containing foods or drugs.

Missed Doses. If you miss a dose, skip the missed dose and go back to your regular dosage regimen. Do not double the dose. If you miss two or more doses contact your physician.

Pharmacokinetics. *Fate.* Milk and calcium salts reduce oral bioavailability by forming nonabsorbable calcium complexes. Dephosphorylated during absorption to estradiol and estrone congeners. (*See* Estradiol, Estrone.)

Adverse Reactions. Emetic potential is low. The major side effects are caused by estrogenic actions. These include very frequent gynecomastia, cardiovascular effects (frequent edema, occasional leg cramps, or thrombophlebitis, and rare pulmonary embolism and infarction), and GI effects (frequent nausea without vomiting, diarrhea, and occasional anorexia). Laboratory abnormalities are minimal; there is no consistent hematologic suppression and only mild increases in AST or LDH in about 30% of patients.[164]

Contraindications. Thrombophlebitis or thromboembolic conditions (except when tumor is the cause).

Precautions. Use with caution in patients with severe underlying cardiovascular diseases. Poorly controlled CHF can also be exacerbated by estrogen-induced fluid retention. Type 1 diabetics and patients on antihypertensive medications may have increased medication requirements for these diseases.

Drug Interactions. Dairy products or calcium salts may reduce estramustine bioavailability.

Parameters to Monitor. Responses in prostate cancer are predominantly subjective, including reduced pain and less urinary retention. Objective responses can be followed with serial acid phosphatase determinations. Attention to cardiovascular or thromboembolic signs and symptoms is important.

Notes. Estramustine phosphate is principally used in the palliative treatment of advanced prostate cancer. Objective partial response rates of 20% are common. The drug can be safely combined with cytotoxic agents.[164]

GONADOTROPIN-RELEASING HORMONE ANALOGUES:

GOSERELIN ACETATE   Zoladex

LEUPROLIDE ACETATE   Lupron

Pharmacology. Goserelin and leuprolide are synthetic peptide analogues of the natural hypothalamic hormone, gonadotropin-releasing hormone (GnRH). This hormone controls the release of pituitary luteinizing hormone (LH) and follicle-stimulating hormone (FSH) to stimulate sex hormone production in the testes (testosterone) and ovaries (estradiol, others). Both synthetic agents have D-amino acid and other substitutions to increase stimulatory potency. FSH and LH are initially stimulated, followed by profound inhibition of circulating sex hormones to castration levels. This retards the growth of hormonally dependent organs including the prostate, breast, endometrium, and ovaries.[165,166]

Administration and Adult Dosage. **SC for prostatic carcinoma** (goserelin) insert 3.6 mg implant into upper abdominal wall q 28 days; (leuprolide aqueous) 1 mg/day. **IM for prostatic carcinoma** (leuprolide depot) 7.5 mg of 1-month formulation q 28–33 days or 22.5 mg of the 3-month formulation q 3 months. **SC for endometriosis** (goserelin) insert 3.6 mg implant into upper abdominal wall q 28 days for 6 months; **IM for endometriosis** (leuprolide depot) 3.75 mg monthly for 6 months.

Special Populations. *Pediatric Dosage.* **SC for central precocious puberty (CPP)** (leuprolide aqueous) 50 µg/kg/day initially, increasing in 10 µg/kg/day increments until total down-regulation is achieved. **IM for CPP** initial dosage is (≤25 kg) 7.5 mg monthly; (25–37.5 kg) 11.25 mg monthly; (>37.5 kg) 15 mg monthly. Increase in 3.75 mg/month increments until total down-regulation is achieved.

Geriatric Dosage. (Prostatic carcinoma) same as adult dosage.

Dosage Forms. (Goserelin) **Implant** 3.6 mg. (Leuprolide) **Inj (aqueous)** 5 mg/mL; **Inj (depot, 1-month formulations)** 3.75, 7.5, 11.25, 15 mg; **(3-month formulation)** 22.5 mg/1.5 mL. (*Note:* do not use a partial dose of the 3-month formulation in place of a 1-month formulation.)

Patient Instructions. Instruct in proper method of aseptic preparation of vials and syringes, proper technique for SC administration, and proper disposal of syringes and needles. (Prostate cancer) Disease symptoms such as bone pain and urinary retention may become worse briefly upon initiation of therapy. (Endometriosis) Do not become pregnant while on this drug; always use a barrier contraceptive. Notify your physician if regular menstruation continues. Because therapy may cause a loss of bone density, calcium supplementation is recommended. (Pediatric CPP) A slight increase in pubertal signs and symptoms may occur initially. Adherence to therapy is critical; symptoms such as menses or breast or testicular development may indicate inadequate therapy.

Pharmacokinetics. *Fate.* Both drugs are inactive orally. The SC, IM, and IV routes provide comparable bioavailability. The metabolism of these compounds has not been described. (Goserelin) Goserelin is slowly absorbed over the first 8 days. Thereafter, absorption is steady for the remaining 28 days with no evidence of dose-to-dose accumulation. Goserelin serum levels of about 2.5 μg/L occur on days 15–16 in males with prostate cancer. (Leuprolide) The absorption profile of leuprolide 3-month formulation is similar to the 7.5 mg 1-month formulation. Leuprolide serum levels after a 7.5 mg depot injection are 20 μg/L at 4 hr and 0.36 μg/L at 4 weeks.

$t_{1/2}$. (Goserelin) 4.2 hr with Cl_{cr} >70 mL/min; 12.1 hr with Cl_{cr} <20 mL/min. (Leuprolide) 2.9 hr.

Adverse Reactions. Emetic potential is low; nausea occurs in <5% of patients. Prostate cancer symptoms flare initially, causing bone pain or urinary retention. Sexual dysfunction and decreased erections are reported in about 20% of males. Hot flashes may initially occur in up to 80% of patients with endometriosis, who may also experience calcium loss and estrogen deficiency side effects including decreased libido, vaginal discomfort, dizziness, general malaise, emotional lability, or depression. Mild injection site reactions are rare, unless the patient is sensitive to benzyl alcohol (leuprolide aqueous only).

Contraindications. Pregnancy, because of an established teratogenic activity in animals. Do not initiate therapy for endometriosis until after negative pregnancy test.

Precautions. Monitor carefully initially in prostate cancer patients. Those with severe metastatic vertebral lesions are subject to spinal cord compression, and those with severe urinary retention may develop renal impairment.

Drug Interactions. None known.

Parameters to Monitor. (Prostate cancer) Monitor serum LH, FSH, estradiol, and testosterone; concentrations should fall to castrate levels with adequate GnRH analogue therapy. Close initial monitoring of disease symptom severity (bone pain, urinary retention) is required. Serum PSA levels should fall and remain low in patients who respond. (Endometriosis) Monitor pain and menstrual symptoms.

Notes. In prostate cancer, these drugs are often combined with an androgen receptor antagonist (eg, bicalutamide, flutamide) to provide complete hormonal blockade.

| **TAMOXIFEN CITRATE** | Nolvadex, Various |

Pharmacology. Tamoxifen is a synthetic, nonsteroidal antiestrogen that binds to cytosol or nuclear estrogen receptor (ER) proteins in hormonally sensitive organs including the breast, prostate, uterus, and ovary.[167] The tamoxifen-receptor complex binds to chromatin in the cell nucleus, stopping estrogen-dependent growth-stimulatory mRNA synthesis.

Administration and Adult Dosage. **PO for breast cancer** usually 20 mg bid in premenopausal patients and 10 mg bid in postmenopausal patients. To rapidly achieve steady-state levels, an initial 2-week course of 40 mg/m^2 bid followed by the standard maintenance dosage has been recommended.[168]

Special Populations. *Geriatric Dosage.* Same as adult dosage.

Dosage Forms. **Tab** 10 mg.

Patient Instructions. In premenopausal patients the chance of becoming pregnant is increased and a barrier contraceptive should be used. You should have regular gynecologic examinations after taking this drug and report any menstrual irregularities, abnormal vaginal discharge or bleeding, or pelvic pain or pressure. Lactation may occur while on tamoxifen.

Missed Doses. If you miss a dose, skip the missed dose and go back to your regular dosage regimen. Do not double the dose. If you miss two or more doses contact your physician.

Pharmacokinetics. *Onset and Duration.* Therapeutic levels are attained in 7 or more days with 10–20 mg/m^2/day, but in 3 hr after the loading dose regimen of 40 mg/m^2 or more bid.[168]

Serum Levels. There does not appear to be a direct relationship between serum levels and response or time to response, but all responders have tamoxifen levels over 180 μg/L (0.48 μmol/L) at the time of remission.

Fate. Well absorbed orally, with a peak of 42 μg/L (0.11 μmol/L; 12 μg/L is N-desmethyl metabolite) achieved 3–4 hr after a 20 mg dose.[169] Initially, the N-desmethyl concentration is only 50% of the tamoxifen level, but after 21 days the metabolite level is higher because of its longer half-life. With low-dose continuous therapy, mean steady-state tamoxifen levels of 260 μg/L (0.7 μmol/L) or more are achieved after 16 weeks. Tamoxifen is slowly but extensively metabolized, mainly to N-desmethyltamoxifen, which is equally antiestrogenic to tamoxifen. Neither is readily conjugated, and both undergo hepatic hydroxylation and conjugation followed by elimination into the bile and feces; levels are measurable for up to 6 weeks after drug discontinuation.[168]

t$_{1/2}$. (Tamoxifen) 4 days; (N-desmethyltamoxifen) 9 days.[169] With long-term use, these half-lives increase slightly.[168]

Adverse Reactions. Emetic potential is moderately low. Well tolerated, producing rare minor myelosuppression (usually in heavily pretreated patients). Menopausal symptomatology, including hot flashes, nausea, and rarely vomiting, is produced in one-third of patients. Menstrual difficulties include irregularity, vaginal bleeding, and pruritus vulvae. A serious disease "flare" occurs occasionally during initial therapy involving hypercalcemia and an increase in bone or soft tissue pain;[170] the flare often subsides even with continued therapy and may indicate early tumor response. Retinopathy has occurred, most commonly after very large dosages, but also with usual dosages. The drug appears to produce estrogen-like effects in the bone; thus, skeletal demineralization is not a problem with long-term therapy. An increased risk of secondary uterine cancer has been reported.

Precautions. Pregnancy. Use with caution in patients with pre-existing leukopenia and thrombocytopenia.

Drug Interactions. Aminoglutethimide may decrease tamoxifen serum levels. Tamoxifen may attenuate the cytotoxic activities of fluorouracil and doxorubicin.[1]

Notes. The response rate in breast cancer is about 50–70% in ER-positive patients, whereas the rate in ER-negative patients is only about 5–10%.[171] Tamoxifen has been used in endometrial, stage D prostatic, and renal cell cancers as well as in melanoma.[1] It has also been used investigationally to decrease the size and pain of gynecomastia.

TOREMIFENE CITRATE   Fareston

Pharmacology. Toremifene is a chloro derivative of tamoxifen that binds to high-affinity estrogen receptors in hormonally dependent tissues. Like tamoxifen, it has both antiestrogenic and estrogenic activity in different tissues. Effects on serum lipids are similar to tamoxifen (reduced total and LDL cholesterol), but toremifene also slightly increases HDL levels. In estrogen receptor-positive breast cancer, toremifene is comparable to tamoxifen, but has minimal activity in tamoxifen-refractory patients. Unlike **tamoxifen**, toremifene does not produce DNA/genotoxic effects or hepatocellular carcinoma in animals, suggesting a possibly improved long-term safety profile.[158,172,173]

Administration and Adult Dosage. PO for breast cancer 50 mg/day.

Special Populations. *Geriatric Dosage.* Same as adult dosage.

Dosage Forms. Tab 60 mg.

Patient Instructions. (*See* Tamoxifen.)

Pharmacokinetics. *Fate.* Peak serum levels occur 1.5–4.5 hr after a single dose, but the time to reach steady-state with long-term oral administration ranges from 1–5 weeks. Steady-state levels with a dosage of 60 mg/day average 900 μg/L. The drug is extensively metabolized in the liver, primarily by CYP3A4. Major metabolites are N-desmethyl- and 4-hydroxytoremifene, both of which are active antiestrogens. However, only the N-desmethyl derivative is detectable in plasma with a dosage of 60 mg/day.[158,172]

$t_{1/2}$. (Toremifene) 5 days; (N-desmethyltoremifene) 6 days.[172]

Adverse Reactions. Toremifene is generally well tolerated with hot flashes (in 34%) the most frequent side effect. Vaginal discharge or bleeding occurs in 13% of patients, dizziness in 9%, and edema in 5%. It causes minimal GI toxicity, consisting of nausea in 14% and vomiting in 4% of patients. Sweating, vaginal discharge or bleeding, dizziness, and edema also occur frequently. Acute tumor flare occurs in 16%, marked by transient increases in bone or musculoskeletal pain, cutaneous erythema, and/or hypercalcemia within 2 weeks of starting therapy. Worsening cataracts occur in 10%, which is similar to tamoxifen, and mild corneal keratopathies occur in 4%. All of these ocular effects are reversible upon discontinuation. In a comparative trial, mild liver function abnormalities occurred in the toremifene group, although most were related to progressive metastatic breast cancer.

Drug Interactions. Drugs that induce CYP3A4 may decrease toremifene levels and those that inhibit CYP3A4 may increase levels. Toremifene may increase PT in patients taking warfarin.

Mitotic Inhibitors

DOCETAXEL
Taxotere

Pharmacology. Docetaxel is a semisynthetic derivative of a taxane extracted from the needles of the yew tree, *Taxus baccata*. It binds to microtubule tubulin sites distinct from paclitaxel with the similar result of enhanced microtubule polymerization, causing clumps to form and halting cell division in metaphase. It is active in refractory breast cancer and in non–small cell lung cancer.[174]

Administration and Adult Dosage. **IV for breast cancer** 60–100 mg/m^2 infused over 1 hr q 21 days; premedicate with dexamethasone 16 mg/day for 5 days, starting 1 day prior to docetaxel.

Special Populations. *Pediatric Dosage.* (<16 yr) safety and efficacy not established.

Geriatric Dosage. Same as adult dosage.

Other Conditions. Reduce dosage by 25–50% in patients with elevated hepatic enzymes (and probably also with elevated serum bilirubin).

Dosage Forms. **Inj** 40 mg/mL.

Patient Instructions. Immediately report fever or chills occurring 1–2 weeks after drug administration. This drug may cause swelling of the extremities and tingling sensations.

Pharmacokinetics. *Fate.* Peak serum levels average 3.6 μg/mL following a 1-hr IV infusion of 100 mg/m^2. Over 90% is plasma protein bound. Cl averages 40 L/hr in adults; Cl is reduced by 25% or more in patients with elevated liver function tests (transaminases >1.5 times normal and alkaline phosphatase >2.5 times normal). Most of the drug is metabolized to less active hydroxylated forms and excreted by biliary secretion into the feces; <5% is excreted in urine.

t$_{1/2}$. α phase 5 min; β phase 38 min; γ phase 12 hr.

Adverse Reactions. Emetic potential is moderate. The dose-limiting toxicity is neutropenia, which is more severe with reduced liver function; the onset of febrile neutropenia can be as soon as 5 days after drug administration. Thrombocytopenia also occurs, but is less severe. Anemia and alopecia also occur, but are not dose limiting. Infusion-associated hypersensitivity symptoms (eg, facial flushing) occur in 50% of patients, whereas dyspnea, chest tightness, and low back pain are rare. A pruritic rash on the forearms, hands, and neck occurs in about 40% of patients.

Mucositis and nausea and vomiting occur in about one-third of patients. Peripheral nerve numbness and paresthesia, fluid retention, and edema are cumulative dose-related toxicities. Weight gain initially involves peripheral edema at cumulative dosages over 500 mg/m^2; edema may become prominent after 6 cycles (600 mg/m^2 total dosage) and can proceed to pulmonary edema. Pretreatment with oral dexamethasone (8 mg bid for 5 days, starting 24 hr before docetaxel) retards the development of serious fluid retention.

Contraindications. Severe hypersensitivity to drugs formulated with polysorbate 80; neutropenia <1500/μL; hepatic transaminase levels over 1.5 times the upper limit of normal; hepatic alkaline phosphatase levels over 2.5 times normal; severe pre-existing neutropenia, edema, or peripheral neuropathy.

Precautions. Febrile neutropenia is frequent, necessitating careful followup of infectious signs after administration.

Drug Interactions. In vitro, metabolism of docetaxel to its hydroxy metabolites is reduced by inhibitors of CYP3A such as cimetidine, erythromycin, ketoconazole, and troleandomycin. Barbiturates stimulate metabolism of docetaxel.[175] The clinical importance of these findings is not known.

Parameters to Monitor. WBC count, peripheral edema, liver function tests (ALT, AST, alkaline phosphatase) and signs of infection.

ETOPOSIDE	VePesid, Various
ETOPOSIDE PHOSPHATE	Etopophos

Pharmacology. Etoposide (VP-16) is a substituted epipodophyllotoxin derivative from the May apple plant. The major cytotoxic activity is cell cycle phase specific for G$_2$ and involves the induction of protein-linked DNA strand breaks by inhibiting DNA topoisomerase II enzymes.

Administration and Adult Dosage. IV 200–250 mg/m^2 q 7 weeks, or 70 mg/m^2/day for 5 days. IV of etoposide should be administered over 30–60 min or longer; etoposide phosphate may be administered over 5–210 min. **IV continuous infusion** 125 mg/m^2/day for 5 days.[176] **PO for small cell lung cancer** 2 times the IV dose, rounded to the nearest 50 mg; alternatively, 50 mg/day for 30 days.

Special Populations. *Pediatric Dosage.* Safety and efficacy are not established. However, etoposide has been used in dosages similar to adult body surface area dosages.[177–179]

Geriatric Dosage. Same as adult dosage, but adjust for age-related reduction in renal function.

Other Conditions. With Cl$_{cr}$ ≤20 mL/min give 75% of standard dose; reduced dosage is also required with severe bone marrow compromise. Dosage reduction may also be necessary with altered hepatobiliary function.

Dosage Forms. **Inj** (Etoposide) 20 mg/mL; (etoposide phosphate) 100 mg; **Cap** (etoposide) 50 mg.

Patient Instructions. (*See* Antineoplastics Class Instructions.)

Pharmacokinetics. *Fate.* Oral bioavailability is $52 \pm 17\%$ with inter- and intrapatient variability. CSF levels are <10% of serum levels. V_d is 0.36 ± 0.13 L/kg;[10] Cl is 1.1–1.7 L/hr/m² or 0.04 ± 0.014 L/hr/kg.[176,180] Inactive metabolites include the hydroxyacid and cis-lactones. Up to 16% of a dose may be eliminated in bile; $30 \pm 5\%$ is eliminated in urine, about 70% of this is unchanged drug.

$t_{½}$. 8.1 ± 4.3 hr, increased in uremia.[176,180]

Adverse Reactions. Emetic potential is low. Myelosuppression occurs, with a nadir at 7–10 days (longer with daily regimens), principally affecting the granulocytes, but also affecting platelets, with a nadir at 9–16 days. Myelosuppression may be less frequent with the phosphate form. Mild mucositis and alopecia can occur. Diarrhea is more frequent with oral administration. Hypotension occurs rarely with rapid IV bolus injections. There is one report of radiation recall skin injury in 13 of 23 patients with small cell lung cancer. Long-term administration may result in development of acute leukemia.

Precautions. Pregnancy; decrease dosage in severe renal dysfunction; avoid rapid IV bolus injection.

Drug Interactions. Anaphylaxis and possible synergistic neuropathy with vincristine and/or cardiomyopathy with anthracyclines have been reported. Cyclosporine may increase serum etoposide levels and toxicity. Phenytoin, phenobarbital, and possibly other CYP3A inducers may decrease etoposide serum levels.

Parameters to Monitor. Obtain peripheral granulocyte counts immediately prior to administration on repetitive courses. Nadir counts (1–2 weeks after dose) are optional.

Notes. Etoposide is indicated in the combination treatment of small cell carcinoma of the lung and refractory nonseminomatous testicular cancer. The drug is also active in lymphomas and in acute leukemias (both lymphoblastic and myeloblastic varieties). Etoposide is not a vesicant. Store capsules under refrigeration. Etoposide and cisplatin are compatible for 24 hr in the same container. Concentrated etoposide solutions (>1 mg/mL) may cause cracking of ABS plastic infusion system components and have short stability times of 2 hr. More dilute solutions in NS or D5W of 0.4–0.6 mg/mL have longer stability times of 8 hr and 48 hr, respectively.

IRINOTECAN   Camptosar

Pharmacology. Irinotecan is a water-soluble derivative of camptothecin. It is a prodrug for the despiperidine metabolite SN-38, which is an inhibitor of topoisomerase-1 enzymes. This causes single strand breaks in DNA. Irinotecan is approved for the treatment of patients with advanced colorectal cancer who have failed therapy with fluorouracil. The overall response rate in advanced fluorouracil-refractory colon cancer is about 15%, with a 5.2 month median duration of response.[181]

Adult Dosage. IV 125 mg/m² administered in 500 mL of D5W over 90 min once weekly for 4 consecutive weeks. If no toxicity occurs, subsequent doses are increased by 25–50 mg/m^2; if severe toxicity occurs, dosage is decreased by 25–50 mg/m^2.

Dosage Forms. *Inj* 20 mg/mL.

Pharmacokinetics. The half-lives of irinotecan and the active SN-38 metabolite are 5.7 and 9.8 hr, respectively, with peak SN-38 levels (2–5% of irinotecan) achieved 1 hr after administration. Renal excretion accounts for <10% of a dose as irinotecan and <1% as SN-38; hepatic elimination predominates.

Adverse Reactions. Diarrhea occurs in 90% of patients and can be severe, requiring aggressive prophylaxis with fluids and multiple doses of loperamide. Leukopenia occurs in one-third of patients, although moderate to severe myelosuppression occurs in only 15 and 11% of patients, respectively.

PACLITAXEL Taxol, Various

Pharmacology. Paclitaxel is a naturally occurring diterpene taxane obtained from the bark of the Pacific yew tree *Taxus brevifolia*. It binds to tubulin proteins to cause abnormal microtubule polymerization and cell cycle arrest in metaphase.[182,183]

Administration and Adult Dosage. *IV* 135–175 mg/m^2 over 3 or 24 hr q 3 weeks. Doses up to 250 mg/m^2 have been used with hematopoietic colony stimulation factors. Use non-PVC infusion systems.

Special Populations. *Pediatric Dosage.* Safety and efficacy not established.

Geriatric Dosage. Same as adult dosage.

Dosage Forms. *Inj* 6 mg/mL.

Patient Instructions. (*See* Antineoplastics Class Instructions.)

Pharmacokinetics. *Fate.* Erratic oral bioavailability precludes oral administration. Cl is 18 L/hr/m^2. It is metabolized to a much less active hydroxylated species by CYP3A. Eliminated 30–40% by hepatobiliary excretion; only 1–5% excreted in urine.[184]

$t_{1/2}$. α phase 0.2 hr; β phase 1.9 hr (range 0.5–2.8); γ phase 20.7 hr (range 4–65).[184]

Adverse Reactions. Emetic potential is low. The usual dose-limiting toxicity is neutropenia, with an 8- to 11-day nadir; more severe with prolonged infusion. Dose-limiting toxicity in combination regimens with doxorubicin include neutropenia, inflammation of the cecum (typhlitis) and, with cisplatin, neuropathy. Peripheral neuropathy (eg, numbness, paresthesias) is cumulative, dose related, and more severe with prior vinca alkaloid or concurrent cisplatin therapy. Alopecia can involve all body hair, with an abrupt onset of 2 weeks. Mucositis is dose dependent. Cardiotoxicity, primarily bradycardia, occurs in 10–30% of patients, but rarely requires treatment. Myalgia and arthralgia are common, but usually transient. Hypersensitivity reactions, thought to be caused by Cremophor, may occur within the first few minutes of infusion; symptoms include chest pain, hypotension, bronchospasm, urticaria, and flushing, and can rapidly progress to anaphylaxis. (*See* Precautions.)

Contraindications. Hypersensitivity to Cremophor vehicle; neutropenia (<1500/μL).

Precautions. Recommended premedications include dexamethasone PO 20 mg at 12 and 6 hr before paclitaxel, and diphenhydramine IV 50 mg, plus either cimetidine 300 mg, ranitidine 50 mg, or famotidine 20 mg, 30 min before paclitaxel. Ensure that emergency resuscitation equipment is available at the start of infusion. Use cautiously in patients with heart rhythm disturbances.

Drug Interactions. Ketoconazole may decrease paclitaxel clearance and enhance toxicity. Although their effect is not well studied, use other CYP3A inhibitors with caution. (*See also* Adverse Reactions.)

Parameters to Monitor. Neutrophil count prior to administration.

Notes. Highly effective as a first-line or refractory treatment for ovarian cancer; typically used in platinum-containing regimens; also active in breast cancer, non–small cell lung cancer, lymphoma, and malignant melanoma.[183]

TENIPOSIDE   Vumon

Pharmacology. Teniposide is a semisynthetic podophyllum derivative that has cell cycle S and G_2 phase specific cytotoxic activities similar to etoposide. Teniposide is active in acute leukemias and in children with relapsed acute leukemia or neuroblastoma.[180,185,186]

Pediatric Dosage. IV for acute leukemias 165–200 mg/m^2/week or 165 mg/m^2 twice weekly.

Dosage Forms. Inj 10 mg/mL.

Pharmacokinetics. Teniposide is over 90% plasma protein bound and is eliminated much more slowly than etoposide. Teniposide half-lives are α phase 45 min, β phase 4 hr, and γ phase 11–30 hr (average 20); 40% of a dose is eliminated in the feces; CSF drug levels are high (27% of serum levels).

Adverse Reactions. The dose-limiting side effect of teniposide is myelosuppression, with the leukopenic nadir at 10–14 days. Emetic potential is low; nausea and vomiting are typically mild (more severe after oral etoposide). Hypotension is reported with rapid drug infusions. Rarely severe hypersensitivity reactions (including anaphylaxis), alopecia, and chemical phlebitis during infusion occur.

TOPOTECAN   Hycamtin

Pharmacology. Topotecan is a topoisomerase I inhibitor that causes single strand breaks in DNA. It is a semisynthetic derivative of camptothecin, which is derived from the bark of the Chinese tree, *Camptotheca acuminata*. Topotecan is approved as a second-line treatment for metastatic ovarian carcinoma after failure of a primary agent and is also being studied in breast and colon cancer.[1]

Adult Dosage. IV 1.5 mg/m^2/day administered over 30 min for 5 days, starting on day 1 of a 21-day course of therapy for a minimum of 4 courses. With a Cl_{cr} between 20–39 mL/min, the dosage is reduced to 0.75 mg/m^2/day; no guidelines exist for Cl_{cr} <20 mL/min. If severe neutropenia occurs, either reduce further doses by 0.25 mg/m^2/day or administer filgrastim with subsequent courses.

Dosage Forms. Inj 4 mg.

Pharmacokinetics. Topotecan is rapidly hydrolyzed in plasma. About 70% of the drug is excreted renally as metabolites.

Adverse Reactions. The primary dose-limiting side effect of topotecan is neutropenia with a nadir at a mean of 11 days; severe neutropenia occurs in 80% of patients. Severe anemia in 40% of patients and severe thrombocytopenia in 26% have also been reported. Nausea and vomiting occur in most patients; other GI effects include frequent diarrhea, constipation, and abdominal pain. Alopecia occurs in about 60% of patients; fatigue and fever of 101°F or greater are also frequent. Topotecan is contraindicated in pregnancy, breastfeeding, or severe bone marrow depression.

VINCA ALKALOIDS:	
VINBLASTINE SULFATE	Velban, Various
VINCRISTINE SULFATE	Oncovin, Various
VINORELBINE TARTRATE	Navelbine

Pharmacology. The vinca alkaloids are *Vinca rosea* (periwinkle) plant-derived antimitotic agents; cytotoxic activity is related to specific binding to the microtubule protein tubulin, causing microtubule dissolution. This blocks formation of the mitotic spindle apparatus necessary for cell division. The vincas are lethal to cells at high concentrations and, at lower concentrations, dividing cells are arrested in the metaphase portion of mitosis.

Administration and Dosage.

	VINBLASTINE	**VINCRISTINE**	**VINORELBINE**
Administration	IV push, infusion.	IV push.	IV short infusion.
Adult Dosage	IV push 4–12 mg/m^2 as a single agent at monthly intervals; or 1.5–1.7 mg/m^2/ day for 5 days as a continuous infusion.[187]	0.4–1.4 mg/m^2/ week (2.5 mg typical single dose limit).	30 mg/m^2/week.
Pediatric Dosage	IV push 4–10 mg/m^2 q 1–2 weeks.	1.4–2 mg/m^2/week (2 mg typical single dose limit).	Not used in children.
Geriatric Dosage	Same as adult dosage.	Same as adult dosage.	Same as adult dosage.

Special Populations. *Other Conditions.* Vinblastine and vinorelbine require substantial dosage reduction in heavily pretreated patients (ie, drug or radiation therapy). Reduce vinorelbine dosage by 50% in patients in whom over 75% of the liver is replaced by tumor, or for granulocyte levels on the day of treatment of 1000–1499/μL; do not administer at lower WBC levels.[188] Vinca alkaloids are extensively eliminated in the bile, and the dosages of vinblastine and vincristine must be reduced by approximately 50–75% in the presence of severe hepatobiliary dysfunction. Reduce vinorelbine dosage to 15 mg/m^2/week for a serum total bilirubin of 2.1–3 mg/dL, and to 7.5 mg/m^2/week for a bilirubin over 3 mg/dL.

Dosage Forms. (Vinblastine) **Inj** 1 mg/mL. (Vincristine) **Inj** mg/mL. (Vinorelbine) **Inj** 10 mg/mL.

Patient Instructions. (*See* Antineoplastics Class Instructions.)

Pharmacokinetics. *Fate.*

Distribution	Pharmacokinetics can be described by a two-compartment open model: an initial short phase with rapid tissue uptake (V$_d$ approximating total body water) and a long terminal phase of greater than 1 day with a large V$_d$ reflecting slow drug release from tissue binding sites—see below. Vincas do not effectively penetrate into the CNS or other fatty tissues and achieve their highest levels in the liver, gallbladder, and spleen.
Metabolism	Approximately 50% of renally and fecally excreted products are closely related metabolites. An example is the formation of desacetyl vinblastine (which is more active on a weight basis than vinblastine) following vinblastine administration.
Excretion	The vinca alkaloids appear to be eliminated primarily in the bile and feces, some in the urine.

	VINBLASTINE	VINCRISTINE	VINORELBINE
PHARMACOKINETIC PARAMETERS[189–191]			
V$_c$ (L/kg)	0.7	0.33	—
V$_d$ (L/kg)	27.3	8.4	40.1 (V$_{dss}$)
Urinary Excretion	—	10% (24 hr)	—
(cumulative)	33% (72 hr)	13% (72 hr)	21% (21 days)
Fecal Excretion	—	33% (24 hr)	—
(cumulative)	21% (72 hr)	67% (72 hr)	34–58% (21 days)
$t_{1/2}$			
$t_{1/2\,\alpha}$ (min)	<5	<5	<27
$t_{1/2\,\beta}$ (hr)	0.164	2.3	<1.9
$t_{1/2\,\gamma}$ (hr)	25	85	40

Adverse Reactions. Emetic potential is low (vincristine) to moderate (vinblastine and vinorelbine). Myelosuppression is the dose-limiting toxicity for vinblastine and vinorelbine, with the leukopenic nadir at 4–10 days; unless patients have been heavily pretreated with drugs or radiation, recovery from leukopenia is rather prompt, sometimes facilitating weekly or semimonthly drug administration. The major toxicity of vincristine is peripheral neuropathy manifested by paresthesias, constipation, jaw pain, decreased deep tendon reflexes, and rarely bladder atony or paralytic ileus; gut neurotoxicity occurs rarely with vinorelbine. All of these neurologic symptoms slowly resolve over 1 month and necessitate substantial dosage reduction if present at the time of drug administration. Seizures and ocular toxicity presenting as blurred vision or ptosis occur frequently. Mild laxatives or **metoclopramide** may be useful for constipation. The vincas are extremely toxic if inadvertently extravasated; **hyaluronidase** (150 units/mL) may be effective as a local (subcutaneous) antidote. Vinorelbine also causes substantial phlebitis, which may be lessened by a short (6- to 10-min) infusion. Transiently severe pain in tumor masses occurs with vinblastine frequently. Alopecia is frequent with all agents. Inadvertent intrathecal administration of any vinca alkaloid is fatal.

Contraindications. (Vinblastine) severe bone marrow compromise from prior therapy; uncontrolled infection. (Vincristine) severe peripheral nervous system effects from prior doses, particularly paralytic ileus, tingling paresthesias, or decreased deep tendon reflexes; demyelinating form of Charcot-Marie-Tooth syndrome. (Vinorelbine) Pretreatment granulocyte count <1000/μL.

Precautions. Pregnancy. Use with caution in patients with neurologic deficiencies or hepatic disease.

Drug Interactions. Vinca administration (especially vincristine) has been associated with increased cellular retention of methotrexate (increased even in CNS tissues). Concurrent use of vincristine with zalcitabine may increase neuropathy.

Parameters to Monitor. (Vinblastine and vinorelbine) obtain pretreatment and at least monthly WBC and hemoglobin/hematocrit assessments; (vincristine) obtain serial peripheral neurologic assessments; (all drugs) assess biliary function prior to drug administration and before making dosage adjustments for impaired hepatobiliary status.

Notes. Protect these drugs from light and store under refrigeration. Place individual vincristine doses in an overwrap (eg, plastic bag) that is labeled, "Do not remove covering until the moment of injection. Fatal if given intrathecally. For intravenous use only." Useful in hematologic neoplasms (primarily vincristine) and in solid tumors, including non–small cell lung cancer in combination with cisplatin (vinorelbine) and refractory breast cancer and Kaposi's sarcoma (vinblastine).[192]

Monoclonal Antibodies

IODINE I-131 TOSITUMOMAB   Bexxar

Pharmacology. This agent is a mouse-derived monoclonal antibody that binds to the CD-20 receptor of normal and malignant B-lymphocytes. The β particle-emitting isotope ^{131}I is coupled to the antibody, forming a selective radioimmunoconjugate for patients with CD-20 positive non-Hodgkin's lymphoma refractory to chemotherapy.[193,194]

Adult Dosage. In clinical trials, a two-stage dosage schedule has been used. First, patients are administered unlabeled antibody IV to suppress nonspecific binding sites. Next, patients are given trace-labeled doses of ^{131}I-labeled antibody (15–20 mg containing 5 mCi IV) to assess antibody distribution. One week later, patients are given a 685 mg dose of unlabeled antibody IV, followed 1 day later by 2 individualized therapeutic (labeled) doses of 135 mg and 685 mg of antibody to deliver up to 75 cGy of whole-body radiation. A total body irradiation dosage of 55 cGy may be the maximum tolerated in patients who have undergone bone marrow transplantation. Give diphenhydramine 50 mg and acetaminophen 650 mg prior to each infusion.

Adverse Reactions. Nonhematologic toxicities following both labeled and unlabeled infusions are mild, with low-grade fever in 31% of patients and chills or rigors in 1%. Mild fatigue and nausea occur in 6–8% of radiolabeled infusions. The dose-limiting toxicity is hematologic suppression with grade 3 or 4 leukopenia and thrombocytopenia in 66% of patients who receive a whole-body radiation dose of 85 cGy. All patients develop complete or near-complete depletion of CD-19 and CD-20 positive B-cells from peripheral blood, recovering to normal levels in 3 months. Serum immunoglobulin levels are unchanged. Because of the short, single course of therapy, antimouse antibody (HAMA) reactions are uncommon. However, when they occur, they are usually marked by hypotension that can be treated with fluid hydration and vasopressors.

RITUXIMAB   Rituxan

Pharmacology. Rituximab is a chimeric murine/human monoclonal antibody that binds to the CD-20 antigen on the surface of normal and malignant B-lymphocytes. This blocks normal CD-200–dependent signaling of cell cycle initiation and differentiation, leading to apoptosis. After binding to CD-20, the free Fc portion of the antibody can also recruit immune effector functions to cause lysis of B-cells of B-lymphocytes.[195,196]

Administration and Adult Dosage. IV infusion (not bolus) for relapsed or refractory low-grade B-cell non-Hodgkin's lymphoma 375 mg/m^2 once weekly for 4 doses (days 1, 8, 15, and 22), diluted in NS or D5W. Premedicate the patient with diphenhydramine and acetaminophen and begin the first infusion at a rate of 50 mg/hr. Increase the rate by 50 mg/hr q 30 min to a maximum of 400 mg/hr if no hypotension or hypersensitivity develops. Subsequent infusions are started at a rate of 100 mg/hr and increased by 100 mg/hr q 30 min to the maximum rate of 400 mg/hr, if tolerated. If severe hypersensitivity reactions occur, stop the infusion and treat with diphenhydramine, acetaminophen, and a corticosteroid; for life-threatening reactions, add saline, epinephrine, and bronchodilators. If the reaction is not life-threatening, the infusion may be restarted at one-half of the earlier rate after symptoms subside.

Special Populations. *Pediatric Dosage.* Safety and efficacy not established.

Geriatric Dosage. Same as adult dosage.

Dosage Forms. Inj 10 mg/mL.

Patient Instructions. This drug may cause a flu-like syndrome including fever, chills, and weakness shortly after it is given.

Pharmacokinetics. *Fate.* Peak serum levels are inversely correlated with the number of CD-20–positive B-cells. Levels average about 280 mg/L. Major sites of antibody distribution are to lymphoid cells of the thymus gland, white pulp of the spleen, and B-lymphocytes in peripheral blood and lymph nodes. Cl averages 0.054 L/hr; the antibody is still detectable in serum 3–6 months after the last dose.

$t_{1/2}$. Half-life is proportional to the dose with an average of 60 hr after a dosage of 375 mg/m^2 (range 11–105 hr).

Adverse Reactions. Most patients experience an infusion-related symptom complex with fever, chills, and rigors on the first infusion. Other frequent, acute infusion-related symptoms include nausea (18%), vomiting (10%), angioedema (13%), urticaria or pruritus (10%), and bronchospasm and rhinitis (8%). Hypotension and other acute effects are moderate or severe in 10% of the first doses. Overall, the frequency and severity of all reactions diminishes with subsequent injections. Most first-dose reactions occur within 30 min to 2 hr and resolve with slowing of the infusion rate for mild to moderate reactions or temporary halting the infusion and treating with supportive medications for severe reactions. Epinephrine is required only occasionally. Myelosuppression (neutropenia and thrombocytopenia) is typically mild and occurs in only 10% of patients, although long-term depletion of B-cells occurs in 70–80%; a minority will also have decreased serum immunoglobulins. The frequency of grade 3 infections during the 4-week treatment period is 9% and grade 4 infections generally do not occur.

Contraindications. Patients with a known type I hypersensitivity (or anaphylaxis) to mouse proteins.

Precautions. Pregnancy; lactation. Contraception is recommended in women of childbearing potential. The ability to respond immunologically to a vaccination may be compromised after therapy; the safety of live virus vaccination is not known. Consider stopping antihypertensive medications on the day of treatment to reduce hypotensive reactions. Cardiac monitoring is recommended only in patients with pre-existing arrhythmias and angina that have worsened during the infusion.

Drug Interactions. Additive hypotension may occur in patients on antihypertensive therapy. There is no inhibition of cytotoxic activity in patients being treated for lymphoma with CHOP chemotherapy.

Parameters to Monitor. Monitor for allergic reactions and hypotension frequently during the infusion. Monitor CBC after therapy.

TRASTUZUMAB   Herceptin

Pharmacology. Trastuzumab is a humanized monoclonal antibody that binds to the HER2 protein found on the surface of some normal cells and plays a role in regulating cell growth. It is used only to treat tumors having an overexpression of HER2 protein. It is used alone in the treatment of metastatic breast cancer in patients who have been treated with chemotherapy or with paclitaxel in patients who have not had chemotherapy for their metastatic disease.

Adult Dosage. IV for breast cancer in tumors with overexpression of HER2 4 mg/kg over 90 min as a loading dose, then 2 mg/kg weekly. Subsequent doses may be infused over 30 min if the loading dose was well tolerated. Do not administer as an IV push or bolus.

Dosage Forms. Inj 440 mg.

Pharmacokinetics. With the recommended dosage regimen, steady-state peak and trough concentrations are 123 and 79 mg/L, respectively. Trough serum levels are 1.5 times higher when given with paclitaxel, possibly because of inhibition of metabolism. The drug is distributed primarily in serum with a V_d of 0.44 L/kg. Pharmacokinetics appear to be dose related: Cl decreases and half-life increases with increasing dosages. Half-life averages 5.8 days (range 1–32 days) with the recommended regimen. Renal impairment appears not to affect pharmacokinetics.

Adverse Reactions. Side effects are frequent, but usually not severe. Mild to moderate chills with or without fever occur in 40% of patients during the infusion and can usually be treated with acetaminophen, diphenhydramine and/or meperidine. Other common side effects are diarrhea, pain, asthenia, nausea, vomiting, flu-like symptoms, cough, dyspnea, rash, edema, anemia, and leukopenia. Occasional serious reactions include anaphylaxis, thrombosis, pancytopenia, convulsions, apnea, hypoxia, and renal failure. Cardiac dysfunction and CHF have also occurred. Use the drug with caution in pre-existing cardiac dysfunction; monitor cardiac function during therapy and consider discontinuation if clinically important CHF develops.

Miscellaneous Antineoplastics

ASPARAGINASE	Elspar
PEGASPARGASE	Oncaspar

Pharmacology. Asparaginase is the levo isomer of a macromolecular protein, isolated from *Escherichia coli* and other bacteria, which hydrolyzes the essential amino acid asparagine in the serum, thus depriving susceptible lymphocyte-derived malignancies of a necessary element for protein synthesis. Pegaspargase is a PEG-modified form of asparaginase that can be given to patients allergic to asparaginase. The drug is cell cycle G phase specific.

Administration and Adult Dosage. IM (preferably) or IV for combination therapy of acute leukemia (asparaginase) 200 IU/kg/day for 28 days,[197] or 1000–6000 IU/m²/day for 5 days,[198] or 20,000 IU/m²/week;[199] (pegaspargase) 2500 IU/m² q 14 days.

Special Populations. *Pediatric Dosage.* **IM (preferably) or IV for combination therapy of acute leukemia** (asparaginase) 1000–6000 IU/m²/day for 5 days;[198,200] up to 20,000 IU/m²/week; (pegaspargase) 2500 IU/m² q 14 days.

Geriatric Dosage. Same as adult dosage.

Dosage Forms. Inj (Asparaginase) 10,000 IU vial. (Pegaspargase) 750 IU/mL.

Patient Instructions. (*See* Antineoplastics Class Instructions.) Asparaginase often causes allergic reactions, which can be life-threatening. This drug may also alter blood glucose levels and might worsen diabetes mellitus. Report any abdominal pain immediately, because it may be a sign of pancreatitis.

Pharmacokinetics. *Fate.* (Asparaginase) IV and IM produce equivalent serum levels. There is negligible distribution out of the vascular compartment, with minimal urinary and biliary excretion. Clearance is probably immune mediated. Asparaginase remains detectable in serum 13–22 days after administration.[201] (Pegaspargase) asparaginase is slowly released from pegaspargase and is distributed in the body similarly to native asparaginase.

$t_{1/2}$. (Asparaginase) α phase 4–9 hr; β phase 1.4–1.8 days.[201] (Pegaspargase) 3.2 ± 1.8 days in patients hypersensitive to asparaginase; 5.7 ± 3.3 days in nonsensitive patients.

Adverse Reactions. Emetic potential is low. Moderate to severe non–dose-related hypersensitivity reactions occur in about 20–35% of patients. (IM use may reduce and/or delay allergic complications);[197] a prophylactic antihistamine may sometimes be helpful. (*See* Precautions.) The drug is usually not myelotoxic. Transient blood glucose lowering followed by a pancreatitis-induced hyperglycemia may occur. Elevated serum cholesterol, severely elevated hepatic enzymes, steatosis, depressed clotting factors (especially profound for fibrinogen), and decreased albumin synthesis occur frequently. Lethargy and somnolence occur and may be more frequent in adults.[202] Fatal hyperthermia has been reported.

Contraindications. Anaphylactic reaction to commercial *E. coli* preparation; severe pancreatitis or history of pancreatitis.

Precautions. Onset of abdominal pain, serum amylase elevation, any changes in mental status, or severe elevation of prothrombin time require drug discontinuation. Some elevations of liver function tests should be anticipated. Anaphylaxis can occur with any dose; ensure that emergency resuscitation equipment is available at the time of each dose. Intradermal scratch tests and desensitization procedures are not reliably predictive or preventive for anaphylaxis.[197,201]

Drug Interactions. None known.

Parameters to Monitor. Monitor serum hepatic enzymes, amylase, glucose, and prothrombin time routinely, and all vital signs during administration.

Notes. Reconstitute with NS or D5W (2-mL maximum for IM use); stable at least 24 hr; do not filter.

BLEOMYCIN SULFATE   Blenoxane

Pharmacology. Bleomycin is a mixture of 13 glycopeptide fractions produced by *Streptomyces verticillus*. Antineoplastic effects include single and double strand DNA scission, producing excision of thymine bases mediated through binding with ferric iron and subsequent production of highly reactive hydroxyl and superoxide radicals. It is cell cycle phase specific, with maximal activity in the G_2 (premitotic) phase.[203]

Administration and Adult Dosage. **IM test dose** 1–2 units may be useful in malignant lymphoma patients to assess exaggerated hyperpyrexic response. If no reaction occurs in 2–4 hr, give regular dose. **SC, IM, or IV** 10–20 units/m² 1–2 times/week.[203] **IV continuous infusion** 15–20 units/day for 4–5 days.[204] Experimental evidence in animals favors continuous administration to lessen pulmonary toxicity and maximize cell kill. A total lifetime dosage limit of 400 units is recommended to avoid pulmonary fibrosis. **Intracavitary for malignant effusion** 15–240 units (60 units for pleural effusion) in 50–100 mL or NS.[205]

Special Populations. *Pediatric Dosage.* **SC, IM, or IV** 10–20 units/m² 1–2 times a week in combination regimens. **IV continuous infusion** 15–20 units/m²/day for 4–5 days, usually as a single agent.

Geriatric Dosage. Same as adult dosage, but use with caution in patients >70 yr and adjust dosage for age-related reduction in renal function.

Other Conditions. Dosage reduction has been recommended in renal impairment:[206]

SERUM CREATININE (MG/DL)	PERCENTAGE OF DOSE RECOMMENDED
2.5–4	25 (75% reduction)
4–6	20
6–10	5–10 (90–95% reduction)

Dosage Forms. Inj 15 units.

Patient Instructions. (*See* Antineoplastics Class Instructions.) Report any coughing, shortness of breath, or wheezing. Skin rashes, shaking chills, or transient high fever may occur following administration. Hyperpigmentation of skin fold areas, scars, pressure areas, or sites of trauma may occur.

Pharmacokinetics. *Fate.* Poorly absorbed topically; roughly one-half of intracavitary-administered drug may be systemically available (use this fraction to calculate lifetime exposure). Following an IV dose of about 15 units/m^2, serum levels of 10–1000 milliunits/L are obtained.[204] Steady-state levels during continuous infusion of 20 units/day are 50–200 milliunits/L.[207] $V_{d\beta}$ is 0.27 ± 0.04 L/kg; Cl is 0.066 ± 0.018 L/hr/kg.[10] Tissue inactivation is mediated by specific bleomycin-hydrolase, which is low in skin and lung, the two main toxicity targets of the drug.[204,207] From 50–60% of a dose is recovered in the urine, 68% of this as unchanged drug.[10]

$t_{1/2}$. α phase 24 min; β phase 3.1 ± 1.7 hr.[10,204,207]

Adverse Reactions. Emetic potential is moderately low. Alopecia and acute fever and generalized erythema with edema, eventually leading to hyperpigmentation and skin thickening, are frequent. The most serious long-term toxicity is pulmonary fibrosis manifested by dry cough, rales, dyspnea, and bilateral infiltrates. Pulmonary function studies show hypoxemia and reduced CO diffusing capacity. Pulmonary toxicity usually does not occur below 150 units/m^2, but the frequency increases to 55% at doses above 283 units/m^2 and 66% at 360 units/m^2;[208] life-threatening pulmonary fibrosis is rare if dosage limits are observed. Prior chest radiotherapy, age >70 yr, and hyperoxic ventilation predispose patients to toxicity. About 1% of high-dose bleomycin-treated patients die from pulmonary fibrosis. Low-dose hypersensitivity pneumonitis, which may be responsive to a glucocorticoid, also occurs.[209]

Precautions. Use with extreme caution in patients with renal or pulmonary disease, in those with lymphoma, and in those >70 yr.

Drug Interactions. Inspired oxygen concentrations >35% may cause acute respiratory failure in bleomycin-treated patients.

Parameters to Monitor. Calculate cumulative dosage before and after each treatment. Monitor temperature initially, especially in lymphoma patients. Assess renal function prior to administering. Pulmonary damage is best monitored with CO diffusing capacity and forced vital capacity; specific serial pulmonary function studies have been suggested prior to and during therapy. Characteristic x-ray findings include changes suggestive of progressive diffuse bilateral fibrosis.

Notes. One mg of bleomycin equals 1 unit of activity. Reconstituted solution is stable for 1 month under refrigeration and 2 weeks at room temperature. Incompatible with divalent cations (especially copper), ascorbic acid, and compounds with sulfhydryl groups.

TRETINOIN   Vesanoid

Pharmacology. Tretinoin (all-trans-retinoic acid) is a modified form of vitamin A used in the treatment of acute promyelocytic leukemia. It causes immature promyeloblasts to differentiate into mature granulocytes, thereby halting cell division and inducing complete remissions in up to 90% of patients. Resistance rapidly develops during therapy because of accelerated drug catabolism to the 4-oxo metabolite, which is excreted in the urine, increased cellular retinoic acid binding protein (II), and tumors with high levels of a mutated α retinoic acid receptor.[210–212]

Pediatric Dosage. PO 45 mg/m^2/day as a single dose until remission is obtained.

Dosage Forms. Cap 10 mg.

Pharmacokinetics. Peak serum levels of 294 μg/L occur 1–2 hr after a dose; the serum half-life is 0.8 hr.

Adverse Reactions. Hyperleukocytosis and effects typical of hypervitaminosis A—headache, dry skin and mucosa, cheilitis, bone pain, and hypertriglyceridemia—occur. Tolerance to these effects develops rapidly, and skin creams, lip balms, and eye and nasal drops are helpful. Liver and renal function test elevations occur occasionally.

Chemoprotectants

AMIFOSTINE   Ethyol

Pharmacology. Amifostine is a phosphorothiol compound metabolized by membrane-bound alkaline phosphatase to an active sulfhydryl form capable of binding electrophilic metabolites from DNA-binding anticancer agents or ionizing radiation. It is used prophylactically to block cisplatin-induced nephrotoxicity and neurotoxicity without altering antitumor efficacy in patients with advanced ovarian cancer.[213]

Administration and Adult Dosage. IV to block cisplatin toxicity 910 mg/m^2 in NS over ≤15 min, beginning 30 min prior to cisplatin.

Special Populations. *Pediatric Dosage.* Safety and efficacy not established.

Geriatric Dosage. Same as adult dosage, but limited experience exists in patients >70 yr.

Other Conditions. In patients who develop rare symptomatic acute hypocalcemia, reduce dose to 740 mg/m^2 and extend infusion time. Reduce dosage in patients who developed hypotension (drop of 15–20 mm Hg systolic) with prior courses.

When used as a radioprotective agent, the maximally tolerated dosage is 340 mg/m^2 for 4 days/week.[214]

Dosage Forms. **Inj** 50 mg/mL.

Patient Instructions. The severity of chemotherapy-induced nausea and vomiting may increase with amifostine. Drink lots of fluids in the hours prior to receiving this medication to reduce its toxicity.

Pharmacokinetics. *Fate.* The mean peak serum level is 100 μmol/L following an IV dose of 740 mg/m^2. V_{dss} is 6.4 ± 1.5 L; Cl is 2.2 ± 0.4 L/min. Relatively little unchanged drug (1.1% of a dose), actifostine (1.4% of a dose), or disulfide metabolite (4.2% of a dose) is excreted renally.[215]

$t_{1/2}$. α phase 0.88 ± 0.12 min; β phase 8.8 ± 2 min.

Adverse Reactions. Toxic effects are all acute and include transient hypotension during or immediately following drug infusion; nausea; and vomiting.[216] Prophylactic antiemetics before administration can reduce nausea and vomiting. Rapid infusion (≤15 min) and aggressive hydration may lessen or eliminate hypotensive toxicity.[217] Stopping the infusion and placing the patient in the Trendelenberg position usually reverses the hypotension. Other less serious but common reactions include sneezing (27%), a flushed sensation (26%), somnolence (10–20%), a sensation of cold hands, or a metallic taste in the mouth (<5% each).

Contraindications. Allergy to aminothiol compounds or mannitol.

Precautions. Do not administer concurrently with or after cisplatin infusion. Use with caution in patients in whom hypotension or nausea might pose a serious risk. There is limited experience in patients with pre-existing cardiac or cardiovascular conditions such as CHF, angina pectoris, history of stroke, or TIAs.

Drug Interactions. Amifostine may reduce the systemic exposure to paclitaxel, but not to docetaxel, cisplatin, carboplatin, or cyclophosphamide.[218]

Parameters to Monitor. Monitor blood pressure frequently during drug administration and immediately after infusion.

Notes. Amifostine has been safely combined with ionizing radiation, **carboplatin,** and **cyclophosphamide.** Amifostine markedly reduces mucositis when it is combined with carboplatin and radiotherapy in the treatment of head and neck cancer.[219] Amifostine allows dose escalation of **paclitaxel** and it also has hematopoietic activity in the investigational treatment of refractory myelodysplastic syndrome.

DEXRAZOXANE   Zinecard

Pharmacology. Dexrazoxane, a cardioprotectant for anthracyclines, is the water-soluble dextro isomer of razoxane. Dexrazoxane's two piperazinedione rings open to form sites that chelate intracellular ferrous ions, blocking the formation of doxorubicin-iron complexes capable of forming membrane-damaging oxygen free radicals. Dexrazoxane can extend **doxorubicin** cumulative dosage in patients with breast cancer. It also reduces the risk of short-term subclinical cardiotoxicity in pediatric sarcoma patients. It does not alter the pharmacokinetics of doxorubicin.[220–222]

Administration and Adult Dosage. **IV as a cardioprotectant** give in a 10:1 dexrazoxane:doxorubicin mg/m^2 ratio (eg, 500 mg/m^2 dexrazoxane:50 mg/m^2

doxorubicin). Infuse IV over 15 min, beginning not more than 30 min before an IV push dose of doxorubicin.

Special Populations. *Pediatric Dosage.* Safety and efficacy not established, but it has been used in a 20:1 dosage ratio (dexrazoxane:doxorubicin) in children with sarcomas.[222]

Geriatric Dosage. Same as adult dosage.

Patient Instructions. (*See* Antineoplastics Class Instructions.)

Pharmacokinetics. *Fate.* The mean peak serum level after a dose of 500 mg/m^2 given over 15 min is 36.5 mg/L (136 μmol/L). The drug is not protein bound. V_d is 22 L/m^2 or approximately body water; Cl averages 7.9 L/hr/m^2. About 42% is renally eliminated as parent drug, and mono- and diacid amide metabolites.[223]

$t_{1/2}$. α phase 0.2–0.3 hr; β phase 2.1–2.5 hr.[223]

Adverse Reactions. Dexrazoxane has little toxicity, but does slightly increase the myelosuppressive and emetogenic toxicities of doxorubicin-containing regimens. Pain on injection also occurs.

Contraindications. None known.

Precautions. Avoid use with bleomycin. Do not administer *after* doxorubicin.

Drug Interactions. None known.

Parameters to Monitor. WBC counts at nadir (7–11 days) after doxorubicin.

Notes. Dexrazoxane does not reduce the antitumor activity of fluorouracil, doxorubicin, and cyclophosphamide regimens in advanced breast cancer.[220] Effects on other antineoplastics are unknown.

MESNA
Mesnex

Pharmacology. Mesna (2-mercaptoethanesulfonate) is a sulfhydryl compound that minimizes urotoxicity from the alkylating agents cyclophosphamide (CTX) and ifosfamide (IFX) by binding to the irritant metabolite acrolein in the urinary bladder to prevent hemorrhagic cystitis.[35,224]

Administration and Adult Dosage. IV or PO (ampule contents dissolved in water or juice) in 3 doses as a percentage of the dose of ifosfamide or cyclophosphamide:

TIME BEFORE OR AFTER CTX OR IFX	PERCENTAGE OF CTX OR IFX DOSE[225]	
	IV Mesna Route	*PO Mesna Route*
15 min before	20	Not recommended
4 hr after	20	40
8 hr after	20	40

Oral administration is not recommended for patients with poor compliance or those experiencing nausea or vomiting.

Special Populations. *Pediatric Dosage.* Same as adult dosage.[42,226]

Geriatric Dosage. Same as adult dosage.

Dosage Forms. Inj 100 mg/mL.

Patient Instructions. This agent does not have antitumor activity but is essential to reduce or prevent permanent bladder damage from chemotherapy.

Pharmacokinetics. *Fate.* About 48% is orally absorbed.[227] V_d is 0.65 L/kg; Cl is 1.23 L/hr/kg. Mesna is oxidized to the inactive dimer, dimesna, which does not inactivate CTX or IFX metabolites in the serum. About 60% of the dimesna is converted back to mesna in the renal tubule and delivered to the bladder in the active sulfhydryl form. About two-thirds of a dose is excreted in the urine, one-half as mesna and one-half as dimesna.[228]

$t_½$. (Mesna) 22 min; (dimesna) 1.2 hr.[228]

Adverse Reactions. When administered alone, mesna produces little if any serious toxicity.[228] GI effects (eg, diarrhea, nausea, and, rarely, vomiting) of CTX or IFX may be slightly greater when mesna is administered. Other CTX or IFX toxicities such as myelosuppression or alopecia are not altered by mesna. With oral administration, a disagreeable sulfur odor may lessen palatability unless the drug is diluted with cola or juice.

Drug Interactions. Mesna inhibits the antitumor activity of cisplatin and carboplatin, but not other anticancer agents.

Notes. Mesna is compatible with solutions of CTX or IFX and has been administered concurrently as a continuous infusion of both agents at equal doses in the same infusion container.[229] It is stable in D5W or NS for at least 96 hr.

Immunosuppressants

Geneal Precautions for Immunosuppressants. Immunosuppression increases the risk of infectious complications. Serious opportunistic infections can occur during immunosuppressive therapy. Long-term immunosuppression also increases the risk of malignancy or lymphoproliferative disease. Vaccinations may be less effective during immunosuppression. Live or live attenuated vaccines may proliferate excessively in immunosuppressed patients and should be avoided.

ANTITHYMOCYTE GLOBULIN (EQUINE)   Atgam

Pharmacology. Antithymocyte globulin is a concentrated solution of polyclonal IgG purified from serum of horses immunized with human thymus lymphocytes. Antithymocyte globulin is an immunosuppressant that primarily inhibits cell-mediated immunity. The immunosuppressive effects of antithymocyte globulin may be secondary to clearance of alloreactive T-lymphocytes from the plasma; however, the exact pharmacologic mechanism of action has not been elucidated. (*See* Notes.)

Administration and Adult Dosage. **Intradermal sensitivity testing** to identify patients at risk for anaphylaxis is *strongly* recommended prior to administration of the initial dose. Give 1:1000 (5 µg in 0.1 mL NS) freshly diluted antithymocyte globulin intradermally on the medial aspect of one forearm, with intradermal administration of 0.1 mL NS on the other forearm as a control. Observe q 15–20 min for swelling, urticaria, pruritus, and wheal and/or erythema. A positive skin test is defined as local wheal or erythema formation ≥10 mm in diameter. A systemic reaction to the skin test usually precludes further administration of antithymocyte globulin. Administration following a positive skin test or systemic reaction to the skin test should only be done in a facility capable of supporting life-threatening allergic reactions. The skin test is not 100% predictive of subsequent hypersensitivity reactions; allergic reactions and anaphylaxis have occurred following negative skin tests. **IV for prevention of renal allograft rejection** 15 mg/kg/day for 14 doses, followed by the same dose every other day for an additional 14 days. The first dose of antithymocyte globulin is administered within 24 hr preceding or following surgery. **IV for treatment of renal allograft rejection** same dosage regimen as above with administration of the first dose when the initial rejection episode is diagnosed. **IV for prevention of acute graft-versus-host disease** in allogeneic bone marrow transplant recipients, 7–10 mg/kg administered every other day for 6 doses. **IV for treatment of moderate to severe steroid-refractory acute graft-versus-host disease** 7–15 mg/kg for a total of 6 doses or as indicated by the patient's clinical status. **IV to facilitate skin allograft survival in patients with full-thickness burns** 10–15 mg/kg every other day is usually used; however, dosages range from 5 mg/kg every other day to 40 mg/kg/day. The duration of therapy is generally 40–60 days, ending when skin allografts cover <20% of body surface area. **IV for treatment of aplastic anemia** 10–30 mg/kg/day for 8–14 days followed by the same dose every other day for 14 days for a total of 21 doses in 28 days. Alternatively, 40 mg/kg/day IV for 4 days q 3 weeks has been used.[230] **The maximum tolerated cumulative dosage** has not been determined. A total of 50 doses has been administered during a 4-month period, and four 28-day courses have been administered in renal allograft recipients without changing the frequency, severity, or character of adverse drug reactions. **IV administration** is achieved by slow infusion of the dose over 4–8 hr, diluted in ½NS or NS to a final concentration ≤4 mg/mL. The admixture should be infused through an in-line filter with pore size of 0.22–1 μ. **Premedication and prn administration** of acetaminophen and a corticosteroid is a common practice to reduce infusion-related adverse effects.

Special Populations. *Pediatric Dosage.* Same as adult dosage.

Geriatric Dosage. Same as adult dosage.

Dosage Forms. **Inj** 50 mg/mL.

Patient Instructions. This medicine can cause serious allergic symptoms, especially in people allergic to horses and horse products. You will receive a skin test to check for allergy to this product. You may experience fevers, shaking, and chills when this medication is being given. You may be given additional medications to reduce these side effects.

Pharmacokinetics. *Fate.* Peak concentrations of 727 ± 310 μg/mL occur with repeated IV doses of 10 mg/kg. Systemic distribution of equine immune globulin is not well defined. In vitro studies predict binding to circulating lymphocytes, granulocytes, and platelets. Binding to bone marrow cells, plus thymus and testis cell membranes, occurs in vitro.

$t_{½}$. 3–9 days.

Adverse Reactions. Anaphylaxis can occur at anytime during therapy. If signs or symptoms of anaphylaxis occur, the infusion must be stopped immediately and appropriate management must be initiated. Serum sickness occurs frequently; the onset is typically 6–18 days after initiation of therapy. The morbilliform rash of the serum sickness reaction generally starts as a truncal distribution of faint macules with subsequent progression to the extremities. The macules may become confluent. Erythema may spread to involve palms of the hands and soles of the feet. Antihistamines are helpful for pruritus associated with serum sickness. Although not clearly shown to reduce serum sickness–related adverse effects, corticosteroids have been used. Antithymocyte globulin may bind formed elements in the blood, other than T-lymphocytes, and promote clearance of these blood constituents. Subsequently, patients may experience acute normochromic normocytic anemia, thrombocytopenia, or leukopenia which is reversible upon drug discontinuation. Less frequent adverse effects include periorbital edema, seizures, headache, hypertension, edema, CHF, bradycardia, myocarditis, and hyperglycemia.

Contraindications. Allergy to antithymocyte globulin, horse serum, or horse products.

Precautions. Pregnancy; lactation. (*See also* General Precautions for Immunosuppressants.)

Drug Interactions. None known.

Parameters to Monitor. Observe for anaphylaxis during infusion, and for serum sickness for 6–18 days following initiation of therapy. Monitor CBC with platelet count q 1–3 days during therapy.

Notes. Antithymocyte globulin is also known as ATG, lymphocyte immune globulin, antithymocyte gamma globulin, antithymocyte immunoglobulin, and horse antihuman thymocyte gamma globulin. T-cell receptor binding of antithymocyte globulin is indirectly tested by in vitro inhibition of red blood cell rosette formation. A test for immunosuppressive potency has not been developed. Subsequently, lot-to-lot variation of immunosuppressive potency may occur with the commercial product. Antithymocyte globulin raised in nonequine species are investigational products.

AZATHIOPRINE   Imuran

Pharmacology. Azathioprine is a thiopurine prodrug of 6-mercaptopurine (6-MP). Conversion to 6-MP with subsequent phosphoribosylation yields antimetabolites capable of inhibiting DNA and RNA synthesis. The metabolite 6-methylmercaptopurine ribotide is a potent inhibitor of de novo purine synthesis. T-lymphocytes are sensitive to inhibition of de novo purine synthesis because these cells lack efficient salvage pathways to maintain adequate intracellular stores.

Administration and Adult Dosage. **PO or IV for immunosuppression following solid organ transplantation** 3–5 mg/kg/day as a single daily dose beginning the day of, or 1–3 days preceding, transplantation. **Maintenance dosage** is 1–3 mg/kg/day as a single daily dose. **PO for rheumatoid arthritis** 1 mg/kg/day in 1 or 2 doses. The dosage may be increased after 6–8 weeks if indicated by disease response and patient tolerance. Increase the dosage in increments of 0.5 mg/kg/day q 4 weeks to a maximum of 2.5 mg/kg day. (*See* Drug Interactions.)

Special Populations. *Pediatric Dosage.* **PO or IV for immunosuppression following renal transplantation** same as adult dosage.

Geriatric Dosage. Same as adult dosage.

Dosage Forms. **Tab** 50 mg; **Inj** 100 mg.

Patient Instructions. This medication may be taken with food to reduce stomach upset. Notify your physician if any of the following symptoms occur: unusual bleeding or bruising, fever, sore throat, mouth sores, abdominal pain, yellowing of the eyes, pale stools, or dark urine, or if nausea, vomiting, diarrhea, skin rash, or joint pains become severe or persist.

Missed Doses. Take a missed dose as soon as possible. If you take the drug once daily and it is time for the next dose, take it at the regular time. Do not double the dose. If you take two or more doses daily, and it is time for the next dose, take both doses together. If two or more doses are missed contact your physician.

Pharmacokinetics. *Onset and Duration.* Onset of immunosuppression occurs within days to weeks. Immunosuppression continues for days to weeks following drug discontinuation.

Serum Levels. No correlation between serum concentrations and efficacy or toxicity has been defined.

Fate. Following oral absorption, conversion to 6-MP occurs rapidly.[1] (*See* Mercaptopurine.)

$t_{1/2}$. (Azathioprine) 9.6 ± 4.2 min; (6-MP) 0.9 ± 0.37 hr.[1,10]

Adverse Reactions. Dose-related bone marrow suppression, which may include leukopenia, thrombocytopenia, and anemia, occurs frequently. Macrocytic anemia, with megaloblastic features, or selective erythrocyte aplasia can occur with long-term azathioprine administration. Skin rash is a common adverse effect. Mouth sores can occur. Dose-related nausea and vomiting are frequent, and can be reduced by administration in divided doses. Rare GI hypersensitivity characterized by severe nausea and vomiting, diarrhea, hyperpyrexia, malaise, myalgia, and liver function test abnormalities can occur early in the course of therapy. GI hypersensitivity is reversible with discontinuation of azathioprine, and can recur with rechallenge. Hepatic veno-occlusive disease of the liver, secondary lymphomas, and other malignancies can occur with long-term administration. Azathioprine is teratogenic. Rare adverse effects include pancreatitis, constrictive lung disease, renal failure, alopecia, arthralgia, and retinopathy.

Contraindications. Pregnancy in patients treated for rheumatoid arthritis.

Precautions. Pregnancy; lactation. (*See also* General Precautions for Immunosuppressants.)

Drug Interactions. To reduce the risk of life-threatening myelosuppression, azathioprine dosage must be reduced to 25–33% of the normal dosage in patients receiving allopurinol. Enhanced bone marrow suppression can occur with concurrent use of drugs that inhibit hematopoiesis. Concurrent corticosteroids used for immunosuppression may mask fever.

Parameters to Monitor. Monitor CBC and platelets weekly for 1 month following initiation of therapy or any dosage increase. Then, for patients with stable hemograms, the CBC and platelet count may be monitored twice monthly for 2 months, then monthly for the duration of therapy. Monitor serum transaminases, alkaline phosphatase, and total bilirubin periodically. Observe for signs of infection.

Notes. Azathioprine is used in combination with other immunosuppressants as an adjunct in the prevention of renal allograft rejection and for the prevention of solid organ rejection for cardiac and hepatic allografts. It is rarely used for the management of acute or chronic graft-versus-host disease in allogeneic bone marrow transplant recipients because it markedly increases the risk for infections.[231]

CYCLOSPORINE   Neoral, Sandimmune

Pharmacology. Cyclosporine is a cyclic polypeptide immunosuppressant produced by the fungus *Tolypocladium inflatum Gams.* The intracellular drug-ligand complex formed by cyclosporine and cyclophilin indirectly blocks T-lymphocyte activation by inhibiting calcineurin-mediated dephosphorylation of transcription factors necessary for interleukin-2 transcription.

Administration and Adult Dosage. PO for prophylaxis of organ rejection or graft-versus-host disease (GVHD) 8–12 mg/kg/day in 2 divided doses depending on the type of transplant and the other immunosuppressants being given. To hasten achievement of an immunosuppressive blood level, **an oral loading dose** of cyclosporine 15 mg/kg may be administered. Cyclosporine is usually started 4–12 hr before surgery. **Maintenance dosage** is based on cyclosporine blood levels, the risk for organ rejection or GVHD, and patient tolerance. **An IV loading dose** of 3–4 mg/kg may be useful in patients with a low cyclosporine level during periods of moderate-to-severe diarrhea with oral maintenance therapy. **IV for patients unable to take oral medication** 2–6 mg/kg/day in 1 or 2 divided doses. **IV for prevention of GVHD** 3–4 mg/kg/day in 2 divided doses q 12 hr. Cyclosporine is generally started 1–2 days prior to bone marrow transplantation. Drug-induced mucositis or diarrhea usually necessitate use of IV cyclosporine in allogeneic bone marrow transplant recipients. Dilute IV cyclosporine in a glass container with D5W or NS to a concentration of 50 mg/20–100 mL. Doses may be infused over 2–6 hr or given as a continuous infusion. **Conversion from IV to PO administration** the ratio of IV:PO doses is typically 1:3 to 1:4 for Sandimmune capsules or solution or 1:1 to 1:2 for Neoral capsules or solution. Absorption may be reduced in allogeneic bone marrow transplant patients because of residual gut damage from intensive chemotherapy, radiation, or GVHD. **Conversion from PO Sandimmune to Neoral** give the same daily dosage initially with prompt dosage adjustment based on subsequent blood levels. A cyclosporine blood level should be drawn 48 hr following dosage form conversion. Because of better bioavailability, maintenance Neoral dosages are usually lower than Sandimmune dosages. **Discontinuation** cyclosporine may eventually be discontinued in certain renal or allogeneic bone marrow transplant recipients. Cyclosporine dosage must be decreased gradually over time to reduce the risk of reactive immune stimulation and graft rejection or GVHD.

Special Populations. *Pediatric Dosage.* Same as adult dosage.

Geriatric Dosage. Same as adult dosage. Age-related loss of renal function and co-morbid conditions may predispose geriatric patients to cyclosporine-induced nephrotoxicity and hypertension.

Other Conditions. Use ideal body weight to calculate initial dosage in obese patients.

Dosage Forms. **Cap** (Neoral) 25, 100, mg, (Sandimmune) 25, 50, 100 mg; **Soln** (Neoral, Sandimmune) 100 mg/mL; **Inj** 50 mg/mL.

Patient Instructions. Take this medication on a regular schedule in relation to the time of day and meals. Do not discontinue it unless directed to do so. The oral solution may taste better if mixed with another liquid. Sandimmune may be mixed with milk, chocolate milk, or orange juice. Neoral may be mixed with orange juice or apple juice. Using a glass container, mix the cyclosporine solution with the milk or juice well and drink immediately. Fill the glass container a second time with milk or juice, stir well, and drink immediately to ensure that the entire cyclosporine dose is swallowed. Do *not* refrigerate the oral solution. Use the oral solution within 2 months after opening. Grapefruit juice can interact with cyclosporine. Talk to your physician before drinking grapefruit juice and before starting, stopping, or changing the dose of any medication.

Missed Doses. Take a missed dose as soon as possible if you remember within 12 hours. If it is within 2 hours of the next dose, skip the missed dose and do not double the next dose. If you miss 2 or more doses, contact your physician.

Pharmacokinetics. *Serum Levels.* The serum (blood) concentration-response relationship is not completely defined. Trough blood or serum concentrations are monitored for toxicity. Therapeutic and toxic concentrations vary with assay, biologic fluid, and time post-transplant. Therapeutic serum concentrations are: polyclonal radioimmunoassay (RIA) 100–250 µg/L; monoclonal RIA 50–125 µg/L; high-performance liquid chromatography (HPLC) 50–125 µg/L. Therapeutic whole blood concentrations are: polyclonal RIA 200–800 µg/L; monoclonal RIA 150–400 µg/L; HPLC 150–400 µg/L.[232] In routine clinical practice, spurious serum drug concentrations may result from in vitro drug redistribution.[233] Artifactually elevated serum concentrations may occur when blood is drawn through the same central venous line used for IV cyclosporine administration.[234]

Fate. Oral absorption is formulation dependent. Sandimmune absorption is incomplete and variable. The mean bioavailability of Sandimmune is 34%; however, the reported range is 5–90%. Absorption of Sandimmune is improved following a high-fat meal. Peak concentrations occur 2–6 hr following ingestion of Sandimmune capsules or oral solution. Neoral absorption is independent of food intake; peak concentrations occur 1.5–2 hr following ingestion of Neoral capsules or oral solution. Factors that may decrease cyclosporine absorption include diarrhea, gastroenteritis, and short small bowel. Systemic cyclosporine distributes to erythrocytes (45%), leukocytes (15%), and plasma lipoproteins (35%). Marked elevations of plasma lipoproteins may increase measured cyclosporine concentrations without a proportional increase in therapeutic or toxic effects. V_{dss} (whole blood, HPLC) is 4 ± 0.8 L/kg in renal transplant patients and 5.3 ± 2.9 L/kg in bone marrow transplant patients. Cl (whole blood, HPLC) is 0.4 ± 0.2 L/hr/kg in renal or liver transplant recipients and 0.6 ± 0.04 L/hr/kg in allogeneic bone marrow transplant recipients. Cyclosporine is extensively metabolized by CYP3A. At least 25 metabolites, some with immunosuppressant activity, have been identified. Cyclosporine and its metabolites are cleared primarily in the bile. Approximately 3% is excreted in the urine as cyclosporine and metabolites. Less than 1% is excreted unchanged in the urine.

$t_{1/2}$. (Whole blood, HPLC) 10 ± 3.5 hr, possibly prolonged in hepatic failure.[236]

Adverse Reactions. Acute nephrotoxicity, which generally occurs within the first month of treatment, is characterized by Cr_s increasing by ≥ 0.3 mg/dL/24 hr and frequently abates with interruption of drug therapy. Dosage reduction may be required for continued administration. Chronic progressive renal toxicity is characterized by a slow continual increase in Cr_s and BUN, mild proteinuria, and tubular dysfunction.[232] Cr_s >2 mg/dL in adult patients, or doubling of Cr_s is an indication for interruption of therapy or dosage reduction. Electrolyte abnormalities, including hypomagnesemia, hypokalemia, hyperkalemia, and renal tubular acidosis are consequences of cyclosporine-induced nephrotoxicity. Concurrent administration of nephrotoxic drugs increases the likelihood of renal dysfunction. Hypertension occurs frequently. **Calcium-channel blockers** and **clonidine** are suitable agents for cyclosporine-induced hypertension because they do not have deleterious effects on renal blood flow. Fine tremors occur frequently and can persist and worsen after drug discontinuation. Neurotoxicity can also present as seizures, cortical blindness, paresthesias, hyperesthesia, or headache. Patients with low serum cholesterol may be at increased risk of neurotoxicity. Anaphylactoid reactions to cyclosporine or the solubilizing agent, polyoxyethylated castor oil, may occur. Cyclosporine-induced cholestasis is dose related and transient. Elevated serum transaminases and hypertriglyceridemia can occur. Additional side effects include hemolytic-uremic syndrome, pancreatitis, hirsutism, gingival hyperplasia, nausea, vomiting, acne, and gynecomastia. Leukopenia, anemia, and thrombocytopenia occur rarely.

Contraindications. Allergy to cyclosporine or polyoxyethylated castor oil.

Precautions. Pregnancy; lactation. Use with caution in patients at risk for renal dysfunction. (*See also* General Precautions for Immunosuppressants.)

Drug Interactions. Numerous important drug interactions have been identified. Additive or synergistic renal toxicity may occur with concurrent administration of nephrotoxic drugs. Potassium-sparing diuretics may exacerbate hyperkalemia. Concurrent use of the following drugs frequently increases cyclosporine blood levels: corticosteroids, erythromycin and other macrolide antibiotics, itraconazole, and ketoconazole. Other drugs that may increase cyclosporine blood levels include: acetazolamide, alcohol, allopurinol, calcium-channel blockers, cimetidine, colchicine, oral contraceptives, fluconazole, imipenem/cilastatin, metoclopramide, norfloxacin, and sulindac. Enzyme-inducing drugs, such as carbamazepine, phenobarbital, phenytoin, and rifampin reduce cyclosporine blood levels. Octreotide may decrease cyclosporine oral absorption. Additional drugs that may reduce cyclosporine blood levels include: co-trimoxazole, nafcillin, and sulfonamides. Cyclosporine reduces the clearance of lovastatin and may increase the risk of drug-induced rhabdomyolysis.

Parameters to Monitor. Observe for anaphylaxis with IV administration. Monitor Cr_s q 2–7 days, and daily in patients at risk of acute renal dysfunction. Monitor blood pressure regularly. Monitor liver function tests weekly, triglycerides and amylase monthly. Monitor blood or serum cyclosporine concentrations q 2–3 days when starting therapy. As the patient's clinical condition and renal function allow, reduce frequency to once or twice weekly, then monthly during the first year of therapy. After the first year of therapy, blood or serum concentration monitoring may be reduced to q 1–2 months in stable patients. Monitor for signs and symptoms of graft rejection or GVHD, especially following dosage reduction.

Notes. Admix injectable cyclosporine in glass containers, because it may leach plasticizers from PVC containers. Cyclosporine is generally used in combination with other immunosuppressant drugs for the prevention of graft rejection or GVHD. Cyclosporine is used in the management of various immunologic diseases, including aplastic anemia, rheumatoid arthritis, psoriasis, atopic dermatitis, acute ocular Behçet's syndrome, endogenous uveitis, primary biliary cirrhosis, and acute Crohn's disease. High-dose cyclosporine is administered with certain cancer chemotherapy regimens as a modulator of p-glycoprotein–mediated drug resistance.[236] Optimmune (cyclosporine) ophthalmic (University of Georgia College of Veterinary Medicine) has orphan drug status for treatment of severe keratoconjunctivitis sicca with Sjögren's syndrome. Sandimmune 2% ophthalmic ointment (Allergan) has orphan drug status for patients at high risk for graft rejection following penetrating keratoplasty, and for treatment of corneal melting syndrome. Comparative clinical trials found greater nephrotoxicity and neurotoxicity with tacrolimus than with cyclosporine.[237] Case reports describe resolution of certain drug-induced toxicities following replacement of cyclosporine with tacrolimus,[238] and resolution of cyclosporine-refractory GVHD with initiation of tacrolimus.[239]

INTERLEUKIN-2 RECEPTOR ANTAGONISTS:

BASILIXIMAB	Simulect
DACLIZUMAB	Zenapax

Pharmacology. Basiliximab and daclizumab (formerly dacliximab) are immunosuppressive, humanized, recombinant IgG1 monoclonal antibodies that bind specifically to the alpha subunit (p55 alpha, CD25, or Tac subunit) of the human high-affinity interleukin-2 (IL-2) receptor present on the surface of activated lymphocytes. They act as IL-2 receptor antagonists by preventing IL-2 binding to lymphocytes, subsequently reducing IL-2–mediated immune activation. Both drugs are indicated for prevention of renal allograft rejection in a regimen that includes cyclosporine and a corticosteroid.

Administration and Adult Dosage. **IV for prevention of renal allograft rejection** (basiliximab) 20 mg infused over 30 min for 2 doses. The initial dose should be given about 2 hr before transplantation, the second dose is given on the fourth day following the transplant. (Daclizumab) 1 mg/kg for 5 doses at 14-day intervals. The initial dose should be infused within 24 hr preceding surgery. The remaining 4 doses should be administered at 14-day intervals following surgery. Dilute each dose in 50 mL NS and infuse over 15 min through a peripheral or central venous line.

Special Populations. *Pediatric Dosage.* (Basiliximab) 12 mg/m^2 to a maximum of 20 mg/dose, given as adult dosage above. (Daclizumab) same as adult dosage. Information about use in pediatric patients is limited.

Geriatric Dosage. Same as adult dosage. Information about use in patients >65 yr is limited.

Other Conditions. No dosage adjustment is necessary for patients with severe renal dysfunction.

Dosage Forms. **Inj** (basiliximab) 20 mg; (daclizumab) 25 mg.

Patient Instructions. This drug is being used as part of combination therapy to prevent rejection of your transplanted kidney.

Pharmacokinetics. *Onset and Duration.* (Basiliximab) receptor saturation is maintained for 36 ± 14 days with the recommended regimen. (Daclizumab) receptor saturation is maintained for about 120 days with the recommended regimen.

Serum Levels. (Basiliximab) >200 μg/L maintains complete binding to IL-2 receptor and maintains effective T-lymphocyte suppression. (Daclizumab) 5–10 mg/L inhibits activated T-lymphocytes.

Fate. (Basiliximab) peak serum levels of 9.3 ± 4.5 mg/L are attained with the recommended dosage regimen. (Daclizumab) following the first dose of 1 mg/kg, a peak of 21 ± 14 mg/L occurs, and after the 5th dose, a peak of 32 ± 22 mg/L results. The trough is 7.6 ± 4 mg/L following repeated doses of 1 mg/kg in adult renal transplant recipients.

t$_{1/2}$. (Basiliximab) about 14 days; (daclizumab) 11–38 days.

Adverse Reactions. Both drugs are well tolerated. The frequency and type of adverse events were similar between renal transplant patients receiving these drugs or placebo, along with a corticosteroid and cyclosporine.[240,241] Hypertension and dehydration with daclizumab may be more frequent in children than in adults.

Precautions. Pregnancy; lactation. (*See also* General Precautions for Immunosuppressants.)

Drug Interactions. None known.

Parameters to Monitor. Monitor signs and symptoms of infection and graft rejection periodically.

Notes. After preparation, these drugs should be used within 4 hr if stored at room temperature or within 24 hr if refrigerated. Although basiliximab and daclizumab have not been directly compared, their efficacy appears to be similar.

MUROMONAB-CD3   Orthoclone OKT3

Pharmacology. Muromonab-CD3 is a murine monoclonal antibody which recognizes the zeta chain of the CD3 protein complex associated with the T-cell receptor (TCR). CD3 protein complex is an integral component of TCR signal transduction. Muromonab-CD3 binding to CD3 blocks allograft rejection by inhibition of T-lymphocyte function. Muromonab-CD3 is used to treat acute renal allograft rejection or steroid-resistant heart or liver allograft rejection.

Administration and Adult Dosage. **IV for the treatment of allograft rejection** 5 mg/day as an IV push for 10–14 days. Administration of methylprednisolone 8 mg/kg IV 1–4 hr prior to muromonab is strongly recommended by the manufacturer to reduce the frequency and severity of reactions with the first dose. Acetaminophen and diphenhydramine are also often used to control symptoms. The manufacturer recommends that the patient's temperature be <37.8°C (<100°F) prior to infusion of muromonab-CD3.

Special Populations. *Pediatric Dosage.* Safety and efficacy is not established; however, children have received dosages of ≤5 mg/day.

Geriatric Dosage. Same as adult dosage.

Dosage Forms. **Inj** 1 mg/mL.

Patient Instructions. This medication may cause shortness of breath, fever, and chills during the initial days of treatment.

Pharmacokinetics. *Serum Levels.* Levels ≥0.8 mg/L block cytotoxic T-lymphocyte function in vitro and in vivo.

Adverse Reactions. Cytokine release syndrome (CRS) occurs frequently with the initial 2–3 doses; it is related to cytokine release from activated lymphocytes. CRS may present as mild flu-like symptoms, or as a life-threatening, shock-like reaction. Onset of CRS is usually 30–60 min following drug administration, although it may be delayed for hours. CRS may last for hours. Pretreatment and symptomatic treatment (*see* Administration and Adult Dosage) may reduce the frequency and severity of reactions with the first dose. Common symptoms include fever, headache, rigors, chills, tremor, nausea, vomiting, abdominal pain, myalgia, arthralgia, and rash. CRS may include CNS and cardiovascular adverse effects. CNS side effects include headache, seizures, encephalopathy, and aseptic meningitis. Cardiovascular side effects include angina, acute MI, CHF, hypertension, hypotension, and arrhythmias. Arterial and venous thrombosis of allograft and other vascular beds has occurred. Consider coadministration of prophylactic antithrombotic agents in patients with a history of thrombotic events or underlying vascular disease. Pulmonary edema occurs frequently. Additional respiratory side effects include dyspnea, bronchospasm, wheezing, tachypnea, adult respiratory distress syndrome, and respiratory arrest. Hypersensitivity, including anaphylaxis and Stevens-Johnson syndrome, has been reported. Leukopenia, thrombocytopenia, pancytopenia, and lymphopenia have also occurred. Transient elevations of Cr_s and serum transaminases may occur 1–3 days after initiation of treatment.

Contraindications. Human antimouse antibody titer ≥1:1000.

Precautions. Pregnancy; lactation. Use with caution in patients with volume overload or a history of thrombotic events or vascular disease. (*See also* General Precautions for Immunosuppressants.)

Drug Interactions. Concurrent use of indomethacin has been associated with encephalopathy and other CNS side effects.

Parameters to Monitor. A chest x-ray obtained ≤24 hr before starting muromonab should be free of evidence of volume overload or heart failure. Obtain human antimouse antibody before initiating treatment. (*See* Contraindications.) Obtain Cr_s q 2 days, AST and ALT q 3 days, CBC including differential and platelets q 3 days. Monitor one of the following immunologic tests during therapy: serum muromonab concentrations or quantitative T-lymphocyte surface phenotyping (target: CD3+ T-lymphocytes <25 cells/μL blood).

Notes. Transfer muromonab into a syringe through a 0.2-μ low-protein–binding filter. Do not dilute with IV fluids for administration. Flush IV line with NS before and after injection.

| **MYCOPHENOLATE MOFETIL** | Cellcept |

Pharmacology. Mycophenolate mofetil is an ester prodrug of mycophenolic acid. Mycophenolic acid, which was isolated from the mold *Penicillium glaucum,* inhibits de novo purine synthesis by potent inhibition of inosine monophosphate dehydrogenase. Lymphocyte proliferation and antibody formation are subsequently inhibited by purine deficiency, because lymphocytes lack an efficient salvage pathway for biosynthesis of purine bases. Mycophenolate is used in combination with cyclosporine and corticosteroids to prevent renal allograft rejection. Mycophenolate mofetil has also been used in combination with other immunosuppressants for the prevention of heart and liver allograft rejection.[242]

Administration and Adult Dosage. **PO for prophylaxis of kidney or heart transplant rejection** 1 g bid beginning within 72 hr of transplantation. **IV for prophylaxis of kidney transplant rejection** 1 g bid over at least 2 hr. **IV for prophylaxis of heart transplant rejection** 1.5 g bid over at least 2 hr.

Special Populations. *Pediatric Dosage.* Pediatric renal transplant patients have received mycophenolate mofetil in 2 divided doses (3 months–18 yr) 30 mg/kg/day; (12–18 yr) 46 mg/kg/day.

Geriatric Dosage. Same as adult dosage.

Other Conditions. With a chronic Cl_{cr} <25 mL/min, the dosage should not exceed 1 g bid. This does not apply to the immediate post-transplant period for renal transplant patients.

Dosage Forms. **Cap** 250; **Susp** 100 mg/mL; **Tab** 500 mg; **Inj** 500 mg.

Patient Instructions. Do not stop this medication without consulting your physician.

Missed Doses. Take a missed dose as soon as possible if you remember within 12 hours. If it is within 2 hours of next dose, skip the missed dose and do not double the next dose. If you miss 2 or more doses, contact your physician.

Pharmacokinetics. *Serum Levels.* Not established; but one study found that dosage adjustment to a blood level of 2.5–4 mg/L decreased heart transplant rejection rate.[243]

Fate. Bioavailability is 94% in normal, healthy volunteers. Food decreases the peak serum concentration by 40%, but not bioavailability. Bioavailability is decreased immediately after renal transplantation. Peak serum concentrations after 1 g PO bid are 8.2 ± 4.5 mg/L during the first 40 days post-transplant and 24 ± 12 mg/L after 3 months post-transplant (similar to normal volunteers). The mean time to peak is prolonged to 1.3 ± 0.8 hr during the first 40 days post-transplant compared to 0.9 ± 0.2 hr after 3 months. AUC is also reduced by 42% during the first 40 days post-transplant; AUC is increased approximately 1.5-fold in patients with severe renal impairment. Alcoholic cirrhosis appears not to affect AUC. Mycophenolic acid is 97% bound to albumin. V_d in normal healthy volunteers is 4 ± 1.2 L/kg; Cl is 0.17 ± 0.04 L/hr/kg. Mycophenolate mofetil is rapidly hydrolyzed to mycophenolic acid, which is subsequently glucuronidated to an inactive metabolite. Enterohepatic recirculation may contribute to the mycophenolic acid AUC. Less than 1% of the dose is excreted in the urine as mycophenolic acid.

$t_{1/2}$. 16.6 ± 5.8 hr.

Adverse Reactions. Hematologic adverse effects include leukopenia, anemia, thrombocytopenia, and pancytopenia. Adverse effects of mycophenolate rarely necessitate discontinuation of therapy, but the drug should be stopped temporarily if neutropenia (ANC <1300/μL) develops during therapy. GI effects, including nausea, vomiting, dyspepsia, abdominal pain, constipation, and diarrhea, occur frequently. GI side effects may be reduced by giving the drug in 3–4 divided doses.

Contraindications. Allergy to mycophenolate mofetil.

Precautions. Pregnancy; lactation. Use with caution in patients with renal dysfunction. (*See also* General Precautions for Immunosuppressants.)

Drug Interactions. Concurrent administration of aluminum- or magnesium-containing antacids reduces absorption. Cholestyramine reduces the serum concentration of mycophenolate mofetil. In vitro, salicylate increases the unbound fraction of mycophenolic acid.

Parameters to Monitor. Monitor CBC, including differential and platelet count, weekly during the first 1–2 months of therapy, q 2 weeks during the 2–4 months of therapy, and monthly thereafter. Monitor for signs and symptoms of infection, graft rejection, and graft-versus-host disease.

Notes. A dosage of 3 g/day does not confer a therapeutic advantage, and is associated with more adverse effects. IV mycophenolate mofetil is an investigational drug.

SIROLIMUS (Investigational—Wyeth-Ayerst)   Rapamune

Pharmacology. Sirolimus (formerly rapamycin) is a macrolide antibiotic isolated from *Streptomyces hygroscopicus* that is structurally related to tacrolimus. However, sirolimus inhibits immunologic stimulation by a different pathway. Intracellular sirolimus complexes with the immunophilin FK binding protein 25 (FKBP25), and a protein known as FKBP-rapamycin–associated protein (FRAP). The sirolimus-FKBP25-FRAP complex indirectly inhibits T-lymphocyte activation through inhibition of cytokine-mediated intracellular signal transduction.[244]

Adult Dosage. PO phase II trials have used 0.5–3 mg/m^2/day in combination with corticosteroids in renal transplant recipients.

Pharmacokinetics. Oral bioavailability of sirolimus is 15%. Peak concentrations occur in 0.8–3 hr. V_d is 5.6–16.7 L/kg. Sequestration in erythrocytes occurs. Metabolism is by CYP3A.

Adverse Reactions. Adverse effects include dose-dependent thrombocytopenia. Leukopenia, hypercholesterolemia, and triglyceridemia have been reported. (*See also* General Precautions for Immunosuppressants.)

TACROLIMUS   Prograf

Pharmacology. Tacrolimus (formerly FK506) is a macrolide antibiotic produced by *Streptomyces tsukubaensis*. The intracellular drug–ligand complex of tacrolimus and FK506 binding protein (FKBP-12) indirectly blocks T-lymphocyte activation. It inhibits calcineurin-mediated dephosphorylation of factors necessary for interleukin-2 transcription.

Administration and Adult Dosage. **PO for prophylaxis of organ rejection or graft-versus-host disease (GVHD)** 0.15–0.3 mg/kg initially, depending on the type of transplant and coadministration of other immunosuppressants. Tacrolimus is usually started 4–12 hr before surgery and administered on a bid schedule. **Maintenance dosage** is based on tacrolimus blood concentrations, the magnitude of risk for organ rejection or GVHD, and patient tolerance. **IV for patients unable to take medication orally** 0.03–0.1 mg/kg/day as a continuous infusion diluted in D5W or NS in a glass container to a concentration of 2 mg/100–500 mL (final concentration 4–20 mg/L).[245] Mucositis generally necessitates initial use of IV tacrolimus for allogeneic bone marrow transplant recipients. Tacrolimus is generally started 1 or 2 days prior to bone marrow transplantation. **To convert from IV to PO tacrolimus** the IV:PO dosage ratio is typically 1:3. A tacrolimus blood level should be drawn 48 hr following dosage form conversion. Absorption of oral medications may be reduced in allogeneic bone marrow transplant patients due to residual gut damage from intensive chemotherapy or radiation, or GVHD. **Discontinuation** tacrolimus may be eventually discontinued in certain renal or allogeneic bone marrow transplant recipients. However, it must be decreased gradually to reduce the risk of reactive immune stimulation and consequent graft rejection or GVHD.

Special Populations. *Pediatric Dosage.* Same as adult dosage.

Geriatric Dosage. Same as adult dosage. Age-related reduction in renal function and co-morbid conditions may predispose elderly patients to tacrolimus-induced nephrotoxicity and hypertension.

Special Populations. Use ideal body weight to calculate initial dosage in obese patients.

Dosage Forms. **Cap** 1, 5 mg; **Soln** 100 mg/mL; **Inj** 5 mg/mL.

Patient Instructions. Take this medication on a regular schedule in relation to the time of day and meals. Do not discontinue it unless directed to do so. Grapefruit juice can interact with cyclosporine. Talk to your physician before drinking grapefruit juice and before starting, stopping or changing the dose of any medication.

Missed Doses. Take a missed dose as soon as possible if you remember within 12 hours. If it is within 2 hours of next dose, skip the missed dose and do not double the next dose. If you miss 2 or more doses, contact your physician.

Pharmacokinetics. *Serum Levels.* The serum (blood) concentration–response relationship is not completely defined. Trough blood or serum concentrations are monitored to reduce the risk of toxicity. Therapeutic and toxic concentrations vary with assay, biologic fluid, and time post-transplant. Artifactually elevated serum concentrations may occur when blood is drawn through the same central venous line used for IV tacrolimus administration. Whole blood trough levels of 10–20 μg/L are often considered therapeutic.

Fate. The mean absorption of tacrolimus capsules in normal healthy volunteers is $17 \pm 7\%$. In liver transplant patients absorption is $22 \pm 6\%$. Factors that may decrease absorption include diarrhea, gastroenteritis, and short small bowel. Food does not affect bioavailability, but decreases and delays peak serum levels. Whole blood peak concentrations in liver transplant patients after 0.15 mg/kg is 52.4 μg/L fasting and 27.5 μg/L with food. Tacrolimus is extensively bound to erythrocytes and plasma proteins, primarily albumin and α_1-acid glycoprotein. V_d (whole blood) is 0.85 ± 0.3 L/kg in liver transplant patients; Cl (whole blood) is 0.053 ± 0.017 L/hr/kg in liver transplant recipients. Tacrolimus is extensively metabolized by CYP3A. At least 10 metabolites, some with immunosuppressant activity, have been identified. Less than 1% is excreted unchanged in the urine.

$t_{\frac{1}{2}}$. (whole blood) 21.2 ± 8.5 hr in normal healthy volunteers; 11.7 ± 3.9 hr in liver transplant patients.

Adverse Reactions. Acute nephrotoxicity, which usually occurs within 1 month post-transplant and is characterized by Cr_s increasing ≥ 0.3 mg/mL/24 hr, frequently abates with interruption of drug therapy. Dosage reduction may be required for continued administration. Chronic progressive renal toxicity is characterized by a slow, continual increase in Cr_s and BUN, mild proteinuria, and tubular dysfunction. Cr_s >2 mg/dL in adult patients, or doubling of Cr_s, is an indication for interruption of therapy or dosage reduction. Electrolyte abnormalities, including hypomagnesemia, hypokalemia or hyperkalemia, and renal tubular acidosis are consequences of tacrolimus-induced nephrotoxicity. Concurrent administration of nephrotoxic drugs increases the likelihood of renal dysfunction. Hypertension occurs frequently. **Calcium-channel blockers** and **clonidine** are suitable agents for the management of tacrolimus-induced hypertension because these agents do not have a deleterious effect on renal blood flow. Fine tremors occur frequently and can persist and worsen after drug discontinuation. Neurotoxicity includes headache, seizures, encephalopathy, confusion, insomnia, cortical blindness, expressive dysphagia, paraesthesia, hyperaesthesia, and myoclonic reactions. Anaphylactoid reactions to tacrolimus or the solubilizing agent, polyoxyethylated castor oil, may occur. Following an allergic reaction to IV tacrolimus, patients may receive a trial of oral tacrolimus capsules under close observation. Hyperbilirubinemia, increased γ-glutamyltranspeptidase, serum alkaline phosphatase, and serum transaminases occur frequently. Additional adverse effects include photophobia, rash, hirsutism, pleural effusion, gingival hyperplasia, diarrhea, nausea, vomiting, and hypertriglyceridemia.

Contraindications. Allergy to tacrolimus or polyoxyethylated castor oil.

Precautions. Pregnancy; lactation. Use with caution in patients at risk for renal dysfunction. (*See also* General Precautions for Immunosuppressants.)

Drug Interactions. Additive or synergistic renal toxicity may occur with concurrent administration of nephrotoxic drugs. Potassium-sparing diuretics may exacerbate hyperkalemia. Because tacrolimus is metabolized by CYP3A, numerous drug interactions are possible with concurrent administration of drugs that affect this enzyme system. The following drugs may increae tacrolimus blood levels: corticosteroids, itraconazole, ketoconazole, erythromycin and other macrolide antibiotics, oral contraceptives, fluconazole, calcium-channel blockers, cimetidine, danazol, and metoclopramide. Enzyme-inducing drugs, such as carbamazepine, phenobarbital, phenytoin, rifabutin, and rifampin, may decrease tacrolimus blood levels. Tacrolimus may decrease the clearance of lovastatin and increase the risk of drug-induced rhabdomyolysis.

Parameters to Monitor. Observe for anaphylaxis with IV administration. Monitor Cr_s q 2–7 days, and daily in patients at risk for acute renal dysfunction. Monitor liver function tests weekly, triglycerides monthly, and blood pressure regularly. Monitor blood or serum concentrations q 2–3 days when starting therapy. As the patient's clinical condition and renal function allow, reduce frequency to 1–2 times weekly, then monthly during the first year of therapy. After the first year of therapy, blood or serum concentration monitoring may be reduced q 1–2 months in stable patients. Monitor for signs and symptoms of graft rejection or GVHD, especially following dosage reduction.

Notes. Admix the injectable formulation in a glass container because tacrolimus may leach plasticizers from PVC containers. The manufacturer recommends a minimum of 24 hr between the last **cyclosporine** dose and the first tacrolimus dose when changing drugs. Comparative clinical trials found greater nephrotoxicity and neurotoxicity with tacrolimus than with cyclosporine.[237] Case reports describe resolution of drug-induced toxicity following replacement of cyclosporine with tacrolimus and resolution of cyclosporine-refractory acute GVHD or chronic GVHD with tacrolimus.[238,239]

■ REFERENCES

1. Dorr RT, Von Hoff DD, eds. *Cancer chemotherapy handbook*, 2nd ed. Norwalk CT: Appleton & Lange; 1994.
2. Lindley CM et al. Incidence and duration of chemotherapy-induced nausea and vomiting in the outpatient oncology population. *J Clin Oncol* 1989;7:1142–9.
3. Wharton JT et al. Hexamethylmelamine: an evaluation of its role in the treatment of ovarian cancer. *Am J Obstet Gynecol* 1979;133:833–44.
4. Manetta A et al. Hexamethylmelamine as a single second-line agent in ovarian cancer. *Gynecol Oncol* 1990;36:93–6.
5. Ames MM et al. Phase I and clinical pharmacological evaluation of a parenteral hexamethylmelamine formulation. *Cancer Res* 1990;50:206–10.
6. Sawitsky A et al. Comparison of daily versus intermittent chlorambucil and prednisone therapy in the treatment of patients with chronic lymphocytic leukemia. *Blood* 1977;50:1049–59.
7. Alexanian R, Dreicer R. Chemotherapy of multiple myeloma. *Cancer* 1984;53:583–8.
8. Adair CG et al. Renal function in the elimination of oral melphalan in patients with multiple myeloma. *Cancer Chemother Pharmacol* 1986;17:185–8.
9. Hoogstraten B et al. Intermittent melphalan therapy in multiple myeloma. *JAMA* 1969;209:251–3.

280   ANTINEOPLASTICS

10. Benet LZ et al. Design and optimization of dosage regimens: pharmacokinetic data. In, Hardman JG et al., eds. *Goodman and Gilman's the pharmacological basis of therapeutics.* 9th ed. New York: McGraw-Hill; 1996:1707–92.
11. McLean A et al. Pharmacokinetics and metabolism of chlorambucil in patients with malignant disease. *Cancer Treat Rev* 1979;6(suppl):33–42.
12. Adair CG et al. Can food affect the bioavailability of chlorambucil in patients with hematological malignancies? *Cancer Chemother Pharmacol* 1986;17:99–102.
13. Alberts DS et al. Oral melphalan kinetics. *Clin Pharmacol Ther* 1979;26:737–45.
14. Alberts DS et al. Kinetics of intravenous melphalan. *Clin Pharmacol Ther* 1979;26:73–80.
15. Taetle R et al. Pulmonary histopathologic changes associated with melphalan therapy. *Cancer* 1978; 42:1239–45.
16. Heard BE, Cooke RA. Busulfan lung. *Thorax* 1968;23:187–93.
17. Lane SD et al. Fatal interstitial pneumonitis following high-dose intermittent chlorambucil therapy for chronic lymphocytic leukemia. *Cancer* 1981;47:32–6.
18. Micetich KC et al. A comparative study of the cytotoxicity and DNA-damaging effects of cis-(diammino) (1,1-cyclobutanedicarboxylato)-platinum(II) and cis-diamminedichloroplatinum(II) on L1210 cells. *Cancer Res* 1985;45:4043–7.
19. Curt GA et al. A phase I and pharmacokinetic study of diamminecyclobutane-dicarboxylatoplatinum (NSC 241240). *Cancer Res* 1983;43:4470–3.
20. Meyers FJ et al. Infusion carboplatin treatment of relapsed and refractory acute leukemia: evidence of efficacy with minimal extramedullary toxicity at intermediate doses. *J Clin Oncol* 1989;7:173–8.
21. Smit E et al. Continuous infusion carboplatin on a 21-day schedule: a phase I and pharmacokinetic study. *J Clin Oncol* 1991;9:100–10.
22. Allen JC et al. Carboplatin and recurrent childhood brain tumors. *J Clin Oncol* 1987;5:459–63.
23. Calvert AH et al. Carboplatin dosage: prospective evaluation of a simple formula based on renal function. *J Clin Oncol* 1989;7:1748–56.
24. Chatelut E et al. Prediction of carboplatin clearance from standard morphological and biological patient characteristics. *J Natl Cancer Inst* 1995;87:573–80.
25. Newell DR et al. Plasma free platinum pharmacokinetics in patients treated with high dose carboplatin. *Eur J Cancer Clin Oncol* 1987;23:1399–405.
26. Calvert AH et al. Early clinical studies with cis-diammine-1,1-cyclobutane dicarboxylate platinum(II). *Cancer Chemother Pharmacol* 1982;9:140–7.
27. Einhorn LH, Donahue J. Cis-diamminedichloroplatinum, vinblastine, and bleomycin combination chemotherapy in disseminated testicular cancer. *Ann Intern Med* 1977;87:293–8.
28. Belt RJ et al. Pharmacokinetics of non-protein-bound platinum species following administration of cis-dichlorodiammineplatinum (II). *Cancer Treat Rep* 1979;63:1515–21.
29. DeConti RC et al. Clinical and pharmacological studies with cis-diammine-dichloroplatinum (II). *Cancer Res* 1973;33:1310–5.
30. Gonzalez-Vitale JC et al. Acute renal failure after cis-dichlorodiammineplatinum (II) and gentamicin-cephalothin therapies. *Cancer Treat Rep* 1978;62:693–8.
31. Macaulay VM et al. Prophylaxis against hypomagnesemia induced by cisplatinum combination therapy. *Cancer Chemother Pharmacol* 1982;9:179–81.
32. Brock N et al. Activation of cyclophosphamide in man and animals. *Cancer* 1971;6:1512–29.
33. Grochow LB, Colvin M. Clinical pharmacokinetics of cyclophosphamide. *Clin Pharmacokinet* 1979;4:380–94.
34. Bagley CM et al. Clinical pharmacology of cyclophosphamide. *Cancer Res* 1973;33:226–33.
35. Scheef W et al. Controlled clinical studies with an antidote against the urotoxicity of oxazophosphorines: preliminary results. *Cancer Treat Rep* 1979;63:501–5.
36. Carter SK, Friedman MA. 5-(3,3-dimethyl-1-triazeno)-imidazole-4-carboxamide (DTIC, DIC, NSC-45388)— a new antitumor agent with activity against malignant melanoma. *Eur J Cancer* 1972;8:85–92.
37. Loo TL et al. Mechanism of action and pharmacology studies with DTIC (NSC-45388). *Cancer Treat Rep* 1976;60:149–52.
38. Zalupski M, Baker LH. Ifosfamide. *J Natl Cancer Inst* 1988;80:556–66.
39. Araujo C, Tessler J. Treatment of ifosfamide-induced urothelial toxicity by oral administration of sodium 2-mercaptoethane sulphonate (mesna) to patients with inoperable lung cancer. *Eur J Cancer Clin Oncol* 1983;19:195–201.
40. Stuart-Harris RC et al. High-dose alkylation therapy using ifosfamide infusion with mesna in the treatment of adult advanced soft tissue sarcoma. *Cancer Chemother Pharmacol* 1983;11:69–72.

41. Sangster G et al. Failure of 2-mercaptoethane sulphonate sodium (mesna) to protect against ifosfamide nephrotoxicity. *Eur J Cancer Clin Oncol* 1984;20:435–6.

42. Pratt CB et al. Phase II trial of ifosfamide in children with malignant solid tumors. *Cancer Treat Rep* 1987;71:131–5.

43. Miser JS et al. Ifosfamide with uroprotection and etoposide: an effective regimen in the treatment of recurrent sarcomas and other tumors of children and young adults. *J Clin Oncol* 1987;5:1191–8.

44. Creaven PJ et al. Clinical pharmacology of ifosfamide. *Clin Pharmacol Ther* 1974;16:77–86.

45. Colvin M. The comparative pharmacology of cyclophosphamide and ifosfamide. *Semin Oncol* 1982;9(suppl 1):2–7.

46. Allen LM et al. Studies on the human pharmacokinetics of ifosfamide (NSC-109724). *Cancer Treat Rep* 1976;60:451–8.

47. Wheeler BM et al. Ifosfamide in refractory male germ cell tumors. *J Clin Oncol* 1986;4:28–34.

48. Fossa SK, Talle K. Treatment of metastatic renal cancer with ifosfamide and mesnum with and without irradiation. *Cancer Treat Rep* 1980;64:1103–8.

49. Stuart-Harris RC et al. High dose alkylation therapy using ifosfamide infusion with mesna in the treatment of adult advanced soft tissue sarcoma. *Cancer Chemother Pharmacol* 1983;11:69–72.

50. Meanwell CA et al. Phase II study of ifosfamide in cervical cancer. *Cancer Treat Rep* 1986;70:727–30.

51. Goren MP et al. Dechlorethylation of ifosfamide and neurotoxicity. *Lancet* 1986;2:1219–20.

52. DeVita VT et al. Combination chemotherapy in the treatment of advanced Hodgkin's disease. *Ann Intern Med* 1970;73:881–95.

53. Taylor JR, Halprin KM. Topical use of mechlorethamine in the treatment of psoriasis. *Arch Dermatol* 1972;106:362–4.

54. Taylor JR et al. Mechlorethamine hydrochloride solutions and ointment. *Arch Dermatol* 1980;116:783–5.

55. Van Scott EJ, Kalmanson JD. Complete remissions of mycosis fungoides lymphoma induced by topical nitrogen mustard (HN$_2$). *Cancer* 1973;32:18–30.

56. Crooke ST, Bradner WT. Mitomycin C: a review. *Cancer Treat Rev* 1976;3:121–39.

57. Buice RG et al. Pharmacokinetics of mitomycin C in non–oat cell carcinoma of the lung. *Cancer Chemother Pharmacol* 1984;13:1–4.

58. Dorr RT et al. Mitomycin C skin toxicity studies in mice. *J Clin Oncol* 1986;4:1399–1404.

59. DeFuria MD et al. Phase I-II study of mitomycin C topical therapy for low-grade, low-stage transitional cell carcinoma of the bladder: an interim report. *Cancer Treat Rep* 1980;64:225–30.

60. Sponzo RW et al. Physiologic disposition of 1-(2-chloroethyl)-3-cyclohexyl-1-nitrosourea (CCNU) and 1-(2-chloroethyl)-3-(4-methyl cyclohexyl)-1-nitrosourea (MeCCNU) in man. *Cancer* 1973;31:1154–9.

61. De Vita VT et al. Clinical trials with 1,3-bis(2-chloroethyl)-3-cyclohexyl-1-nitrosourea, NSC-409962. *Cancer Res* 1965;25:1876–81.

62. Oliverio VT. Toxicology and pharmacology of the nitrosoureas. *Cancer Chemother Pharmacol* 1973;4(part 3):13–20.

63. Aronin PA et al. Prediction of BCNU pulmonary toxicity in patients with malignant gliomas. *N Engl J Med* 1980;303:183–8.

64. Durant JR et al. Pulmonary toxicity associated with bischloroethylnitrosourea (BCNU). *Ann Intern Med* 1979;90:191–4.

65. Brem H et al. Placebo-controlled trial of safety and efficacy of intraoperative controlled delivery by biodegradable polymers of chemotherapy for recurrent gliomas. *Lancet* 1995;345:1008–12.

66. Tamargo RJ et al. Interstitial chemotherapy of the 9L gliosarcoma: controlled release polymers for drug delivery in the brain. *Cancer Res* 1993;53:329–33.

67. Spivack SD. Procarbazine. *Ann Intern Med* 1974;81:795–800.

68. Schein PS et al. Clinical antitumor activity and toxicity of streptozotocin (NSC-85998). *Cancer* 1974;34:993–1000.

69. Cohen BE et al. Human plasma pharmacokinetics and urinary excretion of thiotepa and its metabolites. *Cancer Treat Rep* 1986;70:859–64.

70. Beutler E. Cladribine (2-chlorodeoxyadenosine). *Lancet* 1992;340:952–6.

71. Saven A et al. Treatment of hairy cell leukemia. *Blood* 1992;79:1111–20.

72. Sipe JC et al. Cladribine in treatment of chronic progressive multiple sclerosis. *Lancet* 1994;344:9–13.

73. Liliemark J et al. On the bioavailability of oral and subcutaneous 2-chloro-2'-deoxyadenosine in humans: alternative routes of administration. *J Clin Oncol* 1992;10:1514–8.

74. Grant S. Ara-C: cellular and molecular pharmacology. *Adv Cancer Res* 1998;72:197–233.

75. Rudnick SA et al. High dose cytosine arabinoside (HDARAC) in refractory acute leukemia. *Cancer* 1979;44:1189–93.

76. Wan SH et al. Pharmacokinetics of 1-b-D-arabinofuranosylcytosine in humans. *Cancer Res* 1974;34:392–7.

77. Harris AL et al. Pharmacokinetics of cytosine arabinoside in patients with acute myeloid leukaemia. *Br J Clin Pharmacol* 1979;8:219–27.

78. van Prooijen R et al. Pharmacokinetics of cytosine arabinoside in acute myeloid leukemia. *Clin Pharmacol Ther* 1977;21:744–50.

79. Ho DHW, Frei E. Clinical pharmacology of 1-b-D-arabinofuranosylcytosine. *Clin Pharmacol Ther* 1971;12:944–54.

80. Chabner BA et al. Clinical pharmacology of anticancer drugs. *Semin Oncol* 1977;4:165–91.

81. Ritch PS et al. Ocular toxicity from high-dose cytosine arabinoside. *Cancer* 1983;51:430–2.

82. Lazarus HM et al. Central nervous system toxicity of high-dose systemic cytosine arabinoside. *Cancer* 1981;48:2577–82.

83. Ahmed I et al. Cytosine arabinoside-induced vasculitis. *Mayo Clin Proc* 1998;73:239–42.

84. Guilhot F et al. Interferon alfa-2b combined with cytarabine versus interferon alone in chronic myelogenous leukemia. French Chronic Myeloid Leukemia Study Group. *N Engl J Med* 1997;337:223–9.

85. Kemeny N et al. Intrahepatic or systemic infusion of fluorodeoxyuridine in patients with liver metastases from colorectal carcinoma. *Ann Intern Med* 1987;107:459–65.

86. Ensminger WD et al. A clinical pharmacological evaluation of hepatic arterial infusions of 5-fluoro-2'-deoxyuridine and 5-fluorouracil. *Cancer Res* 1978;38:3784–92.

87. Jacobs EM et al. Treatment of cancer with weekly 5-fluorouracil; study by the Western Cooperative Cancer Chemotherapy Group (WCCCG). *Cancer* 1971;27:1302–5.

88. Horton J et al. 5-Fluorouracil in cancer: an improved regimen. *Ann Intern Med* 1970;73:897–900.

89. Seifert P et al. Comparison of continuously infused 5-fluorouracil with bolus injection in treatment of patients with colorectal adenocarcinoma. *Cancer* 1975;36:123–8.

90. Cohen JL et al. Clinical pharmacology of oral and intravenous 5-fluorouracil (NSC-19893). *Cancer Chemother Rep* 1974;58(part 1):723–31.

91. Kirkwood JM et al. Comparison of pharmacokinetics of 5-fluorouracil and 5-fluorouracil with concurrent thymidine infusions in a phase I trial. *Cancer Res* 1980;40:107–13.

92. Abbruzzese JL et al. A phase I clinical, plasma, and cellular pharmacology study of gemcitabine. *J Clin Oncol* 1991;9:491–8.

93. Kaye SB. Gemcitabine: current status of phase I and II trials. *J Clin Oncol* 1994;12:1527–31.

94. Rothenberg ML et al. Gemcitabine: effective palliative therapy for pancreas cancer patients failing 5-FU. *Proc Am Soc Clin Oncol* 1995;14:198.

95. Mullarkey MF et al. Long-term methotrexate treatment in corticosteroid-dependent asthma. *Ann Intern Med* 1990;112:577–81.

96. Hedman J et al. Controlled trial of methotrexate in patients with severe chronic asthma. *Eur J Clin Pharmacol* 1996;49:347–9.

97. Henry MA, Gentry WL. Single injection of methotrexate for treatment of ectopic pregnancies. *Am J Obstet Gynecol* 1994;171:1584–7.

98. Corsan GH et al. Identification of hormonal parameters for successful systemic single-dose methotrexate therapy in ectopic pregnancy. *Hum Reprod* 1995;10:2719–22.

99. Wiebe ER. Abortion induced with methotrexate and misoprostol. *Can Med Assoc J* 1996;154:165–70.

100. Creinin MD. A randomized trial comparing misoprostol three and seven days after methotrexate for early abortion. *Am J Obstet Gynecol* 1995;173:1578–84.

101. Weibe ER. Abortion induced with methotrexate and misoprostol: a comparison of various protocols. *Contraception* 1997;55:159–63.

102. Bonadonna G et al. Combination chemotherapy as an adjuvant treatment in operable breast cancer. *N Engl J Med* 1976;294:405–10.

103. Bleyer WA. Clinical pharmacology of intrathecal methotrexate II. An improved dosage regimen derived from age-related pharmacokinetics. *Cancer Treat Rep* 1977;61:1419–25.

104. Evans WE, Pratt CB. Effect of pleural effusion on high-dose methotrexate kinetics. *Clin Pharmacol Ther* 1978;24:68–72.

105. Campbell MA et al. Methotrexate: bioavailability and pharmacokinetics. *Cancer Treat Rep* 1985;69:833–8. Dosages in the table were derived using the nomogram of Rowland M, Tozer TN. *Clinical pharmacokinetics: concepts and applications.* Philadelphia: Lea & Febiger; 1980:233.

106. Isacoff WH et al. Pharmacokinetics of high-dose methotrexate with citrovorum factor rescue. *Cancer Treat Rep* 1977;61:1665–74.

107. Shen DD, Azarnoff DL. Clinical pharmacokinetics of methotrexate. *Clin Pharmacokinet* 1978;3:1–13.

108. O'Dwyer PJ et al. 2'-deoxycoformycin (pentostatin) for lymphoid malignancies. *Ann Intern Med* 1988;108:733–43.

109. Malspeis L et al. Clinical pharmacokinetics of 2'-deoxycoformycin. *Cancer Treat Symp* 1984;2:7–15.

110. Wiernik PH, Serpick AA. A randomized clinical trial of daunorubicin and a combination of prednisone, vincristine, 6-mercaptopurine, and methotrexate in adult acute nonlymphocytic leukemia. *Cancer Res* 1967;32:2023–6.

111. Lin S-N et al. Quantitation of plasma azathioprine and 6-mercaptopurine levels in renal transplant patients. *Transplantation* 1980;29:290–4.

112. Bach JF, Dardenne M. The metabolism of azathioprine in renal failure. *Transplantation* 1971;12:253–9.

113. Zimm S et al. Variable bioavailability of oral mercaptopurine. *N Engl J Med* 1983;308:1005–9.

114. Duttera MJ et al. Hematuria and crystalluria after high-dose 6-mercaptopurine administration. *N Engl J Med* 1972;287:292–4.

115. Penn I, Starzl TE. A summary of the status of de novo cancer in transplant recipients. *Transplant Proc* 1972;4:719–32.

116. Ho DH et al. Clinical pharmacology of combined oral uracil and ftorafur. *Drug Metab Disp* 1992;20:936–40.

117. Salz LB et al. A fixed-ratio combination of uracil and ftorafur (UFT) with low dose leucovorin. *Cancer* 1995;75:782–5.

118. Rosenberg SA et al. Observations on the systemic administration of autologous lymphokine-activated killer cells and recombinant interleukin-2 to patients with metastatic cancer. *N Engl J Med* 1985;313:1485–92.

119. Winkelhake JL, Gauny SS. Human recombinant interleukin-2 as an experimental therapeutic. *Pharmacol Rev* 1990;42:1–28.

120. Konrad MW et al. Pharmacokinetics of recombinant interleukin-2 in humans. *Cancer Res* 1990;50:2009–17.

121. Goldstein D, Laszlo J. Interferon therapy in cancer: from imaginon to interferon. *Cancer Res* 1986;46:4315–29.

122. Krown SE. The role of interferon in the therapy of epidemic Kaposi's sarcoma. *Semin Oncol* 1987;14:27–33.

123. Perrillo RP et al. A randomized controlled trial of interferon alfa-2b alone and after prednisone withdrawal for the treatment of chronic hepatitis B. *N Engl J Med* 1990;323:295–301.

124. Spiegel RJ. Intron A (interferon alfa-2b): clinical overview. *Cancer Treat Rev* 1985;12(suppl B):5–16.

125. Wills RJ et al. Interferon kinetics and adverse reactions after intravenous, intramuscular, and subcutaneous injection. *Clin Pharmacol Ther* 1984;35:722–7.

126. Quesada JR et al. Antitumor activity of recombinant-derived interferon alpha in metastatic renal cell carcinoma. *J Clin Oncol* 1985;3:1522–8.

127. Berman E et al. Idarubicin in acute leukemia: results of studies at Memorial Sloan-Kettering Cancer Center. *Semin Oncol* 1989;16:30–44.

128. Lambertenghi-Deliliers G et al. Idarubicin plus cytarabine as first-line treatment of acute nonlymphoblastic leukemia. *Semin Oncol* 1989;16:16–20.

129. Blum RH, Carter SK. Adriamycin: a new anticancer drug with significant clinical activity. *Ann Intern Med* 1974;80:249–59.

130. Legha SS et al. Reduction of doxorubicin cardiotoxicity by prolonged continuous intravenous infusion. *Ann Intern Med* 1982;96:133–9.

131. Weiss AJ et al. Studies on adriamycin using a weekly regimen demonstrating its clinical effectiveness and lack of cardiac toxicity. *Cancer Treat Rep* 1976;60:813–22.

132. Von Hoff DD et al. Daunomycin-induced cardiotoxicity in children and adults: a reviw of 110 cases. *Am J Med* 1977;62:200–8.

133. Benjamin RS et al. Adriamycin chemotherapy—efficacy, safety, and pharmacologic basis of an intermittent single high-dosage schedule. *Cancer* 1974;33:19–27.

134. Smith DB et al. Clinical pharmacology of oral and intravenous 4-demethoxydaunorubicin. *Cancer Chemother Pharmacol* 1987;19:138–42.

135. Robert J et al. Pharmacokinetics of idarubicin after daily intravenous administration in leukemic patients. *Leuk Res* 1987;11:961–4.

136. Huffman DH et al. Daunorubicin metabolism in acute nonlymphocytic leukemia. *Clin Pharmacol Ther* 1972;13:895–905.

137. Lu K et al. Clinical pharmacology of 4-demethoxydaunorubicin (DMDR). *Cancer Chemother Pharmacol* 1986;17:143–8.

138. Dean JC et al. Scalp hypothermia: a comparison of ice packs and the Kold Kap in the prevention of doxorubicin-induced alopecia. *J Clin Oncol* 1983;1(1):33–7.

139. Von Hoff DD et al. Risk factors for doxorubicin-induced congestive heart failure. *Ann Intern Med* 1979;91:710–7.

140. Lipshultz SE et al. Late effects of doxorubicin therapy for acute lymphoblastic leukemia in childhood. *N Engl J Med* 1991;324:808–15.

141. Bartlett NL et al. Phase I trial of doxorubicin with cyclosporine as a modulator of multidrug resistance. *J Clin Oncol* 1994;12:835–42.
142. Dorr RT. Anthracycline update: stability and compatibility of adriamycin in solution. *Highlights on Antineoplastic Drugs* 1985;3(2):6–7.
143. Speyer JL et al. Protective effect of the bispiperazinedione ICRF-187 against doxorubicin-induced cardiac toxicity in women with advanced breast cancer. *N Engl J Med* 1988;319:745–52.
144. Olver IN et al. A prospective study of topical dimethylsulfoxide for treating anthracycline extravasation. *J Clin Oncol* 1988;6:1732–5.
145. Gill PS et al. Phase I/II clinical and pharmacokinetic evaluation of liposomal daunorubicin. *J Clin Oncol* 1995;13:996–1003.
146. Forssen EA et al. Selective in vivo localization of daunorubicin small unilamellar vesicles in solid tumors. *Cancer Res* 1992;52:3255–61.
147. Northfelt DW et al. Doxorubicin encapsulated in liposomes containing surface-bound polyethylene glycol: pharmacokinetics, tumor localization, and safety in patients with AIDS-related Kaposi's sarcoma. *J Clin Pharmacol* 1996;36:55–63.
148. Harrison M et al. Liposomal-entrapped doxorubicin: an active agent in AIDS-related Kaposi's sarcoma. *J Clin Oncol* 1995;13:914–20.
149. Frei E. The clinical use of actinomycin. *Cancer Chemother Rep* 1974;58:49–54.
150. Tattersall MHN et al. Pharmacokinetics of actinomycin D in patients with malignant melanoma. *Clin Pharmacol Ther* 1975;17:701–8.
151. Shenkenberg TD, Von Hoff DD. Mitoxantrone: a new anticancer drug with significant clinical activity. *Ann Intern Med* 1986;105:67–81.
152. Vietti TJ et al. Mitoxantrone in children with advanced malignant disease. In, Rozencweig M et al., eds. *New anticancer drugs: mitoxantrone and bisantrene.* New York: Raven Press; 1983:93–102.
153. Savaraj N et al. Pharmacology of mitoxantrone in cancer patients. *Cancer Chemother Pharmacol* 1982;8:113–7.
154. Slayton RE et al. New approach to the treatment of hypercalcemia: the effect of short-term treatment with mithramycin. *Clin Pharmacol Ther* 1971;12:833–7.
155. Kennedy BJ. Metabolic and toxic effects of mithramycin during tumor therapy. *Am J Med* 1970;49:494–503.
156. Asbury RF et al. Treatment of metastatic breast cancer with aminoglutethimide. *Cancer* 1981;47:1954–8.
157. Plourde PV. Arimidex: a potent and selective fourth-generation aromatase inhibitor. *Breast Cancer Res Treat* 1994;30:103–11.
158. Anon. Toremifene and letrozole for advanced breast cancer. *Med Lett Drugs Ther* 1998;40:43–5.
159. Newling DWW et al. The response of advanced prostatic cancer to a new non-steroidal antiandrogen: results of a multicenter open phase II study of Casodex. *Eur Urol* 1990;18:18–21.
160. Cockshott ID et al. The pharmacokinetics of Casodex in prostate cancer patients after single and during multiple dosing. *Eur Urol* 1990;18:10–7.
161. Katchen B, Buxbaum S. Disposition of a new nonsteroid antiandrogen, alpha, alpha, alpha-trifluoro-2-methyl-4'-nitro-m-propionotoluidide (flutamide) in men following a single oral 200 mg dose. *J Clin Endocrinol Metab* 1975;41:373–9.
162. Symchowicz S et al. Single and multiple dose pharmacokinetics of flutamide (Eulexin) in normal geriatric volunteers. *Acta Pharmacol Toxicol (Copenh)* 1986;58:301. Abstract.
163. Yagoda A. Flutamide-induced diarrhea secondary to lactose intolerance. *J Natl Cancer Inst* 1989;81:1839–40. Letter.
164. Hauser AR, Marryman R. Estramustine phosphate sodium. *Drug Intell Clin Pharm* 1984;18:368–74.
165. Ahmann FR et al. Zoladex: a sustained-release, monthly luteinizing hormone-releasing hormone analogue for the treatment of advanced prostate cancer. *J Clin Oncol* 1987;5:912–7.
166. Leuprolide Study Group. Leuprolide versus diethylstilbestrol for metastatic prostate cancer. *N Engl J Med* 1984;311:1281–6.
167. Patterson JS, Battersby LA. Tamoxifen: an overview of recent studies in the field of oncology. *Cancer Treat Rep* 1980;64:775–8.
168. Fabian C et al. Clinical pharmacology of tamoxifen in patients with breast cancer: comparison of traditional and loading dose schedules. *Cancer Treat Rep* 1980;64:765–73.
169. Adam HK et al. Studies on the metabolism and pharmacokinetics of tamoxifen in normal volunteers. *Cancer Treat Rep* 1980;64:761–4.
170. Plotkin D et al. Tamoxifen flare in advanced breast cancer. *JAMA* 1978;240:2644–6.
171. Lippman ME, Allegra JC. Receptors in breast cancer: estrogen receptor and endocrine therapy of breast cancer. *N Engl J Med* 1978;299:930–3.

172. Wiebe VJ et al. Pharmacokinetics of toremifene and its metabolites with advanced breast cancer. *Cancer Chemother Pharmacol* 1990;25:247–51.

173. Saarto T et al. Antiatherogenic effects of adjuvant antiestrogens: a randomized trial comparing the effects of tamoxifen and toremifene on plasma lipid levels in postmenopausal women with node-positive breast cancer. *J Clin Oncol* 1996;14:429–33.

174. Cortes JE et al. Docetaxel. *J Clin Oncol* 1995;13:2643–55.

175. Royer I. Metabolism of docetaxel by human cytochromes P450: interactions with paclitaxel and other antineoplastic drugs. *Cancer Res* 1996;56:58–65.

176. O'Dwyer PJ et al. Etoposide (VP-16–213): current status of an active anticancer drug. *N Engl J Med* 1985;312:692–700.

177. Rivera GK et al. Epipodophyllotoxins in the treatment of childhood cancer. *Cancer Chemother Pharmacol* 1994;34(suppl):S89–95.

178. Chamberlain MC, Grafe MR. Recurrent chiasmatic-hypothalamic glioma treated with oral etoposide. *J Clin Oncol* 1995;13:2072–6.

179. Snyder DS et al. Fractionated total-body irradiation and high-dose etoposide as a preparatory regimen for bone marrow transplantation for 94 patients with chronic myelogenous leukemia in chronic phase. *Blood* 1994;84:1672–9.

180. Allen LM, Creaven PJ. Comparison of the human pharmacokinetics of VM-26 and VP-16, two antineoplastic epipodophyllotoxin glucopyranoside derivatives. *Eur J Cancer* 1975;11:697–707.

181. Wiseman LR, Markham A. Irinotecan. A review of its pharmacological properties and clinical efficacy in the management of advanced colorectal cancer. *Drugs* 1996;52:606–23.

182. Holmes FA et al. Phase II study of taxol in patients with metastatic breast cancer. *Proc Am Soc Clin Oncol* 1991;10:60. Abstract.

183. McGuire WP et al. Taxol: a unique antineoplastic agent with significant activity in advanced ovarian epithelial neoplasms. *Ann Intern Med* 1989;111:273–9.

184. Huizing MT et al. Pharmacokinetics of paclitaxel and metabolites in a randomized comparative study in platinum-pretreated ovarian cancer patients. *J Clin Oncol* 1993;11:2127–35.

185. Rozencweig M et al. VM-26 and VP 16-213: a comparative analysis. *Cancer* 1977;40:334–42.

186. Grem JL et al. Teniposide in the treatment of leukemia: a case study of conflicting priorities in the development of drugs for fatal diseases. *J Clin Oncol* 1988;6:351–79.

187. Yap H-Y et al. Vinblastine given as a continuous 5-day infusion in the treatment of refractory advanced breast cancer. *Cancer Treat Rep* 1980;64:279–83.

188. Robieux I et al. Pharmacokinetics of vinorelbine in patients with liver metastases. *Clin Pharmacol Ther* 1996;59:32–40.

189. Owellen RJ et al. Pharmacokinetics of vindesine and vincristine in humans. *Cancer Res* 1977;37:2603–7.

190. Nelson RL et al. Comparative pharmacokinetics of vindesine, vincristine and vinblastine in patients with cancer. *Cancer Treat Rev* 1980;7(suppl):17–24.

191. Wargin WA, Lucas VS. The clinical pharmacokinetics of vinorelbine (Navelbine). *Semin Oncol* 1994;21(5 suppl 10):21–7.

192. Le Chevalier T et al. Randomized study of vinorelbine and cisplatin versus vindesine and cisplatin versus vinorelbine alone in advanced non-small-cell lung cancer: results of a European multicenter trial including 612 patients. *J Clin Oncol* 1994;12:360–7.

193. Kaminski MS et al. Radioimmunotherapy of B-cell lymphoma with [^{131}I]-anti-B1(anti-CD-20) antibody. *N Engl J Med* 1993;329:459–65.

194. Kaminski MS et al. Iodine-131–anti-B1 radioimmunotherapy for B-cell lymphoma. *J Clin Oncol* 1996;14:1974–81.

195. Maloney DG et al. IDEC-C2B8: results of a phase I multiple-dose trial in patients with relapsed non-Hodgkin's lymphoma. *J Clin Oncol* 1997;15:3266–74.

196. Maloney DG et al. Phase I clinical trial using escalating single-dose infusion of chimeric anti-CD20 monoclonal antibody (IDEC-C2B8) in patients with recurrent B-cell lymphoma. *Blood* 1994;84:2457–66.

197. Clarkson B et al. Clinical results of treatment with *E. coli* 1-asparaginase in adults with leukemia, lymphoma and solid tumors. *Cancer* 1970;25:279–305.

198. Sutow WW et al. Evaluation of dose and schedule of 1-asparaginase in multidrug therapy of childhood leukemia. *Med Pediatr Oncol* 1976;2:387–95.

199. Pratt CB et al. Comparison of daily versus weekly 1-asparaginase for the treatment of childhood acute leukemia. *J Pediatr* 1970;77:474–83.

200. Nesbit M et al. Evaluation of intramuscular versus intravenous administration of 1-asparaginase in childhood leukemia. *Am J Pediatr Hematol Oncol* 1979;1:9–13.

201. Ohnuma T et al. Biochemical and pharmacological studies with asparaginase in man. *Cancer Res* 1970;30:2297–305.

202. Haskell CM et al. L-asparaginase: therapeutic and toxic effects in patients with neoplastic disease. *N Engl J Med* 1969;281:1028–35.

203. Bennett JM, Reich SD. Bleomycin. *Ann Intern Med* 1979;90:945–8.

204. Alberts DS et al. Bleomycin pharmacokinetics in man. *Cancer Chemother Pharmacol* 1978;1:177–81.

205. Paladine W et al. Intracavitary bleomycin in the management of malignant effusions. *Cancer* 1976;38:1903–8.

206. Crooke ST et al. Effects of variations in renal function on the clinical pharmacology of bleomycin administered as an IV bolus. *Cancer Treat Rep* 1977;61:1631–6.

207. Kramer WG et al. The pharmacokinetics of bleomycin in man. *J Clin Pharmacol* 1978;18:346–52.

208. Sostman HD et al. Cytotoxic drug-induced lung disease. *Am J Med* 1977;62:608–15.

209. Yagoda A et al. Bleomycin, an antitumor antibiotic: clinical experience in 274 patients. *Ann Intern Med* 1972;77:861–70.

210. Muindi JRF et al. Clinical pharmacology of oral all-trans retinoic acid in patients with acute promyelocytic luekemia. *Cancer Res* 1992;52:2138–42.

211. Warrell RP et al. Differentiation therapy of acute promyelocytic leukemia with tretinoin (all-trans-retinoic acid). *N Engl J Med* 1991;324:1385–90.

212. Fenaux P et al. Effect of all transretinoic acid in newly diagnosed acute promyelocytic leukemia. Results of a multicenter randomized trial. European APL 91 Group. *Blood* 1993;82:3241–9.

213. Glick J et al. A randomized trial of cyclophosphamide and cisplatin ± amifostine in the treatment of advanced epithelial ovarian cancer. *Proc Am Soc Clin Oncol* 1994;13:432.

214. Kligerman MM et al. Final report on phase I trial of WR-2721 before protracted fractionated radiation. *Int J Radiat Oncol Biol Phys* 1988;14:1119–22.

215. Shaw LM et al. Pharmacokinetics of WR-2721. *Pharmacol Ther* 1988;39:195–201.

216. Kligerman MM et al. Phase I clinical studies with WR-2721. *Cancer Clin Trials* 1980;3:217–21.

217. Turrisi AT et al. Final report of the phase I trial of single-dose WR-2721 [S-2-(3-aminopropylamono)ethylphosphorothiolic acid]. *Cancer Treat Rep* 1986;70:1389–93.

218. Korst AEC et al. Influence of amifostine (AMI) on the pharmacokinetics (PK) of carboplatin (CARBO) in patients with solid tumors. *Proc Am Soc Clin Oncol* 1995;14:172. Abstract.

219. Büntzel J et al. Selective cytoprotection by amifostine in the treatment of head and neck cancer with simultaneous radiochemotherapy. *Proc Am Soc Clin Oncol* 1997;16:393a. Abstract.

220. Speyer JL et al. ICRF-187 permits longer treatment with doxorubicin in women with breast cancer. *J Clin Oncol* 1992;10:117–27.

221. Swain SM et al. Cardioprotection with dexrazoxane for doxorubicin-containing therapy in advanced breast cancer. *J Clin Oncol* 1997;15:1318–32.

222. Wexler LH et al. Randomized trial of the cardioprotective agent ICRF-187 in pediatric sarcoma patients treated with doxorubicin. *J Clin Oncol* 1996;14:362–72.

223. Hochster H et al. Pharmacokinetics of the cardioprotector ADR-529 (ICRF-187) in escalating doses combined with high-dose doxorubicin. *J Natl Cancer Inst* 1992;84:1725–30.

224. Burkert H. Clinical overview of mesna. *Cancer Treat Rev* 1983;10:175–81.

225. Antman KH et al. Phase II trial of ifosfamide with mesna in previously treated metastatic sarcoma. *Cancer Treat Rep* 1985;69:499–504.

226. Pratt CB et al. Phase II trial of ifosfamide in children with malignant solid tumors. *Cancer Treat Rep* 1987;71:131–5.

227. Burkert H et al. Bioavailability of orally administered mesna. *Arzneimittelforschung* 1984;34:1597–600.

228. Pohl J et al. Toxicology, pharmacology and interactions of sodium 2-mercaptoethanesulfonate (mesna). *Curr Chemother* 1981;2:1387–9.

229. Stuart-Harris RC et al. High-dose alkylation therapy using ifosfamide infusion with mesna in the treatment of adults advanced soft-tissue sarcoma. *Cancer Chemother Pharmacol* 1983;11:69–72.

230. Bodenstein H. Successful treatment of aplastic anemia with high-dose immunoglobulin. *N Engl J Med* 1991;324:1368–9.

231. Sullivan KM et al. Prednisone and azathioprine compared with prednisone and placebo for treatment of chronic graft-v-host disease: prognostic influence of prolonged thrombocytopenia after allogenic marrow transplantation. *Blood* 1988;72:546–54.

232. Yee GC, Salomon DR. Cyclosporine. In, Evans WE et al., eds. *Applied pharmacokinetics. Principles of therapeutic drug monitoring.* 3rd ed. Vancouver, WA: Applied Therapeutics; 1992;28:1–40.

233. Ptachcinski RJ et al. Cyclosporine concentration determinations for monitoring and pharmacokinetic studies. *J Clin Pharmacol* 1986;26:358–66.

234. Brinch L. Fooled by cyclosporin levels. *Bone Marrow Transplant* 1992;9:77–8.

235. Yee GC et al. Effect of hepatic dysfunction on oral cyclosporine pharmacokinetics in marrow transplant patients. *Blood* 1984;64:1277–9.

236. List AF et al. Phase I/II trial of cyclosporine as a chemotherapy-resistance modifier in acute leukemia. *J Clin Oncol* 1993;11:1652–60.

237. US Multicenter FK506 Liver Study Group. A comparison of tacrolimus (FK506) and cyclosporine for immunosuppression in liver transplantation. *N Engl J Med* 1994;331:1110–5.

238. Pratschke J et al. Treatment of cyclosporine-related adverse effects by conversion to tacrolimus after liver transplantation. *Transplantation* 1997;64:938–40.

239. Ohashi Y et al. Successful treatment of steroid-resistant severe acute GVHD with 24-h continuous infusion of FK506. *Bone Marrow Transplant* 1997;19:625–7.

240. Vincenti F et al. Interleukin-2 receptor blockade with daclizumab to prevent acute rejection in renal transplantation. Daclizumab Triple Therapy Study Group. *N Engl J Med* 1998;338:161–5.

241. Nashan B et al. Randomised trial of basiliximab versus placebo for control of acute cellular rejection in renal allograft recipients. *Lancet* 1997;350:1193–8.

242. Sievers TM et al. Mycophenolate mofetil. *Pharmacotherapy* 1997;17:1178–97.

243. Meiser BM et al. Mycophenolate mofetil dose adjustments based on trough levels improve outcome after heart transplantation. *J Heart Lung Transplant* 1998;17:85, abstract.

244. Kelly PA et al. Sirolimus, a new, potent immunosuppressive agent. *Pharmacotherapy* 1997;17:1148–56.

245. Przepiorka D et al. Tacrolimus and minidose methotrexate for prevention of acute graft-versus-host disease after matched unrelated donor marrow transplantation. *Blood* 1996;88:4383–9.

Cardiovascular Drugs

Antiarrhythmic Drugs

ADENOSINE
Adenocard

Pharmacology. Adenosine is a purinergic agonist, acting on the purine P_1 and P_2 receptors (although P_1 receptors are more sensitive to adenosine). Pharmacologic effects include coronary and peripheral vasodilation, negative inotropic actions, and depression of sinus node and AV nodal conduction. It is used most frequently for supraventricular tachycardia caused by re-entry (ie, AV nodal re-entry or AV re-entry associated with an extranodal pathway). In these instances, restoration of sinus rhythm occurs in 85–95% of patients. The drug may also be helpful in diagnosing wide-QRS tachycardias believed to be supraventricular in origin.[1–4]

Adult Dosage. IV for supraventricular tachycardia administer over 1–2 sec through an IV line with minimal dead space, followed by a saline flush; **initial dose** is 6 mg (3 mg if administered through a central line); if this is ineffective, 12 mg can be given 2 min later and repeated again if necessary. An average effective dose of 1 mg has been reported in patients receiving concurrent dipyridamole.

Pediatric Dosage. IV 50 μg/kg increased in increments of 50 μg/kg q 2 min prn, to a maximum of 250 μg/kg.

Dosage Forms. Inj 3 mg/mL.

Pharmacokinetics. Adenosine is rapidly metabolized in blood to inactive adenosine monophosphate and inosine; elimination half-life is about 1–10 seconds.

Adverse Reactions. Frequent, but short-lived, subjective complaints include chest discomfort, dyspnea, flushing, and headache. Postconversion arrhythmias are also frequent, but transient, and include ventricular ectopy, sinus bradycardia, AV block, atrial fibrillation, and rapid reinitiation of supraventricular tachycardia. Adenosine is contraindicated in patients with pre-existing sinus node dysfunction or second- or third-degree heart block without a functioning pacemaker, because of the risk of prolonged sinus arrest or AV block. Also use adenosine with caution in asthmatics because it may precipitate bronchospasm, and in patients with atrial fibrillation with an accessory AV pathway because it may accelerate ventricular response.

Drug Interactions. Dipyridamole blocks the cellular uptake of adenosine, enhancing the pharmacologic effect; theophylline, a purine antagonist, inhibits the therapeutic actions of adenosine.

AMIODARONE HYDROCHLORIDE
Cordarone, Pacerone

Pharmacology. Amiodarone is a type III antiarrhythmic that prolongs the effective refractory period of atrial and ventricular tissue by blocking potassium conductance. It decreases sinus rate and slows conduction through the AV node by β-adrenergic blockade. Amiodarone also blocks sodium and calcium channels. The antiarrhythmic actions may be caused by interruption of re-entrant substrate or abolition of premature beats that trigger re-entry.

Administration and Adult Dosage. **PO loading dosage** 800–1600 mg/day in divided doses for 1–2 weeks. Loading dosages are usually toward the lower end of this range for atrial arrhythmias and toward the upper end of the range for ventricular arrhythmias. **PO maintenance dosage** 100–600 mg/day (usually 300–400 mg/day for recurrent ventricular tachycardia and 100–200 mg/day for supraventricular tachycardias such as atrial fibrillation). Some suggest a 600–800 mg/day priming dosage for 1–2 months after the initial loading period and prior to maintenance therapy.[5] **IV for treatment or prevention of refractory ventricular tachycardia or fibrillation** 150 mg over 10 min, then 360 mg over the next 6 hr, followed by 540 mg over the next 18 hr. Initiate amiodarone only during hospitalization for the first several days of the loading phase.

Special Populations. *Pediatric Dosage.* Safety and efficacy not established. **PO** 10–15 mg/kg/day for 10 days, then 5 mg/kg/day maintenance therapy has been used.[6]

Geriatric Dosage. Same as adult dosage.

Dosage Forms. **Tab** 200 mg; **Inj** 50 mg/mL.

Patient Instructions. Report any shortness of breath, tiredness, abdominal discomfort, or visual abnormalities. Avoid intense sunlight; use sunscreen. Divided daily dosage during loading- or maintenance-dosage phases may reduce GI upset.

Missed Doses. Take this drug at regular intervals. If you miss a dose do *not* take it. If it is about time for the next dose, take that dose only. Do not double the dose or take extra.

Pharmacokinetics. *Onset and Duration.* Onset is variable, from several days to a month; full effect may not occur for several months.[7]

Serum Levels. 1–2.5 mg/L (1.6–4 μmol/L) is proposed, although the therapeutic range is not well established.[8] Desethylamiodarone accumulates to serum levels similar to or greater than the parent drug.

Fate. Oral absorption is erratic and incomplete; bioavailability is 46 ± 22%. Peak serum concentrations occur in 3–7 hr. The drug is 99.9% plasma protein bound;[7,9] V_d is 66 ± 44 L/kg; Cl is 0.11 ± 0.024 L/hr/kg.[7,9,10] Amiodarone is primarily hepatically eliminated with at least one active metabolite, desethylamiodarone. No unchanged amiodarone or desethylamiodarone is found in urine.[7]

$t_{1/2}$. α phase 4–12 hr; β phase varies with duration of therapy and study sampling. Reported variously as 25 ± 12 days and 53 ± 23 days.[7,9,10] Similar for desethylamiodarone.[7,10]

Adverse Reactions. Corneal microdeposits occur in virtually all patients and are no reason for stopping treatment; however, visual disturbances are reported in about 5%.[10] Neurologic effects occur frequently and include tremor, ataxia, paresthesias, and nightmares, which may be more common during the loading phase.[10] Anorexia, nausea, vomiting, and/or constipation occur frequently. Transient elevations in hepatic enzymes occur in over 50% of patients, but clinical hepatitis occurs only occasionally.[11] Photosensitivity occurs frequently, and a blue-gray skin pigmentation (sometimes irreversible) develops in 2–4% of patients.[10] Hypothyroidism (low-T_3 syndrome) or hyperthyroidism may occur frequently.[12] Proximal muscle weakness and myopathy have been reported occasionally. Symptomatic pulmonary fibrosis has been reported in 1–6% of patients; it is probably not immunologic in etiology and seems to occur more often in patients with underlying lung disease.[10,13] Pulmonary symptoms usually improve upon drug discontinuation, but up to 10% of cases result in death.[10,13] Aggravation of ventricular tachycardia and drug-induced torsades de pointes may occur.[10,14] Severe sinus bradycardia (requiring a pacemaker) or AV block has been reported occasionally.

Contraindications. Sick sinus syndrome or second- or third-degree heart block in the absence of a ventricular pacemaker; patients in whom bradycardia has caused syncope; long-QT syndrome.

Precautions. Electrophysiologic studies may not predict the long-term efficacy of amiodarone.[15]

Drug Interactions. Amiodarone increases cyclosporine, digoxin, flecainide, phenytoin, procainamide, and quinidine serum levels, and potentiates warfarin's anticoagulant effects; the initial dosage of warfarin should be reduced by one-third to one-half.

Parameters to Monitor. Monitor ECG daily during loading phase for heart rate, PR, QRS, and QT duration. Baseline and periodic thyroid function tests and liver enzymes (especially if symptoms present). Obtain baseline pulmonary function tests; repeat chest x-ray and clinical examination q 3–6 months.[10,13]

Notes. After the results of CAST,[16] many clinicians use type III antiarrhythmics (eg, amiodarone, sotalol) as first-line therapy in both supraventricular and ventricular arrhythmias.

BRETYLIUM TOSYLATE   Bretylol, Various

Pharmacology. Bretylium is a type III antiarrhythmic with actions thought to be caused by an initial catecholamine release and subsequent catecholamine depletion and/or direct effect independent of the adrenergic nervous system. Direct actions may be mediated by blockade of potassium channels. Bretylium causes an initial increase in blood pressure, heart rate, and myocardial contractility (catecholamine release) followed by hypotension (neuronal blockade). Its greatest usefulness is in severe ventricular tachyarrhythmias resistant to other antiarrhythmics. Bretylium can be effective for ventricular fibrillation, but is usually ineffective against ventricular tachycardia.

Administration and Adult Dosage. IV loading dose 5 mg/kg push with additional dose of 10 mg/kg if no response. **Maintenance dosage** can be given as IM or IV (over 8 min or more) 5–10 mg/kg q 6 hr, or as an IV infusion of 1–2 mg/min.

Special Populations. *Pediatric Dosage.* Not well established, although the following has been suggested. **IV loading dosage for ventricular fibrillation** 5 mg/kg, followed by 10 mg/kg at 15- to 30-min intervals, to a maximum total dosage of 30 mg/kg, then **IV maintenance dosage** 5–10 mg/kg q 6 hr.

Geriatric Dosage. Same as adult dosage.

Other Conditions. In renal impairment, lower dosages may be required.[17] A nomogram for dosage in renal insufficiency has been described.[18]

Dosage Forms. **Inj** 50 mg/mL.

Pharmacokinetics. *Onset and Duration.* IV onset usually 5–10 min, but may be delayed to 20–60 min; myocardial levels increase gradually over 6–12 hr.[17,19] Duration is usually 6–12 hr after a single dose. Because of persistent myocardial levels, duration after multiple doses may be much longer.[19]

Fate. 23 ± 9% is orally absorbed.[9,17] The drug is not bound to plasma proteins.[17,20] V_d is 5.9 ± 0.8 L/kg;[21] Cl is 0.61 ± 0.11 L/hr/kg.[9] After IV administration, bretylium is primarily cleared renally, with 77 ± 15% excreted in the urine unchanged.[21] Disposition is probably route and concentration dependent.[17,22]

$t_{1/2}$ α phase about 25 min; β phase 8.9 ± 1.8 hr,[17,21] mean of 33.4 hr in renal insufficiency.[18]

Adverse Reactions. Hypotension (usually orthostatic) via adrenergic blockade occurs in up to 50% of patients. The drop in mean arterial pressure is usually not more than 20 mm Hg; however, sometimes it can be severe, necessitating drug discontinuation. Nausea and vomiting occur frequently after rapid IV administration.

Contraindications. Suspected digitalis-induced ventricular tachycardia (may increase the rate of ventricular tachycardia or the likelihood of ventricular fibrillation).

Precautions. Use with caution if hypotension exists prior to administration. Keep patient supine until tolerance to hypotension develops. Prolonged effects may occur, and dosage reduction in patients with impaired renal function may be required.

Drug Interactions. The pressor effects of catecholamines are enhanced by bretylium.

Parameters to Monitor. Close monitoring of blood pressure and constant ECG monitoring is required.

DIGOXIN   Lanoxin, Various

Pharmacology. Digitalis glycosides exert positive inotropic effects through improvement of availability of calcium to myocardial contractile elements, thereby increasing cardiac output in CHF. Antiarrhythmic actions of digitalis glycosides are primarily caused by an increase in AV nodal refractory period via increased vagal tone, sympathetic withdrawal, and direct mechanisms. Additionally, digitalis exerts a moderate direct vasoconstrictor action on arterial venous smooth muscle.

Administration and Adult Dosage. IV loading dosage 10–15 μg/kg in divided doses over 12–24 hr at intervals of 6–8 hr.[23] **PO loading dosage** adjust dosage for percent oral absorption. (*See* Fate.) Usually, 0.5–0.75 mg is given initially, then 0.125–0.375 mg q 6–8 hr until desired effect or total digitalizing dosage is achieved. **Maintenance dosage** = (total body stores) × (% lost/day), where total body stores is the original calculated loading dosage and % lost/day is 14 + ($Cl_{cr}/5$). Usual maintenance dosage ranges from 0.125–0.5 mg/day.[23] A dosage nomogram has also been described.[24] **IM** not recommended.

Special Populations. *Pediatric Dosage.* Base all dosages on ideal body weight. **Total digitalizing dosage (TDD) PO** (premature newborn) 20–30 μg/kg; (full-term newborn) 25–35 μg/kg; (1–24 months) 35–60 μg/kg; (2–5 yr) 30–40 μg/kg; (5–10 yr) 20–35 μg/kg; (>10 yr) 10–15 μg/kg. Give ½ TDD initially, then ¼ TDD q 8–18 hr twice. **PO maintenance dosage** (premature newborn) 5–7.5 μg/kg/day; (full-term newborn) 6–10 μg/kg/day; (1–24 months) 10–15 μg/kg/day; (2–5 yr) 7.5–10 μg/kg/day; (5–10 yr) 5–10 μg/kg/day; (>10 yr) 2.5–5 μg/kg/day. In children <10 yr, give in 2 divided doses per day. **IV** (all ages) 75% of PO dosage.

Geriatric Dosage. Maintenance dosage may be lower because of age-related decrease in renal function.[25,26]

Other Conditions. Decrease loading and maintenance dosage in renal impairment. Base dosage on ideal body weight in obese individuals.

Dosage Forms. **Cap** 0.05, 0.1, 0.2 mg; **Elxr** 50 μg/mL; **Tab** 0.0625, 0.125, 0.1875, 0.25, 0.375, 0.5 mg; **Inj** 0.1, 0.25 mg/mL.

Patient Instructions. Report feelings of tiredness, appetite loss, nausea, abdominal discomfort, or visual disturbances such as hazy vision, light sensitivity, spots, halos, or red-green blindness.

Missed Doses. Take this drug at regular intervals. If you miss a dose and it has been less than 12 hours since your dose was due, take it as soon as you remember. If it is about time for the next dose, take that dose only. Do not double the dose or take extra.

Pharmacokinetics. *Onset and Duration.* IV onset 14–30 min; peak 1.5–5 hr; somewhat slower after oral administration.

Serum Levels. Therapeutic 0.5–2 μg/L (0.6–2.5 nmol/L); toxic, greater than 3 μg/L (3.8 nmol/L). Considerable overlap exists between therapeutic and toxic ranges.[27] Signs or symptoms of digitalis toxicity may be evident below 3 μg/L, especially if other risk factors are present.[27] Obtain blood samples for digoxin levels at least 4 hr after an IV dose and 6–8 hr after an oral dose to allow central and tissue compartment equilibration. Digoxin concentrations (digitalis-like immunoreactive substance) have been detected in patients with renal failure, neonates, pregnant women, and those with severe liver disease not receiving digitalis glycosides.[28]

Fate. Oral absorption is 70 ± 13% from tablets; 85% from elixir; 95% from capsules.[29] Enterohepatic recycling of digoxin may be as high as 30%.[30] Protein binding to albumin is 25 ± 5%; V_d is 7–8 L/kg; Cl is 0.16 ± 0.036 L/hr/kg; both are dependent on renal function.[29] The drug is excreted $60 \pm 11\%$ unchanged in the urine in patients with normal renal function.[29] Active metabolites include digitoxigenin, bisdigitoxoside, digoxigenin monodigitoxoside, and dihydrodigoxin.[29]

$t_{\frac{1}{2}}$ α phase 0.5–1 hr; β phase 39 ± 13 hr;[9,29] β phase 3.5–4.5 days in anephric patients.[23]

Adverse Reactions. Arrhythmias, listed by decreasing prevalence, are premature ventricular beats, second- and third-degree heart block, AV junctional tachycardia, atrial tachycardia with block, ventricular tachycardia, and SA nodal block.[31] Visual disturbances are serum level related and occur in up to 25% of patients with digoxin intoxication. They include blurred vision, yellow or green tinting, flickering lights or halos, or red-green color blindness. GI symptoms occur frequently and include abdominal discomfort, anorexia, nausea, and vomiting. CNS side effects occur frequently, yet are nonspecific, such as weakness, lethargy, disorientation, agitation, and nervousness. Hallucinations and psychosis have been reported. Rare reactions include gynecomastia, hypersensitivity, and thrombocytopenia.

Contraindications. Hypertrophic obstructive cardiomyopathy; suspected digitalis intoxication; second- or third-degree heart block in the absence of mechanical pacing; atrial fibrillation with accessory AV pathway; ventricular fibrillation.

Precautions. Electrolyte abnormalities predisposing to digitalis toxicity include hypokalemia, hypomagnesemia, and hypercalcemia. Hypothyroidism may reduce digoxin requirements because of lower V_d and clearance.[29] Direct current cardioversion carries little risk in the absence of digitalis toxicity.[32] Use with caution in patients with pulmonary disease, because hypoxia may sensitize the myocardium to arrhythmias and increase the risk of toxicity.[33] Serious bradyarrhythmias may occur with sick sinus syndrome, but controversy exists concerning the clinical importance of its effects on the SA node. Digitalis glycosides may increase infarct size in the nonfailing heart.

Drug Interactions. β-Blockers may worsen CHF or digitalis-induced bradycardia. Potassium loss caused by amphotericin B or diuretics may contribute to digoxin toxicity. Spironolactone may decrease digoxin renal elimination. ACE inhibitors, amiodarone, bepridil, diltiazem, nitrendipine, quinidine, and verapamil may increase digoxin levels. Oral antacids, kaolin-pectin, oral neomycin, and sulfasalazine may reduce digoxin absorption. Penicillamine may decrease serum digoxin levels.

Parameters to Monitor. Digitalis glycoside serum levels need only be obtained when compliance, effectiveness, or systemic availability is questioned or toxicity is suspected.[34,35] (*See* Serum Levels.) Monitor heart rate, ECG for digitalis-induced arrhythmias, subjective complaints of toxicity, renal function; serum electrolytes (especially potassium) should be monitored frequently initially, then q 1–2 months when stabilized.

Notes. Treatment of severe or life-threatening digitalis (eg, digoxin) toxicity should include IV **digoxin immune Fab** (Digibind). About 40 mg (one vial) of digoxin-specific Fab fragments bind 0.6 mg of the glycoside. Exact dosage can be calculated based on estimated total body stores.

DISOPYRAMIDE PHOSPHATE   Norpace, Various

Pharmacology. Disopyramide has qualitatively the same electrophysiologic actions as procainamide and quinidine and is effective for both ventricular and (unlabeled) supraventricular tachycardia. It causes an increase in systemic vascular resistance through vasoconstriction; additionally, it may exert a profound negative inotropic effect and has marked anticholinergic properties systemically and on the heart. Disopyramide's isomers have stereospecific pharmacologic actions.[36,37]

Administration and Adult Dosage. PO loading dosage 300–400 mg. PO maintenance dosage 400–800 mg/day, to a maximum of 1.6 g/day. Give daily dosage in 4 equally divided doses q 6 hr with non-SR Cap, or in 2 equally divided doses q 12 hr with SR Cap. Initiate disopyramide during hospitalization.

Special Populations. *Pediatric Dosage.* PO (<1 yr) 10–30 mg/kg/day, (1–4 yr) 10–20 mg/kg/day, (4–12 yr) 10–15 mg/kg/day, (12–18 yr) 6–15 mg/kg/day. Daily dosage is divided into 4 equal doses q 6 hr. (*See* Notes.)

Geriatric Dosage. Decreased dosage is probably necessary because the elderly may not tolerate anticholinergic side effects.

Other Conditions. In patients who weigh less than 50 kg, or with hepatic disease or moderate renal insufficiency (Cl_{cr} >40 mL/min), load with 150–200 mg, then give 400 mg/day in 2 or 4 divided doses, depending on the dosage form used. Initial daily dosage in patients with hepatic disease is about 4.4 mg/kg/day.[38,39] In patients with severe renal insufficiency, give maintenance dosages as follows (non-SR Cap):

CREATININE CLEARANCE	DAILY MAINTENANCE DOSAGE
30–40 mL/min	300 mg
15–30 mL/min	200 mg
<15 mL/min	100 mg

Dosage Forms. Cap 100, 150 mg; **SR Cap** 100, 150 mg. (*See* Notes.)

Patient Instructions. Report any symptoms such as difficulty in urination, constipation, blurred vision, or dry mouth. Report shortness of breath, weight gain, or edema also. Do not crush or chew SR capsules. SR capsule core may appear in the stool, but this does not mean there was a lack of absorption.

Missed Doses. Take this drug at regular intervals. If you miss a dose, take it as soon as you remember. If it is about time for the next dose, take that dose only. Leave a minimum of 4 hours between regular capsule doses and 6–8 hours between sustained-release capsule doses. Do not double the dose or take extra.

Pharmacokinetics. *Onset and Duration.* PO onset is within 1 hr. Duration varies with individual differences in drug disposition, but is usually 6–12 hr.

Serum Levels. Usual range is 2–5 mg/L, (6–15 μmol/L),[39,40] with toxicity more likely over 4 mg/L. Therapeutic range of unbound drug is 0.5–2 mg/L (1.5–6 μmol/L).[38] Monitoring unbound concentrations eliminates variability caused by concentration-dependent disposition.[39,41]

Fate. Oral absorption is rapid; systemic availability is $83 \pm 11\%$.[39,40] Unbound drug in serum varies from 19–46% over a serum concentration range of 2–8 mg/L and is also age dependent.[42] V_d (unbound) is 1.4–1.7 L/kg in normal subjects;[9,39] Cl (unbound) is about 0.25 L/hr/kg;[39] Cl is stereospecific.[43] The major metabolite is a mono-N-dealkylated form that has weak antiarrhythmic but potent anticholinergic activity; $55 \pm 6\%$ is excreted unchanged in the urine.[9]

$t_{½}$. α phase 2–4 min (IV);[47] β phase is concentration dependent, usually 6 ± 1 hr,[9] 11–17 hr in renal impairment, depending on severity.[42]

Adverse Reactions. Nausea or anorexia occur frequently. Dry mouth, urinary retention, blurred vision, and constipation are dose-related anticholinergic effects that may occur in up to 70% of patients, and result in drug discontinuation in about 20%.[44] Through its vagolytic action, disopyramide may cause sinus tachycardia. Severe bradycardia, AV nodal block, or asystole may also occur, especially in patients with SA or AV nodal disease. Exacerbation of CHF is most prevalent (20–40%) in patients with left ventricular systolic dysfunction.[36] Torsades de pointes, similar to quinidine syncope, has been reported. Rarely, rash, hepatic cholestasis, psychosis, or peripheral neuropathy occur. Hypoglycemia has also been reported.

Contraindications. History of disopyramide-induced heart block or serious ventricular arrhythmias; second- or third-degree heart block in the absence of a ventricular pacemaker; long-QT syndrome; cardiogenic shock or severe CHF.

Precautions. In atrial fibrillation or flutter, give digitalis or drugs that slow AV nodal conduction prior to disopyramide. Use very cautiously, if at all, in patients with CHF, because of negative inotropic and vasoconstrictive actions.[36] The drug may worsen sick sinus syndrome or aggravate underlying ventricular arrhythmias. If possible, use other antiarrhythmics in patients with prostatic hypertrophy or preexisting urinary retention. Disopyramide may exacerbate glaucoma or myasthenia gravis.

Drug Interactions. Erythromycin inhibits disopyramide metabolism. Phenytoin may decrease disopyramide serum levels and increase its anticholinergic effects. Rifampin, barbiturates, and other enzyme inducers may decrease disopyramide serum levels. Concurrent use of disopyramide and quinidine may increase disopyramide serum levels or decrease quinidine serum levels.

Parameters to Monitor. Because of concentration-dependent protein binding, total drug levels unreliably reflect active drug concentration, and monitoring unbound drug concentrations is preferable. Monitor serum levels and symptoms or signs of toxicity closely in patients with altered states of drug disposition such as renal dysfunction. When initiating therapy, observe ECG daily for 3–4 days for QT, QRS, or PR prolongation. Obtain frequent vital signs initially for evidence of adverse hemodynamic effects (eg, CHF), and less frequently when a maintenance dosage is attained. Question the patient about anticholinergic manifestations, such as urinary and visual abnormalities.

Notes. A 1–10 mg/mL suspension, prepared from capsules, in cherry syrup is stable for 1 month under refrigeration in an amber bottle.

DOFETILIDE (Investigational—Pfizer)   Xelide

Pharmacology. Dofetilide is a class III antiarrhythmic drug that selectively prolongs atrial and ventricular repolarization by blocking the delayed rectifier (rapid component) potassium current. It is being investigated for both the acute treatment (IV) and prevention (PO) of supraventricular and ventricular arrhythmias.[45,46] Other type III antiarrhythmic drugs under clinical investigation that block potassium channels include **azimilide, ambasilide, almokalant, sematilide,** and **terikalant.**

Adult Dosage. PO 125–500 mg bid and IV 4–8 μg/kg bid have been used in preliminary clinical trials.

Pharmacokinetics. Oral bioavailability is 99% and peak concentrations occur 2.5 hr after oral administration. V_d is 3.9 ± 1.3 L/kg. About 50% of dofetilide is eliminated renally as unchanged drug and 50% is metabolized hepatically. Elimination half-life is 9.7 ± 2.7 hr.

Adverse Reactions. The major side effect is drug-induced torsades de pointes. Dofetilide should not be given in hypokalemia or pre-existing QT prolongation.

FLECAINIDE ACETATE   Tambocor

Pharmacology. Flecainide is a type Ic antiarrhythmic that predominantly slows conduction velocity with minimal effect on refractoriness. (*See* Electrophysiologic Actions of Antiarrhythmics Comparison Chart.) Compared to type Ia or Ib antiarrhythmics, it binds to and dissociates from the sodium channel very slowly. It can decrease cardiac output by a negative inotropic action.

Administration and Adult Dosage. PO 50 mg q 12 hr initially, then increase in 50 mg increments q 12 hr q 4–7 days until desired response. **Usual maintenance dosage** is 100 mg PO q 12 hr, to a maximum of 300 mg/day. Initiate flecainide during hospitalization.

Special Populations. *Pediatric Dosage.* Safety and efficacy not established. **PO** 100–200 mg/m²/day (average 140 mg/m²/day) in 2 divided doses has been used.[47]

Geriatric Dosage. Same as adult dosage.

Other Conditions. Lower maintenance dosage requirements are expected in patients with CHF, liver disease, or renal insufficiency. Start these patients with 50–100 mg q 12–24 hr and cautiously increase dosage as required with the aid of serum levels.[39,48]

Dosage Forms. Tab 50, 100, 150 mg.

Patient Instructions. Report any symptoms of dizziness, extra or rapid heart beats, or visual disturbances. Report symptoms of worsening shortness of breath or exercise intolerance.

Missed Doses. Take this drug at regular intervals. If you miss a dose and it has been less than 4 hours since your dose was due, take it as soon as you remember.

If it is about time for the next dose, take that dose only. Do not double the dose or take extra.

Pharmacokinetics. *Onset and Duration.* Onset 1–6 hr (average 3); duration 12–30 hr.[48]

Serum Levels. (Therapeutic trough) 0.2–1 mg/L (0.5–2.5 μmol/L).[48,49]

Fate. Oral bioavailability is 70 ± 11%.[9,49] From 37–55% is plasma protein bound, but the percentage may be higher (61%) post-MI because of increases in $α_1$-acid glycoprotein.[48] V_d is 8–10 L/kg;[48] Cl is reported as 0.34 ± 0.1 L/hr/kg,[9] and 0.61 ± 0.23 L/hr/kg;[39,48] Cl decreases in CHF, renal failure, and liver disease. Flecainide is about 60% stereoselectively metabolized by the liver through the CYP2D6 isozyme[50] and about 30% excreted unchanged in urine.

$t_{1/2}$. α phase 3–8 min; β phase 14 ± 5 hr. β phase is 20 ± 4 hr with ventricular ectopy; 37.8 ± 39.7 hr in patients with severe renal dysfunction.[51]

Adverse Reactions. Neurologic side effects, which include dizziness and visual abnormalities, occur frequently. Exacerbation of CHF in patients with underlying left ventricular dysfunction occurs frequently. Nausea, dyspnea, and headache may also occur frequently. Flecainide has proarrhythmic effects, which may result in new sustained ventricular tachycardia or aggravation of underlying ventricular arrhythmias. These reactions occur more frequently in patients with left ventricular dysfunction, coronary disease, or ventricular arrhythmias.[16,52] Risk may be sustained over time and not limited to the several days after initiation of therapy. Flecainide-induced ventricular tachycardia may be unresponsive to cardioversion or pacing, but may respond to lidocaine therapy or sodium bicarbonate. Aggravation of underlying conduction disturbances may also occur.

Contraindications. Second- or third-degree AV block or bifasicular block in the absence of a ventricular pacemaker; severe CHF; history of type Ic–induced arrhythmia.

Precautions. Use with caution in patients with sick sinus syndrome and in combination with other negative inotropic drugs, such as calcium-channel blockers or β-blockers, or following recent therapy with a type Ia antiarrhythmic. Flecainide may increase pacemaker capture threshold.[53] (*See* Notes.)

Drug Interactions. Amiodarone and cimetidine may increase flecainide serum concentrations; flecainide slightly elevates serum digoxin levels.

Parameters to Monitor. Frequent or continuous (preferred) ECG when therapy initiated, then periodically on an ambulatory basis. Obtain a baseline evaluation of left ventricular function prior to starting flecainide. Obtain periodic trough serum levels (particularly in those with renal or liver disease and CHF) once an individual's effective level is determined. Observe closely for neurologic toxicities and CHF symptoms when initiating therapy.

Notes. Because the results of CAST show an increase in mortality in patients with asymptomatic ventricular arrhythmias post-MI given flecainide,[16] it should be reserved for individuals with life-threatening ventricular arrhythmias such as sustained ventricular tachycardia refractory to other drugs.

IBUTILIDE FUMARATE   Corvert

Pharmacology. Ibutilide is a class III antiarrhythmic that selectively prolongs atrial and ventricular repolarization by increasing sodium influx (the window current). It may also block potassium channels. It is indicated for the acute termination of atrial fibrillation or atrial flutter of recent onset. In these arrhythmias, sinus rhythm is restored in about 50% of patients.[46,54]

Adult Dosage. IV (≥60 kg) 1 mg over 10 min; (<60 kg) 0.01 mg/kg. If the tachycardia is not terminated 10 min after the end of the initial infusion, the dose may be repeated.

Dosage Forms. Inj 0.1 mg/mL.

Pharmacokinetics. Ibutilide has a V_d of 11 ± 4 L/kg and is approximately 40% bound to plasma proteins. It is primarily metabolized by the liver. Although many metabolites have been identified, only a hydroxylated form has shown activity. Less than 10% is excreted unchanged in urine. Elimination half-life is about 6 hr (range 2–12).

Adverse Reactions. The major side effect is drug-induced proarrhythmia; torsades de pointes (sustained or nonsustained) occurs in 4–5% of patients. Risk factors are hypokalemia and underlying left ventricular dysfunction. Monitor QT interval closely, and do not give ibutilide with other drugs known to delay repolarization or prolong QT interval (eg, astemizole). Heart block and heart failure have occurred rarely. Patients with atrial fibrillation of more than 2 days' duration must be anticoagulated with warfarin for 3 weeks prior to the administration of ibutilide. Normalize serum magnesium and potassium concentrations prior to the administration of ibutilide.

LIDOCAINE HYDROCHLORIDE   Xylocaine, Various

Pharmacology. Lidocaine's electrophysiologic actions differ in healthy and diseased cardiac tissues. (*See* Electrophysiologic Actions of Antiarrhythmics Comparison Chart.) Most of its antiarrhythmic activity is caused by frequency-dependent blockade of the fast sodium channel in Purkinje fibers. In comparison to other antiarrhythmics, lidocaine binds to and dissociates from the sodium channel very quickly. It is used in the acute treatment of ventricular arrhythmias associated with MI or digitalis intoxication. Effectiveness in the treatment of supraventricular arrhythmia is limited.

Administration and Adult Dosage. **IV loading dose for ventricular tachycardia or fibrillation** 100 mg (1–1.5 mg/kg) over 1 min; if ineffective, may repeat with 50–100 mg q 5–10 min, to a maximum of 300 mg.[55] **IV maintenance** 2–4 mg/min infusion.[55] **IV for neuropathic pain** 5 mg/kg/hr for 60–90 min has been used.[56] (*See* Notes.)

Special Populations. *Pediatric Dosage.* **IV (or intratracheal) loading dose** 1 mg/kg, may repeat q 10–15 min, to a maximum of 5 mg/kg. **IV maintenance dosage** 20–50 µg/kg/min infusion.

Geriatric Dosage. Same as adult dosage. Elderly may be at increased risk of toxicity because of decreased clearance.

Other Conditions. In CHF, use one-half of IV loading dose. In liver disease or CHF, initial maintenance infusion is 1 mg/min, to a maximum of 2–3 mg/min.[55] In MI without CHF, maintenance infusion rate may need to be decreased by 30–50% in 24 hr;[55] however, empiric dosage alterations in MI are not recommended because of increases in α_1-acid glycoprotein and lidocaine binding.[57]

Dosage Forms. **Inj** 10, 20, 40, 100, 200 mg/mL. Also available premixed in D5W in concentrations of 2, 4, 8 mg/mL.

Patient Instructions. Report side effects such as drowsiness, perioral numbness or tingling, dizziness, and nausea during maintenance infusion.

Pharmacokinetics. *Onset and Duration.* IV onset is immediate; duration after initial IV bolus is 10–20 min. IM onset is 10 min; duration is 3 hr.[58]

Serum Levels. Therapeutic (total) 1.5–6 mg/L (7–28 μmol/L);[40] (unbound) 0.5–1.5 mg/L (2–7 μmol/L).[57] Toxic reactions are more likely at total concentrations >5 mg/L (22 μmol/L).[55] (*See* Adverse Reactions.)

Fate. The drug is well absorbed orally; however, a large hepatic first-pass effect limits systemic availability to 35 ± 11%.[59] IM absorption half-life is 12–28 min.[55] The drug is 70 ± 5% plasma protein bound;[55] V_d is 1.3 ± 0.4 L/kg in normals, 0.9 ± 0.2 L/kg in CHF.[60] Cl is 0.55 ± 0.14 L/hr/kg, decreased in CHF, liver disease, and during long-term infusion.[55,60,61] Lidocaine is primarily metabolized in the liver, with 2 ± 1% excreted unchanged in the urine.[60] The major metabolites, monoethylglycinexylidide (MEGX) and glycinexylidide (GX), both have neurotoxic[62] and antiarrhythmic[63] actions. Accumulation of these metabolites in renal impairment or during prolonged infusions may contribute to lidocaine toxicity.

$t_{1/2}$. α phase about 8 min;[58,60] β phase 98 ± 24 min.[55,60] The β phase in CHF or liver disease may be prolonged to 4.5 ± 2.4 hr and 6.6 ± 1.1 hr, respectively.[55,60] Elimination half-life of total lidocaine increases to an average of 3.2 ± 0.5 hr, 24 hr after MI without CHF, and up to 10.2 ± 2 hr after MI with CHF.[64] In MI, the rise in total lidocaine half-life is greater than that of unbound lidocaine.[65]

Adverse Reactions. Serum level–related neurologic side effects including dizziness, nausea, drowsiness, speech disturbances, perioral numbness, muscle twitching, confusion, vertigo, and tinnitus are frequent at total serum levels over 5 mg/L. Serious toxicities including psychosis, seizures, and respiratory depression occur at serum levels over 9 mg/L.[55] Sinus arrest or severe bradycardia is associated with sinus node disease, toxic drug levels, or concomitant therapy with other antiarrhythmics. Complete AV block may occur, especially in patients with preexisting bifasicular bundle branch block, AV nodal block, or inferior wall MI.[66,67]

Contraindications. History of hypersensitivity to any amide-type local anesthetic (rare); second- or third-degree heart block unless the site of block can be localized to the AV node itself[66] or ventricular pacemaker is functional; severe sinus node dysfunction; Stokes-Adams syndrome; atrial fibrillation in association with Wolff-Parkinson-White syndrome.

Precautions. Lidocaine administered to prevent ventricular fibrillation in acute myocardial infarction is no longer recommended.[67] Toxicity during bronchoscopy because of tracheal lidocaine absorption has been reported.

Drug Interactions. Propranodol decreases lidocaine clearance, so close monitoring is necessary with concomitant administration of these drugs. Cimetidine may decrease lidocaine clearance, but empiric dosage reduction with concomitant cimetidine is not recommended.[68] Phenytoin may decrease lidocaine serum levels and also increase myocardial depression.

Parameters to Monitor. Monitor serum levels and signs or symptoms of toxicity closely in patients with altered drug disposition such as CHF, hepatic disease, acute MI, or prolonged IV infusion (>24 hr). Monitoring unbound levels is preferable post-MI. Minor subjective and objective toxicities are extremely important because they are often subtle and may forecast more serious toxicities (eg, psychosis or seizures). Continuously observe ECG for therapeutic and/or toxic actions. Monitor vital signs such as blood pressure, heart rate, and respiration frequently.

Notes. IV lidocaine has been used to treat pain of peripheral origin such as neuropathies and burns.[56,69] Oral mexiletine has been used for ongoing treatment if lidocaine is successful. (*See* Mexiletine.)

MEXILETINE HYDROCHLORIDE   Mexitil, Various

Pharmacology. Mexiletine has electrophysiologic actions similar to lidocaine and tocainide. Depression of conduction is accentuated in ischemic/hypoxic tissue. It also has a slight negative inotropic action. It is used in the treatment of ventricular arrhythmias; effectiveness in supraventricular tachycardias is limited.

Administration and Adult Dosage. PO loading dose 400 mg once, followed by maintenance dosage in 8 hr; **PO maintenance dosage** 200–300 mg q 8 hr, to a maximum of 400 mg q 8 hr. **PO for neuropathic pain** 450 mg/day;[70] dosages as high as 10 mg/kg/day have been used to treat the thalmic pain syndrome.[71] (*See* Notes.) Initiate mexiletine during hospitalization.

Special Populations. *Pediatric Dosage.* Safety and efficacy not established.

Geriatric Dosage. Same as adult dosage.

Other Conditions. Reduce maintenance dosage by 30–50% in patients with hepatic disease or severe CHF.[39,72] Dosage may also need to be decreased with Cl_{cr} <10 mL/min.[73]

Dosage Forms. Cap 150, 200, 250 mg.

Patient Instructions. Report numbness, drowsiness, dizziness, or tingling. Nausea or loss of appetite may occur and may be reduced by taking the drug with food. Report any abnormal bruising.

Missed Doses. Take this drug at regular intervals. If you miss a dose and it has been less than 4 hours since your dose was due, take it as soon as you remember. If it is about time for the next dose, take that dose only. Do not double the dose or take extra.

Pharmacokinetics. *Onset and Duration.* PO onset 1–4 hr (average 2); duration 8–16 hr.

Serum Levels. 0.5–2 mg/L (3–11 μmol/L), although not well correlated with therapeutic or toxic effects.[74]

Fate. Oral bioavailability is 87 ± 13%, and, unlike lidocaine, mexiletine undergoes less than 10% first-pass hepatic elimination.[74,75] Absorption can be incomplete in MI patients receiving narcotic analgesics.[74,75] The drug is 63 ± 3% plasma protein bound;[9] V_d is large and variably reported as 6.6 ± 0.9 L/kg and 10.8 ± 7.2 L/kg.[74,75] Cl is variable, ranging from 0.4–0.6 L/hr/kg,[43] decreasing in both CHF and liver disease.[74] Mexiletine is predominantly metabolized in the liver, where it undergoes polymorphic metabolism, primarily via the CYP2D6 isozyme;[76] 10–20% is excreted unchanged in urine, depending on urinary pH.[74,75]

$t_{1/2}.$ α phase 3–12 min; β phase 9.2 ± 2.1 hr,[77] 18.5 hr in poor metabolizers.[76] β phase 15.7 ± 4.9 hr in severe renal dysfunction,[73] 15 ± 0.6 hr in CHF with or without MI,[78,79] and may be prolonged in cirrhosis.

Adverse Reactions. Neurologic toxicities are frequent and include tremor, ataxia, drowsiness, confusion, paresthesias, and occasionally psychosis or seizures. Minor CNS side effects may occur in up to 40% of patients.[80] Nausea, vomiting, and anorexia are frequent. Mexiletine may aggravate underlying ventricular arrhythmias or conduction disturbances. Thrombocytopenia has been reported rarely.[80] Mexiletine is an ether analogue of lidocaine, so cross-sensitivity between mexiletine and tocainide or lidocaine is not expected.[81]

Contraindications. Second- or third-degree AV block in the absence of a ventricular pacemaker; cardiogenic shock.

Precautions. Worsening of sick sinus syndrome may occur. Mexiletine can increase pacemaker capture threshold and alter the effectiveness of internal defibrillators.[52]

Drug Interactions. Mexiletine increases theophylline concentrations by 30–50% by decreasing theophylline metabolism.[82] Phenytoin and rifampin may increase mexiletine metabolism. Quinidine and theophylline occasionally increase serum mexiletine levels.

Parameters to Monitor. ECG for 3–5 days when therapy is initiated, then q 3–6 months on an ambulatory basis. Obtain periodic serum levels once an individual's effective level is determined. Observe closely for neurologic toxicities when initiating therapy.

Notes. The efficacy of mexiletine for ventricular tachycardia can be increased by the addition of a type Ia antiarrhythmic, such as **quinidine**.[83] Mexiletine has been used to treat neuropathic pain such as diabetic neuropathy and for thalmic pain syndrome.[70,71]

MORICIZINE HYDROCHLORIDE   Ethmozine

Pharmacology. Moricizine is a phenothiazine-like type I (probably Ic)[84] antiarrhythmic that (in normal tissue) slows conduction velocity by blocking sodium channels in a frequency-dependent manner. Its effects appear to be accentuated by ischemia.

Administration and Adult Dosage. PO 200 q 8 hr initially, then increase daily dosage q 3 days by 150 mg until desired effect or toxicity occurs, to a usual maintenance dosage of 200–300 mg q 8 hr. Initiate moricizine during hospitalization.

Special Populations. *Pediatric Dosage.* Safety and efficacy not established. **PO** 200–600 mg/m^2/day has been used.[85]

Geriatric Dosage. Same as adult dosage.

Other Conditions. Not well studied; patients with hepatic disease may require a lower dosage.

Dosage Forms. **Tab** 200, 250, 300 mg.

Patient Instructions. Report any dizziness, rapid heartbeat, or gastrointestinal upset.

Missed Doses. Take this drug at regular intervals. If you miss a dose and it has been less than 4 hours since your dose was due, take it as soon as you remember. If it is about time for the next dose, take that dose only. Do not double the dose or take extra.

Pharmacokinetics. *Onset and Duration.* Onset is variable, from 2–20 hr after multiple doses; duration is 12–36 hr after long-term use.[86]

Serum Levels. Correlation between serum levels and therapeutic effect is not well established, but 0.2–3.6 mg/L (0.5–8.4 μmol/L) has been suggested.[87]

Fate. Moricizine is well absorbed after oral administration, but the large hepatic first-pass metabolism limits bioavailability to 34–38%. About 81–90% is bound to plasma proteins.[88] V_d is 5.9 ± 3.2 and 11.6 ± 6.7 L/kg after 1 and 13 days of therapy, respectively.[89] Cl is 3.8 ± 1.8 to 4.7 ± 2.3 L/hr/kg, depending on length of therapy.[90] Moricizine undergoes extensive hepatic metabolism and appears to induce its own metabolism. Over 40 metabolites appear in small quantities systemically.[90] At least two, including moricizine sulfoxide, are active and probably account for some of the drug's antiarrhythmic activity and for its long duration of action. Less than 1% appears in the urine unchanged.[89,90]

t$_{1/2}$. α phase 4–20 min; β phase 1.6 ± 0.2 hr.[89,90]

Adverse Reactions. Frequent noncardiac side effects include nausea, anorexia, and dizziness. Dizziness may be lessened by administering more frequent, smaller doses. Moricizine has proarrhythmic actions, which result in new or worsened ventricular tachycardia in 2–5% of patients. Exacerbation of CHF occurs occasionally. Worsening of underlying conduction disturbances such as AV block, ventricular conduction defects, or sick sinus syndrome may occur. Drug fever has been reported.[91]

Contraindications. Second- or third-degree AV block or bifasicular block in the absence of a ventricular pacemaker; cardiogenic shock; hypersensitivity to phenothiazines.

Precautions. Use with caution in patients with sick sinus syndrome. Because of the final results of CAST II,[92] moricizine is indicated only for life-threatening ventricular arrhythmias such as sustained ventricular tachycardia, where there is a clear benefit to therapy.

Drug Interactions. Cimetidine may increase moricizine serum levels. Moricizine decreases theophylline levels.

Parameters to Monitor. Daily ECG for the first 2–4 days when therapy is initiated, then q 3–6 months on an ambulatory basis, observing for PR and QRS lengthening. Observe for GI side effects and dizziness.

Notes. Limited data exist on the use of moricizine in supraventricular tachycardias.

PROCAINAMIDE HYDROCHLORIDE   Procanbid, Pronestyl, Various

Pharmacology. Procainamide is a class Ia antiarrhythmic that alters conduction in normal and ischemic tissues by sodium-channel blockade in a fashion similar to quinidine. It may decrease systemic blood pressure by causing peripheral ganglionic blockade;[93] it also has weak anticholinergic action and a slight negative inotropic action. The active metabolite N-acetylprocainamide (NAPA) has primarily type III antiarrhythmic activity, predominantly delaying repolarization by blocking potassium conductance.

Administration and Adult Dosage. **PO loading dose** (Cap, Tab) 1 g over 2 hr in 2 divided doses. **PO maintenance dosage** (Cap, Tab) 1–6 g/day in 4–6 divided doses, to a maximum of 9 g/day;[94] (SR Tab) may be given q 6–8 hr (Pronestyl-SR) or q 12 hr (Procanbid), to a maximum of 50 mg/kg/day. **IV loading dose** 1–1.5 g at 20–50 mg/min,[93] alternatively, 15–20 mg/kg. **IV maintenance dosage** 1.5–5 mg/min (20–80 μg/kg/min) infusion.[93] **Intermittent IV or IM** 1–6 g/day in 4–6 divided doses, to a maximum of 9 g/day. Initiate procainamide during hospitalization.

Special Populations. *Pediatric Dosage.* Safety and efficacy not established. **PO** 15–50 mg/kg/day in 4–8 divided doses, to a maximum of 4 g/day; **IV loading dose** 3–6 mg/kg over 5 min (up to 100 mg/dose), may repeat q 5–10 min, to a maximum of 15 mg/kg. **IV maintenance dosage** 20–80 μg/kg/min infusion, to a maximum of 2 g/day. **IM maintenance dosage** 20–30 mg/kg/day in 4–6 divided doses, to a maximum of 4 g/day.[95]

Geriatric Dosage. Same as adult dosage, but adjust for age-related decrease in renal function.

Other Conditions. Reduce maintenance dosage in liver disease. In renal insufficiency, procainamide and its active metabolite accumulate, necessitating a lower maintenance dosage.[39] Recent data imply no need for decreasing loading and maintenance dosages in CHF and MI.[96]

Dosage Forms. **Cap, Tab** 250, 375, 500 mg; **SR Tab** (6-hr; Pronestyl-SR, various) 250, 500, 750, 1000 mg; (12-hr; Procanbid) 500, 1000 mg; **Inj** 100, 500 mg/mL.

Patient Instructions. Report any symptoms such as nausea, vomiting, fever, sore throat, joint pain, rash, chest or abdominal pain, and shortness of breath. Do not chew, split, or crush SR tablets. The SR tablet shell may appear in the stool, but this does not mean there was a lack of absorption.

Missed Doses. Take this drug at regular intervals. If you miss a dose, take it as soon as you remember. If it is about time for the next dose, take that dose only.

Leave a minimum of 2 hours between regular capsule or tablet doses and 4–6 hours between sustained-release tablet doses. Do not double the dose or take extra.

Pharmacokinetics. *Onset and Duration.* IV onset is immediate; PO and IM onset within 1 hr; SR Tab preparations are somewhat slower. Duration is usually 3–6 hr.

Serum Levels. Therapeutic range is 4–10 mg/L (17–43 μmol/L);[40] toxicity is more likely at serum levels over 12 mg/L (51 μmol/L).[97] In some arrhythmias (eg, recurrent ventricular tachycardia), levels of 20 mg/L (85 μmol/L) or greater may be required for prevention of arrhythmias, with average effective levels of 13 mg/L.[94] Effective serum levels of NAPA are 15–25 mg/L (53–88 μmol/L), with overlap between the toxic and therapeutic ranges.[98]

Fate. Oral bioavailability is 83 ± 16%;[9] about 16 ± 5% is bound to plasma proteins; V_d is 1.9 ± 0.3 L/kg.[9] The drug is 67 ± 8% excreted in the urine as unchanged drug; the remainder is metabolized, mostly to active NAPA by the liver, with smaller amounts excreted as para-aminobenzoic acid. Cl is highly variable depending upon acetylator status and renal function. The total quantity of NAPA produced depends on liver function and acetylator phenotype.[9, 99]

$t_{1/2}$. (Procainamide) α phase about 6 min; β phase in normals 3 ± 0.6 hr, 5.3–20.7 hr in renal dysfunction, with anephric patients averaging 12.5 ± 1.4 hr. (NAPA) 7 ± 1 hr, 41.5 ± 7.8 hr in renal failure.[9,98,99]

Adverse Reactions. About 50–80% of patients develop a positive ANA, with 30–50% developing SLE symptoms; genetically slow acetylators more rapidly develop positive ANA and SLE symptoms.[100] Common SLE symptoms or signs are rash, arthralgias, fever, pericarditis, and pleuritis. Although drug cessation usually reverses these symptoms in about 2 weeks, some patients have prolonged manifestations and for others the SLE syndrome may be initially life-threatening.[100] Hypotension may occur frequently after rapid IV administration. Severe bradycardia, AV nodal block, or asystole have been reported. Procainamide can aggravate underlying ventricular arrhythmias and cause torsades de pointes.[101] GI symptoms occur frequently and include nausea and vomiting; drug fever and dermatologic reactions may occur occasionally.[101] Agranulocytosis is reported occasionally and is potentially fatal. Whether the SR product carries a higher risk of neutropenia than the fast-release preparation is controversial.[102] Hepatitis has been reported rarely.

Contraindications. SLE (including drug-induced); second- or third-degree heart block in the absence of a ventricular pacemaker; long-QT syndrome; severe sinus node dysfunction or torsades de pointes caused by other type Ia antiarrhythmics.

Precautions. In atrial fibrillation or flutter, procainamide may paradoxically increase ventricular rate; administer digoxin or other drugs that slow AV nodal conduction prior to procainamide. Procainamide may worsen symptoms of sick sinus syndrome; it may also exacerbate myasthenia gravis.

Drug Interactions. Amiodarone, trimethoprim, cimetidine, and, to a lesser extent, ranitidine may increase procainamide levels; alcohol may decrease levels.

Parameters to Monitor. Monitor serum levels and symptoms or signs of toxicity in patients with suspected altered drug disposition such as hepatic disease or renal dysfunction. Monitor ECG continuously (with IV) or daily initially (with PO) for QRS, QT, or PR prolongation; monitor oral therapy less frequently once maintenance dosage is established. Monitor blood pressure frequently when therapy is initiated (especially with IV), and less frequently once a maintenance dosage is established. Periodically monitor WBC counts and signs of infection for the development of drug-induced agranulocytosis. Observe closely for symptoms of drug-induced SLE.

PROPAFENONE HYDROCHLORIDE   Rhythmol

Pharmacology. Propafenone is a sodium-channel blocker that predominantly slows atrial and ventricular conduction velocity without appreciably prolonging repolarization. It is therefore classified as a type Ic antiarrhythmic, similar to flecainide. Propafenone is administered as a racemate; the enantiomers and the 5-hydroxy metabolite are all equipotent sodium-channel blockers. Propafenone, particularly the (S)-enantiomer, and its active 5-hydroxy metabolite also have variable, nonselective β-blocking actions.[103]

Administration and Adult Dosage. **PO** 150 mg q 8 hr initially, increasing q 3–4 days to desired effect or toxicity. **PO maintenance** 150–200 mg q 8 hr, to a maximum of 1.2 g/day.[104] Initiate propafenone during hospitalization.

Special Populations. *Pediatric Dosage.* Safety and efficacy not established. **PO** 10–20 mg/kg/day in 2–3 divided doses has been used.[105]

Geriatric Dosage. Same as adult dosage. Lower initial dosages have been suggested.[106]

Other Conditions. Bioavailability and half-life are increased in patients with hepatic disease and dosage reduction of 50% has been suggested,[107] but this has been questioned.[104] Lower initial dosages have been suggested for patients with renal dysfunction.[104]

Dosage Forms. **Tab** 150, 225, 300 mg.

Patient Instructions. Report any symptoms of dizziness, rapid heartbeat, blurred vision, or shortness of breath.

Missed Doses. Take this drug at regular intervals. If you miss a dose, take it as soon as you remember. If it is about time for the next dose, take that dose only. Leave a minimum of 4 hours between doses. Do not double the dose or take extra.

Pharmacokinetics. *Onset and Duration.* Onset 2–4 hr; peak 2–6 hr; duration 4–22 hr.[104,106]

Serum Levels. No established therapeutic range. Levels of parent compound and metabolite are highly variable, depending on genetically determined variations in hepatic metabolism. Mean minimal effective concentration was 0.2 mg/L (6 μmol/L) in one study.[108] Side effects are more frequent when trough propafenone level exceeds 0.9 mg/L (26 μmol/L).[109]

Fate. Completely absorbed after oral administration, but large hepatic first-pass metabolism limits bioavailability to 12.1 ± 11%. First-pass elimination appears saturable, so bioavailability is highly variable and increases with larger oral doses and long-term therapy.[104,106,109] About 85–95% is bound to plasma proteins, primarily α_1-acid glycoprotein.[104] V_d is 3.6 ± 2.6 L/kg.[110] The parent drug undergoes polymorphic hepatic metabolism via the CYP2D6 isozyme. Extensive metabolizers (EMs, about 90% of patients) form clinically important quantities of the active metabolite 5-hydroxypropafenone; poor metabolizers (PMs, about 10% of patients) form little of this compound.[106,109] Another active metabolite, N-desethyl-propafenone, is not subject to genetic polymorphism.[104,109] Cl is 0.96 ± 1.08 L/hr/kg in EMs and 0.23 ± 0.042 L/hr/kg in PMs.[111] Cl is also stereospecific.

$t_{1/2}$. α phase 5 min; β phase (EMs) 5.5 ± 2 hr, (PMs) 17 ± 8 hr.[109]

Adverse Reactions. Frequent noncardiac side effects include metallic or bitter taste in 15–20% of patients, and nausea and CNS toxicity such as dizziness and headache in 10–15% of patients.[110] Because of the β-blocking activity of propafenone, worsening of asthma or obstructive lung disease may occur.[103,110] Propafenone has proarrhythmic actions (sometimes life-threatening), which may result in new or worsened ventricular tachycardia. This may occur in 5–15% of patients, particularly in those with poor left ventricular function caused by structural heart disease or with underlying ventricular tachycardia. Worsening of existing CHF or underlying conduction disturbances, such as AV block or sick sinus syndrome, may occur. Cholestatic jaundice occurs rarely.[112]

Contraindications. Second- or third-degree AV block or bifasicular block in the absence of a ventricular pacemaker; history of type Ic–induced arrhythmia; bronchospastic disorders; uncontrolled CHF; cardiogenic shock; marked hypotension; sick sinus syndrome; bradycardia; electrolyte imbalance.

Precautions. Propafenone may increase pacemaker capture threshold and affect the efficacy of internal defibrillators.[52] Because of the results of CAST (although not studied in this trial), propafenone is indicated only for arrhythmias where there is a clear benefit to therapy.

Drug Interactions. Propafenone inhibits hepatic enzymes and reportedly increases the serum concentrations of digoxin, theophylline, warfarin, and β-blockers.[106]

Parameters to Monitor. Daily or continuous (preferred) ECG for 3–4 days initially, then q 3–6 months on an ambulatory basis. Observe closely for CNS symptoms such as dizziness.

Notes. Although not a labeled indication, propafenone can be effective for some supraventricular arrhythmias.

QUINIDINE SULFATE	Various
QUINIDINE GLUCONATE	Duraquin, Quinaglute, Quinora, Various

Pharmacology. Quinidine is a class Ia antiarrhythmic that slows conduction velocity, prolongs effective refractory period, and decreases automaticity of normal and diseased fibers. (*See* Electrophysiologic Actions of Antiarrhythmics Comparison Chart.) The cellular mechanism appears to be frequency-dependent blockade of the fast sodium channel. Quinidine also blocks potassium conductance, particularly at low concentrations. AV nodal conduction may be increased reflexly through vasodilation, attributed to peripheral α-adrenergic blockade or vagolytic action. Slight negative inotropic action may be clinically important in patients with severe CHF.

Administration and Adult Dosage. **IM and PO loading doses** not recommended. **PO maintenance dosage** generally 200–400 mg q 6–8 hr; **SR products** (gluconate) may be given q 12 hr, (polygalacturonate) may be given q 8 hr. **IV loading dose** (gluconate) 5–8 mg/kg (3.75–6 mg/kg in CHF) at a rate of 0.3 mg/kg/min. (*See* Notes.) Initiate quinidine during hospitalization.

Special Populations. *Pediatric Dosage.* PO (gluconate salt) 15–60 mg/kg/day in 4 divided doses. **IV and IM** not recommended.

Geriatric Dosage. (>60 yr) use lower initial dosages and adjust maintenance dosage based on side effects, therapeutic response, and serum levels.

Other Conditions. In liver disease, CHF, or renal disease, use lower initial dosages and adjust maintenance dosages based on side effects, therapeutic response, and serum levels.[39,113]

Dosage Forms. **Cap** (sulfate) 200, 300 mg; **Tab** (sulfate) 100, 200, 300 mg; (polygalacturonate) 275 mg; **SR Tab** (gluconate) 324, 330 mg; (sulfate) 300 mg; **Inj** (gluconate) 80 mg/mL. (*See* Notes.)

Patient Instructions. Report any symptoms such as blurred vision, dizziness, tinnitus, diarrhea, abnormal bleeding or bruising, rash, or fainting episodes. Do not crush or chew SR tablets. The SR tablet shell may appear in the stool, but this does not mean there was a lack of absorption.

Missed Doses. Take this drug at regular intervals. If you miss a dose and it has been less than 2 hours since your dose was due, take it as soon as you remember. If it is about time for the next dose, take that dose only. Do not double the dose or take extra.

Pharmacokinetics. *Onset and Duration.* PO onset of sulfate within 1 hr, SR gluconate and polygalacturonate salts 2–4 hr. IM onset within 1 hr; IV is immediate. Duration (sulfate) 6–8 hr;[114] SR (gluconate) 12 hr; (polygalacturonate) 8–12 hr.

Serum Levels. Therapeutic range about 2–6 mg/L (6–18 μmol/L), depending on assay. Toxicity is more likely with serum levels over 6 mg/L.[39,40]

Fate. Oral sulfate and gluconate are 80 ± 15% and 71 ± 17% bioavailable, respectively, with some first-pass elimination; bioavailability is increased in the elderly; IM absorption is incomplete.[9,114] The drug is 87 ± 3% bound to plasma proteins.[9] V_d is 2.7 ± 1.2 L/kg, 1.8 ± 0.5 L/kg in patients with CHF; Cl is 0.28 ± 0.11 L/hr/kg.[9,115] The elderly and patients with liver disease or CHF are likely to have decreased clearance.[9] Quinidine is primarily metabolized in the liver to two active metabolites, 3-hydroxyquinidine and 2′-quinidinone, and 18 ± 5% of a dose is excreted unchanged in the urine.

$t_{1/2}$. α phase about 7 min; β phase in normals 6.2 ± 1.8 hr.[9] In CHF, Cl is decreased and V_d is less than normal, so elimination half-life remains about the same.[115] Half-life in alcoholic cirrhosis is prolonged to 9 ± 1 hr.[116]

Adverse Reactions. Diarrhea occurs in up to 30% of patients receiving quinidine, and may be treated with **aluminum hydroxide gel** or by using the polygalacturonate salt. Nausea or vomiting occurs frequently. Cinchonism may occur at high quinidine levels; symptom complex includes tinnitus, blurred vision, headache, and nausea; it may progress in severe cases to delirium and psychosis. Hypotension may occur, especially after IV administration. Quinidine may aggravate underlying ventricular arrhythmias or CHF. Non–dose-related syncope, attributed to drug-induced torsades de pointes, may occur in 1–8% of patients, usually during the first week of therapy; it may occur in association with hypokalemia and/or hypomagnesemia.[117] Asystole or AV nodal block has been reported. Rare or occasional idiosyncratic reactions include hepatitis, drug fever, anaphylactoid reactions, SLE, thrombocytopenia, and hemolytic anemia. IM use may cause pain and muscle damage.[114]

Contraindications. History of past immunologic reaction to quinidine or quinine; previous occurrence of quinidine syncope; second- or third-degree heart block in the absence of a ventricular pacemaker; severe sinus node dysfunction or long-QT syndrome; digitalis intoxication; myasthenia gravis.

Precautions. In atrial fibrillation or flutter, administer digoxin or other drugs that decrease AV nodal conduction prior to quinidine. Chronic quinidine use in patients with atrial fibrillation is associated with increased mortality,[118] which may be caused by torsades de pointes occurring late in therapy.[119]

Drug Interactions. Quinidine is an inhibitor of CYP2D6 and may alter the disposition of many drugs that undergo genetically determined polymorphic metabolism through this pathway. Use care with concurrent digitalis and quinidine therapy, because quinidine increases digoxin or digitoxin serum levels approximately 2-fold. Urinary alkalinization (eg, with acetazolamide or antacids) can decrease quinidine clearance. Phenytoin may increase quinidine metabolism. Amiodarone and cimetidine may reduce quinidine clearance. Quinidine occasionally increases warfarin response and tricyclic antidepressant serum levels.

Parameters to Monitor. Monitor serum levels and signs or symptoms of toxicity in patients with altered drug disposition such as CHF or liver disease. ECG, observing for QT, QRS, or PR prolongation daily for first 2–4 days of therapy, then q 3–6 months on an ambulatory basis. Monitor blood pressure (especially with IV) frequently when therapy is initiated. These may be done less frequently when a maintenance dosage is determined. Monitor liver enzymes during the first 4–8 weeks of therapy. Monitor other parameters, such as platelet count and hematocrit, only if idiosyncratic reactions are suspected.

Notes. Adjust dosage when switching from one salt form to another; sulfate salt contains 83% quinidine, gluconate 62%, and polygalacturonate 60%. The gluconate and polygalacturonate forms are slowly dissociating salts of quinidine.

SOTALOL HYDROCHLORIDE   Betapace

Pharmacology. Sotalol is a type III antiarrhythmic that is commercially available as a racemate: the l-isomer has nonselective β-blocking actions, and both the D- and L-isomers delay repolarization by blockade of potassium channels. (*See* Electrophysiologic Actions of Antiarrhythmics Comparison Chart.) Sotalol is effective for both ventricular and (unlabeled) supraventricular arrhythmias.

Administration and Adult Dosage. PO 80 mg bid initially, increasing at 2- to 3-day intervals, to a maximum of 640 mg/day in 2 or 3 divided doses. Reserve high dosages (480–640 mg/day) for drug-refractory ventricular arrhythmias. Initiate sotalol during hospitalization.

Special Populations. *Pediatric Dosage.* Safety and efficacy not established. **PO** 2–8 mg/kg/day in 2 divided doses has been used.[120]

Geriatric Dosage. Same as adult dosage.

Other Conditions. Reduce frequency of administration in patients with renal insufficiency as follows: Cl_{cr} 30–60 mL/min, q 24 hr; Cl_{cr} 10–30 mL/min, q 36–48 hr.[121] Use with caution, if at all, in patients with Cl_{cr} <10 mL/min.

Dosage Forms. **Tab** 80, 160, 240 mg.

Patient Instructions. Report any symptoms of fainting, dizziness, shortness of breath, or fatigue.

Missed Doses. Take this drug at regular intervals. If you miss a dose and your next dose is more than 8 hours away, take it as soon as you remember. If it is about time for the next dose, take that dose only. Do not double the dose or take extra.

Pharmacokinetics. *Onset and Duration.* PO onset 1–3 hr; duration 12–18 hr.

Serum Levels. 1–3 mg/L (3.7–11 μmol/L), although not well correlated with therapeutic effect. Concentrations required to achieve delay in repolarization may be greater than for β-blockade.[120]

Fate. Bioavailability is 90–100% with negligible first-pass metabolism.[121] AUC is decreased 20% by food.[121] The drug is not bound to plasma proteins. V_d is 1.2–2.4 L/kg; Cl is 0.13 ± 0.04 L/hr/kg;[121–123] 80–90% is excreted unchanged in urine.[121] The disposition of the d-isomer is similar to that of the racemate.[122,123]

$t_{1/2}$. α phase 3–5 min; β phase variously reported as 7.5 ± 0.8 to 17.5 ± 9.7 hr.[123,124] Half-life is highly dependent on renal function: 22.7 ± 6.4 hr for Cl_{cr} 30–80 mL/hr; 64 ± 27 hr for Cl_{cr} 10–30 mL/hr; and 98 ± 57 hr for Cl_{cr} <10 mL/min.[124]

Adverse Reactions. Fatigue, dyspnea, and bradycardia occur frequently, probably caused by the β-blocking actions of sotalol.[125] Exacerbation of CHF (1.7%) and asthma may also occur. (*See* Propranolol.) Sotalol induces arrhythmias, usually torsades de pointes, in 4.6% of patients.[125] Risk factors for torsades de pointes are hypokalemia, hypomagnesemia, concurrent diuretic usage, and high sotalol dosages.[126]

Contraindications. Asthma; symptomatic sinus tachycardia; second- and third-degree AV block in the absence of a ventricular pacemaker; long-QT syndrome; uncontrolled CHF.

Precautions. Use with caution in sinus node dysfunction. Because of its β-blocking actions, use sotalol with caution in patients with diabetes, depressed left ventricular function, obstructive pulmonary disease, or peripheral vascular disease. Do not abruptly discontinue the drug in patients with coronary artery disease. Use with caution with electrolyte disorders, other drugs that prolong QT interval, or pre-existing QT prolongation. Escalate dosage only after perceived steady state (2–3 days).[127]

Drug Interactions. Because of its β-blocking actions, observe β-blocker interaction precautions. (*See* Propranolol.)

Parameters to Monitor. Baseline and daily ECG for first 2–5 days when therapy is initiated or dosage adjusted, then q 3–6 months on an ambulatory basis. QT prolongation to over 550 msec is an indication to discontinue sotalol because of the risk of torsades de pointes.

Notes. After the results of CAST,[16] many clinicians use type III antiarrhythmics (eg, amiodarone, sotalol) as first-line therapy in both supraventricular and ventricular arrhythmias. Most antiarrhythmics currently under investigation are similar to sotalol in structure and electrophysiologic actions.[54]

TOCAINIDE   Tonocard

Pharmacology. Tocainide has electrophysiologic actions similar to lidocaine and mexiletine. Depression of conduction is accentuated in ischemic/hypoxic tissue. Antiarrhythmic actions are somewhat stereospecific. It also has a slight negative inotropic action. It is used in the treatment of ventricular arrhythmias, but it has limited effectiveness in supraventricular tachycardias. There may be a concordance of response (and nonresponse) between tocainide and lidocaine.[128]

Administration and Adult Dosage. PO 400 mg q 8 hr initially; **usual maintenance dosage** is 1.2–1.8 g/day, to a maximum of 2.4 g/day in 2–3 divided doses. **PO during lidocaine to tocainide conversion** 600 mg q 6 hr for 3 doses, then 600 mg q 12 hr; discontinue lidocaine infusion at the time of the second oral dose of tocainide.[129] Initiate tocainide during hospitalization.

Special Populations. *Pediatric Dosage.* Safety and efficacy not established.

Geriatric Dosage. Same as adult dosage.

Other Conditions. Reduce initial maintenance dosage by 50% in severe liver disease, by 25% in patients with Cl_{cr} of 10–30 mL/min, and by 50% in patients with Cl_{cr} <10 mL/min.[130] Dosages may have to be slightly reduced in CHF, but more data are needed.[131]

Dosage Forms. **Tab** 400, 600 mg.

Patient Instructions. Report any symptoms of numbness, drowsiness, dizziness, or tingling. Nausea or loss of appetite may occur and may be reduced by taking the drug with food. Report sore throat, mouth sores, fever, or abnormal bruising.

Missed Doses. Take this drug at regular intervals. If you miss a dose, take it as soon as you remember. If it is about time for the next dose, take that dose only. Leave a minimum of 4–6 hours between doses. Do not double the dose or take extra.

Pharmacokinetics. *Onset and Duration.* PO onset 1–2 hr (delayed by food); duration 12–24 hr.

Serum Levels. 3–10 mg/L (16–52 μmol/L), although not well correlated with therapeutic or toxic effects.[40,132]

Fate. Oral bioavailability is 89 ± 5% with negligible first-pass metabolism.[130–132] The drug is 10 ± 15% plasma protein bound.[9,133] V_d is 3 ± 0.2 L/kg, slightly lower in CHF;[130,131] Cl is 0.16 ± 0.03 L/hr/kg[9]; 38 ± 7% of the drug is excreted unchanged in urine, and 50–60% is hepatically eliminated.[130,132] Renal clearance is dependent on urine pH; hepatic metabolism is stereospecific, with the (S)-enantiomer eliminated more quickly.[134]

$t_{1/2}$. α phase 5–10 min;[133] β phase 13.5 ± 2.3 hr, 14–19 hr with ventricular arrhythmia or CHF,[132] 22 ± 3.1 hr in severe renal insufficiency.[135]

Adverse Reactions. Neurologic toxicities, which include dizziness, tremor, ataxia, drowsiness, confusion, and paresthesias, are frequent (30–50%); psychosis and seizures occur occasionally. The neurologic toxicities of lidocaine and tocainide may be additive.[136] Nausea, vomiting, and anorexia occur frequently. Tocainide may exacerbate underlying ventricular arrhythmias or conduction disturbances. Agranulocytosis and other forms of bone marrow depression have been reported in up to 0.18% of patients.[132] Pulmonary fibrosis or interstitial pneumonitis occurs in 0.03–0.11% of patients.[129] Rash and fever occur occasionally, with cross-sensitivity between lidocaine and tocainide possible.[81]

Contraindications. Second- or third-degree AV block in the absence of a ventricular pacemaker.

Precautions. Worsening of sick sinus syndrome may occur. May worsen CHF.

Drug Interactions. Cimetidine may decrease tocainide serum levels; rifampin may decrease levels.

Parameters to Monitor. Monitor ECG daily for 2–4 days when therapy is initiated, then q 3–6 months on an ambulatory basis. Obtain periodic serum levels once an individual's effective level is determined. Observe closely for neurologic toxicities when initiating therapy. Monitor WBC counts frequently, particularly during the first 3 months of therapy.[132] Obtain baseline chest x-ray; repeat if pulmonary symptoms arise.

Notes. Because of reports of bone marrow toxicity, pulmonary fibrosis, and hypersensitivity reactions, the indications for tocainide are restricted to patients with life-threatening ventricular arrhythmias.

ELECTROPHYSIOLOGIC ACTIONS OF ANTIARRHYTHMICS COMPARISON CHART

CLASS AND DRUG[a,b]	CONDUCTION VELOCITY	REFRACTORY PERIOD	AUTOMATICITY	AV NODAL CONDUCTION
IA (INTERMEDIATE SODIUM-CHANNEL BLOCKERS)				
Disopyramide	↓↓	↑↑	↓↓	↑
Procainamide	↓↓	↑↑	↓↓	↑/↓
Quinidine	↓↓	↑↑	↓↓	↑/↓
IB (FAST ON-OFF SODIUM-CHANNEL BLOCKERS)				
Lidocaine				
Normal Tissue	0	→↓	→↓↓	0
Ischemic Tissue	↓↓	→↑	→	0
Mexiletine	0	→	→	0
Phenytoin				
Normal Tissue	0	→↓	→↓↓	←↑
Ischemic Tissue	↓↓	→↑	→	←↑
Tocainide	0	→	→	0
IC (SLOW ON-OFF SODIUM-CHANNEL BLOCKERS)				
Flecainide	↓↓↓	0	→	0
Moricizine[c]	↓↓↓	↓/0	→	0
Propafenone[e]	↓↓↓	0	→	0
II (β-BLOCKERS)				
Propranolol[d]	→	↓ (acute) ↑ (chronic)	→	↓↓

(continued)

CLASS AND DRUG[a,b]	CONDUCTION VELOCITY	REFRACTORY PERIOD	AUTOMATICITY	AV NODAL CONDUCTION
III (POTASSIUM-CHANNEL BLOCKERS)				
Amiodarone[e,g]	0/↓	↑↑	0	↓
Bretylium	0	↑↑	↑/0	↑/0
Ibutilide	0	↑↑	0	0
Sotalol[e,f]	0	↑	0	↓
IV (CALCIUM-CHANNEL BLOCKERS)				
Diltiazem	0	0	0	↓
Verapamil	0	0	0	↓↓

↑ = increase, ↓ = decrease, 0 = minimal or no effect, ↑/↓ = variable.

[a]Classification system from references 137 and 138.

[b]Type I antiarrhythmics are subdivided into Ia, Ib, and Ic based on their actions on repolarization in normal ventricular tissue and their binding characteristics to the sodium channel: type Ia prolongs repolarization; type Ib shortens repolarization; type Ic causes no change in repolarization.

[c]Classification of moricizine is controversial; it also has type Ia characteristics.

[d]When caused by sympathetic stimulation.

[e]Amiodarone, propafenone, and sotalol also have type II or β-adrenergic–blocking activity.

[f]Most investigational antiarrhythmics are potassium-channel blockers, many of which are analogues of sotalol. (*See* reference 46.)

[g]Amiodarone also has type Ib sodium-channel–blocking activity.

313

Antihypertensive Drugs

Class Instructions: Antihypertensives. This medication can control hypertension, but it will not cure the disease. Long-term treatment is necessary to control hypertension and prevent damage to several body systems. Do not start or stop taking medications or change the dosage without medical supervision, and avoid running out of medications. Some prescription and nonprescription medications may interact with medications for hypertension; make sure that your physician and pharmacist know the names of any other medications that you are taking.

Missed Doses. Take this drug at regular intervals. If you miss a dose, take it as soon as you remember. If it is about time for the next dose, take that dose only. Do not double the dose or take extra.

α_1-ADRENERGIC–BLOCKING DRUGS:	
DOXAZOSIN MESYLATE	Cardura
PRAZOSIN HYDROCHLORIDE	Minipress, Various
TERAZOSIN HYDROCHLORIDE	Hytrin

Pharmacology. Doxazosin, prazosin, and terazosin are closely related quinazoline derivatives that selectively block postsynaptic α_1-adrenergic receptors. Total peripheral resistance is reduced through both arterial and venous dilation. Reflex tachycardia that occurs with other vasodilators is infrequent because of the absence of presynaptic, α_2-receptor blockade. The drugs also decrease total cholesterols, increase HDL cholesterol, and may improve glucose tolerance and reduce left ventricular mass during long-term therapy. They increase urine flow in BPH by relaxing smooth muscle tone in the bladder neck and prostate.[139,140]

Administration and Adult Dosage. The initial dose, and the first dose of all increased dosage regimens, should be given hs, and the patient observed closely for syncope. **PO for hypertension** (doxazosin) 1 mg/day initially, double the dose at 1- to 2-week intervals, to a maximum of 16 mg/day in a single dose, although dosages over 4 mg/day are more likely to cause postural side effects. (Prazosin) 1 mg bid or tid initially, increase dosage slowly, based on response, to the usual dosage of 6–15 mg/day; although the maximum effective dosage is usually 20 mg/day, dosages up to 40 mg/day may be effective in some patients who fail to respond to lower dosages. (Terazosin) 1 mg/day initially, increase to 2, 5, or 10 mg/day in 1–2 doses, to a maximum of 20 mg/day. **PO for benign prostatic hypertrophy** (doxazosin) 1 mg/day initially, double the dose at 1- to 2-week intervals, to a maximum of 8 mg/day. (Terazosin) 1 mg/day initially, increase to 2, 5, and finally 10 mg/day in 1–2 divided doses.

Special Populations. *Pediatric Dosage.* **PO for hypertension** (prazosin) 0.05–0.4 mg/kg/day in 2–3 divided doses. Do not exceed single doses of 7 mg and a total daily dosage of 15 mg.[141] (Doxazosin, terazosin) safety and efficacy not established.

Geriatric Dosage. Same as adult dosage, although the dosage of doxazosin should be increased at longer intervals because of its longer half-life in the elderly.[142]

Dosage Forms. (Doxazosin) **Tab** 1, 2, 4, 8 mg. (Prazosin) **Cap** 1, 2, 5 mg; **Cap** 1, 2, 5 mg with polythiazide 0.5 mg (Minizide). (Terazosin) **Cap** 1, 2, 5, 10 mg.

Patient Instructions. (*See* Antihypertensives Class Instructions.) Take the initial dose of this drug at bedtime. Dizziness or drowsiness may occur with this medication, especially after the first dose or when the dosage is being increased. Do not arise suddenly, stand for long periods, or exercise too vigorously, especially in hot weather. Alcohol may worsen all of these effects.

Pharmacokinetics. *Onset and Duration.* (Doxazosin) onset 1–2 hr, duration 24 hr for hypertension; full effect for BPH may not occur for 1–2 weeks. (Prazosin) onset 1–2 hr, duration about 6–12 hr, up to 4–6 weeks may be required for full antihypertensive effect. (Terazosin) onset 15 min, duration 24 hr, but up to 6–8 weeks may be required for full antihypertensive effect. In BPH, a minimum of 4–6 weeks may be required to fully evaluate response to 10 mg/day dosage.

Serum Levels. No established correlation between serum levels and clinical effect.[9,140]

Fate. (Doxazosin) oral bioavailability is $63 \pm 14\%$; absorption is slowed, but bioavailability is not affected by food; 98–99% is plasma protein bound. V_d is 1.5 ± 0.3 L/kg; Cl is 0.1 ± 0.024 L/kg/hr. Extensively metabolized and excreted primarily in the feces, with only about 9% excreted in urine as unchanged drug and metabolites.[9,140] (Prazosin) bioavailability is $68 \pm 17\%$, $48 \pm 16\%$ in the elderly; food may delay, but does not affect the extent of absorption. About 95% is plasma protein bound, decreased in cirrhosis and uremia. V_d is 0.63 ± 0.14 L/kg and Cl is 0.24 ± 0.04 L/hr/kg in young patients; V_d is 0.89 ± 0.26 L/kg and Cl is 0.21 ± 0.06 L/hr/kg in the elderly; Cl is lower in CHF and pregnancy. Prazosin is metabolized in the liver by demethylation and conjugation; metabolites have about 20% of the activity of the drug. It is excreted renally as metabolites and 3.4% or less as unchanged drug.[143] (Terazosin) pharmacokinetics do not appear to be affected by uremia, CHF, or aging. Oral bioavailability is about 90%. From 90–94% is plasma protein bound. V_d is 0.8 ± 0.18 L/kg; Cl is 0.066 ± 0.012 L/hr/kg.[9] It is extensively metabolized in the liver, with 18% excreted unchanged in feces, 10% unchanged in urine, and the remainder excreted as metabolites.[144]

t½. (Doxazosin) 10.5 ± 2.4 hr in young adults, 11.9 ± 4.7 hr in the elderly. (Prazosin) 2.1 ± 0.3 hr in young adults, 3.2 ± 0.6 hr in the elderly; also prolonged in CHF and pregnancy. (Terazosin) 13.5 ± 3.5 hr in young adults, 16.2 ± 2.2 hr in the elderly.[142]

Adverse Reactions. The most important adverse effect is first-dose syncope, which is more likely in patients being treated with other antihypertensive drugs, especially diuretics. During long-term treatment, the most frequent reactions are dizziness, headache, drowsiness, lack of energy or weakness, palpitations, or nausea, all of which occur in 5–20% of patients. Occasionally reported are rash, vomiting, diarrhea, edema, orthostatic hypotension, syncope, dyspnea, blurred vision, nasal congestion, or urinary frequency. Rarely, allergic reactions, priapism, or impotence occur.[145]

Contraindications. Allergy to a quinazoline derivative.

Precautions. Syncope may occur after the first dose (doxazosin, 2–6 hr; prazosin, 30–90 min; terazosin, 1–2 hr), but may also occur during rapid upward dosage titration or when adding an additional antihypertensive drug. Hold doses of diuretics for 1 day before starting an α_1-blocker. Increase dosage gradually and reduce dosage when adding another antihypertensive, then retitrate dosage. Use doxazosin with caution in patients with hepatic impairment.

Drug Interactions. β-Blockers and verapamil may enhance postural effects of prazosin; NSAIDs may decrease the hypotensive effect of prazosin. The α_1-blockers may decrease the hypotensive effect of clonidine.

Parameters to Monitor. Monitor blood pressure regularly.

Notes. α_1-Antagonists may be particularly useful for hypertension in men with BPH, in those with hyperlipidemia or renal disease, in diabetics, in physically active young patients (no decrease in cardiac output), and in the elderly.[139,142] However, drugs in this class have not been shown to decrease long-term mortality of hypertension.[140] **Tamsulosin** (Flomax) is a selective α_{1a}-receptor blocker, specific for adrenoreceptors in the prostate. Tamsulosin is not indicated for hypertension, but rather for signs and symptoms of BPH. The initial oral dosage is 0.4 mg/day, increasing as needed up to 0.8 mg/day.

CAPTOPRIL
Capoten, Various

Pharmacology. Captopril is an ACE inhibitor pharmacologically similar to enalapril. Captopril's rapid onset and short duration of action are advantageous initially to assess patient tolerance to ACE inhibitors, but are inconvenient during long-term use.[146–149] (*See* ACE Inhibitors Comparison Chart.)

Adult Dosage. **PO for hypertension** 12.5–25 mg bid–tid initially, increasing after 1–2 weeks to 50 mg bid–tid, to a maximum of 450 mg/day. **PO for CHF** 6.25–25 mg tid initially, then increase over several days based on patient tolerance to a dosage of 50 mg tid. Delay further dosage increases, if possible, for at least 2 weeks to evaluate response. Most patients respond to 50–100 mg tid. **For hypertension or CHF** reduce initial dosages by 50–75% and increase slowly in patients on diuretic therapy, with sodium restriction or with renal impairment. **PO for left ventricular dysfunction post-MI** 6.25 mg once at 3 or more days post-MI, then 12.5 mg tid; increase to 25 mg tid over several days to a target of 50 mg tid over several weeks as tolerated. **PO for diabetic nephropathy** 25 mg tid.

Pediatric Dosage. **PO for hypertension** (neonates) 0.01 mg/kg bid–tid initially; (children) up to 0.3 mg/kg tid initially.[146]

Dosage Forms. **Tab** 12.5, 25, 50, and 100 mg, and 25 or 50 mg in combination with hydrochlorothiazide 15 or 25 mg (Capozide, various).

Pharmacokinetics. Oral bioavailability is about 65%; food decreases absorption, so the drug should be taken on an empty stomach. About 30% is plasma protein bound and its $V_{d\beta}$ is 2 ± 0.09 L/kg; Cl is 0.76 L/hr/kg in normals, 0.31 L/hr/kg in mild renal dysfunction, and 0.096 L/hr/kg in dialysis patients between dialyses. Approximately 50% of a dose is metabolized, primarily to captopril disulfide, which can be converted back to active captopril in vivo. Urinary excretion of unchanged captopril is 24–38% over 24 hr. Its half-life is estimated to be 1.7 ± 0.02 hr in healthy subjects, and is prolonged in renal dysfunction or CHF.[147]

Adverse Reactions. Adverse reactions are similar to enalapril's, although skin rashes and taste impairment may be more prevalent, and cough may be less prevalent.[148]

CLONIDINE HYDROCHLORIDE   Catapres, Various

Pharmacology. Clonidine stimulates postsynaptic α_2-adrenergic receptors in the CNS, activating inhibitory neurons to produce a decrease in sympathetic outflow. Since clonidine is not a complete agonist, some of its effects may also result from antagonist actions at presynaptic α-receptors.[150] These actions result in a reduction in peripheral vascular resistance, renal vascular resistance, heart rate, and blood pressure.

Administration and Adult Dosage. PO for hypertension 0.1 mg bid initially, increasing weekly in increments of 0.1 mg/day until the desired response is achieved. **Maintenance dosage for monotherapy** is usually 0.2–0.6 mg/day, to a maximum of 2.4 mg/day. If rapid blood pressure lowering is desired (eg, hypertensive urgency), give 0.1–0.2 mg initially, then 0.1 mg q 1 hr until desired response is achieved or a total of 0.8 mg has been given. **SR patch for hypertension** initially apply one #1 (0.1 mg/24 hr) patch weekly; dosage may be increased at 1- to 2-week intervals up to a #3 patch that delivers 0.3 mg/24 hr. Dosages in excess of two #3 patches/week do not produce additional efficacy. **PO for opiate withdrawal** 1.25–1.5 mg/day in 3–4 divided doses, decreasing over 14 days by 0.1–0.2 mg/day.[151] **PO for smoking cessation** 0.1–0.3 mg/day in divided doses.[152] **SR patch for smoking cessation** apply one #1 (0.1 mg/24 hr) patch weekly.[152] (*See* Notes.)

Special Populations. *Pediatric Dosage.* Safety and efficacy not established.

Geriatric Dosage. Lower oral dosages may be required, but decreased skin permeability may require higher transdermal dosages.[153]

Other Conditions. In renal impairment, lower oral dosages may be required, but decreased skin permeability may require higher transdermal dosages.[153]

Dosage Forms. Tab 0.1, 0.2, 0.3 mg; **Tab** 0.1, 0.2, 0.3 mg with chlorthalidone 15 mg (Combipres, various); **SR Patch** 0.1, 0.2, 0.3 mg/24 hr.

Patient Instructions. (*See* Antihypertensives Class Instructions.) Do not abruptly discontinue this drug or interrupt therapy unless under medical supervision. Apply transdermal patches weekly to a clean, hairless area of the upper arm or torso that is free of irritation, abrasions, or scars. Do not touch the adhesive surface. Apply patch to a different location with each application. If the system loosens during the 7 days, apply the adhesive overlay directly over the system. If a generalized rash or moderate to severe redness or vesicles appear at the site of application, notify the prescriber. Dispose of the patch by folding the sides together and placing in a disposal site inaccessible to children.

Missed Doses. Take this drug at regular intervals. If you miss a dose, take it as soon as you remember. If it is about time for your next dose, take that dose only. Do not double the dose or take extra. Contact your physician if you miss two or more doses or if you are late in changing the transdermal system by 3 or more days.

Pharmacokinetics. *Onset and Duration.* (Hypertension) PO onset 30–60 min; peak 2–5 hr; duration 6–8 hr, but may increase to 12–24 hr with long-term use.[153] Transdermally, maximal reduction in blood pressure occurs in 2–3 days and persists throughout the 7-day application period. After removal, the blood pressure rapidly increases toward baseline initially, followed by a slower rate of increase, and returns to pretreatment levels over several days.[150]

Serum Levels. (Hypotensive effect) 0.2–2 μg/L (0.9–9 nmol/L); (dry mouth, sedation) 1.5–2 μg/L.[153]

Fate. Oral bioavailability is 75–95%.[153] Transdermally, maximum serum levels are reached in 3–4 days and remain constant throughout the 7-day application period.[150] Rate of release is a zero-order process and primarily controlled by the delivery system. Serum concentrations remain constant when a patch is removed and another is immediately applied to a different site.[150] Clonidine is 20% plasma protein bound; V_d is 2.1 ± 0.4 L/kg; Cl is 0.186 ± 0.072 L/hr/kg.[9] It is metabolized in the liver, with drug and metabolites excreted primarily in urine; remaining drug may undergo enterohepatic recycling. About 62% is excreted unchanged in urine.[9]

$t_{\frac{1}{2}}$ (PO) α phase 10.8 ± 4.7 min; β phase 12 ± 7 hr.[9] (Transdermal) 14 hr, but may be up to 26 hr, reflecting continued absorption from a skin depot.[150]

Adverse Reactions. Frequent adverse reactions include dry mouth (40%), drowsiness (33%), dizziness (16%), constipation (10%), weakness (10%), sedation (10%), nausea or vomiting (5%), nervousness and agitation (3%), orthostatic hypotension (3%), and sexual dysfunction (3%). Occasionally rash, weight gain, anorexia, transient abnormalities in liver function tests, insomnia or vivid dreams, palpitations, tachycardia or bradycardia, or urinary retention occur. Rarely hepatitis, thrombocytopenia, parotitis, elevations of blood glucose or CPK, or cardiac conduction disturbances occur. Allergic contact dermatitis occurs in up to 50% of patients treated with patches.[154] Abrupt withdrawal of oral therapy may result in a withdrawal reaction characterized by rapid reversal of antihypertensive effect within 24–48 hr up to or above pretreatment levels, a rise of blood pressure >40 mm Hg systolic or >25 mm Hg diastolic, or a blood pressure >225/125 mm Hg. Subjective symptoms of sweating, palpitations, anxiety, and insomnia may also occur, even in the absence of marked blood pressure changes. The frequency and severity of symptoms appear to be greater in patients treated with high dosages for >3 months and in those with more severe hypertension.[155]

Precautions. Use with caution in patients with severe coronary insufficiency, conduction disturbances, recent MI, cerebrovascular disease, or chronic renal failure. Patients who develop a rash from the transdermal system may develop a generalized skin rash if oral clonidine is substituted.[154] Inadvertent person-to-person transfer of the patches has been reported; check application site frequently and dispose of patch by folding adhesive sides together and placing in a container inaccessible to children.[156]

Drug Interactions. Heterocyclic antidepressants may decrease the hypotensive effect of clonidine. Clonidine may inhibit the antiparkinson effect of levodopa. Clonidine use with propranolol may cause *hyper*tension, especially if clonidine is abruptly discontinued. Direct-acting sympathomimetics may have an exaggerated effect during clonidine use. Prazosin may decrease the effects of clonidine. Synergistic hypotension and conduction disturbances may occur with verapamil.

Parameters to Monitor. Monitor blood pressure regularly; check patient compliance.

Notes. Clonidine has been used to suppress symptoms of withdrawal of opiates and to reduce craving and other symptoms in alcohol and tobacco withdrawal.[151,152,157] It has also been used in a variety of psychiatric applications including treatment of mania, anxiety, panic disorders, schizophrenia, and in the treatment of antipsychotic-induced tardive dyskinesia.[157] As an aid in the diagnosis of pheochromocytoma, a single 0.3 mg dose has been administered after determination of baseline catecholamine levels, followed by three subsequent determinations at hourly intervals.[158] Other conditions for which it may be effective include diabetic diarrhea (0.1–0.6 mg q 12 hr), menopausal flushing (0.1–0.2 mg bid), and premenstrual syndrome.[159–161] **Apraclonidine** (Iopidine) is a clonidine derivative for control of intraocular pressure following laser trabeculostomy or iridotomy.

DIAZOXIDE
Hyperstat I.V., Proglycem, Various

Pharmacology. Diazoxide is a nondiuretic thiazide that reduces total peripheral resistance via direct relaxation of arteriolar smooth muscle. It also increases heart rate, cardiac output, and renal blood flow. Diazoxide increases blood glucose by inhibiting insulin release and by inhibiting peripheral utilization.

Administration and Adult Dosage. **IV for severe hypertension** 1–3 mg/kg, to a maximum single dose of 150 mg administered undiluted over less than 30 sec q 5–15 min, until adequate blood pressure reduction is achieved. (*See* Notes.) Repeat q 4–24 hr as needed to maintain blood pressure control. A slow infusion of 15–30 mg/min, to a total dosage of 5 mg/kg or until an adequate blood pressure reduction is achieved, is also effective and may avoid excessive reduction in blood pressure.[162] Administration for longer than 10 days is not recommended. **PO for hypoglycemia** 3–8 mg/kg/day in 2–3 equal doses q 8–12 hr, titrated to response.

Special Populations. *Pediatric Dosage.* **IV for severe hypertension** same as adult dosage. **PO for hypoglycemia** (neonates and infants) 8–15 mg/kg/day in 2–3 divided doses q 8–12 hr, titrated to response; (children) same as adult dosage.

Geriatric Dosage. Same as adult dosage.

Other Conditions. Uremic patients may be particularly sensitive to hypotensive effects.

Dosage Forms. **Inj** 15 mg/mL (Hyperstat I.V.); **Cap** 50 mg (Proglycem); **Susp** 50 mg/mL (Proglycem).

Patient Instructions. (*See* Antihypertensives Class Instructions.) Remain in the supine position during and immediately following IV administration.

Pharmacokinetics. *Onset and Duration.* (Hypertension) onset in 2–4 min; peak within 5 min; duration is 3–12 hr. (Hypoglycemia) onset within 1 hr; duration 8 hr.

Serum Levels. 35 mg/L (152 μmol/L) produces a 20–25% reduction in MAP.[9,163] Levels required for the hyperglycemic effect are not known.

Fate. Oral bioavailability is 86–96%; 94 ± 14% is plasma protein bound at typical concentrations, decreased at higher concentrations and in uremia. V_d is 0.21 ± 0.02 L/kg with normal renal function; Cl is 0.0036 ± 0.0012 L/hr/kg. The drug is metabolized by oxidation and sulfate conjugation and excreted slowly in urine as unchanged drug (20–50%) and metabolites.[9,163]

t½. β phase 48 ± 12 hr, prolonged in renal failure in proportion to Cl_{cr}.[9,163]

Adverse Reactions. (Hypertension) with the previous 300 mg bolus dose regimen, hypotension (7%), nausea and vomiting (4%), and dizziness and weakness (2%) are the most frequent reactions. Use of the currently recommended regimen, which has replaced the 300 mg bolus dose, produces similar but less frequent and/or severe adverse effects. Sodium and water retention, and hyperglycemia may occur, especially with repeated administration. Hypotension may lead to cerebral or myocardial ischemia. (Hypoglycemia) frequent adverse reactions include sodium and fluid retention, which may precipitate CHF; hyperglycemia or glycosuria, which may require dosage reduction; hirsutism of the lanugo type and distribution, which subsides upon drug discontinuation; tachycardia; palpitations; increases in uric acid; thrombocytopenia with or without purpura, which requires discontinuation of the drug; neutropenia, which is transient, is not associated with an increased susceptibility to infection, and usually does not require discontinuation; eosinophilia; decreased hemoglobin and hematocrit; increased AST levels; a reversible nephrotic syndrome; hematuria; and albuminuria. Rarely, diabetic ketoacidosis or hyperosmolar, nonketotic coma may develop rapidly.

Contraindications. Hypersensitivity to thiazides or other sulfonamide derivatives; compensatory hypertension, such as that seen secondary to coarctation of the aorta or arteriovenous shunts; functional hypoglycemia; dissecting aortic aneurysm.

Precautions. Use with caution in patients with impaired cerebral or cardiac circulation in whom rapid reduction of blood pressure may be detrimental. Avoid extravasation of the IV drug because of its alkalinity. Highly protein bound drugs may be displaced; recent or co-administration of other antihypertensive drugs may produce excessive blood pressure reduction with the IV route. Some patients may attain higher drug levels with the oral suspension than with the capsules; when switching from one oral dosage form to another, it may be necessary to retitrate the dosage.

Drug Interactions. Diazoxide and hydantoins may be mutually antagonistic. Use with a thiazide diuretic may potentiate hyperuricemia and hypotensive effects.

Phenothiazines may potentiate the effects of oral diazoxide. Diazoxide may antagonize the effects of sulfonylureas.

Parameters to Monitor. (Hypertension) frequent measurements of blood pressure until stable, then hourly; blood glucose and uric acid with repeated doses. Monitor for signs of cerebral or myocardial ischemia. (Hypoglycemia) frequent blood glucose and urine glucose and ketones initially, and when dosage adjustments or dosage form changes are made, then regularly during stabilization. Because of the long half-life, up to 7 days of monitoring may be required in patients who develop hyperglycemia.

Notes. Previous antihypertensive dosage recommendations used rapid IV push administration to allow for drug effect before extensive protein binding occurred. However, the recognition that diazoxide has a greater affinity for arterial wall binding sites than for serum albumin has led to the use of short infusion regimens.[164] Concomitant diuretic therapy may be necessary with repeated administration to counteract diazoxide-induced sodium and water retention and to avoid precipitating CHF.

ENALAPRIL MALEATE	Vasotec
ENALAPRILAT	Vasotec

Pharmacology. Enalapril is a prodrug rapidly converted to its active metabolite, enalaprilat, by ester hydrolysis in the liver. Enalaprilat is a competitive ACE inhibitor. It also reduces serum aldosterone, leading to decreased sodium retention, potentiates the vasodilator kallikrein-kinin system, and may alter prostanoid metabolism, inhibit the sympathetic nervous system, and inhibit the tissue renin-angiotensin system. The net effect is reduction in total peripheral resistance and blood pressure in hypertensive patients, especially those with high pretreatment plasma renin activity and increased renal plasma flow, and reduction of elevated afterload in patients with CHF.[148]

Administration and Adult Dosage. **PO for hypertension** 5 mg/day initially. **Usual maintenance dosage** is 10–40 mg/day in 1–2 doses. If the patient has recently been receiving a diuretic, discontinue the diuretic for 2–3 days or start with a lower initial enalapril dose of 2.5 mg; bid administration may be necessary in some individuals to achieve adequate 24-hr blood pressure control. A diuretic may be added if blood pressure control is inadequate with enalapril monotherapy. **PO for CHF** 2.5 daily, bid initially, using the lower dosage for patients taking a diuretic. **Usual maintenance dosage** is 5–20 mg/day, to a maximum of 40 mg; bid administration is preferred. **IV for hypertension** 1.25 mg (0.625 mg initially if patient is taking a diuretic) over 5 min q 6 hr. Dosages as high as 5 mg q 6 hr may be tolerated for up to 36 hr, but there is inadequate experience with dosages over 20 mg/day. For patients converting from PO to IV, 5 mg/day PO is about equivalent to 1.25 mg IV q 6 hr.

Special Populations. *Pediatric Dosage.* Safety and efficacy not established.

Geriatric Dosage. No change required necessarily, but observe cautions for impaired renal function.

Other Conditions. For patients with $Cl_{cr} \leq 30$ mL/min, $Cr_s > 3$ mg/dL, or CHF with a serum sodium <130 mEq/L, use lower initial doses (2.5 mg PO; 0.625 mg IV). For patients on dialysis, the initial dose should be 0.625 mg IV q 6 hr or PO 2.5 mg on dialysis days.

Dosage Forms. **Tab** 2.5, 5, 10, 20 mg (Enalapril); **Tab** 5 mg with hydrochlorothiazide 12.5 mg, 10 mg with hydrochlorothiazide 25 mg (Vaseretic); **SR Tab** 5 mg with diltiazem 180 mg (Teczem), 5 mg with 5 mg felodipine (Lexxel); **Inj** 1.25 mg/mL (enalaprilat).

Patient Instructions. (*See* Antihypertensives Class Instructions.) Use potassium supplements or salt substitutes only under medical supervision. Report any signs or symptoms of the following: infection (eg, sore throat or fever); angioedema (eg, swelling of face, eyes, lips, tongue, larynx, extremities, or hoarseness or difficulty in swallowing); or excessive fluid loss (eg, vomiting, diarrhea, or excessive perspiration). Report any skin rash, taste disturbance, or persistent, dry cough. If you become pregnant while taking this drug, contact your prescriber immediately.

Pharmacokinetics. *Onset and Duration.* PO onset is 1 hr; peak in 4–6 hr; duration is up to 24 hr.[165] The onset of action and maximal hemodynamic response correspond to the appearance of enalaprilat in serum. IV onset is 15–30 min; peak is within 1 hr; duration is usually 4–6 hr with recommended doses, but may be as long as 12 hr in some patients.[166]

Serum Levels. (Enalaprilat) 5–20 μg/L (13–52 nmol/L) is the EC_{50} for ACE inhibition; 40 μg/L (104 nmol/L) produces a mean blood pressure reduction of 12 mm Hg.[9,167]

Fate. Oral bioavailability is $41 \pm 15\%$, is not altered by meals, but is decresed in cirrhosis.[9] Peak enalapril and enalaprilat serum levels after a 10 mg oral dose occur at about 1 hr and 4 hr, and range from 40–50 μg/L (104–130 nmol/L) and 30–40 μg/L (78–104 nmol/L), respectively.[167] About 60% of a dose is converted to enalaprilat; conversion may be reduced in patients with cirrhosis.[9,167] Enalapril and enalaprilat levels are increased in renal dysfunction. Less than 50% of enalaprilat is bound to plasma protein.[167] $V_{d\beta}$ is 1.7 ± 0.7 L/kg; Cl is 0.294 ± 0.09 L/hr/kg.[168] Clearance is decreased in uremia, CHF, the elderly, and neonates.[9] After IV administration, 88% is excreted unchanged in urine,[9] after oral administration, 33% of the dose is recovered in the feces (6% as enalapril, 27% as enalaprilat), and 61% in the urine (18% as enalapril, 43% as enalaprilat).[167,169] Enalapril may be actively secreted into the urine; fecal recovery may represent unabsorbed drug or biliary excretion.[169]

$t_{1/2}$. (Enalapril) estimated to be 11 hr; (enalaprilat) about 30–35 hr in normals, increased in CHF, renal dysfunction, cirrhosis, and uremia.[9,167]

Adverse Reactions. ACE inhibitors have a common side effect profile. Most adverse effects are related to dosage and renal function. A dry, nonproductive cough occurs in 1–3% or more (up to 20% in some surveys) of treated patients, most frequently in women and nonsmokers.[149] The cough is caused by potentiation of tissue kinins or prostaglandins in the lung. It may be more frequent with longer-acting drugs, but is usually not resolved by switching to another ACE inhibitor. Taste disturbances occur in 2–7%, but may resolve despite continued therapy.[145,149]

Skin rashes occur in 1–7%, usually within a few days to weeks after starting.[170] Rashes often resolve with continued therapy and do not appear to cross-react among ACE inhibitors.[149] Angioedema is an occasional serious, potentially fatal reaction, possibly more frequent with longer-acting ACE inhibitors and possibly in blacks.[149] Hypotension may occur, especially with the first dose, in vigorously diuresed patients, those who are hyponatremic or hypovolemic, those with severe hypertension, and the elderly. In salt-restricted patients with CHF receiving ACE inhibitors and continuous diuretic therapy, up to one-third may experience worsening of renal function, which may improve when sodium is replenished.[149] Hyperkalemia occurs in 1–4% of patients, most often in those with diabetes mellitus or renal dysfunction. Proteinuria occurs occasionally with normal renal function and frequently with pre-existing renal disease,[148] although patients with progressive renal insufficiency tolerate the drug well and many experience a reduction in proteinuria despite transient reductions in renal function.[171] Neutropenia may occur, usually in the first 3 months of therapy; it is rare in normal patients, but is more frequent with high doses or in renal impairment.[149] Cholestatic hepatotoxicity is reported rarely and it may cross-react among ACE inhibitors;[149] it is reversible with drug discontinuation, but fatalities have been reported. Serious fetal harm, including renal failure and face or skull abnormalities and increased risk of miscarriage occurs with ACE-inhibitor use during the second and third trimesters of pregnancy.[149]

Contraindications. Angioedema caused by any ACE inhibitor.

Precautions. Pregnancy. It is best to avoid ACE inhibitors in women of childbearing potential who are not actively avoiding pregnancy. Monitor patients on dietary salt restriction, diuretic therapy, or dialysis (salt or volume depletion) for hypotensive episodes following the initial dose. If possible, discontinue these therapies prior to treatment. Titrate dosage slowly to the minimal effective dosage in patients with impaired renal function or collagen vascular disorders, or in patients receiving drugs altering WBC count or immune function.[171,172] Patients with aortic stenosis may develop decreased coronary perfusion when treated with afterload reducers such as the ACE inhibitors. Elevations in Cr_s and BUN may require dosage reduction or drug discontinuation. Patients with unilateral or bilateral renal artery stenosis may be more prone to increases in Cr_s and BUN. Hypotension responsive to volume expansion may occur during surgical procedures.

Drug Interactions. Hyperkalemia may develop with concomitant use of potassium-sparing diuretics, potassium supplements, or potassium-containing salt substitutes, particularly with pre-existing renal impairment.[149] Sodium and volume depletion because of a loop diuretic may cause postural hypotension when an ACE inhibitor is begun. ACE inhibitors may cause increased lithium levels. ACE inhibitors may potentiate oral hypoglycemic drugs and may increase neutropenia caused by azathioprine and hypotensive reactions when used with IV plasma protein solutions. NSAIDs may antagonize the hypotensive effect of ACE inhibitors. Phenothiazines may increase the effects of ACE inhibitors and rifampin may decrease the effects of enalapril. ACE inhibitors may increase serum digoxin concentrations.

Parameters to Monitor. Monitor blood pressure regularly. Obtain baseline Cr_s and BUN to assess the potential for adverse effects and titrate dosages accordingly; thereafter, monitor periodically. Obtain WBC count with differential q 2 weeks for the first 3 months, then periodically in renally impaired patients or if signs of infection occur. Obtain baseline serum potassium, then monitor periodically, especially in patients receiving potassium-sparing diuretics, potassium supplements, or salt substitutes. Obtain periodic urinary protein estimates (morning urines) by dipstick in patients with renal impairment.

Notes. ACE inhibitors are considered first-line drugs, along with diuretics, β-blockers, and calcium-channel blockers for the treatment of hypertension.[162] They are also first-line treatment for CHF in combination with digoxin and a diuretic, because their use is associated with prolonged survival.[148,173] Regression or attenuation of left ventricular hypertrophy occurs in patients with hypertension and in post-MI patients.[148] Additional advantages of ACE inhibitors are their renal protective effects and improved insulin sensitivity in type 1 diabetics, their lack of adverse effects on serum lipid profile, an improvement in quality of life in hypertensive patients (with one study favoring **captopril** over **enalapril**), and possibly prevention of structural changes in the heart, systemic vasculature, and kidneys.[148,165] ACE inhibitors with greater tissue ACE inhibition (eg, **benazepril, quinapril, ramipril**) may be more effective in this latter regard, but studies are lacking.[148] (*See* ACE Inhibitors Comparison Chart.)

FENOLDOPAM   Corlopam

Pharmacology. Fenoldopam is a dopamine D_1-receptor agonist that dilates renal and mesenteric vascular beds causing a reduction in total peripheral resistance and increases in renal blood flow and sodium excretion. Stimulation of postsynaptic D_1-receptors leads to smooth muscle relaxation through activation of adenylate cyclase and a subsequent increase in intracellular cyclic AMP. Unlike dopamine, fenoldopam has no α- or β-adrenergic receptor activity, stimulation of which causes increases in blood pressure and heart rate, respectively.[174]

Administration and Adult Dosage. **IV for the in-hospital, short-term (up to 48 hr) management of severe hypertension** 0.03–0.1 μg/kg/min initially, increasing in increments of 0.05–0.1 μg/kg/min at intervals of ≥20 min to a maximum of 1.7 μg/kg/min.[175] Bolus injections should not be used. Lower initial infusion rates and slower titration results in less reflex tachycardia. When the desired effect is achieved, the infusion may be stopped either gradually or abruptly, because rebound elevation of blood pressure has not been observed.[175]

Special Populations. *Pediatric Dosage.* Safety and efficacy not established.

Geriatric Dosage. Same as adult dosage.

Other Conditions. Dosage adjustments are not necessary for renal or hepatic disease or continuous ambulatory peritoneal dialysis. The effects of hemodialysis have not been evaluated.

Dosage Forms. **Inj** 10 mg/mL.

Pharmacokinetics. *Onset and Duration.* Onset <15 min; peak 2–6 hr. BP returns to baseline 2 hr after infusion discontinuation.[176]

Serum Levels. Plasma fenoldopam concentrations ≥3.5 μg/L are required for demonstrable BP reduction. Each 1 μg/L increase in plasma fenoldopam concentration causes a 0.8% decrease in diastolic blood pressure (DBP). A concentration of 18 μg/L is required for each 10 mm Hg reduction in DBP.[175]

Fate. Fenoldopam displays nonlinear increases in V_d with increases in dosage. V_{dss} are 0.23, 0.66, and 0.67 L/kg at infusion rates of 0.025, 0.25, and 0.5 μg/kg/min, respectively.[175] Cl is dose dependent, increasing from 1.49 L/hr/kg at an infusion rate of 0.025 μg/kg/min to 2.29 L/hr/kg at a rate of 0.5 μg/kg/min.[177] Fenoldopam is about 88% bound to plasma proteins. Elimination is primarily due to conjugation to inactive metabolites. About 90% is excreted in the urine (4% unchanged), 10% in feces.

$t_{1/2}$. 5–10 min.

Adverse Reactions. Fenoldopam causes dose-related reduction in BP and reflex tachycardia; excessive decreases in BP and vasodilation are responsible for most adverse effects. Frequent adverse effects are headache (11–36%), flushing (7–11%), nausea (about 20%), asymptomatic ST-segment abnormalities (6–33%), and hypotension (>5%).[176] Most adverse events occur during the first 24 hr of therapy. Hypokalemia, elevated BUN, serum glucose, transaminase, and LDH have been reported in 0.5–5% of patients. Fenoldopam may cause a reversible, dose-related increase in intraocular pressure.[178]

Contraindications. None known.

Precautions. Use with caution in patients with glaucoma or intraocular hypertension. Fenoldopam causes hypotension and reflex tachycardia, which may lead to increased myocardial oxygen demand and possibly ischemia. Patients with low serum potassium concentrations should be closely monitored, especially during the first 6 hr of fenoldopam therapy.

Drug Interactions. IV allopurinol may attenuate fenoldopam-induced increases in renal blood flow. Concomitant use of β-blockers may cause excessive hypotension and inhibition of reflex responses to fenoldopam and should be avoided if possible.

Parameters to Monitor. Monitor BP and heart rate at least q 15 min because of the rapid onset and termination of effects. Monitor serum potassium frequently during fenoldopam therapy, especially during the first 24 hr.

Notes. Fenoldopam causes reductions in BP similar to **nitroprusside.**[179–181] Fenoldopam may be preferred to nitroprusside in patients with renal dysfunction or in patients requiring prolonged therapy, due to the accumulation of thiocyanate with nitroprusside.[181,182] The infusion solution should be prepared using either NS or D5W and is stable for 24 hr under normal light and temperature conditions.

GUANABENZ ACETATE   Wytensin, Various

Pharmacology. Guanabenz is a central α_2-adrenergic receptor agonist structurally and pharmacologically similar to clonidine.[183]

Adult Dosage. PO for hypertension 4 mg bid initially; dosage may be increased in 4–8 mg/day increments q 1–2 weeks, to a maximum of 32 mg bid.

Dosage Forms. Tab 4, 8 mg.

Pharmacokinetics. Onset is within 60 min, peak effect is in 2–4 hr; effect is reduced appreciably by 6–8 hr; and blood pressure approaches baseline within 12 hr after a single dose. It is about 75% orally bioavailable and 90% bound to plasma proteins. Hydroxylation followed by glucuronidation appears to be the major metabolic pathway; the major metabolite is inactive. Renal clearance of unchanged guanabenz is 5.4 and 7.9 L/hr following 16 and 32 mg doses, respectively. Only 1.4% of unchanged drug is recovered in the urine. Its half-life is 6 hr.[184]

Adverse Reactions. Adverse reactions and drug interactions are similar to clonidine, with drowsiness or sedation (39%), dry mouth (28%), dizziness (17%), weakness (10%), and headache (5%) being the most frequent side effects. Use with caution in conjunction with other sedating medications and in patients with severe coronary insufficiency, recent MI, cerebrovascular disease, or renal or hepatic dysfunction.

GUANADREL SULFATE   Hylorel

Pharmacology. Guanadrel is a postganglionic adrenergic-blocking drug that is structurally and pharmacologically related to guanethidine. Its antihypertensive effect is comparable to guanethidine in mild to moderate hypertension, but it has a faster onset and shorter duration of action.[185,186]

Adult Dosage. PO for hypertension 5 mg bid, increasing in 10–40 mg/day increments at 1- to 4-week intervals to the usual dosage of 20–75 mg/day; dosages in excess of 150 mg/day are rarely needed, but up to 600 mg/day has been used. Higher dosages may require tid or qid administration.

Dosage Forms. Tab 10, 25 mg.

Pharmacokinetics. The onset of action of 30–120 min correlates with the appearance of peak serum levels; peak blood pressure lowering occurs in 4–6 hr; the duration of action is approximately 14 hr. The drug is 20% plasma protein bound; 85% is eliminated in the urine in 24 hr, 40% of a dose as unchanged drug. The elimination half-life varies widely but averages 10 hr.

Adverse Reactions. Adverse reactions are similar to, but less frequent than, those that occur with guanethidine, and include orthostatic hypotension (10–20%), diarrhea or increased bowel movements (5–30%), drowsiness (8–20%), fatigue (20–30%), ejaculation disturbances (7–20%), and impotence (1–5%). Peripheral edema, nasal stuffiness, cough, palpitations, and shortness of breath occur in 5–30% of patients; 21–43% of patients report leg cramps and aching limbs. Contraindications, precautions, drug interactions, and patient instructions are similar to those for guanethidine.

GUANETHIDINE SULFATE   Ismelin

Guanethidine is a postganglionic adrenergic-blocking drug that produces a selective block of efferent, peripheral sympathetic pathways. Its long-term antihypertensive effects are caused by a reduction in total peripheral resistance secondary to norepinephrine depletion from adrenergic nerve endings and inhibition of norepinephrine release in response to sympathetic stimulation.[187]

Administration and Adult Dosage. **PO in ambulatory patients** 10 mg/day initially, increased in 10–12.5 mg/day increments at 5- to 7-day intervals based on patient response to an average dosage of 25–50 mg/day. **PO in hospitalized patients** 25–50 mg initially, increased in 25–50 mg/day increments daily or every other day as indicated. The entire dose may be given once daily.

Special Populations. *Pediatric Dosage.* PO 0.2 mg/kg/day or 6 mg/m^2/day initially as a single dose, increasing q 1–2 weeks in increments equal to the initial dose, to a maximum of 3 mg/kg/day.

Geriatric Dosage. Same as adult dosage, but the elderly may tolerate postural hypotension less well.

Dosage Forms. **Tab** 10, 25 mg; **Tab** 10 mg with hydrochlorothiazide 25 mg (Esimil).

Patient Instructions. (*See* Antihypertensives Class Instructions.) Avoid sudden or prolonged standing; arise slowly, especially in the morning, and avoid the use of alcohol to reduce the chance for a sudden drop in blood pressure. Avoid the use of nonprescription products containing ephedrine, phenylpropanolamine, or pseudoephedrine.

Missed Doses. Take this medication exactly as instructed. If a dose is missed, take only the next scheduled dose (without doubling it).

Pharmacokinetics. *Onset and Duration.* Maximum hypotensive response may not occur for up to 1–3 weeks after initiating or changing the dosage. Upon discontinuation, blood pressure remains depressed for 3–4 days and gradually returns to pretreatment levels in 1–3 weeks.

Serum Levels. Adrenergic blockade occurs at 8 μg/L (40 nmol/L) or greater.[188]

Fate. Bioavailability is 3–50%; guanethidine is metabolized to inactive metabolites and ecreted in urine by glomerular filtration and tubular secretion as unchanged drug (6.4%) and metabolites.[189]

t½. α phase 1.5 days; β phase 4.1–7.7 days.[189]

Adverse Reactions. Frequently postural or postexercise hypotension manifested as weakness, dizziness, fatigue, and syncope; increased frequency of bowel movements and explosive diarrhea; edema and weight gain, occasionally precipitating CHF; and inhibition of ejaculation (retrograde ejaculation) occur. Occasionally fatigue, anorexia, nausea, vomiting, dermatitis, loss of scalp hair, dry mouth, and increased BUN occur. Rarely myalgia, muscle tremor, mental depression, bradycardia, or complete AV nodal block occur.

Contraindications. Known or suspected pheochromocytoma; frank CHF not caused by hypertension; use of an MAO inhibitor.

Precautions. May potentially aggravate asthma. Use with caution in renal dysfunction (to avoid further worsening caused by a drop in blood pressure), coronary artery disease, recent MI, cerebrovascular disease, encephalopathy, or peptic ulcer disease.

Drug Interactions. With the exception of low-dose doxepin (<150 mg/day), heterocyclic antidepressants and some phenothiazines block the uptake of guanethidine into nerve endings and thus prevent its action. Oral contraceptives, indirect-acting sympathomimetics, drugs with α-blocking properties (eg, phenothiazines, heterocyclic antidepressants, haloperidol), anorexiants (with the exception of fenfluramine), and NSAIDs may decrease the hypotensive effect. Additive hypotensive effects may occur with levodopa and alcohol. Concomitant therapy with minoxidil can result in profound orthostatic hypotension; discontinue guanethidine 1–3 weeks before initiation of oral minoxidil therapy or initiate therapy in the hospital. Consult a comprehensive drug interactions reference before using this drug in combination with any other drug.

Parameters to Monitor. Blood pressure regularly.

Notes. Guanethidine is infrequently used because of poor tolerance and the availability of numerous other drugs. Occasionally useful in patients who are not controlled by, or do not tolerate, other antihypertensives.[187]

GUANFACINE HYDROCHLORIDE   Tenex, Various

Pharmacology. Guanfacine is a central α_2-adrenergic receptor agonist pharmacologically similar to clonidine but with greater α_2-receptor selectivity. In equipotent dosages, it is equivalent to clonidine in antihypertensive activity alone or in combination with a diuretic.[190,191]

Adult Dosage. PO 1 mg/day, given hs initially. The dosage can be increased in 1 mg/day increments at 3- to 4-week intervals. Dosages above 3 mg/day are associated with an increase in adverse effects with no evidence of increased efficacy.

Dosage Forms. Tab 1, 2 mg.

Pharmacokinetics. Bioavailability is about 80%; peak serum levels occur at 1–4 hr (average 2.6); about 70% is bound to plasma proteins; V_d is 6.3 L/kg. Approximately 40–75% of a dose is excreted in the urine as unchanged drug; the remainder is eliminated as conjugates of metabolites. The average elimination half-life is 17 hr, but may be 13–14 hr in younger patients.

Adverse Reactions. Dry mouth (30%), sedation (21%), dizziness (11%), constipation (10%), fatigue, headache, and insomnia are the most frequent adverse effects. Rebound hypertension may occur, but may be milder than with clonidine because of guanfacine's longer half-life. Contraindications, precautions, and drug interactions are similar to those for clonidine.

HYDRALAZINE HYDROCHLORIDE   Apresoline, Various

Pharmacology. Hydralazine is a vasodilator that reduces total peripheral resistance by direct action on vascular smooth muscle, with an effect greater on arterioles than on veins. (*See* Notes.)

Administration and Adult Dosage. **PO for hypertension** 10 mg qid for the first 2–4 days, increasing to 25 mg qid for the remainder of the first week; after the first week, the dosage may be increased to 50 mg qid, to a maximum of 300 mg/day; bid administration may be as effective as qid. **PO for CHF** 50–75 mg bid–qid initially. **Usual maintenance dosage** 200–600 mg/day, but dosages as high as 3 g/day have been used.[192] **IM or IV for hypertension and CHF** 10–40 mg prn.

Special Populations. *Pediatric Dosage.* **PO for hypertension and CHF** 0.75 mg/kg/day or 25 mg/m^2/day initially in 4 divided doses; the initial dose should not exceed 25 mg. Increase gradually over 3–4 weeks, to a maximum of 5 (infants) to 7.5 (children) mg/kg/day or 200 mg/day. **IM or IV for hypertension and CHF** 0.1–0.2 mg/kg q 4–6 hr prn; initial parenteral dosage should not exceed 20 mg.

Geriatric Dosage. Lower dosage and slower titration is desirable because of longer half-life in the elderly.

Dosage Forms. **Inj** 20 mg/mL; **Tab** 10, 25, 50, 100 mg; **Tab** 25 mg with hydrochlorothiazide 15 mg (Apresazide); **Cap** 25 mg with hydrochlorothiazide (HCTZ) 25 mg, 50 mg with HCTZ 50 mg, 100 mg with HCTZ 50 mg (Apresazide).

Patient Instructions. (*See* Antihypertensives Class Instructions.) This drug may cause headache, dizziness, or palpitations; report if these symptoms are persistent. Report symptoms of drug-induced SLE such as fever, joint pains, dermatitis, pleuritic chest pain, and generalized malaise.

Pharmacokinetics. *Onset and Duration.* PO onset is in 1 hr; following 300 mg/day, a minimum of 30 hr is required for MAP to return to 50% of baseline value.[193] IV onset is in 10–20 min, peak in 10–80 min; IM onset is in 10–30 min; duration for IV and IM is 3–8 hr.

Serum Levels. 100 μg/L reduces MAP by 10–20 mm Hg.[9]

Fate. Bioavailability is a function of acetylator phenotype and averages 35 ± 4% for slow acetylators and 16 ± 6% for rapid acetylators. Food may enhance the bioavailability; the first-pass effect may be saturable. Plasma protein binding is 87%. V_d is 1.5 ± 1 L/kg; Cl is 3.36 ± 0.78 L/hr/kg, reduced in CHF. The drug is extensively metabolized by acetylation to multiple metabolites, principally hydrazones, at a rate that is genetically determined; only 1–15% of unchanged drug, as well as metabolites, is excreted in the urine.[9]

$t_{1/2}$. β phase 0.96 ± 0.28 hr, longer in CHF.[9]

Adverse Reactions. Frequently headache, anorexia, nausea, vomiting, diarrhea, palpitations, tachycardia, and angina occur. Occasionally hypotension, edema, peripheral neuritis, dizziness, tremors, muscle cramps, urinary retention, nasal congestion, and flushing occur. A syndrome similar to SLE with joint pain and skin rash (only rarely with cerebritis and nephritis) has been reported at an overall frequency of 6.7% in 281 patients over 51 months; daily dosage affects the frequency, with none at 50 mg/day, 5.4% at 100 mg/day, and 10.4% at 200 mg/day. Women had a higher overall frequency than men (11.6 and 2.8%, respectively), and women taking 200 mg/day had a 19.4% rate; slow acetylator phenotype may also increase the risk; the syndrome is reversible upon drug discontinuation, although residual effects may be detected years later.[194] An immune complex glomerulonephritis has been reported in patients with hydralazine-induced SLE.[195]

Contraindications. Coronary artery disease; mitral valvular rheumatic disease.

Precautions. Reflex tachycardia may precipitate anginal attacks or ECG evidence of myocardial ischemia.

Drug Interactions. NSAIDs may antagonize the hypotensive effect of hydralazine.

Parameters to Monitor. Blood pressure and heart rate regularly. Baseline and periodic CBC. ANA titers may become positive after several months of therapy; routine monitoring is generally not warranted because the symptoms of hydralazine-induced SLE are characteristic and reversible upon drug discontinuation.

Notes. Reflex increases in heart rate, cardiac output, and stroke volume, as well as increases in plasma renin activity and retention of sodium and water, can attenuate hydralazine's antihypertensive action; therefore, long-term regimens for hypertension should include a diuretic and a sympatholytic drug. When hydralazine is used as an afterload-reducing drug in the treatment of CHF in patients on maintenance diuretics, the increase in cardiac output usually prevents the development of reflex tachycardia; likewise, hypotension is usually prevented by the increased cardiac output, but may occur if myocardial reserves are inadequate or if the heart cannot respond by increasing output (eg, severe cardiomyopathy or aortic stenosis).[192]

LABETALOL HYDROCHLORIDE   Normodyne, Trandate, Various

Pharmacology. Labetalol is an adrenergic receptor blocking drug that has both selective α_1- and nonselective β-adrenergic receptor blocking action. Although its pharmacologic profile resembles that of other β-blockers and the postsynaptic α_1-adrenergic blocking action of prazosin, its β-blocking activity is approximately 3 times greater than the α-blocking activity following oral administration and 7 times greater following IV administration. During long-term treatment there is a further reduction in relative α-blocking activity.[196,197]

Administration and Adult Dosage. **PO for hypertension** 100 mg bid initially, increasing at 2- to 3-day intervals in 100 mg bid increments until blood pressure is controlled. Usual **maintenance dosage** is 200–400 mg bid, to a maximum of 1.2–2.4 g/day for severe hypertension. **IV for hypertension** 20 mg by slow (2 min) injection, followed by 40–80 mg at 10-min intervals until blood pressure is controlled or to a total of 300 mg. Alternatively, administer a dilute solution by continuous infusion at a rate of 2 mg/min, to a maximum total dosage of 300 mg; the usual effective cumulative dosage is 50–200 mg; the infusion may be repeated q 6–8 hr.[162,196,197]

Special Populations. *Pediatric Dosage.* Safety and efficacy not established; however, the following has been used: **IV for hypertension** 0.2–1 (average 0.55) mg/kg initially, followed by a continuous infusion of 0.25–1.5 (average 0.8) mg/kg/hr.[198]

Geriatric Dosage. Same as adult dosage.

Other Conditions. Titrate dosage to blood pressure control. No dosage adjustment is required in renal impairment. Patients with hepatic dysfunction may require lower than usual dosages.

Dosage Forms. **Tab** 100, 200, 300 mg; **Tab** 100, 200, 300 mg with hydrochlorothiazide 25 mg (Normozide, Trandate HCT); **Inj** 5 mg/mL.

Patient Instructions. (*See* Antihypertensives Class Instructions.) Do not discontinue medication abruptly except under medical supervision. Do not sit up or stand for 3 hours after intravenous administration.

Pharmacokinetics. *Onset and Duration.* PO onset within 2 hr, peak 3 hr, duration 8–12 hr; may be longer with higher dosages. IV injection onset <10 min, peak in 5–15 min, duration 3–6 hr.[162,197]

Fate. Almost completely absorbed, but bioavailability is only $18 \pm 5\%$ because of extensive first-pass metabolism, with the higher values reported in the elderly and patients with cirrhosis.[9,199] Peak serum levels occur within 1–2 hr after oral administration; food delays the time to peak, but may increase bioavailability. Plasma protein binding averages 50%. There is little distribution into the brain because of low lipid solubility. V_d is 9.4 ± 3.4 L/kg; Cl is 1.5 ± 0.6 L/hr/kg, lower in young hypertensive patients and the elderly, and unchanged in cirrhosis. The drug is extensively metabolized primarily in the liver and possibly gut wall to inactive compounds. Unchanged drug (<5%) and metabolites are excreted in urine and feces.[9,196,197,199]

$t_{1/2}$. β phase 4.9 ± 2 hr, independent of route of administration, increased in the elderly.[9,196,199]

Adverse Reactions. These are generally related to α- and β-adrenergic blockade and usually occur during the first few weeks of therapy. Frequently dizziness, fatigue, headache, scalp tingling, nausea, dyspepsia, and nasal congestion occur. Occasionally postural hypotension, edema, taste disturbance, impotence, rash, and blurred vision occur. IV administration causes ventricular arrhythmias rarely.

Contraindications. Bronchial asthma; overt cardiac failure; greater than first-degree heart block; cardiogenic shock; bradycardia.

Precautions. Lower dosages may be required in patients with impaired hepatic function.

Drug Interactions. Cimetidine may increase bioavailability of oral labetalol. Glutethimide may decrease the effect of labetalol by inducing hepatic enzymes. Concurrent use with halothane can produce myocardial depression. Labetalol decreases the reflex tachycardia induced by nitroglycerin and the bronchodilator effects of β2-agonist bronchodilators.

Parameters to Monitor. Monitor blood pressure regularly.

Notes. Labetalol injection is incompatible with 5% sodium bicarbonate.

LOSARTAN POTASSIUM   Cozaar

Pharmacology. Losartan is a selective, reversible, nonpeptide, competitive antagonist of the angiotensin II receptor (AT_1), which is responsible for the physiologic effects of angiotensin II, including vasoconstriction, aldosterone secretion, sympathetic outflow, and stimulation of renal sodium reabsorption. Losartan and other angiotensin II receptor antagonists are highly selective for the AT_1 receptor over the AT_2 receptor, whose physiologic function is unknown. Angiotensin II receptor antagonists have no inhibitory effects on angiotensin converting enzyme and therefore decrease BP with no appreciable effect on kinin metabolism.[200]

Administration and Adult Dosage. *PO for hypertension* 50 mg/day initially; 25 mg/day in patients on diuretics or volume depleted. The usual dosage is 25–100 mg/day given without regard to meals once daily; may increase to bid in patients not adequately controlled with once-daily administration. Most patients respond to 50 mg/day, although further BP reductions are possible with 100 mg/day.[201] Patients who do not respond to 50 mg/day may benefit more with the addition of hydrochlorothiazide than an increased dosage. Dosages >100 mg/day offer little added benefit.[200]

Special Populations. *Pediatric Dosage.* Safety and efficacy not established.

Geriatric Dosage. Same as adult dosage.

Other Conditions. No dosage adjustment is necessary in renal impairment or patients on dialysis. Patients with hepatic insufficiency may require lower doses (eg, starting dose of 25 mg/day) because of decreased losartan clearance.

Dosage Forms. **Tab** 25, 50 mg (Cozaar); **Tab** 50 mg with 12.5 mg hydrochlorothiazide (Hyzaar).

Patient Instructions. (*See* Antihypertensives Class Instructions.) This medication may cause dizziness, especially with the first few doses; do not drive or operate dangerous machinery until you know how you will react to this medicine. Do not use this medicine if you are pregnant or planning on becoming pregnant. If you become pregnant while taking this medicine, contact your prescriber immediately. Report any skin rash or signs or symptoms of angioedema (eg, swelling of face, eyes, lips, tongue, larynx, extremities, or hoarseness or difficulty in swallowing) immediately to your prescriber.

Pharmacokinetics. *Onset and Duration.* PO onset <2 hr; peak 6 hr; duration >24 hrs, may be less with doses ≤25 mg/day.[202] Maximum antihypertensive effect occurs after 1 week in most patients, but may take 3–6 weeks.

Serum Levels. Large interindividual variability, with IC_{50} for AT_1 inhibition occurring at losartan concentrations of 1.4–200 nmol/L.[203]

Fate. Oral absorption is rapid, but extensive first-pass metabolism results in a bioavailability of 33%, which may be doubled in hepatic insufficiency. About 14% of an oral dose is converted to an active carboxylic acid metabolite. Peak concentrations of losartan occur in 1 hr and those of its metabolite in 3–4 hr. The metabolite is approximately 10–40 times more potent than the parent compound and is believed to be responsible for most of the antihypertensive effects of losartan.[204] Losartan and its metabolite are both about 99% protein bound, mainly to albumin. V_d of losartan and its active metabolite are 34 L and 12 L, respectively. Metabolism of losartan occurs through CYP2C9 and CYP3A4 to the active carboxylic acid metabolite and several inactive metabolites. Cl is about 36 L/hr for losartan (12–15% renal Cl) and 3 L/hr for the active metabolite (50% renal Cl). Losartan Cl may be 50% less with hepatic insufficiency.[204] About 4% of an oral losartan dose is excreted unchanged in the urine and 6% of the dose as active metabolite. Following oral administration, 60% of a losartan dose is excreted in the feces.

$t_{1/2}$. (Losartan) 2 hr; (metabolite) 6–9 hr.

Adverse Reactions. Angiotensin II receptor antagonists are generally well tolerated, with adverse reactions occurring at frequencies similar to placebo; adverse events are not dose related. The most frequent reactions are headache (10–20%) and upper respiratory tract infection (1–12%).[205] Nasal congestion, cough, and fatigue occur in <6% of patients.[205,206] Unlike ACE inhibitors, angiotensin II receptor antagonists induce cough about as frequently as placebo, probably because bradykinin concentrations are not elevated as they are with ACE inhibitors. Angiotensin II receptor antagonists are effective alternatives in patients who experience cough with ACEIs.[207,208] Like ACE inhibitors, angiotensin II receptor antagonists may induce reversible renal dysfunction as a consequence of affecting the renin-angiotensin-aldosterone system. Increases in Cr_s and BUN may also occur in patients with unilateral or bilateral renal artery stenosis. Hypersensitivity reactions (eg, angioedema, rash) have been reported in patients receiving losartan or **valsartan.** Angiotensin II receptor antagonists may cause decreases in hemoglobin and hematocrit and increase serum bilirubin, but these changes are rarely of clinical importance. Neutropenia has been reported in 1.8% of patients taking valsartan (0.9% for placebo). Hyperkalemia has been reported in 1.5% of losartan-treated patients (1.3% for ACE inhibitor) and 4.4% of valsartan-treated patients (2.9% for placebo).[206]

Contraindications. Hypersensitivity to any product components.

Precautions. Use of drugs affecting the renin-angiotensin-aldosterone system may cause injury and even death to the developing fetus if used in the second or third trimesters of pregnancy. Increase dosage slowly in patients with liver dysfunction, because of reduced drug clearance (losartan, valsartan) in these patients. Patients taking angiotensin II receptor antagonists whose renal function is dependent on the renin-angiotensin-aldosterone system (eg, CHF patients) may experience oliguria, progressive azotemia, and (rarely) acute renal failure or death. Reversible increases in Cr_s and/or BUN may occur in patients with unilateral or bilateral renal artery stenosis.

Drug Interactions. Inhibitors of the CYP3A4 or 2C9 isoenzymes (eg, ketoconazole) may impair the conversion of losartan to the active metabolite. No important drug–drug interactions have been reported with valsartan or **irbesartan.**

Parameters to Monitor. Monitor for hypersensitivity reactions (eg, flushing, dyspnea, facial swelling, rash) at the start of therapy. Monitor blood pressure regularly. Monitor patients on dietary salt restriction, diuretic therapy, or dialysis (salt or volume depletion) for hypotensive episodes following the initial dose. Obtain baseline and periodic Cr_s and BUN to assess the potential for adverse effects. Obtain baseline serum potassium, WBC count, hemoglobin, and hematocrit. Monitor periodically for hyperkalemia, neutropenia, and anemia.

Notes. Although JNC VI guidelines do not promote this, many clinicians consider angiotensin II receptor antagonists as first-line therapy for hypertension because of their efficacy, safety, and ease of administration.[162,205] Losartan is a uricosuric, which may lower plasma uric acid concentration while increasing the risk of acute uric acid nephropathy or acute gout.[204] Losartan has been shown to improve cardiac output, and reduce peripheral vascular resistance and pulmonary capillary wedge pressure in patients with CHF.[209] The ELITE study found losartan superior to captopril in reducing mortality in patients with CHF, although this was not the primary end point of the study.[210] Numerous other AT_1 antagonists are available or under development. (*See* Angiotensin II Receptor Antagonists Comparison Chart.)

METHYLDOPA   Aldomet, Various

METHYLDOPATE HYDROCHLORIDE   Aldomet

Pharmacology. The action of methyldopa is thought to be mediated through stimulation of central α-adrenergic receptors in a manner similar to clonidine. Stimulation is primarily caused by the metabolite α-methylnorepinephrine.

Administration and Adult Dosage. **PO for hypertension** 250 mg bid–tid initially, increasing at intervals of no less than 48 hr to the usual daily dosage of 500 mg–2 g/day in 2–4 divided doses. **IV for hypertension** usual dosage is 250–500 mg over 30–60 min in 100 mL D5W q 6 hr, to a maximum of 1 g q 6 hr.

Special Populations. *Pediatric Dosage.* **PO** 10 mg/kg/day in 2–4 doses initially, to a maximum of 65 mg/kg/day or 3 g/day, whichever is less. **IV** 20–40 mg/kg/day in divided doses q 6 hr, to a maximum of 65 mg/kg/day or 3 g/day, whichever is less.

Geriatric Dosage. Use lower dosages to avoid causing syncope.

Other Conditions. Patients with renal failure may respond to smaller dosages of methyldopa.

Dosage Forms. **Tab** 125, 250, 500 mg; **Tab** 250 mg with chlorothiazide 150 or 250 mg (Aldoclor); **Tab** 250 or 500 mg with hydrochlorothiazide 15, 25, 30, or 50 mg (Aldoril, various); **Susp** 50 mg/mL; **IV** 50 mg/mL.

Patient Instructions. (*See* Antihypertensives Class Instructions.) Report changes in mood (depression), loss of appetite, yellowing of eyes or skin, abdominal pain, or unexplained fever or joint pains. This drug may cause your urine to darken if it is exposed to air after voiding.

Pharmacokinetics. *Onset and Duration.* PO onset 2 hr, peak within 4–6 hr; duration 12–24 hr. IV onset 4–6 hr, duration 10–16 hr.

Serum Levels. No correlation between serum levels and therapeutic effect.

Fate. Oral bioavailability is 42 ± 16%.[9] Peak serum levels occur in 2–4 hr, but correlate poorly with the hypotensive effect. IV bioavailability is similar to oral, apparently because a large portion of methyldopate ester is not hydrolyzed to methyldopa. From 10 to 15% is plasma protein bound. V_d is 0.46 ± 0.15 L/kg; Cl is 0.22 ± 0.06 L/hr/kg and is decreased in uremia. The drug is excreted in the urine as metabolites, sulfate conjugate, and unchanged drug. About 49% (IV) and 70% (PO) of a dose are excreted in urine as sulfate conjugate and unchanged drug.[9,211]

$t_{1/2}$. α phase 0.21 hr (range 0.16–0.26); β phase 1.8 ± 0.6 hr, increased in uremia and in neonates.[9,211]

Adverse Reactions. Frequently, drowsiness, headache, weight gain, nasal stuffiness, postural hypotension, or dry mouth occur. A positive Coombs' test develops in 10–20% of patients, usually between 6 and 12 months of therapy; hemolytic anemia, however, is rare. Occasionally, depression, sexual dysfunction, diarrhea, or nightmares are reported. Rarely, hepatitis, drug fever, lupuslike syndrome, leukopenia, thrombocytopenia, or granulocytopenia occurs.

Contraindications. Active hepatic disease such as acute hepatitis and active cirrhosis or liver dysfunction associated with previous methyldopa therapy.

Precautions. Use with caution in patients with a prior history of liver disease. A previously positive Coombs' test does not preclude methyldopa use, but early recognition of hemolytic anemia may be more difficult in such patients.

Drug Interactions. Methyldopa may potentiate the effect of tolbutamide and lithium. It may also cause confusion or disorientation when used with haloperidol. An increase in norepinephrine's pressor response may occur with concurrent use. Iron products reduce methyldopa absorption. Amphetamines and heterocyclic antidepressants may decrease the efficacy of methyldopa. Levodopa and methyldopa may enhance each other's effects.

Parameters to Monitor. Obtain direct Coombs' test initially and at 6 and 12 months. Obtain baseline and periodic CBC and liver function tests to monitor for hemolytic anemia, blood dyscrasias, and hepatic dysfunction.

Notes. Methyldopa is not a first-line drug because of its frequent side effects; however, it may be useful in those with ischemic heart disease or with diastolic dysfunction, in whom it reduces left ventricular mass.[187]

MINOXIDIL   Loniten, Rogaine, Various

Pharmacology. Minoxidil is a potent vasodilator that acts by direct relaxation of arteriolar smooth muscle, resulting in a reduction of total peripheral resistance. The vasodilation and associated reduction in blood pressure leads to reflex sympathetic activation, vagal inhibition, and altered renal homeostatic mechanisms manifested as an increase in heart rate and cardiac output, increase in renin secretion, and salt and water retention. Because these responses may attenuate the hypotensive actions, minoxidil should be administered with a sympatholytic drug and a diuretic. Topically, minoxidil stimulates vertex hair growth by an unknown mechanism.

Administration and Adult Dosage. **PO for hypertension** 5 mg/day initially as a single daily dose, increased to 10, 20, then 40 mg/day q 3 days in single or divided doses based on blood pressure response, to a maximum of 100 mg/day; usual dosage is 10–40 mg/day. If a single dose reduces supine diastolic blood pressure by more than 30 mm Hg, divide the total daily dosage into 2 equal doses. **Top for male pattern baldness or female alopecia androgenetica** 1 mL to affected areas bid.

Special Populations. *Pediatric Dosage.* **PO for hypertension** 0.2 mg/kg as a single daily dose, increased in 50–100% increments q 3 days until optimum blood pressure control or a total daily dosage of 50 mg is achieved; usual dosage is 0.25–1 mg/kg/day.

Geriatric Dosage. Same as adult dosage.

Other Conditions. In renal impairment, lower dosages may be required.

Dosage Forms. **Tab** 2.5, 10 mg (Loniten, various); **Top** 10, 20, 50 mg/mL (1, 2, 5%) (Rogaine, various).

Patient Instructions. (*See* Antihypertensives Class Instructions.) If a dose is missed, wait until the next regularly scheduled dose and continue with your regular dose; do not double the next dose. Report any of the following: increase in resting heart rate of greater than 20 beats per minute, rapid weight gain of more than 5 pounds, or the development of edema, increased difficulty in breathing, new or worsening angina, dizziness, lightheadedness, or fainting.

Pharmacokinetics. *Onset and Duration.* PO single dose onset 30 min; peak 2–3 hr; duration up to 75 hr with a gradual return to baseline at a rate of about 30% per day. Time to maximum effect with repeated administration is a function of dose and averages 7 days at 10 mg/day, 5 days at 20 mg/day, and 3 days at 40 mg/day. Top onset 4 or more months; relapse may occur 3–4 months after drug discontinuation.

Serum Levels. No correlation between serum levels and effects.

Fate. Oral absorption is at least 90%, but bioavailability is probably lower. Protein binding is negligible. V_d is 2.7 ± 0.7 L/kg; Cl is 1.4 ± 0.4 L/hr/kg. The drug is primarily metabolized and renally excreted, with about 20% unchanged drug in the urine. The major metabolite, a glucuronide conjugate, is active and may contribute to the drug's effect.[9,187,212]

$t_{1/2}$. 3.1 ± 0.6 hr.[9]

Adverse Reactions. Frequently hypertrichosis (elongation, thickening, and enhanced pigmentation) (80%), transient ECG T-wave changes (60%), temporary edema (7%), or tachycardia occur. Occasionally pericardial effusion with or without tamponade (3%), CHF, or angina occur. Rarely breast tenderness and rashes (including Stevens-Johnson syndrome) occur. Minor dermatologic reactions occur occasionally after topical application.

Contraindications. (Oral) pheochromocytoma, caused by possible stimulation of catecholamine release from the tumor; acute MI; dissecting aortic aneurysm.

Precautions. For hypertension, minoxidil must usually be administered with a diuretic to prevent fluid retention; a loop diuretic is almost always required. Drugs or regimens that provide around-the-clock sympathetic suppression are usually required to prevent tachycardia, which may precipitate or worsen existing angina. Degenerative myocardial lesions reported in animal studies have yet to be confirmed in humans.

Drug Interactions. Concomitant therapy with guanethidine can result in profound orthostatic hypotension; discontinue guanethidine 1–3 weeks before initiation of oral minoxidil therapy or initiate therapy in the hospital.

Parameters to Monitor. Blood pressure, pulse rate, body weight, cardiac and pulmonary function regularly.

Notes. Minoxidil is reserved for use in severe hypertension in combination with other drugs, usually a diuretic and a sympatholytic drug (eg, β-blocker).[187]

NITROPRUSSIDE SODIUM   Nipride, Various

Pharmacology. Nitroprusside is a potent vasodilator that has direct action on vascular smooth muscle to reduce arterial pressure and produce a slight increase in heart rate, a mild decrease in cardiac output, and a moderate reduction in total peripheral resistance (TPR). The decrease in TPR suggests arteriolar dilation (afterload reduction), whereas the reduction in cardiac output may be caused by peripheral pooling of blood (preload reduction). Nitroprusside is somewhat more active on veins than on arteries. The active component of sodium nitroprusside is the free nitroso (NO^-) group.

Administration and Adult Dosage. IV 0.3 μg/kg/min by continuous infusion initially, increasing to an average rate of 3 μg/kg/min based on blood pressure response with a range of 0.5–10 μg/kg/min. Infusion at the maximum rate should never exceed 10 min. Patients receiving other antihypertensives can usually be controlled with a smaller dosage. Control administration rates carefully using a microdrip regulator or an infusion pump; avoid too rapid reduction in blood pressure. Infusion rates greater than 2 μg/kg/min generate more cyanide ion (CN^-) than the body can metabolize or eliminate. Maintain infusions at the lowest possible dosage, for the shortest possible duration to avoid toxicity.[213] (*See* Adverse Reactions.)

Special Populations. *Pediatric Dosage.* IV same as adult dosage.

Geriatric Dosage. Initiate therapy with low infusion rates and titrate the rate and degree of blood pressure lowering carefully to avoid coronary and cerebral hypoperfusion.

Other Conditions. Patients with CHF, stroke victims, and patients receiving other antihypertensive drugs may be particularly sensitive to the blood-pressure–lowering effects of nitroprusside sodium; initiate therapy with low infusion rates and titrate the rate and degree of blood pressure lowering carefully to avoid coronary and cerebral hypoperfusion. Limit the total dosage in renal failure to avoid accumulation of thiocyanate. Caution in hepatic insufficiency.

Dosage Forms. Inj 50 mg.

Pharmacokinetics. *Onset and Duration.* Onset within 1 min; peak 1–2 min; blood pressure usually returns to pretreatment levels in 2–10 min.[162]

Serum Levels. Therapeutic and toxic levels are not established for nitroprusside because of rapid metabolism to cyanide and thiocyanate. Thiocyanate levels >60 mg/L (1 mmol/L) are associated with toxicity.

Fate. Nitroprusside is distributed in a volume that approximates the extravascular space, from which it is rapidly metabolized by a reaction with hemoglobin, yielding cyanmethemoglobin and an unstable intermediate that dissociates, releasing cyanide ion. Cyanide is converted to thiocyanate by the enzyme thiosulfate-cyanide sulfur transferase (rhodanese) in the liver and the kidney. The rate of conversion is principally determined by the availability of sulfur, usually as thiosulfate. Thiocyanate is largely excreted by the kidneys and may accumulate with high infusion rates for prolonged periods or in the presence of renal dysfunction.

$t_{1/2}$. (Nitroprusside) 2 min; (thiocyanate) 2.7 days, up to 9 days in patients with renal dysfunction.[214]

Adverse Reactions. Most adverse reactions are related to excessive or too rapid reduction of blood pressure and include nausea, retching, diaphoresis, apprehension, restlessness, headache, retrosternal discomfort, palpitations, dizziness, and abdominal pain, all of which resolve when the infusion rate is reduced or the infusion is temporarily discontinued. Thiocyanate is not particularly toxic and usually accumulates to toxic levels only with prolonged (>48 hr) or high-dosage (>10 μg/kg/min) infusions, when cyanide elimination is increased by the administration of thiosulfate, or in the presence of renal dysfunction. To limit the risk of thiocyanate toxicity, infuse at <3 μg/kg/min. Manifestations of thiocyanate toxicity include fatigue, anorexia, nausea, disorientation, toxic psychosis, and hallucinations. Cyanide toxicity usually occurs only when large dosages (>10 μg/kg/min) are infused rapidly or for periods >1 hr. Since an early manifestation of cyanide toxicity can be apparent nitroprusside resistance, the need for increasing dosages to achieve the same level of blood pressure control should prompt the clinician to look for metabolic acidosis, an indicator of cyanide toxicity, but one that may not be evident for >1 hr after accumulation of dangerous cyanide levels. Other symptoms of cyanide toxicity include dyspnea, vomiting, dizziness, loss of consciousness, weak pulse, distant heart sounds, areflexia, dilated pupils, shallow breathing, convulsions, and the occasional smell of bitter almonds on the breath. **Hydroxocobalamin** (25 mg/hr by continuous infusion) may facilitate the conversion of cyanide to cyanocobalamin;[215] however, an appropriate hydroxocobalamin dosage form is unavailable. Concurrent **sodium thiosulfate** administration can also prevent cyanide toxicity, but thiocyanate levels may increase.[216] Management of cyanide toxicity includes immediate discontinuation of nitroprusside and the administration of sodium nitrite (0.2 mL/kg of a 3% solution IV over 2–4 min), followed by 12.5 g of sodium thiosulfate infused over 10 min. Methemoglobinemia may develop in patients congenitally unable to convert nitroprusside-induced methemoglobin back to hemoglobin. Management consists of IV administration of **methylene blue** 1–2 mg/kg over several min.

Contraindications. Compensatory hypertension (eg, arteriovenous shunt or coarctation of the aorta); controlled hypotension during surgery in patients with inadequate cerebral circulation; congenital (Leber's) optic atrophy; use of sildenafil. (*See* Drug Interactions.)

Precautions. If an adequate hypotensive response is not achieved after the maximum recommended infusion rate of 10 μg/kg/min for a maximum of 10 min, stop the infusion because these dosages increase the risk of toxicity. Use with caution in renal, hepatic, or thyroid disease, and in vitamin B_{12} deficiency or elevated intracrania pressure.

Drug Interactions. Use during general anesthesia may impair the capacity to compensate for hypovolemia and anemia, and cause abnormal perfusion:ventilation ratio. Use in patients taking sildenafil can result in profound hypotension with serious consequences, including death.

Parameters to Monitor. Monitor blood pressure frequently (eg, every few minutes) because of the rapid onset and offset of effects. Monitor thiocyanate levels after 24–48 hr in patients with normal renal function and daily in patients with impaired renal function or those receiving large dosages. However, these levels are of no value in detecting cyanide toxicity. Monitoring of serum cyanide concentrations has been recommended, but the assay is technically difficult and not readily interpretable if fluids other than packed RBCs are analyzed. Frequent monitoring of acid-base balance, particularly in patients with hepatic dysfunction, is considered by most clinicians to be adequate.

Notes. Protect from light and discard solution after 24 hr or if the color changes from the usual faint brownish tint to blue, green, or dark red. Do not administer IV push medications through the same line or use the solution for the simultaneous administration of any other drug.

RESERPINE Various

Pharmacology. Reserpine is a hypotensive drug that acts primarily by depleting norepinephrine from postganglionic adrenergic neurons. It is a weak antihypertensive that is most effective when used in combination with a diuretic or as an adjunct to other drugs, permitting lower dosages of each drug and possibly minimizing side effects.[162,187] Advantages include proven efficacy, relatively good patient tolerance in low dosages, once-daily administration, and very low cost.

Adult Dosage. **PO for hypertension** 0.5 mg/day for 1–2 weeks, followed by a maintenance dosage of 0.1–0.25 mg/day in a single dose.

Dosage Forms. **Tab** 0.1, 0.25, 1 mg and in combination with diuretics, vasodilators.

Pharmacokinetics. Full effects are usually delayed for 2–3 weeks; the duration of action is up to 24 hr; CNS and cardiac effects may persist longer. The drug is extensively metabolized.

Adverse Reactions. Dose-related mental depression can occur, but this adverse effect is rare at dosages less than 0.25 mg/day. Drowsiness, weakness, GI disturbances (eg, abdominal pain, activation of peptic ulcer disease, diarrhea, epigastric distress), nasal congestion, sexual dysfunction, and bradycardia occur occasionally. Reserpine is contraindicated in patients with a history of mental depression (especially those with suicidal tendencies), active peptic ulcer, or ulcerative colitis, and during electroconvulsive therapy.

ACE INHIBITORS COMPARISON CHART

DRUG	DOSAGE FORMS	DAILY ADULT DOSAGE (MG)[a]	INDICATED FOR CHF	PEAK (HR)	DURATION (HR)	HALF-LIFE (HR)	ELIMINATION ROUTES
Benazepril Lotensin	Tab 5, 10, 20, 40 mg.	10–40	No	2–4	24+	22[b]	Renal, Hepatic.
Captopril Capoten Various	Tab 12.5, 25, 50, 100 mg.	25–150	Yes	1	6–10	1.7	Renal, Hepatic
Enalapril Vasotec	Tab 2.5, 5, 10, 20 mg. Inj 1.25 mg/mL.	PO 10–40; IV 1.25–5 mg q 6 hr.	Yes	4–6	24 (PO)	11[c] (enalaprilat-35)	Renal.
Fosinopril Monopril	Tab 10, 20, 40 mg.	20–80	Yes	3–6	24	12–15[b]	Hepatic, Renal.
Lisinopril Prinivil Zestril	Tab 2.5, 5, 10, 20, 40 mg.	10–40	Yes	2–6	24	13[b]	Renal.
Moexipril Univasc	Tab 7.5, 15 mg.	7.5–30	No	3–8	24	2–9[b]	Hepatic, Renal.
Perindopril Aceon	Tab 2, 4, 8 mg.	4–8	No	4–8	24+	9[b]	Renal.
Quinapril Accupril	Tab 5, 10, 20, 40 mg.	20–80	Yes	2–4	24+	2–3[b]	Renal.

(continued)

ACE INHIBITORS COMPARISON CHART (continued)

DRUG	DOSAGE FORMS	DAILY ADULT DOSAGE (MG)[a]	INDICATED FOR CHF	PEAK (HR)	DURATION (HR)	HALF-LIFE (HR)	ELIMINATION ROUTES
Ramipril Altace	Cap 1.25, 2.5, 5, 10 mg.	2.5–20	Yes[d]	3–8	24+	11–17[b]	Renal, Hepatic.
Spirapril Renomax (Investigational, Schering)	—	—	—	4–8	24+	35[b]	Renal, Hepatic.
Trandolapril Mavik Tarka	Tab 1, 2, 4 mg.	1–4	Yes[d]	6	24+	24[b]	Hepatic, Renal.
Zofenopril Zoprace (Investigational, Bristol-Myers Squibb)	—	—	—	2	24	5.5[b]	Renal, Hepatic.

[a]Usual maintenance dosage range. Initial dosage is often lower, and higher dosages are sometimes effective.
[b]Half-life of active drug.
[c]Half-life of prodrug; active form longer.
[d]Indicated for CHF post-MI.
From references 217–220, and product information.

ANGIOTENSIN II RECEPTOR ANTAGONISTS COMPARISON CHART

DRUG	DOSAGE FORMS	USUAL DAILY ADULT DOSAGE (MG)	PEAK (HR)	DURATION (HR)	HALF-LIFE (HR)	ELIMINATION ROUTES
Candesartan Atacand	Tab 4, 8, 16, 32 mg.	8–32	3–4	24+	9	Hepatic, Renal.
Eprosartan Teveten	—	—	—	24+	5–7	Renal, Hepatic.
Irbesartan Avapro	Tab 75, 150, 300 mg.	150–300	3–6	24+	11–15	Renal, Hepatic.
Losartan Cozaar	Tab 25, 50 mg.	25–100[b]	6	24+	2 6–9[a]	Hepatic. Renal, Hepatic.[a]
Telmisartan Micardis	—	—	—	35	—	—
Valsartan Diovan	Cap 80, 160 mg.	80–320	6	24+	15	Hepatic.

[a]For active metabolite, which is responsible for most or all pharmacologic effects.
[b]Occasionally, the daily dosage must be given in 2 divided doses.
From references 204, 221, 222 and product information.

α₁-ADRENERGIC-BLOCKING DRUGS COMPARISON CHART

DRUG	DOSAGE FORMS	DAILY ADULT DOSAGE (MG)[a]	PEAK (HR)	DURATION (HR)	HALF-LIFE (HR)	ELIMINATION ROUTES
Doxazosin Cardura	Tab 1, 2, 4, 8 mg.	1–16	2–3	18–36	10–12	Hepatic.
Prazosin Minipress Various	Cap 1, 2, 5 mg.	2–20	1–3	6–12	2–3	Hepatic.
Terazosin Hytrin	Tab 1, 2, 5, 10 mg.	1–20	1–2	24	14–16	Hepatic, Renal.
Tamsulosin Flomax	Cap 0.4 mg.	0.4–0.8[b]	—	—	15	Hepatic.

[a]Usual maintenance dosage range; higher dosages are sometimes effective. Dosage is the same in the elderly.
[b]Not for hypertension; for symptoms of benign prostatic hypertrophy only.
From references 142, 223, 224 and product information.

343

DRUGS FOR HYPERTENSIVE URGENCIES AND EMERGENCIES COMPARISON CHART

DRUG	DOSAGE RANGE	ONSET (MIN)	DURATION	COMMENTS
ORAL DRUGS FOR HYPERTENSIVE URGENCIES				
Captopril Capoten Various	PO, SL 12.5–25 mg.	10–30	2–6 hr	Hypotensive effect is particularly large in patients on a diuretic or in hypertensive crisis. Subsequent doses may be less effective unless given with a diuretic. Acute renal failure may occur.
Clonidine Catapres	PO 0.1–0.2 mg initially, then 0.1 mg/hr, to a maximum total dosage of 0.8 mg.	30–120	6–8 hr	Rate of onset is slower after a meal; drowsiness or dry mouth can occur. Rebound hypertension is possible.
Labetalol Normodyne Trandate Various	PO 200–400 mg, may repeat q 2–3 hr.	30–120	6–12 hr	Orthostatic hypotension, bronchoconstriction, and heart block can occur. Avoid in COPD and asthma.
Nifedipine Adalat Procardia	PO 10–20 mg, may repeat in 20 min.	5–20	2–6 hr	Bite and swallow capsule. Precipitous drops in blood pressure may occur. Increases cardiac output; mild flushing, headaches, and palpitations may occur; use with caution in patients with severe arteriosclerotic stenosis because it may precipitate cerebral ischemic symptoms. Nifedipine is not recommended for this use because of unpredictability of the blood pressure response.
Prazosin Minipress Various	PO 1–2 mg, may repeat q 1 hr.	30–90	1–10 hr	Useful in presence of increased circulating catecholamines. First-dose syncope, palpitations, tachycardia, and headache reported.

(continued)

DRUG	DOSAGE RANGE	ONSET (MIN)	DURATION	COMMENTS
INTRAVENOUS DRUGS FOR HYPERTENSIVE EMERGENCIES				
Diazoxide Hyperstat I.V.	IV 1–3 mg/kg (up to 150 mg) over 30 sec, may repeat q 5–15 min. Alternatively, IV infusion 10–30 mg/min. After 300 mg given, give furosemide IV 40 mg before subsequent doses.	2–4	3–12 hr	Useful in hypertensive encephalopathy, malignant hypertension, and eclampsia. Increases cardiac output; requires BP monitoring at hourly intervals. Avoid with ischemic heart disease or intracranial hemorrhage.
Enalaprilat Vasotec	IV 0.625–1.25 mg. (*See* monograph.)	15–30	4–6 hr	Useful in CHF and those at risk for cerebral hypotension. Avoid in severe renal impairment. Blacks may respond poorly. Hypotension may occur.
Esmolol Brevibloc	IV 250–500 μg/kg/min for 1–2 min, then 50–100 μg/kg/min for 4 min; may repeat sequence.	1–2 min	10–20 min	Useful in perioperative patients with aortic dissection. Does not cause tachycardia, but rather decreases heart rate.
Fenoldopam Corlopam	IV 0.1–0.3 μg/kg/min initially by continuous infusion.	<5	30 min	Useful in patients with renal insufficiency who risk cyanide toxicity with nitroprusside. Use with caution in glaucoma.
Hydralazine Apresoline	IM or IV 10–40 mg q 3–6 hr.	10–20	3–8 hr	Limited to treatment of severe pre-eclampsia and eclampsia. Increases cardiac output; many patients sensitive to parenteral doses, resulting in excessive hypotension.
Labetalol Normodyne Trandate	IV push 20 mg initially, then 40–80 mg q 10 min until desired response achieved or a total dose of 300 mg. Alternatively, IV infusion 0.5–2 mg/min.	<10	3–6 hr	Hypotensive effect is predictable; contraindicated in CHF, head trauma, and intracranial hemorrhage; often causes marked postural hypotension. Avoid use in patients with COPD, CHF, or bradycardia.

(*continued*)

DRUGS FOR HYPERTENSIVE URGENCIES AND EMERGENCIES COMPARISON CHART (continued)

DRUG	DOSAGE RANGE	ONSET (MIN)	DURATION	COMMENTS
Nicardipine Cardene	IV infusion 5–15 mg/hr.	<5–15	1–4 hr	Predictable effect. Useful in coronary, cerebral, or peripheral artery disease and in surgical patients. Tachycardia may occur.
Nitroglycerin Various	IV 0.3–6 mg/hr by continuous infusion.	1–5	3–5 min	Useful in myocardial ischemia and hypertension associated with MI. Hypotension, headache, tachycardia, and tachyphylaxis occur. Avoid in constrictive pericarditis, pericardial tamponade, or intracranial hypertension.
Nitroprusside Sodium Nipride Various	IV 0.3–10 μg/kg/min by continuous infusion. Average dosage is 3 μg/kg/min.	0.5–1	1–2 min	Especially useful in ischemic heart disease. Continuous monitoring required; arterial pressure response adjusted by changing infusion rate; hypotensive effect enhanced by elevating head of patient's bed. Decreases cardiac output; cyanide toxicity with prolonged, high infusion rates.

Adapted from references 162, 202, 225 and 226.

β-Adrenergic Blocking Drugs

ESMOLOL HYDROCHLORIDE   Brevibloc

Pharmacology. Esmolol is an ultrashort-acting, cardioselective, β_1-adrenergic blocking agent. It is effective in controlling ventricular response in patients with atrial fibrillation and other supraventricular tachycardias and in slowing heart rate in patients with sinus tachycardia associated with acute MI or cardiac surgery. Esmolol is useful for treating hypertensive emergencies, particularly in patients with tachycardia, because it has a rapid onset, short duration of action, and reduces heart rate. It may also be effective in perioperative hypertension.[162,202,227,228]

Adult Dosage. Dilute injection to a final concentration of 10 mg/mL. **IV** loading dose is 500 μg/kg/min for 1 min, then 50 μg/kg/min. The IV loading dose may be repeated as often as q 5 min with a concomitant increase of infusion rate in 50 μg/kg/min increments, titrated to ventricular response, heart rate, and/or BP. Most patients respond to infusions of 100–200 μg/kg/min. Once the desired endpoint is obtained, the infusion rate may be decreased in 25–50 μg/kg/min increments at 5- to 10-min intervals. Infusions up to 48 hr in duration are well tolerated.

Pediatric Dosage. **IV** 500 μg/kg/min for 1 min, then 25–200 (average 120) μg/kg/min.[228] Weight-adjusted dosages may be higher than in adults because of its more rapid elimination in children; infusion rates as high as 1 mg/kg/min have been required to achieve complete β blockade.[229]

Dosage Forms. **Inj** 10, 250 mg/mL.

Pharmacokinetics. Effective plasma levels are about 1–1.5 mg/L (3.4–5.1 μmol/L). The α half-life is about 2 min; V_d averages 3.5 L/kg (range 2–5). Esmolol is rapidly hydrolyzed by plasma and blood esterases to a metabolite with weak, clinically unimportant β-blocking activity and small amounts of methanol. No unchanged esmolol appears in the urine. The elimination half-life is about 9 min in adults and 3 min in children.[227,228]

Adverse Reactions. The side effect profile is similar to that of other β_1-selective β-blockers. Dose-related hypotension is frequent; IV site phlebitis occurs occasionally. Concurrent IV morphine may increase serum levels by 46%.

PROPRANOLOL HYDROCHLORIDE   Inderal, Various

Pharmacology. Propranolol is a nonselective β-adrenergic blocker used in arrhythmias, hypertension, and angina pectoris. It is also effective in decreasing mortality after MI. The antiarrhythmic mechanism is caused by decreased AV nodal conduction in supraventricular tachycardias and blockade of catecholamine-induced dysrhythmias. The antihypertensive mechanism is unknown, but contributing factors are a CNS mechanism, renin blockade, and decreases in myocardial contractility and cardiac output. Propranolol also lowers myocardial oxygen demand by decreasing contractility and heart rate, which symptomatically alleviates anginal pain and increases exercise tolerance in coronary artery disease. β-Blockers and diuretics are recommended as first-line drugs for hypertension because of demonstrated reductions in morbidity and mortality.[162] (*See* β-Adrenergic Blocking Drugs Comparison Chart.)

Administration and Adult Dosage. PO 10–20 mg q 6 hr initially, increasing gradually to desired effects. In hypertension, over 1 g/day has been used; however, consider adding another drug if 480 mg/day is ineffective. In angina pectoris, the dosage is titrated to pain relief and exercise evidence of β-blockade (bradycardia). The end point for dosage escalation in acute arrhythmias is the return to sinus rhythm or, in atrial fibrillation or flutter, to a ventricular rate <100 beats a min with hemodynamic stability. Twice-daily administration is effective in angina pectoris and hypertension. Administer **SR Cap** in the same daily dosage once or twice daily (not indicated post-MI). **PO for post-MI prophylaxis (non-SR)** 180–240 mg/day in 2–3 divided doses. **IV slow push** 1 mg q 5 min, to a maximum of 0.15 mg/kg; some authors recommend that the first dose be given over 2–10 min.

Special Populations. *Pediatric Dosage.* **PO for hypertension** 0.5 mg/kg/day in 2–4 divided doses, increasing to a maximum of 2 mg/kg/day. **IV slow push** 0.01–0.1 mg/kg/dose over 10 min up to 1 mg (infants) or 3 mg (children), may repeat in 6–8 hr.[95]

Geriatric Dosage. Bioavailability is increased in the elderly, necessitating lower initial doses.

Other Conditions. Therapeutic end points may be achieved with lower dosages in hypothyroidism or liver disease. Begin with lower dosages and titrate to clinical response. Patients with thyrotoxicosis require higher dosages to achieve the desired effect.[230]

Dosage Forms. **Soln** 4, 8, 80 mg/mL; **Tab** 10, 20, 40, 60, 80, 90 mg; **SR Cap** 60, 80, 120, 160 mg; **Inj** 1 mg/mL.

Patient Instructions. Report any symptoms such as shortness of breath, swelling, wheezing, fatigue, depression, nightmares, or inability to concentrate. Do not stop therapy abruptly. Do not crush or chew SR capsule. The SR capsule core may appear in the stool, but this does not mean there was a lack of absorption.

Missed Doses. Take this drug at regular intervals. If you miss a dose take it as soon as you remember. If it is about time for the next dose, take that dose only. Leave a minimum of 4 hours between regular tablet doses and 6–8 hours between extended-release capsule doses. Do not double the dose or take extra.

Pharmacokinetics. *Onset and Duration.* PO onset is variable; the duration varies from 6 to >12 hr.[230]

Serum Levels. No definite relationship has been established between serum concentrations and therapeutic effect in the treatment of arrhythmias, angina pectoris, or hypertension. β-Blockade is associated with serum concentrations >100 μg/L (340 nmol/L).[231]

Fate. Propranolol is rapidly and completely absorbed after oral administration; however, a large hepatic first-pass effect occurs, limiting systemic availability to $26 \pm 10\%$. First-pass elimination is saturable with an oral dose greater than about 30 mg.[231] The drug is $87 \pm 6\%$ bound to α_1-acid glycoprotein and other plasma proteins.[9,230] V_d is 4.3 ± 0.6 L/kg; Cl is 0.96 ± 0.3 L/hr/kg. Unlike most other drugs, displacement from plasma proteins increases elimination half-life and V_d because of high tissue affinity (nonrestrictive elimination). An active metabolite, 4-hydroxypropranolol, is formed after oral, but not IV, administration. Less than 0.5% of a dose is excreted unchanged in urine.[9]

$t_{1/2}$. α phase is about 10 min;[230] β phase after a single PO dose is 3.9 ± 0.4 hr.[9] With long-term oral therapy, β phase is 4–6 hr; however, it may be as long as 10–20 hr in patients with liver disease.[232]

Adverse Reactions. Adverse effects are often not dose related. Depression, nightmares, insomnia, fatigue, and lethargy occur frequently, and, less often, psychotic changes have been reported. CNS side effects probably occur more often with the lipophilic β-blockers (eg, propranolol). The drug may cause occasional life-threatening reactions when therapy (especially IV) is initiated, and acute CHF with pulmonary edema and hypotension or symptomatic bradycardia and heart block may occur. Acute drug cessation in patients with coronary artery disease may precipitate unstable angina pectoris or MI. The drug may precipitate hypoglycemia, but probably more important in diabetics is its ability to mask hypoglycemic symptoms (except for sweating). It may exacerbate symptoms of peripheral vascular disease or Raynaud's disease. β-Blockers may exacerbate previously stable asthma or chronic airway obstruction by causing bronchospasm, or renal dysfunction by further depressing GFR.

Contraindications. Severe obstructive pulmonary disease, asthma or active allergic rhinitis; cardiogenic shock or severe CHF; second- or third-degree heart block; severe sinus node disease.

Precautions. In coronary artery disease, discontinue drug by tapering the dosage over 4–7 days. Use cautiously in patients with Prinzmetal's vasospastic angina to prevent worsening of chest pain. Use caution in peripheral vascular disease or CHF and in patients with brittle diabetes or a history of hypoglycemic episodes. May worsen atrial fibrillation associated with accessory AV pathway.

Drug Interactions. Concurrent digitalis therapy may lessen the β-blocker exacerbation of CHF. When taken with oral hypoglycemics, nonselective β-blockers such as propranolol prolong hypoglycemic episodes and inhibit tachycardia and tremors, which are signs of hypoglycemia (sweating is not inhibited); hypertension may occur during hypoglycemia. Epinephrine may produce hypertensive reactions in patients on propranolol (and probably other nonselective β-blockers); this may also occur with other sympathomimetics such as phenylephrine and phenylpropanolamine. Barbiturates and rifampin may increase metabolism of hepatically eliminated β-blockers such as propranolol. Cimetidine may increase propranolol effects. Combined use of clonidine and propranolol may result in *hypertensive* reactions, especially if clonidine is abruptly discontinued. β-Blockers may increase the first-dose hypotensive effect of prazosin and similar drugs. NSAIDs may blunt the hypotensive response of β-blockers.

Parameters to Monitor. During IV administration, blood pressure and pulse must be taken q 5 min with constant ECG monitoring for signs of AV nodal block (lengthened PR interval) or bradycardia. Evaluate vital signs routinely for hemodynamic end points (eg, blood pressure in hypertension and heart rate or pressure-rate product in angina pectoris). Question the patient about subjective complaints such as nightmares or fatigue. When a patient at risk for adverse reactions is first given propranolol, signs and symptoms of toxicity must be evaluated (eg, CHF, shortness of breath or edema; bronchospasm, wheezing or shortness of breath; diabetes, blood glucose; peripheral vascular disease, painful or cold extremities).

Notes. Propranolol may be beneficial for treatment of symptomatic hypertrophic obstructive cardiomyopathy by increasing end-diastolic volume, producing ventricular relaxation and relieving ventricular outflow obstruction. If a β-blocker must be used in lung disease, β₁-selective drugs (eg, **acebutolol, atenolol,** or **metoprolol**) cause alterations in pulmonary function that are more easily reversed by bronchodilators; these drugs are probably a better choice than propranolol or other nonselective β-blockers. (*See* β-Adrenergic Blocking Drugs Comparison Chart.)

β-ADRENERGIC BLOCKING DRUGS COMPARISON CHART

DRUG	DOSAGE FORMS	CARDIO-SELECTIVITY	β HALF-LIFE (HR)	EXCRETED UNCHANGED IN URINE	PROTEIN BINDING	LABELED USES	STARTING DOSAGE	MAXIMUM DOSAGE
Acebutolol [a] Sectral Various	Cap 200, 400 mg.	+	3–4 (diacetolol) 8–13	30–40%	25%	Hypertension, arrhythmias.	PO 400 mg/day.	PO 1.2 g/day.
Atenolol Tenormin Various	Tab 25, 50, 100 mg Inj 0.5 mg/mL.	+ (up to 100 mg)	6–7	85%	10%	Hypertension. Post-MI prophylaxis.	PO 50 mg/day. IV 5 mg × 2, then PO 100 mg/day.	PO 200 mg/day.
Betaxolol [b] Kerlone	Tab 10, 20 mg.	+	14–20	15%	50%	Hypertension.	PO 10 mg/day.	PO 40 mg/day.
Bevantolol Vantol (Investigational, Parke-Davis)	—	+	1–3	<10%	95%	—	PO 150 mg/day.	PO 400 mg/day.
Bisoprolol Zebeta	Tab 5, 10 mg.	+	9–12	50%	30%	Hypertension.	PO 2–5 mg/day.	PO 20 mg/day.
Bopindolol [a] (Investigational, SKB)	—	0	9–12	—	—	—	PO 0.5– 1 mg/day.	PO 40 mg/day.
Bucindolol [a,c] Bextra (Investigational, Interneuron)	—	0	—	—	—	Hypertension, CHF (Investigational)	—	—

(continued)

β-ADRENERGIC BLOCKING DRUGS COMPARISON CHART (continued)

DRUG	DOSAGE FORMS	CARDIO-SELECTIVITY	β HALF-LIFE (HR)	EXCRETED UNCHANGED IN URINE	PROTEIN BINDING	LABELED USES	STARTING DOSAGE	MAXIMUM DOSAGE
Carteolol[a] Cartrol	Tab 2.5, 5 mg.	0	6–11	60%	15%	Hypertension.	PO 2.5 mg/day.	PO 10 mg/day.
Carvedilol[c] Coreg	Tab 3.125, 6.25, 12.5, 25 mg.	0	6–8	1%	95%	Hypertension, CHF.	PO 3.125 mg bid, increasing q 2 weeks.	PO (<85 kg) 50 mg/day; (>85 kg) 100 mg/day.
Celiprolol[a, c] (Investigational, Rhone-Poulenc Rorer)	—	+	4–8	10–20%	25%	—	PO 200 mg/day.	PO 600 mg/day.
Esmolol Brevibloc	Inj 10, 250 mg/mL.	+	9 min	0%	55%	Supraventricular tachycardia.	IV 50 μg/kg/min.	IV 200 μg/kg/min.
Labetalol[c] Trandate Normodyne Various	Tab 100, 200, 300 mg Inj 5 mg/mL.	0	4–9	5%	50%	Hypertension.	PO 100 mg/day. IV 20 mg, then 40–80 mg q 10 min.	PO 2.4 g/day. IV 300 mg.
Metoprolol Lopressor Toprol XL	Tab 50, 100 mg SR Tab 50, 100, 200 mg Inj 1 mg/mL.	+ (up to 100 mg)	3–7	39%	10%	Hypertension. Hypertension, angina pectoris. Acute MI.	PO 100 mg/day. PO SR 50–100 mg/day. IV 5 mg × 3, then PO 50 mg q 6 hr × 48 hr.	PO 450 mg/day. PO SR 400 mg/day.

(continued)

β-ADRENERGIC BLOCKING DRUGS COMPARISON CHART (continued)

DRUG	DOSAGE FORMS	CARDIO-SELECTIVITY	β HALF-LIFE (HR)	EXCRETED UNCHANGED IN URINE	PROTEIN BINDING	LABELED USES	STARTING DOSAGE	MAXIMUM DOSAGE
Nadolol Corgard Various	Tab 20, 40, 80, 120, 160 mg.	0	17–24	70%	25%	Hypertension, angina pectoris.	PO 40 mg/day.	PO 320 mg/day.
Penbutolol [a] Levatol	Tab 20 mg.	0	4–8	5%	80–90%	Hypertension.	PO 20 mg/day.	PO 80 mg/day.
Pindolol [a] Visken	Tab 5, 10 mg.	0	3–4	40%	57%	Hypertension.	PO 10 mg/day.	PO 60 mg/day.
Propranolol Inderal Various	(*See* monograph.)	0	4–6	<0.5%	87%	Hypertension, angina pectoris, arrhythmias. Post-MI prophylaxis.	PO 40–80 mg/day.	PO 480 mg/day.
Sotalol [d] Betapace	Tab 80, 160, 240 mg.	0	7–15	80–90%	0%	Life-threatening ventricular arrhythmias.	PO 180 mg/day. PO 160 mg/day.	PO 240 mg/day. PO 640 mg/day.
Timolol [b] Blocadren	Tab 5, 10, 20 mg.	0	4–5	20%	<10%	Hypertension. Post-MI prophylaxis.	PO 20 mg/day. PO 20 mg/day.	PO 60 mg/day. PO 20 mg/day.

[a] Acebutolol, bopindolol, bucindolol, carteolol, celiprolol, penbutolol, and pindolol have intrinsic agonist (sympathomimetic) activity (ISA).

[b] Betaxolol is also available as Betoptic ophthalmic drops 0.5%; carteolol is also available as Ocupress 1%; and timolol is also available as Timoptic ophthalmic drops 0.25% and 0.5% for treatment of glaucoma.

[c] Carvedilol and bucindolol have α₁-blocking actions; and celiprolol has weak α₂-blocking actions. Labetalol has potent α₁-blocking actions (ratio of α- to β-blockade 1:3 and 1:7 with PO and IV, respectively).

[d] Sotalol also has type III antiarrhythmic properties.

From references 120, 227, 233–240 and product information.

Calcium-Channel Blocking Drugs

DILTIAZEM HYDROCHLORIDE   Cardizem, Dilacor XR, Tiazac, Various

Pharmacology. Diltiazem is a calcium-channel blocking drug that decreases heart rate, prolongs AV nodal conduction, and decreases arteriolar and coronary vascular tone. It also has negative inotropic properties. Diltiazem is effective in symptomatic angina pectoris, essential hypertension, and supraventricular tachycardias. It may also reduce early reinfarction rates in patients with non-Q-wave MI and normal left ventricular function. (*See* Calcium-Channel Blocking Drugs Comparison Chart.)

Administration and Adult Dosage. **IV loading dose** 0.25 mg/kg (about 20 mg) over 2 min, may repeat in 15 min with 0.35 mg/kg (about 25 mg). **IV infusion** 5–15 mg/hr, titrated to ventricular response. **PO for angina** 30–60 mg q 6–8 hr initially; dosages up to 480 mg/day may be required for symptomatic relief of angina;[241,242] 180–300 mg once daily with Cardizem CD. **PO for hypertension** 120–240 mg/day initially, in 2 divided doses using Cardizem SR, or 180–300 mg once daily using Cardizem CD or Dilacor XR, titrated to clinical response; **maintenance dosages** of 180–480 mg/day are usually necessary.

Special Populations. *Pediatric Dosage.* Safety and efficacy are not established.

Geriatric Dosage. Same as adult dosage, but titrate dosage slowly.

Other Conditions. Patients with liver disease may require lower dosages; titrate to clinical response.

Dosage Forms. **Tab** 30, 60, 90, 120 mg; **SR Cap** (12-hr; Cardizem SR, various) 60, 90, 120 mg; **SR Cap** (24-hr; Cardizem CD) 120, 180, 240, 300 mg; (24-hr; Dilacor XR) 120, 180, 240 mg; (24-hr; Tiazac) 120, 180, 240, 300, 360 mg; **SR Tab** 120, 180, 240 mg (Tiamate); **Inj** 5 mg/mL; **SR Tab** 180 mg with enalapril 5 mg (Teczem).

Patient Instructions. Report dizziness, leg swelling, or shortness of breath. (For angina) Maintain a diary to document the numbers of episodes of chest pain and sublingual nitroglycerin tablets used.

Missed Doses. Take this drug at regular intervals. If you miss a dose take it as soon as you remember. If it is about time for the next dose, take that dose only. Do not double the dose or take extra.

Pharmacokinetics. *Onset and Duration.* PO onset 0.5–3 hr, duration 6–10 hr;[243] 12–24 hr with SR cap, depending on the product.

Serum Levels. Levels over 95 µg/L (230 nmol/L) are necessary to cause hemodynamic changes, but their clinical usefulness is questionable.[244] Levels of desacetyldiltiazem are similar to diltiazem.[245]

Fate. Oral bioavailability is 38 ± 11% with the first dose, but 90 ± 21% during long-term therapy.[245] The drug is 78 ± 3% plasma protein bound; V_d is 5.3 ± 1.7 L/kg;[245] Cl is 0.72 ± 0.3 L/hr/kg.[9] Enterohepatic recycling occurs. The drug is almost entirely metabolized by the liver, with only 1–3% excreted unchanged in urine. One metabolite, desacetyldiltiazem, has 40–50% the activity of diltiazem. Metabolites are excreted primarily in the feces.

$t_{1/2}$. α phase 2–5 min; β phase 4.9 ± 0.4 hr,[243,245] longer in the elderly.[242] β phase for desacetyldiltiazem 6.1 ± 1.2 hr.[245]

Adverse Reactions. Frequency of side effects is dose related. Headache, flushing, dizziness, and edema occur frequently. Sinus bradycardia and AV block occur frequently, often in association with concomitant β-blockers.[242] Worsening of CHF may occur in patients with underlying left ventricular dysfunction. A variety of skin reactions have been occasionally reported.[242] Hepatitis occurs rarely.

Contraindications. Second- or third-degree block or sick sinus syndrome in the absence of a ventricular pacemaker; symptomatic hypotension or severe CHF, acute MI, or pulmonary congestion; atrial fibrillation with accessory AV pathway.

Precautions. Use caution with concomitant use of β-blockers in patients with underlying CHF, especially those with poor left ventricular function.[242]

Drug Interactions. Cimetidine and propranolol increase diltiazem serum levels.[242,246] Diltiazem inhibits the CYP3A metabolism of many drugs, including carbamazepine, cyclosporine, and theophylline.[242]

Parameters to Monitor. Blood pressure, heart rate, and ECG, especially when initiating therapy. Observe for symptoms of hypotension and CHF. Serial treadmill exercise tests can be performed to assess efficacy in angina. Monitor the number of episodes of chest pain and SL nitroglycerin used.

NIFEDIPINE   Adalat, Procardia

Pharmacology. Nifedipine is a dihydropyridine calcium-channel blocking drug with potent arterial and coronary vasodilating properties. A reflex increase in sympathetic tone (in response to vasodilation) counteracts the direct depressant effects on SA and AV nodal conduction. This renders nifedipine ineffective in the treatment of supraventricular tachycardias. It is used for vasospastic and chronic stable angina and in the treatment of hypertension. (*See* Calcium-Channel Blocking Drugs Comparison Chart.)

Administration and Adult Dosage. **PO for angina** (Cap) 10 mg tid initially, increasing to a usual maximum of 20–30 mg tid or qid; dosages over 180 mg/day are not recommended. **PO for hypertension** (SR Tab only) 30–60 mg/day initially, increasing to 120 mg/day prn. **PO for severe hypertension** (non-SR) 10 mg, may repeat prn in 20 min. The capsule may be punctured or bitten and swallowed, usually resulting in a more rapid onset than SL administration.[247]

Special Populations. *Pediatric Dosage.* Safety and efficacy not established. **PO for hypertensive crisis** 0.25–0.5 mg/kg q 6–8 hr.[95]

Geriatric Dosage. Same as adult dosage.

Other Conditions. Patients with liver disease may require lower dosages;[248] titrate to clinical response.

Dosage Forms. **Cap** 10, 20 mg; **SR Tab** 30, 60, 90 mg.

Patient Instructions. Report flushing, edema, dizziness, or increased frequency of chest discomfort. Do not split, chew, or crush sustained-release tablets. The SR tablet core may appear in the stool, but this does not mean there was a lack of absorption. Maintain a diary to document the number of episodes of chest pain and sublingual nitroglycerin tablets used.

Missed Doses. Take this drug at regular intervals. If you miss a dose take it as soon as you remember. If it is about time for the next dose, take that dose only. Do not double the dose or take extra.

Pharmacokinetics. *Onset and Duration.* PO onset 0.5–2 hr; duration (Cap) 4–8 hr; (SR Tab) 12–24 hr. PO (punctured capsule) onset 10–20 min; duration 3–4 hr.

Serum Levels. (Therapeutic) above 90 µg/L (260 nmol/L), although clinical utility is questionable.[249]

Fate. Bioavailability is 52 ± 37% in normals and 91 ± 26% in cirrhosis because of extensive and variable first-pass hepatic elimination.[248] It is 96 ± 1% plasma protein bound; V_d is 0.8 ± 0.2 L/kg.[249,250] Cl is 0.42 ± 0.12 L/hr/kg.[9] Nifedipine is almost all eliminated by hepatic metabolism via the CYP3A4 isozyme, which is present in variable amounts (but is not a true polymorphism).[251] Only traces of drug are excreted unchanged in urine.[249]

$t_{1/2}$. α phase 4–7 min; β phase 2 ± 0.4 hr.[249,250]

Adverse Reactions. Most side effects relate to vasodilatory actions and occur frequently; symptoms include dizziness (with or without hypotension), flushing, and headache. These types of side effects seem less frequent with SR dosage forms.[252] Immediate-release products may increase mortality when used chronically to treat hypertension and should be avoided for this use.[162,253] Edema occurs frequently and is related to venous pooling and usually not exacerbation of CHF. Nifedipine can paradoxically worsen anginal chest pain, possibly because of a reflex increase in sympathetic tone or redistribution of coronary blood flow away from ischemic areas. Acute, reversible renal failure may occur in patients with chronic renal insufficiency;[254] rare reactions include hepatitis and hyperglycemia.

Contraindications. Symptomatic hypotension.

Precautions. Use with caution in unstable angina pectoris when used alone (ie, without a β-blocker) and in patients with CHF caused by systolic dysfunction, because mortality may be increased.[253,255] Do not use immediate-release products to treat hypertension. Nifedipine has an antiplatelet action and may increase bleeding time.[256] Nifedipine may worsen symptoms of obstructive cardiomyopathy.

Drug Interactions. Barbiturates increase nifedipine metabolism. Cimetidine may increase nifedipine serum levels. Nifedipine occasionally increases PT in patients on oral anticoagulants. Nifedipine and IV magnesium sulfate may cause neuromuscular blockade and hypotension.

Parameters to Monitor. Blood pressure and heart rate, especially when initiating therapy. Observe for symptoms of hypotension and edema. Serial treadmill exercise tests can be performed to assess efficacy.

Notes. Other potential uses for nifedipine include migraine prophylaxis, achalasia, and Raynaud's phenomenon.

VERAPAMIL HYDROCHLORIDE   Calan, Covera-HS, Isoptin, Verelan, Various

Pharmacology. Verapamil is a calcium-channel blocking drug that prolongs AV nodal conduction. It is used to convert re-entrant supraventricular tachycardias and to slow ventricular rate in atrial fibrillation or flutter. Because it decreases contractility and arteriolar resistance, it is used in angina caused by coronary obstruction or vasospasm. Verapamil is also effective in the treatment of hypertension and hypertrophic obstructive cardiomyopathy, and in migraine prophylaxis. (*See* Calcium-Channel Blocking Drugs Comparison Chart.)

Administration and Adult Dosage. **PO for angina** 80–120 mg tid initially, increasing at daily (for unstable angina) or weekly intervals, to a maximum of 480 mg/day. Covera-HS is designed to be taken hs. **PO for hypertension** usually 240 mg/day using SR tablet; SR dosages of 120 mg/day to 240 mg bid have been used. Covera-HS is designed to be taken hs. **PO for migraine prophylaxis** 160–320 mg/day. **IV for supraventricular arrhythmias** 5–10 mg (0.075–0.15 mg/kg) over at least 2 min (3 min in elderly), may repeat with 10 mg (0.15 mg/kg) in 30 min if arrhythmia is not terminated or desired end point is not achieved. **IV constant infusion** 5–10 mg/hr.[257]

Special Populations. *Pediatric Dosage.* PO 4–8 mg/kg/day in 3 divided doses. **IV** (<1 yr) 0.1–0.2 mg/kg; (1–15 yr) 0.1–0.3 mg/kg, to a maximum of 5 mg over 2–3 min initially, may repeat with same dose in 30 min if initial response inadequate.[95]

Geriatric Dosage. Same as adult dosage, but administer over 3 min.

Other Conditions. Dosage may need to be decreased in patients with liver disease; titrate to clinical response.

Dosage Forms. **Tab** 40, 80, 120 mg; **SR Tab** 120, 180, 240 mg; **SR Cap** 120, 180, 240 mg; **Inj** 2.5 mg/mL; **SR Tab** 180 mg with trandolapril 2 mg, 240 mg with trandolapril 4 mg (Tarka).

Patient Instructions. Report any dizziness, shortness of breath, or edema. Constipation occurs often. Maintain a diary to document the number of episodes of chest pain and sublingual nitroglycerin used.

Missed Doses. Take this drug at regular intervals. If you miss a dose take it as soon as you remember. If it is about time for the next dose, take that dose only. Do not double the dose or take extra.

Pharmacokinetics. *Onset and Duration.* IV onset immediate; duration 2–6 hr, up to 12 hr with long-term use.[258]

Serum Levels. 50–400 μg/L (100–800 nmol/L), although therapeutic range is not well established.

Fate. Although the drug is well absorbed orally, only 22 ± 8% is bioavailable because of extensive first-pass elimination; bioavailability increases in liver disease.[259] Covera-HS provides a 4- to 5-hr delay before releasing the drug. Verapamil has stereospecific pharmacology and pharmacokinetics; L-verapamil is a more potent AV nodal blocking drug, but it undergoes greater first-pass metabolism.[260] Norverapamil is an active metabolite. Verapamil is about 90 ± 2% plasma protein bound, with the more active L-isomer having a greater unbound fraction.[259,261] V_d is 5 ± 2 L/kg and increases in liver disease;[9,259] Cl is 0.9 ± 0.36 L/hr/kg. About 1% is excreted unchanged in urine.[9]

$t_{\frac{1}{2}}$. (Verapamil) α phase 5–30 min; β phase 4 ± 1.5 hr; may increase during long-term use; 13.6 ± 3.9 hr in severe liver disease; (norverapamil) 8 ± 1.9 hr.[9,259,261]

Adverse Reactions. Constipation occurs frequently (5–40%), particularly in elderly patients. CHF may occur in patients with left ventricular dysfunction. Serious hemodynamic side effects (eg, severe hypotension) and conduction abnormalities (eg, symptomatic bradycardia or asystole) have been reported; these reactions usually occur when the patient is concurrently receiving a β-blocker or has underlying conduction disease.[262] Infants appear to be particularly susceptible to arrhythmias. IV **calcium** (gluconate or chloride salts, 10–20 mL of a 10% solution) and/or **isoproterenol** may, in part, reverse these adverse effects.[262] The administration of IV calcium prior to verapamil may prevent hypotension without abolishing the antiarrhythmic actions.[263]

Contraindications. Shock or severely hypotensive states; second- or third-degree AV nodal block; sick sinus syndrome, unless functioning ventricular pacemaker is in place; hypotension or CHF unless caused by supraventricular tachyarrhythmias amenable to verapamil therapy; atrial fibrillation and an accessory AV pathway.

Precautions. Use caution with any wide-QRS tachycardia; severe hypotension and shock may ensue if the tachycardia is ventricular in origin. Use with caution in combination with oral β-blockers and poor left ventricular function.

Drug Interactions. Verapamil may increase serum levels of several drugs, including carbamazepine, cyclosporine, digoxin, and theophylline. Barbiturates and rifampin may increase verapamil metabolism.

Parameters to Monitor. Blood pressure and constant ECG monitoring during IV administration. Pay particular attention to signs and symptoms of CHF and hypotension. Also, monitor the ECG for PR prolongation and bradycardia.

CALCIUM CHANNEL BLOCKING DRUGS COMPARISON CHART

DRUG	DOSAGE FORMS	ADULT DOSAGE	CONTRACTILITY	HEART RATE	AV NODAL CONDUCTION	VASCULAR RESISTANCE
Amlodipine[a] Norvasc	Tab 2.5, 5, 10 mg.	PO 5–10 mg/day.	0	0	0	↓↓
Bepridil[b] Vasocor	Tab 200, 300, 400 mg.	PO for angina 200–400 mg/day.	0/↓	0/↓	0/↓	→
Diltiazem[c] Cardizem Dilacor XR	(*See* monograph.)	(*See* monograph.)	→	→	→	→
Felodipine[d] Plendil	SR Tab 2.5, 5, 10 mg.	PO for hypertension 2.5–20 mg once daily.	0/↑	0/↑	0/↑	↓↓
Isradipine[d] DynaCirc	Cap 2.5, 5 mg SR Cap 5, 10 mg.	PO for hypertension 2.5–10 mg bid or SR 5–10 mg once daily.	0/↑	0/↑	0/↑	↓↓
Nicardipine[d] Cardene Various	Cap 20, 30 mg SR Cap 30, 45, 60 mg Inj 2.5 mg/mL.	PO for angina or hypertension 20–40 mg tid or SR 30–60 mg q 12 hr. IV for hypertension 5–15 mg/hr.	0/↑	0/↑	0/↑	↓↓
Nifedipine[d] Adalat Procardia	Cap 10, 20 mg SR Tab 30, 60, 90 mg.	(*See* monograph.)	0/↑	0/↑	0/↑	↓↓

(continued)

CALCIUM CHANNEL BLOCKING DRUGS COMPARISON CHART (continued)

DRUG	DOSAGE FORMS	ADULT DOSAGE	CONTRACTILITY	HEART RATE	AV NODAL CONDUCTION	VASCULAR RESISTANCE
Nimodipine[d] Nimotop	Cap 30 mg.	PO postsubarachnoid hemorrhage 60 mg q 4 hr for 21 days.	0/↑	0/↑	0/↑	↓↓
Nisoldipine[d] Sular	SR Tab 10, 20, 30, 40 mg.	PO for hypertension SR 20–40 mg once daily.	0/↑	0/↑	0/↑	↓↓
Verapamil[c] Calan Isoptin Verelan	(*See monograph.*)	(*See monograph.*)	↓↓	↓	↓↓	↓

KEY: ↑ = increase; ↓↓ = marked decrease, ↓ = decrease, 0 = no change.
[a]Selective vascular actions.
[b]Complex pharmacology with probable sodium- and potassium-channel blockade (quinidine-like).
[c]Vascular and eletrophysiologic actions.
[d]Predominantly vascular actions.
From reference 264 and product information.

Hypolipidemic Drugs

Class Instructions: Hypolipidemics. There is a strong relationship between elevated serum cholesterol and death caused by coronary heart disease (CHD). Cholesterol lowering has been demonstrated to decrease events related to CHD and may slow or even reverse atherosclerosis. These effects are associated with a decrease in CHD mortality. Generally, each 1% decrease in serum cholesterol results in a 2% decrease in the risk of coronary events. Hypolipidemic drugs must be taken daily to achieve these results. Drug therapy does not eliminate the need for appropriate diet and other measures such as weight reduction (if appropriate), smoking cessation, and physical activity. Use of estrogen and progestin in postmenopausal women also has beneficial effects on lipoprotein levels. Hypolipidemic drug therapy (with the exception of niacin) has been associated with an increase in cancer in animals, but it is not known if they have this effect in humans.

Missed Doses. Take this drug at regular intervals. If you miss a dose take it as soon as you remember. If it is about time for the next dose, take that dose only. Do not double the dose or take extra.

CHOLESTYRAMINE RESIN   Questran, Various

Pharmacology. Cholestyramine is a bile acid sequestrant that acts as an anion exchange resin, releasing chloride ions and adsorbing bile acids in the intestine to form a nonabsorbable complex that is excreted in the feces. The resulting increase in activity of hepatic low-density lipoprotein cholesterol (LDL-c) receptors leads to the oxidation of cholesterol to form new bile acids. Despite a compensatory increase in hepatic cholesterol synthesis, total serum cholesterol and LDL-c levels are reduced by 15–30%. The increase in cholesterol synthesis sometimes results in an increase in VLDL cholesterol levels, which may increase triglyceride levels by 10–50%.[265,266] Cardioprotective HDL cholesterol levels may increase by 3–8%.[266]

Administration and Adult Dosage. **PO for hyperlipidemia** 4 daily–bid initially, increasing slowly to a maintenance dosage of 8–16 g/day in 1–6 (usually 2) divided doses, to a maximum of 24 g/day. Compliance appears to be best in the range of 8–10 g/day in 1–2 divided doses. **PO for treatment of cholestatic pruritus** 4–8 g/day is usual. **PO for treatment of relapsing enterocolitis caused by** *Clostridium difficile* 4 g tid or qid (with or without vancomycin) has been used.

Special Populations. *Pediatric Dosage.* Limited data are available, especially concerning long-term use. Drug therapy is generally reserved for children 10 yr or older, initiated at the lowest possible dosage, and gradually increased until the desired response is achieved. Base initial dosage on serum LDL-c level rather than body weight, and adjust dosage based on response: **PO for hyperlipidemia** (LDL-c <195 mg/dL) 4 g/day; (LDL-c 195–235 mg/dL) 8 g/day; (LDL-c 236–280 mg/dL) 12 g/day; (LDL-c >280 mg/dL) 16 g/day.[267,268] (*See* Precautions.)

Geriatric Dosage. Initiate therapy at lowest possible dosage, and slowly titrate to desired effect. Maximum dosage may not be required or tolerated.

Other Conditions. In patients with a history of constipation, start at the low end of the dosage range. In patients with GI intolerance, reduce dosage and increase gradually. (*See* Adverse Reactions.)

Dosage Forms. **Pwdr** 4 g resin/9 g powder (Questran); 4 g resin/5 g powder (Questran Light).

Patient Instructions. (*See* Hypolipidemics Class Instructions.) It is preferable to take this drug before meals, but you may adjust the time of the dosages around the scheduling of other oral medications. Take other oral medications at least 1 hour before or 4–6 hours after cholestyramine. Do not take dry; mix each packet or level scoopful with at least 60–180 mL (2–6 fl. oz.) of water or noncarbonated beverage, highly fluid soup, or pulpy fruit such as applesauce or crushed pineapple. You may need to experiment with different products and vehicles to determine your preference based on taste, cost, and caloric restrictions. Mixtures may be refrigerated to improve palatability, but do not cook because the drug may be inactivated. This drug frequently causes constipation. If this becomes a problem, contact your physician or pharmacist to discuss measures to potentially minimize constipation. It may cause other gastrointestinal symptoms, which usually decrease over time.

Pharmacokinetics. *Onset and Duration.* Reduction in cholesterol begins in the first month.

Fate. It is not absorbed from the GI tract. Resin and complex are excreted in the feces.

Adverse Reactions. Almost 70% of patients experience at least one GI side effect.[269] Constipation frequently occurs, especially with higher dosages, in the elderly, and in patients with previous constipation; fecal impaction is rare. Nausea, heartburn, abdominal pain, bloating, steatorrhea, and belching also occur frequently, but tend to decrease over time.[265] GI side effects tend to be milder in children than in adults. Hemorrhoids may be aggravated or develop. Rash may occur. Chloride absorption in place of bicarbonate may lead to hyperchloremic acidosis, especially in children, and calcium excretion may be increased. Absorption of vitamins D and K may be impaired, leading to osteomalacia and bleeding, respectively. Absorption of folic acid may also be impaired, especially in children. Alimentary cancers in rats are somewhat more prevalent with cholestyramine treatment because of enhancement of other carcinogens, but the importance of this in humans is unknown.[270]

Contraindications. Complete biliary obstruction.

Precautions. Pregnancy and lactation, caused by possible malabsorption of fat-soluble vitamins. Avoid constipation in patients with symptomatic coronary artery disease. Constipation may be controlled by reducing dosage, slowly titrating dosage, increasing dietary fiber, or using stool softeners. Avoid use in the presence of diverticular disease and local intestinal tract lesions because constipation may be a problem.[271] Discontinue if a clinically important elevation in serum triglycerides occurs. Vitamin supplementation may be needed with high dosage or long-term therapy. Children particularly may need multivitamins with folate and iron.[268] Patients with osteoporosis may need to restrict dietary chloride to limit calcium excretion.[272] Phenylketonurics should avoid Questran Light because it contains aspartame.

Drug Interactions. Absorption of many drugs may be delayed or reduced, including acetaminophen, coumarin anticoagulants, digitoxin (affected to a greater extent than digoxin), digoxin, furosemide, gemfibrozil, hydrocortisone, oral hypoglycemic drugs,[273] iron, loperamide, methotrexate, naproxen, penicillin G, phenobarbital, oral phosphate supplements, pravastatin, propranolol, tetracyclines, thyroid hormones, thiazides, and vancomycin. Monitor for concurrent drug therapy effects when initiating and altering sequestrant therapy, particularly for drugs with a narrow therapeutic index.

Parameters to Monitor. Monitor LDL-c and triglycerides 4 weeks and 3 months after initiation of therapy. If therapy goals are achieved, monitor q 4 months unless adverse effects are suspected. Periodically monitor hemoglobin and serum folic acid during long-term therapy. Monitor efficacy of and appropriate tests for concurrent drug therapy that may be affected by cholestyramine. In children, monitor serum concentrations of vitamins A, D, and E and erythrocyte folate, liver function tests, and CBC annually.[268]

Notes. Bile acid sequestering resins are indicated as an adjunct to diet for primary hypercholesterolemia (type IIa and IIb) in patients for whom hypertriglyceridemia is not a primary concern (triglyceride levels <300 mg/dL).[272] Bile acid sequestrants produce moderate lowering of LDL-c relative to some of the other hypolipidemic drugs, but are considered to be safer because they are not absorbed. These drugs may be particularly useful with moderately elevated LDL-c and in situations of lower risk of CHD when long-term safety is of concern (eg, primary prevention and in young men and premenopausal women).[265,274] They may be used in combination with other hypolipidemic drugs for additive effects when a larger decrease in LDL-c is required. Long-term use reduces cardiovascular morbidity and mortality, including the incidence of first heart attacks. Because over one-third of patients discontinue bile acid sequestrants in the first year, primarily because of adverse effects, conservative dosage titration as well as education and support is required to manage and avoid adverse effects.[269,275] Maximum dosage is rarely needed.[266] Low-dose therapy (8–10 g/day) appears to be best tolerated[265] and the most cost-effective, either alone or in combination therapy.[276] Increased dosage may increase adverse effects without meaningful increases in cholesterol lowering. Resins are not effective in patients with homozygous familiar hypercholesterolemia.[266] (*See* Recommendations for Initiation of Drug Therapy in Hypercholesterolemia Chart.)

The resins are also used for reduction of pruritus caused by dermal deposition of bile acids in patients with partial biliary obstruction, and cholestyramine has been used to treat relapsing *Clostridium difficile* colitis.[277,278] Interference with digoxin and digitoxin absorption suggests a possible role in managing mild intoxication caused by these drugs; however, do not rely on cholestyramine alone in cases of severe digitalis toxicity.[273] Questran contains 14 kcal/9 g packet or scoop; Questran Light is flavored with aspartame and contains 1.6 kcal and 16.8 mg of phenylalanine/5 g packet or scoop.

COLESTIPOL HYDROCHLORIDE   Colestid

Pharmacology. Colestipol is a bile acid sequestrant similar to cholestyramine with equivalent lipid-lowering effects in most patients. Selection of a bile acid sequestrant is generally based on patient preference and cost. The palatability of cholestyramine-vehicle combinations is often preferred over colestipol granules, although colestipol tablets are well tolerated. A 5 g dose of colestipol provides equivalent cholesterol lowering to 4 g of cholestyramine; a 4 g dose of the tablet is about equivalent to 5 g of the granules.[279–285] (*See* Hypolipidemic Drugs Comparison Chart and Recommendations for Initiation of Drug Therapy in Hypercholesterolemia Chart.)

Adult Dosage. **PO for hypercholesterolemia** (Granules) 5 g bid initially, increasing in 5 g/day increments at 1- to 2-month intervals to a maximum of 30 g/day in 1–4 doses; (tablets) 2 g bid initially, increasing in 2 g/day increments at 1- to 2-month intervals to a maximum of 16 g/day. (*See* Adverse Effects.) **PO for relapsing enterocolitis caused by** *Clostridium difficile* 5 g q 12 hr has been used with oral vancomycin, but avoid coadministration with vancomycin to prevent vancomycin binding.

Dosage Forms. **Granules** 5 g packets and bulk containers; **Tab** 1 g.

Adverse Effects. Adverse effects, precautions, monitoring instructions, and drug interactions are similar to those of cholestyramine. Patients with moderate hypercholesteremia who are unable to tolerate colestipol granules due to GI side effects may benefit from giving one-half the colestipol dose mixed with 2.5 g of **psyllium.**

FENOFIBRATE   TriCor

Pharmacology. Fenofibrate is a fibric acid derivative indicated for the treatment of types IV and V hyperlipidemia. It reduces serum LDL cholesterol by 17–35% and triglycerides by 15–43%, and increases HDL. It appears to act by enhancing lipoprotein lipase activity, inhibiting VLDL synthesis, and reducing cholesterol synthesis, possibly by inhibiting acyltransferase activity. It may also reduce platelet aggregation and decrease serum uric acid.[286–288]

Adult Dosage. **PO for types IV or V hyperlipidemia in those at risk of pancreatitis** 67 mg/day initially, increasing at 4–8-week intervals to a maximum of 201 mg/day. Doses should be taken with a meal.

Dosage Forms. **Cap** 67 mg.

Pharmacokinetics. Following absorption, fenofibrate is hydrolyzed to the active drug, fenofibric acid which is >99% plasma protein bound. It is predominantly excreted unchanged in urine with a half-life of 20 hr, which is prolonged in renal dysfunction.

Adverse Reactions. Side effects include GI disturbances, skin rash, muscle pain, and headache. Elevations in serum transaminases and CPK have occurred. Cholelithiasis has been reported, but it is not clear if the frequency is as great as with clofibrate. Fenofibrate should be avoided in those with liver, gallbladder, or kidney disease.

GEMFIBROZIL

Pharmacology. Gemfibrozil is a fibric acid derivative that decreases triglyceride and VLDL cholesterol (VLDL-c) concentrations and increases HDL cholesterol (HDL-c) concentrations. Effects on LDL-cholesterol (LDL-c) are variable. LDL-c may increase in some patients, especially those with type IV hyperlipoproteinemia. Its exact mechanism is unclear; however, it appears to act through multiple mechanisms. There is an increased secretion of cholesterol into bile, increased affinity of LDL receptors for LDL particles, activation of lipoprotein lipase, inhibition of triglyceride synthesis, suppression of free fatty acid release from adipose tissue, and a change in LDL-c toward a potentially less atherosclerotic form.[266,288]

Administration and Adult Dosage. **PO** as an hypolipidemic 600 mg bid.

Special Populations. *Pediatric Dosage.* Safety and efficacy not established.

Geriatric Dosage. Initiate therapy at lowest possible dosage, and slowly titrate to desired effect. Maximum dosage may not be required or tolerated.

Other Conditions. Some authors advise decreasing dose by one-half with Cl_{cr} of 20–50 mL/min.

Dosage Forms. **Tab** 600 mg.

Patient Instructions. (*See* Hypolipidemics Class Instructions.) Take doses 30 minutes prior to morning and evening meals. Gemfibrozil may cause a slightly increased risk of cancer and is similar to another medication that has been found to increase the risk of cancer, gallstones, and pancreatitis. You and your physician may decide the benefit of reducing the risk of coronary heart disease may be worth these other risks. Report any muscle pain, tenderness, or weakness promptly, especially if you are also taking lovastatin or a similar drug.

Pharmacokinetics. *Onset and Duration.* The maximum decrease in serum triglyceride and total cholesterol occurs within 4–12 weeks; lipids return to pretreatment levels after drug discontinuation.

Fate. The drug is rapidly and completely absorbed after oral administration. Mean peak serum concentrations of 15–25 mg/L (60–100 μmol/L) occur within 1–2 hr after administration of 600 mg bid. Serum concentrations are directly proportional to dose. The drug is 97–98.6% bound to albumin. Cl appears to be independent of renal function, but further study may be needed. Gemfibrozil is metabolized in the liver to a number of compounds. Approximately 70% of a dose is excreted in the urine, primarily as the glucuronide conjugates of the drug and metabolites; less than 2% is excreted renally as unchanged drug.[289–291]

$t_{\frac{1}{2}}$. Reportedly 1.5–2 hr, but may be longer allowing for complete distribution.[289]

Adverse Reactions. Dyspepsia (20%), abdominal pain (10%), diarrhea (7%), fatigue (3%), and nausea and vomiting (3%) are frequent; acute appendicitis, dizziness, eczema, rash, vertigo, constipation, headache, paresthesia (all between 1 and 2%) also occur. Occasional side effects include atrial fibrillation and elevations in liver function tests (AST, ALT, LDH, bilirubin, alkaline phosphatase), which return to normal upon drug discontinuation. Occasional mild decreases in WBCs, hematocrit, and hemoglobin occur, but usually stabilize. However, there are rare reports of severe blood dyscrasias. Serum glucose may be slightly elevated, as may LDL-c in some patients with high triglyceride levels. Gemfibrozil may increase biliary lipogenicity and possibly increase long-term risk of cholelithiasis.[266] Cholelithiasis requiring gallbladder surgery developed in 0.9% of gemfibroziltreated patients, compared to 0.5% of patients in a placebo group. This excess was similar to that which occurs with clofibrate. (*See* Notes.) An acute infectionlike syndrome characterized by arthralgias, myalgia, and myositis has occurred during therapy. Rhabdomyolysis with elevated creatine kinase levels may precipitate acute renal failure, especially with the combination of gemfibrozil and lovastatin.[271] This has occurred as early as after several weeks to months of therapy. Routine monitoring of creatine kinase may not detect rhabdomyolysis in a timely manner. Many recommend avoiding the combination of gemfibrozil and any HMG-CoA reductase inhibitor.[273] Worsening of renal insufficiency has been reported with an initial Cr_s >2 mg/dL. Carcinogenesis, impairment of fertility, and development of cataracts occur in rats. (*See* Precautions and Notes.)

Contraindictions. Hepatic or severe renal dysfunction; primary biliary cirrhosis; pre-existing gallbladder disease.

Precautions. Pregnancy, lactation. Evaluate any reports of muscle pain, tenderness, or weakness for myositis, including a determination of serum creatine kinase. Discontinue if an adequate effect does not occur after 3 months, if cholelithiasis is suspected, or if liver function tests remain elevated.

Drug Interactions. Gemfibrozil may potentiate the effect of oral anticoagulants. Cholesterol-binding resins may decrease absorption of gemfibrozil. Insulin or an oral hypoglycemic may be required.[289,291] Displacement of glyburide from plasma protein binding sites, producing hypoglycemia, has been reported.[292] Gemfibrozil and lovastatin (and possibly other HMG-CoA reductase inhibitors) together may have an increased risk of myotoxicity. (*See* Adverse Reactions.)

Parameters to Monitor. Serum lipids, initially every few weeks, then approximately q 3 months.[274] Liver function tests and CBC q 3–6 months. Monitor serum glucose if patient is receiving insulin or an oral hypoglycemic and prothrombin time if patient is taking an oral anticoagulant.

Notes. Gemfibrozil is not considered a major treatment for hypercholesteremia because of its effects on LDL-c, but it does increase HDL-c and decrease triglycerides, so it is useful in some patients.[265] Gemfibrozil is indicated for the treatment of types IV and V hyperlipidemias with very high serum triglycerides (usually >2000 mg/dL) in patients at risk for pancreatitis and not responding to diet. It is also indicated in type IIb patients (only those without a history or symptoms of CHD) with low HDL-c and an inadequate response to weight loss, diet, exercise, and other drugs that raise HDL-c (eg, bile acid sequestrants, niacin), but is not indicated in type I or IIa hyperlipidemias or in those patients who have a low HDL-c only. The Helsinki Heart Study showed a 34% reduction in the incidence of CHD in middle-aged men (initially without CHD symptoms) treated with gemfibrozil in a 5-yr study, although total death rate was no different between treated and placebo groups.[293,294] A substudy of the Helsinki Heart Study showed an increase in gallstone and gallbladder surgery in gemfibrozil-treated patients. After a 3.5-yr extension of this study, all-cause mortality was slightly higher in the original gemfibrozil group, primarily because of cancer deaths.[294] An ancillary study of the Helsinki Heart Study investigated the use of gemfibrozil in patients with signs or symptoms of CHD.[295] The rate of serious adverse cardiac advents and total mortality with gemfibrozil treatment did not significantly differ from placebo; however, information on key prognostic indicators and their distribution was not known.[295] Gemfibrozil is chemically and pharmacologically similar to **clofibrate.** A 44% relative increase in age-adjusted, all-cause mortality occurred in a study of long-term clofibrate use related to a 33% increase in noncardiovascular disease such as malignancy, gallbladder disease, and pancreatitis. Because of the smaller size of the gemfibrozil studies, the increase in mortality in the gemfibrozil group relative to placebo may not be statistically significantly different from the excess mortality associated with clofibrate use.

HMG-CoA REDUCTASE INHIBITORS:	
ATORVASTATIN	Lipitor
CERIVASTATIN	Baycol
FLUVASTATIN	Lescol
LOVASTATIN	Mevacor
PRAVASTATIN	Pravachol
SIMVASTATIN	Zocor

Pharmacology. Hydroxymethylglutaryl-CoA (HMG-CoA) reductase inhibitors competitively inhibit conversion of HMG-CoA to mevalonate, an early, rate-limiting step in cholesterol synthesis. A compensatory increase in LDL receptors, which bind and remove circulating LDL-cholesterol (LDL-c) results. Production of LDL-c may also be decreased because of decreased production of VLDL or increased VLDL removal by LDL receptors. These drugs produce dose-dependent, maximum reductions in LDL of 30–40% (up to 60% with atorvastatin) and triglycerides of 10–30%, and increases in HDL levels of 2–15%.[266,296,297] Drug effects are dose dependent until the following doses are reached: 80 mg for atorvastatin, 0.3 mg for cerivastatin, 20 mg for fluvastatin and simvastatin, and 40 mg for lovastatin and pravastatin. Fluvastatin is about 30% less effective in lowering lipids than the other drugs.[266,298]

Administration and Adult Dosage. Adjust dosage at no less than 4-week intervals. **PO for hyperlipidemia** (Atorvastatin) 10 mg/day initially, increasing to a maximum of 80 mg/day. (Cerivastatin) 0.2 or 0.3 mg/day in the evening. (Fluvastatin) 20 mg hs initially, increasing to 40 mg/day; a slight increase in fluvastatin LDL-c lowering occurs with a bid schedule. (Lovastatin) 20 mg (40 mg with serum cholesterol >300 mg/dL) with the evening meal initially. Start with 10 mg/day in patients requiring <20% decrease in LDL-c or when concurrent use with cyclosporine is unavoidable. Increase to a maintenance dosage of 20–80 mg/day. Do not exceed a lovastatin dosage of 20 mg/day when used with cyclosporine. (Pravastatin) 10–20 mg hs initially, increasing to 10–40 mg/day hs. (Simvastatin) 5–10 mg/day in the evening initially, increasing to 5–40 mg/day in the evening.

Special Populations. *Pediatric Dosage.* Safety and efficacy not established.

Geriatric Dosage. **PO** (Pravastatin) 10 mg/day initially; (Simvastatin) 5 mg/day initially; the elderly may achieve maximal reductions in LDL-c at doses ≤20 mg/day. Maximum dosage may not be required or tolerated.

Other Conditions. (Atorvastatin) no dosage adjustment necessary in renal impairment. (Cerivastatin) start with 0.2 mg/day in moderate to severe renal impairment. (Lovastatin) start with 10 mg/day when concurrent use with cyclosporine is unavoidable; maximum dosage is 20 mg/day with concurrent immunosuppressant therapy. (Pravastatin) start with 10 mg/day with renal or hepatic impairment and in patients concurrently taking cyclosporine; do not exceed a dose of 20 mg/day in the latter case. (Simvastatin) start with 5 mg/day in patients requring <20% reductions in LDL-c and with severe renal insufficiency. Use dosages >20 mg/day only with extreme caution in patients with a Cl_{cr} <30 mL/min.

Dosage Forms. (*See* Hypolipidemic Drugs Comparison Chart.)

Patient Instructions. (*See* Hypolipidemics Class Instructions.) Atorvastatin may be taken any time of day without regard to meals. Take lovastatin with the evening meal to increase its absorption; other drugs can be taken without regard to meals. Take pravastatin 1 hour before or 4 hours after a dose of a cholesterol-binding resin. Promptly report any unexplained muscle pain or tenderness, especially if accompanied by malaise or fever. Avoid excessive concurrent use of alcohol, but abstinence is not required. Do not take these drugs during pregnancy because of possible harm to the fetus. Inform your physician if you become or intend to become pregnant.

Pharmacokinetics. *Onset and Duration.* Onset is within 2 weeks; peak effect is within 4–6 weeks; cholesterol levels return to baseline after drug discontinuation.

Fate. Absorption is rapid. Lovastatin and simvastatin are prodrugs that undergo extensive first-pass metabolism to active metabolites. Serum concentrations of the active lovastatin metabolite when taken under fasting conditions are two-thirds of that when taken with food. Absorption of other drugs is unaffected by food. Systemic bioavailability of all drugs is low because of extensive (>60%) first-pass extraction. Peak serum concentrations of active inhibitors are achieved in 1–4 hr for all drugs. Protein binding is 98% for atorvastatin, 99% for cerivastatin, 55–60% for pravastatin, 95% for simvastatin, >95% for lovastatin, and 98% for fluvastatin. Atorvastatin, lovastatin, and simvastatin are lipophilic and cross the blood-brain barrier; cerivastatin, fluvastatin, and pravastatin are hydrophilic and do not. All the drugs are primarily (>70%) hepatically metabolized to active and inactive metabolites, which then undergo extensive fecal elimination. Renal elimination accounts for <2% for atorvastatin, 5% for fluvastatin, 10% for lovastatin, 13% for simvastatin, 20% for pravastatin, and 26% for cerivastatin. Severe renal insufficiency (Cl_{cr} 10–30 mL/min) results in a 2-fold increase in serum concentrations of lovastatin inhibitors.[265,297–303]

$t_{1/2}$. (Fluvastatin, lovastatin, pravastatin, simvastatin) <2 hr; (cerivastatin) 2–3 hr; (atorvastatin) 14 hr.[297–298]

Adverse Reactions. The drugs are generally well tolerated, with discontinuation rates less than other hypolipidemic drugs.[275] The frequency of side effects appears to be similar for all drugs.[297–304] GI complaints such as diarrhea, constipation, flatulence, abdominal pain, and nausea occur in about 5% of patients. Headache (4–9%), rash (3–5%), dizziness (3–5%), and blurred vision (1–2%) are other frequent side effects. Myopathy and myositis occur rarely with single therapy and may be associated with mild elevations of CPK. Rhabdomyolysis leading to acute renal failure is a rare complication, but occurs more frequently in combination with gemfibrozil, cyclosporine, or ≥1 g/day of niacin. Pravastatin may cause less myopathy than lovastatin with cyclosporine.[298] Increases in liver function tests >3 times normal occur in up to 2% of patients, but most are asymptomatic and reverse with discontinuation.[266] Anomalies have been reported with intrauterine exposure. Carcinogenicity occurs in mice and rats at higher than human doses, but the clinical implications are unclear.[270,305]

Contraindications. Pregnancy; lactation; active liver disease; unexplained persistent elevations of serum transaminases.

Precautions. Administer to women of childbearing age only when possibility of becoming pregnant is unlikely. Use with caution in patients who consume substantial quantities of alcohol and/or have a history of liver disease. Discontinue therapy if liver function tests are >3 times normal. Consider withholding the drug in any patient with risk factors for renal failure secondary to rhabdomyolysis, such as severe acute infection; hypotension, major surgery or trauma; severe electrolyte, endocrine, or metabolic abnormalities; or uncontrolled seizures.

Drug Interactions. Myositis and rhabdomyolysis may be more common in combination with cyclosporine (lovastatin levels are quadrupled), erythromycin, gemfibrozil, itraconazole, ketoconazole (and possibly other inhibitors of CYP3A4), or lipid-lowering dosages of niacin (>1 g/day).[298] HMG-CoA reductase inhibitors may increase the effect of warfarin. Bile acid sequestrants may markedly decrease pravastatin oral bioavailability when taken together; take pravastatin 1 hr before or 4 hr after resin doses.

Parameters to Monitor. Obtain serum lipid and liver function tests on initiation, 6 and 12 weeks after initiation, after dosage increases, and at least semiannually thereafter. Others recommend more frequent monitoring.[265,266] Increase the frequency of monitoring if adverse effects are suspected. Routine monitoring of muscle enzymes may not adequately identify patients at risk for rhabdomyolysis, but may be warranted in patients with skeletal muscle complaints and risk factors.

Notes. The HMG-CoA reductase inhibitors are indicated for the treatment of type IIa and IIb hyperlipoproteinemias. They are the most effective in decreasing LDL-c, and their effect on decreasing coronary morbidity and mortality is proven.[298] The choice of drug depends on cost, amount of cholesterol lowering desired, and risk factors for CHD. Lovastatin, pravastatin, and simvastatin are more effective than fluvastatin and are therefore preferable when a >25% reduction in LDL-c is required.[398,306] They may have additive effects with the bile acid sequestrants and have been used in combination with niacin and gemfibrozil. (*See* Adverse Reactions and Drug Interactions.) Cholesterol reduction with these agents may reduce the risk of stroke and total mortality.[307] One large study found a reduced CHD risk with lovastatin in men and women with "average" serum cholesterol and no evidence of pre-existing heart disease.[308]

NIACIN   Various

Pharmacology. Niacin (nicotinic acid), in dosages of 1 g/day or more, decreases serum total cholesterol, LDL and VLDL cholesterol, and triglycerides, and increases HDL cholesterol. Mean serum cholesterol and triglyceride levels are reduced by 10% and 26%, respectively. The mechanism for these effects is not entirely known, but may involve inhibition of lipolysis, reduced LDL and VLDL synthesis, and increased lipoprotein lipase activity.[309,310] Niacin consistently decreases lipoprotein (a).[265] **Niacinamide** (nicotinamide) does not have hypolipidemic effects and cannot be substituted for niacin.

Administration and Adult Dosage. PO as a hypolipidemic 250 mg/day with evening meal initially, increasing at 4- to 7-day intervals to 1.5–2 g/day in 3 divided doses. Continue this dosage for 2 months. If necessary, the dosage can then be increased at 2- to 4-week intervals to 1 g tid; the dose can be further increased if necessary to reach the desired clinical effect or the maximum tolerated dosage to a usual maximum of 2 g tid. Use of >3–4 g/day does not appear to increase efficacy appreciably and is associated with increased side effects.[309] If an **SR product** is substituted for an immediate-release form, reduce the dosage by one-half. Risk of hepatotoxicity increases at SR doses >1.5–3 g/day, and these are not recommended.[266]

Special Populations. *Pediatric Dosage.* Safety and efficacy not established. Although niacin is effective in reducing triglycerides and cholesterol in children and adolescents, adverse effects are common and can be severe. Some authors recommend niacin use be avoided in children or used only under close supervision by a lipid specialist if diet and bile acid sequestrants have failed.[267,311] In these cases, niacin should generally be used in combination with diet and a bile acid sequestrant if tolerated.[267] Close monitoring is necessary. (*See* Adverse Reactions and Precautions.)

Geriatric Dosage. Initiate therapy at lowest possible dosage, and slowly titrate to desired effect. Maximum dosage may not be required or tolerated.

Patient Instructions. Use only under medical supervision. Effects may differ with different preparations. Almost everyone experiences some flushing. Tolerance to flushing generally occurs with time. Taking 325 mg of aspirin or 200 mg of ibuprofen (or an equivalent dose of another NSAID) 30–60 minutes before each niacin dose may reduce flushing. Taking niacin with meals may also help minimize flushing and reduce GI upset. Avoid hot liquids or alcohol after taking a dose. Avoid interruptions in therapy; tolerance may be lost if therapy is interrupted, so slow resumption of the usual dosage is recommended. Avoid sudden changes in posture if you are also taking medicine for high blood pressure. Report any persistent nausea.

Dosage Forms. **Tab** 25, 50, 100, 250, 500 mg; **Elxr** 10 mg/mL; **SR Cap** 125, 250, 300, 400, 500 mg; **SR Tab** 250, 500, 750, 1000 mg; **Inj** 100 mg/mL.

Pharmacokinetics. *Onset and Duration.* The onset of triglyceride and cholesterol reductions usually occurs within several days, although some studies have demonstrated a response after a single dose.[309] A return to pretreatment lipid levels occurs 2–6 weeks after drug discontinuation.

Fate. The drug is almost completely absorbed from standard formulations; peak serum levels 30–60 min after 1 g standard formulations are 15–30 μg/L (120–240 μmol/L). Niacin is largely metabolized in the liver to niacinamide (nicotinamide) and its derivatives (eg, nicotinuric acid), which may contribute to the lipid-lowering activity, especially after long-term use. The majority is excreted as unchanged drug or metabolites in urine.[309]

$t_{\frac{1}{2}}$. 20–48 min.[309]

Adverse Reactions. Dose-related flushing of the neck and face (usually in "blush" areas) occurs in almost all patients and is related to the rate of rise of serum levels rather than the absolute serum concentrations. Tolerance may develop, but may be lost if therapy is interrupted. Administration with food, gradual upward dosage titration, use of an SR formulation, or premedication with 325 mg of aspirin or 200 mg of ibuprofen (or equivalent dose of another NSAID) 30–60 min before each dose may reduce flushing. Postural hypotension may occur, especially when niacin is used with antihypertensive drugs or when it is taken with alcohol or hot liquids. Vasodilatory effects may precipitate or aggravate angina. Rash, pruritus, and stomach discomfort also occur frequently; the latter may occur more commonly with SR preparations. Increases in AST, ALT, bilirubin, and LDH concentrations occur frequently and may be related to increasing the daily dosage by more than 2.5 g/month. Severe hepatotoxicity (hepatic necrosis) is rare and tends to occur with abrupt dosage increases, SR forms substituted for immediate-release products without dosage reduction, or brand interchange. Hepatotoxicity can occur at low dosages (≤3 g/day) of SR products and as soon as 2 days after initiation. Discontinue therapy if liver function tests remain over three times pretreatment values.[310]

Contraindications. Arterial hemorrhage; severe hypotension; hepatic dysfunction; unexplained elevations of transaminases, active peptic ulcer disease.

Precautions Pregnancy; lactation. Use with caution in patients with gallbladder disease or a history of liver disease, unstable angina, gout, gouty arthritis, glaucoma, or diabetes.[266,312] Nausea may be a presenting sign of hepatotoxicity.[266] If the SR form is substituted for the immediate-release form, reduce dosage by about one-half. If use with an HMG-CoA reductase inhibitor is unavoidable, use with extreme caution. Some formulations contain tartrazine dye, which may cause allergic reactions in sensitive patients.

Drug Interactions. Concurrent use with HMG-CoA reductase inhibitors may increase the risk of rhabdomyolysis. Concurrent therapy with α-adrenergic blocking antihypertensives may result in hypotension. Diet and/or dosage of oral hypoglycemic drugs or insulin may require adjustment with concurrent niacin use. Hepatotoxic drugs may have additive effects.[265]

Parameters to Monitor. Monitor serum lipids q 2 weeks initially, then q 1–3 months. Periodic liver function tests, blood glucose, and serum uric acid levels are recommended, especially at dosages >1.5 g/day.[265] Obtain liver function tests at baseline and q 6–12 weeks for the first year, then semiannually unless hepatotoxicity is suspected.

Notes. Indicated for types IIa, IIb, III, IV, and V hyperlipoproteinemias. A reduction in sudden cardiac deaths and fatal and nonfatal MI occurs, as well as an 11% decrease in mortality (compared to placebo) in patients treated with niacin.[304] The cost of standard nicacin formulations can be much lower than alternative drugs; the cost of SR products may be higher. SR products appear to have equal efficacy at lowering LDL-c at one-half the dosage of standard products, but the SR form may be less effective in lowering triglycerides or raising HDL at dosages equal to standard forms.[265,311,313] Some advocate avoidance of SR preparations altogether for treatment of hyperlipidemia because of their potentially greater hepatotoxicity.[311,313]

HYPOLIPIDEMIC DRUGS COMPARISON CHART

DRUG	DOSAGE FORMS	ADULT ORAL DOSAGE[a] INITIAL (I) MAINTENANCE (M)	RELATIVE EFFECT ON LIPIDS[b]			INDICATIONS BY WHO CATEGORY[c] TYPE	COMMENTS
			LDL	HDL	TG		
BILE ACID SEQUESTRANTS							
Cholestyramine Questran Questran Light Various	Pwdr 4 g resin/9 g drug packet or scoop Pwdr 4 g resin/5 g packet or scoop.	(I) 4 g daily–bid. (M) 8–16 g/day in 1–6 doses, to a maximum of 24 g/day.[d]	↓↓	↑	↑	IIa	Constipation frequent. May be used in children. Numerous interactions. Decrease in mortality demonstrated. Take before meals.
Colestipol HCl Colestid	Gran 5 g resin/7.5 g packet or scoop Tab 1 g.	(I) (gran) 5 g daily–bid. (M) (gran) 15–30 g/day in 1–4 doses.[e]	↓↓	↑	↑	IIa	Similar to cholestyramine. (*See above.*)
FIBRIC ACID DERIVATIVES							
Fenofibrate Tricor	Cap 67 mg.	(I) 67 mg/day. (M) up to 201 mg/day.	↓↓↓	↑↑	↓↓↓	IV, V	Avoid in liver, gallbladder, or kidney disease. Take with food.
Gemfibrozil Lopid Various	Tab 600 mg.	(M) 600 mg bid.	↑↓	↑↑	↓↓↓	IIb, IV, V	Overall mortality rate with long-term therapy is increased. Take 30 min prior to AM and PM meals.
Clofibrate	Not recommended because of a large increase in overall mortality.						

(*continued*)

373

HYPOLIPIDEMIC DRUGS COMPARISON CHART (continued)

DRUG	DOSAGE FORMS	ADULT ORAL DOSAGE[a] INITIAL (I) MAINTENANCE (M)	RELATIVE EFFECT ON LIPIDS[b] LDL	RELATIVE EFFECT ON LIPIDS[b] HDL	RELATIVE EFFECT ON LIPIDS[b] TG	INDICATIONS BY WHO CATEGORY TYPE[c]	COMMENTS
NICOTINIC ACID							
Niacin Various	Tab 25, 50, 100, 250, 500 mg Inj 100 mg/mL Elxr 10 mg/mL SR Cap 125, 250, 300, 400, 500 mg[e] SR Tab 250, 500, 750 mg.[e]	(I) Titrate slowly. (*See* monograph.) (M) 1.5–3 g/day, to a maximum of 6 g/day.	↓↓	↑↑	↓↓↓	IIa, IIb, III, IV, V	Frequent flushing and GI side effects. Must titrate dosage slowly. Decrease in mortality demonstrated. Avoid SR products. Low cost. Take with food or milk.
HMG-CoA REDUCTASE INHIBITORS							
Atorvastatin Lipitor	Tab 10, 20, 40 mg.	(I) 10 mg/day. (M) 10–80 mg/day.	↓↓↓↓	↑	↓↓↓	IIa, IIb	Take at any time without regard to meals.
Cerivastatin Baycol	Tab 0.2, 0.3 mg	0.2–0.3 mg/day.	↓↓↓	↑	↓↓	IIa, IIb	Take in evening without regard to meals.
Fluvastatin Lescol	Cap 20, 40 mg.	(I) 20 mg q hs. (M) 20–40 mg q hs.	↓↓	↑	↓	IIa, IIb	Take without regard to meals. Monitor for myositis and hepatic dysfunction. Important drug interactions.

(continued)

HYPOLIPIDEMIC DRUGS COMPARISON CHART (continued)

DRUG	DOSAGE FORMS	ADULT ORAL DOSAGE[a] INITIAL (I) MAINTENANCE (M)	RELATIVE EFFECT ON LIPIDS[b] LDL	RELATIVE EFFECT ON LIPIDS[b] HDL	RELATIVE EFFECT ON LIPIDS[b] TG	INDICATIONS BY WHO CATEGORY TYPE[c]	COMMENTS
Lovastatin Mevacor	Tab 10, 20, 40 mg.	(I) 20 mg/day. (M) 20–80 mg/day in 1–2 divided doses.	↓↓↓	↑	↓↓	IIa, IIb	Take with evening meal. (*See* Fluvastatin.)
Pravastatin Pravachol	Tab 10, 20, 40 mg.	(I) 10–20 mg q hs. (M) 10–40 mg q hs.	↓↓↓	↑	↓↓	IIa, IIb	Take without regard to meals. (*See* Fluvastatin.)
Simvastatin Zocor	Tab 5, 10, 20, 40, 80 mg.	(I) 5–10 mg q hs. (M) 5–80 mg/day.	↓↓↓	↑	↓↓	IIa, IIb	Take without regard to meals. (*See* Fluvastatin.)

LDL = serum low-density lipoprotein cholesterol, shown to have a graded, positive relationship with coronary heart disease (CHD); HDL = serum high-density lipoprotein, shown to have a cardioprotective effect against CHD; TG = serum triglycerides, which have a positive relationship to CHD.

[a]Clinical trials in the elderly are limited, but the drugs are considered effective. Base decision on drug treatment on life expectancy, concomitant disease, potential adverse effects, patient desire for treatment, quality of life, assessment of coronary heart disease risk, and cost. A conservative approach is recommended, generally initiating therapy at lowest possible dosage, slowly titrating to desired effect while closely monitoring possible side effects. Maximum dosage may not be required or tolerated.

[b]Arrows represent approximate relative effects based on results achieved with usual dosage. Study results vary because of differences in patient groups, administration schedules, dosage, and degree of hypercholesterolemia.

[c]World Health Organization (WHO) classification by characteristics of dyslipidemia.

[d]All dosages are expressed in terms of anhydrous resin.

[e]Do not substitute SR niacin products for an equal dosage of immediate-release products; use one-half the dosage of immediate-release products.

From references 274, 291, 314, 315 and product information.

RECOMMENDATIONS FOR INITIATION OF DRUG THERAPY IN HYPERCHOLESTEROLEMIA

Evaluate and treat other conditions that may contribute to hyperlipidemia prior to initiation of drug therapy. If possible, avoid drug therapy that may contribute to hyperlipidemia (eg, corticosteroids, isotretinoin, thiazides, anabolic steroids, some β blockers, cyclosporin, and progestins). Patients should generally also receive an adequate trial of diet and other nonpharmacologic measures such as an increase in physical activity and weight reduction (if appropriate). If these methods fail, then drug therapy may be considered based on the patient's age, serum low-density lipoprotein cholesterol (LDL-c) concentrations, and risk factors for coronary heart disease (CHD) according to the following tables.

ADULT

LDL-c	RISK FACTORS[d]	GOAL OF THERAPY

Primary Prevention (patient currently without signs or symptoms of CHD) Consider drug therapy in men ≥35 yr and postmenopausal women[a] with the following LDL-c levels *and* risk factors.[b,c]

LDL-c ≥190 mg/dL (4.9 mmol/L)	Without any two other risk factors	LCL-c ≤160 mg/dL (4.1 mmol/L)
LDL-c ≥160 mg/dL (4.1 mmol/L)	With any two other risk factors	LDL-c ≤130 mg/dL (3.4 mmol/L)

Secondary Prevention (patient currently with signs or symptoms of CHD)[e] Consider drug therapy in patients with the following LDL-c levels *and* risk factors. [b]

LDL-c ≥130 mg/dL (3.4 mmol/L)	Established CHD/atherosclerotic disease	LDL-c ≤100 mg/dL (2.5 mmol/L)

(continued)

RECOMMENDATIONS FOR INITIATION OF DRUG THERAPY IN HYPERCHOLESTEROLEMIA (continued)

PEDIATRIC

LDL-c	RISK FACTORS	MINIMUM GOAL OF THERAPY	IDEAL GOAL OF THERAPY
LDL-c ≥190 mg/dL (4.9 mmol/L)	Any or none	LDL-c ≤130 mg/dL (3.4 mmol/L)	LCL-c ≤110 mg/dL (2.9 mmol/L)
LDL-c ≥160 mg/dL (4.1 mmol/L)	Family history of CVD before age 55; or with two other risk factors[b]	LDL-c ≤130 mg/dL (3.4 mmol/L)	LCL-c ≤110 mg/dL (2.9 mmol/L)

(Children and adolescents ≥10 yr)[f] Consider drug therapy in patients with the following LDL-c levels and risk factors[g]:

[a]Estrogen replacement therapy can be an alternative or addition to hypolipidemic drug therapy in postmenopausal women.

[b]Use clinical judgment to individualize drug therapy in patients who do not meet the upper LDL-c criteria for drug therapy and have not achieved goal LDL-c levels after maximal efforts to decrease cholesterol (with diet, physical activity, and reduction of other risk factors). Consider potential benefit, side effects, degree of LDL-c elevation above goal, and cost. Low-dose bile acid sequestrant therapy may be useful in these patients.

[c]In men under 35 yr and premenopausal women without other risk factors, drug therapy can be delayed if LDL-c is 190–220 mg/dL (4.9–5.7 mmol/L).

[d]Risk factors for CHD include age, family history, smoking history, hypertension, diabetes, and HDL-c <35 mg/dL.

[e]Also screen family members of patients with severe hypercholesteremia.

[f]Use clinical judgment regarding initiation of drug therapy in children <10 yr if cholesterol is extremely high.

[g]Complete a 6 month–1 yr trial of diet therapy before initiating drug therapy. Continue diet therapy even if drug therapy is initiated. Bile acid sequestrants are considered the drugs of choice due to their relative safety. (*See* Cholestyramine.)

[h]Before initiating drug therapy, make rigorous attempts to control risk factors.

From the National Cholesterol Education Program (NCEP), references 267 and 274.

Inotropic Drugs

AMRINONE LACTATE
Inocor, Various

Pharmacology. Amrinone increases cyclic AMP and calcium availability via the inhibition of phosphodiesterase III, which improves cardiac output through vasodilatory and positive inotropic actions.[316]

Administration and Adult Dosage. **IV loading dose** 0.5–1 mg/kg (usually 0.75 mg/kg) over 2–3 min, may repeat in 30 min based on response. **IV maintenance dosage by continuous infusion** 5–10 μg/kg/min.

Special Populations. *Pediatric Dosage.* Safety and efficacy not established;[317] however, the following dosages have been suggested:[141] **IV loading dosage** (neonates and infants) 3–4.5 mg/kg. **IV maintenance dosage by continuous infusion** (neonates) 3–5 μg/kg/min; (infants) 10 μg/kg/min.

Geriatric Dosage. Same as adult dosage.

Dosage Forms. **Inj** 5 mg/mL.

Pharmacokinetics. *Onset and Duration.* IV onset 2–5 min after bolus, peak 10 min, duration 60–90 min.[316]

Serum Levels. A level of 1.5–4 mg/L (8–21.3 μmol/L) is associated with therapeutic response. Although a correlation exists between amrinone levels and increased cardiac output, the clinical usefulness of serum level monitoring is questionable.[318,319]

Fate. Bioavailability is 93 ± 12%. The drug is 20–50% plasma protein bound; V_d is 1.8 ± 0.9 L/kg; Cl is 0.28 ± 0.1 L/hr/kg. The drug is eliminated primarily by hepatic metabolism, with 30 ± 20% excreted in urine unchanged.[318]

$t_{1/2}$. α phase 1–5 min; β phase 4.3 ± 1.3 hr in normals, 7.3 ± 4.6 hr in CHF.[318,319]

Adverse Reactions. Dose-dependent, asymptomatic thrombocytopenia occurs frequently. Platelet counts return to normal within 2–4 days of discontinuing therapy; in some cases, this side effect may be reversible when dosage is maintained or reduced. Thrombocytopenia may be caused primarily by the metabolite N-acetylamrinone.[320] Nausea and vomiting are unusual with IV use.[316] Occasional side effects include nephrogenic diabetes insipidus, liver enzyme elevation, fever, taste disturbances, flu-like syndrome, rash, and aggravation of underlying arrhythmias.[321,322]

Precautions. Caution in hypertrophic obstructive cardiomyopathy. One study suggests a decreased survival rate in patients on long-term amrinone therapy.[322] Use concomitant antiplatelet drugs with caution.

Drug Interactions. None known.

Parameters to Monitor. Continuous ECG and frequent vital signs. Invasive hemodynamic monitoring is necessary in seriously ill patients for adequate dosage titration.

Notes. Do not dilute with dextrose-containing solutions, but may infuse through dextrose-containing IV lines.

DOBUTAMINE HYDROCHLORIDE

Dobutrex, Various

Pharmacology. Dobutamine is a synthetic sympathomimetic amine that exists as the racemic mixture of an L-isomer with predominantly α-adrenergic agonist actions and a D-isomer that has β_1- and β_2-adrenergic agonist actions. The net clinical effect is typically that of a potent β_1-agonist with mild vasodilatory properties. At low dosages, it increases myocardial contractility without markedly increasing heart rate; this specificity is dose dependent and is lost at high dosages. Unlike dopamine, dobutamine does not release stored catecholamines, nor does it have any effect on dopaminergic receptors.[323,324]

Administration and Adult Dosage. **IV for inotropic support, by infusion only** (in any *non*alkaline IV fluid) 2.5 μg/kg/min initially, increasing gradually in 2.5 μg/kg/min increments up to 20 μg/kg/min, adjusting dosage to desired response. Maintenance dosages are typically 2–10 μg/kg/min.[325] Although dosages up to 40 μg/kg/min have been used, use dosages over 20 μg/kg/min with caution because of increased risks of tachycardia, arrhythmias, and myocardial ischemia.[326]

Special Populations. *Pediatric Dosage.* Safety and efficacy not established. However, **IV infusion** 2 μg/kg/min initially, followed by adjustment to desired hemodynamic response, up to 20 μg/kg/min, has been used.[327]

Geriatric Dosage. Same as adult dosage.

Dosage Forms. **Inj** 12.5 mg/mL.

Pharmacokinetics. *Onset and Duration.* Onset <2 min; peak within 10 min; duration <10 min.[328]

Fate. Wide interpatient variability exists, especially between adult and pediatric patients. V_d in CHF is 0.2 ± 0.08 L/kg; Cl in CHF is 3.5 ± 1.3 L/hr/kg. The drug is eliminated primarily in the liver to inactive glucuronide conjugates and 3-O-methyldobutamine.[9,323]

$t_{1/2}$. 2.4 ± 0.7 min.[9]

Adverse Reactions. Precipitation or exacerbation of ventricular ectopy occurs frequently; ventricular arrhythmias may occur (although these are less likely than with other sympathomimetics).[323] Modest increases in heart rate or systolic blood pressure occur frequently; dosage reduction usually reverses these effects rapidly. Occasionally, nausea, headache, angina, nonspecific chest pain, palpitations, and shortness of breath are noted. Patients with atrial fibrillation may be at risk of developing rapid ventricular responses because dobutamine facilitates AV conduction.

Contraindications. Idiopathic hypertrophic subaortic stenosis.

Precautions. Correct hypovolemia before using in patients who are hypotensive. Although most cases of extravasation cause no signs of tissue damage, at least one case of dermal necrosis following extravasation of a 2.5 μg/kg/min infusion has been reported. Dobutamine contains a sulfite preservative, which may be problematic in sensitive individuals, especially asthmatics.

Drug Interactions. Bretylium, guanethidine, and heterocyclic antidepressants may potentiate the pressor response to direct-acting vasopressors. Oxytocics used in obstetrics may cause severe, persistent hypertension when used with vasopressors. Halogenated hydrocarbon anesthetics may predispose patients to serious arrhythmias.

Parameters to Monitor. Monitor heart rate, arterial blood pressure, urine output, pulmonary capillary wedge pressure, cardiac index, ECG for ectopic activity, and infusion rate of solution continuously in the acute care setting and during periods of dosage titration or adjustment.

Notes. The drug is physically incompatible with sodium bicarbonate and other alkaline solutions. Use the reconstituted solution within 24 hr. (*See* Sympathomimetic Drugs for Hemodynamic Support Comparison Chart.)

DOBUTAMINE DILUTION GUIDE

AMOUNT ADDED		VOLUME OF	FINAL
mg	*Volume*	DILUENT	CONCENTRATION[a]
250	1 vial (20 mL)	1000 mL	250 mg/L
250	1 vial (20 mL)	500 mL	500 mg/L
250	1 vial (20 mL)	250 mL	1 g/L

[a]Recommended concentrations, but concentrations up to 5 g/L have been used.

DOPAMINE HYDROCHLORIDE Dopastat, Intropin, Various

Pharmacology. Dopamine is a catecholamine that acts directly, in a dose-dependent fashion, on postsynaptic dopaminergic (DA_1) receptors to produce renal and mesenteric vasodilation as well as on postsynaptic α_1-, α_2-, and β_1-adrenergic receptors. Additionally, it acts indirectly by releasing norepinephrine from sympathetic nerve storage sites. Clinical response varies depending on the patient's clinical condition and baseline sympathetic nervous system activity.[329] Approximate ranges follow: dopaminergic, 0.5–2 μg/kg/min; β_1, 5–10 μg/kg/min; mixed α and β, 10–20 μg/kg/min; predominantly α, >20 μg/kg/min.[323]

Administration and Adult Dosage. **IV for shock, by infusion only** (in any nonalkaline IV fluid) 2.5 μg/kg/min initially, increasing gradually in 5–10 μg/kg/min increments up to 20–50 μg/kg/min, adjusting dosage to desired response. If a dosage over 20 μg/kg/min is required, consider other pressors.[326] Use dosages over 50 μg/kg/min only with careful monitoring of hemodynamic parameters and urine output. **IV for chronic refractory CHF** 2–3 μg/kg/min initially, increasing gradually until desired increases in urine flow, diastolic blood pressure, or heart rate are observed.[330] Dosages over 20 μg/kg/min are rarely used in CHF.[325,329,330]

Special Populations. *Pediatric Dosage.* Safety and efficacy not established. However, **IV for shock** (PALS recommendations) 2–5 μg/kg/min initially, increased to 10–20 μg/kg/min to improve blood pressure, perfusion, and urine output.[327]

Geriatric Dosage. Same as adult dosage.

Dosage Forms. Inj 40, 80, 160 mg/mL.

Pharmacokinetics. *Onset and Duration.* Onset within 5 min, duration <10 min.

Fate. There is large interpatient variability.[323] One evaluation in adult surgery patients derived a V_d of 0.89 ± 0.25 L/kg.[331] Cl is usually 3–4.2 L/hr/kg and was 4.48 ± 0.94 L/hr/kg in adult surgery patients.[323,326] The drug is primarily metabolized to homovanillic acid (HVA) and related metabolites; the remainder is metabolized to norepinephrine and excreted in urine as HVA and metabolites of both HVA and norepinephrine; very little is excreted as unchanged dopamine.[320,332]

$t_{\frac{1}{2}}$. α phase 1–2 min, β phase 6–9 min.[323,328]

Adverse Reactions. Increases in ventricular ectopy and ventricular arrhythmias may occur, particularly at high dosages (although this is less likely than with other sympathomimetics); reduce dosage if increased number of ventricular ectopic beats occurs. Hypertension may occur at high infusion rates. Nausea, vomiting, headache, anxiety, and angina pectoris have also been observed. Gangrene of the extremities has occurred in patients given large dosages of dopamine for long periods of time or in patients with occlusive vascular disease given low dosages.[323,333]

Contraindications. Pheochromocytoma; presence of uncorrected tachyarrhythmias or ventricular fibrillation.

Precautions. Correct hypovolemia before using in patients with shock. If increased diastolic pressure, decreased pulse pressure, or decreased urine flow occurs, decrease infusion rate and observe patient for signs of excessive vasoconstriction. Use with caution in patients with occlusive vascular disease, and extreme caution in patients receiving halogenated hydrocarbon anesthesia. Avoid extravasation of solution; however, if it occurs, the area may be infiltrated with 5–10 mg of phentolamine diluted in 10–15 mL of NS. Dopamine contains a sulfite preservative, which may be problematic in sensitive individuals, especially asthmatics.

Drug Interactions. MAOIs (including furazolidone) may increase the pressor response to dopamine by up to 20-fold; avoid these combinations. Bretylium, guanethidine, and heterocyclic antidepressants may potentiate the pressor response to direct-acting vasopressors. Oxytocics used in obstetrics may cause severe, persistent hypertension when used with vasopressors. IV phenytoin may produce hypotension in severely ill patients receiving IV dopamine. Halogenated hydrocarbon anesthetics may predispose patients to serious arrhythmias.

Parameters to Monitor. In shock, closely monitor heart rate, ECG, pulmonary capillary wedge pressure, cardiac index, arterial blood pressure, arterial blood gases, acid-base balance, toe temperature, urine output, and infusion rate of solution, and watch for signs of vasoconstriction or extravasation (eg, blanching). With low dosages for dopaminergic effects, monitor urine output and ECG.

Notes. The drug is physically incompatible with sodium bicarbonate or other alkaline solutions. (*See* Sympathomimetic Drugs for Hemodynamic Support Comparison Chart.)

DOPAMINE DILUTION GUIDE

| AMOUNT ADDED | | VOLUME OF | FINAL |
mg	Volume	DILUENT	CONCENTRATION[a]
200	5 mL (1 amp, 40 mg/mL)	250 mL	800 mg/L
200	5 mL (1 amp, 40 mg/mL)	500 mL	400 mg/L
400	5 mL (1 amp, 80 mg/mL)	500 mL	800 mg/L
800	5 mL (1 amp, 160 mg/mL)	500 mL	1.6 g/L

[a]Recommended concentrations, but concentrations up to 3.2 g/L have been used.

EPINEPHRINE AND SALTS

Adrenalin, Sus-Phrine, Various

Pharmacology. Epinephrine stimulates α_1-, α_2- (vasoconstriction, pressor effects), β_1- (increased myocardial contractility and conduction), and β_2-adrenergic (bronchodilation and vasodilation) receptors. It is used for reversible bronchospasm, anaphylactic reactions, laryngeal edema (croup), open-angle glaucoma, and cardiac arrest. (*See* Medical Emergencies.)

Administration and Adult Dosage. **SC for anaphylaxis** 0.2–0.5 mg (0.2–0.5 mL of 1:1000 aqueous soln), may repeat q 10–15 min prn; if SC is ineffective, then **IV** 0.1–0.25 mg (1–2.5 mL of 1:10,000) q 5–15 min may be given and followed by an IV infusion if necessary. **SC for asthma** same dosage as SC for anaphylaxis; may repeat q 20 min to 4 hr as needed.[141] **SC aqueous suspension for asthma** 0.5–1.5 mg (0.1–0.3 mL of 1:200), may repeat with 0.5–1.5 mg no sooner than q 6 hr. **IV infusion for hemodynamic support** 1 µg/min (1 mg in 500 mL NS or D5W) initially, adjust to hemodynamic response (usually 2–10 µg/min).[326] **Inhal (metered dose) not recommended** because of low efficacy and ultrashort duration of action.

Special Populations. *Pediatric Dosage.* **SC for anaphylaxis or asthma** 0.01 mL/kg/dose of 1:1000 aqueous solution, to a maximum of 0.5 mL; may repeat q 15–20 min for 2 doses, then q 4 hr prn. **SC aqueous suspension for asthma** (1 month–12 yr) 0.005 mL/kg/dose of 1:200, to a maximum of 0.15 mL/dose for children ≤30 kg, may repeat no sooner than q 6 hr.[141] **Inhal for croup** 0.25–0.5 mL of 2.25% racemic aqueous solution diluted in 1.5–4.5 mL of NS q 1–2 hr prn by nebulizer.[334,335] Alternatively, 5 mL of prediluted L-epinephrine in NS (1:1000) has been used.[335] **IV for hemodynamic support** 0.05–0.3 µg/kg/min initially, adjusted to desired hemodynamic response; avoid dosages >0.3 µg/kg/min if possible, because they are associated with marked vasoconstrictor effects.[327,336]

Geriatric Dosage. Same as adult dosage. (*See* Precautions.)

Dosage Forms. **Inhal Pwdr** 200, 220, 250 µg/spray; **Inhal Pwdr** (bitartrate) 160 µg/spray; **Inhal Soln** (HCl) 1% (1:100); **Inhal Soln** (racepinephrine) 2, 2.25%; **Inj** (aqueous solution as HCl) 0.01 mg/mL (1:100,000), 0.1 mg/mL (1:10,000), 0.5 mg/mL (1:2000), 1 mg/mL (1:1000); **Inj** (aqueous suspension as free base) 5 mg/mL (1:200).

Patient Instructions. (Autoinjectors) periodically familiarize yourself with instructions for use so you maintain an adequate comfort level. Obtain new kit by expiration date, or earlier if precipitate or color change is noted in solution.

Pharmacokinetics. *Onset and Duration.* Onset SC (aqueous soln or susp) 3–10 min; inhal peak 3–5 min. Duration SC (aqueous soln) 0.5–2 hr, (aqueous susp) up to 6–10 hr; inhal 15–60 min.[333,337]

Fate. Parenteral action is terminated by uptake into adrenergic neurons. Metabolism is by MAO and COMT.[323,333] Cl ranges from 2.1–5.3 L/hr/kg.[323]

$t_{1/2}$. About 1 min.[141]

Adverse Reactions. Dose-related restlessness, anxiety, tremor, cardiac arrhythmias, palpitations, hypertension, weakness, dizziness, and headache occur. Cerebral hemorrhage may be caused by a sharp rise in blood pressure from overdosage. Angina may be precipitated when coronary insufficiency is present, and elevation of blood glucose has been reported. Local necrosis from repeated injections and tolerance with prolonged use may also occur.[323,333]

Contraindications. Intra-arterial administration is not recommended because of marked vasoconstriction. Do not use with local anesthetics in fingers or toes, or during general anesthesia with halogenated hydrocarbons. Other contraindications include α-adrenergic blocker-induced (including phenothiazines) hypotension; cerebral arteriosclerosis; organic heart disease; narrow-angle glaucoma; shock; labor.

Precautions. Use with caution in patients with cardiovascular disease, hypertension, diabetes, or hyperthyroidism, and in psychoneurotic patients. Caution is usually recommended in the elderly, because of a higher frequency of cardiovascular intolerance. However, one evaluation of patients suffering from acute asthma attacks found no difference in hemodynamic alterations or arrhythmias between those >40 yr and those <40 yr in response to SC epinephrine.[338] IM injection may produce local tissue necrosis. Epinephrine infusions are preferably administered through a central venous line. Extravasation can cause necrosis; if extravasation occurs, infiltrate the area with **phentolamine** 5–10 mg diluted in 10–15 mL of NS.

Drug Interactions. Bretylium, guanethidine, and heterocyclic antidepressants may potentiate the pressor response to epinephrine. Oxytocics used in obstetrics may cause severe, persistent hypertension when used with vasopressors. Halogenated hydrocarbon anesthetics may predispose patients to serious arrhythmias. A hypertensive reaction may occur when epinephrine is given with nonselective β-adrenergic blockers (eg, propranolol, nadolol).

Parameters to Monitor. (IV infusion) ECG, infusion rate and site; (in the elderly) ECG; (asthma or allergy) blood pressure, heart rate, relief of symptoms.

Notes. Do not use solution if it is brown in color or contains a precipitate. Protect solution from light. Suspension provides a sustained effect; shake suspension well prior to use. Nonprescription inhalers have only a transient effect because of their low dosage.[337] They should be used only by patients who have infrequent symptoms (less than once a week) and obtain total relief of symptoms from administration of two inhalations. Parenteral administration offers no advantage over inhalation for the treatment of acute bronchospasm.[339] (*See* Sympathomimetic Drugs for Hemodynamic Support Comparison Chart.)

MILRINONE LACTATE
Primacor

Pharmacology. Milrinone is a phosphodiesterase inhibitor, positive inotropic agent, and a vasodilator similar to amrinone, but 10–15 times more potent on a weight basis. Milrinone is labeled for temporary use in patients with severe left ventricular dysfunction and CHF. It has also been used for postoperative hemodynamic support and for those awaiting cardiac transplantation.[340,341]

Adult Dosage. IV loading dose 50 μg/kg over 10 min, then **IV continuous infusion** 0.375–0.5 μg/kg/min; adjust dosage depending upon patient response and hemodynamic variables to a maximum of 0.75 μg/kg/min. In renal impairment, reduce dosage as follows: Cl_{cr} 50 mL/min, 0.43 μg/kg/min; 40 mL/min, 0.38 μg/kg/min; 30 mL/min, 0.33 μg/kg/min; 20 mL/min, 0.28 μg/kg/min; 10 mL/min, 0.23 μg/kg/min; 5 mL/min, 0.2 μg/kg/min.

Pediatric Dosage. Safety and efficacy not established, but weight-based dosages similar to adult dosages have been used.

Dosage Forms. Inj 1 mg/mL.

Pharmacokinetics. Although well absorbed orally, milrinone is only available for IV use. 70% bound to plasma proteins; V_d is 0.47 ± 0.3 L/kg. It is 88–90% eliminated as unchanged drug by renal excretion. Elimination half-life in patients with CHF is 2.3 ± 0.1 hr, longer than in normal volunteers. Thrombocytopenia is less frequent (0.4%) with milrinone than with amrinone. Milrinone can cause or worsen existing ventricular and supraventricular arrhythmias. Hypotension and headaches occur frequently. Long-term oral or IV milrinone may lead to increased mortality in patients with CHF.

NOREPINEPHRINE BITARTRATE
Levophed

Pharmacology. Norepinephrine is a catecholamine that directly stimulates β_1-, α_1- and α_2-adrenergic receptors. It has little action on β_2-receptors.[324]

Administration and Adult Dosage. IV for shock, by infusion only (in any nonalkaline IV fluid) 8–12 μg of base/min initially, adjusting rate to maintain a systolic blood pressure of about 80–100 mm Hg or to a specific hemodynamic response; average maintenance dosage ranges from 2–4 μg of base/min. Very large dosages (up to 1.5 μg/kg/min) have been used in patients with septic shock.[323,342]

Special Populations. *Pediatric Dosage.* Safety and efficacy not established. **IV for shock, by infusion only** 0.05–0.1 μg/kg/min of base initially, adjust dosage to blood pressure response, to a maximum of 1.5 μg/kg/min.[323]

Geriatric Dosage. Same as adult dosage. (*See* Precautions.)

Dosage Forms. Inj 1 mg (of base)/mL.

Pharmacokinetics. *Onset and Duration.* Onset 1–2 min; duration 1–2 min after discontinuing infusion.[333]

Fate. Action is primarily terminated by uptake into adrenergic neurons. Free drug is metabolized primarily by catechol-O-methyl transferase (COMT), and to a lesser extent by MAO, to inactive metabolites and their conjugates.

$t_{1/2}$. 2–2.5 min.[323]

Adverse Reactions. Dose-related hypertension (sometimes indicated by headache), reflex bradycardia, increased peripheral vascular resistance, and decreased cardiac output occur. Volume depletion may occur if fluid is not replaced. Arrhythmias may occur in extreme hypoxia or hypercarbia.

Contraindications. Hypotension secondary to uncorrected blood volume deficit; severe visceral or peripheral vasoconstriction; mesenteric or peripheral vascular thrombosis, unless drug is life-saving; halogenated hydrocarbon anesthesia.

Precautions. Use with caution in patients receiving MAO inhibitors or heterocyclic antidepressants. Administer into a large vein (antecubital preferred) to avoid necrosis secondary to vasoconstriction; avoid the leg veins whenever possible, especially in the elderly or in those with occlusive vascular diseases. Avoid extravasation of solution; however, if it occurs, the area may be infiltrated with 5–10 mg of **phentolamine** diluted in 10–15 mL of NS.

Drug Interactions. Bretylium, guanethidine, MAOIs, methyldopa, and heterocyclic antidepressants may potentiate the pressor response to direct-acting vasopressors. Oxytocics used in obstetrics may cause severe, persistent hypertension when used with vasopressors. Halogenated hydrocarbon anesthetics may predispose patients to serious arrhythmias.

Parameters to Monitor. In shock, closely monitor heart rate, pulmonary capillary wedge pressure, cardiac index, arterial blood pressure, arterial blood gases, acid-base balance, urine output, and infusion rate of solution, and watch for signs of vasoconstriction or extravasation (eg, blanching).

Notes. Do not use solution if it has a brown color or precipitate. 2 mg of norepinephrine bitartrate = 1 mg norepinephrine base. (*See* Sympathomimetic Drugs for Hemodynamic Support Comparison Chart.)

NOREPINEPHRINE DILUTION GUIDE

AMOUNT ADDED		VOLUME OF	FINAL
mg (base)	*Volume*	5% DEXTROSE	CONCENTRATION[a]
2 mg	2 mL	500 mL	4 mg/L[a]
4 mg	4 mL	500 mL	8 mg/L
8 mg	8 mL	500 mL	16 mg/L

[a]Recommended pediatric concentration.[343]

SYMPATHOMIMETIC DRUGS FOR HEMODYNAMIC SUPPORT COMPARISON CHART[a]

ADRENERGIC RECEPTOR SELECTIVITY

DRUG	Inotropic Activity (β_1)	Chronotropic Activity (β_1)	Vasodilation (β_2)	Vasoconstriction (α)	Renal/Mesenteric Vasodilation (DA_1)	TOTAL PERIPHERAL RESISTANCE	CARDIAC OUTPUT
Dobutamine Dobutrex Various	++	0/+[b]	+	0/+[b]	0	→	↑
Dopamine Inotropin Various	++	+/++[b,c]	++	+/++	+++	↓/↑[b]	↑
Epinephrine Adrenalin Various	+++	++	++	+++	0	→	↑
Isoproterenol Isuprel Various	+++	+++	++++	0	0	↓	↑
Norepinephrine[d] Levophed	++	++[e]	0	+++	0	↑	0/↓/↑
Phentolamine[f] Regitine	0	g	0	0	0	↓	↑

(continued)

386

SYMPATHOMIMETIC DRUGS FOR HEMODYNAMIC SUPPORT COMPARISON CHART[a] (continued)

DRUG	ADRENERGIC RECEPTOR SELECTIVITY					TOTAL PERIPHERAL RESISTANCE	CARDIAC OUTPUT
	Inotropic Activity (β_1)	Chronotropic Activity (β_1)	Vasodilation (β_2)	Vasoconstriction (α)	Renal/ Mesenteric Vasodilation (DA_1)		
Phenylephrine[h] Neo-Synephrine	0	0[e]	0	++++	0	↑	↓

++++ = Pronounced effect; + = Minimal effect; 0 = No effect; ↓ = Decreased; ↑ = Increased.

[a]This table compares only a few of the many factors important in the treatment of shock. Consult references 323, 325, 344–346 for clinical use. Cross-table comparisons of the adrenergic selectivity properties between this table and the Sympathomimetic Bronchodilators Comparison Chart cannot be made for the following reasons: (1) the rating scale of this table reflects a finer degree of differentiation of effects (hence 0–5+ vs 0–4+); (2) the routes of administration are different; and (3) vascular β_2-receptors appear to respond slightly differently from bronchiolar β_2-receptors.

[b]Dose dependent.

[c]Releases stored norepinephrine via tyraminelike mechanism.

[d]Primarily used to increase peripheral vascular resistance in volume-repleted hypotensive patients.

[e]Decrease in heart rate may result from reflex mechanisms.

[f]α-Adrenergic blocking drug; useful in severe vasoconstriction (eg, extravasation of norepinephrine or dopamine).

[g]Increase in heart rate may result from reflex and direct mechanisms.

[h]Primary use is to increase BP to reflexly increase vagal tone in paroxysmal supraventricular tachycardias. Other pressors are preferred in most shock states because they also have positive inotropic activity. Phenylephrine has no inotropic activity and with its strong α-agonist properties functions as a pure vasopressor (afterload increaser).

Nitrates

Class Instructions: Nitrates. This drug may cause headache, dizziness, and/or flushing; alcohol may worsen these side effects. Tolerance to side effects of long-acting nitrates such as headache may occur with continued therapy. If necessary, a mild analgesic may be used until tolerance to side effects occurs. During an acute angina attack, discontinue activity, assume a sitting position, and dissolve one sublingual tablet under the tongue. If chest discomfort does not improve after use of the tablets, seek medical attention. Keep tablets in the original container, tightly closed. If you have been taking this medication for a long time, do not discontinue it abruptly.

ISOSORBIDE DINITRATE   Isordil, Sorbitrate, Various

Pharmacology. (*See* Nitroglycerin.)

Administration and Adult Dosage. **SL tab for acute anginal attack** 2.5–10 mg q 2–3 hr prn;[347,348] **Chew Tab for acute anginal attack** 5 mg initially, then 5–10 mg q 2–3 hr prn.[348] **PO for prophylaxis of angina and for CHF** 10–60 mg q 4–6 hr; individual doses up to 120 mg have been used.[347,349] (*See* Vasodilators in Heart Failure Comparison Chart.) **SR products for prophylaxis of angina** 40–80 mg q 8–12 hr (once daily–bid at 8 AM and 2 PM preferred). Start the dosage low and adjust upward slowly over a period of several days to weeks to patient tolerance or to the desired therapeutic effect. A daily nitrate-free period of at least 12 hr is desirable in order to minimize tolerance.[349]

Special Populations. *Pediatric Dosage.* Safety and efficacy not established.

Geriatric Dosage. Same as adult dosage. However, some clinicians recommend lower doses, and that initial SL doses be given under medical observation because of an increased likelihood of postural hypotension.[350]

Dosage Forms. **Chew Tab** 5, 10 mg; **SL Tab** 2.5, 5, 10 mg; **SR Cap** 40 mg; **SR Tab** 40 mg; **Tab** 2.5, 5, 10, 20, 30, 40 mg.

Patient Instructions. (*See* Nitrates Class Instructions.) Do not crush or chew sustained-release preparations.

Missed Doses. Take this drug at regular intervals. If you miss a dose take it as soon as you remember. If it is about time for the next dose, take that dose only. Leave a minimum of 2 hours between regular tablet doses and 6 hours between sustained-release tablet or capsule doses. Do not double the dose or take extra.

Pharmacokinetics. *Onset and Duration.* Onset is 5–20 min after SL and Chew Tab administration, 15–45 min after PO tab administration, up to 4 hr in rare cases or with SR products; peak occurs 15–60 min after SL administration, 45–120 min after PO tab administration.[347,348] Duration is 1–3 hr after SL or Chew Tab, 2–6 hr after PO tab, up to 8 hr after SR.[347,351] Although PO administration may improve exercise tolerance for 4–8 hr after the first dose, with long-term, around-the-clock administration, the duration of action declines to 2–3 hr, probably because of nitrate tolerance.[351]

Fate. Oral bioavailability is 22 ± 14%. There is extensive first-pass metabolism by liver after oral administration to less active isosorbide mononitrate metabolites

(2-ISMN, 5-ISMN). Larger doses and long-term administration saturate metabolic processes, with appreciable increases in serum concentrations of the parent compound and metabolites.[352] The drug is 28 ± 12% bound to plasma proteins; V_d is 1.5 ± 0.8 L/kg; Cl is 2.7 ± 1.2 L/hr/kg.[9] (*See* Isosorbide Mononitrate *Fate*.)

*t*½ (Isosorbide dinitrate) 50 ± 20 min; (2-ISMN) 1.9 ± 0.5 hr; (5-ISMN) 4.6 ± 0.7 hr.[9,353]

Adverse Reactions. (*See* Nitroglycerin.)

Contraindications. (*See* Nitroglycerin.)

Precautions. (*See* Nitroglycerin.)

Drug Interactions. (*See* Nitroglycerin.)

Parameters to Monitor. Observe for headache, orthostatic hypotension, and dizziness. In angina, monitor frequency of angina. In CHF, monitor hemodynamic and functional measurements.

Notes. Because of their slower onset of action, reserve SL and chewable isosorbide dinitrate (ISDN) for acute anginal attacks only in patients intolerant of or unresponsive to nitroglycerin. ISDN is a mainstay of antianginal and CHF therapy because of its long record of efficacy in these disorders. It is also less expensive than other long-term nitrate preparations. However, patients must take multiple doses daily on an eccentric schedule to achieve and maintain efficacy.

ISOSORBIDE MONONITRATE   Imdur, ISMO, Monoket

Pharmacology. Isosorbide mononitrate (ISMN) is the active 5-mononitrate metabolite of isosorbide dinitrate. (*See* Nitroglycerin.)

Administration and Adult Dosage. PO for prophylaxis of angina (ISMO, Monoket) 20 mg bid, doses 7 hr apart. **SR for prophylaxis of angina** (Imdur) 30–60 mg once daily in the morning, may increase to 120 mg once daily, to a maximum (rarely) of 240 mg once daily. There may be some attenuation of antianginal efficacy after 6 weeks of therapy with the 30 and 60 mg doses, but not with the 120 mg dose.[351,354]

Special Populations. *Pediatric Dosage.* Safety and efficacy not established.

Geriatric Dosage. Same as adult dosage.

Other Conditions. For persons of particularly small stature, the manufacturer of Monoket recommends an alternative initial dosage of 5 mg bid, but to increase it to at least 10 mg bid by the second or third day of therapy.

Dosage Forms. SR Tab (Imdur) 30, 60, 120 mg; **Tab** (ISMO, Monoket) 10, 20 mg.

Patient Instructions. (*See* Nitrates Class Instructions.) Follow the prescribed administration schedule closely. Do not crush the sustained-release product.

Missed Doses. Take this drug at regular intervals. If you miss a dose take it as soon as you remember. If it is about time for the next dose, take that dose only. Leave a minimum of 6 hours between regular tablet doses and 12 hours between sustained-release tablet doses. Do not double the dose or take extra.

Pharmacokinetics. *Onset and Duration.* Non-SR tablet onset 30–60 min;[354] peak 1–2 hr, duration 12–14 hr with bid administration.[351] SR Tab onset within 4 hr; peak 4 hr; duration about 12 hr.[351,354]

Fate. The tablet is rapidly absorbed and essentially 100% bioavailable; SR Tab bioavailability is 78–86%.[354] The drug is distributed into total body water with negligible plasma protein binding and a V_d of 0.62 ± 0.05 L/kg.[353,355] Cl is 0.094 $\pm$ 0.005 L/hr/kg.[353] It is primarily hepatically metabolized by denitration and glucuronidation to inactive products that are renally eliminated; less than 2% of a dose is excreted unchanged in urine.[355]

$t_{1/2}$. 4.6 ± 0.7 hr.[353]

Adverse Reactions. (*See* Nitroglycerin.)

Contraindications. (*See* Nitroglycerin.)

Precautions. (*See* Nitroglycerin.)

Drug Interactions. (*See* Nitroglycerin.)

Parameters to Monitor. Observe for headache, orthostatic hypotension, and dizziness; antianginal efficacy; and compliance with 7-hr dosage regimen for non-SR tablet.

Notes. ISMN is an effective nitrate with dosage schedules proven to avoid tolerance. Patient compliance is favored with the use of ISMN because the products are administered once (Imdur) or twice (ISMO, Monoket) daily. Although the available preparations are comparable to each other in cost at relatively low dosages (ie, 20 mg bid for the immediate-release products and 60 mg/day or less of the SR products), they are much more expensive than generic ISDN, which is also effective when taken properly. Compliance and cost factors must be carefully assessed in the individual patient when choosing an oral nitrate product.

NITROGLYCERIN   Various

Pharmacology. Nitroglycerin and other organic nitrates are believed to be converted to nitric oxide (NO) by vascular endothelium. NO activates guanylate cyclase, increasing cyclic GMP, which in turn decreases intracellular calcium, resulting in direct relaxation of vascular smooth muscle.[347,349,356] The venous (capacitance) system is affected to a greater degree than the arterial (resistance) system. Venous pooling, decreased venous return to the heart (preload), and decreased arterial resistance (afterload) reduce intracardiac pressures and left ventricular size, thereby decreasing myocardial oxygen consumption and ischemia. In myocardial ischemia, nitrates dilate large epicardial vessels, enhance collateral size and flow, and reduce coronary vasoconstriction.[347] The various organic nitrate preparations have the same pharmacologic effects and differ only in bioavailability and pharmacokinetics.[330]

Administration and Adult Dosage. SL Tab for acute anginal attack 150–600 μg prn, up to 3 doses in 15 min; **SL aerosol for acute anginal attack** 400–800 μg prn, up to 1200 μg/15 min; **Buccal for acute anginal attack and/or prophylaxis and treatment of angina pectoris or CHF** 1–3 mg q 4–6 hr; **PO SR for prophylaxis of angina or CHF** 2.5–19.5 mg bid or tid;[347,351] **Top ointment for prophylaxis and treatment of angina pectoris or CHF** 1.3–5 cm (0.5–2 in.)

q 6–8 hr.[347,351] Start the dosage low and adjust slowly upward over a period of several days to weeks to patient tolerance or to the desired therapeutic effect. **SR Patch for prophylaxis and treatment of angina pectoris** 0.2–0.8 mg/hr, patch applied once daily, dosage adjusted to patient response.[347] Greater antianginal efficacy has been noted with patches delivering 0.4 mg/hr or greater.[347,357] A daily nitrate-free period of 12 hr is desirable in order to minimize nitrate tolerance.[349,351] **IV for CHF, post-MI, angina pectoris, perioperative blood pressure control, or hypotensive anesthesia** 5 μg/min initially by constant infusion using an infusion pump. Dosage must be adjusted to the individual patient's response. Increase dosage initially in 5 μg/min increments q 3–5 min until response noted. If no response occurs at 20 μg/min, increments of 10 μg/min, and later, 20 μg/min, can be used. Once partial blood pressure response occurs, decrease incremental increases and increase intervals. (*See* Notes.)

Special Populations. *Pediatric Dosage.* Safety and efficacy not established. **IV** 0.5–20 μg/kg/min has been suggested.[358]

Geriatric Dosage. Same as adult dosage. However, some clinicians recommend lower doses, and that initial SL doses be given under medical observation because of an increased likelihood of postural hypotension.[350]

Doasage Forms. **Buccal Tab** 1, 2, 3 mg; **Oint** 2%; **SL Aerosol** 400 μg/spray; **SL Tab** 300, 400, 600 μg; **SR Cap** 2.6, 6.5, 9 mg; **SR Tab** 2.5, 6.5, 9, 13 mg; **SR Patch** 0.1, 0.2, 0.3, 0.4, 0.6, 0.8 mg/hr; **Inj** 0.5, 5 mg/mL.

Patient Instructions. (*See* Nitrates Class Instructions.)

Pharmacokinetics. *Onset and Duration.* Onset immediate after IV, 2–5 min after SL or buccal, 20–45 min after SR Cap or Tab, 15–60 min after topical ointment, and 30–60 min after transdermal administration.[347] Peak 4–8 min after SL, 4–10 min after buccal, 45–120 min after SR Cap or Tab, 30–120 min after topical ointment, and 1–3 hr after transdermal administration.[347] Duration 10–30 min after IV and SL, 0.5–5 hr after buccal, 2–6 hr after oral, 4–8 hr after SR, and 3–8 hr after topical administration.[347,351] Although the SR patch may act for a longer duration after the first application, long-term continuous therapy limits the duration of action to 4 hr or less, probably because of tolerance.[359] With sustained intermittent therapy (removal of patch after 12 hr), duration is 8–12 hr.[351]

Fate. Bioavailability of SL and Top are 38 ± 26% and 72 ± 20%, respectively.[9,360] Extensive first-pass metabolism occurs after oral administration. The drug is 87 ± 1% plasma protein bound. V_d is 3.3 ± 1.2 L/kg; Cl is 13.8 ± 5.4 L/hr/kg.[9,360] It is metabolized in the liver to less active dinitro and inactive mononitro metabolites. Larger doses and long-term administration may saturate metabolism and result in increased serum concentrations of drug and metabolites.[360]

$t_{½}$. β phase estimated to be 2.3 ± 0.6 min.[9]

Adverse Reactions. Headache occurs very frequently; dizziness occurs frequently, especially with oral or topical administration. Occasionally flushing, weakness, nausea, vomiting, palpitations, tachycardia, and postural hypotension occur. Many of these effects are dose related and may be minimized by increasing the dosage slowly. Tolerance and dependence may occur with prolonged use. Contact dermatitis occurs in up to 40% of patients using transdermal patches.[361]

Contraindications. Severe anemia; severe hypotension or uncompensated hypovolemia; increased intracranial pressure; purported hypersensitivity or idiosyncrasy to nitroglycerin, nitrates, or nitrites; use of sildenafil. (*See* Drug Interactions.) Constrictive pericarditis, pericardial tamponade, and inadequate cerebral circulation are also considered contraindications by some authors.[351]

Precautions. Some tolerance and cross-tolerance with other nitrates may occur with long-term or excessive use.[351] Use with caution in patients with severe renal or hepatic disease, those with low or normal pulmonary capillary wedge pressure, and those receiving drugs that lower blood pressure. With intermittent therapy, anginal episodes may increase during the nitrate-free interval.[362]

Drug Interactions. Nitrates can produce additive vasodilation and severe postural hypotension when combined with alcohol or hypotensive drugs. Use in patients taking sildenafil can result in profound hypotension with serious consequences, including death.

Parameters to Monitor. Observe for headache, dizziness, and other side effects. Monitor for orthostatic hypotension, especially with first SL dose in elderly. (Angina) monitor frequency of angina. (CHF) obtain hemodynamic and functional measurements. (IV use) monitor blood pressure and heart rate constantly in all patients; pulmonary capillary wedge pressure may also be useful in some patients.

Notes. Large and unpredictable amounts of nitroglycerin are lost through PVC containers, most IV administration sets and tubing, and certain IV filters.[363,364] The manufacturers recommend IV nitroglycerin infusions be prepared and stored in glass bottles and infused via special non-PVC tubing, avoiding the use of in-line filters. However, because nitroglycerin infusion rate is usually adjusted to response rather than by a μg/kg dosage, the need for special tubing has been questioned.[347] Some institutions have discontinued use of nitroglycerin tubing as part of cost-savings efforts, and have achieved good results clinically when using PVC tubing to infuse nitroglycerin.[365,366] However, because substantial amounts of nitroglycerin are adsorbed onto PVC tubing, special attention to patient response is advisable at the time of IV tubing changes. Stored in glass containers, the diluted injection is stable for 48 hr at room temperature and 7 days under refrigeration. When administration sets with large dead spaces are used, flush the line whenever the concentration of solution is changed. (*See* Vasodilators in Heart Failure Comparison Chart.)

APPROXIMATE EQUIVALENT DOSAGES OF NITRATES

PRODUCT	LOW DOSAGE	HIGH DOSAGE
Nitroglycerin Ointment	≤1 inch q 6 hr	1–2 inches q 6 hr
Nitroglycerin Patch	0.4 mg/hr	0.4–0.6 mg/hr
Isosorbide Dinitrate	20 mg tid	20–40 mg tid
Isosorbide Mononitrate		
Immediate-Release	10–20 mg bid	20 mg bid
Sustained-Release	30–60 mg/day	60–120 mg/day

VASODILATORS IN HEART FAILURE COMPARISON CHART

DRUG	DOSAGE[a]	DURATION	SITE OF ACTION[b]	HR	MAP	PCWP	CI	SVR
ACE INHIBITORS								
Captopril Capoten	PO 25–100 mg tid.	HOURS	A, V	0/↓	↓	↓	↑	↓
Enalapril Vasotec	PO 2.5–10 mg bid; IV 0.625–5 mg q 6–12 hr.							
Lisinopril Prinivil Zestril	PO 5–20 mg/day.							
Quinapril Accupril	PO 5–20 mg q 12 hr.							
HYDRALAZINE								
Hydralazine Apresoline Various	PO 50–75 mg q 6–8 hr; usual maintenance 200–600 mg/day.	hours	A	0/↑	sl↓	sl↓	↑	↓
NITRATES								
Isosorbide Dinitrate Isordil Sorbitrate Various	PO 10–60 mg q 4–6 hr.	hours	V,(A)	sl↑/↓	↓	↓	↑/↓	sl↓

(continued)

VASODILATORS IN HEART FAILURE COMPARISON CHART

DRUG	DOSAGE[a]	DURATION	SITE OF ACTION[b]	HR	MAP	PCWP	CI	SVR
Nitroglycerin Various	(See monograph.)	minutes	V,(A)	sl↑/↓	↓	↓	↑/↓	sl↓
NITROPRUSSIDE **Nitroprusside Sodium** Various	IV 0.1–3 µg/kg/min.	minutes	A,V	0	sl↓	↓	↑	↓

A = arterial; V = venous; HR = heart rate; MAP = mean arterial pressure; PCWP = pulmonary capillary wedge pressure; CI = cardiac index; SVR = systemic vascular resistance; ↑ = increase; ↓ = decrease; sl = slight; 0 = no change

[a]Start with low dosages of these drugs and increase gradually with continuous hemodynamic monitoring. To avoid adverse rebound effects, carefully taper the dosages of these drugs if they are to be discontinued. (See Nitroglycerin Notes.)

[b]Predominant site of action. Parentheses denote lesser activity.

From references 330, 367–371 and product information.

■ REFERENCES

1. Parker RB, McCollam PL. Adenosine in the episodic treatment of paroxysmal supraventricular tachycardia. *Clin Pharm* 1990;9:261–71.
2. Camm AJ, Garratt CJ. Adenosine and supraventricular tachycardia. *N Engl J Med* 1991;325:1621–9.
3. DiMarco JP et al. Adenosine for paroxysmal supraventricular tachycardia: dose ranging and comparison with verapamil. *Ann Intern Med* 1990;113:104–10.
4. McIntosh-Vellin NL et al. Safety and efficacy of central intravenous bolus administration of adenosine for termination of supraventricular tachycardia. *J Am Coll Cardiol* 1993;22:741–5.
5. Pedrid PJ. Amiodarone: reevaluation of an old drug. *Ann Intern Med* 1995;122:689–700.
6. Gilette PC et al. Amiodarone for children. *Clin Prog Electrophysiol Pacing* 1986;4:328–30.
7. Roden DM. Pharmacokinetics of amiodarone: implications for drug therapy. *Am J Cardiol* 1993;72:45F–50F.
8. Rotmensch HH et al. Steady-mate serum amiodarone concentrations: relationship with antiarrhythmic efficacy and toxicity. *Ann Intern Med* 1984;101:462–9.
9. Benet LZ et al. Design and optimization of dosage regimens; pharmacokinetic data. In, Hardman JG et al., eds. *Goodman and Gilman's the pharmacological basis of therapeutics.* 9th ed. New York: McGraw-Hill; 1996:1707–92.
10. Gill J et al. Amiodarone. An overview of its pharmacologic properties, and review of its therapeutic use in cardiac arrhythmias. *Drugs* 1992;43:69–110.
11. Rigas B et al. Amiodarone hepatotoxicity. A clinicopathologic study of five patients. *Ann Intern Med* 1986;104:348–51.
12. Figge HL, Figge J. The effects of amiodarone on thyroid hormone function: a review of the physiology and clinical manifestations. *J Clin Pharmacol* 1990;30:588–95.
13. Dusman RE et al. Clinical features of amiodarone-induced pulmonary toxicity. *Circulation* 1990;82:51–9.
14. Hohnloser SH et al. Amiodarone-associated proarrhythmic effects. A review with special reference to torsade de pointes tachycardia. *Ann Intern Med* 1994;121:529–35.
15. Roberts SA et al. Invasive and noninvasive methods to predict the long-term efficacy of amiodarone: a compilation of clinical observations using meta-analysis. *PACE Pacing Clin Electrophysiol* 1994;17:1590–602.
16. Echt DS et al. Mortality and morbidity in patients receiving encainide, flecainide, or placebo. The Cardiac Arrhythmia Suppression Trial. *N Engl J Med* 1991;324:781–8.
17. Rapeport WG. Clinical pharmacokinetics of bretylium. *Clin Pharmacokinet* 1985;10:248–56.
18. Adir J et al. Nomogram for bretylium dosing in renal impairment. *Ther Drug Monit* 1985;7:265–8.
19. Anderson JL et al. Kinetics of antifibrillatory effects of bretylium: correlation with myocardial drug concentrations. *Am J Cardiol* 1980;46:583–92.
20. Anderson JL et al. Oral and intravenous bretylium disposition. *Clin Pharmacol Ther* 1980;28:468–78.
21. Narang PK et al. Pharmacokinetics of bretylium in man after intravenous administration. *J Pharmacokinet Biopharm* 1980;8:363–73.
22. Anderson JL et al. Clinical pharmacokinetics of intravenous and oral bretylium tosylate in survivors of ventricular tachycardia or fibrillation: clinical application of a new assay for bretylium. *J Cardiovasc Pharmacol* 1981;3:485–99.
23. Jelliffe RW. An improved method of digoxin therapy. *Ann Intern Med* 1968;69:703–17.
24. Jelliffe RW, Brooker G. A nomogram for digoxin therapy. *Am J Med* 1974;57:63–8.
25. Mooradian AD, Wynn EM. Pharmacokinetic prediction of serum digoxin concentration in the elderly. *Arch Intern Med* 1987;147:650–3.
26. Cusack B et al. Digoxin in the elderly: pharmacokinetic consequences of old age. *Clin Pharmacol Ther* 1979;25:772–6.
27. Doherty JE et al. Clinical pharmacokinetics of digitalis glycosides. *Prog Cardiovasc Dis* 1978;21:141–58.
28. Soldin SJ. Digoxin—issues and controversies. *Clin Chem* 1986;32:5–12.
29. Iisalo E. Clinical pharmacokinetics of digoxin. *Clin Pharmacokinet* 1977;2:1–16.
30. Caldwell JH, Cline CT. Biliary excretion of digoxin in man. *Clin Pharmacol Ther* 1976;19:410–5.
31. Ewy GA et al. Digitalis intoxication—diagnosis, management and prevention. *Cardiol Clin* 1974;6:153–74.
32. Mann DL et al. Absence of cardioversion-induced ventricular arrhythmias in patients with therapeutic digoxin levels. *J Am Coll Cardiol* 1985;5:882–8.
33. Green LH, Smith TW. The use of digitalis in patients with pulmonary disease. *Ann Intern Med* 1977;87:459–65.
34. Slaughter RL et al. Appropriateness of the use of serum digoxin and digitoxin assays. *Am J Hosp Pharm* 1978;35:1376–9.
35. Weintraub M. Interpretation of the serum digoxin concentration. *Clin Pharmacokinet* 1977;2:205–19.
36. Podrid PJ et al. Congestive heart failure caused by oral disopyramide. *N Engl J Med* 1980;302:614– 7.

37. Lima JJ et al. Antiarrhythmic activity and unbound concentrations of disopyramide enantiomers in patients. *Ther Drug Monit* 1990;12:23–8.
38. Lima JJ. Disopyramide. In, Taylor WJ, Caviness MHD, eds. *A textbook for the clinical application of therapeutic drug monitoring.* Irving, TX: Abbott Diagnostics; 1986:97–108.
39. Bauman JL et al. Practical optimisation of antiarrhythmic drug therapy using pharmacokinetic principles. *Clin Pharmacokinet* 1991;20:151–66.
40. Latini R et al. Therapeutic drug monitoring of antiarrhythmic drugs: rationale and current status. *Clin Pharmacokinetic* 1990;18:91–103.
41. Piscitelli DA et al. Bioavailability of total and unbound disopyramide: implications for clinical use of the immediate and controlled-release forms. *J Clin Pharmacol* 1994;34:823–8.
42. Siddoway LA, Woosley RL. Clinical pharmacokinetics of disopyramide. *Clin Pharmacokinet* 1986; 11:214–22.
43. Hasselstrom J et al. Enantioselective steady-state kinetics of unbound disopyramide and its dealkylated metabolite in man. *Eur J Clin Pharmacol* 1991;41:481–4.
44. Bauman JL et al. Long-term therapy with disopyramide phosphate: side effects and effectiveness. *Am Heart J* 1986;111:654–60.
45. Rasmussen HS et al. Dofetilide, a novel class III antiarrhythmic agent. *J Cardiovasc Pharmacol* 1992;20 (suppl 2):S96–105.
46. Roden DM. Current status of class III antiarrhythmic drug therapy. *Am J Cardiol* 1993;72:44B–9B.
47. Perry JC, Garson A. Flecainide acetate for treatment of tachyarrhythmias in children: review of world literature on efficacy, safety and dosing. *Am Heart J* 1992;124:1614–21.
48. Holmes B, Heel RC. Flecainide. A preliminary review of its pharmacodynamic properties and therapeutic efficacy. *Drugs* 1985;29:1–33.
49. Conrad GJ, Ober RE. Metabolism of flecainide. *Am J Cardiol* 1984;53:41B–51B.
50. Gross AS et al. Polymorphic flecainide disposition under conditions of uncontrolled urine flow and pH. *Eur J Clin Pharmacol* 1991;40:155–62.
51. Forland SC et al, Flecainide pharmacokinetics after multiple dosing in patients with impaired renal function. *J Clin Pharmacol* 1988;28:727–35.
52. McCollam P et al. Proarrhythmia: a paradoxical response to antiarrhythmic drugs. *Pharmacotherapy* 1989;9:144–53.
53. Tworek DA et al. Interference by antiarrhythmic agents with function of electrical cardiac devices. *Clin Pharm* 1992;11:48–56.
54. Anon. Ibutilide. *Med Lett Drugs Ther* 1996;38:38.
55. Benowitz NL, Meister W. Clinical pharmacokinetics of lignocaine. *Clin Pharmacokinet* 1978;3:177–201.
56. Galer BS et al. Response to intravenous lidocaine infusion differs based on clinical diagnosis and site of nervous system injury. *Neurology* 1993;43:1233–5.
57. Routledge PA et al. Control of lidocaine therapy: new perspectives. *Ther Drug Monit* 1982;4:265–70.
58. Rowland M et al. Disposition kinetics of lidocaine in normal subjects. *Ann N Y Acad Sci* 1971;179:383–98.
59. Boyes RN et al. Pharmacokinetics of lidocaine in man. *Clin Pharmacol Ther* 1971;12:105–16.
60. Thomson PD et al. Lidocaine pharmacokinetics in advanced heart failure, liver disease, and renal failure in humans. *Ann Intern Med* 1973;78:499–508.
61. Bauer LA et al. Influence of long-term infusions on lidocaine kinetics. *Clin Pharmacol Ther* 1982;31:433–7.
62. Blumer J et al. The convulsant potency of lidocaine and its N-dealkylated metabolites. *J Pharmacol Exp Ther* 1973;186:31–6.
63. Burney RG et al. Anti-arrhythmic effects of lidocaine metabolites. *Am Heart J* 1974;88:765–9.
64. LeLorier J et al. Pharmacokinetics of lidocaine after prolonged intravenous infusions in uncomplicated myocardial infarction. *Ann Intern Med* 1977;87:700–2.
65. Routledge PA et al. Increased alpha-1-acid glycoprotein and lidocaine disposition in myocardial infarction. *Ann Intern Med* 1980;93:701–4.
66. Gupta PK et al. Lidocaine-induced heart block in patients with bundle branch block. *Am J Cardiol* 1974;33:187–92.
67. Singh BN. Routine prophylactic lidocaine administration in acute myocardial infarction, An idea whose time is all but gone? *Circulation* 1992;86:1033–5. Editorial.
68. Berk SI et al. The effect of oral cimetidine on total and unbound serum lidocaine concentrations in patients with suspected myocardial infarction. *Int J Cardiol* 1987;14:91–4.
69. Jonsson A et al. Inhibition of burn pain by intravenous lignocaine infusion. *Lancet* 1991;338:151–2.
70. Stracke H et al. Mexiletine in the treatment of diabetic neuropathy. *Diabetes Care* 1992;15:1550–5.
71. Awerbuch GI, Sandyk R. Mexiletine for thalamic pain syndrome. *Int J Neurosci* 1990;55:129–33.

72. Bauman JL. Mexiletine. In, Taylor WJ, Caviness MHD, eds. *A textbook for the clinical application of therapeutic drug monitoring.* Irving, TX: Abbott Diagnostics; 1986:125–30.

73. Allaf et al. Pharmacokinetics of mexiletine in renal insufficiency. *Br J Clin Pharmacol* 1982;14:431–5.

74. Schrader BJ, Bauman IL. Mexiletine: a new type I antiarrhythmic agent. *Drug Intell Clin Pharm* 1986;20:255–60.

75. Woosley RL et al. Pharmacology, electrophysiology, and pharmacokinetics of mexiletine. *Am Heart J* 1984;107:1058–65.

76. Lledo P et al. Influence of debrisoquine hydroxylation phenotype on the pharmacokinetics of mexiletine. *Eur J Clin Pharmacol* 1993;44:63–7.

77. Campbell NPS et al. The clinical pharmacology of mexiletine. *Br J Clin Pharmacol* 1978;6:103–8.

78. Leahey EB et al. Effect of ventricular failure on steady state kinetics of mexiletine. *Clin Res* 1982;31:239A. Abstract.

79. Pentikainen PJ et al. Pharmacokinetics of oral mexiletine in patients with acute myocardial infarction. *Eur J Clin Pharmacol* 1983;25:773–7.

80. Campbell NPS et al. Long-term oral antiarrhythmic therapy with mexiletine. *Br Heart J* 1978;40:796–801.

81. Duff HJ et al. Molecular basis for the antigenicity of lidocaine analogs: tocainide and mexiletine. *Am Heart J* 1984;107:585–9.

82. Hurwitz A et al. Mexiletine effects on theophylline disposition. *Clin Pharmacol Ther* 1991;50:299–307.

83. Duff HJ et al. Mexiletine in the treatment of resistant ventricular arrhythmias: enhancement of efficacy and reduction of dose-related side effects by combination with quinidine. *Circulation* 1983;67:1124–8.

84. Vaughan Williams EM. Classification of the antiarrhythmic action of moricizine. *J Clin Pharmacol* 1991;31:216–21.

85. Moak JP et al. Newer antiarrhythmic drugs in children. *Am Heart J* 1987;61:179–85.

86. Morganroth J. Dose effect of moricizine on suppression of ventricular arrhythmias, *Am J Cardiol* 1990;65:26D–31.

87. Giardina EG et al. Moricizine concentration to guide arrhythmia treatment with attention to elderly patients. *J Clin Pharmacol* 1994;34:725–33.

88. Yang JM et al. Distribution of moricizine in human blood: binding to plasma proteins and erythrocytes. *Ther Drug Monit* 1990;12:59–64.

89. Sidddoway LA et al. Clinical pharmacokinetics of moricizine. *Am J Cardiol* 1990;65:21D–5D.

90. Carnes CA, Coyle JD. Moricizine: a novel antiarrhythmic agent. *DICP* 1990;24:745–53.

91. Miura DS et al. Ethmozine toxicity: fever of unknown origin. *J Clin Pharmacol* 1986;26:153–5.

92. The Cardiac Arrhythmia Suppression Trial II Investigators. Effect of the antiarrhythmic agent moricizine on survival after myocardial infarction. *N Engl J Med* 1992;327:227–33.

93. Hoffman BF et al. Electrophysiology and pharmacology of cardiac arrhythmias. VII. Cardiac effects of quinidine and procaine amide. A. *Am Heart J* 1975;89:804–8.

94. Greenspan AM et al. Large dose procainamide therapy for ventricular tachyarrhythmia. *Am J Cardiol* 1980;46:453–62.

95. Johnson KB ed. *The Harriet Lane handbook.* 13th ed. Mosby-Year Book: St. Louis; 1993.

96. Kessler KM et al. Procainamide pharmacokinetics in patients with acute myocardial infarction or congestive heart failure. *J Am Coll Cardiol* 1986;7: 1131–9.

97. Koch-Weser J. Serum procainamide levels as therapeutic guides. *Clin Pharmacokinet* 1977;2:389–402.

98. Connolly SJ, Kates RE. Clinical pharmacokinetics of N-acetylprocainamide. *Clin Pharmacokinet* 1982;7:206–20.

99. Karlsson E. Clinical pharmacokinetics of procainamide. *Clin Pharmacokinet* 1978;3:97–107.

100. Henningsen NC et al. Effects of long-term treatment with procaine amide. A prospective study with special regard to ANF and SLE in fast and slow acetylators. *Acta Med Scand* 1975;198:475–82.

101. Strasberg B et al. Procainamide-induced polymorphous ventricular tachycardia. *Am J Cardiol* 1981;47:1309–14.

102. Meyers DG et al. Severe neutropenia associated with procainamide: comparison of sustained release and conventional preparations. *Am Heart J* 1985;109:1393–5.

103. Lee JT et al. The role of genetically determined polymorphic drug metabolism in the beta-blockade produced by propafenone. *N Engl J Med* 1990;322:1764–8.

104. Funck-Brentano C et al. Propafenone. *N Engl J Med* 1990;322:518–25.

105. Musto et al. Electrophysiological effects and clinical efficacy of propafenone in children with recurrent paroxysmal supraventricular tachycardia. *Circulation* 1988;78:863–9.

106. Hii JTY et al. Clinical pharmacokinetics of propafenone. *Clin Pharmacokinet* 1991;21:1–10.

107. Lee JT et al. Influence of hepatic dysfunction on the pharmacokinetics of propafenone. *J Clin Pharmacol* 1987;27:384–9.

108. Capucci A et al. Minimal effective concentration values of propafenone and 5-hydroxy-propafenone in acute and chronic therapy. *Cardiovasc Drugs Ther* 1990;4:281–7.
109. Siddoway LA et al. Polymorphism of propafenone metabolism and disposition in man: clinical and pharmacokinetic consequences. *Circulation* 1987;75:785–91.
110. Parker RB et al. Propafenone: a novel type Ic antiarrhythmic agent. *DICP* 1989;23:196–202.
111. Bryson HM et al. Propafenone. A reappraisal of its pharmacology, pharmacokinetics and therapeutic use in cardiac arrhythmias. *Drugs* 1993;45:85–130.
112. Mondardini A et al. Propafenone-induced liver injury: report of a case and review of the literature. *Gastroenterology* 1993;104:1524–6.
113. Verme CN et al. Pharmacokinetics of quinidine in male patients. A population analysis. *Clin Pharmacokinet* 1992;22:468–80.
114. Greenblatt DJ et al. Pharmacokinetics of quinidine in humans after intravenous, intramuscular and oral administration. *J Pharmacol Exp Ther* 1977;202:365–78.
115. Ueda CT, Dzindzio BS. Quinidine kinetics in congestive heart failure. *Clin Pharmacol Ther* 1978;23:158–64.
116. Kessler KM et al. Quinidine pharmacokinetics in patients with cirrhosis or receiving propranolol. *Am Heart J* 1978;96:627–35.
117. Bauman JL et al. Torsade de pointes due to quinidine: observations in 31 patients. *Am Heart J* 1984;107:425–30.
118. Coplen SE et al. Efficacy and safety of quinidine therapy for maintenance of sinus rhythm after cardioversion. *Circulation* 1990;82:1106–16.
119. Oberg KC et al. "Late" proarrhythmia due to quinidine. *Am J Cardiol* 1994;74:192–4.
120. Nappi JM, McCollam PL. Sotalol: a breakthrough antiarrhythmic? *Ann Pharmacother* 1993;27:1359–68.
121. Hanyok JJ. Clinical pharmacokinetics of sotalol. *Am J Cardiol* 1993;72:19A–26A.
122. Fiset C et al. Stereoselective disposition of (±)-sotalol at steady-state conditions. *Br J Clin Pharmacol* 1993;36:75–7.
123. Poirer M et al. The pharmacokinetics of d-sotalol and d,l-sotalol in healthy volunteers. *Br J Clin Pharmacol* 1990;38:579–82.
124. Dumas M et al. Variations of sotalol kinetics in renal insufficiency. *Int J Clin Pharmacol Ther Toxicol* 1989;27:486–9.
125. MacNeil D et al. Clinical safety profile of sotalol in the treatment of arrhythmias. *Am J Cardiol* 1993;72:44A–50A.
126. Campbell RWF, Furniss SS. Practical considerations in the use of sotalol for ventricular tachycardia and ventricular fibrillation. *Am J Cardiol* 1993;72:80A–5A.
127. Kehoe RF et al. Safety and efficacy of oral sotalol for sustained ventricular tachyarrhythmias refractory to other antiarrhythmic agents. *Am J Cardiol* 1993;72:56A–66A.
128. Winkle RA et al. Tocainide for drug-resistant ventricular arrhythmias: efficacy, side effects, and lidocaine responsiveness for predicting tocainide success. *Am Heart J* 1980;100:1031–6.
129. Kutalek SP et al. Tocainide: a new oral antiarrhythmic agent. *Ann Intern Med* 1985;103:387–91.
130. Routledge PA. Tocainide. In, Taylor WJ, Caviness MHD, eds. *A textbook for the clinical application of therapeutic drug monitoring.* Irving, TX: Abbott Diagnostics; 1986:175–80.
131. Mohiuddin SM et al. Tocainide kinetics in congestive heart failure. *Clin Pharmacol Ther* 1983;34:596–603.
132. Roden DM, Woosley RL. Tocainide. *N Engl J Med* 1986;315:41–5.
133. Holmes B et al. Tocainide. A review of its pharmacological properties and therapeutic efficacy. *Drugs* 1983;26:93–123.
134. Hoffmann K-J et al. Analysis and stereoselective metabolism after separate oral doses of tocainide enantiomers to healthy volunteers. *Biopharm Drug Dispos* 1990;11:351–63.
135. Braun J et al. Pharmacokinetics of tocainide in patients with severe renal failure. *Eur J Clin Pharmacol* 1985;28:665–70.
136. Forrence E et al. A seizure induced by concurrent lidocaine-tocainide therapy—is it just a case of additive toxicity? *Drug Intell Clin Pharm* 1986;20:56–9.
137. Vaughan Williams ED. A classification of antiarrhythmic actions reassessed after a decade of new drugs. *J Clin Pharmacol* 1984;24:129–47.
138. Task Force of the Working Group on Arrhythmias of the European Society of Cardiology. The Sicilian gambit. A new approach to the classification of antiarrhythmic drugs based on their actions on arrhythmogenic mechanisms. *Circulation* 1991;84:1831–51.
139. Cauffield JS et al. Alpha blockers: a reassessment of their role in therapy. *Am Fam Physician* 1996;54:263–70.
140. Fulton B et al. Doxazosin. An update of its clinical pharmacology and therapeutic applications in hypertension and benign prostatic hypertrophy. *Drugs* 1995;49:295–320.
141. Advice for the patient, Vol II. In, *USP DI,* 15th ed. Rockville, MD: US Pharmacopeal Convention; 1995.

142. Studer JA, Piepho RW. Antihypertensive therapy in the geriatric patient: II. A review of the alpha₁-adrenergic blocking agents. *J Clin Pharmacol* 1993;33:2–13.

143. Vincent J et al. Clinical pharmacokinetics of prazosin—1985. *Clin Pharmacokinet* 1985;10:144–54.

144. Titmarsh S, Monk JP. Terazosin. A review of its pharmacodynamic and pharmacokinetic properties, and therapeutic efficacy in essential hypertension. *Drugs* 1987;33:461–77.

145. Carruthers SG. Adverse effects of α_1-adrenergic blocking drugs. *Drug Saf* 1994;11:12–20.

146. O'Dea RF et al. Treatment of neonatal hypertension with captopril. *J Pediatr* 1988;113:403–6.

147. Duchin KL et al. Pharmacokinetics of captopril in healthy subjects and in patients with cardiovascular diseases. *Clin Pharmacokinet* 1988;14:241–59.

148. Burris JF. The expanding role of angiotension converting enzyme inhibitors in the management of hypertension. *J Clin Pharmacol* 1995;35:337–42.

149. Alderman CP. Adverse effects of the angiotensin-converting enzyme inhibitors. *Ann Pharmacother* 1996; 30:55–61.

150. Langely MS, Heel RC. Transdermal clonidine: a preliminary review of its pharmacodynamic properties and therapeutic efficacy. *Drugs* 1988;35:123–42.

151. Guthrie SK. Pharmacologic interventions for the treatment of opioid dependence and withdrawal. *DICP* 1990;24:721–34.

152. Nunn-Thompson CL, Simon PA. Pharmacotherapy for smoking cessation. *Clin Pharm* 1989;8:710–20.

153. Lowenthal DT el al. Clinical pharmacokinetics of clonidine. *Clin Pharmacokinet* 1988;14:287–310.

154. Holdiness MR. A review of contact dermatitis associated with transdermal therapeutic systems. *Contact Dermatitis* 1989;20:3–9.

155. Reid JL et al. Withdrawal reactions following cessation of central α-adrenergic receptor agonist. *Hypertension* 1984;6(suppl II): 71II–5II.

156. Harris JM. Clonidine patch toxicity. *DICP* 1990;24:1191–4.

157. Bond WS. Psychiatric indications for clonidine: the neuropharmacologic and clinical basis. *J Clin Psychopharmacol* 1986;6:81–7.

158. Bravo EL et al. Clonidine-suppression test: a useful aid in the diagnosis of pheochromocytoma. *N Engl J Med* 1981;305:623–6.

159. Fedorak RN. Treatment of diabetic diarrhea with clonidine. *Ann Intern Med* 1985;102:197–9.

160. Hammer M, Berg G. Clonidine in the treatment of menopausal flushing. *Acta Obstet Gynecol Scand Suppl* 1985;132:29–31.

161. Nilsson LC et al. Clonidine for the relief of premenstrual syndrome. *Lancet* 1985;2:549–50.

162. Joint National Committee on Prevention, Detection, Evaluation, and Treatment of High Blood Pressure. The sixth report of the Joint National Committee on Prevention, Detection, Evaluation, and Treatment of High Blood Pressure. *Arch Intern Med* 1997;157:2413–46.

163. Ogilvie RI et al. Diazoxide concentration-response relation in hypertension. *Hypertension* 1982;4:167–73.

164. Andreasen F et al. The biological relevance of the protein binding of diazoxide. *Acta Pharmacol Toxicol (Copenh)*1985;57:30–5.

165. Leonetti G, Cuspidi C. Choosing the right ACE inhibitors. A guide to selection. *Drugs* 1995;49:516–35.

166. DiPette DJ et al. Enalaprilat, an intravenous angiotensin-converting enzyme inhibitor, in hypertensive crisis. *Clin Pharmacol Ther* 1985;38:199–204.

167. Todd PA, Heel RC. Enalapril: a review of its pharmacodynamic and pharmacokinetic properties and therapeutic use in hypertension and congestive heart failure. *Drugs* 1986;31:198–248.

168. Till AE et al. Pharmacokinetics of repeated oral doses of enalapril maleate (MK-421) in normal volunteers. *Biopharm Drug Dispos* 1984;5:273–80.

169. Ulm EH et al. Enalapril maleate and a lysine analogue (MK-521): disposition in man. *Br J Clin Pharmacol* 1982;14:357–62.

170. Brogden RN et al. Captopril. An update of its pharmacodynamic and pharmacokinetic properties, and therapeutic use in hypertension and congestive heart failure. *Drugs* 1988;36:540–600.

171. Keane WF et al. Angiotension converting enzyme inhibitors and progressive renal insufficiency; current experience and future directions. *Ann Intern Med* 1989;111:503–16.

172. Cooper RA. Captopril-associated neutropenia: who is at risk? *Arch Intern Med* 1983;143:659–60.

173. CONSENSUS Trial Study Group. Effects of enalapril on mortality in severe congestive heart failure. *N Engl J Med* 1987;316:1430–5.

174. Murphy MB, Elliott WJ. Dopamine and dopamine receptor agonists in cardiovascular therapy. *Crit Care Med* 1990;18:S14–8.

175. Brogden RN, Markham A. Fenoldopam. *Drugs* 1997;54:634–50.

176. White WB, Halley SE. Comparative renal effects of intravenous administration of fenoldopam mesylate and sodium nitroprusside in patients with severe hypertension. *Arch Intern Med* 1989;149:870–4.

177. Allison NL et al. The effect of fenoldopam, a dopaminergic agonist, on renal hemodynamics. *Clin Pharmacol Ther* 1987;41:282–8.

178. Everitt DE et al. Effect of intravenous fenoldopam on intraocular pressure in ocular hypertension. *J Clin Pharmacol* 1997;37:312–20.

179. Pilmer BL et al. Fenoldopam mesylate versus sodium nitroprusside in the accute management of severe systemic hypertension. *J Clin Pharmacol* 1993;33:549–53.

180. Panacek EA et al. Randomized, prospective trial of fenoldopam vs sodium nitroprusside in the treatment of acute severe hypertension. *Acad Emerg Med* 1995;2:959–65.

181. Bednarczyk EM et al. Comparative acute blood pressure reduction from intravenous fenoldopam mesylate versus sodium nitroprusside in severe systemic hypertension. *Am J Cardiol* 1989;63:993–6.

182. Reisin E et al. Intravenous fenoldopam versus sodium nitroprusside in patients with severe hypertension. *Hypertension* 1990;15(suppl I):I-59–I-62.

183. Holmes B et al. Guanabenz: a review of its pharmacodynamic properties and therapeutic efficacy in hypertension. *Drugs* 1983;26:212–29.

184. Meacham RH et al. Disposition of ^{14}C gaunabenz in patients with essential hypertension. *Clin Pharmacol Ther* 1980;27:44–52.

185. Palmer JD, Nugent CA. Guanadrel sulfate: a postganglionic sympathetic inhibitor for the treatment of mild to moderate hypertension. *Pharmacotherapy* 1983;3:220–9.

186. Finnerty FA, Brogden RN. Guanadrel: a review of its pharmacodynamic and pharmacokinetic properties and therapeutic use in hypertension. *Drugs* 1985;30:22–31.

187. Oates JA. Antihypertensive agents and drug therapy of hypertension. In, Hardman JG et al., eds. *Goodman and Gilman's the pharmacological basis of therapeutics*. 9th ed. New York: McGraw-Hill 1996:780–808.

188. Walter IE et al. The relationship of plasma guanethidine levels to adrenergic blockade. *Clin Pharmacol Ther* 1975;18:571–80.

189. Hengstmann JH, Falkner FC. Disposition of guanethidine during chronic oral therapy. *Eur J Clin Pharmacol* 1979;15:121–5.

190. Jerie P. Clinical experience with guanfacine in long-term treatment of hypertension. Part I: efficacy and dosage. *Br J Clin Pharmacol* 1980;10:37S–47S.

191. Sorkin EM, Heel RC. Guanfacine: a review of its pharmacodynamic and pharmacokinetic properties, and therapeutic efficacy in the treatment of hypertension. *Drugs* 1986;31:301–36.

192. Mulrow JP, Crawford MH. Clinical pharmacokinetics and therapeutic use of hydralazine in congestive heart failure. *Clin Pharmacokinet* 1989;16:86–99.

193. O'Malley K et al. Duration of hydralazine action in hypertension. *Clin Pharmacol Ther* 1975;18:581–6.

194. Cameron HA, Ramsay LE. The lupus syndrome induced by hydralazine: a common complication with low-dose treatment. *Br Med J* 1984;289:410–2.

195. Shapiro KS et al. Immune complex glomerulonephritis in hydralazine-induced SLE. *Am J Kidney Dis* 1984;3:270–4.

196. Goa KL et al. Labetalol: a reappraisal of its pharmacology, pharmacokinetics and therapeutic use in hypertension and ischaemic heart disease. *Drugs* 1989;37:583–627.

197. MacCarthy EP, Bloomfield SS. Labetalol: a review of its pharmacology, pharmacokinetics, clinical uses and adverse effects. *Pharmacotherapy* 1983;3:193–219.

198. Bunchman TE et al. Intravenously administered labetalol for treatment of hypertension in children. *J Pediatr* 1992;120:140–4.

199. McNeil JJ, Louis WJ. Clinical pharmacokinetics of labetalol. *Clin Pharmacokinet* 1984;9:157–67.

200. Oliverio MI, Coffman TM. Angiotensin-II receptors: new targets for antihypertensive therapy. *Clin Cardiol* 1997;20:3–6.

201. Weber MA et al. Blood pressure effects of the angiotensin II receptor blocker, losartan. *Arch Intern Med* 1995;115:405–11.

202. Abdelwahab W et al. Management of hypertensive urgencies and emergencies. *J Clin Pharmacol* 1995;35:747–62.

203. Timmermans PBMWM et al. Angiotensin II receptors and angiotensin II receptor antagonists. *Pharmacol Rev* 1993;45:205–51.

204. Csajka C et al. Pharmacokinetic-pharmacodynamic profile of angiotensin II receptor antagonists. *Clin Pharmacokinet* 1997;32:1–29.

205. Gavras HP, Salerno CM. The angiotensin II type I receptor blocker losartan in clinical practice: a review. *Clin Ther* 1996;18:1058–67.

206. Ellis ML, Patterson JH. A new class of antihypertensive therapy: angiotensin II receptor antagonists. *Pharmacotherapy* 1996:16:849–60.

207. Benz J et al. Valsartan, a new angiotensin II receptor antagonist: a double-blind study comparing the incidence of cough with lisinopril and hydrochlorothiazide. *J Clin Pharmacol* 1997;37:101–7.

208. Lacourcière Y et al. Effects of modulators of the renin-angiotensin-aldosterone system on cough. *J Hypertens* 1994;12:1387–93.

209. Crozier I et al. Losartan in heart failure. Hemodynamic effects and tolerability. *Circulation* 1995;91:691–7.

210. Pitt B et al. Randomised trial of losartan versus captopril in patients over 65 with heart failure (Evaluation of Losartan in the Elderly Study, ELITE). *Lancet* 1997;349:747–52.

211. Myhre E et al. Clinical pharmacokinetics of methyldopa. *Clin Pharmacokinet* 1982;7:221–33.

212. Fleishaker JC et al. The pharmacokinetics of 2.5 to 10 mg oral doses of minoxidil in healthy volunteers. *J Clin Pharmacol* 1989;29:162–7.

213. Vesey CJ, Cole PV. Blood cyanide and thiocyanate concentrations produced by long-term therapy with sodium nitroprusside. *Br J Anaesth* 1985;57:148–55.

214. Schultz V et al. Kinetics of elimination of thiocyanate in 7 healthy subjects and in 8 subjects with renal failure. *Klin Wochenschr* 1979;57:243–7.

215. Cottrell JE et al. Prevention of nitroprusside induced cyanide toxicity with hydroxocobalamin. *N Engl J Med* 1978;298:809–11.

216. Pasch TH et al. Nitroprusside-induced formation of cyanide and its detoxification with thiosulphate during deliberate hypotension. *J Cardiovasc Pharmacol* 1983;5:77–82.

217. McAreavey D, Robertson JI. Angiotensin-converting enzyme inhibitors and moderate hypertension. *Drugs* 1990;40:326–45.

218. Frank GJ et al. Overview of quinapril, a new ACE inhibitor. *J Cardiovasc Pharmacol* 1990;15(suppl 2): S14–23.

219. Salvetti A. Newer ACE inhibitors: a look at the future. *Drugs* 1990;40:800–28.

220. Anon. Moexipril: another ACE inhibitor for hypertension. *Med Lett Drugs Ther* 1995;37:75–6.

221. Tenero D et al. Effect of hepatic disease on the pharmacokinetics and plasma protein binding of eprosartan. *Pharmacotherapy* 1998;18:42–50.

222. McClellan KJ, Balfour JA. Eprosartan. *Drugs* 1998;55:713–8.

223. Donnelly R et al. Pharmacokinetic-pharmacodynamic relationships of α-adrenoreceptor antagonists. *Clin Pharmacokinet* 1989;17:264–74.

224. Frishman WH et al. Terazosin: a new long-acting α₁-adrenergic antagonist for hypertension. *Med Clin North Am* 1988;72:441–8.

225. Stumpf JL. Drug therapy of hypertensive crises. *Clin Pharm* 1988;7:582–91.

226. Hirschl MM. Guidelines for the drug treatment of hypertensive crisis. *Drugs* 1995;50:991–1000.

227. Angaran DM et al. Esmolol hydrochloride: an ultrashort-acting β-adrenergic blocking agent. *Clin Pharm* 1986;5:288–303.

228. Cuneo BF et al. Pharmacodynamics and pharmacokinetics of esmolol, a short-acting β-blocking agent, in children. *Pediatr Cardiol* 1994;15:296–301.

229. Trippel DL et al. Cardiovascular and antiarrhythmic effects of esmolol in children. *J Pediatr* 1991;119(1,Pt 1):142–7.

230. Routledge PA, Shand DG. Clinical pharmacokinetics of propranolol. *Clin Pharmacokinet* 1979;4:73–90.

231. Nies AS, Shand DG. Clinical pharmacology of propranolol. *Circulation* 1975;52:6–15.

232. Johnsson G, Regardh CG. Clinical pharmacokinetics of β-adrenoreceptor blocking drugs. *Clin Pharmacokinet* 1976;1:233–63.

233. McTavish D et al. Carvedilol. A review of its pharmacodynamic and pharmacokinetic properties, and therapeutic efficacy. *Drugs* 1993;45:232–58.

234. Milne RJ, Buckley MM-T. Celiprolol. An updated review of its pharmacodynamic and pharmacokinetic properties, and therapeutic efficacy in cardiovascular disease. *Drugs* 1991;41:941–69.

235. MacCarthy EP, Bloomfield SS. Labetalol. A review of its pharmacology, pharmacokinetics, clinical uses and adverse effects. *Pharmacotherapy* 1983;3:193–219.

236. Ryan JR. Clinical pharmacology of acebutolol. *Am Heart J* 1985;109:1131–6.

237. Harron DWG et al. Bopindolol. A review of its pharmacodynamic and pharmacokinetic properties and therapeutic efficacy. *Drugs* 1991;41:130–49.

238. Frishman WH, Covey S. Penbutolol and carteolol: two new beta-adrenergic blockers with partial agonism. *J Clin Pharmacol* 1990;30:412–21.

239. Frishman WH et al. Bevantolol. A preliminary review of its pharmacodynamic and pharmacokinetic properties, and therapeutic efficacy in hypertension and angina pectoris. *Drugs* 1988;35:1–21.

240. Lancaster SG, Sorkin EM. Bisoprolol. A preliminary review of its pharmacodynamic and pharmacokinetic properties, therapeutic efficacy in hypertension and angina pectoris. *Drugs* 1988;36:256–85.

241. Petru MA et al. Long-term efficacy of high-dose diltiazem for chronic stable angina pectoris: 16-month serial studies with placebo controls. *Am Heart J* 1985;109:99–103.

242. Markham A, Brogden RN. Diltiazem. A review of its pharmacology and therapeutic use in older patients. *Drugs Aging* 1993;3:363–90.

243. Zelis RF, Kinney EL. The pharmacokinetics of diltiazem in healthy American men. *Am J Cardiol* 1982;49:529–32.

244. Joyal M et al. Pharmacodynamic aspects of intravenous diltiazem administration. *Am Heart J* 1986;111:54–60.

245. Smith MS et al. Pharmacokinetic and pharmacodynamic effects of diltiazem. *Am J Cardiol* 1983;51:1369–74.

246. Winship LC et al. The effect of ranitidine and cimetidine on single-dose diltiazem pharmacokinetics. *Pharmacotherapy* 1985;5:16–9.

247. McAllister RG. Kinetics and dynamics of nifedipine after oral sublingual doses. *Am J Med* 1986;81(suppl 6A):2–5.

248. Kleinbloesem CH et al. Nifedipine: kinetics and hemodynamic effects in patients with liver cirrhosis after intravenous and oral administration. *Clin Pharmacol Ther* 1986;40:21–8.

249. Sorkin EM et al. Nifedipine. A review of its pharmacodynamic and pharmacokinetic properties, and therapeutic efficacy, in ischemic heart disease, hypertension and related cardiovascular disorders. *Drugs* 1985;30:182–274.

250. Kleinbloesem CH et al. Nifedipine: kinetics and dynamics in healthy subjects. *Clin Pharmacol Ther* 1984;36:742–9.

251. Breimer DD et al. Nifedipine: variability in its kinetics and metabolism in man. *Pharmacol Ther* 1989;44:445–54.

252. Vetrovec GW et al. Comparative dosing and efficacy of continuous release nifedipine versus standard nifedipine for angina pectoris: clinical response, exercise performance and plasma nifedipine levels. *Am Heart J* 1988;115:793–8.

253. Opie LH. Calcium channel blockers for hypertension: dissecting the evidence for adverse effects. *Am J Hypertens* 1997;10(5 pt 1):565–77.

254. Diamond JR et al. Nifedipine-induced renal dysfunction. Alterations in renal hemodynamics. *Am J Med* 1984;77:905–9.

255. Elkayam U et al. A prospective, randomized, double-blind, crossover study to compare the efficacy and safety of chronic nifedipine therapy with that of isosorbide dinitrate and their combination in the treatment of chronic congestive heart failure. *Circulation* 1990;82:1954–61.

256. Dale J et al. The effects of nifedipine, a calcium antagonist, on platelet function. *Am Heart J* 1983;105:103–5.

257. Barbarash RA et al. Verapamil infusions in the treatment of atrial tachyarrhythmias. *Crit Care Med* 1986;14:886–8.

258. Schwartz JB et al. Prolongation of verapamil elimination kinetics during chronic oral administration. *Am Heart J* 1982;104:198–203.

259. Hamann SR et al. Clinical pharmacokinetics of verapamil. *Clin Pharmacokinet* 1984;9:26–41.

260. Hoon TJ et al. The pharmacodynamic and pharmacokinetic differences of the D- and L-isomers of verapamil: implications in the treatment of paroxysmal supraventricular tachycardia. *Am Heart J* 1986;112:396–403.

261. McTavish D, Sorkin EM. Verapamil. An updated review of its pharmacodynamic and pharmacokinetic properties, and therapeutic use in hypertension. *Drugs* 1989;38:19–76.

262. Singh BN et al. New perspectives in the pharmacologic therapy of cardiac arrhythmias. *Prog Cardiovasc Dis* 1980;22:243–301.

263. Schoen MD et al. Evaluation of the pharmacokinetics and electrocardiographic effects of intravenous verapamil with intravenous calcium chloride pretreatment in normal subjects. *Am J Cardiol* 1991;67:300–4.

264. Singh BN et al. Second generation calcium antagonists: search for greater selectivity and versatility. *Am J Cardiol* 1985;55:214B–21B.

265. Bays HE, Dujovne CA. Drugs for treatment of patients with high cholesterol blood levels and other dyslipidemias. *Prog Drug Res* 1994;43:9–41.

266. Larsen ML, Illingworth DR. Drug treatment of dyslipoproteinemia. *Med Clin North Am* 1994;78:225–45.

267. National Cholesterol Education Program. Report of the Expert Panel on Blood Cholesterol Levels in Children and Adolescents. *Pediatrics* 1992;89:S525–70.

268. Kwiterovich PO. Diagnosis and management of familial dyslipoproteinemia in children and adolescents. *Pediatr Clin North Am* 1990;37:1489–521.

269. Lipid Research Clinics Program. Lipid research clinics coronary primary prevention trial results. I. Reduction in incidence of coronary heart disease. *JAMA* 1984;251:351–64.

270. Newman TB, Hulley SB. Carcinogenicity of lipid-lowering drugs. *JAMA* 1996;275:55–60.

271. Smellie WAS, Lorimer AR. Adverse effects of the lipid-lowering drugs. *Adverse Drug React Toxicol Rev* 1992;11:71–92.

272. Ast M, Frishman WH. Bile acid sequestrants. *J Clin Pharmacol* 1990;30:99–106.

273. Farmer JA, Gotto AM Jr. Antihyperlipidaemic agents. Drug interactions of clinical significance. *Drug Saf* 1994;11:301–9.

274. Expert Panel on Detection, Evaluation and Treatment of High Blood Cholesterol in Adults. Summary of the second report of the National Cholesterol Education Program (NCEP) Expert Panel on Detection, Evaluation, and Treatment of High Blood Cholesterol in Adults (Adult Treatment Panel II). *JAMA* 1993;269:3015–23.

275. Andrade SE et al. Discontinuation rates of antihyperlipidemic drugs—do rates reported in clinical trials reflect rates in primary care settings? *N Engl J Med* 1995;332:1125–31.

276. Hilleman DE et al. Comparative cost-effectiveness of bile acid sequestering resins, HMG Co-A reductase inhibitors, and their combination in patients with hypercholesterolemia. *J Managed Care Pharm* 1995;1:188–92.

277. Bartlett JG. Antibiotic-associated diarrhea. *Clin Infect Dis* 1992;15:573–81.

278. Kelly CP et al. *Clostridium difficile* colitis. *N Engl J Med* 1994;330:257–62.

279. Jungnickel PW et al. Blind comparison of patient preference for flavored Colestid granules and Questran Light. *Ann Pharmacother* 1993;27:700–3.

280. Shaefer MS et al. Acceptability of cholestyramine or colestipol combinations with six vehicles. *Clin Pharm* 1987;6:51–4.

281. Shaefer MS et al. Sensory/mixability preference evaluation of cholestyramine powder formulations. *DICP* 1990;24:472–4.

282. Ito MK, Morreale AP. Acceptability of cholestyramine and colestipol formulations in three common vehicles. *Clin Pharm* 1991;10:138–40.

283. Insull W Jr et al. The effects of colestipol tablets compared with colestipol granules on plasma cholesterol and other lipids in moderately hypercholesterolemic patients. *Atherosclerosis* 1995;112:223–35.

284. Spence JD et al. Combination therapy with colestipol and psyllium mucilloid in patients with hyperlipidemia. *Ann Intern Med* 1995;123:493–9.

285. Superko HR et al. Effectiveness of low-dose colestipol therapy in patients with moderate hypercholesterolemia. *Am J Cardiol* 1992;70:135–40.

286. Balfour JA et al. Fenofibrate. *Drugs* 1990;40:260–90.

287. Adkins JC, Faulds D. Micronized fenofibrate. *Drugs* 1997;54:615–33.

288. Sheperd J. Mechanism of action of fibrates. *Postgrad Med J* 1993;69:S34–41.

289. Todd PA, Ward A. Gemfibrozil. A review of its pharmacodynamic and pharmacokinetic properties, and therapeutic use in dyslipidemia. *Drugs* 1988;36:314–39.

290. Evans JR et al. Effect of renal function on the pharmacokinetics of gemfibrozil. *J Clin Pharmacol* 1987;27:994–1000.

291. Shen D et al. Effect of gemfibrozil treatment in sulfonylurea-treated patients with noninsulin-dependent diabetes mellitus. *J Clin Endocrinol Metab* 1991;73:503–10.

292. Lozada A, Dujovne CA. Drug interactions with fibric acids. *Pharmacol Ther* 1994;63:163–76.

293. Frick MH et al. Helsinki heart study: primary prevention trial with gemfibrozil in middle-aged men with dyslipidemia. *N Engl J Med* 1987;317:1237–45.

294. Heinonen OP et al. Helsinki heart study: coronary heart disease incidence during an extended follow-up. *J Intern Med* 1994;235:41–9.

295. Frick MH et al. Efficacy of gemfibrozil in dyslipidaemic subjects with suspected heart disease. An ancillary study in the Helsinki heart study frame population. *Ann Med* 1993;25:41–5.

296. Furberg CD et al. Effect of lovastatin on early carotid atherosclerosis and cardiovascular events. *Circulation* 1994;90:1679–87.

297. Davignon J et al. HMG-CoA reductase inhibitors: a look back and a look ahead. *Can J Cardiol* 1992;8:843–64.

298. Hsu I et al. Comparative evaluation of the safety and efficacy of HMG-CoA reductase inhibitor monotherapy in the treatment of primary hypercholesterolemia. *Ann Pharmacother* 1995;29:743–59.

299. Henwood JM, Heel RC. Lovastatin. A preliminary review of its pharmacodynamic properties and therapeutic use in hyperlipidaemia. *Drugs* 1988;429–54.

300. McTavish D, Sorkin EM. Pravastatin. A review of its pharmacological properties and therapeutic potential in hypercholesterolemia. *Drugs* 1991;65–89.

301. Todd PA, Goa KL. Simvastatin. A review of its pharmacological properties and therapeutic potential in hypercholesterolemia. *Drugs* 1990;40:583–607.

302. Mauro VF, MacDonald JL. Simvastatin: a review of its pharmacology and clinical use. *DICP* 1991;25:257–64.

303. Jungnickel PW et al. Pravastatin: a new drug for the treatment of hypercholesterolemia. *Clin Pharm* 1992;11:677–89.

304. Canner PL et al. Fifteen year mortality in coronary drug project patients: long-term benefit with niacin. *J Am Coll Cardiol* 1986;8:1245–55.

305. Dalen JE, Dalton WS. Does lowering cholesterol cause cancer? *JAMA* 1996;275:67–9. Commentary.

306. Scandinavian Simvastatin Survival Study Group. Randomised trial of cholesterol lowering in 4444 patients with coronary artery disease: the Scandinavian Simvastatin Survival Study (4S). *Lancet* 1994;344:1383–9.

307. Blauw GJ et al. Stroke, statins, and cholesterol. A meta-analysis of randomized, placebo-controlled, double-blind trials with HMG-CoA reductase inhibitors. *Stroke* 1997;28:946–50.

308. Downs JR et al. Primary prevention of acute coronary events with lovastatin in men and women with average cholesterol levels. *JAMA* 1998;279:1615–22.

309. Figge HL et al. Nicotinic acid: a review of its clinical use in the treatment of lipid disorders. *Pharmacotherapy* 1988;8:287–94.

310. ASHP Therapeutic Position Statement on the safe use of niacin in the management of dyslipidemias. *Am J Health-Syst Pharm* 1997;54:2815–9.

311. Colletti RB et al. Niacin treatment of hypercholesterolemia in children. *Pediatrics* 1993;92:78–82.

312. Hunninghake DB. Diagnosis and treatment of lipid disorders. *Med Clin North Am* 1994;78:247–57.

313. McKenney JM et al. A comparison of the efficacy and toxic effects of sustained- vs immediate-release niacin in hypercholesterolemic patients. *JAMA* 1994;271:672–7.

314. Chong PH, Seeger JD. Atorvastatin calcium: an addition to HMG-CoA reductase inhibitors. *Pharmacotherapy* 1997;17:1157–77.

315. Anon. Cerivastatin for hypercholesterolemia. *Med Lett Drugs Ther* 1998;40:13–4.

316. Wynne J, Braunwald E. New treatment for congestive heart failure: amrinone and milrinone. *J Cardiovasc Med* 1984;9:393–405.

317. Lawless ST et al. The acute pharmacokinetics and pharmacodynamics of amrinone in pediatric patients. *J Clin Pharmacol* 1991;31:800–3.

318. Rocci ML, Wilson H. The pharmacokinetics and pharmacodynamics of newer inotropic agents. *Clin Pharmacokinet* 1987;13:91–109.

319. Edelson J et al. Relationship between amrinone plasma concentration and cardiac index. *Clin Pharmacol Ther* 1981;29:723–8.

320. Ross MP et al. Amrinone-associated thrombocytopenia: pharmacokinetic analysis. *Clin Pharmacol Ther* 1993;53:661–7.

321. Dunkman WB et al. Adverse effects of long-term amrinone administration in congestive heart failure. *Am Heart J* 1983;105:861–3.

322. Packer M et al. Hemodynamic and clinical limitations of long-term inotropic therapy with amrinone in patients with severe chronic heart failure. *Circulation* 1984;70:1038–47.

323. Zaritsky AL. Catecholamines, inotropic medications, and vasopressor agents. In, Chernow B et al., eds. *The pharmacologic approach to the critically ill patient.* 3rd ed. Baltimore: Williams & Wilkins; 1994;387–404.

324. Kulka PJ, Tryba M. Inotropic support of the critically ill patient. A review of the agents. *Drugs* 1993;45:654–67.

325. Trujillo MH, Bellorin-Font E. Drugs commonly administered by intravenous infusion in intensive care units: a practical guide. *Crit Care Med* 1990;18:232–8.

326. American College of Cardiology, American Heart Association Task Force. Adult advanced cardiac life support. *JAMA* 1992;268:2199–241.

327. American College of Cardiology, American Heart Association Task Force. Pediatric advanced life support. *JAMA* 1992;268:2262–75.

328. Bhatt-Mehta V, Nahata MC. Dopamine and dobutamine in pediatric therapy. *Pharmacotherapy* 1989;9:303–14.

329. Murphy MB, Elliott WJ. Dopamine and dopamine receptor agonists in cardiovascular therapy. *Crit Care Med* 1990;18:S14–8.

330. Geraci SA. Pharmacologic approach in patients with heart failure. In, Chernow B et al., eds. *The pharmacologic approach to the critically ill patient.* 3rd ed. Baltimore: Williams & Wilkins; 1994:80–94.

331. Jarnberg P-O et al. Dopamine infusion in man. Plasma catecholamine levels and pharmacokinetics. *Acta Anaesthesiol Scand* 1981;25:328–31.

332. Cedarbaum JM, Schleifer LS. Drugs for Parkinson's disease, spacticity, and acute muscle spasms. In, Gilman AG et al., eds. *Goodman and Gilman's the pharmacological basis of therapeutics.* 8th ed. New York: Pergamon Press; 1990:463–84.

333. Hoffman BB, Lefkowitz RJ. Catecholamines and sympathomimetic drugs. In, Gilman AG et al., eds. *Goodman and Gilman's the pharmacological basis of therapeutics.* 8th ed. New York: Pergamon Press; 1990:187–220.

334. Skolnik NS. Treatment of croup. A critical review. *Am J Dis Child* 1989;143:1045–9.

335. Waisman Y et al. Prospective randomized double-blind study comparing L-epinephrine and racemic epinephrine aerosols in the treatment of laryngotracheitis (croup). *Pediatrics* 1992;89:302–6.

336. Zaritsky A, Chernow B. Use of catecholomines in pediatrics. *J Pediatr* 1984;105:341–50.

337. Tashkin DP, Jenne JW. Alpha and beta adrenergic agonists. In, Weiss EB et al., eds. *Bronchial asthma: mechanisms and therapeutics.* 2nd ed. Boston: Little, Brown; 1985:604–39.

338. Cydulka R et al. The use of epinephrine in the treatment of older adult asthmatics. *Ann Emerg Med* 1988;17:322–6.

339. Kelly HW. New β₂-adrenergic agonist aerosols. *Clin Pharm* 1985;4:393–403.

340. Edelson J et al. Pharmacokinetics of the bipyridines amrinone and milrinone. *Circulation* 1986;73(suppl III):145-III–52-III.

341. Young RA, Ward A. Milrinone. A preliminary review of its pharmacological properties and therapeutic use. *Drugs* 1988;36:158–92.

342. Martin C et al. Norepinephrine or dopamine for the treatment of hyperdynamic septic shock? *Chest* 1993;103:1826–31.

343. Notterman DA. Pediatric pharmacotherapy. In, Chernow B et al., eds. *The pharmacologic approach to the critically ill patient.* 3rd ed. Baltimore: Williams & Wilkins; 1994:139–55.

344. Neugebauer E et al. Pharmacotherapy of shock. In, Chernow B et al., eds. *The pharmacologic approach to the critically ill patient.* 3rd ed. Baltimore: Williams & Wilkins; 1994:1104–21.

345. Rackow EC, Astiz ME. Mechanisms and management of septic shock. *Crit Care Clin* 1993;9(2):219–37.

346. Zaloga GP et al. Pharmacologic cardiovascular support. *Crit Care Clin* 1993;9:335–62.

347. Abrams J. Nitroglycerin and long-acting nitrates. P&T 1992;59–64, 67–9.

348. Parker JO. Nitrate therapy in stable angina pectoris. *N Engl J Med* 1987;316:1635–42.

349. Elkayam U. Tolerance to organic nitrates: evidence, mechanisms, clinical relevance, and strategies for prevention. *Ann Intern Med* 1991;114:667–77.

350. Cannon LA, Marshall JM. Cardiac disease in the elderly population. *Clin Geriatr Med* 1993;9:499–525.

351. Thadani U, Opie LH. Nitrates. In, Opie LH ed. *Drugs for the heart.* 4th ed. Philadelphia: WB Saunders; 1995:31–48.

352. Sporl-Radun S et al. Effects and pharmacokinetics of isosorbide dinitrate in normal man. *Eur J Clin Pharmacol* 1980;18:237–44.

353. Abshagen WWP et al. Pharmacokinetics of intravenous and oral isosorbide-5-mononitrate. *Eur J Clin Pharmacol* 1981;20:269–75.

354. Frishman WH et al. Mononitrates: defining the ideal long-acting nitrate. *Clin Ther* 1994;16:130–9.

355. Abshagen WWP. Pharmacokinetics of isosorbide mononitrate. *Am J Cardiol* 1992;70:61G–6G.

356. Fung H-L. Clinical pharmacology of organic nitrates. *Am J Cardiol* 1993;72:9C–15C.

357. Fletcher A. Transdermal nitroglycerin. Does it really work in the treatment of angina? *Drugs Aging* 1991;1:6–16.

358. Friedman WF, George BL. New concepts and drugs in the treatment of congestive heart failure. *Pediatr Clin North Am* 1984;31:1197–226.

359. Anon. Nitroglycerin patches—do they work? *Med Lett Drugs Ther* 1989;31:65–6.

360. Abrams J. Pharmacology of nitroglycerin and long-acting nitrates and their usefulness in the treatment of chronic congestive heart failure. In, Gould L, Reddy CVR, eds. *Vasodilator therapy for cardiac disorders.* Mount Kisco, NY: Futura Publishing; 1979:129–67.

361. Schrader BJ et al. Acceptance of transcutaneous nitroglycerin patches by patients with angina pectoris. *Pharmacotherapy* 1986;6:83–6.

362. DeMots H, Glasser SPP. Intermittent transdermal nitroglycerin therapy in the treatment of chronic stable angina. *J Am Coll Cardiol* 1989;13:786–93.

363. Baaske DM et al. Nitroglycerin compatibility with intravenous fluid filters, containers, and administration sets. *Am J Hosp Pharm* 1980;37:201–5.

364. Amann AH et al. Plastic I.V. container for nitroglycerin. *Am J Hosp Pharm* 1980;37:618. Letter.

365. Haas CE et al. Effect of using a standard polyvinyl chloride intravenous infusion set on patient response to nitroglycerin. *Am J Hosp Pharm* 1992;49:1135–7.

366. Altavela JL et al. Clinical response to intravenous nitroglycerin infused through polyethylene or polyvinyl chloride tubing. *Am J Hosp Pharm* 1994;51:490–4.

367. Mulrow CD et al. Relative efficacy of vasodilator therapy in chronic congestive heart failure. Implications of randomized trials. *JAMA* 1988;259:3422–6.

368. Chaterjee K et al. Vasodilator therapy in chronic congestive heart failure. *Am J Cardiol* 1988;62:46A–54A.

369. Cohn JN et al. A comparison of enalapril with hydralazine-isosorbide dinitrate in the treatment of chronic congestive heart failure. *N Engl J Med* 1991;325:303–10.

370. Parillo JE. Vasodilator therapy. In, Chernow B et al., eds. *The pharmacological approach to the critically ill patient.* 3rd ed. Baltimore: Williams & Wilkins; 1994:470–83.

371. Johnson JA, Lalonde Rl. Congestive heart failure. In, DiPiro JT et al., eds. *Pharmacotherapy: a pathophysiologic approach.* 2nd ed. East Norwalk, CT: Appleton & Lange; 1993:160–93.

Central Nervous System Drugs

Anticonvulsants

Class Instructions: Anticonvulsants. It is important to take this medication as prescribed to control seizures; stopping it suddenly may cause an increase in seizures. This medication may cause drowsiness. Until the extent of this effect is known, use caution when driving, operating machinery, or performing other tasks requiring mental alertness. Avoid concurrent use of alcohol or other drugs that cause drowsiness. Report unusual or bothersome side effects. Always use an effective contraceptive; contact your physician if you plan to become or become pregnant.

CARBAMAZEPINE   Carbatrol, Tegretol, Various

Pharmacology. Carbamazepine is an iminostilbene compound related structurally to the tricyclic antidepressants. In animals, carbamazepine acts presynaptically to block firing of action potentials, which decreases the release of excitatory neurotransmitters, and postsynaptically by blocking high-frequency repetitive discharge initiated at cell bodies.

Administration and Adult Dosage. **PO for epilepsy** 100–200 mg bid with meals initially, increase in increments of up to 200 mg/day at weekly intervals to effective dosage. **Usual maintenance dosage** is 10–30 mg/kg/day or 600–1600 mg/day in 2–4 divided, doses;[1,2] tid or qid administration is recommended when enzyme-inducing antiepileptic drugs are administered concurrently. **SR** product may be given bid. **PO for trigeminal neuralgia** 100 mg bid initially, increasing in 200 mg/day increments until relief of pain, to a maximum of 1.2 g/day. **Usual maintenance dosage** is 400–800 mg/day in 2–3 divided doses. **PO loading dose** 8 mg/kg in a single dose achieves therapeutic levels in 2 hr (with suspension) or 5 hr (with tablets) and is well tolerated. **Rectal administration** has been reported. (*See* Fate.)

Special Populations. *Pediatric Dosage.* **PO for epilepsy** (<6 yr) (10–20 mg/kg/day in 3–4 divided doses with the chewable tablets or in 4 divided doses with the suspension; (6–12 yr) 10–20 mg/kg/day with meals initially, increasing weekly in 100 mg/day increments as needed to achieve optimal clinical response. **Usual maintenance dosage** is 15–35 mg/kg/day or 400–800 mg/day in 3–4 divided doses. (>12 yr) same as adult dosage.[2]

Geriatric Dosage. Clearance of carbamazepine is reduced in some elderly patients; therefore, a lower maintenance dosage may be required.[3]

Other Conditions. During pregnancy, increases in carbamazepine clearance may occur; dosage increases guided by serum levels and patient status may be necessary.[2]

Dosage Forms. **Chew Tab** 100 mg; **Susp** 20 mg/mL; **Tab** 200 mg; **SR Cap** 200, 300 mg (Carbatrol); **SR Tab** 100, 200, 400 mg (Tegretol XR).

Patient Instructions. (*See* Anticonvulsants Class Instructions.) Sore throat, fever, mouth ulcers, or easy bruising may be an early sign of a severe, but rare, blood disorder and should be reported immediately.

Missed Doses. Take this drug at regular intervals. If you miss a dose, take it as soon as you remember. If it is about time for the next dose, take that dose only. Do not double the dose or take extra. If you miss more than one dose in a day, call your physician.

Pharmacokinetics. *Onset and Duration.* Steady-state serum levels are attained within 2–4 days and may subsequently decline because of autoinduction of metabolism.[2] (*See* Fate.)

Serum Levels. (Anticonvulsant) 4–12 mg/L (17–50 μmol/L). Variability exists in the relationship between serum levels and CNS side effects. (*See* Notes.)

Fate. Absorption from tablets is slow and erratic, with a bioavailability of 75–85%; peak serum levels occur 4–8 hr after a dose of immediate-release product and 19 ± 7 hr after a dose of SR product.[2] Absorption is rapid with the suspension, with a peak serum level of 7.9 ± 1.9 mg/L at 1.6 ± 1.3 hr in the fasting state or 3.4 ± 3.4 hr with concomitant enteral tube feeding after a 500 mg oral dose.[4] A peak serum level of 5.1 ± 1.6 mg/L occurs 6.3 ± 1.5 hr after rectal administration of 6 mg/kg oral suspension (100 mg/5 mL) diluted with an equal volume of water.[5] The drug is 75–78% plasma protein bound.[2,6] V_d is 0.88 ± 0.06 L/kg in adults[4] and 1.2 ± 0.2 L/kg in children.[7] Large differences in Cl occur because of autoinduction of liver enzymes; autoinduction is completed within 1–2 weeks of monotherapy; Cl is 0.052 ± 0.04 L/hr/kg at end of week 1, 0.04 ± 0.02 L/hr/kg at week 2, and 0.054 ± 0.04 L/hr/kg at week 4.[8] Carbamazepine is metabolized to pharmacologically active carbamazepine-10,11-epoxide; the epoxide metabolite (CBZ-E) serum level ratio at steady state is 0.19 ± 0.06 at a carbamazepine level of 6.9 ± 1.5 mg/L and 0.28 ± 1.4 at a carbamazepine level of 10.5 ± 2.6 mg/L.[9] (*See* Notes.) Only about 2% of drug is excreted unchanged in the urine.[2,6]

$t_{\frac{1}{2}}$. There are large interindividual differences because of autoinduction of liver enzymes. (Adults) 31.3 ± 5.9 hr after a single dose,[4] 14.5 ± 5.3 hr after 2 months;[9] (children) 29.4 ± 3.6 hr after a single dose, 15.2 ± 5.2 hr after 5 months.[7]

Adverse Reactions. Dizziness, drowsiness, headache, diplopia, nausea, and vomiting occur frequently with initiation of therapy and are minimized by slow titration of dosage. Mild, transient, morbilliform rash and thrombocytopenia also occur frequently. Occasionally, confusion, stomatitis, or rash occur. Hyponatremia and water intoxication occur, and risk factors include carbamazepine monotherapy, elevated serum levels, patient age >25 yr, vomiting, or diarrhea.[2] Transient leukopenia has been observed in 10–20% of patients; persistent leukopenia occurs in 2% of patients.[2] Discontinue drug if leukopenia (absolute neutrophil count less than 1500/μL) persists or any evidence of bone marrow depression develops. Rare effects include aplastic anemia, agranulocytosis, hepatitis, lenticular opacities, and arrhythmias.

Contraindications. History of bone marrow depression; hypersensitivity to tricyclic antidepressants.

Precautions. Pregnancy; history of liver disease. Abrupt withdrawal of the drug in patients with epilepsy may precipitate status epilepticus. Exacerbation of atypical absence seizures may occur in children receiving carbamazepine for mixed seizure disorders.[2] Use carbamazepine cautiously in patients with a history of severe hypersensitivity reactions to phenytoin or phenobarbital.

Drug Interactions. Because of structural similarities to tricyclic antidepressants, discontinue MAOIs for a minimum of 14 days before carbamazepine is begun. Carbamazepine can stimulate the metabolism of many drugs metabolized by CYP3A4, including oral anticoagulants, oral contraceptives, corticosteroids, cyclosporine, doxycycline, haloperidol, heterocyclic antidepressants, and theophylline. Many drugs inhibit carbamazepine metabolism, including cimetidine, clarithromycin, danazol, erythromycin, fluoxetine, isoniazid, propoxyphene, quinine, troleandomycin, verapamil, and diltiazem.

Parameters to Monitor. Baseline CBC and platelet counts; monitor more frequently if a decrease in WBC or platelet counts occurs. Monitor liver function tests periodically during long-term therapy. Monitor serum levels at least weekly during the first month of therapy because of autoinduction. Periodic serum level monitoring is useful in evaluating therapeutic efficacy or potential for adverse effects.[2]

Notes. The contribution of the carbamazepine-10,11-epoxide (CBZ-E) metabolite to the therapeutic or adverse effects of carbamazepine (CBZ) is uncertain. In one study, there was no significant correlation between toxicity score or seizure frequency and serum levels of CBZ, CBZ-E, or their sum in patients receiving CBZ monotherapy, or combination therapy with phenytoin or valproic acid.[9] (*See* Anticonvulsants Comparison Chart.) **Oxcarbazepine** (Trileptal), the 10-keto analogue of CBZ, is an investigational anticonvulsant.

CLONAZEPAM   Klonopin

Pharmacology. Clonazepam is a benzodiazepine anticonvulsant that limits the spread of seizure activity, possibly by enhancing the postsynaptic effect of the inhibitory neurotransmitter, γ-aminobutyric acid (GABA).

Administration and Adult Dosage. **PO for epilepsy** initial dosage should not exceed 0.5 mg tid; increase in 0.5–1 mg/day increments q 3 days to effective dosage, or to a maximum of 20 mg/day. **Usual maintenance dosage** is 4–8 mg/day.[1] **PO for panic disorder** 0.25 mg bid initially, increasing to 1 mg/day after 3 days. **Usual maintenance dosage** is 1 mg/day; some patients require up to 4 mg/day. (*See* Notes.) **Rectal administration** has been reported. (*See* Fate.)

Special Populations. *Pediatric Dosage.* **PO for epilepsy** (≤10 yr or ≤30 kg) 0.01–0.03 mg/kg/day initially in 2–3 divided doses, increase in 0.25–0.5 mg/day increments q 3 days to effective dosage, to a maximum of 0.2 mg/kg/day in 3 divided doses. Rectal administration has been reported. (*See* Fate.)

Geriatric Dosage. **PO for epilepsy and as an antipanic agent** same as adult dosage initially. **Maintenance dosage** requirements may be lower in elderly patients because of reduced drug clearance and enhanced pharmacodynamic response.[10]

Dosage Forms. **Tab** 0.5, 1, 2 mg.

Patient Instructions. (*See* Anticonvulsants Class Instructions.)

Missed Doses. Take this drug at regular intervals. If you miss a dose take it as soon as you remember. If it is about time for the next dose, take that dose only. Do not double the dose or take extra.

Pharmacokinetics. *Onset and Duration.* Steady-state serum levels are attained in 4–8 days.[2] (*See* Notes.)

Serum Levels. 13–72 μg/L (40–230 nmol/L); however, some patients controlled with clonazepam may have levels below this range. There is a poor correlation between serum levels and efficacy or adverse effects.[2]

Fate. Rapidly absorbed orally; peak serum levels occur 1–3 hr after a dose. Serum levels of 18–40 μg/L occur 20–120 min following rectal administration of a 0.1 mg/kg dose of clonazepam suspension.[11] The drug is 86 ± 0.5% plasma protein bound;[2] V_d is 3.1 ± 1.2 L/kg; Cl is 0.059 ± 0.011 L/hr/kg.[12] The principal metabolite, 7-aminoclonazepam, is inactive. Less than 0.5% of clonazepam is excreted unchanged in urine.[2]

$t_{1/2}$. 34.1 ± 7.5 hr.[12]

Adverse Reactions. Drowsiness, ataxia, behavior disturbances, and personality changes (hyperactivity, restlessness, irritability; especially in children) occur frequently and require dosage reduction.[2] Occasionally, hypersalivation and bronchial hypersecretion occur and may cause respiratory difficulties. Rarely, anemia, leukopenia, thrombocytopenia, and respiratory depression occur. Nearly 50% of patients receiving long-term clonazepam may experience transient exacerbations of seizures, dysphoria, restlessness, or autonomic signs during clonazepam withdrawal.[13] An increased seizure frequency and status epilepticus occur rarely, possibly associated with supratherapeutic serum levels.[2]

Contraindications. Severe liver disease; acute narrow-angle glaucoma.

Precautions. Pregnancy; lactation; patients with chronic respiratory disease. May increase frequency of generalized tonic-clonic seizures in patients with mixed seizure types. Abrupt withdrawal of the drug in patients with epilepsy may precipitate status epilepticus. Absence status has been reported in patients receiving valproic acid concurrently.

Drug Interactions. Concurrent use with other CNS depressants may potentiate the sedation caused by clonazepam.

Parameters to Monitor. Periodic serum level monitoring is of limited value. Close attention to changes in patient's seizure frequency is necessary to monitor for the development of tolerance to the therapeutic effect. (*See* Notes.)

Notes. Tolerance to the anticonvulsant effect of clonazepam occurs in approximately one-third of patients within 3–6 months of starting the drug. Taper and discontinue clonazepam if therapeutic benefit cannot be demonstrated. Because of prominent CNS adverse effects and the development of tolerance, it is considered an alternative to **valproic acid** for myoclonic seizures and an alternative to **ethosuximide** or valproic acid for absence seizures.[16] (*See* Anticonvulsants Comparison Chart.) Clonazepam has also become an alternative to **alprazolam** for treatment of panic disorder. For patients who experience interdose symptom recurrence or morning rebound with alprazolam, clonazepam offers an equally effective alternative with the benefit of a longer duration of effect. When switching a patient from alprazolam to clonazepam, an equivalent dosage of clonazepam is one-half that of alprazolam.[14–16]

ETHOSUXIMIDE   Zarontin

Pharmacology. Ethosuximide is a succinimide that produces an anticonvulsant effect by direct modification of membrane function in excitable cells and/or alteration of inhibitory neurotransmitters. In humans, it suppresses three cycle per second spike and wave activity. (*See* Notes.)

Administration and Adult Dosage. PO for epilepsy 250 mg bid initially; increase in 250 mg/day increments at 4- to 7-day intervals to an effective dosage, to a maximum of 1.5 g/day. **Usual maintenance dosage** 750–1250 mg/day in 1–2 doses.[1,2]

Special Populations. *Pediatric Dosage.* PO for epilepsy (3–6 yr) 250 mg/day initially; increase in 250 mg/day increments q 4–7 days to effective dosage, to a maximum of 1 g/day. **Usual maintenance dosage** 20–40 mg/kg/day in 1–2 doses.[1,2] (>6 yr) same as adult dosage.

Geriatric Doses. Same as adult dosage.

Dosage Forms. **Cap** 250 mg; **Syrup** 50 mg/mL.

Patient Instructions. (*See* Anticonvulsants Class Instructions.) This drug may be taken with food or milk to minimize stomach upset.

Missed Doses. Take this drug at regular intervals. If you miss a dose take it as soon as you remember. If it is about time for the next dose, take that dose only. Do not double the dose or take extra.

Pharmacokinetics. *Onset and Duration.* Steady-state serum levels are attained in 7–12 days.[2]

Serum Levels. 40–100 mg/L (280–710 μmol/L).[2]

Fate. The drug is well absorbed orally, with peak serum level in 3–7 hr in adults and children. Plasma protein binding is less than 10%. V_d is 0.69 L/kg;[17] Cl is 0.01 ± 0.04 L/hr/kg, greater in children.[2] Ethosuximide is metabolized to three inactive metabolites. About 20% of drug is excreted unchanged in the urine.[2,6]

$t_{\frac{1}{2}}$. (Adults) 52.6 hr;[18] (children) 31.6 ± 5.4 hr.[17]

Adverse Reactions. Nausea, vomiting, drowsiness, headache, hiccups, and dizziness occur frequently during initiation of therapy and usually are dose related. Occasionally, behavior changes or rashes occur. Rarely, SLE, leukopenia, aplastic anemia, or Stevens-Johnson syndrome occur.

Precautions. Pregnancy; patients with known liver or renal disease. Generalized tonic-clonic seizures may occur in patients with mixed seizure types who are treated with ethosuximide alone. Abrupt withdrawal of the drug may precipitate absence status epilepticus.

Contraindications. None known.

Drug Interactions. Ethosuximide may increase phenytoin serum levels and decrease levels of primidone (and its phenobarbital metabolite).

Parameters to Monitor. Periodic serum level monitoring, after attaining steady state (7–12 days), is useful in evaluating therapeutic efficacy or potential adverse effects.[2] Periodically monitor CBC, urinalysis, and liver function tests.

Notes. Ethosuximide is only indicated for treatment of absence seizures. Because of the drug's low potential for serious or long-term toxicity and its proven efficacy, it is considered the drug of choice for absence seizures. (*See* Anticonvulsants Comparison Chart.)

FELBAMATE   Felbatol

Pharmacology. Felbamate is a dicarbamate structurally related to meprobamate; its mechanism of action is not known, but may involve inhibition of N-methyl-D-aspartate responses and potentiation of γ-aminobutyric acid-a ($GABA_a$) receptor chloride currents.[19]

Administration and Adult Dosage. **PO for epilepsy** 1.2 g/day initially in 3–4 divided doses while reducing the dosage of concomitant antiepileptic drugs (phenytoin, carbamazepine, valproic acid, or phenobarbital) by 20–30%. Increase in 1200 mg/day increments at weekly intervals to a maximum of 3.6 g/day. Further reduction in the dosage of concomitant antiepileptic drugs may be required during felbamate titration.

Special Populations. *Pediatric Dosage.* **PO for epilepsy** 15 mg/kg/day initially in 3–4 divided doses while reducing the dosage of concomitant antiepileptic drugs (phenytoin, carbamazepine, valproic acid, or phenobarbital) by 20–30%. Increase in 15 mg/kg/day increments at weekly intervals to a maximum of 45 mg/kg/day. Further reduction in the dosage of concomitant antiepileptic drugs may be required during felbamate titration.

Geriatric Dosage. Dosage reduction may be required in patients with reduced hepatic or renal function and should be guided by clinical response.

Dosage Forms. **Tab** 400, 600 mg; **Susp** 120 mg/mL.

Patient Instructions. (*See* Anticonvulsants Class Instructions.) Felbamate has been associated with severe blood and liver disorders that can be fatal. Report signs of infection, bleeding, easy bruising, or signs of anemia (fatigue, weakness) immediately; also report abdominal pain or yellowing of the skin immediately. Give the patient the information/consent section of the Felbatol prescribing information and obtain informed consent at the time of initial prescribing.

Missed Doses. Take this drug at regular intervals. If you miss a dose take it as soon as you remember. If it is about time for the next dose, take that dose only. Do not double the dose or take extra.

Pharmacokinetics. *Onset and Duration.* Steady-state serum levels are attained in 2–3 days.[2]

Serum Levels. A therapeutic range has not been established. Serum concentrations reported in clinical studies range from 20–137 mg/L.[20,21]

Fate. Rapidly absorbed with over 90% bioavailability; peak serum levels occur 1–4 hr after an oral dose.[22] Food and antacids have no appreciable effect on absorption.[2] The drug is 22–25% plasma protein bound, primarily to albumin. V_d is 0.76 ± 0.08 L/kg; Cl is 0.030 ± 0.008 L/hr/kg in adults. From 40–50% is excreted unchanged in urine; 5% is excreted unchanged in feces; the remainder is excreted as inactive metabolites.[2]

$t_{1/2}$. 20.2 hr in normal volunteers;[22] 14.7 ± 2.8 hr in epileptic patients on concomitant enzyme-inducing antiepileptic drugs.[23]

Adverse Reactions. Anorexia, vomiting, insomnia, nausea, headache, weight loss, dizziness, and somnolence occur frequently. Adverse reaction frequency is lower when felbamate is used as monotherapy, and reactions often resolve during long-term therapy. Adverse reactions during adjunctive therapy may be the result of drug interactions. Felbamate is occasionally associated with aplastic anemia and hepatic failure (*see* Precautions), with fatality rates of 20–30%. It is not known whether the risks of aplastic anemia and hepatic failure are related to the duration of felbamate exposure.[24]

Contraindications. History of any blood dyscrasia or hepatic dysfunction.

Precautions. Do not use felbamate as a first-line antiepileptic drug. Because of the risk of aplastic anemia and hepatic failure, use felbamate only in patients whose seizures cannot be controlled with other antiepileptic drugs and in patients whose epilepsy is so severe that the risks are deemed acceptable. Fully inform patients of the risks of felbamate therapy. (*See* Patient Instructions.)

Drug Interactions. Felbamate increases serum concentrations of phenytoin, carbamazepine epoxide (the active metabolite of carbamazepine), and valproate; therefore, reduce the dosage of these antiepileptics by 20–30% when felbamate is initiated.

Parameters to Monitor. Close monitoring of CBC, platelets, liver function tests, and clinical signs or symptoms of infection, bruising, bleeding, or hepatitis is essential. Monitor liver function tests (AST, ALT, bilirubin) q 1–2 weeks while treatment continues. The acceptable frequency of hematologic monitoring is not established. Routine monitoring of serum levels is of limited value because of the lack of a well-defined therapeutic range.

Notes. Felbamate is effective for the treatment of partial and secondarily generalized seizures in adults and for partial and generalized seizures associated with the Lennox-Gastaut syndrome in children.

FOSPHENYTOIN   Cerebyx

Pharmacology. Fosphenytoin is a phosphate ester prodrug that is rapidly and completely converted to phenytoin in vivo by phosphatases after parenteral administration Fosphenytoin has no pharmacologic activity prior to its conversion to phenytoin. (*See* Phenytoin.)

Administration and Adult Dosage. **IV loading dose** 15–20 mg phenytoin equivalents (PE)/kg at a maximum rate of 150 mg PE/min. **IM loading dose** 10–20 mg PE/kg in 1 or more injection sites. **IV or IM maintenance dosage** 4–6 mg PE/kg/day in 1 or 2 divided doses. Safety and effectiveness have not been established for therapy lasting more than 5 days. **IV or IM substitution for oral phenytoin therapy** use same total daily dosage in PEs.

Special Populations. *Pediatric Dosage.* Safety and efficacy not established.

Geriatric Dosage. Advanced age has no effect on fosphenytoin pharmacokinetics. However, phenytoin clearance and protein binding may be reduced. (*See* Phenytoin.)

Other Conditions. In patients with renal or hepatic disease, fosphenytoin conversion to phenytoin may be increased because of protein binding changes.[25] Because of an increased fraction of unbound phenytoin in patients with renal or hepatic diseases or hypoalbuminemia, dosage adjustments should be guided by patient status and measurement of unbound phenytoin concentrations.

Dosage Forms. **Inj** 50 mg PE/mL.

Patient Instructions. Itching or tingling may occur during intravenous infusion, particularly in the facial and groin areas. These sensations are usually mild and disappear within minutes of stopping the infusion. These symptoms do not indicate an allergic reaction to either fosphenytoin or phenytoin.

Pharmacokinetics. *Onset and Duration.* Therapeutic concentrations of unbound phenytoin (≥ 1 μg/mL) are attained within 8–10 min after the start of an IV infusion of fosphenytoin (administered at a rate of 100–150 mg PE/min) and are similar to those attained after an equivalent dose of phenytoin administered at 50 mg/min. Therapeutic concentrations of unbound phenytoin are attained within 30 min after IM injection of fosphenytoin.

Serum Levels. Fosphenytoin serum concentration monitoring is not clinically useful. Phenytoin serum concentrations correlate with efficacy and toxicity. (*See* Phenytoin.)

Fate. Fosphenytoin is completely converted to phenytoin by phosphatases. Peak free phenytoin concentrations occur 30 min after completion of fosphenytoin infusion administered at rates of 100–150 mg PE/min and occur 3 hr after an IM dose of fosphenytoin. (*See* Onset and Duration.) Fosphenytoin is 95–99% bound to plasma proteins, primarily albumin. Fosphenytoin binding is saturable and V_d of fosphenytoin ranges from 4.3–10.8 L depending upon plasma concentration. Fosphenytoin displaces phenytoin from protein binding sites. The free (unbound) fraction of phenytoin ranges from 0.30 (in the presence of fosphenytoin) to 0.12 (after complete conversion of fosphenytoin to phenytoin).[26,27] (*See* Phenytoin.)

$t_{1/2}$. (Conversion to phenytoin) 15 min.

Adverse Reactions. Fosphenytoin commonly causes burning, itching, or paresthesias during IV infusion, particularly in the groin and facial areas. These symptoms usually disappear within minutes and can be minimized by slowing or stopping the infusion. The frequency and severity of these symptoms increase with fosphenytoin dose and infusion rate and may be related to the phosphate load. Venous irritation including pain, erythema, swelling, tenderness, and cording (hardening of the vessel) occurs less often than with phenytoin.[28] IM fosphenytoin injections are well tolerated and no significant differences in local symptoms were reported when compared with IM saline injections.[29] No significant differences between fosphenytoin and phenytoin have been reported with regard to adverse cardiovascular effects with IV infusion. CNS adverse effects are common and likely represent reactions to phenytoin. (*See* Phenytoin.)

Contraindications. Sinus bradycardia; sino-atrial block; second- and third-degree AV block; Adams-Stokes syndrome.

Precautions. The phosphate load of fosphenytoin (0.0037 mmol phosphate/mg PE fosphenytoin) should be considered in patients with renal insufficiency and those requiring phosphate restriction. (*See* Phenytoin.)

Drug Interactions. No drugs are known to affect the conversion of fosphenytoin to phenytoin. (*See* Phenytoin.)

Parameters to Monitor. Common immunoassays (eg, TDx, TDx/FLx) overestimate phenytoin concentrations when fosphenytoin is present. Determine serum phenytoin concentrations no earlier than 2 hr after an IV infusion or 4 hr after an IM dose of fosphenytoin. Obtain samples in EDTA-containing tubes to minimize the ex vivo conversion of fosphenytoin to phenytoin. Monitor BP and ECG during and 1–2 hr after IV fosphenytoin infusion.

Notes. Unlike parenteral phenytoin, fosphenytoin is not formulated with propylene glycol and is compatible with most common IV solutions (including those containing dextrose). Fosphenytoin, either undiluted or admixed in NS or D5W, is stable for 30 days at room temperature.[30]

GABAPENTIN   Neurontin

Pharmacology. Gabapentin is a cyclohexane compound structurally related to γ-aminobutyric acid (GABA); its mechanism of action is not known. Gabapentin does not interact with GABA receptors, nor does it alter the formation, release, degradation, or reuptake of GABA.

Administration and Adult Dosage. **PO for epilepsy** 300 mg hs on day 1; 300 mg bid on day 2; 300 mg tid on day 3. Dosage may be increased further according to clinical response. **Usual maintenance dosage** 900–2400 mg/day in 3 divided doses.[1] Dosages of 3.6–4.8 g/day have been well tolerated in some patients.[31] Give dosages ≥3.6 g/day in 4 divided doses qid. (*See* Notes.)

Special Populations. *Pediatric Dosage.* (<12 yr) safety and efficacy not established.

Geriatric Dosage. Lower dosages may be required due to normal age-related decreases in renal function.

Other Conditions. Reduce dosage in patients with compromised renal function as indicated below:

CL$_{CR}$ (ML/MIN)	TOTAL DAILY DOSAGE	DOSAGE REGIMEN
>60	1200 mg	400 mg tid
30–60	600 mg	300 mg bid
15–30	300 mg	300 mg daily
<15	150 mg	300 mg every other day
Hemodialysis	—	200–300 mg after dialysis

Dosage Forms. Cap 100, 300, 400 mg.

Patient Instructions. (*See* Anticonvulsants Class Instructions.) Do not take this drug with antacids.

Missed Doses. Take this drug at regular intervals. If you miss a dose take it as soon as you remember. If it is about time for the next dose, take that dose only. Do not double the dose or take extra.

Pharmacokinetics. *Onset and Duration.* Steady-state serum levels are attained in 1–2 days in patients with normal renal function.[32]

Serum Levels. A therapeutic range has not been established. In one study, a therapeutic effect correlated with serum concentrations greater than 2 mg/L.[33]

Fate. Rapidly absorbed and food has no effect on absorption. Absorption occurs via a saturable transport mechanism; therefore, bioavailability decreases with dosages greater than 1.8 g/day. At this dosage it is 60%, but at a dosage of 4.8 g/day, bioavailability is 35%.[32] The drug is not bound to plasma proteins. V$_d$ is 58 ± 6 L in adults; Cl is 0.17 ± 0.05 L/kg/hr in adults with normal renal function; Cl is linearly related to Cl$_{cr}$. Gabapentin is not appreciably metabolized, but is eliminated unchanged in urine and normal renal function.[34]

t$_{½}$. 4.8 ± 1.4 hr in adults with epilepsy and normal renal function.[34]

Adverse Reactions. Somnolence, dizziness, ataxia, nystagmus, and headache occur frequently. Symptoms are of mild to moderate severity and resolve within 2 weeks with continued treatment.[35] Weight gain (mean, 4.9% of body weight) and peripheral edema also occur frequently.[36] Occasionally, rash occurs. Rarely, behavioral changes in children occur.[37]

Contraindications. None known.

Precautions. Abrupt withdrawal of gabapentin in patients with epilepsy may precipitate status epilepticus. In vivo carcinogenicity studies demonstrate a high incidence of pancreatic acinar cell tumors in male rats; however, the relevance of this observation to humans is not known.

Drug Interactions. Gabapentin does not induce or inhibit hepatic microsomal enzymes and does not affect the metabolism of other antiepileptic drugs or oral contraceptives. Antacids decrease the oral bioavailability of gabapentin by about 20%.

Parameters to Monitor. Serum level monitoring is of limited value because of the lack of a well-defined therapeutic range. Routine monitoring of clinical laboratory parameters during gabapentin therapy is not indicated.

Notes. Gabapentin is indicated as adjunctive treatment for partial and secondarily generalized seizures in adults. Preliminary studies indicate that the drug may be efficacious as an adjunct in children with refractory partial seizures.[38] Gabapentin may not be effective as monotherapy.[39] Preliminary evidence suggests efficacy in the prophylaxis of migraine headache and in the treatment of neuropathic pain states (eg, trigeminal neuralgia, peripheral neuropathy, and postherpetic neuralgia), often at doses lower than those used for refractory epilepsy.[40–42]

LAMOTRIGINE   Lamictal

Pharmacology. Lamotrigine is a phenyltriazine derivative unrelated to other marketed antiepileptic drugs. Lamotrigine inhibits voltage-dependent sodium channels, thereby stabilizing neuronal membranes and reducing the release of excitatory neurotransmitters such as glutamate and aspartate. (*See* Notes.)

Administration and Adult Dosage. Adjust starting dosages, titration schedules, and maintenance dosage based on concomitant therapy. **PO for epilepsy in patients receiving enzyme-inducing antiepileptic drugs** (eg, carbamazepine, phenytoin, phenobarbital, and primidone) 50 mg/day for 2 weeks, then increase to 50 mg bid for 2 more weeks. Thereafter, increase dosage in 100 mg/day increments at weekly intervals to a maintenance dosage of 300–500 mg/day in 2 divided doses. **PO for epilepsy in patients receiving enzyme-inducing antiepileptic drugs with valproic acid** 25 mg every other day for 2 weeks, then increase to 25 mg/day for 2 more weeks. Thereafter, increase dosage in 25–50 mg/day increments at 1- to 2-week intervals to a **maintenance dosage** of 100–200 mg/day in 2 divided doses. Dosage recommendations are not available for patients receiving valproic acid alone, but dosages are expected to be lower due to prolonged half-life.

Special Populations. *Pediatric Dosage.* (<16 yr) safety and efficacy not established.

Geriatric Dosage. Dosage reduction may be required in patients with reduced hepatic or renal function and should be guided by clinical response.

Other Conditions. Patients with chronic renal failure or liver disease may require lower dosages of lamotrigine; however, specific dosage guidelines are not available.

Dosage Forms. **Chew Tab** 5, 25 mg; **Tab** 25, 100, 150, 200 mg.

Patient Instructions. (*See* Anticonvulsants Class Instructions.) Inform your physician if a skin rash develops.

Missed Doses. Take this drug at regular intervals. If you miss a dose take it as soon as you remember. If it is about time for the next dose, take that dose only. Do not double the dose or take extra.

Pharmacokinetics. *Onset and Duration.* Steady-state serum levels are attained in 2–3 days.[2]

Serum Levels. A therapeutic range has not been established. In most clinical trials, trough serum concentrations of lamotrigine ranged from 1–3 mg/L.[43]

Fate. The drug is rapidly absorbed, with a bioavailability of 98 ± 5%; peak serum levels occur 2.8 ± 1.3 hr after an oral dose. Food does not affect absorption. Lamotrigine is 56% bound to plasma proteins. V_d is 1.2 ± 0.12 L/kg;[44] Cl is 0.049 ± 0.028 L/hr/kg in adults.[45] From 7–30% is excreted unchanged in urine; 80–90% is excreted as the inactive glucuronide conjugate.[44]

$t_{1/2}$. 24.1 ± 5.7 hr in normal volunteers taking no other medications;[44] 14.3 ± 6.9 hr in patients taking enzyme-inducing antiepileptic drugs; 29.6 ± 10 hr in patients taking enzyme-inducing antiepileptic drugs with valproic acid;[45] 59 hr in patients taking valproic acid alone.[44]

Adverse Reactions. Dose-related dizziness, ataxia, somnolence, headache, diplopia, nausea, vomiting, and rash occur frequently. Rash occurs in about 10% of patients, usually within 4–6 weeks of treatment initiation. The rash is usually maculopapular and erythematous. Potentially life-threatening rashes (including Stevens-Johnson syndrome and toxic epidermal necrolysis) are reported in 1:1000 adults and as many as 1:50 to 1:100 children. Risk factors for rash include concomitant valproic acid therapy, high initial dosage of lamotrigine, and rapid escalation of lamotrigine dosage. Discontinue lamotrigine at the first sign of rash.

Contraindications. None known.

Precautions. Initiate lamotrigine cautiously in patients taking valproic acid because of a higher risk of rash. (*See* Administration and Adult Dosage.)

Drug Interactions. Dizziness, diplopia, and ataxia are more common in patients taking carbamazepine concomitantly and appear to be the result of a pharmacodynamic interaction.[46] Lamotrigine has no important effect on blood levels of phenytoin, carbamazepine, or carbamazepine-10,11-epoxide. Lamotrigine reduces steady-state valproic acid levels by 25%. Valproic acid increases lamotrigine levels by about 2-fold, and carbamazepine, phenobarbital, primidone, and phenytoin each decrease lamotrigine serum levels.

Parameters to Monitor. Serum level monitoring is of limited value because of the lack of a well-defined therapeutic range. Routine monitoring of clinical laboratory parameters during lamotrigine therapy is not necessary.

Notes. Lamotrigine is indicated as adjunctive treatment for partial and secondarily generalized seizures in adults and for the treatment of the Lennox-Gastaut syndrome.[47] Lamotrigine may be effective as monotherapy and appears to be better tolerated than carbamazepine monotherapy at dosages that are equally effective for the treatment of partial epilepsy.[48] (*See* Anticonvulsants Comparison Chart.)

PHENOBARBITAL
Various

Pharmacology. Phenobarbital is a barbiturate that exerts an anticonvulsant effect by depressing excitatory postsynaptic seizure discharge and increasing the convulsive threshold for electric and chemical stimulation.

Administration and Adult Dosage. PO or IM for epilepsy 60–90 mg/day initially, increase in 30–60 mg/day increments q 7–14 days to an effective dosage. **Usual maintenance dosage** 90–240 mg/day or 1–3 mg/kg/day hs.[1] **IV for status**

epilepticus 20 mg/kg at a rate of 100 mg/min.[49] **Rectal administration** has been reported. (*See* Fate.) (*See also* Adverse Reactions and Notes.)

Special Populations. *Pediatric Dosage.* **PO or IM for epilepsy** initially, titrate dosage to minimize sedation. **Usual maintenance dosage** is 2–5 mg/kg/day or 125 mg/m^2/day given at bedtime.[2] **IV for status epilepticus** 20 mg/kg at a rate of 50–100 mg/min.[50] (*See* Adverse Reactions and Notes.)

Geriatric Dosage. Clearance of phenobarbital is reduced in the elderly, so lower maintenance dosages may be required.[3]

Other Conditions. During pregnancy, phenobarbital clearance may increase. Dosage increases may be necessary and should be guided by serum levels and patient status.[2]

Dosage Forms. **Cap** 16 mg; **Tab** 15, 16, 30, 60, 100 mg; **Elxr** 3, 4 mg/mL; **Inj** 30, 60, 65, 130 mg/mL.

Patient Instructions. (*See* Anticonvulsants Class Instructions.)

Missed Doses. Take this drug at regular intervals. If you miss a dose take it as soon as you remember. If it is about time for the next dose, take that dose only. Do not double the dose or take extra.

Pharmacokinetics. *Onset and Duration.* Steady-state serum levels are attained in about 21 days.[2]

Serum Levels. (Anticonvulsant) 15–35 mg/L (65–150 μmol/L); dysarthria, ataxia, and nystagmus appear as serum level approaches 40 mg/L (172 μmol/L).[1,2,51]

Fate. The drug is slowly absorbed orally with 95–100% bioavailability; peak serum level occurs 2–4 hr after a PO or IM dose.[2] Rectal bioavailability is 90%, with a peak of 7.2 ± 0.8 mg/L (31 ± 3.4 μmol/L) 4.4 ± 0.6 hr after rectal administration of a 5 mg/kg dose of parenteral phenobarbital sodium solution.[52] The drug is 45–60% plasma protein bound. V_d is 0.61 ± 0.05 L/kg; Cl is 0.004 ± 0.0008 L/hr/kg in adults,[53] with 50–80% metabolized in the liver to *p*-hydroxyphenobarbital (inactive). The drug is 20–50% excreted unchanged in urine; alkalinization of urine increases renal phenobarbital clearance.[2,6]

$t_{1/2}$. (Adults) 100 ± 17 hr;[54] (cirrhosis) 130 ± 15 hr;[53] (children 1–5 yr) 69 ± 3.2 hr.[55]

Adverse Reactions. (*See* Serum Levels.) Sedation is frequent and dose related; tolerance usually develops with long-term administration. In adults, phenobarbital can impair cognition, reaction time, and motor performance.[56] Loss of concentration, mental dulling, depression of affect, insomnia, and hyperkinetic activity occur frequently with long-term therapy in children and the elderly.[51] Connective tissue disorders associated with barbiturates occur in 6% of patients, usually within the first year of treatment.[57] Occasionally, skin rashes or folate deficiency occur. Rarely, megaloblastic anemia, hepatitis, exfoliative dermatitis, or Stevens-Johnson syndrome are reported. Patients may be at risk for similar hypersensitivity reactions if rechallenged with phenytoin or carbamazepine.[58] Neonatal hemorrhage has been reported in newborns whose mothers were taking phenobarbital. SC or intra-arterial injection may produce tissue necrosis. IV administration, especially when given after IV benzodiazepines, may produce severe respiratory depression and provision for respiratory support should be made.

Contraindications. History of porphyria or severe respiratory disease where dyspnea or obstruction is present.

Precautions. Pregnancy; lactation. Use with caution in patients with marked liver or renal disease because drug clearance is slowed. Abrupt withdrawal of the drug in patients with epilepsy may precipitate status epilepticus.

Drug Interactions. Concurrent use with other CNS depressants may potentiate the sedation caused by phenobarbital. Numerous drugs may increase phenobarbital serum levels, possibly requiring phenobarbital dosage reduction; phenobarbital may stimulate CYP2D6 and CYP3A, and increase metabolism of many drugs.

Parameters to Monitor. Periodic serum level monitoring, after attaining steady state (about 21 days), is useful in guiding dosage changes or evaluating adverse effects.[2] Monitor CBC and liver function tests periodically during long-term therapy.

Notes. In tonic-clonic status epilepticus, phenobarbital is usually considered a third agent after IV phenytoin plus IV diazepam or lorazepam have failed to control seizures.[49] Considering clinical efficacy and patient tolerance, phenobarbital is a third- or fourth-line choice for single-drug therapy of partial or generalized tonic-clonic seizures compared to the drugs of first choice: carbamazepine, phenytoin, or valproic acid.[2] (*See* Anticonvulsants Comparison Chart.)

PHENYTOIN   Dilantin, Various

Pharmacology. Phenytoin is a hydantoin that suppresses the spread of seizure activity mainly by inhibiting synaptic post-tetanic potentiation and blocking the propagation of electric discharge. Phenytoin may decrease sodium transport and block calcium channels at the cellular level to produce these actions.

Administration and Adult Dosage. **PO maintenance dosage** 300 mg/day in 1–3 doses initially. Using serum levels as a guide, increase in 30–100 mg/day increments q 10–21 days to effective dosage.[2] Because of dose-dependent, saturable metabolism, small increases in dosage may produce disproportionate increases in serum levels. **Usual maintenance dosage** 300–400 mg/day or 4–8 mg/kg/day in 1 or 2 doses.[1] Only extended-release phenytoin sodium capsules are approved for once-daily administration. **PO loading dosage** 15 mg/kg in 3 divided doses, administered at 2-hr intervals. Using serum levels as a guide, a maintenance dosage can be initiated within 24 hr of starting the loading dosage. **IV loading dose** 15–20 mg/kg by direct IV injection, at a rate not greater than 50 mg/min or 0.75 mg/kg/min in adults.[51] Therapeutic serum levels persist for 12–24 hr in most patients.[59] Alternatively, dilute the loading dose in 50–150 mL of 0.45% or 0.9% NaCl and infuse through an IV volume control set with an in-line filter at a rate not greater than 50 mg/min.[2,60] In nonemergency situations, an IV dose of 5 mg/kg q 2 hr for 3 doses at a rate of 50 mg/min results in phenytoin serum levels of 10–20 mg/L 12 hr after the third dose.[61] (*See* Adverse Reactions and Notes.) **IM administration** is painful and results in slow, but complete, absorption because of deposition of phenytoin crystals in muscle.[2] The IM route is not recommended. The IV route is preferred in patients unable to take phenytoin by mouth. (*See* Fosphenytoin.)

Special Populations. *Pediatric Dosage.* **PO maintenance dosage** 5 mg/kg/day initially in 2–3 divided doses. Increase initial dosage in small increments q 7–10 days to effective dosage.[2] Because of dose-dependent metabolism, small increases in dosage may produce disproportionate increases in serum levels. **Usual maintenance dosage** 4–8 mg/kg/day in 2–3 divided doses.[1] **IV loading dose** (neonates) 15–20 mg/kg given at a rate of 0.5 mg/kg/min; (older infants and children) same as adult dosage.

Geriatric Dosage. **PO maintenance dosage** 200–300 mg/day in 1–3 doses. Advanced age may be associated with a decrease in phenytoin clearance and a reduction in albumin concentration.[62] Dosage adjustment should be guided by phenytoin levels and patient status. (*See* Serum Levels.)

Other Conditions. During pregnancy or febrile illness, or following acute traumatic injury, phenytoin clearance may increase; dosage adjustment may be necessary and should be guided by serum levels and patient status.[63–65] Renal disease and hypoalbuminemia can alter phenytoin binding to plasma proteins, resulting in a change in the usual ratio of free to total phenytoin levels; renal disease alters phenytoin protein binding because of decreased affinity of plasma proteins. Increases in fraction unbound are most pronounced in patients with Cl_{cr} <25 mL/min. Ideally, dosage adjustment should be guided by patient status and actual measurement of unbound and total phenytoin levels. (*See* Serum Levels.)

Dosage Forms. (Phenytoin) **Chew Tab** 50 mg; **Susp** 6, 25 mg/mL. (Phenytoin sodium) **Cap** (extended or prompt) 30, 100 mg; **Inj** 50 mg/mL. Phenytoin sodium is 92% phenytoin.

Patient Instructions. (*See* Anticonvulsants Class Instructions.) Good dental hygiene and regular dental visits may minimize gum tenderness, bleeding, or enlargement (especially in children). Shake oral suspension well prior to each dose and use a calibrated measuring device. (*See* Notes.) Call physician if skin rash develops.

Missed Doses. Take this drug at regular intervals. If you miss a dose, take it as soon as you remember. If it is about time for the next dose, take that dose only. When taking multiple daily doses, leave a minimum of 4–6 hours between doses. If you are taking the drug only once daily and you do not remember until the next day, skip the missed dose and return to your normal schedule. Do not double the dose or take extra. If doses are missed for 2 or more days in a row, consult your physician.

Pharmacokinetics. *Onset and Duration.* Time to steady state increases with increasing dosage and serum level. Steady state is usually attained within 7–14 days, but may take as long as 28 days.[2]

Serum Levels. 10–20 mg/L (40–80 μmol/L) in patients with normal renal function and serum albumin concentration. Nystagmus, slurred speech, ataxia, or dizziness appear in most patients as serum level approaches 20 mg/L; drowsiness, diplopia, behavioral changes, and cognitive impairment above 30 mg/L (120 μmol/L).[2] The equation $C_{normal} = C_{observed}/([0.2 \times albumin] + 0.1)$ is used to estimate the concentration of phenytoin that would be expected if the albumin concentration were normal (C_{normal}) from the measured total phenytoin concentration in a hypoalbuminemic patient ($C_{observed}$) and the patient's albumin concentration in g/dL (albumin). In patients with end-stage renal disease (Cl_{cr} <10 mL/min), the equation $C_{normal} = C_{observed}/([0.1 \times albumin] + 0.1)$ is used.[66] (*See also* Special Populations, Other Conditions.)

Fate. Oral phenytoin absorption is very slow and incomplete in infants ≤3 months of age.[2] Bioavailability of the suspension is decreased in patients receiving concomitant enteral feedings. (*See* Precautions.) IM injection is slowly absorbed over several days because of deposition of phenytoin crystals in muscle. Peak serum levels occur 4–8 hr after a single dose of an extended-release capsule;[2] after oral loading given in divided doses, the time to reach a serum level of 10 mg/L is 4.5 ± 2.1 hr for prompt-release capsules and 9.6 ± 2.5 hr for extended-release capsules.[67] Time to peak serum level increases with increasing oral dosages.[68] About 90% is plasma protein bound.[2] Hypoalbuminemia, chronic liver or renal disease, nephrotic syndrome, AIDS, or acute traumatic injury alter protein binding and increase the fraction of unbound phenytoin.[2,63] V_d is 0.83 ± 0.2 L/kg in adults with acute seizures[60]; 0.79 ± 0.25 L/kg in critically ill adults following trauma.[63] Hepatic metabolism is capacity limited, exhibiting Michaelis-Menten pharmacokinetics; therefore, Cl decreases as serum level increases. Mean apparent V_{max} is 0.45 mg/L/hr; mean apparent K_m is 6.2 mg/L in adults.[2] About 70% of phenytoin is excreted in urine as the inactive metabolite, 5-(p-hydroxyphenyl)-5-phenylhydantoin (HPPH). Less than 5% of the parent drug is excreted unchanged in urine.[2,6]

$t_{1/2}$. Phenytoin has no true half-life, but its apparent half-life increases as serum level increases; at phenytoin serum level of 1 mg/L, predicted mean phenytoin half-life is 13 hr, 26 hr at 10 mg/L, 40 hr at 20 mg/L, and 69 hr at 40 mg/L.[2,69]

Adverse Reactions. (*See* Serum Levels.) Erythematous morbilliform rash occurs frequently. Do not resume phenytoin if rash is exfoliative, purpuric, bullous, or accompanied by fever. With long-term administration, hirsutism, gingival hypertrophy (especially in children and adolescents), coarsening of facial features, acneiform eruption, osteomalacia, and folate deficiency with mild macrocytosis occur frequently.[2,51] Bradycardia or hypotension caused by rapid IV administration are reported occasionally; slowing the rate of administration may minimize these complications.[49,59] Severe soft tissue injury following IV phenytoin is more likely in elderly (>70 yr) women who receive 2 or more infusions through small (20 gauge or smaller) IV devices.[70] Hepatotoxicity occurs occasionally, usually within the first 6 weeks, and presents with fever, rash, lymphadenopathy, and hepatomegaly.[71] Other idiosyncratic reactions are rare, may occur together within the first 2 months, and include fever, lymphoid hyperplasia, eosinophilia, erythema multiforme, exfoliative dermatitis, Stevens-Johnson syndrome, leukopenia, anemia, thrombocytopenia, serum sickness, and SLE.[2] These patients are at risk for similar hypersensitivity reactions if rechallenged with phenobarbital or carbamazepine.[58] Concurrent cranial irradiation predisposes patients to the development of erythema multiforme.[72] A syndrome of anomalies in infants of phenytoin-exposed mothers has been described (fetal hydantoin syndrome).

Contraindications. (Parenteral phenytoin) sinus bradycardia; sino-atrial block; second- and third-degree AV block; Adams-Stokes syndrome.

Precautions. Pregnancy; lactation. Use with caution in patients with severe liver disease or diabetes, or those with a history of severe hypersensitivity reactions to carbamazepine or phenobarbital. Abrupt withdrawal of the drug in patients with epilepsy may precipitate status epilepticus. If the patient's nutritional status allows, interrupt tube feeding 2 hr before and after the dose and irrigate the feeding tube to improve absorption; nevertheless, the patient may require an increase in phenytoin dosage. If the feedings are discontinued after the phenytoin dosage is increased, the dosage must be adjusted to prevent toxic serum levels from occurring.[73]

Drug Interactions. Chronic alcohol use, barbiturates, rifampin, and some other drugs may stimulate phenytoin metabolism and increase phenytoin dosage requirements. Numerous drugs may increase phenytoin serum levels, possibly requiring phenytoin dosage reduction; phenytoin may stimulate CYP2D6 and CYP3A, and may increase metabolism of many drugs. IV phenytoin may produce hypotension in severely ill patients receiving IV dopamine. The antiparkinson effect of levodopa may be inhibited by phenytoin. Signs of lithium toxicity may occur in the absence of increased serum lithium in patients on phenytoin.

Parameters to Monitor. Serum level monitoring, after attaining steady state (10–21 days), is useful in evaluating therapeutic efficacy or potential for adverse effects.[2] Patient and serum level monitoring are recommended when changing phenytoin dosage form or brand; monitor serum levels q 5–7 days to assess trend in concentrations. Monitor CBC and liver function tests periodically with long-term therapy.

Notes. Agitation or shaking is needed to resuspend phenytoin suspension; settling occurs 5 weeks after resuspension.[74] In tonic-clonic status epilepticus, phenytoin's anticonvulsant effect appears 20–30 min after start of the infusion. Thus, in this situation, concurrent use of phenytoin with a rapid-acting injectable benzo-diazepine (**diazepam** or **lorazepam**) is recommended.[49] Phenytoin is recommended, as is **carbamazepine**, as a drug of first choice for single-drug therapy of partial or generalized tonic-clonic seizures.[75] (*See* Anticonvulsants Comparison Chart.)

PRIMIDONE
Mysoline, Various

Pharmacology. Primidone (desoxyphenobarbital) is structurally related to the barbiturates. Primidone and its metabolites, phenylethylmalonamide (PEMA) and phenobarbital, all exert anticonvulsant activity. (*See* Phenobarbital.)

Administration and Adult Dosage. PO for epilepsy 50–100 mg hs initially; increase in 100–125 mg/day increments q 2–3 days to effective dosage, to a maximum of 2 g/day. **Usual maintenance dosage** 250–500 mg tid.[1]

Special Populations. *Pediatric Dosage.* **PO for epilepsy** (<8 yr) 50 mg hs initially; increase by 50 mg in 3 days and thereafter in 100–125 mg/day increments q 3 days to effective dosage. **Usual maintenance dosage** 125–250 mg tid or 10–20 mg/kg/day in 3 divided doses. (≥8 yr) same as adult dosage.

Geriatric Dosage. Clearance of primidone is unchanged in elderly patients; however, phenobarbital clearance is reduced. Lower maintenance dosages may be required.

Dosage Forms. **Susp** 50 mg/mL; **Tab** 50, 250 mg.

Patient Instructions. (*See* Anticonvulsants Class Instructions.)

Missed Doses. Take this drug at regular intervals. If you miss a dose take it as soon as you remember. If it is about time for the next dose, take that dose only. Do not double the dose or take extra.

Pharmacokinetics. *Onset and Duration.* Steady-state serum levels are attained in about 3 days.[2]

Serum Levels. (Primidone) 6–12 mg/L (28–55 μmol/L).[1,2,51] (*See also* Phenobarbital.) During monotherapy, primidone to phenobarbital serum level ratios are about 1:1.[2] During polytherapy with enzyme-inducing agents, this ratio increases to 4:1.[2] During monotherapy, the PEMA to primidone serum level ratio at steady state is 0.74 ± 0.38 for samples drawn before the first morning dose.[2]

Fate. The drug is rapidly absorbed with 90–100% bioavailability; peak serum levels occur 2–6 hr after an oral dose. The drug is 0–20% plasma protein bound; V_d is 0.86 ± 0.22 L/kg;[76] C1 with monotherapy is 0.035 ± 0.02 L/hr/kg; with concomitant anticonvulsants, it is 0.052 ± 0.02 L/hr/kg;[2] in monotherapy with concomitant acute viral hepatitis, it is 0.042 ± 0.14 L/hr/kg.[76] Primidone is metabolized in the liver to PEMA and phenobarbital; 76% of the drug is excreted into the urine within 5 days after a single dose as 64% primidone, 7% PEMA, 2% phenobarbital, and 3% unidentified products.[2]

$t_{1/2}$. (Primidone) 15.2 ± 4.8 hr (monotherapy); 8.3 ± 2.9 hr (with concomitant enzyme-inducing anticonvulsants); 18 ± 3.1 hr (with acute viral hepatitis).[76] (PEMA) 21 ± 3 hr (primidone monotherapy); 17 ± 4.3 hr (with concomitant anticonvulsants).[77] (*See also* Phenobarbital.)

Adverse Reactions. Drowsiness, ataxia, nausea, weakness, and dizziness occur frequently during first month of therapy and may become tolerable with time. Behavioral disturbances, depression of affect, and cognitive impairment occur frequently with long-term therapy in children and the elderly.[2] Occasionally, skin rashes and rarely, impotence, leukopenia, thrombocytopenia, megaloblastic anemia, or lymphadenopathy occur.[2,51]

Contraindications. History of porphyria; hypersensitivity to phenobarbital.

Precautions. Pregnancy; lactation. Use with caution in patients with severe liver or renal disease. Abrupt withdrawal of the drug may precipitate status epilepticus. (*See* Phenobarbital Notes.)

Drug Interactions. Concurrent use with other CNS depressants may potentiate the sedation caused by phenobarbital. Primidone levels may be decreased by concurrent acetazolamide, carbamazepine, or succimides. Primidone levels may be increased by concurrent hydantoins, isoniazid, or niacinamide.

Parameters to Monitor. Periodic serum level monitoring of primidone and phenobarbital, after attaining steady state (primidone, 3 days; phenobarbital, 21 days), is useful in guiding dosage changes, detecting noncompliance, or evaluating adverse effects.[2] Monitor CBC, electrolytes, and liver function tests periodically during long-term therapy.

Notes. Considering comparative efficacy and good patient tolerance of **carbamazepine, phenytoin,** and **valproic acid,** primidone is a fourth- or fifth-line choice for single-drug therapy of generalized tonic-clonic seizures. In a large, multicenter trial comparing carbamazepine, phenytoin, phenobarbital, and primidone, primidone was least successful in controlling seizures with acceptable adverse effects.[75]

TIAGABINE   Gabatril

Pharmacology. Tiagabine is a nipecotic acid derivative unrelated to other marked antiepileptic drugs. It interacts with the γ-aminobutyric acid (GABA) uptake carrier and is thought to enhance the inhibitory effect of GABA by preventing its reuptake into neurons. Tiagabine is indicated in adults and adolescents (>12 yr) as adjunctive therapy for patients with partial-onset seizures.[78,79]

Administration and Adult Dosage. PO for epilepsy in patients taking enzyme-inducing antiepileptic drugs (eg, carbamazepine, phenytoin, phenobarbital, primidone), initiate at 4 mg/day for 1 week, increasing in increments of 4–8 mg/day at weekly intervals according to clinical response. **Usual maintenance dosage** is 32–56 mg/day. The daily dosage is given in 2–4 divided doses; with dosages >32 mg/day, tid or qid administration may be required. Patients taking only non-enzyme-inducing antiepileptic drugs (eg, gabapentin, lamotrigine, valproate) may require lower doses or a slower titration schedule.

Special Populations. *Pediatric Dosage.* (≤12 yr) safety and efficacy not established; (>12 yr) same as adult dose.

Geriatric Dosage. Same as adult dosage.

Other Conditions. No apparent need to adjust tiagabine dosage in renal impairment. Patients with liver disease may require lower dosages of tiagabine; however, specific dosage guidelines are not available.

Dosage Forms. **Tab** 4, 12, 16, 20 mg.

Patient Instructions. (*See* Anticonvulsants Class Instructions) Take this medication with food.

Missed Doses. Take this drug at regular intervals. If you miss a dose, take it as soon as you remember. If it is about time for the next dose, take that dose only. Do not double the dose or take extra.

Pharmacokinetics. *Onset and Duration.* Steady-state serum levels are attained within 2 days.

Serum Levels. A therapeutic range has not been established.

Fate. Rapidly absorbed with a bioavailability of 89.9 ± 9.7%.[80,81] Food slows the rate, but not the extent, of tiagabine absorption. Peak serum concentrations of 241 ± 79 μg/L occur 1.3 ± 1 hr after a single 12 mg dose in healthy volunteers.[82] Tiagabine is 96% bound to plasma proteins, primarily albumin and α_1-acid glycoprotein. V_d is 1.07 ± 0.22 L/kg;[82] Cl is 6.5 ± 1.5 L/hr in healthy volunteers.[81] Cl is increased in patients taking enzyme-inducing antiepileptic drugs. Tiagabine is metabolized by oxidation (primarily CYP3A) and glucuronidation; approximately 2% is excreted unchanged in urine.

$t_{½}$. 7–9 hr in healthy subjects taking no other medications; reduced by 50–65% in patients with epilepsy taking enzyme-inducing antiepileptic drugs.[81,82]

Adverse Reactions. Dizziness, asthenia/lack of energy, somnolence, nausea, nervousness, tremor, abdominal pain, and difficulty with concentration occur frequently. Tremor, difficulty with concentration, and asthenia appear to be dose related. The most common reasons for discontinuation are dizziness, somnolence, depression, confusion, and asthenia. Moderate to severe generalized weakness occurs occasionally.

Contraindications. None known.

Precautions. Dosage reduction may be required in hepatic impairment.

Drug Interactions. Carbamazepine, phenytoin, and phenobarbital reduce tiagabine levels by 60% compared with noninduced patients. Valproate has no important effect on tiagabine levels. Tiagabine has no effect on serum concentrations of phenytoin, carbamazepine, phenobarbital, or primidone. Valproate concentrations decrease approximately 10% during tiagabine therapy. Tiagabine has no effect on the pharmacokinetics of warfarin, theophylline, digoxin, or oral contraceptives.

Parameters to Monitor. Serum level monitoring is of limited value because of the lack of a well-defined therapeutic range. No routine laboratory test monitoring is required during therapy.

TOPIRAMATE   Topamax

Pharmacology. Topiramate, a derivative of the naturally occurring monosaccharide D-fructose, reduces the frequency of action potentials elicited by depolarizing currents in a manner suggestive of sodium channel blocking action. Topiramate also increases γ-aminobutyric acid (GABA)-induced chloride flux, although the drug has no direct effect on GABA binding sites. It also inhibits kainate activation of a subtype of the excitatory glutamate receptor. Topiramate inhibits carbonic anhydrase; however, this action may not contribute to the drug's anticonvulsant effect. (*See* Notes.)

Administration and Adult Dosage. PO for epilepsy 50 mg/day initially, increasing in 50 mg/day increments at weekly intervals to 200–400 mg/day in 2 divided doses. **Usual maintenance dosage** 400 mg/day. Higher dosages have not been shown to be more effective; however, individual patients may require ≥1 g/day.[83] (*See* Notes.)

Special Populations. *Pediatric Dosage.* Safety and efficacy not established.

Geriatric Dosage. Same as adult dosage.

Other Conditions. With Cl_{cr} <70 mL/min/1.73 m^2, reduce dosage by 50%. Topiramate clearance increases during hemodialysis to a rate 4–6 times greater than a normal person. Additional doses of topiramate may be required depending upon the dialysis method and duration.

Dosage Forms. **Tab** 25, 100, 200 mg.

Patient Instructions. (*See* Anticonvulsants Class Instructions.) Maintain adequate fluid intake to minimize the formation of kidney stones. If you are taking oral contraceptives, report any change in menstrual bleeding patterns to your health care provider.

Missed Doses. Take this drug at regular intervals. If you miss a dose take it as soon as you remember. If it is about time for the next dose, take that dose only. Do not double the dose or take extra.

Pharmacokinetics. *Onset and Duration.* Steady-state serum concentrations are attained in 4 days in patients with normal renal function.

Serum Levels. A therapeutic range has not been established.[84]

Fate. The bioavailability of oral tablets is 80% compared to an oral solution and peak concentrations occur 3.5 ± 0.6 hr after a 400 mg dose.[2] Administration with food delays absorption (by approximately 2 hr), but does not affect extent of absorption.[2] Topiramate is 13–17% bound to plasma proteins and binds to a saturable, low-capacity binding site on or in erythrocytes.[78] V_d is 0.6–0.8 L/kg in healthy volunteers.[2] Cl is 0.021 ± 0.004 L/kg/hr in adults on topiramate monotherapy after tapering of valproic acid.[84] Approximately 70% is eliminated unchanged in urine. Six metabolites (each <5% of the administered dose) have been identified.

$t_{1/2}$. 23 hr after a single 400 mg dose in healthy adults.[2]

Adverse Reactions. Somnolence, dizziness, ataxia, speech problems, psychomotor slowing, nystagmus, and paresthesias occur commonly and are not dose related. Common dose-related adverse effects include fatigue, nervousness, difficulty with concentration or attention, confusion, depression, weight loss, and tremor. These adverse effects are minimized by slow dose titration. Psychomotor slowing and difficulty with concentration are the most common reasons for topiramate discontinuation. Kidney stones occur in 1.5% of patients and may be related to carbonic anhydrase inhibition.

Contraindications. None known.

Precautions. Avoid concomitant use of other carbonic anhydrase inhibitors (eg, acetazolamide) because of the potential increased risk of kidney stones.

Drug Interactions. Concomitant phenytoin and carbamazepine cause reductions in topiramate concentrations of 48% and 40%, respectively. Concomitant valproate reduces topiramate concentrations by 17%.[84] Topiramate variably affects phenytoin concentrations (0–25% decrease) and has no important effect on other anticonvulsants. Topiramate may reduce the effectiveness of oral contraceptives; consider using products containing $\geq$35 μg of ethinyl estradiol.[85]

Parameters to Monitor. Serum level monitoring is of limited value because of the lack of a well-defined therapeutic range. Routine monitoring of clinical laboratory parameters during topiramate therapy is not indicated.

Notes. Topiramate is indicated as adjunctive treatment for partial and secondarily generalized seizures in adults. Preliminary evidence suggests that topiramate may also be effective for generalized-onset seizures,[86] as monotherapy for partial-onset seizures,[87] as adjunctive therapy for children with partial-onset seizures,[88] and as adjunctive treatment of the Lennox-Gastaut syndrome.[89]

VALPROIC ACID	Depakene, Depacon, Various
DIVALPROEX SODIUM	Depakote

Pharmacology. Valproic acid is a carboxylic acid compound whose anticonvulsant activity may be mediated by an inhibitory neurotransmitter, γ-aminobutyric acid (GABA). Valproic acid may increase GABA levels by inhibiting GABA metabolism or by enhancing postsynaptic GABA activity. Valproic acid also limits repetitive neuronal firing through voltage- and usage-dependent sodium channels. Divalproex is comprised of sodium valproate and valproic acid. (*See* Notes.)

Administration and Adult Dosage. **PO for epilepsy** (valproic acid) 15 mg/kg/day initially in 2–3 divided doses, increasing in 5–10 mg/kg/day increments at weekly intervals to an effective dosage, to a maximum of 60 mg/kg/day. **Usual maintenance dosage** 15–40 mg/kg/day in 3 divided doses.[90] In patients receiving valproic acid, divalproex can be substituted at the same daily dosage, and in selected patients, it can be given bid. **PO for migraine prophylaxis** (divalproex) 250 mg bid, to a maximum of 1 g/day. **PO for mania** (divalproex) 750 mg/day in divided doses, increasing as rapidly as possible to the lowest dosage that produces the desired effect, to a maximum of 60 mg/kg/day. (*See* Serum Levels.) Long-term experience with this use is minimal and characterized by a high drop-out rate. **IV for epilepsy** (valproic acid) same as oral dosage. Administer infusion over 60 min or at a rate of $\leq$20 mg/min. **Rectal administration** has been reported. (*See* Fate.)

Special Populations. *Pediatric Dosage.* Same as adult dosage.

Geriatric Dosage. Reduce the starting dosage in the elderly. Protein binding and unbound clearance of valproic acid are reduced in the elderly, and the desired clinical response may be achieved with a lower dosage than in younger adults. Dosage adjustments should be guided by valproic acid levels (preferably free levels in patients with low serum albumin) and patient status.[3]

Dosage Forms. (Valproic acid) **Cap** 250 mg; **Syrup** 50 mg/mL; **Inj** 100 mg/mL; (divalproex) **EC Tab** 125, 250, 500 mg; **Cap** (EC granules) 125 mg.

Patient Instructions. (*See* Anticonvulsants Class Instructions). This drug may be taken with food or milk to minimize stomach upset. Do not chew, break, or crush the tablet or capsule, because this may irritate your mouth or throat. Sprinkle capsule may be swallowed whole or administered by sprinkling the entire contents on small amount (1 teaspoonful) of soft food such as pudding or applesauce; swallow the drug/food mixture immediately (avoid chewing). Polymer from the sprinkles may appear in the stools, but does not indicate a lack of absorption. Weakness, tiredness, repeated vomiting, or loss of seizure control may be an early sign of severe, but rare, liver disorder and should be reported immediately.

Missed Doses. Take this drug at regular intervals. If you miss a dose take it as soon as you remember. If it is about time for the next dose, take that dose only. Leave a minimum of 6 hours between doses. Do not double the dose or take extra.

Pharmacokinetics. *Onset and Duration.* Steady-state serum levels are attained in 2–4 days.[2] Several weeks may be required for attainment of maximal therapeutic effect.[90] For mania, levels should be above 45 mg/L for efficacy and below 125 mg/L to minimize adverse effects.

Serum Levels. 50–120 mg/L (350–830 μmol/L) for epilepsy and mania. Some patients require and can tolerate serum levels up to 150 mg/L.[90] Tremor, irritability, confusion, and restlessness may be observed with levels >100–150 mg/L.[2]

Fate. The bioavailability of the oral capsule is 93 ± 13%, with peak levels occurring 1–2 hr after dose. The bioavailability of the EC divalproex tablet is 90 ± 14%, with peak levels in 4 hr.[2,91] The peak time of both is delayed by food: (cap) 5.2 ± 1.7 hr; (EC divalproex tab) 8.1 ± 3.6 hr.[92] Bioavailability is 80 ± 7% after a 250 mg suppository.[93] Peak serum levels of 40–50 mg/L (280–350 μmol/L) occur 2–4 hr after a 15–20 mg/kg dose of syrup diluted 1:1 with water as a retention enema.[11] V_d is 0.19 ± 0.05 L/kg in adults and 0.26 ± 0.09 L/kg in children.[2] Plasma protein binding is about 90%.[91] Increasing serum concentrations, hypoalbuminemia, severe liver disease, renal disease, or pregnancy reportedly increase the unbound fraction and may alter clearance. Cl is (healthy adults) 0.0066 ± 0.0005 L/hr/kg; (epileptic adults) 0.018 ± 0.011 L/hr/kg; (children) 0.027 ± 0.015 L/hr/kg.[2] Over 96% is metabolized to at least 10 metabolites. Only 1.8–3.2% of drug is excreted unchanged in urine.[2]

$t_{1/2}$. (Healthy adults) 13.9 ± 3.4 hr; (epileptic adults) 8.5 ± 3.3 hr; (children) 7.2 ± 2.3 hr.[2]

Adverse Reactions. (*See* Serum Levels.) Nausea, vomiting, diarrhea, and abdominal cramps occur frequently during initiation of therapy and are minimized by slow titration of valproic acid or substitution of EC divalproex for valproic acid. Transient elevations in liver function tests occur frequently. The risk of valproate-exposed women having children with spina bifida is approximately 1–2%. Drowsiness, ataxia, tremor, behavioral disturbances, transient hair loss, asymptomatic hyperammonemia, or weight gain occur occasionally. Drowsiness and ataxia are more prominent in patients taking valproic acid together with other anticonvulsants.[2] Rarely, thrombocytopenia, acute pancreatitis, abnormal coagulation parameters, or hyperglycinemia occur. Liver failure occurs rarely; the greatest risk is during the first 6 months of therapy and in children <2 yr who receive multiple anticonvulsants.[94]

Contraindications. Hepatic dysfunction or disease.

Precautions. Pregnancy; lactation. The drug may alter results of urine ketone test.

Drug Interactions. Valproate levels may be decreased by concurrent carbamazepine, lamotrigine, phenytoin, or rifampin. Valproate levels may be increased by concurrent aspirin, chlorpromazine, cimetidine, or felbamate. Lamotrigine and phenobarbital levels may be increased by valproate.

Parameters to Monitor. Baseline liver function tests (LFTs) and platelets; repeat LFTs frequently, especially during the first 6 months. Monitor coagulation tests prior to surgery. Periodic serum level monitoring is useful for guiding dosage changes and evaluating potential adverse effects. Serum levels fluctuate considerably during a 24-hr period, making a single random measurement of limited value. Predose blood sampling at standard times is recommended.[2,91]

Notes. Valproic acid and ethosuximide are equally effective for treating absence seizures, although **ethosuximide** is sometimes preferred as a first-line agent because of its lower risk of serious toxicity. Valproic acid is preferred for patients with both absence and generalized tonic-clonic seizures. Many clinicians in the United States use valproic acid as a second-line agent (after **phenytoin** or **carbamazepine**) for the treatment of partial seizures. Valproic acid is as effective as phenytoin and carbamazepine for tonic-clonic seizures and is a drug of choice for atonic and myoclonic seizures.[2,90,95] (*See* Anticonvulsants Comparison Chart.)

Divalproex is equivalent to **lithium** in bipolar disorder and is more effective than lithium for rapid-cycling bipolar patients (4 or more episodes in 1 yr) and comorbid substance abuse. Carbamazepine is more effective as an adjunctive treatment with lithium to enhance partial efficacy than with lithium alone.[96–98]

For migraine prophylaxis, divalproex is effective and well tolerated. It may be more effective in those having frequent migraines than in those characterized as having tension headaches.[99,100]

VIGABATRIN (Investigational—HMR)   Sabril

Pharmacology. Vigabatrin, a synthetic amino acid, is a γ-vinyl analogue of γ-aminobutyric acid (GABA), an inhibitory neurotransmitter. Vigabatrin irreversibly inhibits GABA transaminase, the primary degradative enzyme for GABA, resulting in increases in GABA in the CSF. Vigabatrin is effective as adjunctive therapy for medically refractory partial seizures. In clinical trials, 33–66% of patients had a ≥50% reduction in the frequency of seizures. Vigabatrin also appears to be effective for infantile spasms and as monotherapy in patients with newly diagnosed epilepsy; however, it may worsen absence and myoclonic seizures.[2,101–106] In 1983, clinical trials of vigabatrin in the U.S. were suspended due to reports of microscopic vacuoles in the brain white matter of rats, mice, and dogs. However, neuropathologic evaluation of surgery and autopsy specimens uncovered no evidence of similar changes in humans, and clinical trials have resumed.

Adult Dosage. PO maintenance dosage 2–4 g/day in 1–2 divided doses. Dosage reduction is recommended in patients with a $Cl_{cr} < 60$ mL/min.

Pharmacokinetics. The duration of therapeutic effect outlasts the presence of the drug in serum and is affected by the rate of resynthesis of GABA transaminase. CSF concentrations of GABA return to baseline within 2 weeks after drug discontinuation. Vigabatrin is rapidly absorbed after oral administration with peak concentrations reached within 2 hr. However, due to vigabatrin's mechanism of action, there is no correlation between serum concentrations and therapeutic effect. Food has little effect on the rate of absorption. Vigabatrin does not bind to plasma proteins. V_d is 0.81 L/kg; renal Cl is 0.076 ± 0.019 L/hr/kg; vigabatrin is not metabolized. In healthy volunteers, the half-life of the S(+)-enantiomer is 7.5 ± 2.2 hr, increasing to 13.2 ± 8.4 hr in the elderly, probably reflecting age-related reduction in Cl_{cr}.[107,108]

Adverse Reactions. Common adverse effects include drowsiness, fatigue, dizziness, tremor, and weight gain. Behavioral changes including anxiety, depression, and psychosis are reported, and are more common in patients with a history of psychiatric disturbance. Photophobia, retinal disorders, and visual field abnormalities, including a few cases of severe, persistent tunnel vision, have been reported. Visual testing should be performed at baseline and during therapy.

Drug Interactions. Vigabatrin has no effect on serum concentrations of carbamazepine or valproic acid, but phenytoin concentrations are reduced by 20% during vigabatrin therapy.

ZONISAMIDE (Investigational—Athena)   Zonagen

Pharmacology. Zonisamide is a 1,2-benzisoxazole derivative chemically unrelated to other antiepileptic drugs. It blocks seizure spread and inhibits epileptic foci in animals. The anticonvulsant effect is likely related to blockade of voltage-sensitive sodium and T-type calcium channels. It is also a weak carbonic anhydrase inhibitor. In placebo-controlled studies of adults with medically refractory partial seizures, zonisamide reduces the frequency of seizures by ≥50% in 30–40% of patients as adjunctive therapy. The drug also appears to be effective for the generalized and progressive myoclonic epilepsies.[2]

Adult Dosage. **PO as adjunctive therapy for partial seizures** 200–400 mg/day in 1–3 divided doses.

Pharmacokinetics. No clear relationship exists between serum concentration and therapeutic effect. Zonisamide is rapidly absorbed after oral administration. Absolute bioavailability is unknown. Food does not affect the rate or extent of absorption. Peak serum concentrations occur 2.8 ± 1.4 hr after a dose in healthy volunteers. Zonisamide is 40–60% bound to plasma proteins, mainly albumin. In healthy volunteers, V_d/F is 1.47 ± 0.39 L/kg; Cl/F is 0.019 ± 0.004 L/kg/hr and half-life is 54 hr after a single oral dose. Elimination is by hepatic metabolism; however, the metabolites and their activity have not been fully characterized in humans.[2,81]

Adverse Reactions. Frequent adverse effects include somnolence, ataxia, anorexia, confusion, abnormal thinking, and nervousness. Kidney stones occur in 2.6% of patients.[2]

Drug Interactions. Enzyme-inducing antiepileptic drugs (carbamazepine, phenytoin, barbiturates) enhance zonisamide's metabolism and reduce its half-life to 27–36 hr. Zonisamide has no apparent effect on the pharmacokinetics of other antiepileptic drugs.[81]

ANTICONVULSANTS COMPARISON CHART

DRUG	CHOICE OF ANTICONVULSANT FOR CLINICAL SEIZURE TYPE[a]					ANTICONVULSANT DOSAGE RANGE AND SERUM LEVELS			
	Generalized Seizures				Partial Seizures[b]	Dosage Range (mg/kg/day)		Therapeutic Serum Levels	
	Tonic-Clonic	Absence	Myoclonic	Atonic		Adult	Pediatric	(mg/L)	(µmol/L)
Carbamazepine	1	W	—	—	1	10–30	15–35	4–12	17–50
Clonazepam	W	3	2	1	—	0.01–0.2	0.01–0.2	13–72 µg/L	40–230 nmol/L
Ethosuximide	—	1	—	—	—	10–30	20–40	40–100	280–710
Gabapentin	—	—	—	—	4	15–35	—	—	—
Lamotrigine	—	—	—	—	4	1.5–7	—	—	—
Phenytoin	1	—	—	—	1	4–8	4–8	10–20	40–80
Tiagabine	—	—	—	—	4	0.5–0.8	—	—	—
Topiramate	—	—	—	—	4	4–8	—	—	—
Valproic Acid[c]	1	2	1	1	2	15–60	15–60	50–120	350–830

1 = Drug of first choice; initial agent; given as monotherapy.

2 = Drug of second choice; alternative to first choice; given as monotherapy or in combination with agent of first choice.

3 = Drug of third choice; alternative to first or second choice; given as monotherapy or in combination with another agent.

4 = Useful as adjunctive therapy after failure of monotherapy with preferred agents.

W = May worsen clinical seizure type.

[a]Choice of anticonvulsant based on relative and comparative efficacy and potential for adverse effects. Choice of agent should consider individual patient factors. (See references 1, 75, 90, and 95.)

[b]Includes simple-partial, complex-partial, and secondarily generalized tonic-clonic seizures.

[c]Drug of first choice when both generalized tonic-clonic and absence seizures are present.

431

Antidepressants

Class Instructions: Antidepressants. This drug may cause drowsiness. Until the extent of this effect is known, use caution when driving, operating machinery, or performing other tasks requiring mental alertness. Avoid excessive concurrent use of alcohol or other drugs that cause drowsiness.

BUPROPION   Wellbutrin, Zyban

Pharmacology. Bupropion is a monocyclic antidepressant, unique as a mild dopamine and norepinephrine uptake inhibitor with no direct effect on serotonin receptors, or on MAO. It is essentially devoid of anticholinergic, antihistaminic, and peripheral adrenergic effects. In contrast with heterocyclic antidepressants, bupropion produces no clinically important effect on cardiac conduction, no orthostatic hypotension, minimal anticholinergic effects, and it is not associated with weight gain. Compared to SSRIs, bupropion offers a similar side effect profile without sexual dysfunction. Its lack of sedation and its activating effect may be advantageous for patients with decreased psychomotor activity and lethargy. Disadvantages of bupropion include seizures and the necessity of multiple daily doses.[109-112] (*See* Antidepressants Comparison Chart.)

Adult Dosage. Small initial doses and gradual dosage escalation is necessary to minimize the risk of seizures. **PO for depression** (immediate-release) 100 mg bid initially, increasing to 100 mg tid no sooner than 3 days after the start of therapy. The maximum daily dosage is 450 mg, with a maximum single dose of 150 mg; (sustained-release) 150 mg given in the morning initially, increasing to 150 mg bid no sooner than 4 days after the start of therapy, to a maximum of 200 mg bid. **PO as an aid to smoking cessation** (sustained-release) Zyban is identical to Wellbutrin SR and is given in the same dosage regimen as Wellbutrin SR is for depression for 7–12 weeks.

Dosage Forms. **Tab** 75, 100 mg (Wellbutrin); **SR Tab** 100, 150 mg (Wellbutrin SR, Zyban).

Pharmacokinetics. Elimination half-life is 11–14 hr, but an active hydroxy metabolite has a half-life of >24 hr.

Adverse Reactions. Frequent adverse effects include insomnia, agitation, headache, and nausea. With dosages of ≤450 mg/day, seizures occur in 0.4% of patients, with a 1-yr cumulative incidence of 0.5%. Bupropion is contraindicated in patients with psychotic disorders (its dopamine agonist effect may cause increased psychotic symptoms), seizure disorders, anorexia, or bulimia, and in those receiving MAOIs. Bupropion seems to offer better safety in overdose than heterocyclic antidepressants.

Drug Interactions. Bupropion may increase levodopa side effects. Phenelzine may increase bupropion's acute adverse reactions.

CLOMIPRAMINE
Anafranil, Various

Pharmacology. Clomipramine is a 3-chloro analogue of imipramine that is a potent inhibitor of serotonin reuptake and, unlike other tricyclic antidepressants, also antagonizes dopaminergic neurotransmission. It has a specific indication for treatment of obsessive-compulsive disorder (OCD). Few patients experience complete OCD symptom relief; typically, about 40–50% of patients have marked symptom improvement. Although it is an effective antidepressant, its adverse effect profile makes other antidepressants preferred for this indication.[113–115] (*See* Antidepressants Comparison Chart.)

Adult Dosage. **PO for obsessive-compulsive disorder** 25 mg/day initially, increasing to 100 mg/day during the first 2 weeks, then gradually increasing over several weeks to a maximum of 250 mg/day. **PO as an antidepressant** 100–150 mg/day. Clomipramine can be given safely once daily at bedtime.

Dosage Forms. **Cap** 25, 50, 75 mg.

Pharmacokinetics. Antiobsessional effects are first seen at week 4, with maximum effects between weeks 10 and 18. Clomipramine is a highly lipophilic drug with a large first-pass effect and oral bioavailability of 36–62%. The major route of elimination is metabolism by demethylation, then hydroxylation and conjugation, with an elimination half-life of 20–24 hr.

Adverse Reactions. Clomipramine's adverse effect profile is similar to that of amitriptyline (ie, frequent sedation, anticholinergic effects, orthostatic hypotension, tremor, nausea, and sweating), but it has a much higher prevalence of sexual dysfunction and seizures. In controlled studies, 42% of patients experienced ejaculatory failure and 20% were impotent. Frequency of sexual dysfunction increases to >90% of patients when asked directly rather than relying on self-reporting.[116] Seizures occur in 0.5% of patients receiving 250 mg/day or less, and 2% of patients experience seizures with dosages above 250 mg/day. Clomipramine is contraindicated in patients who have received MAOIs within the past 14 days. Use with caution in patients with cardiovascular disease (eg, arrhythmias, angina, recent MI).

Drug Interactions. Drug interactions are the same as other TCAs. (*See* Heterocyclic Antidepressants.)

FLUOXETINE
Prozac

Pharmacology. Fluoxetine is a bicyclic antidepressant that is a selective and potent inhibitor of presynaptic reuptake of serotonin (an SSRI). It does not affect reuptake of norepinephrine or dopamine, and has a relative lack of affinity for muscarinic, histamine, α_1- and α_2-adrenergic, and serotonin receptors.[117]

Administration and Adult Dosage. (*See* Antidepressants Comparison Chart.) **PO for depression or OCD** 20 mg/day initially, administered in the morning. Increase dosage no more frequently than q 3–5 weeks. Divide higher dosages, with the last dose given in early afternoon. Although the maximum labeled dosage is 80 mg/day, 20 mg is equal in efficacy for major depression to higher dosages with the benefit of fewer adverse effects.[117,118] **PO for bulimia** 60 mg/day in the morning.

Special Populations. *Pediatric Dosage.* (<18 yr) safety and efficacy not established.

Geriatric Dosage. Reduce initial dosage and rate of dosage increase in the elderly. Single-dose studies suggest no difference in maintenance dosage in the elderly, but data from multiple-dose studies are needed. (*See* Notes.)

Other Conditions. Reduce initial dosage and rate of dosage increase in patients with hepatic impairment. Dosage adjustment in renal impairment is unnecessary.[117]

Dosage Forms. **Cap** 10, 20 mg; **Soln** 4 mg/mL.

Patient Instructions. This drug requires at least 2 weeks for a noticeable response in mood, and up to 4 weeks for full therapeutic benefit. Take fluoxetine in the morning or early afternoon. Inform your physician of any other medications you are taking.

Pharmacokinetics. *Onset and Duration.* Onset is delayed 2–4 weeks, which is similar to other antidepressants.

Serum Levels. Not established.

Fate. Oral bioavailability is 95%. It is 94% plasma protein bound with a V_d of 35 ± 21 L/kg; Cl is 0.58 ± 0.41 L/hr/kg, decreasing with repeated administration. The primary active metabolite is norfluoxetine; the metabolic rate may be under polygenic control.

$t_{\frac{1}{2}}$. (Fluoxetine) 1–3 days after a single oral dose, increasing with multiple doses to 4–5 days; (norfluoxetine) 7–15 days. Half-lives do not appear to be altered in the elderly or in patients with renal impairment. Patients with alcohol-induced cirrhosis have fluoxetine half-life increased by 100% and norfluoxetine half-life increased by 60% compared to controls.[117,119]

Adverse Reactions. Nausea, anxiety, insomnia, nervousness, diarrhea, anorexia, dry mouth, headache, and tremor occur with a frequency of over 10%. Delayed ejaculation and anorgasmia occurs with fluoxetine and all SSRIs in at least 30–55% of patients.[120,121] Unlike TCAs, which typically cause weight gain, fluoxetine dosages over 40 mg/day cause a weight loss of 1–2 kg within the first 6 weeks of treatment.[122] Fluoxetine rarely causes sedation except at dosages over 40 mg/day, and has no adverse cardiovascular or anticholinergic effects.[123] Initial case reports of patients developing new and intense suicidal preoccupation, agitation, and impulsiveness after several weeks of fluoxetine therapy have been adequately evaluated and found not to be directly drug related.[124]

Contraindications. Pregnancy. Concurrent use of an MAOI; 5 weeks must elapse between discontinuation of fluoxetine and starting an MAOI.[125]

Precautions. Use cautiously in the elderly and in patients with hepatic impairment. Use fluoxetine with caution in depressed patients with psychomotor agitation and anxiety, or anorexia and weight loss.

Drug Interactions. Fluoxetine is a potent inhibitor of CYP2D6, causing decreased metabolism and increased serum levels and adverse effects of many drugs, including most other antidepressants, antipsychotics, β-blockers, and type Ic antiarrhythmics. Fluoxetine's effect on other P450 isoenzymes has not yet been well defined.

Parameters to Monitor. Monitor liver function tests periodically during long-term therapy.

Notes. Fluoxetine is a useful alternative to tricyclic antidepressants because of its greater safety in overdose and relative lack of anticholinergic and cardiovascular effects. For severely depressed elderly patients, fluoxetine has been shown to be less effective than **nortriptyline.**[126] Fluoxetine and other SSRIs have demonstrated efficacy for obsessive-compulsive disorder and panic disorder. (*See* Antidepressants Comparison Chart.)

FLUVOXAMINE   Luvox

Pharmacology. Fluvoxamine has a selective and potent inhibitory effect on serotonergic presynaptic reuptake similar to fluoxetine. Although it is also an effective antidepressant, fluvoxamine has been marketed for use in obsessive-compulsive disorder (OCD). Fluvoxamine is equal in efficacy to **clomipramine** in OCD, causing fewer anticholinergic effects and sexual dysfunction, but more headache and insomnia.[127–129] (*See* Antidepressants Comparison Chart.)

Adult Dosage. PO for obsessive-compulsive disorder 50 mg/day initially, with a **maintenance dosage** of 100–300 mg/day. Give dosages over 100 mg/day in 2 divided doses. The elderly and those with hepatic impairment may require a lower starting dosage and slower dosage titration.

Pediatric Dosage. PO for obsessive-compulsive disorder (<8 yr) safety and efficacy not established; (8–17 yr) 25 mg hs initially, increasing in 25 mg/day increments q 4–7 days to a **usual maintenance dosage** of 50–200 mg/day. Dosages >50 mg/day should be divided into 2 doses, either equal or with a greater portion given hs.

Dosage Forms. Tab 25, 50, 100 mg.

Pharmacokinetics. Bioavailability is about 50% and not affected by food. Fluvoxamine is the least protein bound of the SSRIs (77%). On the same dosage, elderly patients have 40% higher serum concentrations than younger patients. Fluvoxamine is metabolized to inactive metabolites. Elimination half-life is about 16 hr in adults and 26 hr in the elderly.

Adverse Reactions. Frequent adverse effects include nausea, somnolence or insomnia, dry mouth, and sexual dysfunction.

Drug Interactions. Unlike other SSRIs, fluvoxamine is a potent inhibitor of CYP1A2, so increased levels and adverse effects are possible with warfarin, propranolol, metoprolol, caffeine, and theophylline. As with all SSRIs, do not administer fluvoxamine with MAOIs.

HETEROCYCLIC ANTIDEPRESSANTS

Pharmacology. Heterocyclic antidepressants (**tricyclic antidepressants** [TCAs], **amoxapine,** and **maprotiline**) are not general CNS stimulants, but rather have a very specific effect on neurotransmitters and receptor sensitivity. The primary pharmacologic effect of heterocyclic antidepressants is blockade of presynaptic reuptake of norepinephrine, with subsequent down-regulation of adrenergic receptors. Amoxapine, a metabolite of **loxapine,** retains some postsynaptic dopamine reuptake inhibition. Heterocyclic antidepressants have less effect on serotonergic activity than on other neurotransmitters.[130,131]

Administration and Adult Dosage. (*See* Antidepressants Comparison Chart for dosage ranges.) **PO for depression** initiate dosage at lower limit of range. Administer in divided doses to assess tolerance to side effects, then once daily hs can be used.[130,132] **Maintenance dosage** should be the same as the dosage necessary to treat the acute depressive episode.[133] **IM** rarely used (eg, surgical patient NPO for 1–2 days). **PO for chronic pain (amitriptyline** or **imipramine)** 10–25 mg/day initially; most patients respond to a dosage of 25–75 mg/day, although dosages up to 200 mg/day have been used.[134,135] (*See* Notes.)

Special Populations. *Pediatric Dosage.* Not recommended <12 yr except for childhood enuresis. **PO for enuresis (imipramine)** (<12 yr) 25–50 mg/day; (≥12 yr) up to 75 mg/day.[136] Imipramine maximum dosage in children is 2.5 mg/kg/day; however, use in prepubertal major depression disorder often requires up to 5 mg/kg/day with serum levels over 150 µg/L.[137]

Geriatric Dosage. (>65 yr) reduce initial dosage by at least 50% of adult dosage, and increase the dosage slowly.[138]

Other Conditions. Reduce initial dosage and rate of titration in patients with cardiovascular or hepatic disease.[139] During the last trimester of pregnancy, the mean dosage of TCAs required is 1.6 times that of nonpregnant women.[140]

Dosage Forms. (*See* Antidepressants Comparison Chart.)

Patient Instructions. (*See* Antidepressants Class Instructions.) These drugs usually take 2 weeks for a noticeable response in mood and up to 4 weeks for full therapeutic benefit. If you have small children, be sure to keep this medication in a secure place.

Pharmacokinetics. *Onset and Duration.* Physiologic symptoms of depression (eg, sleep and appetite disturbance, decreased energy) should show some improvement after 1 week, but mood (pessimism, hopelessness, anhedonia) often requires 2–4 weeks for response.

Serum Levels. **Nortriptyline** has a well-established therapeutic range and a curvilinear relationship of serum levels and response ("therapeutic window"). Other antidepressants show a linear response relationship.[141] (*See* Antidepressants Comparison Chart.)

Fate. Bioavailability is variable (30–70%) because of first-pass metabolism. Major metabolites for TCAs are desmethyl (for tertiary amines) and hydroxy compounds; rate may be genetically determined and result in 30-fold variation in steady-state levels in patients given the same dosage.[142]

$t_{1/2}$. (Tertiary amine TCAs) 10–25 hr; (secondary amine TCAs) 12–44 hr.[141]

Adverse Reactions. Sedation, postural hypotension, anticholinergic effects (dry mouth, blurred near vision, constipation, urinary retention, aggravation of narrow-angle glaucoma, and prostatic hypertrophy), weight gain, and cardiac effects (ECG changes and slowed AV conduction) are frequent. **Nortriptyline** is least likely to cause postural hypotension among the TCAs. *See* Antidepressants Comparison Chart for relative differences in frequency of common adverse reactions. Occasionally, fine hand tremor, seizures, cardiac arrhythmia, or cholestasis occur, as well as hypomanic or manic episodes in bipolar patients. Seizures and blood dyscrasias are rare.[143,144]

Contraindications. Cardiac arrhythmias, especially bundle-branch block.

Precautions. Use with caution in the elderly, in pregnancy, or in patients with CHF and angina pectoris, epilepsy, glaucoma, prostatic hypertrophy, or renal or liver disease. When discontinuing therapy, taper the heterocyclic antidepressant dosage to prevent cholinergic rebound. Cases of sudden cardiac death have been reported in children with attention deficit disorder who received **desipramine** in therapeutic or subtherapeutic dosages.[145] Ingestion of ≥ 1 g of a heterocylic antidepressant constitutes a life-threatening medical emergency. Limit the quantities dispensed to depressed patients with suicidal ideation. **Maprotiline** has an increased frequency of seizures at dosages >225 mg/day. **Amoxapine** has a metabolite with dopamine-blocking activity, resulting in possible extrapyramidal effects, tardive dyskinesia, endocrine effects, and neuroleptic malignant syndrome. Neither amoxapine nor maprotiline offers greater efficacy or safety in overdose than TCAs.

Drug Interactions. Many drug interactions occur. Use with caution with MAOIs. The antihypertensive effect of guanethidine, clonidine, and closely related drugs may be reduced.

Parameters to Monitor. Monitor hepatic and renal function tests periodically during long-term therapy. Obtain ECG in the elderly, children, and those with pre-existing heart disease. With **amoxapine,** monitor carefully for signs of tardive dyskinesia.

Notes. TCAs are commonly used in treating pain associated with diabetic neuropathy and postherpetic neuralgia; **amitriptyline, desipramine,** and **nortriptyline** have proven efficacy, but **SSRIs** are less effective.[134,135] (*See* Antidepressants Comparison Chart.)

MIRTAZAPINE   Remeron

Pharmacology. Mirtazapine is an antidepressant that antagonizes presynaptic α_2-adrenergic auto- and heteroreceptors that are responsible for controlling release of norepinephrine and serotonin (5-HT). It is also a potent antagonist of postsynaptic 5-HT$_2$ and 5-HT$_3$ receptors. The net outcome of these effects is increased noradrenergic activity and enhanced 5-HT activity, especially at 5-HT$_{1A}$ receptors. This unique mechanism of action preserves antidepressant efficacy, but minimizes many of the adverse effects common to both heterocyclic antidepressants and

SSRIs. Mirtazapine is effective in both moderate and severe major depression.[146,147] (*See* Antidepressants Comparison Chart.)

Adult Dosage. **PO for depression** 15 mg/day at bedtime initially, increasing at 1–2-week intervals to a maximum of 45 mg/day.

Dosage Forms. **Tab** 15, 30 mg.

Pharmacokinetics. Mirtazapine has an onset of clinical effect in 2–4 weeks, similar to other antidepressants. It has an elimination half-life of 20–40 hr, allowing once-daily administration at bedtime.

Adverse Reactions. Sedation, increased appetite, and weight gain are the most frequent side effects. Sedation is most frequent at lower doses (15 mg), decreasing in frequency with increasing dosage. Although two cases of agranulocytosis occurred in clinical trials, no specific or additional blood count monitoring is required. Mirtazapine has minimal cardiovascular and anticholinergic effects, and essentially lacks adverse GI effects, insomnia, and sexual dysfunction. Mirtazapine should not be used within 14 days of an MAOI. Cases of overdose up to 975 mg in combination with a benzodiazepine caused marked sedation, but no difficulty with cardiovascular or respiratory effects.

MONOAMINE OXIDASE INHIBITORS

Pharmacology. MAOIs are thought to exert their antidepressant action because of alterations in adrenergic and serotonergic receptor sensitivity. The most consistent findings during long-term MAOI therapy include down-regulation of β-adrenergic and adenyl cyclase activity. **Isocarboxazid** and **phenelzine** are hydrazine derivatives; **tranylcypromine** is a nonhydrazine.

Administration and Adult Dosage. **PO for depression** (isocarboxazid) 20–30 mg/day; (phenelzine) 45–90 mg/day; (tranylcypromine) 30–60 mg/day. Initiate dosage at the lower limit and titrate upward depending on tolerance to side effects. Dosage schedule should remain divided, usually bid or tid. Avoid bedtime administration because MAOIs can delay onset of sleep.

Special Populations. *Pediatric Dosage.* (<16 yr) not recommended.

Geriatric Dosage. Limited information, but decrease initial dosage by 50% because of orthostatic hypotension. Contraindicated in patients >60 yr.

Other Conditions. Reduce the initial dosage and rate of upward titration if the patient has taken a heterocyclic antidepressant within 7–10 days.

Dosage Forms. (Isocarboxazid) **Tab** 10 mg; (Phenelzine) **Tab** 15 mg; (tranylcypromine) **Tab** 10 mg.

Patient Instructions. (*See* Antidepressants Class Instructions.) This drug usually takes 2 weeks for noticeable response in mood and up to 4 weeks for full therapeutic benefit to occur. This drug may cause faintness or dizziness, especially after rising suddenly or standing for prolonged periods, or after exertion or alcohol intake. Nausea, vomiting, sweating, severe occipital headache, and stiff neck may be signs of a serious adverse effect and should be reported immediately. Avoid concurrent use of diet pills and cough and cold remedies, and restrict consumption of aged foods high in tyramine. (*See* Foods That Interact with MAO Inhibitors Chart.)

Pharmacokinetics. *Onset and Duration.* Onset 2 weeks; maximum improvement occurs after 3–4 weeks.[148]

Serum Levels. Not used clinically.

Fate. Termination of drug action is dependent on MAO regeneration, because the drugs or their active metabolites chemically combine with the MAO enzyme.

Adverse Reactions. Autonomic effects are frequent and not necessarily dose dependent; these include postural hypotension, dry mouth, and constipation. Drowsiness is more frequent with phenelzine; while overstimulation and agitation are more likely with tranylcypromine; isocarboxazid is mildly stimulating. Occasionally, delayed ejaculation, edema, skin rash, urinary retention, and blurred vision occur. MAOIs are much less likely than (TCAs) to cause weight gain, with tranylcypromine the least likely.[149]

Contraindications. Patients >60 yr; patients with confirmed or suspected cerebrovascular defect; cardiovascular disease; pheochromocytoma; history of liver disease or abnormal liver function tests.

Precautions. Always consider the possibility of suicide in depressed patients and take adequate precautions. Like other antidepressant drugs, MAOIs may switch bipolar patients to a hypomanic or manic state.

Drug Interactions. Postural hypotension may be increased with coadministration of antipsychotic, heterocyclic antidepressant, or antihypertensive drugs, and in patients with CHF. Avoid concurrent use with buspirone, heterocyclic antidepressants, meperidine, sympathomimetic drugs, SSRIs, and other MAOIs. A 1–2-week drug-free interval is necessary when switching from an MAOI to a TCA, but a drug-free interval is not necessary when switching from a TCA to an MAOI.[150] Although uncommon, hypertensive crisis may result from concurrent use of sympathomimetic amines or ingestion of high–tyramine-content food and drinks.[151,152] Avoid diets high in tyramine content. (*See* Foods That Interact with MAO Inhibitors Chart.)

Parameters to Monitor. Monitor blood pressure frequently.

Notes. MAOIs are excellent alternatives to heterocyclic antidepressants in major depressive disorder, are very effective in panic disorder, and are drugs of choice for atypical depression.[151,153]

FOODS THAT INTERACT WITH MAO INHIBITORS

Many fermented foods contain tyramine as a byproduct formed by the bacterial breakdown of the amino acid tyrosine; it can also be formed by parahydroxylation of phenylethylamine or dehydroxylation of DOPA and dopamine. Tyramine and some other amines found in food can cause hypertensive reactions in patients taking MAO inhibitors. MAO found in the GI tract inactivates tyramine; when drugs prevent this, exogenous tyramine and other monoamines are absorbed and release norepinephrine from sympathetic nerve endings and epinephrine from the adrenal gland. If sufficient quantities of these pressor compounds are released, palpitations, severe headache, and hypertensive crisis can result.

(*continued*)

FOODS THAT INTERACT WITH MAO INHIBITORS

FOOD CONTAINING TYRAMINE

Avocados	Particularly if overripe.
Bananas	Reactions can occur if eaten in large amounts; tyramine levels high in peel.
Bean curd	Fermented bean curd, fermented soya bean, soya bean pastes, soy sauces, and miso soup, prepared from fermented bean curd, all contain tyramine in large amounts; miso soup has caused reactions.
Beer and ale	Major domestic brands do not contain appreciable amounts; some imported brands have had high levels. Nonalcoholic beer may contain tyramine and should be avoided.
Caviar	Safe if vacuum-packed and eaten fresh or refrigerated only briefly.
Cheese	Reactions possible with most, except unfermented varieties such as cottage cheese. In others, tyramine concentration is higher near rind and close to fermentation holes.
Figs	Particularly if overripe.
Fish	Safe if fresh; dried products should not be eaten. Caution required in restaurants. Vacuum-packed products are safe if eaten promptly or refrigerated only briefly.
Liver	Safe if very fresh, but rapidly accumulates tyramine; caution required in restaurants.
Meat	Safe if known to be fresh; caution required in restaurants.
Milk products	Milk and yogurt appear to be safe.
Protein extracts	See also soups; avoid liquid and powdered protein dietary supplements.
Sausage	Fermented varieties such as bologna, pepperoni, and salami have a high tyramine content.
Shrimp paste	Contains large amounts of tyramine.
Soups	May contain protein extracts and should be avoided.
Soy sauce	Contains large amounts of tyramine; reactions have occurred with teriyaki.
Wines	Generally do not contain tyramine, but many reactions have been reported with Chianti, champagne, and other wines.
Yeast extracts	Dietary supplements (eg, Marmite) contain large amounts. Yeast in baked goods, however, is safe.

FOOD NOT CONTAINING TYRAMINE

Caffeine	A weak pressor agent; large amounts may cause reactions.
Chocolate	Contains phenylethylamine, a pressor agent that can cause reactions in large amounts.
Fava beans	(Broad beans, "Italian" green beans) Contain dopamine, a pressor amine, particularly when overripe.
Ginseng	Some preparations have caused headache, tremulousness, and manic-like symptoms.

(continued)

FOODS THAT INTERACT WITH MAO INHIBITORS

Liqueurs	Reactions reported with some (eg, Chartreuse, Drambuie); cause unknown.
New Zealand prickly spinach	Single case report; patient ate large amounts.
Whiskey	Reactions have occurred; cause unknown.

For further information, consult Lippman SB, Nash K. Monoamine oxidase inhibitor update. Potential adverse food and drug interactions. *Drug Saf* 1990;5:195–204.
Anon. Foods interacting with MAO inhibitors. Med Lett Drugs Ther *1989;31:11–2, reproduced with permission.*

NEFAZODONE   Serzone

Pharmacology. Nefazodone is a postsynaptic serotonin 5-HT_{2A} antagonist and presynaptic serotonin reuptake inhibitor. These two serotonergic effects make it different from SSRIs and tricyclic antidepressants (TCAs).[154–157] (*See* Antidepressants Comparison Chart.)

Adult Dosage. PO for depression 100 mg bid initially (50 mg bid in the elderly), increasing q 4–7 days to the effective dosage range of 150–300 mg bid.

Dosage Forms. Tab 50, 100, 150, 200, 250 mg.

Pharmacokinetics. Nefazodone has an oral bioavailability of about 20%. Single-dose studies in the elderly show a 100% larger AUC, and with multiple doses, the AUC differences decrease to 10–20% above younger populations. It is >99% protein bound and extensively metabolized, with a dose-dependent elimination half-life ranging from about 1–2.3 hr in young patients, modestly prolonged in the elderly and 2–3 times longer in hepatic disease. The major active metabolite, hydroxynefazodone, has a half-life ranging from 1.2–1.6 hr in young and elderly patients, increasing to 2–4 hr with hepatic disease. Renal impairment does not markedly affect nefazodone pharmacokinetics.

Adverse Reactions. Although chemically similar to trazodone, it causes less sedation and orthostatic hypotension, and its lower α-adrenergic blockade makes priapism much less likely (no cases reported). Frequent adverse effects include sedation, dry mouth, nausea, and dizziness. Unlike SSRIs, nefazodone's effects on sexual function, agitation, tremor, insomnia, and weight are no different from placebo.

Drug Interactions. Nefazodone is a potent inhibitor of the CYP3A4 isoenzyme and a weak inhibitor of the CYP2D6 isoenzyme. Drug interactions of concern thus include astemizole and the triazolobenzodiazepines (ie, alprazolam, triazolam, midazolam). A 1- to 2-week washout period is recommended when converting a patient to or from a MAOI and nefazodone.

PAROXETINE   Paxil

Pharmacology. Paroxetine is a highly selective and potent inhibitor of serotonin reuptake (an SSRI) similar to fluoxetine.[127,158–164] (*See* Antidepressants Comparison Chart.)

Adult Dosage. PO for depression 20 mg/day; a few patients require 30–50 mg/day for full efficacy. **PO for panic disorder** 10 mg/day initially. **PO for obsessive-compulsive disorder** 20 mg/day initially. The starting dosage for all uses in elderly patients and those with marked renal or hepatic impairment is 10 mg/day. **Maintenance dosage** for both panic and obsessive-compulsive disorders is 40 mg/day to a maximum of 60 mg/day, preferably as a single dose in the morning or evening. For the elderly or those with severe renal or hepatic impairment, the maximum dosage is 40 mg/day.

Dosage Forms. Tab 10, 20, 30, 40 mg; **Susp** 2 mg/mL.

Pharmacokinetics. Paroxetine is completely orally bioavailable; protein binding is 93–95%. Unlike fluoxetine, paroxetine is metabolized to inactive metabolites and has an elimination half-life of 24 hr.

Adverse Reactions. Paroxetine causes the typical SSRI adverse effects of nausea, sexual dysfunction, and headache, but is more likely to cause sedation than insomnia and may cause more delay of orgasm or ejaculation and more impotence than other SSRIs.[165] Like the other SSRIs, it is much safer in overdose than tricyclic antidepressants.

Drug Interactions. Paroxetine is a potent inhibitor of CYP2D6, so most other antidepressants, antipsychotics, β-blockers, and type Ic antiarrhythmics may have increased serum levels and adverse effects when paroxetine is combined with these drugs. Do not use paroxetine within 14 days of using an MAOI.

SERTRALINE   Zoloft

Pharmacology. Sertraline is an SSRI similar to fluoxetine, which indirectly results in a down-regulation of β-adrenergic receptors. It has no clinically important effect on noradrenergic or histamine receptors and no effect on MAO. It lacks stimulant, cardiovascular, anticholinergic, and convulsant effects. Sertraline has antidepressant effects equal to tricyclic antidepressants (TCAs) and fluoxetine, and may have anorectic effects and efficacy in obsessive-compulsive disorder.[131,166–168] (*See* Antidepressants Comparison Chart.)

Adult Dosage. PO for depression 50 mg/day initially, increasing if necessary at weekly intervals to a maximum of 200 mg/day in a single dose in the morning or evening.

Dosage Forms. Tab 25, 50, 100 mg.

Pharmacokinetics. Sertraline has an oral bioavailability of 36%, and, when it is taken with food, both peak serum concentrations and total absorption increase by 30–40%. Peak serum concentrations are reached in 6–8 hr. Sertraline concentrations in breast milk are the lowest of the SSRIs and produce minimal serum levels in the breastfed infant.[169] Its primary metabolite is N-desmethylsertraline, which has 5–10 times less activity than sertraline as an SSRI and has no demonstrated antidepressant activity. Cl is decreased by up to 40% in the elderly. Steady-state half-life is 27 hr.

Adverse Reactions. Frequent adverse effects include nausea, diarrhea, ejaculatory delay, tremor, and increased sweating. It causes less agitation, anxiety, and insomnia than fluoxetine and is a less potent inhibitor of the CYP2D6 isoenzyme at a dosage of 50 mg/day. Use with caution in patients with renal or hepatic impairment, and do not use it within 14 days of using an MAOI. SIADH has been reported.[170]

TRAZODONE HYDROCHLORIDE
Desyrel, Various

Pharmacology. Trazodone shares some effects with other antidepressants, but it causes selective inhibition of serotonin reuptake and blocks postsynaptic serotonin-$5HT_2$ and α-adrenergic receptors.

Administration and Adult Dosage. **PO as an antidepressant** 150 mg/day initially, increasing in 50 mg/day increments q 3–4 days. Trazodone is less potent than most antidepressants; therefore, do not abandon a trial of trazodone without reaching a dosage of 400–600 mg/day for inpatients. Maximum dosage in outpatients is 400 mg/day. Administration after meals minimizes sedation and postural hypotension.[171,172] **PO as a hypnotic** 50–100 mg is commonly used, often in combination with an SSRI.[173]

Special Populations. *Pediatric Dosage.* (<18 yr) safety and efficacy not established.

Geriatric Dosage. Sedation and orthostatic hypotension require initial dosage reduction by 33–50% and slower rate of titration.

Other Conditions. Dosage adjustments in patients with hepatic or renal impairment may be prudent, although limited experience, thus far, does not suggest that major dosage adjustments are necessary.[142,172] Base dosage on ideal body weight in obese patients.

Dosage Forms. **Tab** 50, 100, 150, 300 mg.

Patient Instructions. (*See* Antidepressants Class Instructions.) Take trazodone after a meal.

Pharmacokinetics. *Onset and Duration.* Onset is delayed, similar to heterocyclic antidepressant drugs.

Serum Levels. Not established.

Fate. The drug is well absorbed after oral administration; relative bioavailability is 72–91%. The rate of absorption is decreased with food, but the total amount absorbed is unchanged. V_d is 1–2 L/kg; Cl is 0.13 ± 0.04 L/hr/kg. V_d is larger and Cl lower in the elderly and in obesity. Metabolism is extensive, with one active metabolite.[119,141]

$t_{1/2}$. 5.9 ± 1.9 hr, prolonged in the elderly and obesity.[119]

Adverse Reactions. Sedation and postural hypotension are frequent. Trazodone does not affect AV conduction, nor does it cause tachycardia as do heterocyclic antidepressants. Rarely, trazodone may aggravate ventricular arrhythmias[123] and cause nonsexual penile tumescence and priapism. Priapism can be treated with an α-adrenergic agonist; surgery is not required if treated promptly.[174] Trazodone is much safer in overdose than heterocyclic antidepressants; overdoses of 9 g of trazodone alone have been survived without medical sequelae.

Contraindications. Pregnancy; cardiac ventricular arrhythmia; initial recovery phase of myocardial infarction.

Precautions. Always consider the possibility of suicide in depressed patients and take adequate precautions. Use with caution or avoid in patients immediately post-MI, or with pre-existing cardiac disease.

Drug Interactions. Concurrent use with other CNS depressants may potentiate the sedation caused by trazodone. Use with MAOIs is not well studied, so the combination is best avoided.

Parameters to Monitor. Obtain WBC count and differential in any patient who develops fever, sore throat, or other sign of infection.

Notes. Trazodone is a useful choice for patients who cannot tolerate anticholinergic effects or who have CHF, angina pectoris, or bundle-branch block in which heterocyclic antidepressants are contraindicated. Trazodone is used rarely as an antidepressant, but commonly as a hypnotic.[175] (*See* Antidepressants Comparison Chart.)

VENLAFAXINE   Effexor

Pharmacology. Venlafaxine is a potent reuptake inhibitor of both serotonin and norepinephrine like many of the tricyclic antidepressants, but lacks effects on muscarinic, α-adrenergic, or histamine receptors.[176–179] (*See* Antidepressants Comparison Chart.)

Adult Dosage. **PO for depression** (immediate-release) 75 mg bid or tid initially, increasing q 4–7 days to an effective antidepressant dosage of 225–375 mg/day in 2 or 3 divided doses; (sustained-release) 75 mg once daily initially, increasing in increments of up to 75 mg/day at intervals of 4 or more days to a maximum of 225 mg/day. The sustained-release preparation does not reduce side effects, but allows once-daily administration. Patients with renal impairment or on hemodialysis require a 25–50% dosage reduction.

Dosage Forms. **Tab** 25, 37.5, 50, 75, 100 mg; **SR Cap** 37.5, 75, 100 mg (Effexor XR).

Pharmacokinetics. Venlafaxine is well absorbed orally; food has no effect on absorption. Serum concentrations in elderly patients are no different from those in younger patients. Unlike SSRIs, venlafaxine has minimal protein binding (27–30%). It undergoes extensive hepatic metabolism. Venlafaxine has an elimination half-life of 5 hr, and one major active metabolite has an 11-hr half-life. Venlafaxine exhibits linear pharmacokinetics over the recommended dosage range, and steady-state is reached in 3 days.

Adverse Reactions. Frequent adverse effects include expected serotonin-related effects (eg, nausea, headache, insomnia or somnolence, and sexual dysfunction). At higher dosages (375 mg/day), venlafaxine is unique in causing a consistent but mild elevation in diastolic blood pressure (6 mm Hg). Regular blood pressure monitoring is required for all patients.

Drug Interactions. Venlafaxine is not a potent inhibitor of the cytochrome P450 enzyme system, making it different from most of the SSRIs. It should not be used in patients who have received MAOIs within the past 14 days.

ANTIDEPRESSANTS COMPARISON CHART

CLASS AND DRUG	DOSAGE FORMS	USUAL DAILY ADULT DOSAGE RANGE (MG)	THERAPEUTIC SERUM LEVELS (μG/L)	RELATIVE FREQUENCY OF SIDE EFFECTS		
				Sedation	Anticholinergic	Orthostatic Hypotension
α₂-ADRENERGIC BLOCKERS						
Mirtazapine Remeron	Tab 15, 30 mg.	15-45	a	Moderate	None	None
CHLOROPROPIOPHENONES						
Bupropion Wellbutrin Zyban	Tab 75, 100 mg SR Tab 100, 150 mg.	300-450	a	None	None	None
DIBENZOXAZEPINES^B						
Amoxapine Asendin Various	Tab 25, 50, 100, 150 mg.	300-600	a	Low	Low	Low
MONOAMINE OXIDASE INHIBITORS (MAOIS)						
Phenelzine Nardil	Tab 15 mg.	45-90	a	Moderate	Low	Very High
Tranylcypromine Parnate	Tab 10 mg.	30-60	a	Low	Low	Very High
SELECTIVE SEROTONIN REUPTAKE INHIBITORS (SSRIS)						
Citalopram Celexa	Tab 20, 40 mg.	20-60	a	Very Low	Very Low	None

(continued)

ANTIDEPRESSANTS COMPARISON CHART (continued)

CLASS AND DRUG	DOSAGE FORMS	USUAL DAILY ADULT DOSAGE RANGE (MG)	THERAPEUTIC SERUM LEVELS (μG/L)	RELATIVE FREQUENCY OF SIDE EFFECTS		
				Sedation	Anticholinergic	Orthostatic Hypotension
Fluoxetine Prozac	Cap 10, 20 mg Soln 4 mg/mL.	10–80	a	None	Very Low	None
Fluvoxamine Luvox	Tab 25, 50, 100 mg.	100–300[c]	a	None	None	None
Paroxetine Paxil	Tab 10, 20, 30, 40 mg Susp 2 mg/mL.	20–50	a	Low	Low	Very Low
Sertraline Zoloft	Tab 25, 50, 100 mg.	50–200	a	None	None	None
SEROTONIN NOREPINEPHRINE REUPTAKE INHIBITORS (SNRIS)						
Venlafaxine Effexor Effexor XR	Tab 25, 37.5, 50, 75, 100 mg. SR Cap 37.5, 75, 100 mg.	225–375	a	Very Low	Very Low	Very Low
TETRACYCLICS[B]						
Maprotiline Ludiomil Various	Tab 25, 50, 75 mg.	150–225	200–300[a]	Moderate	Moderate	Moderate
TRIAZOLOPYRIDINES						
Trazodone Desyrel Various	Tab 50, 100, 150, 300 mg.	200–400	a	High	Very Low	High

(continued)

ANTIDEPRESSANTS COMPARISON CHART (continued)

CLASS AND DRUG	DOSAGE FORMS	USUAL DAILY ADULT DOSAGE RANGE (MG)	THERAPEUTIC SERUM LEVELS (μG/L)	RELATIVE FREQUENCY OF SIDE EFFECTS		
				Sedation	Anticholinergic	Orthostatic Hypotension
Nefazodone Serzone	Tab 50, 100, 150, 200, 250 mg.	300–600	a	Moderate	Very low	Moderate
TRICYCLICS (TCAs)[c]						
Amitriptyline Elavil Various	Tab 10, 25, 50, 75, 100, 150 mg Inj 10 mg/mL.	150–300	75–175[d]	High	High	High
Clomipramine Anafranil Various	Cap 25, 50, 75 mg.	100–250[c] 100–150[e]	a	High	High	High
Desipramine Norpramin Various	Cap 25, 50 mg Tab 10, 25, 50, 75, 100, 150 mg.	150–300	100–160	Low	Low	Moderate
Doxepin Adapin Sinequan Various	Cap 10, 25, 50, 75, 100, 150 mg Soln 10 mg/mL.	150–300	110–250[d]	High	Moderate	High
Imipramine Tofranil Janimine Various	Tab 10, 25, 50 mg Inj 12.5 mg/mL Cap (as pamoate) 75, 100, 125, 150 mg.	150–300	>200[d]	Moderate	Moderate	High

(continued)

447

ANTIDEPRESSANTS COMPARISON CHART (continued)

CLASS AND DRUG	DOSAGE FORMS	USUAL DAILY ADULT DOSAGE RANGE (MG)	THERAPEUTIC SERUM LEVELS (µG/L)	RELATIVE FREQUENCY OF SIDE EFFECTS		
				Sedation	Anticholinergic	Orthostatic Hypotension
Nortriptyline Aventyl Pamelor Various	Cap 10, 25, 50, 75 mg Soln 2 mg/mL.	100–200	50–150	Moderate	Moderate	Low
Protriptyline Vivactil Various	Tab 5, 10 mg.	30–60	70–260[a]	Very Low	Moderate	Moderate
Trimipramine Surmontil	Cap 25, 50, 100 mg.	150–300	[a]	Moderate	Moderate	High

[a]Not well established.
[b]Amoxapine, maprotiline, and the tricyclic antidepressants are categorized together here as heterocyclic antidepressants because their therapeutic and side effect profiles are similar.
[c]For obsessive-compulsive disorder.
[d]Includes active metabolites.
[e]Major depression.
From references 109, 114, 123, 127, 128, 141, 142, 146, 147, 149, 154, 159, 160, 171, 178, 180, and 181.

Antipsychotic Drugs

Class Instructions: Antipsychotics. This drug may cause drowsiness. Until the extent of this effect is known, use caution when driving, operating machinery, or performing other tasks requiring mental alertness. Avoid excessive concurrent use of alcohol or other drugs which cause drowsiness.

ANTIPSYCHOTIC DRUGS

Pharmacology. Antipsychotic efficacy is most likely related to blockade of post-synaptic dopaminergic receptors in the mesolimbic and prefrontal cortex of the brain, although other neurotransmitter systems are also involved.[182]

Administration and Adult Dosage. (*See* Antipsychotic Drugs Comparison Chart for oral dosage ranges.) Initiate therapy with divided doses until therapeutic dosage is found, then, for most patients, once-daily hs administration is preferred. For maintenance therapy, decrease acute dosage by 25% q 3 months, with a target maintenance dosage being 50–67% of the acute treatment dosage.[183] Recent concern has focused on the need to establish a minimum effective dosage for antipsychotic drugs, and treatment regimens at the low end of the dosage range are preferred. Oral dosages of high-potency antipsychotics (eg, **fluphenazine, haloperidol**) in the range of 5–20 mg/day are better tolerated and equal in efficacy to dosages above 20 mg/day.[184] Most patients can be given a maintenance dosage of one-half the acute dosage by the end of 1 yr, although 10–15% of chronically ill patients require a maintenance dosage of more than 15 mg/day of **haloperidol** or its equivalent.[185,186] For manic episodes, no additional benefit is achieved with dosages over 10 mg/day of haloperidol.[187]

Special Populations. *Pediatric Dosage.* As with adults, dosage is determined primarily by titration to individual response. No precise dosage range exists, but in general, the initial dosage is lower and should be increased more gradually in children.

Geriatric Dosage. Initial dosage is 20–25% of the dosage used in younger adults. Typical starting dosages in the elderly are **haloperidol** 0.5–2 mg/day, or **thioridazine** 10–50 mg/day. Dosage adjustments must also be done more slowly than in younger adults.[188]

Other Conditions. Dosages in the lower range are sufficient for most elderly patients, and the rate of dosage titration should be slower.

Dosage Forms. (*See* Antipsychotic Drugs Comparison Chart.)

Patient Instructions. (*See* Antipsychotics Class Instructions.) These drugs usually take several weeks for clinical response and up to 8 weeks for full therapeutic response.

Pharmacokinetics. *Onset and Duration.* Onset of antipsychotic activity is variable, with noticeable response requiring days to weeks.

Serum Levels. Correlation of serum levels with clinical response is not yet consistently established. The best evidence exists for **haloperidol,** with serum concentrations of 5–15 μg/L (13–40 nmol/L) correlating well with therapeutic effects in adult psychotic patients, and an increasing risk of adverse effects and decreased efficacy when steady-state concentrations exceed 15 μg/L.[189,190]

Fate. **Haloperidol** is well absorbed; peak serum levels are achieved 2–6 hr after liquid or tablets, and within 30 min after IM. Oral bioavailability of haloperidol is 60–70%. Haloperidol is extensively metabolized, with one active hydroxy metabolite. **Chlorpromazine** and other phenothiazines are well absorbed, but undergo extensive and variable presystemic metabolism in the gut wall and liver; over 20 chlorpromazine metabolites with varying activity have been identified in human plasma.

t½. Serum half-lives have no clinical correlation with biologic half-lives for antipsychotic drugs. **Chlorpromazine** serum half-life is 30 hr, **thioridazine** 4–10 hr, **thiothixene** 34 hr, and **haloperidol** 12–24 hr. Of more clinical importance is that steady-state CNS levels and tissue saturation allow once-daily administration of all antipsychotic drugs.[142]

Adverse Reactions. (*See* Antipsychotic Drugs Comparison Chart for relative frequency of common adverse reactions.) Frequently, sedation, extrapyramidal effects (eg, parkinsonism, dystonic reactions, akathisia), tardive dyskinesia, anticholinergic effects (eg, dry mouth, blurred vision, constipation, urinary retention), photosensitivity, and postural hypotension occur. Occasionally, weight gain, amenorrhea, galactorrhea, ejaculatory disturbance, neuroleptic malignant syndrome, agranulocytosis, skin rash, cholestatic jaundice, and skin or eye pigmentation occur. Rarely, seizures, thermoregulatory impairment, and slowed AV conduction occur. Low-potency drugs are more likely to cause sedation, anticholinergic effects, and orthostatic hypotension, whereas high-potency drugs cause more extrapyramidal effects. Tardive dyskinesia is a long-term adverse effect, untreatable, and sometimes irreversible. Tardive dyskinesia occurs at a 4% yearly incidence for at least the first 5–6 yr of treatment. Neuroleptic malignant syndrome (ie, fever, extrapyramidal rigidity, autonomic instability, alterations in consciousness) occurs more frequently with high-potency antipsychotics, with a prevalence of 1.4% and a fatality rate of 4%.[184,191,192]

Contraindications. Coma; circulatory collapse or severe hypotension; bone marrow depression; history of blood dyscrasia.

Precautions. Use cautiously in patients with myasthenia gravis, Parkinson's disease, seizure disorders, or hepatic disease.

Drug Interactions. Barbiturates may enhance phenothiazine metabolism; carbamazepine may enhance haloperidol metabolism. Phenothiazines may decrease efficacy of guanethidine or guanadrel or may have additive hypotensive effects with hypotensive drugs. Phenothiazines may inhibit the antiparkinson activity of levodopa. Haloperidol may increase the CNS toxicity of lithium. Combined use of haloperidol and methyldopa may result in dementia.

Notes. (*See also* Prochlorperazine Salts in the Antiemetics section for antiemetic uses.)

CLOZAPINE
Clozaril

Pharmacology. Clozapine is an atypical antipsychotic drug that is chemically similar to loxapine and has unique pharmacologic effects and indications, as well as very serious adverse effects. Whereas typical antipsychotic drugs exert their effects primarily via blockade of dopamine-D_2 receptors, clozapine has effects on several dopamine and serotonin receptors. Its high serotonin-$5HT_2$ to dopamine-D_2 ratio is the likely explanation for its unique efficacy. Compared to traditional antipsychotic drugs, clozapine is more effective for negative symptoms of schizophrenia, is more effective in treatment-resistant patients, and rarely causes extrapyramidal effects.[193–196]

Adult Dosage. PO 100–200 mg tid is effective for most patients, but some may require up to 900 mg/day. A therapeutic trial of 12–24 weeks is required for the full therapeutic effect to become apparent.

Dosage Forms. **Tab** 25, 100 mg.

Pharmacokinetics. Clozapine is nearly completely absorbed after oral administration, with about 30% oral bioavailability because of extensive first-pass metabolism. Clozapine is 95% plasma protein bound; with multiple doses, its elimination half-life is 12 hr.[197]

Adverse Reactions. Frequent adverse effects include sedation, orthostatic hypotension, anticholinergic effects, fever, and excessive salivation. Seizures are dose related, with a frequency up to 5% in the therapeutic dosage range and a 1-yr cumulative incidence of 10%. Agranulocytosis is the major adverse effect of concern, occurring in 0.8% of patients after 1 yr.[198] Most cases of agranulocytosis occur within the first 3 months of therapy. Patients must have a baseline WBC count and differential before initiating therapy, and mandatory weekly WBC monitoring for the first 6 months, then q 2 weeks throughout treatment and for 4 weeks after discontinuation. Substantial weight gain has been reported in most patients receiving clozapine. (*See* Antipsychotic Drugs Comparison Chart.)

HALOPERIDOL DECANOATE
Haldol Decanoate, Various

Pharmacology. Haloperidol decanoate (HD) is the preferred long-acting depot antipsychotic drug. Depot antipsychotics are indicated only for patients who demonstrate good response, but who are consistently drug-noncompliant with resultant frequent psychotic relapses. Depot antipsychotics provide fewer relapses and hospitalizations, stable serum drug levels, and side effects equal to oral antipsychotic drugs. HD can be given q 4 weeks; **fluphenazine decanoate** (FD) is similar in efficacy and adverse effects, but it must be administered q 2 weeks. Do not use HD or FD to treat acute psychotic symptoms, but rather, only after a patient is stabilized on an oral antipsychotic drug.[199–203]

Adult Dosage. IM do not exceed an initial HD dosage of 100 mg, with a target monthly dosage 20 times the oral haloperidol daily dosage. An IM loading dose technique has been described that gives 20 times the daily oral dosage, using 100–200 mg of depot q 3–7 days to reach the calculated amount, with a maximum of 450 mg. In geriatric or hepatically impaired patients, use a monthly HD dose of

15 times the oral haloperidol dosage. Experience with HD doses greater than 500 mg is limited, and injections >5 mL should be divided into 2 equal portions given at two sites. Oral haloperidol supplementation may be necessary between monthly injections to treat re-emergence of psychotic symptoms until steady-state concentrations are reached.

Dosage Forms. Inj 50, 100 mg/mL.

Pharmacokinetics. After IM administration of HD, esterases cleave the decanoate chain to release the active drug. Peak serum concentrations of haloperidol occur in 3–9 days, with an apparent half-life of 3 weeks; steady-state levels are reached after 12–16 weeks.

Adverse Reactions. There is no evidence that HD causes adverse effects with a frequency different from oral haloperidol.

OLANZAPINE   Zyprexa

Pharmacology. Olanzapine is an atypical antipsychotic agent that is a potent serotonin-5HT$_2$ and dopamine-D$_2$ antagonist. It also has anticholinergic and histamine H$_1$-receptor antagonistic effects which may account for some of its side effects. (*See* Antipsychotic Drugs Comparison Chart.)

Adult Dosage. **PO for psychotic disorders** 5–10 mg/day initially (5 mg/day in patients >65 yr, debilitated patients, or those with a predisposition to hypotensive reactions). Increase in 5 mg/day increments at ≥7-day intervals. **Usual maintenance dosage** 10–15 mg/day, although dosages >10 mg/day are generally no more effective than 10 mg/day.

Dosage Forms. Tab 2.5, 5, 7.5, 15 mg.

Pharmacokinetics. Olanzapine is well absorbed orally; food has no effect, but bioavailability is about 60% because of a first-pass effect. It is 93% plasma protein bound and has a V$_d$ of about 1000 L. The drug is hepatically metabolized, probably by CYP1A2 and CYP2D6. Only 7% is excreted unchanged in urine. Half-life is 30 hr.

Adverse Reactions. Frequent adverse effects include drowsiness, agitation, nervousness, orthostatic hypotension, dizziness, tachycardia, headache, rhinitis, constipation, akathisia, and weight gain. As with other atypical antipsychotic drugs, weight gain is the most troublesome long-term adverse effect, often affecting compliance.

Drug Interactions. Inducers of CYP2D6 may decrease olanzapine serum levels. Olanzapine does not appear to affect cytochrome P450 enzymes.

PIMOZIDE   Orap

Pharmacology. Pimozide is indicated for the treatment of Tourette's disorder. Although structurally different from other antipsychotic drugs, pimozide shares their ability to block dopaminergic receptors. Its lack of effect on norepinephrine receptors led to the hope that pimozide would have a more favorable adverse effect profile than other antipsychotic drugs. **Haloperidol** is the drug of choice for Tourette's disorder.[204,205]

Adult Dosage. PO 1–2 mg/day in divided doses initially, with dosage increased every other day up to a maximum of 20 mg/day. Most patients who respond require 10 mg/day or less. Periodically attempt to decrease the dosage and withdraw treatment.

Pediatric Dosage. 0.05 mg/kg/day initially (preferably hs), increasing q 3 days to a maximum of 0.2 mg/kg or 10 mg daily.

Dosage Forms. Tab 2 mg.

Pharmacokinetics. Pimozide is about 50% absorbed orally. It undergoes extensive first-pass metabolism in the liver to two metabolites with unknown activity. The elimination half-life averages 55 hr.

Adverse Reactions. The relative frequency of adverse effects of pimozide and haloperidol is similar, and pimozide remains an alternative to haloperidol for Tourette's disorder.

RISPERIDONE   Risperdal

Pharmacology. Risperidone is a potent serotonin-5-HT_2 antagonist with dopamine-D_2 antagonism. Whereas typical antipsychotics are dopamine antagonists, the additional serotonin antagonism increases efficacy for negative symptoms of schizophrenia and reduces the likelihood of extrapyramidal symptoms. Initial evidence also suggests that risperidone is more effective than traditional antipsychotic drugs for treatment-resistant schizophrenic patients.[206–209] (*See* Antipsychotic Drugs Comparison Chart.)

Adult Dosage. PO 1 mg bid initially (0.5 mg bid in the elderly or patients with severe renal or hepatic impairment), increasing q 2–4 days to the usual effective dosage of 4–6 mg/day in 1 or 2 doses. Occasionally, dosages above 6 mg/day may be necessary, but adverse effects increase and efficacy can be less. The solution may be mixed with water, coffee, orange juice, or low-fat milk; it should not be mixed with cola or tea.

Dosage Forms. Tab 1, 2, 3, 4 mg; Soln 1 mg/mL.

Pharmacokinetics. Risperidone is well absorbed orally. The free fraction of risperidone in serum increases in hepatic disease, necessitating lower dosages. It is metabolized by CYP2D6 to an active metabolite. Risperidone's elimination half-life is 3 hr; its active metabolite has a half-life of 24 hr. The half-lives of one or both are prolonged in patients with renal disease.[210]

Adverse Reactions. Frequent dose-related adverse effects include extrapyramidal effects, orthostatic hypotension, headache, rhinitis, and insomnia.

Drug Interactions. Inhibitors of CYP2D6 can increase risperidone levels and adverse effects.

ANTIPSYCHOTIC DRUGS COMPARISON CHART

DRUG AND CLASS	DOSAGE FORMS	ADULT ORAL DOSAGE RANGE (MG/DAY)	ORAL EQUIVALENT ANTIPSYCHOTIC DOSE (MG)	USUAL SINGLE IM DOSE	RELATIVE FREQUENCY OF SIDE EFFECTS			
					Sedation	Anticholinergic	Extrapyramidal	Orthostatic Hypotension
LOW POTENCY								
Chlorpromazine Thorazine Various	Soln 30, 100 mg/mL Syrup 2 mg/mL Tab 10, 25, 50, 100, 200 mg Inj 25 mg/mL Supp 25, 100 mg SR Cap not recommended.	50–1200	100	25–50	High	Moderate	Moderate	High
Thioridazine Mellaril Various	Soln 30, 100 mg/mL Susp 5, 20 mg/mL Tab 10, 15, 25, 50, 100, 150 200 mg.	50–800	100	—	High	High	Low	High
INTERMEDIATE POTENCY								
Loxapine Loxitane Various	Cap 5, 10, 25, 50 mg Soln 25 mg/mL Inj 50 mg/mL.	20–250	10	12.5–50	Low	Low	Moderate	Low

(continued)

ANTIPSYCHOTIC DRUGS COMPARISON CHART (continued)

DRUG AND CLASS	DOSAGE FORMS	ADULT ORAL DOSAGE RANGE (MG/DAY)	ORAL EQUIVALENT ANTIPSYCHOTIC DOSE (MG)	USUAL SINGLE IM DOSE	RELATIVE FREQUENCY OF SIDE EFFECTS			
					Sedation	Anticholinergic	Extrapyramidal	Orthostatic Hypotension
Molindone Moban	Tab 5, 10, 25, 50, 100 mg Soln 20 mg/mL.	25–225	10	—	Very Low	Low	Moderate	Low
ATYPICAL								
Clozapine Clozaril	Tab 25, 100 mg.	300–900	50	—	High	High	Very Low	High
Olanzapine Zyprexa	Tab 2.5, 5, 7.5, 10 mg.	10–15	—	—	Low	Low	Very Low	Low
Quetiapine Seroquel	Tab 25, 100, 200 mg.	150–500	—	—	Moderate	Low	Very Low	Low
Risperidone Risperdal	Tab 1, 2, 3, 4 mg Soln 1 mg/mL.	4–6[a]	—	—	Very Low	Very Low	Low[a]	Moderate
HIGH POTENCY								
Fluphenazine Permitil Prolixin Various	Elxr 0.5 mg/mL Soln 5 mg/mL Tab 1, 2.5, 5, 10 mg Inj 2.5 mg/mL.	2–40	2	2–5	Low	Low	Very High	Low

(continued)

ANTIPSYCHOTIC DRUGS COMPARISON CHART (continued)

DRUG AND CLASS	DOSAGE FORMS	ADULT ORAL DOSAGE RANGE (MG/DAY)	ORAL EQUIVALENT ANTIPSYCHOTIC DOSE (MG)	USUAL SINGLE IM DOSE	RELATIVE FREQUENCY OF SIDE EFFECTS			
					Sedation	Anticholinergic	Extrapyramidal	Orthostatic Hypotension
Fluphenazine Decanoate Prolixin Various	Inj 25 mg/mL.	—	—	12.5–75 q 2 weeks	Low	Low	Very High	Low
Haloperidol Haldol Various	Soln 2 mg/mL Tab 0.5, 1, 2, 5, 10, 20 mg Inj 5 mg/mL.	2–100	2	2–5	Very Low	Very Low	Very High	Very Low
Haloperidol Decanoate Haldol Decanoate	Inj 50, 100 mg/mL.	—	—	50–450 monthly	Very Low	Very Low	Very High	Very Low
Perphenazine Trilafon Various	Soln 3.2 mg/mL Tab 2, 4, 8, 16 mg Inj 5 mg/mL.	12–64	8	5–10	Low	Low	High	Low

(continued)

ANTIPSYCHOTIC DRUGS COMPARISON CHART (continued)

DRUG AND CLASS	DOSAGE FORMS	ADULT ORAL DOSAGE RANGE (MG/DAY)	ORAL EQUIVALENT ANTIPSYCHOTIC DOSE (MG)	USUAL SINGLE IM DOSE	RELATIVE FREQUENCY OF SIDE EFFECTS			
					Sedation	Anticholinergic	Extrapyramidal	Orthostatic Hypotension
Trifluoperazine Stelazine Various	Soln 10 mg/mL Tab 1, 2, 5, 10 mg Inj 2 mg/mL.	5–40	5	1–2	Low	Low	High	Low
Thiothixene Navane Various	Cap 1, 2, 5, 10, 20 mg Soln 5 mg/mL Inj 2, 5 mg/mL.	5–60	4	2–4	Low	Low	High	Low

[a]At dosages over 6 mg/day, nausea and insomnia are limiting side effects; extrapyramidal symptoms markedly increase at dosages over 6 mg/day.
From references 182–184, 193, 197, 200, 201, 207, and 211–215.

Anxiolytics, Sedatives, and Hypnotics

Class Instructions: Sedatives and Hypnotics. This drug causes drowsiness and may produce sleep. Do not exceed prescribed dosage, and use caution when driving, operating machinery, or performing other tasks requiring mental alertness. Avoid concurrent use of alcohol or other drugs that cause drowsiness or sleep. Do not abruptly stop taking this medication; the dosage must be slowly decreased.

Missed Doses. If you miss a dose, take it as soon as you remember. If it is almost time for your next dose, skip it and resume your normal schedule. Do not double doses.

ALPRAZOLAM   Xanax, Various

Pharmacology. Alprazolam is a triazolobenzodiazepine that is equal in efficacy to other benzodiazepines for generalized anxiety disorder, but more effective in the treatment of panic disorder. Although alprazolam has some efficacy in major depression, it is less effective than heterocyclic antidepressants.[216,217] (*See also* Clonazepam, and the Benzodiazepines and Related Drugs Comparison Chart.)

Adult Dosage. **PO for generalized anxiety disorder** 0.25 mg tid, which may be gradually increased to 4 mg/day. **PO for panic disorder** 0.5 mg tid is recommended initially; most panic patients require 5–6 mg/day, and occasionally 10 mg/day may be needed for full response. **SL** alprazolam tablets can be administered SL with no difference from oral administration in onset, peak, or pharmacokinetics.[218] **Discontinuation** decrease the daily dosage by no more than 0.5 mg/day q 3 days until the daily dosage reaches 2 mg, then decrease dosage in 0.25 mg/day increments q 3 days.

Dosage Forms. **Tab** 0.25, 0.5, 1, 2 mg; **Soln** 0.1, 1 mg/mL.

Pharmacokinetics. Like diazepam, alprazolam has a rapid onset of effect after oral administration, but its shorter half-life requires tid administration. The half-life is 11 hr in adults; the elderly may have a decreased clearance and an increased half-life of 21 hr.[217–219]

Adverse Reactions. (*See* Benzodiazepines.) Patients do not show complete cross-tolerance between triazolobenzodiazepines and other benzodiazepines, but **clonazepam** has been shown to be an effective long–half-life substitute drug for use in alprazolam withdrawal.[220]

BENZODIAZEPINES

Pharmacology. Benzodiazepines have a more specific anxiolytic effect than other sedatives. Benzodiazepines facilitate the inhibitory effect of γ-aminobutyric acid on neuronal excitability by increasing membrane permeability to chloride ions.[221]

Administration and Adult Dosage. (*See* Benzodiazepines and Related Drugs Comparison Chart.) Optimal oral use requires individual dosage titration to clinical response. The long-acting drugs can be administered once daily hs; the short-acting drugs require multiple daily doses. (*See* Benzodiazepines and Related Drugs Comparison Chart.) Determine the dosage schedule by the individual patient's relative degree of dysfunction from daytime anxiety compared to insomnia. Despite physiologic dependence, benzodiazepines may need to be used for months and sometimes years for treatment of panic disorder and generalized anxiety disorder; situational anxiety, adjustment disorders, and anxiety secondary to other causes require only days to weeks of drug treatment.[222] **PO for alcohol withdrawal** evidence suggests no superiority of any benzodiazepine in alcohol withdrawal, although **chlordiazepoxide** has been most adequately studied; **(chlordiazepoxide)** 25–100 mg for agitation, anxiety, and tremor; on the first day, up to 400 mg may be given in divided doses with gradual dosage reductions over 4 days; **(diazepam)** 5–20 mg for agitation, anxiety, and tremor; alternatively, it may be given in 20 mg doses q 2 hr until complete suppression of signs and symptoms is achieved. After this loading dose, further administration is unnecessary;[223] **(oxazepam)** 15–60 mg q 4–6 hr for agitation, anxiety, and tremor. Oxazepam is preferred in patients with severe liver disease. **IM chlordiazepoxide** is not recommended because of slow, erratic absorption; however, **lorazepam** is suitable for IM administration.[142,223] Diazepam injectable solution (Valium, various) can be administered **IM or IV;** the injectable emulsion (Dizac) is for **IV use only** (do not administer IM or SC); neither the solution nor the emulsion should be administered faster than 5 mg/min into a peripheral vein, and small veins should be avoided; neither product is recommended to be added to other drugs or solutions. (*See* Fate.) **PR diazepam for seizures** 0.2 mg/kg of Diastat rectal gel, rounded up to the next dosage size (2.5, 5, 10, 15, 20 mg); an additional dose may be given 4–12 hr after the first dose. No more than 1 episode every 5 days or 5 episodes/month should be treated with Diastat.

Special Populations. *Pediatric Dosage.* **PO** (diazepam, >6 months) 1–2.5 mg tid or qid. Most benzodiazepines are not recommended in children because of insufficient clinical experience and concern about the stimulating and paradoxical effects that occur because of disinhibition. **Midazolam** is commonly used in children for preanesthetic sedation. (*See* Midazolam.) **PR diazepam for seizures** (2–5 yr) 0.5 mg/kg of Diastat rectal gel, rounded up to the next dosage size (2.5, 5, 10, 15, 20 mg); (6–11 yr) 0.3 mg/kg of Diastat rectal gel, rounded up to the next dosage size. An additional dose may be given 4–12 hr after the first dose. No more than 1 episode every 5 days or 5 episodes/month should be treated with Diastat.

Geriatric Dosage. The elderly may have reduced clearance and enhanced CNS sensitivity, which requires initial dosage to be reduced by 33–50%.[224]

Other Conditions. Higher dosages may be needed in heavy smokers. Patients with liver disease may have reduced clearance and/or enhanced CNS sensitivity, which requires reduction of initial and subsequent doses. Alcoholic patients with reduced plasma proteins may require a lower dosage because of decreased protein binding.

Dosage Forms. (*See* Benzodiazepines and Related Drugs Comparison Chart.)

Patient Instructions. (*See* Sedatives and Hypnotics Class Instructions.)

Pharmacokinetics. *Serum Levels.* Not used clinically.

Fate. Diazepam and chlordiazepoxide are absorbed faster and more completely orally than intramuscularly. Lorazepam and midazolam have rapid and reliable IM absorption.[142,225] (*See* Benzodiazepines and Related Drugs Comparison Chart.)

Adverse Reactions. Frequent effects include drowsiness, dizziness, ataxia, and disorientation; these effects rarely require drug discontinuation and are easily managed by dosage reduction. Anterograde amnesia is frequent.[142] Occasionally, agitation and excitement may occur.[226] With parenteral therapy, hypotension and respiratory depression occur occasionally. Rarely, hepatotoxicity or blood dyscrasias occur. Diazepam emulsion is associated with less venous thrombosis and phlebitis than the solution, which can be very irritating to veins.

Contraindications. Acute narrow-angle glaucoma; (diazepam emulsion injection) hypersensitivity to soy protein.

Precautions. Pregnancy; impaired hepatic function. Abrupt drug withdrawal may result in rebound insomnia, abstinence syndrome similar to barbiturate withdrawal, seizures, or, rarely, psychosis. Patients do not show complete cross-tolerance between triazolobenzodiazepines and other benzodiazepines. Past history of substance abuse may indicate an increased likelihood of benzodiazepine misuse.[221]

Drug Interactions. Concurrent use with other CNS depressants may potentiate the sedation caused by benzodiazepines. Nefazodone inhibits alprazolam and triazolam metabolism; fluoxetine and fluvoxamine increase levels of alprazolam and diazepam; omeprazole increases serum diazepam levels.

Parameters to Monitor. Periodically reassess the need for therapy during long-term use.

BUSPIRONE HYDROCHLORIDE   BuSpar, Various

Pharmacology. Buspirone is the first of a class of selective serotonin-5-HT_{1A} receptor partial agonists. It also has some effect on dopamine-D_2 autoreceptors and, like antidepressants, can downregulate β-adrenergic receptors. Unlike benzodiazepines, it lacks amnestic, anticonvulsant, muscle relaxant, and hypnotic effects. Its exact anxiolytic mechanism of action is complex and not yet clearly defined.[227,228]

Administration and Adult Dosage. **PO for anxiety** 5 mg tid or 7.5 mg bid for 1 week, increasing in 5 mg/day increments q 2–3 days to a maximum of 60 mg/day in 2 or 3 divided doses. Most patients require 20–30 mg/day in divided doses.

Special Populations. *Pediatric Dosage.* Safety and efficacy not established.

Geriatric Dosage. Same as adult dosage.

Other Conditions. Decrease the initial dose to 5 mg bid in patients with hepatic or renal impairment.[227,229]

Dosage Forms. **Tab** 5, 10, 15 mg.

Patient Instructions. This drug requires several weeks of continuous use for therapeutic effect and is not effective when used intermittently.

Pharmacokinetics. *Onset and Duration.* Onset of anxiolytic effect several weeks.

Fate. The drug is well absorbed; oral bioavailability is $3.9 \pm 4.3\%$. Administration after meals increases bioavailability by 80%. It is extensively metabolized by oxidative dealkylation pathways.[230]

$t_{½}$. 2.1 ± 1.2 hr.[230]

Adverse Reactions. Dosages >60 mg/day may cause dysphoria.[221] Frequent nausea, dizziness, headache, and insomnia occur. Unlike benzodiazepines, buspirone does not cause dependence or withdrawal effects.[227,231]

Contraindications. None known.

Precautions. Buspirone has no cross-tolerance with benzodiazepines, so patients being switched from a benzodiazepine should have their dosage of the benzodiazepine decreased slowly.

Drug Interactions. Unlike benzodiazepines, buspirone does not interact with alcohol.[227,231] Buspirone may increase haloperidol serum levels. Avoid concurrent buspirone and an MAOI because the combination may cause hypertension.

Parameters to Monitor. Monitor renal and hepatic function initially and periodically during long-term therapy.

Notes. Buspirone is indicated only for the treatment of generalized anxiety disorder and is not effective as a prn medication or hypnotic. Buspirone's anxiolytic effect without sedation or respiratory depression has led to its use in agitation and anxiety, in dementia, mental retardation, and spinal cord injury. Its unique effect on the 5-HT$_{1A}$ receptor has led to uncontrolled studies and clinical use for premenstrual tension syndrome and to decrease craving in smoking cessation.[232]

CHLORAL HYDRATE   Noctec, Various

Pharmacology. Chloral hydrate is a chlorinated aliphatic alcohol that is a useful alternative hypnotic to benzodiazepines for prn use or for brief treatment of situational insomnia; hypnotic efficacy is lost by the second week of continuous use. Unlike barbiturates, chloral hydrate causes no enzyme induction or effect on REM sleep or REM rebound.[233,234]

Adult Dosage. PO or PR as a hypnotic 500 mg–1.5 g. Instruct patients to take the capsule with a full glass of liquid, and to mix the syrup in at least one-half glass of water or juice. (*See also* Sedatives and Hypnotics Class Instructions.)

Pediatric Dosage. PO or PR as a sedative 25 mg/kg/day in 3–4 divided doses, to a maximum of 500 mg as a single dose. PO or PR as a hypnotic 50 mg/kg to a maximum of 1 g.

Dosage Forms. Cap 250, 500 mg; Supp 325, 500, 650 mg; Syrup 50, 100 mg/mL.

Pharmacokinetics. Onset of hypnotic effect is 30–60 min. Chloral hydrate is rapidly reduced to the active hypnotic, trichloroethanol, which has a half-life of 8 hr.

Adverse Reactions. Frequent adverse effects include gastric irritation and nausea; rarely, excitement, delirium, disorientation, and erythematous and urticarial allergic reactions may occur. Chloral hydrate is genotoxic and a potential carcinogen, so some investigators caution against its routine use. The drug is contraindicated in marked hepatic or renal impairment and is best avoided in pregnancy and in patients with gastritis or ulcers. (*See* Sedatives and Hypnotics Comparison Chart.)

FLUMAZENIL   Romazicon

Pharmacology. Flumazenil is a selective inhibitor of the CNS effects of benzodiazepine sedatives. It competitively blocks the effect of benzodiazepines and zolpidem on γ-aminobutyric acid (GABA)-mediated inhibitory pathways within the CNS. Flumazenil finds its greatest use in the reversal of benzodiazepine sedation following medical and surgical procedures and occasionally in the management of benzodiazepine overdose.[235–237]

Adult Dosage. IV for reversal of conscious sedation 0.2 mg over 15 sec; this dose may be repeated after 45 sec and every minute thereafter prn, to a total dosage of 1 mg. **IV for benzodiazepine overdose** 0.2 mg over 30 sec, followed, if necessary, by 0.3 mg after 30 sec. Further doses of 0.5 mg over 30 sec may be given at 1-min intervals to a cumulative dosage of 3 mg. Rarely, patients who respond partially to 3 mg respond more completely to a dosage of 5 mg. If resedation occurs after either use, additional doses of up to 1 mg can be given at 20-min intervals to a maximum of 3 mg/hr. Flumazenil does not consistently reverse benzodiazepine amnesia, so patients should be given written instructions to avoid operation of motor vehicles or hazardous equipment, or ingestion of alcohol or nonprescription medications for 18–24 hr, or longer if benzodiazepine effects persist.

Dosage Forms. Inj 0.1 mg/mL.

Pharmacokinetics. Reversal of benzodiazepine coma may occur within 1–2 min and last 1–5 hr, depending on the dosages of the benzodiazepine and flumazenil. First-pass hepatic metabolism limits the bioavailability of oral flumazenil, so the drug is administered by IV injection. It is rapidly hydroxylated in the liver to inactive metabolites. V_d is 0.6–1.6 L/kg; its elimination half-life is 0.7–1.3 hr.

Adverse Reactions. Frequent side effects have been minimal and are usually limited to nausea and vomiting, anxiety, and agitation. However, seizures have occurred, most often in patients on long-term benzodiazepine therapy or following overdose with heterocyclic antidepressants or other potentially convulsant drugs (eg, bupropion, cocaine, cyclosporine, isoniazid, lithium, methylxanthines, MAOIs, propoxyphene). Be prepared to manage seizures before giving flumazenil.[238]

MIDAZOLAM HYDROCHLORIDE   Versed

Pharmacology. Midazolam is a short-acting triazolobenzodiazepine for use in anesthesia. It is unique in its physicochemical properties; at a pH under 4 the drug exists as a highly water-soluble, stable compound, but at physiologic pH, it becomes lipophilic. This allows IV administration of a water-soluble, rapidly acting drug with a very low frequency of venous irritation. Midazolam is given IM for preoperative sedation and IV for induction of anesthesia or for conscious sedation for endoscopy and other procedures.[239–241]

Pharmacokinetics. Midazolam is >90% absorbed after IM injection; peak serum levels occur within 30 min. IM onset is about 15 min. Peak levels after IM administration are about 50% of IV levels. The drug is 97% plasma protein bound and has a V_d of 1–3 L/kg; Cl is 0.25–0.54 L/hr/kg. Midazolam is hepatically metabolized via CYP3A4 to the 1-hydroxy- and 4-hydroxy-metabolites; the 1-hydroxy-metabolite is at least as active as midazolam. Midazolam's half-life is 1.8–6.4 hr.

Adult Dosage. **IM for preoperative sedation** 0.07–0.08 mg/kg (about 5 mg) 1 hr before surgery. **IV for endoscopy and other conscious sedation procedures** dosage must be individualized and not administered by rapid bolus. Titrate slowly to desired effect; some patients may respond to as little as 1 mg. Give no more than 2.5 mg over at least 2 min as the 1 mg/mL (or more dilute) solution; in elderly, debilitated, or chronically ill patients, limit the initial dose to 1.5 mg. Further small doses may be given after waiting at least 2 min. Do not give the drug IV without oxygen and resuscitation equipment immediately available.

Pediatric Dosage. **PO for sedation** 0.25–1 mg/kg to a maximum of 20 mg. **PR for preanesthetic sedation** 0.3 mg/kg as a solution diluted in 5 mL of saline is a safe and effective alternative to IM administration.[242]

Dosage Forms. **Inj** 1, 5 mg/mL; **Syrup** 2mg/mL.

Adverse Reactions. Respiratory depression and respiratory arrest occur frequently. Impairment of psychomotor skills continues after acute sedation has passed, so patients should not drive or operate machinery until it is clear that they have recovered fully.

TRIAZOLAM
Halcion, Various

Pharmacology. Triazolam is a triazolobenzodiazepine hypnotic whose effect is likely related to its facilitation of γ-aminobutyric acid (GABA)-mediated neurotransmission, but its exact mechanism is unknown.

Administration and Adult Dosage. (*See* Benzodiazepines and Related Drugs Comparison Chart.) **PO as a hypnotic** 0.25 mg hs initially; do not exceed 0.5 mg.

Special Populations. *Pediatric Dosage.* (<18 yr) safety and efficacy not established.

Geriatric Dosage. **PO** decrease initial dose to 0.125 mg, increase if necessary to 0.25 mg hs.[243,244]

Other Conditions. **PO** 0.125 mg initially in debilitated patients and those with a low body weight or with hepatic impairment.

Dosage Forms. **Tab** 0.125, 0.25 mg.

Patient Instructions. (*See* Sedatives and Hypnotics Class Instructions.)

Pharmacokinetics. *Onset and Duration.* Onset of hypnotic effect is 0.5–1 hr, with peak serum levels achieved within 2 hr.

Fate. Oral bioavailability 44%, SL 53%, because of nonhepatic presystemic metabolism. V_d is 1.2 ± 0.5 L/kg; Cl is 0.34 ± 0.2 L/hr/kg. Cl is decreased with increasing age (attributed to reduced hepatic oxidizing capacity in the elderly). Triazolam undergoes hydroxylation and rapid conjugation. Smoking does not affect elimination.[119,245] Accumulation does not occur with multiple doses.

$t_{1/2}$. 2.6 ± 1 hr. Half-life is not affected by end-stage renal disease or liver disease.[119,245,246]

Adverse Reactions. Frequently anterograde amnesia,[247] daytime anxiety, and ataxia may occur. Occasionally agitation, confusion, or mood disturbance occur. Rarely respiratory depression, depersonalization, and derealization, or psychosis occur. Unlike other benzodiazepines, several fatalities have been reported in elderly patients who overdosed on traizolam.[248,249]

Contraindications. Pregnancy.

Precautions. Pregnancy; impaired hepatic function. Abrupt drug withdrawal may result in rebound insomnia, abstinence syndrome similar to barbiturate withdrawal, seizures, or, rarely, psychosis. Patients do not show complete crosstolerance between triazolam and other benzodiazepines. Past history of substance abuse may indicate an increased likelihood of triazolam misuse.[221] Do not prescribe the drug for more than 7–10 days of consecutive therapy or in quantities greater than a 30-day supply.

Drug Interactions. Concurrent use with other CNS depressants may potentiate the sedation caused by benzodiazepines. Nefazodone inhibits triazolam metabolism.

Notes. Compared to other benzodiazepine hypnotics, traizolam is equally effective in reducing sleep latency and less likely to cause daytime sedation; however, it is less likely to prevent early morning awakening and more likely to cause rebound insomnia. Hypnotic drugs are most effective when used to treat transient situational insomnia (1–3 days) and short-term insomnia (1–3 weeks maximum).[249,250]

ZOLPIDEM TARTRATE   Ambien

Pharmacology. Zolpidem is the first in a class of short-acting nonbenzodiazepine hypnotics indicated for the short-term treatment of insomnia. Most benzodiazepines bind to all γ-aminobutyric acid (GABA)-benzodiazepine (omega) receptor complexes, but zolpidem selectively binds only to the omega-1 receptor. This difference suggests a more selective sedative-hypnotic effect without anxiolytic, anticonvulsant, or muscle relaxant effects.[251–253] (*See* Benzodiazepines and Related Drugs Comparison Chart.)

Adult Dosage. **PO** as a hypnotic 10 mg immediately before bedtime. In the elderly, patients with hepatic impairment, or patients taking other CNS depressants, the dose is 5 mg.

Dosage Forms. **Tab** 5, 10 mg.

Pharmacokinetics. After oral administration, zolpidem reaches peak serum concentrations in 1.6 hr, is highly protein bound (93%), has no active metabolites, and has an elimination half-life of 1.5–4 hr (average 2.5). Half-life is increased by one-third in the elderly, and greatly increased in patients with hepatic impairment (9.9 hr).

Adverse Reactions. Dose-related side effects include daytime drowsiness, dizziness, and diarrhea. Clinical trials with 20 mg doses report headache, nausea, memory problems, and CNS stimulation. Tolerance has not been reported, nor has rebound insomnia following therapeutic doses. Psychomotor performance is impaired when zolpidem is combined with alcohol. Efficacy has been demonstrated for 35 nights at doses of 10 mg without affecting sleep stages or psychomotor performance.

BENZODIAZEPINES AND RELATED DRUGS COMPARISON CHART

DRUG AND SCHEDULE[a]	DOSAGE FORMS	ADULT ORAL DOSAGE RANGE	PEAK ORAL SERUM LEVELS (HR)	HALF-LIFE (HR)[b]
SHORT-ACTING ANXIOLYTICS				
Alprazolam (C-IV) Xanax Various	Tab 0.25, 0.5, 1, 2 mg Soln 0.1, 1 mg/mL.	0.75–4 mg/day[c] 5–10 mg/day[d]	0.7–1.6	11–21
Lorazepam[e] (C-IV) Ativan Various	Tab 0.5, 1, 2 mg Soln 2 mg/mL Inj 2, 4 mg/mL.	2–10 mg/day	2	10–20
Oxazepam (C-IV) Serax Various	Cap 10, 15, 30 mg Tab 15 mg.	30–120 mg/day	1–2	5–15
LONG-ACTING ANXIOLYTICS				
Chlordiazepoxide (C-IV) Librium Libritabs Various	Cap 5, 10, 25 mg Tab 5, 10, 25 mg Inj 100 mg.	15–100 mg/day	2–4	>24
Clorazepate (C-IV) Tranxene Various	Cap 3.75, 7.5, 15 mg Tab 3.75, 7.5, 15 SR Tab 11.25, 22.5 mg.	15–60 mg/day	1–2[f]	>24
Diazepam (C-IV) Dizac Valium Various	SR Cap 15 mg Tab 2, 5, 10 mg Soln 1, 5 mg/mL Inj 5 mg/mL.	6–40 mg/day	1–2	>24
Halazepam (C-IV) Paxipam	Tab 20, 40 mg.	60–160 mg/day	1–3	>24
Prazepam (C-IV) Various	Cap 5, 10, 20 mg Tab 5, 10 mg.	20–60 mg/day	6	>24
SHORT-ACTING HYPNOTICS				
Midazolam[e] (C-IV) Versed	Inj 1, 5 mg/mL.	—	—	1.5–3
Triazolam (C-IV) Halcion Various	Tab 0.125, 0.25 mg.	0.125–0.25 mg	0.5–2	1.5–3.6
Zolpidem[g] (C-IV) Ambien	Tab 5, 10 mg.	5–20 mg	2	1.5–4

(continued)

BENZODIAZEPINES AND RELATED DRUGS COMPARISON CHART (continued)

DRUG AND SCHEDULE[a]	DOSAGE FORMS	ADULT ORAL DOSAGE RANGE	PEAK ORAL SERUM LEVELS (HR)	HALF-LIFE (HR)[b]
INTERMEDIATE-ACTING HYPNOTICS				
Estazolam (C-IV) Pro-Som Various	Tab 1, 2 mg.	1–2 mg	1–2	12–15
Temazepam (C-IV) Restoril Various	Cap 7.5, 15, 30 mg.	7.5–30 mg	2–3	10–15
LONG-ACTING HYPNOTICS				
Flurazepam (C-IV) Dalmane Various	Cap 15, 30 mg.	15–30 mg	h	>24[b]
Quazepam (C-IV) Doral	Tab 7.5, 15 mg.	7.5–15 mg	1–2	>24[b]

[a]Controlled substance schedule designated after each drug (in parentheses).
[b]Parent drug plus active metabolites.
[c]For generalized anxiety disorder.
[d]For panic disorder.
[e]Also used as an IV anesthetic; well absorbed IM.
[f]Hydrolyzed to nordazepam (desmethyldiazepam) before absorption.
[g]Not a benzodiazepine chemically, but an imidazopyridine, which is a selective benzodiazepine-1 receptor agonist.
[h]Rapidly and completely metabolized to desalkylflurazepam.
From references 217, 218, 221, 225, 23/9, 245, 247, and 253–256.

SEDATIVES AND HYPNOTICS COMPARISON CHART

DRUG AND SCHEDULE[a]	DOSAGE FORMS	ADULT ORAL DOSAGE	HALF-LIFE (HR)
SEDATIVES			
Meprobamate (C-IV) Equanil Miltown Various	Tab 200, 400, 600 mg SR Cap 200, 400 mg.	400 mg tid or qid or 600 mg bid	6–16
Phenobarbital (C-IV) Various	Cap 16 mg Elxr 3, 4 mg/mL Tab 8, 15, 30, 60, 100 mg Inj 30, 60, 65, 130 mg/mL Pwdr for Inj 120 mg.	15–30 mg bid–qid	48–120
HYPNOTICS			
Chloral Hydrate (C-IV) Noctec Various	Cap 250, 500 mg Supp 325, 500, 650 mg Syrup 50, 100 mg/mL.	500 mg– 1.5 g	8 (Trichloro-ethanol)
Ethchlorvynol (C-IV) Placidyl Various	Cap 200, 500, 750 mg.	500 mg–1 g	6
Glutethimide (C-II) Various	Tab 250 mg.	250–500 mg	5–22
Pentobarbital (C-II) Nembutal Various	Cap 50, 100 mg Elxr 4 mg/mL Supp 30, 60, 120, 200 mg (C-III) Inj 50 mg/mL.	100–200 mg	21–42
Secobarbital (C-II) Seconal Various	Cap 100 mg Inj 50 mg/mL.	100–200 mg	19–34

[a]Controlled substance schedule designated after each drug (in parentheses).
From references 249, 250, and 257.

Lithium

LITHIUM CARBONATE	Various
LITHIUM CITRATE	Cibalith-S, Lithonate-S

Pharmacology. Lithium's mechanism of antimanic effect is unknown; it alters actions of several second messenger systems (eg, adenylate cyclase and phosphoinositol).[258,259]

Administration and Adult Dosage. Individualize dosage according to serum levels and clinical response. Acute manic episodes typically require **PO** 1.2–2.4 g/day; **maintenance therapy** requires 900 mg–1.5 g/day. A **loading dose** of 30 mg/kg, in 3 divided doses, can be given to achieve the desired serum level within 12 hr.[260] A number of predictive dosage techniques have been developed based on estimated steady state after one serum level.[261,262]

Special Populations. *Pediatric Dosage.* **PO** (<12 yr) 15–20 mg (0.4–0.5 mEq)/kg/day in 2–3 divided doses; (12–18 yr) same as adult dosage.[263]

Geriatric Dosage. (>65 yr) decrease adult dosage by 33–50%.[264]

Other Conditions. Adjust the dosage more carefully in patients with decreased renal function and in patients receiving thiazide diuretics or NSAIDs.

Dosage Forms. **Cap** 150, 300, 600 mg; **Tab** 300 mg; **SR Tab** 300, 450 mg; **Syrup** 1.6 mEq/mL (as citrate).

Patient Instructions. This drug may be taken with food, milk, or antacid to minimize stomach upset. Report immediately if signs of toxicity occur, such as persistent diarrhea, vomiting, coarse hand tremor, drowsiness, or slurred speech, or prior to beginning any diet. In hot weather, ensure adequate water and salt intake.

Pharmacokinetics. *Onset and Duration.* Onset 7–10 days for therapeutic effect.[142]

Serum Levels. (Acute mania or hypomania) 0.8–1.5 mEq/L; (prophylaxis) 0.6–1.2 mEq/L, although concern about long-term renal effects suggests most patients should be maintained <0.9 mEq/L. Levels >1.5 mEq/L are regularly associated with some signs of toxicity, and levels >2 mEq/L result in serious toxicity.[265] (*See* Adverse Reactions.)

Fate. Absorption is virtually complete within 8 hr after oral administration, with peak levels occurring in 2–4 hr. Distribution is throughout total body water, but tissue uptake is not uniform. The drug is not protein bound or metabolized, but freely filtered through the glomerulus, with about 80% being reabsorbed.

$t_{1/2}$. 18–20 hr; up to 36 hr in the elderly.[142]

Adverse Reactions. Frequent, dose-related effects with therapeutic serum levels include nausea, diarrhea, polyuria, polydipsia, fine hand tremor, and muscle weakness. Signs of toxicity include coarse hand tremor, persistent GI effects, muscle hyperirritability, slurred speech, confusion, stupor, seizures, increased deep tendon reflexes, irregular pulse, and coma. Frequent, non–dose-related effects include nontoxic goiter, hypothyroidism, nephrogenic diabetes insipidus–like syndrome, folliculitis, aggravation of acne or psoriasis, leukocytosis, hypercalcemia, and weight gain.[266,267]

Contraindications. Pregnancy; fluctuating renal function; severe renal or cardiovascular disease.

Precautions. Use with caution in patients with cardiac disease, dehydration, sodium depletion, diuretic therapy, or dementia, in nursing mothers, and in the elderly. (*See* Special Populations.)

Drug Interactions. ACE inhibitors may increase serum lithium concentrations. Theophylline or excess sodium enhance renal lithium clearance; sodium deficiency may promote lithium retention and increase risk of toxicity. Long-term diuretic or NSAID use may result in decreased lithium elimination. Haloperidol may increase the CNS toxicity of lithium; with methyldopa or phenytoin, signs of lithium toxicity may occur in the absence of increased serum lithium.

Parameters to Monitor. Prelithium workup should include thyroid function tests, Cr_s, BUN, CBC (for baseline WBC count), urinalysis (for baseline specific gravity), electrolytes, and ECG (if >40 yr). During therapy, obtain serum lithium levels (drawn 12 hr after last dose) weekly during initiation and monthly during maintenance.[268,269]

Notes. **Divalproex sodium** is equivalent in efficacy to lithium for bipolar disorder and more effective than lithium for rapid-cycling bipolar illness.[270–272]

Neurodegenerative Disease Drugs

AMANTADINE   Symmetrel, Various

Pharmacology. Amantadine is an antiviral compound that prevents the release of viral nucleic acid into the host cell. In Parkinson's disease, the drug increases presynaptic dopamine release, blocks the reuptake of dopamine into the presynaptic neurons, and exerts anticholinergic effects.

Administration and Adult Dosage. PO for Parkinson's disease, give 100 mg/day initially, increasing in 100 mg/day increments q 7–14 days to effective dosage, or to a maximum of 400 mg/day in 2 divided doses. **Usual maintenance dosage** 100 mg bid. **PO for extrapyramidal reactions** 100 mg bid, to a maximum of 300 mg/day in 3 divided doses. **PO for prophylaxis of influenza A** 200 mg/day in 1–2 divided doses continuing for at least 10 days following exposure, for 2–3 weeks after giving influenza A vaccine, or for up to 90 days when vaccine is unavailable or contraindicated. **PO for treatment of influenza A** 200 mg/day in 1–2 divided doses starting within 24–48 hr after onset of illness and continuing for 24–48 hr after symptoms disappear.

Special Populations. *Pediatric Dosage.* **PO for prophylaxis or treatment of influenza A** (<1 yr) safety and efficacy not established; (1–9 yr) 4.4–8.8 mg/kg/day in 2 divided doses, to a maximum of 150 mg/day; (9–12 yr) 100 mg bid. For prophylaxis, continue therapy for at least 10 days following exposure, for 2–3 days after giving influenza A vaccine, or for up to 90 days when vaccine is unavailable or contraindicated. For treatment, continue for 24–48 hr after symptoms disappear.

Geriatric Dosage. **PO for influenza prophylaxis or treatment** (<65 yr) 100 mg/day. **PO for Parkinson's disease** same as adult dosage, adjusting for renal impairment.

Other Conditions. Reduce dosage in renal impairment as follows: with Cl_{cr} of 30–50 mL/min give 200 mg first day, then 100 mg/day; with Cl_{cr} of 15–29 mL/min give 200 mg first day, then 100 mg every other day; with Cl_{cr} <15 mL/min or for patients on hemodialysis give 200 mg q 7 days.

Dosage Forms. **Cap** 100 mg; **Syrup** 10 mg/mL.

Patient Instructions. This medication may cause dizziness, confusion, or difficulty in concentrating. Until the extent of these effects is known, use caution when driving, operating machinery, or performing other tasks requiring mental alertness. Avoid excessive concurrent use of alcohol. **Parkinson's disease.** Stopping this medication suddenly may cause your Parkinson's disease to worsen.

Missed Doses. Take this drug at regular intervals. If you miss a dose take it as soon as you remember. If it is about time for the next dose, take that dose only. Do not double the dose or take extra.

Pharmacokinetics. *Onset and Duration.* Loss of antiparkinson effects occurs in most patients after 6–12 weeks of therapy.[273]

Serum Levels. (Therapeutic trough, antiviral) 300 μg/L (2 μmol/L).

Fate. Peak serum levels occur in 1–4 hr in young adults, 4.5–7 hr in older adults. Steady-state serum levels occur in healthy volunteers and Parkinson's patients within 4–7 days;[274] V_d is 6.6 ± 1.5 L/kg; Cl is 0.39 ± 0.13 L/hr/kg with normal renal function. From 78–88% is excreted unchanged in urine.[275]

$t_{1/2}$. (Healthy young adults) 11.8 ± 2.1 hr,[276] (elderly adults) 31 ± 7.2 hr,[277] (during chronic hemodialysis) 8.3 ± 1.5 days.[276]

Adverse Reactions. Nausea, dizziness, insomnia, confusion, hallucinations, anxiety, restlessness, depression, irritability, peripheral edema, orthostatic hypotension, or livedo reticularis occur frequently. Occasionally, CHF, psychosis, urinary retention, or reversible elevation of liver enzymes may occur. Rarely, seizures, corneal opacities, or leukopenia are reported.

Drug Interactions. Amantadine can potentiate the CNS effects of anticholinergic agents.

Precautions. Pregnancy; lactation. Use with caution in patients with CHF, seizures, renal or hepatic disease, peripheral edema, orthostatic hypotension, psychosis, or a history of eczematoid rash, or in those receiving CNS stimulants. Abrupt drug discontinuation in patients with Parkinson's disease may result in rapid clinical deterioration.

Parameters to Monitor. Monitor renal function and disease symptoms periodically in parkinsonian patients.

Notes. In Parkinson's disease, amantadine is indicated as initial treatment alone or in combination with **levodopa.** Amantadine produces clinical improvements in akinesia and rigidity, but to a lesser degree than levodopa.[273,274] There is no evidence that amantadine alters the course of Parkinson's disease. **Anticholinergics** appear to reduce tremor to a greater degree than amantadine. Concomitant administration of anticholinergics and amantadine may worsen side effects. **Rimantadine** (Flumadine) is an antiviral compound with efficacy similar to amantadine against influenza A. It appears to be slightly better tolerated than amantadine. Dosage is 100 mg bid in adults and 5 mg/kg/day in one dose for children under 10 yr.[278,279] Available as 100 mg tablets and 10 mg/mL syrup.

BENZTROPINE MESYLATE   Cogentin

Pharmacology. Benztropine is a synthetic competitive antagonist of acetylcholine. In Parkinson's disease, the drug reduces the relative excess of cholinergic activity in the basal ganglia that develops because of absolute dopamine deficiency in this area.

Administration and Adult Dosage. PO, IM, or IV for Parkinson's disease 0.5–1 mg/day initially, increasing in 0.5 mg/day increments q 5–6 days to effective dosage, to a maximum of 6 mg/day. **Usual maintenance dosage** 1–2 mg/day in 2–3 divided doses. When used concurrently with levodopa, the dosages of both drugs may require reduction. **PO, IM, or IV for drug-induced extrapyramidal disorders** 1–4 mg/day in 1–2 doses.

Special Populations. *Pediatric Dosage.* (<3 yr) contraindicated; (>3 yr) 0.02–0.05 mg/kg/dose once or twice daily.

Geriatric Dosage. Same as adult dosage, although older patients can often be controlled with 1–2 mg/day.

Dosage Forms. Tab 0.5, 1, 2 mg; **Inj** 1 mg/mL.

Patient Instructions. This drug may cause constipation, difficult or painful urination, dry mouth, blurred vision, or drowsiness. Use caution when driving, operating machinery, or performing other tasks requiring mental alertness. Avoid excessive concurrent use of alcohol and other drugs that cause drowsiness.

Missed Doses. Take this drug at regular intervals. If you miss a dose take it as soon as you remember. If it is about time for the next dose, take that dose only. Do not double the dose or take extra.

Pharmacokinetics. *Onset and Duration.* Onset of resolution of drug-induced extrapyramidal symptoms is within 15 minutes following IV or IM administration, and 1–2 hr after oral administration. Duration is 24 hr.[263]

Fate. Benztropine pharmacokinetics are not well studied, but the drug apparently is hepatically metabolized to conjugates and may undergo enterohepatic recycling.[280]

Adverse Reactions. Frequent adverse effects are dose related and include dry mouth, blurred vision, nausea, dizziness, constipation, nervousness, and urinary retention. Confusional states, impairment of recent memory, and hallucinations occur with use of high doses and in patients with advanced age and underlying dementia. Rarely, paralytic ileus, parotitis, hyperthermia, or skin rash occur.

Contraindications. Children <3 yr; narrow-angle glaucoma; pyloric or duodenal obstruction; stenosing peptic ulcers; achalasia; bladder-neck obstructions; myasthenia gravis.

Precautions. Pregnancy. Use with caution in hot weather or during exercise and in patients with tachycardia, prostatic hypertrophy, open-angle glaucoma, or obstructive diseases of the GI tract.

Drug Interactions. Carefully observe patients given concomitant phenothiazines and/or heterocyclic antidepressants, because intensification of mental symptoms, paralytic ileus, or hyperthermia may occur. Anticholinergics may decrease the effectiveness of phenothiazines. Use with amantadine may result in increased CNS anticholinergic effects. Anticholinergics may decrease digoxin absorption from digoxin tablets.

Parameters to Monitor. Intraocular pressure monitoring and gonioscope evaluation periodically. Monitor for Parkinson's disease symptoms periodically.

Notes. Anticholinergic agents are considered useful for the initial treatment of parkinsonism in patients ≤60 yr with a rest tremor and without akinesia or rigidity.[273,274] The drug does not alleviate the symptoms of tardive dyskinesia.

CARBIDOPA AND LEVODOPA   Sinemet

Pharmacology. Levodopa is centrally converted to dopamine by DOPA decarboxylase and replenishes dopamine, which is deficient in the basal ganglia of patients with Parkinson's disease. Carbidopa, which does not cross the blood-brain barrier, inhibits peripheral DOPA decarboxylase, thereby increasing the amount of levodopa available to the brain for conversion to dopamine while limiting peripheral side effects. Addition of carbidopa decreases levodopa-induced nausea and vomiting, but does not decrease adverse reactions caused by the central effects of levodopa.[281]

Administration and Adult Dosage. **PO for Parkinson's disease in patients not receiving levodopa (standard formulation)** 25 mg carbidopa/100 mg levodopa tid initially, increasing in 1 tablet/day increments q 1–2 days to effective dosage, to a maximum of 8 tablets/day. Alternatively, 10 mg carbidopa/100 mg levodopa tid or qid initially, to a maximum of 8 tablets/day. Initial use of 10 mg carbidopa/100 mg levodopa may result in more nausea and vomiting, because 70–100 mg/day of carbidopa is needed to saturate peripheral DOPA decarboxylase. If initial dosage maximum is reached with 10/100 tablets and further titration is necessary, substitute 25 mg carbidopa/250 mg levodopa tid or qid, increasing in 0.5–1 tablet/day increments q 1–2 days to effective dosage, to a maximum of 8 tablets/day. **SR Tab** (patients already taking non-SR tablets) start with a dosage that provides 10% more levodopa daily. Initially, divide dosage bid or tid with an interval of 4–8 hr between doses while awake. Ultimately, dosages up to 30% greater may be needed, depending on patient response; (patients not receiving carbidopa/levodopa) 1 tablet bid initially, at least 6 hr apart, and allow 3 days between dosage adjustments. **Usual dosage** 2–8 tablets/day. If given in combination with a dopamine agonist or selegiline, lower dosages may be effective.

Special Populations. *Pediatric Dosage.* (<18 yr) safety and efficacy not established.

Geriatric Dosage. Same as adult dosage.

Dosage Forms. **Tab** 10 mg carbidopa/100 mg levodopa, 25 mg carbidopa/100 mg levodopa, 25 mg carbidopa/250 mg levodopa; **SR Tab** 25 mg carbidopa/100 mg levodopa, 50 mg carbidopa/200 mg levodopa. (*See* Notes.)

Patient Instructions. Stopping this medication suddenly may cause Parkinson's disease to worsen quickly. Report bothersome or unexpected side effects. Unless prescribed, do not take levodopa in addition to this drug. Avoid pyridoxine (vitamin B_6) if you are taking levodopa alone, but it may be taken with carbidopa/levodopa. Avoid high-protein meals for maximum absorption. If you are taking the sustained-release tablet, swallow a whole or one-half tablet without chewing or crushing it.

Missed Doses. Take this drug at regular intervals. If you miss a dose take it as soon as you remember. If it is about time for the next dose, take that dose only. Do not double the dose or take extra.

Pharmacokinetics. *Onset and Duration.* Up to 50% of patients experience a reduction in efficacy after 5 yr.[282] (*See* Notes.)

Fate. Carbidopa's inhibition of peripheral levodopa decarboxylation doubles the oral bioavailability of levodopa and decreases its clearance by one-half.[282–284] Dietary proteins compete with levodopa for intestinal absorption and decrease its effectiveness. (Rapid-release 50 mg carbidopa/200 mg levodopa) levodopa bioavailability is 99 ± 21%. A peak of 3.2 ± 1.1 mg/L occurs in 0.7 ± 0.3 hr.[285] (SR 50 mg carbidopa/200 mg levodopa) levodopa bioavailability is 71 ± 24%, increased in the presence of food. A peak of 1.14 ± 0.42 mg/L occurs in 2.4 ± 1.2 hr.[285] Levodopa V_d is 1.09 ± 0.59 L/kg; Cl is 0.28 ± 0.06 L/hr/kg; 90% of clearance is nonrenal.[286]

$t_{1/2}$. (Carbidopa) 2.1 ± 0.6 hr;[285] (levodopa alone) 1.4 ± 0.3 hr; (levodopa with carbidopa) 2 ± 1.3 hr.[286]

Adverse Reactions. Anorexia, nausea, vomiting, and involuntary muscle movements (dyskinesias) occur frequently and are generally reversible with dosage reduction. Occasionally mental changes, depression, dementia, palpitations, or orthostatic hypotensive episodes occur. Rarely, psychosis, hemolytic anemia, leukopenia, or agranulocytosis are reported. Compared to levodopa alone, carbidopa/levodopa has markedly reduced GI and cardiovascular side effects. However, mental disturbances are not eliminated and dyskinesias may appear earlier in therapy. These dyskinesias may require a decrease in dosage or dosage interval.[282,284] Side effects may be more pronounced in patients receiving **selegiline** or a dopamine agonist as adjunctive therapy.

Contraindications. Lactation; nonselective MAO inhibitors concurrently or 2 weeks prior to carbidopa/levodopa; narrow-angle glaucoma; undiagnosed skin lesions; history of melanoma.

Precautions. Pregnancy. Use with caution in patients with history of MI complicated by arrhythmias; peptic ulcer disease; severe cardiovascular, pulmonary, renal, hepatic, or endocrine disease; open-angle glaucoma; bronchial asthma; urinary retention; or psychosis. Also, use caution in patients receiving antihypertensives. Symptoms resembling neuroleptic malignant syndrome may occur when carbidopa/levodopa in combination with other antiparkinson agents is reduced abruptly or discontinued.

Drug Interactions. Ferrous sulfate may decrease levodopa absorption. Selegiline may increase levodopa side effects and levodopa/carbidopa dosage may need to be reduced 10–30% when selegiline is started.

Parameters to Monitor. Monitor CBC, renal, cardiovascular, and liver function periodically during long-term therapy. Monitor symptoms of Parkinson's disease periodically. In patients with open-angle glaucoma, monitor intraocular pressure.

Notes. Levodopa produces sustained improvement in rigidity and bradykinesia in 50–60% of patients.[282] Tremor is variably affected, and postural stability is unresponsive.[273,274] Loss of therapeutic effect is manifested by fluctuations in motor performance. Patients may experience periods of lack of drug effect ("off" periods) alternating with periods of therapeutic efficacy ("on" periods). Response may be predictable where the effect fades before the next dose ("wearing-off" or "end-of-dose"), or unpredictable ("yo-yo") where there is no relationship to the time of dose.[281] SR carbidopa/levodopa reduces "off" time an average of 30–40 min/day and allows a mean 33% reduction in the frequency of administration; the lower bioavailability of the SR product necessitates a 25% median increase in the daily dosage of levodopa compared with non-SR carbidopa/levodopa.[287] With disease progression, adjunctive therapy with an MAO-B inhibitor, a dopamine agonist, or a COMT inhibitor (tolcapone) may be required to decrease the frequency of fluctuations caused by dyskinesia or dystonia.

DONEPEZIL   *Aricept*

Pharmacology. Donepezil enhances the action of acetylcholine by reversibly inhibiting acetylcholinesterase (AChE), the enzyme responsible for its hydrolysis. It has a high degree of selectivity for AChE in the CNS, which may account for the relative lack of peripheral side effects. Donepezil is indicated for the treatment of mild to moderate dementia of the Alzheimer's type.

Administration and Adult Dosage. **PO for Alzheimer's disease** 5 mg every other day initially, gradually increasing as indicated by clinical response to 5 mg/day at bedtime. The **usual maintenance dosage** is 5–10 mg/day at bedtime. An increase in GI side effects has been noted with rapid titration; therefore, maintain a dosage of 5 mg/day for at least 4–6 weeks before increasing to 10 mg/day.

Special Populations. *Geriatric Dosage.* Same as adult dosage.

Other Conditions. No dosage adjustment is necessary in patients with renal or hepatic disease.

Dosage Forms. **Tab** 5, 10 mg.

Patient Instructions. This drug may be taken with food. Side effects may occur when you first start taking donepezil, but frequently subside after 1–2 weeks. The maximum benefits of the drug may not occur until 4–8 weeks after starting the drug. Because there is variability in the way patients respond to donepezil, the decision of how long to take donepezil should be made with your doctor. Do not abruptly discontinue donepezil on your own.

Missed Doses. Take this drug at regular intervals. If you miss a dose take it as soon as you remember. If it is about time for the next dose, take that dose only. Do not double the dose or take extra.

Pharmacokinetics. *Onset and Duration.* Onset is in about 3 weeks, with maximum benefits occurring in 4–8 weeks.[288] The manufacturer recommends waiting 3 months before evaluating the full effects of the drug.[289]

Fate. Donepezil is completely absorbed and is 96% protein bound. About 60% is eliminated as hepatic metabolites including products of CYP2D6 and CYP3A4 and glucuronides. About 17% is excreted unchanged in urine.[290,291]

$t_{1/2}$. >70 hr.

Adverse Reactions. Occasionally, nausea, vomiting, muscle cramps, fatigue, anorexia, and headache occur.

Contraindications. Hypersensitivity to donepezil or piperidine derivatives.

Precautions. Use with caution in peptic ulcer disease, syncope, sick sinus syndrome or bradycardia, altered supraventricular cardiac conduction, asthma, or COPD.

Drug Interactions. There are few in vivo studies. In vitro, ketoconazole and quinidine decrease donepezil metabolism; there is speculation that enzyme inducers may increase its metabolism. Although highly protein bound, donepezil does not interact with warfarin or furosemide, nor does it interact with cimetidine or digoxin.

Parameters to Monitor. Monitor mental status and improvements in activities of daily living initially and periodically during therapy.

Notes. Because Alzheimer's disease is a neurodegenerative disorder, patients may either improve or show no change in their cognitive function.

DOPAMINE AGONISTS:	
BROMOCRIPTINE	Parlodel
PERGOLIDE	Permax
PRAMIPEXOLE	Mirapex
ROPINIROLE	Requip

Pharmacology. Bromocriptine and pergolide are ergot-derived dopamine agonists that stimulate dopamine-D_2 receptors; additionally, pergolide stimulates and bromocriptine partially antagonizes D_1 receptors. Pramipexole and ropinirole are nonergot-derived dopamine subtype selective agonists that exert activity in the central nervous system at D_2 and D_3 receptors but have no activity at the D_1 receptor.[292–294] D_2 receptors are thought to play an important role in improving the akinesia, bradykinesia, rigidity, and gait disturbances of Parkinson's disease. Pramipexole, unlike other dopamine agonists, binds with 7-fold greater affinity to

D_3 receptors than to D_2 receptors and may affect mood. Although bromocriptine may also inhibit prolactin secretion, it is no longer indicated for the prevention of postpartum lactation. Other uses of bromocriptine include the treatment of acromegaly, prolactin-secreting pituitary adenomas, and amenorrhea/galactorrhea secondary to hyperprolactinemia in the absence of a primary tumor. (*See* Dopamine Agonists Comparison Chart).

Administration and Adult Dosage. (Bromocriptine) **PO for acromegaly** 1.25 mg/day or bid with food initially, increasing in 1.25–2.5 mg/day increments q 3–7 days to a **usual maintenance dosage** of 2.5 mg bid–tid. **Maximum dosage** is 100 mg/day. **PO for hyperprolactinemia** 2.5 mg tid. **PO for Parkinson's disease** (*See* Dopamine Agonists Comparison Chart.)

Special Populations. *Pediatric Dosage.* Safety and efficacy not established.

Geriatric Dosage. Same as adult dosage.

Other Conditions. (Pramipexole) adjust for renal impairment as follows: Cl_{cr} 35–59 mL/min, give 1.5 mg bid initially, to a maximum of 1.5 mg bid; Cl_{cr} 15–34 ml/min, give 0.125 mg/day initially, to a maximum of 1.5 mg/day.

Dosage Forms. (*See* Dopamine Agonists Comparison Chart.)

Patient Instructions. This medication may improve the symptoms of Parkinson's disease, but it will not cure it. Take this drug with food to minimize stomach upset. This drug may cause dizziness, drowsiness, or fainting, especially after the first dose. Until the extent of these effects is known, use caution when driving, operating machinery, or performing tasks requiring mental alertness. Mental disturbances, including vivid dreams, confusion, and paranoid delusions can occur even with low doses, especially when added to levodopa therapy. Avoid concurrent use of alcohol. Inform your physician and pharmacist of any other prescription or over-the-counter medications you may be taking because these may interact with your antiparkinsonian medications. Do not abruptly stop taking this medication or change your dosage without medical supervision. (Bromocriptine) women taking this drug to induce ovulation should use a barrier contraceptive.

Missed Doses. Take this drug at regular intervals. If you miss a dose, take it as soon as you remember. If it is about time for the next dose, take that dose only. Do not double the dose or take extra.

Pharmacokinetics. *Onset and Duration.* Onset (bromocriptine) 0.5–1 hr;[295,296] (pergolide and pramipexole) 1–2 hr; (ropinirole) 1–2 hr on an empty stomach, 3–4 hr with food.[297] Duration (bromocriptine, ropinirole) 3–6 hr; (pergolide, pramipexole) 8–12 hr.[298] (Bromocriptine in amenorrhea) normal menstrual function may return within 6–8 weeks.

Fate. (Bromocriptine) bioavilability is about 28%; it is 90% plasma protein bound. Peak serum concentrations occur in 1.2 ± 0.4 hr, and detectable concentrations are found for up to 12 hr following discontinuation of drug;[295] Cl is 4.4 ± 2.6 L/hr/kg.[296] The majority (98%) is excreted in the feces via bile.[295] (Pergolide) bioavailability is about 60%; it is 90% plasma protein bound. Approximately 40–50% of a dose is excreted in feces over 7 days as at least 10 metabolites.[299] (Pramipexole) bioavailability is about 90%; it is 15% plasma protein bound. V_d is 7 L/kg; renal Cl is about 0.4 L/hr/kg and markedly exceeds the GFR. About

90% of a dose is excreted unchanged in urine. (Ropinirole) although completely absorbed, bioavailability is 55% because of first-pass metabolism. It is 36% plasma protein bound and undergoes extensive metabolism in the liver to inactive metabolites. The N-despropyl metabolite is the major metabolite; the drug is also hydroxylated and glucuronidated.

$t_{\frac{1}{2}}$. (*See* Dopamine Agonists Comparison Chart.)

Adverse Reactions. Nausea, headache, hallucinations, dyskinesias, somnolence, vomiting, symptomatic hypotension, dizziness, fatigue, constipation, and light-headedness occur frequently. Occasionally, abdominal cramps and diarrhea may occur. (Bromocriptine, pergolide) rarely, hypertension, stroke, seizures, rhinor-rhea, or erythromelalgia are reported. Pleuropulmonary disease is rare and usually occurs in men, especially in smokers receiving 20–100 mg/day of bromocriptine for 3–6 months; it presents with dyspnea and improves with drug discontinuation.[300]

Contraindications. (Bromocriptine, pergolide) pregnancy; lactation; uncontrolled hypertension; pre-eclampsia; concurrent use of other ergot alkaloids; hypersensitivity to ergot alkaloids.

Precautions. (Bromocriptine, pergolide) use with caution in patients with symptoms of peptic ulcer disease, history of pulmonary disease, MI, liver disease, severe angina, or psychiatric disease. (Bromocriptine) use a barrier contraceptive during treatment for amenorrhea, galactorrhea, or infertility. If pregnancy is detected, discontinue the drug.

Drug Interactions. When used with carbidopa/levodopa, it may be necessary to reduce the dosage of levodopa by as much as 30% to reduce the potential for developing dyskinesias. Drugs that antagonize dopamine (eg, phenothiazines, buty-rophenones, metoclopramide) may reduce the effectiveness of these drugs. (Bromocriptine) erythromycin may increase bromocriptine serum levels. (Bromocriptine, pergolide) other ergot alkaloids may exacerbate cardiotoxic effects. (Pramipexole) pramipexole may result in an earlier and higher peak serum level of levodopa. Drugs that interfere with renal tubular secretion of cations (eg, cimetidine, ranitidine, verapamil, quinidine) may decrease pramipexole renal elimination. (Ropinirole) ropinirole is metabolized by CYP1A2; therefore, it may interact with inhibitors or inducers of this isozyme; ciprofloxacin markedly increases AUC and peak serum concentrations. Ropinirole may require dosage reduction with coadministration of estrogen.

Parameters to Monitor. Monitor blood pressure frequently during the first few days of therapy and periodically thereafter. Periodically evaluate hepatic, hematopoietic, cardiovascular, and renal function during long-term therapy. Monitor symptoms of Parkinson's disease periodically.

Notes. These drugs may be used as single agents for the treatment of early Parkinson's disease and as adjunctive agents in moderate- to late-stage disease.[298,301–305] As first-line agents, dopamine agonists may offer neuroprotection by regulating dopamine turnover and by delaying the introduction of levodopa. However, as single agents they are less effective than **levodopa.**

DOPAMINE AGONISTS COMPARISON CHART

DRUG	DOSAGE FORMS	ADULT DOSAGE	DOPAMINE RECEPTOR SELECTIVITY[b]			EFFECT ON CYTOCHROME P450 ISOZYMES	HALF-LIFE (HR)
			D_1	D_2	D_3		
Bromocriptine[a] Parlodel	Cap 5 mg. Tab 2.5 mg.	PO 1.25 mg bid initially, increasing in 2.5 mg/day increments q 2 weeks to a usual dosage of 10–40 mg/day.	0/+	++	+	*Inhibits* CYP3A4	4
Pergolide[a] Permax	Tab 0.05, 0.25 mg.	PO 0.05 mg/day for 2 days initially, increasing in 0.1–0.15 mg/day increments q 3 days for 12 days, then in 0.25 mg/day increments q 3 days to a usual dosage of 1–4 mg/day.	0/+	++	++	*Inhibits* CYP2D6	27

(continued)

DOPAMINE AGONISTS COMPARISON CHART

DRUG	DOSAGE FORMS	ADULT DOSAGE	DOPAMINE RECEPTOR SELECTIVITY D_1	D_2	D_3	EFFECT ON CYTOCHROME P450 ISOZYMES	HALF-LIFE (HR)
Pramipexole Mirapex	Tab 0.125, 0.25, 1, 1.5 mg.	PO 0.125 mg tid initially, increasing in increments of 0.75 mg/day at weekly intervals to a usual dosage of 1.5–4.5 mg/day in 3 divided doses.	0	++	++++	No effect.	12
Ropinirole Requip	Tab 0.25, 1, 2 mg.	PO 0.25 mg tid initially, increasing in increments of 0.75 mg/day at weekly intervals for 4 weeks, then in increments of 1.5–3 mg/day at weekly intervals to a usual dosage of 3–12 mg/day in 3 divided doses.	0	++	+++	*Inhibits* CYP2D6	4–6

0 = none; 0/+ = minimal; + = mild; ++ = moderate; +++ = potent; ++++ = very potent.

^aErgot alkaloid.

From references 295, 296, 298, 299, 301 and product information.

RILUZOLE

Rilutek

Pharmacology. In the treatment of amyotrophic lateral sclerosis, riluzole is hypothesized to protect motor neurons from degeneration and death. Although the exact mechanism of action is unknown, there are three pharmacologic properties of the drug that are thought to be relevant: inhibition of glutamate release, inactivation of voltage-dependent sodium channels, and interference with intracellular events that follow activation of excitatory amino acid receptors.

Administration and Adult Dosage. **PO for amyotrophic lateral sclerosis** 50 mg bid.

Special Populations. *Geriatric Dosage.* Same as adult dosage.

Dosage Forms. **Tab** 50 mg.

Patient Instructions. Take this medication at the same time each day on an empty stomach. It may cause dizziness, drowsiness, or vertigo. Until the extent of these effects is known, use caution when driving, operating machinery, or performing tasks requiring mental alertness. Do not drink alcohol while taking this medication. Contact your doctor if fever or flu-like symptoms occur. Protect the drug from exposure to light.

Missed Doses. Take this drug at regular intervals. If you miss a dose take it as soon as you remember. If it is about time for the next dose, take that dose only. Do not double the dose or take extra.

Pharmacokinetics. *Fate.* Riluzole is rapidly absorbed with about 90% absorbed, but absolute bioavailability is 60 ± 9% because of a first-pass effect. Peak serum concentrations occur within 60–90 min.[306] A high-fat meal decreases the AUC by about 20%. About 96% is bound to serum proteins, mainly albumin and lipoproteins; it is extensively distributed throughout the body with a V_d of about 3.4 L/kg. Cl is 0.7 L/hr/kg in male Caucasians. Riluzole is extensively metabolized in the liver to at least six major metabolites, mainly by CYP1A2 (hydroxylated derivatives) and P450-dependent glucuronidation.[307] Its metabolism is slower by 32% in women and by 50% in Japanese subjects native to Japan than in male Caucasians. Glucuronides account for about 85% of urine metabolites.[306–308]

$t_{1/2}$. 12 ± 1.8 hr.

Adverse Reactions. Frequently nausea, constipation, vomiting, abdominal pain, elevations in AST/ALT, asthenia, dizziness, diarrhea, vertigo, and circumoral paresthesia occur. Decreased lung function, pneumonia, and somnolence occur occasionally. Rarely neutropenia occurs (3 in 4000 during clinical trials).

Precautions. Use with caution in patients with renal or hepatic disease, especially the elderly.

Drug Interactions. Riluzole may potentially interact with other drugs that are also metabolized by CYP1A2 including theophylline, caffeine, fluoroquinolones, and amitriptyline. Enzyme inducers and cigarette smoking increase the metabolism of riluzole.[308]

Parameters to Monitor. Monitor liver function tests and CBC periodically as well as response to therapy.

Notes. In amyotrophic lateral sclerosis, riluzole prolongs the time to tracheostomy or death (a 21% risk reduction) compared to placebo.[309,310] The difference in rates of muscle deterioration between riluzole and placebo was significant in some studies but not in others.

SELEGILINE HYDROCHLORIDE   Eldepryl

Pharmacology. Selegiline (formerly l-deprenyl) is a selective irreversible MAO-B inhibitor used as adjunctive therapy in the management of Parkinson's disease. MAO-B is found in the brain and plays a role in the catabolism of dopamine.[311,312] By preventing the breakdown of dopamine by MAO-B, selegiline increases the net amount of dopamine available in the brain. Selegiline may also exert a protective effect by preventing the accumulation of neurotoxic free radicals generated by dopamine metabolism.[313-317] However, the exact mechanism of the beneficial effects of selegiline is unclear and may be symptomatic, neuroprotective, or both.

Administration and Adult Dosage. **PO for Parkinson's disease** 5 mg bid taken at breakfast and lunch. Alternatively, give an initial dosage of 2.5 mg/day and slowly increase to 10 mg/day over several weeks to minimize side effects.[311] There is no evidence that dosages >10 mg/day increase efficacy, and they may lead to nonspecific inhibition of MAO-A.

Special Populations. *Pediatric Dosage.* Safety and efficacy not established.

Geriatric Dosage. Same as adult dosage.

Dosage Forms. **Cap** 5 mg; **Tab** 5 mg.

Patient Instructions. Take this medication with morning and midday meals to minimize nausea and nighttime insomnia. At a dosage of 10 mg per day or less, tyramine-containing foods and medications containing amines are safe to consume. Initiation of selegiline may require a reduction of carbidopa/levodopa dosage. Report immediately any severe headache or other unusual or unexpected symptoms.

Missed Doses. Take this drug at regular intervals. If you miss a dose take it as soon as you remember. If it is about time for the next dose, take that dose only. Do not double the dose or take extra.

Pharmacokinetics. *Onset and Duration.* Recovery of platelet MAO-B activity after a single oral dose is 2–4 days; after long-term treatment, >90% of platelet MAO-B remains inhibited after 5 days.[318] With continual use, clinical efficacy lasts 6–12 months in most patients, to a maximum of 12–24 months.[313-316]

Fate. Selegiline is readily absorbed from the GI tract, with a peak at 0.5–2 hr; 94% is plasma protein bound.[318] It is metabolized by the liver to N-desmethylselegiline, L-amphetamine, and L-methamphetamine; these isomers, however, are only 10% as potent as the D-isomers. After long-term therapy with 10 mg/day in 2 divided doses, mean trough serum levels of selegiline and N-desmethylselegiline are undetectable, L-amphetamine is 5.9 ± 2.7 µg/L (22 ± 10 nmol/L), and L-methamphetamine is 14.9 ± 6.8 µg/L (100 ± 45 nmol/L). The concentrations of these metabolites are probably too low to contribute to the drug's clinical efficacy, but may contribute to adverse effects. About 86% is excreted in urine as inactive metabolites.[311,312]

$t_{1/2}$. (N-desmethylselegiline) 2 ± 1.2 hr; (L-amphetamine) 17.7 ± 16.3 hr; (L-methamphetamine) 20.5 ± 11.4 hr.[311,312]

Adverse Reactions. Nausea, abdominal pain, dry mouth, confusion, hallucinations, dizziness, insomnia, lightheadedness, and/or fainting occur frequently. Occasionally vivid dreams, dyskinesias, and headache occur. In decreasing order of frequency, nausea, hallucinations, confusion, depression, loss of balance, and insomnia may lead to discontinuation of the drug. Mild, asymptomatic elevations in liver function tests may occur.

Precautions. Pregnancy; lactation. Concurrent use with meperidine. Do not use at dosages exceeding 10 mg/day.

Drug Interactions. Concurrent administration of selegiline and serotonin reuptake inhibitors (eg, SSRIs, nefazondone, venlafaxine) may cause serotonin syndrome; they should not be given concurrently within 1–2 weeks of each other (5 weeks after stopping fluoxetine).

Parameters to Monitor. Evaluate cardiovascular status and monitor liver function tests periodically. Monitor Parkinson's disease symptoms periodically.

Notes. Selegiline is indicated as adjunctive treatment with **carbidopa/levodopa** in Parkinson's disease. Although selegiline's efficacy is not superior to other adjunctive drugs such as dopamine agonists, it appears to be better tolerated.[292,293] Approximately 60% of patients who receive selegiline experience a modest (10% or less) reduction in "off" periods and are able to reduce their levodopa dosage by 20%.[315] A role for the drug as an initial agent in patients with mild disease is supported by results of a study comparing selegiline 10 mg/day to placebo in patients with early (<5 yr) untreated Parkinson's disease; selegiline delayed the onset of disease-related disability by nearly 1 yr.[313] **Zelepar** (Athena) is a rapid-dissolving form of selegiline in phase III clinical trials.

TOLCAPONE   Tasmar

Pharmacology. Tolcapone reversibly inhibits at least 80% of the activity of catechol-O-methyltransferase (COMT). This action prevents the metabolism of levodopa to 3-O-methyldopa and thus prolongs its duration of action, especially with co-administration of carbidopa.[319,320] Tolcapone increases plasma levodopa bioavailability by about 2-fold and variably prolongs the terminal half-life of levodopa (given with carbidopa) in the elderly from 2 hr to as long as 3.5 hr, but has no effect on the peak serum levels of levodopa or the time at which they occur. (*See* Notes.)

Administration and Adult Dosage. PO for Parkinson's disease 100–200 mg tid as effective and as tolerated. No dosage titration is necessary.

Special Populations. *Geriatric Dosage.* Same as adult dosage.

Dosage Forms. Tab 100, 200 mg.

Patient Instructions. This drug may lower blood pressure, and may cause unsteadiness, nausea, or sweating initially. Do not rise rapidly after sitting or lying down. It may also cause drowsiness. Until the extent of these effects is known, use caution when driving, operating machinery, or performing tasks that require mental alertness. This drug may also worsen dyskinesias or dystonia when it is first started and may require adjustment of the amount of carbidopa/levodopa you are taking.

Missed Doses. Take this drug at regular intervals. If you miss a dose, take it as soon as you remember. If it is about time for the next dose, take that dose only. Do not double the dose or take extra.

Pharmacokinetics. *Onset and Duration.* Onset 1–2 hr; duration 12–24 hr.

Fate. About 65% is orally absorbed. A peak serum concentration of 6.3 ± 2.9 mg/L occurs 1.8 ± 1.3 hr after a 200 mg dose. Food increases the peak time and decreases the peak and AUC of tolcapone. About 99.9% is bound to plasma proteins, mainly albumin. The predominant metabolic pathway is glucuronidation. Major metabolites that are a product of oxidative processes include 3-O-methyltolcapone, and carboxylic acid derivatives, metabolized by CYP2A6 and CYP3A4. Those that are a product of reductive processes include amines and N-acetyl derivatives. Cl is about 0.1 L/kg/hr. About 40% of an orally administered dose is excreted in the urine and feces in 24 hr and >95% in 7–9 days. Less than 0.5% of tolcapone is excreted unchanged in urine.[319,320]

t½. (Tolcapone) 2 ± 0.8 hr; (3-O-methyltolcapone) 32 ± 7 hr.[319,320]

Adverse Reactions. Adverse reactions consistent with increased levodopa exposure include worsening dyskinesia, nausea, sleep disorders, dystonia, somnolence, anorexia, hallucinations, and postural hypotension. They may be lessened by reducing levodopa dosage. Urine discoloration also occurs and is attributable to the yellow color of tolcapone and its metabolites. Other tolcapone-related side effects include headache, abdominal pain, and diarrhea. The most common reason for drug discontinuation from clinical studies was severe diarrhea in 3% of patients. The onset is often delayed and usually occurs within 0.5–3 months after initiation of therapy. The drug may elevate hepatic enzymes, including AST and ALT.

Precautions. Orthostatic hypotension, hallucinations, diarrhea, or dyskinesias may occur at the initiation of therapy. Use with caution in renal or hepatic impairment. Discontinue if jaundice occurs or if ALT reaches 5 times the upper normal limit.

Drug Interactions. Tolcapone may inhibit the metabolism of other drugs also metabolized by COMT (eg, dobutamine, isoproterenol) and exacerbate the dopaminergic side effects of other antiparkinsonian agents. It does not interact with ephedrine or with desipramine (a substrate for CYP2D6), but has in vivo affinity for CYP2C9 (although the clinical relevance is undetermined).

Parameters to Monitor. Monitor transaminases monthly for the first 3 months, then q 6 weeks for the next 3 months. Monitor response to therapy and tolerability periodically.

Notes. Tolcapone may be administered on a scheduled basis (three times daily) and does not need to be administered with each dose of levodopa. The increase in "on time" in both nonfluctuating and fluctuating patients ranged from 1.7–2.9 hr over baseline (compared to 0.7–1 hr for placebo).[321–323] In clinical trials, the average decrease in daily levodopa dosage was about 30% in about 70% of patients.

TRIHEXYPHENIDYL HYDROCHLORIDE
Artane, Various

Pharmacology. Trihexyphenidyl is a competitive antagonist of acetylcholine at central muscarinic receptors. In Parkinson's disease, it is an adjunctive treatment that balances cholinergic and dopaminergic activity in cerebral synapses.

Adult Dosage. PO for Parkinson's disease 1 mg/day initially, increasing in 2 mg/day increments q 3–5 days, to a maximum of 12–15 mg/day. **Usual maintenance dosage** 6–10 mg/day in 3 divided doses or 3–6 mg/day in 3 divided doses concurrent with levodopa. SR caps may be given bid, once the maintenance dosage is determined. **PO for drug-induced extrapyramidal disorders** 1 mg initially, increasing in 1 mg increments every few hours until symptoms are controlled, usually 5–15 mg/day in 3–4 divided doses.

Dosage Forms. Elxr 0.4 mg/mL; **Tab** 2, 5 mg; **SR Cap** 5 mg.

Pharmacokinetics. The onset of action is within 1 hr, and the peak effect lasts 2–3 hr; the duration of action is 6–12 hr. The majority of the drug is excreted in the urine probably unchanged, and the elimination half-life is 10.2 ± 4.7 hr.

Adverse Reactions. Adverse reactions, precautions, contraindications, and drug interactions are the same as for benztropine. When trihexyphenidyl is used concurrently with levodopa, the dosages of both drugs may require reduction.

■ REFERENCES

1. Anon. Drugs for epilepsy. *Med Lett Drugs Ther* 1995;37:37–40.
2. Levy RH et al., eds. *Antiepileptic drugs.* 4th ed. New York: Raven Press; 1995.
3. Cloyd JC et al. Antiepileptics in the elderly: pharmacoepidemiology and pharmacokinetics. *Arch Fam Med* 1994;3:589–98.
4. Bass J et al. Effects of enteral tube feedings on the absorption and pharmacokinetic profile of carbamazepine suspension. *Epilepsia* 1989;30:364–9.
5. Graves NM et al. Relative bioavailability of rectally administered carbamazepine suspension in humans. *Epilepsia* 1985;26:429–33.
6. Morrow JI, Richens A. Disposition of anticonvulsants in childhood. *Clin Pharmacokinet* 1989;17(suppl 1): 89–104.
7. Bertilsson L et al. Autoinduction of carbamazepine metabolism in children examined by a stable isotope technique. *Clin Pharmacol Ther* 1980;27:83–8.
8. Mikati MA et al. Time course of carbamazepine autoinduction. *Neurology* 1989;39:592–4.
9. Theodore WH et al. Carbamazepine and its epoxide: relation of plasma levels to toxicity and seizure control. *Ann Neurol* 1989;25:194–6.
10. Greenblatt DJ et al. Clinical pharmacokinetics of anxiolytics and hypnotics in the elderly: therapeutic considerations (Part I). *Clin Pharmacokinet* 1991;21:165–77.
11. Graves NM, Kriel RL. Rectal administration of antiepileptic drugs in children. *Pediatr Neurol* 1987;3:321–6.
12. Berlin A. Dahlstrom H. Pharmacokinetics of the anticonvulsant drug clonazepam evaluated from single oral and intravenous doses and by repeated oral administration. *Eur J Clin Pharmacol* 1975;9:155–9.
13. Specht U et al. Discontinuation of clonazepam after long-term treatment. *Epilepsia* 1989;30:458–63.
14. Pollack MH et al. Long-term outcome after acute treatment with alprazolam or clonazepam for panic disorder. *J Clin Psychopharmacol* 1993;13:257–63.
15. Herman JB et al. The alprazolam to clonazepam switch for the treatment of panic disorder. *J Clin Psychopharmacol* 1987;7:175–8.
16. Beauclair L et al. Clonazepam in the treatment of panic disorder: a double-blind, placebo-controlled trial investigating the correlation between clonazepam concentrations in plasma and clinical response. *J Clin Psychopharmacol* 1994;14:111–8.
17. Buchanan RA et al. Absorption and elimination of ethosuximide in children. *J Clin Pharmacol* 1969;9:393–8.
18. Goulet JR et al. Metabolism of ethosuximide. *Clin Pharmacol Ther* 1976;20:213–8.

19. Rho JM et al. Mechanism of action of the anticonvulsant felbamate: opposing effects on N-methyl-D-aspartate and γ-aminobutyric acid$_A$ receptors. *Ann Neurol* 1994;35:229–34.

20. Sachdeo R et al. Felbamate monotherapy: controlled trial in patients with partial onset seizures. *Ann Neurol* 1992;32:386–92.

21. Espe-Lillo J et al. Safety and efficacy of felbamate in treatment of infantile spasms. *Epilepsia* 1993;34:110.

22. Perhach JL et al. Felbamate. In, Meldrum BS, Porter RJ, eds. *New anticonvulsant drugs.* London: John Libby; 1986:117–23.

23. Wilensky AJ et al. Pharmacokinetics of W-554 (ADD 03055) in epileptic patients. *Epilepsia* 1985;26:602–6.

24. Pellock JM, Brodie MJ. Felbamate: 1997 update. *Epilepsia* 1997;38:1261–4.

25. Aweeka F et al. Conversion of ACC-9653 to phenytoin in patients with renal or hepatic diseases. *Clin Pharmacol Ther* 1989;45:152. Abstract.

26. Gerber N et al. Safety, tolerance and pharmacokinetics of intravenous doses of the phosphate ester of 3-hydroxymethyl-5,5-diphenylhydantoin: a new prodrug of phenytoin. *J Clin Pharmacol* 1988;28:1023–32.

27. Leppik IE et al. Pharamcokinetics and safety of a phenytoin prodrug given IV or IM in patients. *Neurology* 1990;40:456–60.

28. Jamerson BD et al. Venous irritation related to intravenous administration of phenytoin versus fosphenytoin. *Pharmacotherapy* 1994;14:47–52.

29. Wilder BJ et al. Safety and tolerance of multiple doses of intramuscular fosphenytoin substituted for oral phenytoin in epilepsy or neurosurgery. *Arch Neurol* 1996;53:764–8.

30. Fischer JH et al. Stability of fosphenytoin sodium with intravenous solutions in glass bottles, polyvinyl chloride bags, and polypropylene syringes. *Ann Pharmacother* 1997;31:553–9.

31. Crockett JG et al. Open-label follow-on study of gabapentin (GBP; Neurontin) monotherapy in patients with refractory epilepsy. *Epilepsia* 1995;36:69. Abstract.

32. McLean MJ. Clinical pharmacokinetics of gabapentin. *Neurology* 1994;44(suppl 5): S17–22.

33. Sivenius J et al. Double-blind study of gabapentin in the treatment of partial seizures. *Epilepsia* 1991;32:539–42.

34. Hooper WD et al. Lack of a pharmacokinetic interaction between phenobarbitone and gabapentin. *Br J Clin Pharmacol* 1991;31:171–4.

35. Ramsay RE. Clinical efficacy and safety of gabapentin. *Neurology* 1994;44(suppl 5): S23–30.

36. Asconape J, Collins T. Weight gain associated with the use of gabapentin. *Epilepsia* 1994;36(suppl 4):72. Abstract.

37. Wolf SM et al. Gabapentin toxicity in children manifesting as behavioral changes. *Epilepsia* 1996;36:1203–5.

38. Mikati M et al. Efficacy of gabapentin in children with refractory partial seizures. *Neurology* 1995;45(suppl 4):A201–2. Abstract.

39. Beydoun A et al. Gabapentin monotherapy: II. A 26-week, double-blind, dose-controlled, multicenter study of conversion from polytherapy in outpatients with refractory complex partial or secondarily generalized seizures. *Neurology* 1997;49:746–52.

40. Mathew NT, Lucker C. Gabapentin in migraine prophylaxis: a preliminary open label study. *Neurology* 1996;46(suppl):A169. Abstract.

41. Sist T et al. Gabapentin for idiopathic trigeminal neuralgia: report of two cases. *Neurology* 1997;48:1467.

42. Rosenberg JM et al. The effect of gabapentin on neuropathic pain. *Clin J Pain* 1997;13:251–5.

43. Btaiche IF, Woster PS. Gabapentin and lamotrigine: novel antiepileptic drugs. *Am J Health-Syst Pharm* 1995;52:61–9.

44. Rambeck B, Wolf P. Lamotrigine clinical pharmacokinetics. *Clin Pharmacokinet* 1993;25:433–43.

45. Jawad S et al. Lamotrigine: single-dose pharmacokinetics and initial 1 week experience in refractory epilepsy. *Epilepsy Res* 1987;1:194–201.

46. Besage FMC et al. Carbamazepine toxicity with lamotrigine: pharmacokinetic or pharmacodynamic interaction. *Epilepsia* 1998;39:183–7.

47. Motte J et al. Lamotrigine for generalized seizures associated with the Lennox-Gastaut syndrome. *N Engl J Med* 1997;337:1807–12.

48. Brodie MJ et al. Double-blind comparison of lamotrigine and carbamazepine in newly diagnosed epilepsy. *Lancet* 1995;345:476–9.

49. Working Group on Status Epilepticus. Treatment of convulsive status epilepticus. *JAMA* 1993;270:854–9.

50. Dunn DW. Status epilepticus in infancy and childhood. *Neurol Clin* 1990;8:647–57.

51. Scheuer ML, Pedley TA. The evaluation and treatment of seizures. *N Engl J Med* 1990;323:1468–74.

52. Graves NM et al. Relative bioavailability of rectally administered phenobarbital sodium parenteral solution. *DICP* 1989;23:565–8.

53. Alvin J et al. The effect of liver disease in man on the disposition of phenobarbital. *J Pharmacol Exp Ther* 1975;192:224–35.

54. Wilensky AJ et al. Kinetics of phenobarbital in normal subjects and epileptic patients. *Eur J Clin Pharmacol* 1982;23:87–92.

55. Heimann G, Gladtke E. Pharmacokinetics of phenobarbital in childhood. *Eur J Clin Pharmacol* 1977;12: 305–10.

56. Meador KJ et al. Comparative cognitive effects of phenobarbital, phenytoin, and valproate in healthy adults. *Neurology* 1995;45:1494–99.

57. Mattson RH et al. Barbiturate-related connective tissue disorders. *Arch Intern Med* 1989;149:911–4.

58. Alldredge BK et al. Anticonvulsant hypersensitivity syndrome: in vitro and clinical observations. *Pediatr Neurol* 1994;10:169–71.

59. Ramsay RE. Pharmacokinetics and clinical use of parenteral phenytoin, phenobarbital, and paraldehyde. *Epilepsia* 1989;30(suppl 2):S1–3.

60. Dela Cruz FG et al. Efficacy of individualized phenytoin sodium loading doses administered by intravenous infusion. *Clin Pharm* 1988;7:219–24.

61. Blaser KU et al. Intravenous phenytoin: a loading scheme for desired concentrations. *Ann Intern Med* 1989;110:1029–31.

62. Bauer LA, Blouin RA. Age and phenytoin kinetics in adult epileptics. *Clin Pharmacol Ther* 1982;31:301–4.

63. Boucher BA et al. Phenytoin pharmacokinetics in critically ill trauma patients. *Clin Pharmacol Ther* 1988;44:675–83.

64. Levy RH, Yerby MS. Effects of pregnancy on antiepileptic drug utilization. *Epilepsia* 1985;26(suppl 1): S52–7.

65. Leppik IE et al. Altered phenytoin clearance with febrile illness. *Neurology* 1986;36:1367–70.

66. Tozer TN, Winter ME. Phenytoin. In, Evans WE et al., eds. *Applied pharmacokinetics: principles of therapeutic drug monitoring.* 3rd ed. Vancouver: Applied Therapeutics; 1992.

67. Goff DA et al. Absorption characteristics of three phenytoin sodium products after administration of oral loading doses. *Clin Pharm* 1984;3:634–8.

68. McCauley DL et al. Time for phenytoin concentration to peak: consequences of first-order and zero-order absorption. *Ther Drug Monit* 1989;11:540–42.

69. Browne TR et al. Estimation of the elimination half-life of a drug at any serum concentration when the K_m and V_{max} of the drug are known: calculations and validation with phenytoin. *J Clin Pharmacol* 1987;27:318–20.

70. Spengler RF et al. Severe soft-tissue injury following intravenous infusion of phenytoin—patient and drug administration risk factors. *Arch Intern Med* 1988;148:1329–33.

71. Smythe MA, Umstead GS. Phenytoin hepatotoxicity: a review of the literature. *DICP* 1989;23:13–8.

72. Delattre JY et al. Erythema multiforme and Stevens-Johnson syndrome in patients receiving cranial irradiation and phenytoin. *Neurology* 1988;38:194–8.

73. Haley CJ, Nelson J. Phenytoin-enteral feeding interaction. *DICP* 1989;23:796–8.

74. Sarkar MA et al. The effects of storage and shaking on the settling properties of phenytoin suspension. *Neurology* 1989;39:207–9.

75. Mattson RH et al. Comparison of carbamazepine, phenobarbital, phenytoin and primidone in partial and secondarily generalized tonic-clonic seizures. *N Engl J Med* 1985;313:145–51.

76. Pisani F et al. Single dose kinetics of primidone in acute viral hepatitis. *Eur J Clin Pharmacol* 1984;27:465–9.

77. Cottrell PR et al. Pharmacokinetics of phenylethylmalonamide (PEMA) in normal subjects and in patients treated with antiepileptic drugs. *Epilepsia* 1982;23:307–13.

78. Rosenfeld WE. Topiramate: a review of preclinical, pharmacokinetic, and clinical data. *Clin Therapeutics* 1997;19:1294–308.

79. Markind JE. Topiramate: a new antiepileptic drug. *Am J Health-Syst Pharm* 1998;55:554–62.

80. Jansen JA et al. Absolute bioavailability of tiagabine. *Epilepsia* 1995;36(suppl 3):S159. Abstract.

81. Perucca E, Bialer M. The clinical pharmacokinetics of the newer antiepileptic drugs: focus on topiramate, zonisamide and tiagabine. *Clin Pharmacokinet* 1996;31:29–46.

82. Gustavson LE, Mengel HB. Pharmacokinetics of tiagabine, a γ-aminobutyric acid-uptake inhibitor, in healthy subjects after single and multiple doses. *Epilepsia* 1995;36:605–11.

83. Privitera M et al. Dose-ranging trial with higher doses of topiramate in patients with resistant partial seizures. *Epilepsia* 1995;36(suppl 4):33. Abstract.

84. Rosenfeld WE et al. Comparison of the steady-state pharmacokinetics of topiramate and valproate in patients with epilepsy during monotherapy and concomitant therapy. *Epilepsia* 1997;38:324–33.

85. Rosenfeld WE et al. Effect of topiramate on the pharmacokinetics of an oral contraceptive containing norethindrone and ethinyl estradiol in patients with epilepsy. *Epilepsia* 1997;38:317–23.

86. Biton V et al. Efficacy and safety of topiramate in generalized seizures of non-focal origin. *Epilepsia* 1997;38(suppl 8):206–7. Abstract.

87. Sachdeo SK et al. Topiramate double-blind trial as monotherapy. *Epilepsia* 1996;36(suppl 4):33. Abstract.

88. Elterman R et al. Topiramate as adjunctive therapy in pediatric patients with partial-onset seizures. *Epilepsia* 1997;38(suppl 8):98. Abstract.

89. Glauser TA et al. Topiramate as adjunctive therapy in Lennox-Gastaut syndrome. *Epilepsia* 1997;38(suppl 8):207. Abstract.

90. Brodie MJ, Dichter MA. Antiepileptic drugs. *N Engl J Med* 1996;334:168–75.

91. Zaccara G et al. Clinical pharmacokinetics of valproic acid—1988. *Clin Pharmacokinet* 1988;15:367–89.

92. Fischer JH et al. Effect of food on the serum concentration profile on enteric-coated valproic acid. *Neurology* 1988;38:1319–22.

93. Holmes GB et al. Absorption of valproic acid suppositories in human volunteers. *Arch Neurol* 1989;46:906–9.

94. Dreifuss FE et al. Valproic acid hepatic fatalities—II. US experience since 1984. *Neurology* 1989;39:201–7.

95. Mattson RH et al. A comparison of valproic acid with carbamazepine for the treatment of complex partial seizures and secondarily generalized tonic-clonic seizures in adults. *N Engl J Med* 1992;327:765–71.

96. APA Practice Guideline for the Treatment of Patients with Bipolar Disorder. *Am J Psychiatry* 1994;12 (suppl):1–36.

97. Bowden CL et al. Efficacy of divalproex vs lithium and placebo in the treatment of mania. *JAMA* 1994; 271:918–24.

98. Bowden CL. Predictors of response to divalproex and lithium. *J Clin Psychiatry* 1995;56(suppl 3):25–30.

99. Rothrock JF et al. A differential response to treatment with divalproex sodium in patients with intractable headache. *Cephalalgia* 1994;14:241–4.

100. Mathew NT et al. Migraine prophylaxis with divalproex. *Arch Neurol* 1995;52:281–6.

101. French JA et al. A double-blind, placebo-controlled study of vigabatrin three g/day in patients with uncontrolled complex partial seizures. *Neurology* 1996;46:54–61.

102. Kalviainen R et al. Vigabatrin vs carbamazepine monotherapy in patients with newly diagnosed epilepsy. *Arch Neurol* 1995;52:989–96.

103. Connelly JF. Vigabatrin. *Ann Pharmacother* 1993;27:197–204.

104. Panayiotopoulos CP et al. Vigabatrin aggravates absences and absence status. *Neurology* 1997;49:1467.

105. Luna D et al. Vigabatrin in the treatment of childhood epilepsies: a single-blind placebo-controlled study. *Epilepsia* 1989;30:430–7.

106. Appleton RE, Thornton L. Double blind comparison of vigabatrin vs placebo in newly diagnosed and previously untreated infantile spasms. *Epilepsia* 1996;37(suppl 5):125. Abstract.

107. Haegele KD, Schechter PJ. Kinetics of the enantiomers of vigabatrin after an oral dose of the racemate or the active S-enantiomer. *Clin Pharmacol Ther* 1986;40:581–6.

108. Haegele KD et al. Pharmacokinetics of vigabatrin: implications of creatinine clearance. *Clin Pharmacol Ther* 1988;44:558–65.

109. Preskorn SH, Othmer SC. Evaluation of bupropion hydrochloride: the first of a new class of atypical antidepressants. *Pharmacotherapy* 1984;4:20–34.

110. Davidson J. Seizures and bupropion: a review. *J Clin Psychiatry* 1989;50:256–61.

111. Cooper BR et al. Evidence that the acute behavioral and electrophysiological effects of bupropion (Wellbutrin) are mediated by a noradrenergic mechanism. *Neuropsychopharmacology* 1994;11:133–41.

112. Walker PM et al. Improvement in fluoxetine-associated sexual dysfunction in patients switched to bupropion. *J Clin Psychiatry* 1993;54:459–65.

113. Jermain DM et al. Pharmacotherapy of obsessive-compulsive disorder. *Pharmacotherapy* 1990;10:175–98.

114. Peters MD et al. Clomipramine: an antiobsessional tricyclic antidepressant. *Clin Pharm* 1990;9:165–78.

115. Stokes PE. Fluoxetine: a five-year review. *Clin Ther* 1993;15:216–43.

116. Monteiro WO et al. Anorgasmia from clomipramine in obsessive-compulsive disorder: a controlled trial. *Br J Psychiatry* 1987;151:107–12.

117. Sommi RW et al. Fluoxetine: a serotonin-specific second-generation antidepressant. *Pharmacotherapy* 1987;7:1–15.

118. Schweizer E et al. What constitutes an adequate antidepressant trial for fluoxetine? *J Clin Psychiatry* 1990;51:8–11.

119. Benet LZ et al. Design and optimization of dosage regimens: pharmacokinetic data. In, Hardman JG et al., eds. *Goodman and Gilman's the pharmacological basis of therapeutics.* 9th ed. New York: McGraw-Hill; 1996:1707–92.

120. Balon R. The effects of antidepressants on human sexuality: diagnosis and management update 1996. *Primary Psychiatry* 1997;4:32–44.

121. Gitlin MJ. Psychotropic medications and their effects on sexual function: diagnosis, biology, and treatment approaches. *J Clin Psychiatry* 1994;55:406–13.

122. Kinney-Parker JL et al. Fluoxetine and weight: something lost and something gained? *Clin Pharm* 1989; 8:727–33.

123. Jefferson JW. Cardiovascular effects and toxicity of anxiolytics and antidepressants. *J Clin Psychiatry* 1989; 50:368–78.

124. Tollefson GD et al. Absence of a relationship between adverse events and suicidality during pharmacotherapy for depression. *J Clin Psychopharmacol* 1994;14:163–9.

125. Feighner JP et al. Adverse consequences of fluoxetine-MAOI combination therapy. *J Clin Psychiatry* 1990; 51:222–5.

126. Roose SP et al. Comparative efficacy of selective serotonin reuptake inhibitors and tricyclics in the treatment of melancholia. *Am J Psychiatry* 1994;151:1735–9.

127. Grimsley SR, Jann MW. Paroxetine, sertraline, and fluvoxamine: new selective serotonin reuptake inhibitors. *Clin Pharm* 1992;11:930–57.

128. Wilde MI et al. Fluvoxamine: an updated review of its pharmacology and therapeutic use in depressive illness. *Drugs* 1993;46:895–924.

129. Freeman CPL et al. Fluvoxamine versus clomipramine in the treatment of obsessive-compulsive disorder: a multi-center, randomized, double-blind, parallel group comparison. *J Clin Psychiatry* 1994;55:301–5.

130. Potter WZ et al. The pharmacologic treatment of depression. *N Engl J Med* 1991;325:633–42.

131. Preskorn SH. Recent pharmacologic advances in antidepressant therapy for the elderly. *Am J Med* 1993; 94(suppl 5A):2S–12S.

132. Baldessarini RJ. Current status of antidepressants: clinical pharmacology and therapy. *J Clin Psychiatry* 1989; 50:117–26.

133. Frank E et al. Comparison of full-dose versus half-dose pharmacotherapy in the maintenance treatment of recurrent depression. *J Affect Disord* 1993;27:139–45.

134. Wright JM. Review of the symptomatic treatment of diabetic neuropathy. *Pharmacotherapy* 1994;14:689–97.

135. Max MB. Treatment of post-herpetic neuralgia: antidepressants. *Ann Neurol* 1994;35:S50–3.

136. Rappoport JL et al. Childhood enuresis II. Psychopathology, tricyclic concentration in plasma, and antienuretic effect. *Arch Gen Psychiatry* 1980;37:1146–52.

137. Puig-Antich J et al. Imipramine in prepubertal major depressive disorders. *Arch Gen Psychiatry* 1987; 44:81–9.

138. Salzman C. Pharmacologic treatment of depression in the elderly. *J Clin Psychiatry* 1993;54(suppl 2):23–8.

139. Salzman C. Practical considerations in the pharmacologic treatment of depression and anxiety in the elderly. *J Clin Psychiatry* 1990;51(suppl 1):40–3.

140. Wisner KL, et al. Tricyclic dose requirements across pregnancy. *Am J Psychiatry* 1993;150:1541–2.

141. Preskorn SH. Pharmacokinetics of antidepressants. *J Clin Psychiatry* 1993;54(suppl 9):14–34.

142. DeVane CL. *Fundamentals of monitoring psychoactive drug therapy.* Baltimore: Williams & Wilkins; 1990.

143. Cole JO, Bodkin A. Antidepressant drug side effects. *J Clin Psychiatry* 1990;51(suppl 1):21–6.

144. Rosenstein DL et al. Seizures associated with antidepressants: a review. *J Clin Psychiatry* 1993;54:289–99.

145. Anon. Sudden death in children treated with a tricyclic antidepressant. *Med Lett Drugs Ther* 1990;32:53.

146. Stimmel GL et al. Mirtazapine: an antidepressant with noradrenergic and specific serotonergic effects. *Pharmacotherapy* 1997;17:10–21.

147. Stimmel GL et al. Mirtazapine safety and tolerability: analysis of the clinical trials database. *Primary Psychiatry* 1997;4:82–96.

148. Goodman WK, Charney DS. Therapeutic applications and mechanisms of action of monoamine oxidase inhibitors and heterocyclic antidepressant drugs. *J Clin Psychiatry* 1985;46(10, sec 2):6–22.

149. Cantú TG, Korek JS. Monoamine oxidase inhibitors and weight gain. *Drug Intell Clin Pharm* 1988;22:755–9.

150. Kahn D et al. The safety of switching rapidly from tricyclic antidepressants to monoamine oxidase inhibitors. *J Clin Psychopharmacol* 1989;9:198–202.

151. Brown CS, Bryant SG. Monoamine oxidase inhibitors: safety and efficacy issues. *Drug Intell Clin Pharm* 1988;22:232–5.

152. Shulman KI et al. Dietary restriction, tyramine, and the use of monoamine oxidase inhibitors. *J Clin Psychopharmacol* 1989;9:397–402.

153. Nierenberg AA, Amsterdam JD. Treatment-resistant depression: definition and treatment approaches. *J Clin Psychiatry* 1990;51(suppl 6):39–47.

154. Dopheide JA et al. Focus on nefazodone: a serotonergic drug for major depression. *Hosp Formul* 1995;30:205–12.

155. Fontaine R et al. A double-blind comparison of nefazodone, imipramine, and placebo in major depression. *J Clin Psychiatry* 1994;55:234–41.

156. Barbhaiya RH et al. Single-dose pharmacokinetics of nefazodone in healthy young and elderly subjects and in subjects with renal or hepatic impairment. *Eur J Clin Pharmacol* 1995;49:221–8.

157. Barbhaiya RH et al. Steady-state pharmacokinetics of nefazodone in subjects normal and impaired renal function. *Eur J Clin Pharmacol* 1995;49:229–35.

158. DeWilde J et al. A double-blind, comparative, multicentre study comparing paroxetine with fluoxetine in depressed patients. *Acta Psychiatr Scand* 1993;87:141–5.

159. Dechant KL, Clissold SPP. Paroxetine. *Drugs* 1991;41:225–53.

160. DeVane CL. Pharmacokinetics of the selective serotonin reuptake inhibitors. *J Clin Psychiatry* 1992;53(suppl 2): 13–20.

161. Tollefson GD et al. A multicenter investigation of fixed dose fluoxetine in the treatment of obsessive-compulsive disorder. *Arch Gen Psychiatry* 1994;51:559–67.

162. Greist J et al. Double-blind parallel comparison of three dosages of sertraline and placebo in outpatients with obsessive-compulsive disorder. *Arch Gen Psychiatry* 1995;52;289–95.

163. Johnson MR et al. Panic disorder: pathophysiology and drug treatment. *Drugs* 1995;49:328–44.

164. Sheehan DV, Harnett-Sheehan K. The role of SSRIs in panic disorder. *J Clin Psychiatry* 1996;57(suppl 10): 51–8.

165. Montejo-Gonzalez AL et al. SSRI-induced sexual dysfunction: fluoxetine, paroxetine, sertraline, and fluvoxamine in a prospective, multicenter, and descriptive clinical study of 344 patients. *J Sex Marital Ther* 1997;23:176–94.

166. Heym J, Koe BK. Pharmacology of sertraline: a review. *J Clin Psychiatry* 1988;49(suppl 8):40–5.

167. Doogan DP, Caillard V. Sertraline: a new antidepressant. *J Clin Psychiatry* 1988;49(suppl 8):46–51.

168. Aguglia E et al. Double-blind study of the efficacy and safety of sertraline versus fluoxetine in major depression. *Int Clin Psychopharmacol* 1993;8:197–202.

169. Wisner KL et al. Serum sertraline and *N*-desmethylsertraline levels in breast-feeding mother-infant pairs. *Am J Psychiatry* 1998;155:690–2.

170. Bradley ME et al. Sertraline-associated syndrome of inappropriate antidiuretic hormone: case report and review of the literature. *Pharmacotherapy* 1996;16:680–3.

171. Bryant SG, Ereshefsky L. Antidepressant properties of trazodone. *Clin Pharm* 1982;1:406–17.

172. Georgotas A et al. Trazodone hydrochloride: a wide spectrum antidepressant with a unique pharmacological profile. *Pharmacotherapy* 1982;2:255–65.

173. Nierenberg AA et al. Trazodone for antidepressant-associated insomnia. *Am J Psychiatry* 1994;151:1069–72.

174. Dittrich A et al. Treatment of pharmacological priapism with phenylephrine. *J Urol* 1991;146:323–4.

175. Nierenberg AA et al. Trazodone for antidepressant-associated insomnia. *Am J Psychiatry* 1994;151:1069–72.

176. Cunningham LA. Once-daily venlafaxine extended release (XR) and venlafaxine immediate release (IR) in outpatients with major depression. *Ann Clin Psychiatry* 1997;9:157–64.

177. Schweizer E et al. Placebo-controlled trial of venlafaxine for the treatment of major depression. *J Clin Psychopharmacol* 1991;11:233–236.

178. Montgomery SA. Venlafaxine: a new dimension in antidepressant pharmacotherapy. *J Clin Psychiatry* 1993; 54:119–26.

179. Cunningham LA et al. A comparison of venlafaxine, trazodone, and placebo in major depression. *J Clin Psychopharmacol* 1994;14:99–106.

180. Milne RJ, Goa KL. Citalopram. *Drugs* 1991;41:450–77.

181. Montgomery SA et al. The optimal dosing regimen for citalopram—a meta-analysis of nine placebo-controlled studies. *Int Clin Psychopharmacol* 1994;9(suppl 1):35–40.

182. Ereshefsky L et al. Pathophysiologic basis for schizophrenia and the efficacy of antipsychotics. *Clin Pharm* 1990;9:682–707.

183. Coyle JT. The clinical use of antipsychotic medications. *Med Clin North Am* 1982;66:993–1009.

184. Kane JM. The current status of neuroleptic therapy. *J Clin Psychiatry* 1989;50:322–8.

185. Heresco-Levy U et al. Trial of maintenance neuroleptic dose reduction in schizophrenic outpatients: two year outcome. *J Clin Psychiatry* 1993;54:59–62.

186. Brotman AW et al. A role for high-dose antipsychotics. *J Clin Psychiatry* 1990;51:164–6.

187. Rifkin A et al. Dosage of haloperidol for mania. *Br J Psychiatry* 1994;165:113–6.

188. Zaleon CR, Guthrie SK. Antipsychotic drug use in older adults. *Am J Hosp Pharm* 1994;51:2917–43.

189. Palao DJ et al. Haloperidol: therapeutic window in schizophrenia. *J Clin Psychopharmacol* 1994;14:303–10.

190. Khot V et al. The assessment and clinical implications of haloperidol acute-dose, steady-state, and withdrawal pharmacokinetics. *J Clin Psychopharmacol* 1993;13:120–7.

191. Pearlman CA. Neuroleptic malignant syndrome: a review of the literature. *J Clin Psychopharmacol* 1986;6:257–73.

192. Gardos G et al. Ten year outcome of tardive dyskinesia. *Am J Psychiatry* 1994;151:836–41.

193. Ereshefsky L et al. Clozapine: an atypical antipsychotic agent. *Clin Pharm* 1989;8:691–709.

194. Lieberman JA et al. Clozapine: guidelines for clinical management. *J Clin Psychiatry* 1989;50:329–38.

195. Meltzer HY. An overview of the mechanism of action of clozapine. *J Clin Psychiatry* 1994;55(suppl 9): 47–52.

196. Lieberman JA et al. Clinical effects of clozapine in chronic schizophrenia: response to treatment and predictors of outcome. *Am J Psychiatry* 1994;151:1744–52.

197. Jann MW et al. Pharmacokinetics and pharmacodynamics of clozapine. *Clin Pharmacokinet* 1993;24:161–76.

198. Alvir JMJ, Lieberman JA. Agranulocytosis: incidence and risk factors. *J Clin Psychiatry* 1994;55(suppl 9):137–8.

199. Chouinard G et al. A randomized clinical trial of haloperidol decanoate and fluphenazine decanoate in the outpatient treatment of schizophrenia. *J Clin Psychopharmacol* 1989;9:247–53.

200. Hemstrom CA et al. Haloperidol decanoate: a depot antipsychotic. *Drug Intell Clin Pharm* 1988;22:290–5.

201. Gerlach J. Oval versus depot administration of neuroleptics in relapse prevention. *Acta Psychiatr Scand* 1994;89(suppl 382):28–32.

202. Inderbitzin LB et al. A double-blind dose-reduction trial of fluphenazine decanoate for chronic, unstable schizophrenic patients. *Am J Psychiatry* 1994;151:1753–9.

203. Ereshefsky L et al. A loading-dose strategy for converting from oral to depot haloperidol. *Hosp Community Psychiatry* 1993;44:1155–61.

204. Colvin CL, Tankanow RM. Pimozide: use in Tourette's syndrome. *Drug Intell Clin Pharm* 1985;19:421–4.

205. Tueth MJ, Cheong JA. Clinical uses of pimozide. *South Med J* 1993;86:344–9.

206. Ereshefsky L, Lacomb S. Pharmacological profile of risperidone. *Can J Psychiatry* 1993;38(suppl 3):S80–8.

207. Cohen LJ. Risperidone. *Pharmacotherapy* 1994;14:253–65.

208. Livingston MG. Risperidone. *Lancet* 1994;343:457–60.

209. Marder SR, Meibach RC. Risperidone in the treatment of schizophrenia. *Am J Psychiatry* 1994;151:825–35.

210. Heykants J et al. The pharmacokinetics of risperidone in humans: a summary. *J Clin Psychiatr* 1994;55(suppl 5):13–7.

211. American Psychiatric Association. Practice guideline for the treatment of patients with schizophrenia. *Am J Psychiatry* 1997;154(suppl 4):1–63.

212. Beasley CM et al. Safety of olanzapine. *J Clin Psychiatry* 1997;58(suppl 10):13–7.

213. Small JG et al. Quetiapine in patients with schizophrenia. *Arch Gen Psychiatry* 1997;54:549–57.

214. Anon. Quetiapine for schizophrenia. *Med Lett Drugs Ther* 1997;39:117–8.

215. Arvanitis LA et al. Multiple fixed doses of Seroquel (quetiapine) in patients with acute exacerbation of schizophrenia: a comparison with haloperidol and placebo. *Biol Psychiatry* 1997;42:233–46.

216. Jonas JM, Cohon MS. A comparison of the safety and efficacy of alprazolam versus other agents in the treatment of anxiety, panic, and depression: a review of the literature. *J Clin Psychiatry* 1993;54(suppl 10):25–45.

217. Fawcett JA, Kravitz HM. Alprazolam: pharmacokinetics, clinical efficacy, and mechanism of action. *Pharmacotherapy* 1982;2:243–54.

218. Scavone JM et al. Alprazolam kinetics following sublingual and oral administration. *J Clin Psychopharmacol* 1987;7:332–4.

219. Kroboth et al. Alprazolam in the elderly: pharmacokinetics and pharmacodynamics during multiple dosing. *Psychopharmacology* 1990;100:477–84.

220. Patterson JF. Alprazolam dependency: use of clonazepam for withdrawal. *South Med J* 1988;81:830–2.

221. Dubovsky SL. Generalized anxiety disorder: new concepts and psychopharmacologic therapies. *J Clin Psychiatry* 1990;51(suppl 1):3–10.

222. Gorman JM, Papp LA. Chronic anxiety: deciding the length of treatment. *J Clin Psychiatry* 1990;51 (suppl 1):11–5.

223. Kranzler HR, Orrok B. The pharmacotherapy of alcoholism. In, Tasman A et al., eds. *Review of psychiatry*. vol. 8. Washington DC: American Psychiatric Press; 1989:359–80.

224. Roy-Byrne PP, Cowley DS. *Benzodiazepines in clinical practice: risks and benefits*. Washington DC: American Psychiatric Press; 1991:213–27.

225. Greenblatt DJ et al. Benzodiazepines: a summary of pharmacokinetic properties. *Br J Clin Pharmacol* 1981;11:11S–6S.

226. Dietch JT, Jennings RK. Aggressive dyscontrol in patients treated with benzodiazepines. *J Clin Psychiatry* 1988;49:184–8.

227. Jann MW. Buspirone: an update on a unique anxiolytic agent. *Pharmacotherapy* 1988;8:100–16.

228. Sussman N. The uses of buspirone in psychiatry. *J Clin Psychiatry Monogr* 1994;12:3–19.

229. Gammans RE et al. Pharmacokinetics of buspirone in elderly subjects. *J Clin Pharmacol* 1989;29:72–8.

230. Gammans RE et al. Metabolism and disposition of buspirone. *Am J Med* 1986;80(suppl 3B):41–51.

231. Newton RE et al. Review of the side-effect profile of buspirone. *Am J Med* 1986;80(suppl 3B):17–21.

232. Schweizer E, Rickels K. New and emerging clinical uses for buspirone. *J Clin Psychiatry Monogr* 1994; 12:46–54.

233. Kales A et al. Comparative effectiveness of nine hypnotic drugs: sleep laboratory studies. *J Clin Pharmacol* 1977;17:207–13.

234. Salmon AG et al. Potential carcinogenicity of chloral hydrate—a review. *J Toxicol Clin Toxicol* 1995;33: 115–21.

235. Brogden RN, Goa KL. Flumazenil. A preliminary review of its benzodiazepine antagonist properties, intrinsic activity and therapeutic use. *Drugs* 1988;35:448–67.

236. Longmire AW, Seger DL. Topics in clinical pharmacology: flumazenil, a benzodiazepine antagonist. *Am J Med Sci* 1993;306:49–52.

237. Hoffman EJ, Warren EW. Flumazenil: a benzodiazepine antagonist. *Clin Pharm* 1993;12:641–56.

238. Spivey WH. Flumazenil and seizures: analysis of 43 cases. *Clin Ther* 1992;14:292–305.

239. Kanto JH. Midazolam: the first water-soluble benzodiazepine. *Pharmacotherapy* 1985;5:138–55.

240. Bell GD et al. Intravenous midazolam for upper gastrointestinal endoscopy: a study of 800 consecutive cases relating dose to age and sex of patient. *Br J Clin Pharmacol* 1987;23:241–3.

241. Daneshmend TK, Logan RFA. Midazolam. *Lancet* 1988;1:389. Letter.

242. Saint-Maurice C et al. The pharmacokinetics of rectal midazolam for premedication in children. *Anesthesiology* 1986;65:536–8.

243. Yakabowich MR. Hypnotics in the elderly: appropriate usage guidelines. *J Geriatr Drug Ther* 1992;6:5–21.

244. Weiss KJ. Management of anxiety and depression syndromes in the elderly. *J Clin Psychiatry* 1994;55 (suppl 2):5–12.

245. Garzone PD, Kroboth PD. Pharmacokinetics of the newer benzodiazepines. *Clin Pharmacokinet* 1989;16: 337–64.

246. Robin DW et al. Triazolam in cirrhosis: pharmacokinetics and pharmacodynamics. *Clin Pharmacol Ther* 1993;54:630–7.

247. Scharf MB et al. Comparative amnestic effects of benzodiazepine hypnotic agents. *J Clin Psychiatry* 1988; 49:134–7.

248. Roth T et al. Pharmacology and hypnotic efficacy of triazolam. *Pharmacotherapy* 1983;3:137–48.

249. Gillin JC, Byerley W. The diagnosis and management of insomnia. *N Engl J Med* 1990;322:239–48.

250. Treatment of sleep disorders of older people. *NIH Consensus Dev Conf Consens Statement* 1990;8 (March):26–8.

251. Scharf MB et al. A multi-center placebo-controlled study evaluating zolpidem in the treatment of chronic insomnia. *J Clin Psychiatry* 1994;55:192–9.

252. Jonas JM et al. Comparative clinical profiles of triazolam versus other shorter-acting hypnotics. *J Clin Psychiatry* 1992;53(suppl 12):19–31.

253. Langtry HD, Benfield P. Zolpidem: a review of its pharmacodynamic and pharmacokinetic properties and therapeutic potential. *Drugs* 1990;40:291–313.

254. Mitler MM. Evaluation of temazepam as a hypnotic. *Pharmacotherapy* 1981;1:3–13.

255. Kales A. Quazepam: hypnotic efficacy and side effects. *Pharmacotherapy* 1990;10:1–12.

256. Scherf MB et al. Estazolam and flurazepam: a multicenter, placebo-controlled comparative study in outpatients with insomnia. *J Clin Pharmacol* 1990;30:461–7.

257. Breimer DD. Clinical pharmacokinetics of hypnotics. *Clin Pharmacokinet* 1977;2:93–109.

258. Post RM, Weiss SRB, Chuang DM. Mechanisms of action of anticonvulsants in affective disorders: comparisons with lithium. *J Clin Psychopharmacol* 1992;12:23S–35S.

259. Baldessarini RJ. Drugs and the treatment of psychiatric disorders. In, Hardman JG et al., eds. *Goodman and Gilman's the pharmacological basis of therapeutics.* 9th ed. New York: McGraw-Hill; 1996:431–59.

260. Kook KA et al. Accuracy and safety of a priori lithium loading. *J Clin Psychiatry* 1985;46:49–51.

261. Lobeck F. A review of lithium dosing methods. *Pharmacotherapy* 1988;8:248–55.

262. Gutierrez MA et al. Evaluation of a new steady-state lithium prediction method. *Lithium* 1991;2:57–9.

263. *USP-DI,* Vol I. Rockville, MD. The United States Pharmacopoeal Convention, 1996.

264. Hardy BG et al. Pharmacokinetics of lithium in the elderly. *J Clin Psychopharmacol* 1987;7:153–8.

265. Jefferson JW. Lithium: a therapeutic magic wand. *J Clin Psychiatry* 1989;50:81–6.

266. Jefferson JW. Lithium: the present and the future. *J Clin Psychiatry* 1990;51(suppl 8):4–8.

267. Gitlin MJ et al. Maintenance lithium treatment: side effects and compliance. *J Clin Psychiatry* 1989;50: 127–31.

268. Salem RB. Recommendations for monitoring lithium therapy. *Drug Intell Clin Pharm* 1983;17:346–50.

269. Gitlin MJ. Lithium-induced renal insufficiency. *J Clin Psychopharmacol* 1993;13:276–9.

270. American Psychiatric Association. Practice guideline for the treatment of patients with bipolar disorder. *Am J Psychiatry* 1994;151(suppl 12):1–36.

271. Bowden CL et al. Efficacy of divalproex vs lithium and placebo in the treatment of mania. *JAMA* 1994;271:918–24.

272. Bowden CL et al. Relation of serum valproate concentrations to response in mania. *Am J Psychiatry* 1996; 153:765–70.

273. Koller WC et al. An algorithm for managing Parkinson's disease. *Neurology* 1994;44(suppl 1):S1–52.

274. Stern MB. Contemporary approaches to the pharmacotherapeutic management of Parkinson's disease: an overview. *Neurology* 1997;49(suppl 1):S2–9.

275. Aoki FY, Sitar DA. Clinical pharmacokinetics of amantadine hydrochloride. *Clin Pharmacokinet* 1988;14:35–51.

276. Hordam VW et al. Pharmacokinetics of amantadine hydrochloride in subjects with normal and impaired renal function. *Ann Intern Med* 1981;94(part 1):454–8.

277. Aoki FY, Sitar DS. Amantadine kinetics in healthy elderly men: implications for influenza prevention. *Clin Pharmacol Ther* 1985;37:137–44.

278. Brady MT et al. Safety and prophylactic efficacy of low-dose rimantadine in adults during an influenza A epidemic. *Antimicrob Agents Chemother* 1990;34:1633–6.

279. Tominack RL, Hayden FG. Rimantadine hydrochloride and amantadine hydrochloride use in influenza A virus infections. *Infect Dis Clin North Am* 1987;1:459–78.

280. He H et al. Development of a sensitive and specific radioimmunoassay for benztropine. *J Pharm Sci* 1993;82:1027–32.

281. Nutt JG et al. The effect of carbidopa on the pharmacokinetics of intravenously administered levodopa: the mechanism of action in the treatment of parkinsonism. *Ann Neurol* 1985;18:537–43.

282. Juncos JL. Levodopa: pharmacology, pharmacokinetics, and pharmacodynamics. *Neurol Clin* 1992;10: 487–509.

283. Yeh KC et al. Pharmacokinetics and bioavailability of Sinemet CR: a summary of human studies. *Neurology* 1989;39(suppl 2):S25–38.

284. LeWitt PA. Treatment strategies for extension of levodopa effect. *Neurol Clin* 1992;10:511–26.

285. Koller WC, Hubble JP. Levodopa therapy in Parkinson's disease. *Neurology* 1990;40(suppl 3):S40–7.

286. Cedarbaum JM. Pharmacokinetic and pharmacodynamic considerations in management of motor response fluctuations in Parkinson's disease. *Neurol Clin* 1990;8:31–49.

287. Hutton JT et al. Multicenter controlled study of Sinemet CR vs Sinemet (25/100) in advanced Parkinson's disease. *Neurology* 1989;39(suppl 2):S67–72.

288. Rogers SL, Friedhoff LT, and the Donepezil Study Group. The efficacy and safety of donepezil in patients with Alzheimer's disease. Results of a US multicentre, randomized, double-blind, placebo-controlled trial. *Dementia* 1996;7:293–303.

289. Rogers SL et al. A 24-week, double-blind, placebo-controlled trial of donepezil in patients with Alzheimer's disease. *Neurology* 1998;50:136–45.

290. Rogers SL et al. The pharmacokinetics and pharmacodynamics of E2020 (R,S)-1-benzyl-4-((5,6 dimethoxyl-1-indanon)-2 yl)-methylpiperidine hydrochloride, a novel inhibitor of acetylcholinesterase: implications for use in the treatment of Alzheimer's disease. *Neurobiol Aging* 1992;13:496.

291. Rogers SL, Friedhoff LT. The pharmacokinetic and pharmacodynamic profile of donepezil HCl (E2020) following single and multiple oral doses. *Clin Pharmacol Ther* 1997;61:181. Abstract.

292. Watts RL. The role of dopamine agonists in early Parkinson's disease. *Neurology* 1997;49(suppl 1):S34–48.

293. Goetz CG, Diederich NJ. Dopaminergic agonists for the treatment of Parkinson's disease. *Neurol Clin* 1992; 10:527–40.

294. Piercey MF et al. Functional roles for dopamine-receptor subtypes. *Clin Neuropharmacol* 1995;18(suppl 1): S34–42.

295. Schran HF et al. The pharmacokinetics of bromocriptine in man. In, Goldstein M et al., eds. *Ergot compounds and brain function.* New York: Raven Press; 1980:125–39.

296. Friis ML et al. Pharmacokinetics of bromocriptine during continuous oral treatment of Parkinson's disease. *Eur J Clin Pharmacol* 1979;15:275–80.

297. Thalamas C et al. Effect of food on the pharmacokinetics of ropinirole in patients with Parkinson's disease. *Mov Disor* 1996;2(suppl 1):138. Abstract.

298. Gottwald MD et al. New pharmacotherapy for Parkinson's disease. *Ann Pharmacother* 1997;31:1205–17.

299. Rubin A et al. Physiologic disposition of pergolide. *Clin Pharmacol Ther* 1981;30:258–65.

300. McElvaney NG et al. Pleuropulmonary disease during bromocriptine treatment of Parkinson's disease. *Arch Intern Med* 1988;148:2231–6.

301. Langtry HD, Clissold SPP. Pergolide. A review of its pharmacological properties and therapeutic potential in Parkinson's disease. *Drugs* 1990;39:491–506.

302. Mizuno Y et al. Pergolide in the treatment of Parkinson's disease. *Neurology* 1995;45(suppl 3):S13–21.

303. Hubble JP et al. Pramipexole in patients with early Parkinson's disease. *Clin Neuropharmacol* 1995;18:338–47.

304. Parkinson Study Group. Safety and efficacy of pramipexole in early Parkinson disease. *JAMA* 1997;278:125–30.

305. Lieberman A et al. Clinical evaluation of pramipexole in advanced Parkinson's disease: results of a double-blind, placebo-controlled, parallel-group study. *Neurology* 1997;49:162–8.

306. Bryson HM et al. Riluzole. A review of its pharmacodynamic and pharmacokinetic properties and therapeutic potential in amyotrophic lateral sclerosis. *Drugs* 1996;52:549–63.

307. Sanderink GJ et al. Involvement of human CYP1A isoenzymes in the metabolism and drug interactions of riluzole in vitro. *J Pharmacol Exp Ther* 1997;282:1465–72.

308. Bruno E et al. Population pharmacokinetics of riluzole in patients with amyotrophic lateral sclerosis. *Clin Pharmacol Ther* 1997;62:518–26.

309. Practice advisory on the treatment of amyotrophic lateral sclerosis with riluzole: report of the Quality Standards Subcommittee of the American Academy of Neurology. *Neurology* 1997;49:657–9.

310. Bensimon G, Lacomblez L, Meninger V and the ALS/Riluzole Study Group. A controlled trial of riluzole in amyotrophic lateral sclerosis. *N Engl J Med* 1994;330:585–91.

311. Youdim MBH, Finberg JPM. Pharmacological actions of l-deprenyl (selegiline) and other selective monoamine oxidase B inhibitors. *Clin Pharmacol Ther* 1994;56:725–33.

312. Mahmood I. Clinical pharmacokinetics and pharmacodynamics of selegiline. *Clin Pharmacokinet* 1997; 33:99–102.

313. Olanow CW. Attempts to obtain neuroprotection in Parkinson's disease. *Neurology* 1997;49(1 suppl 1): S26–33.

314. The Parkinson Study Group. Effects of tocopherol and deprenyl on the progression of disability in early Parkinson's disease. *N Engl J Med* 1993;328:176–83.

315. The Parkinson Study Group. Effect of deprenyl on the progression of disability in early Parkinson's disease. *N Engl J Med* 1989;321:1364–71.

316. Parkinson Study Group. Impact of deprenyl and tocopherol treatment on Parkinson's disease in DATATOP patients requiring levodopa. *Ann Neurol* 1996;39:37–45.

317. Parkinson Study Group. Impact of deprenyl and tocopherol treatment on Parkinson's disease in DATATOP subjects not requiring levodopa. *Ann Neurol* 1996;39:29–36.

318. Heinonen EH et al. Pharmacokinetics and metabolism of selegiline. *Acta Neurol Scand* 1989;80(suppl 126): 93–9.

319. Dingemanse J et al. Integrated pharmacokinetics and pharmacodynamics of the novel catechol-O-methyltransferase inhibitor tolcapone during first administration to humans. *Clin Pharmacol Ther* 1995;57:508–17.

320. Jorga KM et al. Optimizing levodopa pharmacokinetics with multiple tolcapone doses in the elderly. *Clin Pharmacol Ther* 1997;62:300–10.

321. Kurth MC et al. Tolcapone improves motor function and reduces levodopa requirement in patients with Parkinson's disease experiencing motor fluctuations: a multicenter, double-blind, randomized, placebo-controlled trial. *Neurology* 1997;48:81–7.

322. Waters CH. Tolcapone in stable Parkinson's disease: efficacy and safety of long-term treatment. The Tolcapone Stable Study Group. *Neurology* 1997;49:665–71.

323. Rajput AH et al. Tolcapone improves motor function in parkinsonian patients with the "wearing-off" phenomenon: a double-blind, placebo-controlled, multicenter trial. *Neurology* 1997;49:1066–71.

Gastrointestinal Drugs

Acid-Peptic Therapy

ANTACIDS

Pharmacology. Antacids are weakly basic inorganic salts whose primary action is to neutralize gastric acid; pH >4 inhibits the proteolytic activity of pepsin. Aluminum-containing antacids suppress, but do not eradicate, *Helicobacter pylori* and may promote ulcer healing in peptic ulcer disease (PUD) by enhancing mucosal defense mechanisms.[1,2] Aluminum salts also bind phosphate and bile salts in the GI tract, decreasing serum phosphate and serum bile salt levels. Antacids may increase urine pH.

Administration and Adult Dosage. PO for symptomatic relief of indigestion, nonulcer dyspepsia, epigastric pain in PUD or heartburn in gastroesophageal reflux disease (GERD) 10–30 mL prn or 1 and 3 hr after meals and hs.[1,2] **PO for treatment of PUD** 100–160 mEq of acid-neutralizing capacity per dose, given 1 and 3 hr after meals and hs for 4–8 weeks or until healing is complete. Additional doses may be taken if epigastric pain persists. There is evidence that lower dosages may heal peptic ulcers.[1,2] **PO or NG for prevention or treatment of upper GI bleeding in critically ill patients** titrate to maintain intragastric pH above 4.0.[3] **PO for phosphate binding in renal failure** (aluminum hydroxide) 1.9–4.8 g tid or qid, or (calcium carbonate) 8–12 g/day; titrate dosage based on serum phosphate.[1]

Special Populations. *Pediatric Dosage.* **PO for treatment of PUD or GERD** (≤12 yr) at least 5–15 mL up to q 1 hr; (>12 yr) same as adult dosage.

Geriatric Dosage. Avoid using magnesium-containing antacids in renal impairment.

Other Conditions. Avoid using magnesium-containing antacids in patients with Cl_{cr} <30 mL/min.

Dosage Forms. (*See* Antacid Products Comparison Chart, page 498.)

Patient Instructions. If antacids do not relieve symptoms of indigestion, upset stomach, or heartburn within 2 weeks, contact your health care practitioner. Diarrhea may occur with magnesium-containing antacids; decrease the daily dosage, alternate doses with, or switch to an aluminum- or calcium-containing antacid. Constipation may occur with aluminum-containing antacids; decrease the daily dosage, alternate doses with, or switch to, a magnesium-containing antacid. Refrigerating liquid antacids may improve their palatability. Antacids may interfere with other medications; take other medications 1–2 hours before or after antacids unless otherwise directed. If tablets are used, chew thoroughly before swallowing and follow with a glass of water.

Missed Doses. If your health care practitioner has told you to take this medicine on a regular schedule and you miss a dose, take it as soon as possible. If it is almost time for your next dose, skip the missed dose and return to your usual dosage schedule. Do not double doses.

Pharmacokinetics. *Onset and Duration.* Onset of acid neutralizing is immediate; duration is 30 ± 10 min in the fasted state and 1–3 hr if ingested after meals.[1]

Fate. Antacid cations are absorbed to varying degrees. Sodium is highly soluble and readily absorbed; calcium absorption is generally less than 30%, but may decrease with increasing age, intake, achlorhydria, and estrogen loss at menopause; magnesium is generally about 30% absorbed, but percent absorption may vary inversely with intake; aluminum is slightly absorbed. Calcium, magnesium, and aluminum are excreted renally with normal renal function.[1] The unabsorbed portion is excreted in the feces.

Adverse Reactions. Long-term use of sodium- or calcium-containing antacids can cause systemic alkalosis. Hypercalcemia may occur with ingestion of large amounts of calcium; soluble antacids plus a diet high in milk products may result in milk-alkali syndrome, which can lead to nephrolithiasis.[1] Magnesium-containing antacids cause a dose-related laxative effect; hypermagnesemia occurs in patients with renal impairment.[1] Aluminum-containing antacids cause dose-related constipation, especially in the elderly. Prolonged administration or large dosages of aluminum hydroxide or carbonate can result in hypophosphatemia, particularly in the elderly and in alcoholics; encephalopathy has been reported in dialysis patients receiving aluminum-containing antacids alone or with sucralfate.[1-3]

Precautions. Avoid magnesium-containing products in renal impairment. Use others with caution in patients with chronic renal failure, edema, hypertension, or CHF. Because antacids are particulate and elevate intragastric pH, they may predispose critically ill patients to nosocomial pneumonia.[3]

Drug Interactions. Antacids reduce the absorption of numerous drugs, the most important of which are digoxin, oral iron (calcium carbonate, sodium bicarbonate, and possibly magnesium trisilicate), isoniazid (aluminum-containing), ketoconazole, oral quinolones, and oral tetracyclines (di- and trivalent cations). Antacids may reduce salicylate levels and increase quinidine levels because of urinary pH changes. Large dosages of calcium antacids may produce hypercalcemia in the presence of thiazides. Sodium polystyrene sulfonate resin can bind magnesium and calcium ions from the antacid in the gut, resulting in systemic alkalosis.

Parameters to Monitor. Monitor for relief of dyspepsia, epigastric pain or heartburn, and diarrhea or constipation. Monitor serum phosphate during long-term use of aluminum-containing products in patients with chronic renal impairment. Monitor for drug interactions.

Notes. Aggressive antacid therapy is at least as effective as the H_2-receptor antagonists or sucralfate when treating PUD or preventing stress-related mucosal bleeding; however, do not use antacids as first-line agents because large, frequent doses are inconvenient and associated with an increased risk of adverse effects.[1-3] Magaldrate is a chemical mixture of magnesium and aluminum hydroxides. **Alginic**

acid has foaming and floating properties that may be beneficial in GERD. Most antacid products have been reformulated to contain low amounts of sodium; some antacid products contain considerable amounts of sugar or artificial sweetener. Antacid tablets, if chewed and swallowed, may be as effective as equivalent doses of liquid formulations. Although gastrin is stimulated by calcium, gastric acid rebound with calcium-containing antacids is of questionable clinical importance.[1]

BISMUTH PREPARATIONS	Pepto-Bismol, Tritec, Various

Pharmacology. Bismuth salts are used to treat nausea, indigestion, diarrhea, gastritis, and peptic ulcers. The precise method by which bismuth heals gastritis and ulcers is uncertain, but possible mechanisms include a local gastroprotective effect, stimulation of endogenous prostaglandins, and antimicrobial activity against *Helicobacter pylori*. Given alone, bismuth salts suppress *H. pylori,* but long-term eradication requires combination therapy with antibiotics. **Bismuth subsalicylate** (BSS; Pepto-Bismol, various) is the bismuth salt used most frequently in the United States. **Ranitidine bismuth citrate** (RBC) is a complex of ranitidine, trivalent bismuth, and citrate.[1,2,4–6]

Adult Dosage. PO for the control of nausea, abdominal cramps, and diarrhea (BSS) 525 mg (305 mg elemental bismuth) qid, to a maximum of 4.2 g/day. When given with antibiotics to eradicate *H. pylori,* treatment is usually limited to 1–2 weeks. (*See also* Eradication of *Helicobacter pylori* Infection.)

Dosage Forms. Susp (Bismuth subsalicylate) 17.5, 35 mg/mL; **Tab** (Ranitidine bismuth citrate) 262 mg; **Tab** 400 mg (containing ranitidine 150 mg and bismuth citrate 240 mg) (Tritec).

Pharmacokinetics. Following oral administration, BSS (58% bismuth, 42% salicylate) is converted in the GI tract to bismuth oxide and salicylic acid. Bismuth is less than 0.2% absorbed with more than 99% of an oral dose excreted in the feces. Over 90% of the salicylate dose is absorbed and excreted in urine. RBC dissociates in intragastric fluid to ranitidine and soluble and insoluble forms of bismuth. Oral absorption of bismuth from RBC is variable.

Adverse Reactions. BSS and bismuth derived from RBC may cause temporary darkening of the tongue and stool. Use BSS with caution in children; in the elderly; in patients with renal impairment, salicylate sensitivity, or bleeding disorders; in those receiving high-dosage salicylate therapy; or when potentially interacting medications are taken. Salicylic acid is less likely than aspirin to cause gastric mucosal damage and blood loss. Prolonged BSS therapy and the use of other salts (subgallate and subnitrate) have been associated with neurotoxicity. Bismuth concentrations may be elevated in the elderly and patients with renal impairment because of decreased renal elimination. RBC should not be used as a single agent for the treatment of active duodenal or gastric ulcers.

ANTACID PRODUCTS COMPARISON CHART[a]

| | ACID NEUTRALIZING CAPACITY | | | SODIUM CONTENT | | |
ANTACID	mEq/5 mL	mEq/Tablet	mEq/5 mL	mg/5 mL	mEq/Tablet	mg/Tablet
Aluminum Carbonate, Basic						
Basalgel	11.5	12.5 (Cap/Tab)	0.13	3	0.12	2.8
Aluminum Hydroxide						
ALternaGEL	16	—	0.109	<2.5	—	—
Amphojel	10	8 (300 mg Tab)	0.10	<2.3	0.08	1.8
		16 (600 mg Tab)	—	—	0.13	3
Aluminum Hydroxide with Magnesium Carbonate						
Gaviscon[b]	3.3–4.3	—	0.57	13	—	—
Gaviscon Extra Strength[b]	14.3	5–7.5	0.9	20.7	1.3	29.9
Maalox Heartburn Relief[b]	8.5	7.4	0.11	2.5	0.13	3
Aluminum Hydroxide with Magnesium Hydroxide						
Maalox	13.3	9.7 (Original)	0.04	1	0.04	1
		10.7 (Regular)	—	—	0.03	0.8
Maalox Therapeutic Concentrate	27.2	—	0.03	0.8	—	—
Aluminum Hydroxide with Magnesium Hydroxide and Simethicone						
Di-Gel	9	—	0.07	1.5	—	—
Gelusil	—	11	—	—	<0.22	<5
Maalox Plus[c]	—	10.7	—	—	0.04	<1
Maalox Plus,[d] Extra Strength	29.1	18.6	0.04	<1	0.07	<1.7
Mylanta	12.7	11.5	0.03	0.68	0.03	0.77
Mylanta Double Strength	25.4	23	0.05	1.14	0.06	1.3

(continued)

ANTACID PRODUCTS COMPARISON CHART[a] (continued)

ANTACID	ACID NEUTRALIZING CAPACITY		SODIUM CONTENT			
	mEq/5 mL	mEq/Tablet	mEq/5 mL	mg/5 mL	mEq/Tablet	mg/Tablet
Aluminum Hydroxide with Magnesium Trisilicate and Sodium Bicarbonate						
Gaviscon[b]	—	0.5	—	—	0.8	18.4
Gaviscon-2[b]	—	1	—	—	1.6	36.8
Calcium Carbonate						
Di-Gel[d]	—	10	—	—	0.05	1.25
Titralac	—	8.5	—	—	0.01	0.3
Titralac Extra Strength	—	15.1	—	—	0.03	0.6
Titralac Plus[c]	11	8.5	0.01	0.25	0.04	1
Tums	—	10	—	—	0.09	2
Tums E-X	—	15	—	—	0.13	3
Tums ULTRA	—	20	—	—	0.17	4
Magaldrate						
Riopan	15	13.5	0.013	0.3	0.004	0.1
Riopan Plus[c]	15	13.5	0.013	0.3	0.004	0.1
Riopan Plus Double Strength[c]	30	30	0.013	0.3	0.022	0.5

[a]The product brands listed are representative of numerous brand and generic products on the market. Product formulations, and hence neutralizing capacity and sodium content, are subject to change by the manufacturer.
[b]Contains alginate.
[c]Contains simethicone.
[d]Tablet contains calcium carbonate, magnesium hydroxide, and simethicone.

499

HISTAMINE H$_2$-RECEPTOR ANTAGONISTS:	
CIMETIDINE	Tagamet, Various
FAMOTIDINE	Pepcid
NIZATIDINE	Axid
RANITIDINE	Zantac, Various

Pharmacology. Histamine H$_2$-receptor antagonists competitively inhibit the action of histamine at the H$_2$ receptors of the parietal cell and reduce basal, nocturnal, pentagastrin-, and food-stimulated gastric acid.

	CIMETIDINE	**FAMOTIDINE**	**NIZATIDINE**	**RANITIDINE**
Ring structure	Imidazole	Thiazole	Thiazole	Furan
Relative potency	1	20–50	4–10	4–10

Administration and Adult Dosage.

INDICATION	CIMETIDINE	FAMOTIDINE	NIZATIDINE	RANITIDINE
PO for prevention or symptomatic relief of heartburn or indigestion (OTC)	200 mg/day or 200 mg bid.	10 mg/day or 10 mg bid.	75 mg/day or 75 mg bid.	75 mg/day or 75 mg bid.
PO for short-term treatment of active duodenal ulcer (4–8 weeks)	300 mg qid, 400 mg bid, 800 mg hs, or 1600 mg hs.[a]	20 mg bid or 40 mg hs.	150 mg bid or 300 mg hs.	150 mg bid or 300 mg hs.
PO for maintenance of healed duodenal ulcer	400 mg hs.	20 mg hs.	150 mg hs.	150 mg hs.
PO for short-term treatment of active benign gastric ulcer (6–8 weeks)	300 mg qid or 800 mg hs.	20 mg bid[b] or 40 mg hs.	150 mg bid or 300 mg hs.	150 mg bid or 300 mg hs.[b]

(continued)

INDICATION	CIMETIDINE	FAMOTIDINE	NIZATIDINE	RANITIDINE
PO for maintenance of healed gastric ulcer	400 mg hs.[b]	20 mg hs.[b]	150 mg hs.[b]	150 mg hs.
PO for symptomatic gastroesophageal reflux disease (6–12 weeks)	300 mg qid or 400 mg bid.	20 mg bid.	150 mg bid.	150 mg bid.
PO for healing of erosive esophagitis (6–12 weeks)	400 mg qid or 800 mg bid.	20 or 40 mg bid.	150 mg bid or 300 mg bid.[b]	150 mg qid or 300 mg bid.[b]
PO for maintenance of healed erosive esophagitis	300 mg qid,[b] 400 mg qid,[b] or 800 mg bid.[b]	20 mg bid[b] or 40 mg bid.[b]	150 mg bid[b] or 300 mg bid.[b]	150 mg bid or 300 mg bid.[b]
PO for pathological hypersecretory conditions	300 mg qid, up to 2.4 g/day; or adjust to patient needs.	20 mg q 6 hr, up to 160 mg q 6 hr; or adjust to patient needs.	[b]	150 mg bid, up to 6 g/day; or adjust to patient needs.
IM	300 mg q 6–8 hr.[c]	[d]	[d]	50 mg q 6–8 hr.[c]
IV intermittent	300 q 6–8 hr, up to 2.4 g/day.[c]	20 mg q 12 hr.[c]	[d]	50 mg q 6–8 hr, up to 400 mg/day.[c]
IV intermittent bolus	Dilute to 20 mL; inject over not less than 5 min.[c]	Dilute to 5–10 mL; inject over not less than 2 min.[c]	[d]	Dilute to 20 mL; inject over not less than 5 min.[c]
IV intermittent infusion	Dilute to 50 mL; infuse over 15–20 min.[c]	Dilute to 100 mL; infuse over 15–30 min.[c]	[d]	Dilute to 100 mL; infuse over 15–20 min.[c]
IV continuous infusion	37.5 mg/hr (900 mg/day); adjust to patient needs; up to 600 mg/hr has been given.[c,e]	1.67 mg/hr[b] (40 mg/day); adjust to patient needs.[c,e]	[d]	6.25 mg/hr (150 mg/day); adjust to patient needs; up to 220 mg/hr has been given.[c,e]

(*continued*)

IV for prevention of upper GI bleeding in critically ill patients (cimetidine) 50 mg/hr by continuous infusion;[e] (cimetidine, famotidine, or ranitidine) use standard dosages given by intermittent or continuous infusion.[b,e] In high-risk surgical patients, adjust the dose and/or frequency of intermittent IV therapy or the rate of continuous infusion to maintain the intragastric pH above 4.0.

[a]Heavy smokers with ulcer larger than 1 cm in diameter.
[b]Nonlabeled indication and dosage.
[c]Pathologic hypersecretory states, intractable ulcers, or patients unable to take oral medication.
[d]Nonlabeled route of administration.
[e]Loading dose may be given, but appears to offer little advantage.
From references 2, 3, and 7–12.

Special Populations. *Pediatric Dosage.* Safety and efficacy not well established.

	CIMETIDINE	FAMOTIDINE	NIZATIDINE	RANITIDINE
Neonates	10–20 mg/ kg/day.	1–1.2 mg/kg/ day.	Unknown.	Unknown.
Children (3–16 yr)	20–40 mg/ kg/day.	0.4–1.6 mg/ kg/day.	Unknown.	1–3 mg/kg/ day.

From references 7 and 13–15.

Geriatric Dosage. Reduce dosage based upon renal function.

Other Conditions.

	CIMETIDINE	FAMOTIDINE	NIZATIDINE	RANITIDINE
Renal impairment[a]	Cl_{cr} 15–30 mL/min: 600 mg/day; <15 mL/min: 300–400 mg/ day.	Cl_{cr} <10 mL/ min: 20 mg/day or 20 mg every other day.	Cl_{cr} 20–50 mL/min: 150 mg/day; <20 mL/min: 150 mg every other day.	Cl_{cr} <50 mL/min: PO 150 mg/day or IM/IV 50 mg q 12–24 hr.

[a]Use the lowest dosage that permits an adequate response; further dosage reduction of cimetidine, famotidine, or ranitidine may be necessary with concomitant severe liver disease. Because only small amounts of H_2-receptor antagonists are removed by hemodialysis and peritoneal dialysis, additional doses may not be necessary; adjust dosage schedule so that the time of the scheduled dose coincides with the end of dialysis.
From references 7, 9, and 16.

Dosage Forms.

	CIMETIDINE	FAMOTIDINE	NIZATIDINE	RANITIDINE
	Tab 100, 200, 300, 400,	Tab 10, 20, 40 mg.	Cap 75, 150, 300 mg.	Tab 75, 150, 300 mg.

(continued)

	CIMETIDINE	FAMOTIDINE	NIZATIDINE	RANITIDINE
	800 mg.	Tab (rapid dissolving) 20, 40 mg.		Tab (chewable) 150 mg.
				Tab (effervescent) 150 mg.[a]
				Granules (effervescent) 150 mg.[a]
				Cap 150, 300 mg.
	Soln 60 mg/mL.	Susp 8 mg/mL.[b]		Syrup 15 mg/mL.
	Inj 150 mg/mL.	Inj 10 mg/mL.[c]		Inj 25 mg/mL.

[a]Dissolve dose in approximately 180–240 mL (6–8 fl oz) of water before drinking.
[b]Discard reconstituted suspension after 30 days.
[c]Store at 2–8°C (36–46°F).

Patient Instructions. The effectiveness of H_2-receptor antagonists in peptic ulcer disease may be decreased by cigarette smoking. Discontinue or decrease smoking, or avoid smoking after the last dose of the day. Antacids may be used as needed for relief of epigastric pain. Even though ulcer or gastroesophageal reflux disease (GERD) symptoms may improve, continue treatment for the duration of therapy unless instructed otherwise. If symptomatic relief is not obtained in 2 weeks with over-the-counter medication, contact your health care practitioner. Report any bleeding, vomiting, or severe esophageal or abdominal pain.

Missed Doses. If you miss a dose, take it as soon as possible. If it is almost time for your next dose, skip the missed dose and return to your usual dosage schedule. Do not double doses.

Pharmacokinetics.

	CIMETIDINE	FAMOTIDINE	NIZATIDINE	RANITIDINE
Onset.				
All agents have an oral onset of 1 hr and an IV onset of 15 min.				
Serum Levels.				
EC_{50}[a]	625 ± 375 µg/L	11 ± 2 µg/L	167 ± 13 µg/L	112 ± 52 µg/L
Fate.				
Oral bioavailability	60 ± 20%	41 ± 4%	95 ± 5%; 75% in renal failure.	55 ± 25%
V_d	1 ± 0.2 L/kg	1.2 ± 0.3 L/kg	1.4 ± 0.2 L/kg	1.6 ± 0.4 L/kg
Protein binding	20 ± 6%	16%	30 ± 5%	15%

(*continued*)

	CIMETIDINE	**FAMOTIDINE**	**NIZATIDINE**	**RANITIDINE**
Excreted unchanged in urine	75%	$70 \pm 5\%$	$70 \pm 5\%$	70%
$t_{1/2}$.				
Normal	1.9 ± 0.4 hr	3 ± 0.5 hr	1.4 ± 0.2 hr	2 ± 0.4 hr
Anuric	4.5 ± 0.5 hr	20+ hr	7.2 ± 1.3 hr	7 ± 3 hr

[a]EC_{50} is the serum concentration necessary to inhibit pentagastrin-stimulated secretion of acid by 50%.
From references 2, 7, 8, 16, and 17.

Adverse Reactions. Adverse reactions are generally mild. The most frequent adverse events occur in 1–7% of patients and include headache, diarrhea, constipation, dizziness, drowsiness, and fatigue.[2,7–9] Reversible confusional states, depression, agitation, and other CNS manifestations may occur occasionally with all H_2-receptor antagonists, predominantly in severely ill patients or those with renal and/or hepatic disease.[2,3,7] Reversible dose-dependent increases in ALT have been reported with IV cimetidine and IV ranitidine. Rare cases of fatal hepatic disease with and without jaundice have been reported with cimetidine and ranitidine.[7] H_2-receptor antagonists do not markedly decrease hepatic blood flow.[7] Cardiac arrhythmias, tachycardia, and hypotension may occur following rapid IV bolus administration of cimetidine or ranitidine; bradycardia has been reported with both IV and oral administration of cimetidine and ranitidine. Although a negative inotropic effect has been noted following oral administration of famotidine in healthy subjects and patients with CHF, refined hemodynamic monitoring has failed to demonstrate a clinically important effect;[7] IV famotidine has been given safely to patients undergoing cardiac surgery.[18] Hematologic reactions occur occasionally with all H_2-receptor antagonists and include leukopenia, neutropenia, thrombocytopenia, and pancytopenia; agranulocytosis and aplastic anemia occur rarely.[2,7] Gynecomastia develops in less than 1% of all men receiving cimetidine, but in 4% of men treated for pathologic hypersecretory states. Dose-dependent increases in serum prolactin concentrations have been reported with cimetidine and ranitidine.[7] Hyperuricemia has been reported with nizatidine. All H_2-receptor antagonists may cause a mild, but reversible, increase in fasting serum gastrin.[19] The effects of H_2-receptor antagonist therapy on gastric emptying are unclear.

Precautions. Pregnancy; lactation. Dosage adjustment may be required in severe renal and/or hepatic failure. Symptomatic response to therapy does not preclude the possibility of gastric or esophageal malignancy.

Drug Interactions. Cimetidine inhibits hepatic CYP1A2, CYP2C8–10, CYP2D6, and CYP3A3–5; ranitidine inhibits CYP2D6 and CYP3A3–5 to a much lesser extent. Clinically important interactions with drugs metabolized by these isoenzymes may occur (the most important of which are carbamazepine, chlordiazepoxide, clozapine, diazepam, glipizide, lidocaine, phenytoin, propranolol, theophylline, tolbutamide, tricyclic antidepressants, quinidine, tacrine, and warfarin). Hepatic microsomal enzyme interactions with cimetidine are dose dependent.[20,21] Controversy remains about interactions with ranitidine, although in general they seem less likely and less severe than with cimetidine.[7,20,21] Cimetidine may inhibit the elimination of certain drugs secreted by renal tubules (eg, procainamide).[20,21] Nizatidine has been reported to increase serum salicylate concentrations in patients on high aspirin doses (3.9 g/day). Cimetidine, ranitidine, and nizatidine (but not famotidine) inhibit gastric mucosal alcohol dehydrogenase; the clinical importance of this interaction is uncertain. Elevations in gastric pH could alter the rate or extent of absorption of ketoconazole, itraconazole, and other drugs whose dissolution and absorption are pH dependent.[20,21]

Parameters to Monitor. Improvement in epigastric pain or heartburn. However, pain relief in peptic ulcer disease (PUD) and GERD does not correlate directly with endoscopic evidence of healing. Monitor Cr_s, CBC, AST, ALT, and CNS status periodically. In patients receiving IV doses of cimetidine ($\geq$2.4 g/day) or ranitidine ($\geq$400 mg/day), it is advisable to monitor serum transaminases routinely throughout the duration of IV therapy. When the drug is used to prevent upper GI bleeding in critically ill patients, measure the intragastric pH periodically. Monitor for potential drug interactions.

Notes. In general, the H_2-receptor antagonists are similar in efficacy when conventional dosages are prescribed for the treatment of gastric and duodenal ulcer and for maintenance of healing of duodenal ulcer. Ulcer healing rates are similar to **sucralfate** or aggressive **antacid** therapy.[2,8,9] The H_2-receptor antagonists are often used in combination with a number of antibiotics to eradicate *Helicobacter pylori* in peptic ulcer disease. (*See* Eradication of *Helicobacter pylori* Infection.) Usual dosages of H_2-receptor antagonists are less effective than **misoprostol** or **proton pump inhibitors** in preventing NSAID-induced gastric ulcer.[22,23] However, high-dose famotidine may be effective in preventing and healing NSAID-induced gastric and duodenal ulcers.[24–26] Although all H_2-receptor antagonists provide symptomatic relief and esophageal healing, higher dosages are required in patients with moderate to severe esophagitis than those used in patients with mild GERD symptoms.[8,27] Intermittent administration or continuous infusion of IV cimetidine, ranitidine, or famotidine is more effective than placebo in preventing upper GI bleeding in critically ill patients.[3,10,12] The maintenance of intragastric pH above 4.0 does not conclusively prevent upper GI bleeding.[3,10,12] Although it is easier to maintain the intragastric pH above 4.0 by continuous infusion, the superiority of continuous infusion of the H_2-receptor antagonists in preventing upper GI bleeding in the critically ill patient has not been established; both intermittent administration and continuous infusion are at least as effective as sucralfate or aggressive antacid therapy.[3,10,12] Combination of an H_2-receptor antagonist with sucralfate provides two different mechanisms of drug action and may be of possible benefit. However, enhanced efficacy of two drugs compared to single-drug therapy has not been substantiated in controlled trials in patients with duodenal ulcer, gastric ulcer, or GERD, or when used to prevent or treat upper GI bleeding. Coadministration of an H_2-receptor antagonist with a proton pump inhibitor is without established benefit and may compromise the action of the proton pump inhibitor.[2] Controlled trials have not demonstrated that H_2-receptor antagonists are of benefit in patients with active upper GI bleeding.[7] The relationship of H_2-receptor antagonist therapy to the development of nosocomial pneumonia in critically ill patients is inconclusive.[3,10,12] (*See* Sucralfate.) Cimetidine may augment cell-mediated immunity by blockade of H_2 receptors on suppressor T-lymphocytes; it remains difficult to determine whether this effect is clinically useful or whether it is potentially dangerous, especially following organ transplantation and in autoimmune disorders.[20] Cimetidine may reduce pain and hasten resolution of herpes zoster lesions.[28] Although it is not certain whether this immune system action is class specific or drug specific, it appears to be related to the cimetidine molecule. All H_2-receptor antagonists are stable in D5W, D10W, NS, LR, TPN, or 5% sodium bicarbonate for 48 hr at room temperature.

MISOPROSTOL   Cytotec

Pharmacology. Misoprostol is a synthetic prostaglandin E_1 analogue that inhibits gastric acid secretion and enhances gastric mucosal defense. Antisecretory effects are dose dependent over the range of 50–200 μg; cytoprotective effects occur at doses of 200 μg or more. The gastric ulcer protective effect of misoprostol appears to plateau between 200 μg bid–tid, but no dose–response effect is apparent in preventing duodenal ulcers.[26,29] Co-therapy with misoprostol reduces the frequency of **NSAID**-induced complications, including GI perforation, obstruction, and bleeding, but its cost effectiveness remains controversial.[26,30,31] In most trials of patients receiving long-term NSAID therapy for rheumatoid arthritis, misoprostol 200 μg qid was superior to the **H_2-receptor antagonists** or **sucralfate** in preventing NSAID-induced gastric ulcer; however, misoprostol did not relieve GI pain or discomfort associated with NSAID use.[22,26,32] **Omeprazole** 20 mg/day is associated with a lower relapse rate and is better tolerated than misoprostol 200 μg bid for prophylactic treatment.[33] (See also Proton Pump Inhibitors.)

Adult Dosage. PO for GI protection during NSAID therapy 200 μg qid with food; if this dosage is not tolerated, 100 μg qid can be used. Lower-dosage regimens of misoprostol 200 μg tid or bid appear similar in efficacy and better tolerated for protection against NSAID-induced gastric and duodenal ulcers than the 200 mg qid dosage. Dosage reduction is not required in renal impairment, hepatic failure, or in the elderly.

Dosage Forms. Tab 100, 200 μg. Misoprostol is also available in combination with diclofenac in Arthrotec. (*See* Diclofenac.)

Pharmacokinetics. After oral administration, misoprostol is extensively absorbed and rapidly de-esterified to the active drug, misoprostol acid. Peak serum concentrations of misoprostol acid are reduced when the drug is taken with food. Plasma protein binding of misoprostol acid is <90%. Misoprostol acid undergoes further metabolism; but approximately 80% is excreted unchanged in urine.

Adverse Reactions. Diarrhea is reported to occur within 2 weeks of initiating therapy in 14–40% of patients on NSAIDs receiving 800 μg/day and less frequently with 400–600 μg/day. Diarrhea is usually self-limiting and resolves in about 1 week with continued treatment; rarely, profound diarrhea occurs in patients with inflammatory bowel disease. Abdominal pain occurs in 13–20% of patients on NSAIDs receiving misoprostol 800 μg/day, but there is no consistent difference from placebo. Antacids (except those containing magnesium) may be used for abdominal pain relief. Nausea, flatulence, headache, dyspepsia, vomiting, and constipation occur occasionally. Women who receive misoprostol occasionally develop gynecological disorders including cramps or vaginal bleeding. Misoprostol is contraindicated in pregnancy because of the risk of abortion. Women of childbearing potential should have a negative serum pregnancy test within 2 weeks of beginning therapy, should begin treatment on the second or third day of the next menstrual period, should comply with effective contraceptive measures, and should receive both oral and written warnings of the hazards of misoprostol therapy and the risk of contraceptive failure. Warn patients not to give misoprostol to others. Advise patients (especially those receiving concurrent corticosteroids or anticoagulants) to report bleeding, vomiting, severe abdominal pain, and diarrhea.[35]

Drug Interactions. Misoprostol does not affect the hepatic cytochrome P450 microsomal enzyme system, nor does it interfere with the beneficial effects of NSAIDs in rheumatoid arthritis.

PROTON PUMP INHIBITORS:

LANSOPRAZOLE	Prevacid
OMEPRAZOLE	**Prilosec**

Pharmacology. Proton pump inhibitors (PPIs) are inactive substituted benzimidazoles that, when protonated in the secretory canaliculi of the parietal cells, covalently bind to H^+/K^+-ATPase. The PPIs produce a profound and prolonged antisecretory effect, and inhibit basal, nocturnal, pentagastrin-, and food-stimulated gastric acid secretion. Serum gastrin levels increase during treatment, but return to pretreatment levels within 1–2 weeks of discontinuing therapy.

Administration and Adult Dosage.[a]

INDICATION	LANSOPRAZOLE	OMEPRAZOLE
PO for short-term treatment of active duodenal ulcer (4–8 weeks)	15 mg/day.	20 mg/day.
PO for maintenance of healed duodenal ulcer	15 mg/day.	20 mg/day.[a]
PO for reduction of the risk of duodenal ulcer recurrence	Days 1–10, 30 mg bid.[b] or Days 1–14, 30 mg bid.[b] or Days 1–14, 30 mg tid.[c]	Days 1–14, 40 mg bid,[d] then Days 15–28, 20 mg bid or Days 1–10, 40 mg bid,[b] then Days 11–28, 20 mg bid.
PO for short-term treatment of active benign gastric ulcer (4–8 weeks)	30 mg/day.	40 mg/day.
PO for maintenance of healed gastric ulcer	15–30 mg/day.[a]	20–40 mg/day.[a]
PO for symptomatic gastroesophageal reflux disease (4–8 weeks)	15 mg/day.[a]	20 mg/day.

(continued)

INDICATION	LANSOPRAZOLE	OMEPRAZOLE
PO for erosive esophagitis or poorly responsive symptomatic GERD, or recurrent esophagitis (4–16 weeks)	30 mg/day, or up to 60 mg/day.[a]	20 mg/day, or up to 80 mg/day.[a]
PO for maintenance of healed erosive esophagitis	15 mg/day.	20 mg/day.
PO for pathological hypersecretory conditions	60 mg/day, up to 90 mg bid; adjust to patient needs.[e]	60 mg/day, up to 120 mg tid; adjust to patient needs.[e]
Nasogastric or nasoduodenal for prevention of upper GI bleeding in critically ill patients	Preliminary studies using various omeprazole formulations suggest that PPIs are effective in increasing intragastric pH and preventing upper GI bleeding; however, the optimal dosage and method of administration have not been determined.[36,37]	

[a]Nonlabeled indication and dosage.
[b]Combined with clarithromycin 500 mg bid and amoxicillin 1 g bid.
[c]Combined with amoxicillin 1 g tid.
[d]Combined with clarithromycin 500 mg tid.
[e]Adjust dosage to patient's needs and continue as long as clinically indicated.
From references 2 and 38–42.

Special Populations. *Pediatric Dosage.* Safety and efficacy not established. However, omeprazole has been used in children **PO for esophagitis** (>10 months) 0.7 mg/kg/day initially, increasing as necessary up to 3.5 mg/kg/day; **PO for peptic ulcer disease in combination with antimicrobials for** *Helicobacter pylori* (<10 yr) 0.6 mg/kg/day or 20 mg/day; (>10 yr) 20 mg daily–bid.[43]

Geriatric Dosage. Dosage reduction is not usually necessary; reduce dosage only if the drug is not well tolerated.

Other Conditions. Dosage reduction of omeprazole and lansoprazole is unnecessary in patients with renal impairment, but should be considered in chronic hepatic disease and Asian patients (due to a higher prevalence of poor metabolizers of mephenytoin). Omeprazole and lansoprazole are not readily dialyzable.

Dosage Forms. (Lansoprazole) **Cap** (EC granules) 15, 30 mg. (Omeprazole) **Cap** (EC granules) 10, 20, 40 mg.

Patient Instructions. Swallow capsule whole or open the capsule and sprinkle the granules on applesauce or place in apple or orange juice and take before meals. Swallow capsule or intact granules immediately without chewing. The effectiveness of PPIs in peptic ulcer disease may be decreased by cigarette smoking. Even though symptoms may improve, continue treatment for the duration of therapy unless instructed otherwise.

Missed Doses. If you miss a dose, take it as soon as possible. If it is almost time for your next dose, skip the missed dose and return to your usual dosage schedule. Do not double doses.

Pharmacokinetics. *Onset and Duration.* Onset of antisecretory activity after multiple oral daily doses is within 1 hr for both drugs. Duration of antisecretory effect is dose dependent. Gastric acid inhibition increases with repeated daily doses, reaching a plateau after several days. Gastric secretory activity gradually returns to pretreatment levels 2–5 days after discontinuation. There is no indication that rebound gastric acidity occurs.

Serum Levels. Antisecretory effect correlates with AUC rather than serum levels. Inhibition of gastric acid secretion continues after serum drug concentrations have decreased below the limit of detection, apparently caused by prolonged drug binding to parietal cell H^+/K^+-ATPase.

Pharmacokinetics.

	LANSOPRAZOLE	OMEPRAZOLE
Fate.		
Oral bioavailability	83 ± 2%[a]	35 ± 5%[a]
Protein binding	97%	95%
Excreted unchanged in urine	Very little	Very little
$t_{1/2}$.		
Healthy young adults	1.5 ± 0.2 hr	0.75 ± 0.25 hr
Healthy elderly	2.2 ± 0.7 hr	1 hr
Chronic hepatic disease	5.2 ± 2 hr	3 hr

[a]Bioavailability increases upon repeated administration more extensively in the elderly and patients with chronic hepatic failure.
From references 38–40.

Adverse Reactions. The short- and long-term safety of lansoprazole appears to be similar to that of omeprazole.[38–40,42,44] Headache, diarrhea, nausea, and dizziness occur frequently. Constipation, fatigue, malaise, muscle cramps, joint pain, myalgia, anxiety, skin rash, and taste perversion occur occasionally. Rarely, gynecomastia, hemolytic anemia, thrombocytopenia, and psychic disturbances have been reported. Rare cases of severe skin reactions (eg, Stevens-Johnson syndrome), overt hepatic failure (some fatal), liver necrosis, pancreatitis, interstitial nephritis, and agranulocytosis have occurred with omeprazole. Rarely, gastric polyposis has occurred in patients receiving 20–40 mg of omeprazole for 12 months or longer.[38,44] Long-term PPI use may reduce the absorption of protein-bound vitamin B_{12}.[40,46] Long-term studies indicate that the adverse effects profile of the PPIs is similar to the H_2-receptor antagonists.[42,44] Atrophic gastritis has been observed during long-term PPI use; patients with *H. pylori* may be at increased risk.[45,46] Adverse effects in patients over 65 years of age are similar to that of younger patients.

Precautions. Pregnancy (omeprazole), because of sporadic reports of congenital abnormalities. Symptomatic response to therapy does not preclude the possibility of gastric malignancy.

Drug Interactions. Elevations in gastric pH could increase the extent of absorption of ampicillin, and decrease the rate or extent of absorption of digoxin, itraconazole, iron salts, ketoconazole, and other drugs or dosage forms that are pH dependent. Omeprazole interacts selectively with hepatic CYP2C and may inhibit the metabolism of drugs, such as some benzodiazepines (eg, diazepam), carbamazepine, cyclosporine, phenytoin, and (R)-warfarin, but not lidocaine, propranolol quinidine, or theophylline. Omeprazole and lansoprazole induce CYP1A1/2, which could theoretically potentiate the hepatotoxicity of acetaminophen or lead to an increased risk of cancer in smokers.[21,47] Lansoprazole does not appear to interact with drugs metabolized by CYP2C, but may increase theophylline clearance.[47]

Parameters to Monitor. Improvement in epigastric pain or heartburn; however, pain relief in peptic ulcer disease and gastroesophageal reflux disease does not correlate directly with endoscopic evidence of healing. Monitor for potential drug interactions and adverse effects. Assess the indication, dosage, and duration of PPI therapy especially as it relates to the need for treatment beyond 16 weeks. Consider monitoring serum vitamin B_{12} concentration every several years in patients on long-term PPI therapy.

Notes. The PPIs are the drugs of choice for patients with erosive esophagitis and Zollinger-Ellison syndrome. In most patients with peptic ulcer disease, erosive esophagitis, and Zollinger-Ellison syndrome, recommended dosages of lansoprazole and omeprazole provide similar rates of healing and symptomatic relief.[38–43] Standard PPI dosages provide more rapid relief of symptoms and ulcer or esophageal healing than standard dosages of the **H_2-receptor antagonists;** however, the longer treatment is continued, the smaller the difference between treatments. Patients with gastric or duodenal ulcers or esophagitis refractory to H_2-receptor antagonists are likely to respond to a PPI, but the rate of recurrence following discontinuation is similar to the H_2-receptor antagonists. The PPIs are effective in preventing **NSAID**-induced gastric and duodenal ulcers and appear to be superior to **misoprostol** 200 mg bid or **ranitidine** 150 mg bid.[23,33,48] When prophylactic treatment with omeprazole 20 mg/day was compared with misoprostol 200 mg bid, omeprazole was associated with a lower relapse rate and was better tolerated than misoprostol.[33] When omeprazole 20 mg/day or 40 mg/day was compared to misoprostol 200 mg qid for the treatment of NSAID-induced gastroduodenal mucosal damage in patients requiring continuous NSAID therapy, gastric and duodenal ulcer healing rates at 8 weeks were higher with the omeprazole dosages; healing rates in patients with erosions were higher with misoprostol.[33] In patients taking NSAIDs, omeprazole 20 mg/day healed and prevented ulcers more effectively than did rantidine 150 mg bid.[23] Although omeprazole 20 mg/day appears to be effective in healing NSAID-induced ulcers when the NSAID is continued, a higher PPI dose (eg, omeprazole 40 mg/day) may be indicated in some patients.

The PPIs are formulated in pH-sensitive granules that release the drug at a pH above 6. Crushing the granules destroys the protective coating and may decrease the drug's oral bioavailability; however, the capsule may be opened and the intact granules administered orally (with apple or orange juice or sprinkled on applesauce), through a gastrostomy tube (with orange juice), dispersed in water, or a solution can be made with sodium bicarbonate and administered nasogastrically or nasoduodenally.[36,37,49,50] Proton pump inhibitors should be taken prior to meals because they inhibit only those proton pumps that are actively secreting acid. Coadministration of a PPI with an **H₂-receptor antagonist** or **sucralfate** is without established benefit; the action of a PPI may be compromised if administered with an H₂-receptor antagonist or **octreotide.**[2] PPIs are more cost-effective than the H₂-receptor antagonists when treating patients with moderate to severe esophagitis.[51] (*See* Eradication of *Helicobacter pylori* Infection.) **Pantoprazole** (Protonix, investigational—Wyeth-Ayerst) is a PPI that can be given orally or intravenously. IV and oral dosage is 40 mg once daily; dosage reduction to 20 mg/day in hepatic insufficiency. **Rabeprazole** (Aciphex–Jannsen) is a partially reversible H^+/K^+ ATPase inhibitor given in a dose of 20 mg/day orally. The efficacy and tolerability of pantoprazole and rabeprazole are similar to those of omeprazole and lansoprazole. Neither pantoprazole or rabeprazole appear to affect cytochrome P450 enzymes.[52–56]

SUCRALFATE
Carafate, Various

Pharmacology. Sucralfate is an aluminum hydroxide salt of a sulfated disaccharide. Its exact mechanism of action is not known; however, it forms an ulcer-adherent complex with proteinaceous exudates at the ulcer site, thereby protecting against further attack by acid, pepsin, and bile salts. Adherence to the ulcer crater is enhanced at a pH <3.5. Sucralfate inhibits pepsin activity; a 1 g dose has approximately 14–16 mEq of acid-neutralizing capacity. The aluminum moiety stimulates endogenous prostaglandins and binds bile salts and phosphate in the GI tract.[2,57,58]

Administration and Adult Dosage. **PO for short-term treatment of duodenal ulcer** 1 g qid on an empty stomach, 1 hr before meals and at bedtime or 2 g bid for 4–8 weeks.[2,57,58] **PO for maintenance of healed duodenal ulcer** 1 g bid. **PO for short-term treatment of active benign gastric ulcer** 1 g qid.[2,57,58] **PO for treatment of symptomatic gastroesophageal reflux disease (GERD) or erosive esophagitis** 1 g qid.[57,58] **PO or NG for prevention of upper GI bleeding in critically ill patients** 1 g q 4–6 hr.[3,10,12,58,59] **PO or NG for phosphate binding in renal failure** titrate dosage based on serum phosphate.[2,57]

Special Populations. *Pediatric Dosage.* Safety and efficacy not well established. **PO** 500 mg bid has been used.[60]

Geriatric Dosage. Dosage reduction usually not necessary.

Dosage Forms. **Tab** 1 g; **Susp** 100 mg/mL.

Patient Instructions. Take this drug with water on an empty stomach, 1 hour before each meal and at bedtime. Antacids may be used as needed for pain relief, but do not take them within 30 minutes before or after sucralfate. Take potentially interacting drugs 2 hours before sucralfate in order to avoid or minimize drug interactions. Even though symptoms may decrease, continue treatment for the duration of therapy unless instructed otherwise.

Missed Doses. If you miss a dose, take it as soon as possible. If it is almost time for your next dose, skip the missed dose and return to your usual dosage schedule. Do not double doses.

Pharmacokinetics. *Onset and Duration.* Onset (attachment of sucralfate to ulcer site) is within 1 hr; duration is about 6 hr.

Fate. Sucralfate is only minimally absorbed from the GI tract and is excreted primarily in the feces. About 3–5% (primarily aluminum) is absorbed and excreted in urine.[2,57] Aluminum excretion is decreased in uremia.

Adverse Reactions. Adverse reactions are usually minor and occur in about 5% of patients. Constipation occurs in about 2% of patients. Other effects, including diarrhea, nausea, gastric discomfort, indigestion, dry mouth, rash, pruritus, backache, dizziness, drowsiness, vertigo, and a metallic taste occur occasionally. Aluminum accumulation and toxicity, including osteodystrophy, osteomalacia, encephalopathy, and seizures, have been reported in patients with chronic renal failure. Hypophosphatemia may develop in critically ill patients and those on prolonged sucralfate therapy. Bezoar formation has been reported.[2,57]

Precautions. Use with caution in patients receiving other aluminum-containing drugs or in chronic renal failure and dialysis.

Drug Interactions. Sucralfate may inhibit the absorption of drugs including digoxin, ketoconazole, levothyroxine, phenytoin, quinidine, oral quinolones, tetracyclines, theophylline, and warfarin.[21] In most cases, these interactions can be avoided if the drug is given 2 hr before sucralfate administration.

Parameters to Monitor. Improvement in epigastric pain or heartburn; however, pain relief in peptic ulcer disease and GERD does not correlate directly with endoscopic evidence of healing. Observe for constipation and signs of aluminum toxicity in the elderly, in chronic renal failure, or in patients receiving other aluminum-containing drugs. Obtain serum phosphate periodically in patients receiving concurrent aluminum-containing drugs or with prolonged use. Monitor for potential drug interactions.

Notes. Sucralfate is as effective as standard doses of the **H$_2$-receptor antagonists** in the short-term treatment and maintenance of healed duodenal ulcer.[2,57,58] Sucralfate may overcome the negative effect of cigarette smoking on duodenal ulcer healing and recurrence.[57] Its efficacy in healing erosive esophagitis and in maintenance of esophageal healing is inferior to the **H$_2$-receptor antagonists** or **proton pump inhibitors.** Sucralfate is effective in preventing stress-related mucosal bleeding and may be more cost effective than H$_2$-receptor antagonists.[3,10,12,58,61] Its efficacy as a single agent in preventing NSAID-induced gastric and duodenal ulcer, chemotherapy-induced stomatitis, and stress-related bleeding in high-risk critically ill surgical patients is unsubstantiated. Whether sucralfate is associated with a lower frequency of nosocomial pneumonia in critically ill patients than H$_2$-receptor antagonists remains controversial.[3,10,12,58,62] The value of topical sucralfate after sclerotherapy or in treating proctitis, inflammatory bowel disease, or decubitus ulcers is questionable.[57] Although therapy with sucralfate and an H2-receptor antagonist or proton pump inhibitor provides two different mechanisms of drug action, enhanced efficacy of 2 drugs has not been substantiated for any indication.

ERADICATION OF *HELICOBACTER PYLORI* INFECTION

The eradication of *Helicobacter pylori* is recommended for all infected ulcer patients with an active ulcer, history of ulcer-related complications, or who require maintenance therapy. The value of *H. pylori* eradication in patients with dyspepsia, nonulcer dyspepsia, or to prevent gastric cancer remains controversial. Most patients with gastric or duodenal ulcers who are not taking an NSAID have evidence of *H. pylori* infection and antral gastritis. Drug regimens to eradicate *H. pylori* are considered first-line therapy for *H. pylori*–associated duodenal and gastric ulcers. Eradication of *H. pylori* heals ulcers, reduces ulcer recurrence to less than 10%, and is more cost beneficial than conventional antiulcer treatments. Conventional antiulcer drugs, bismuth salts, and antibiotics are generally ineffective as single agents in eradicating *H. pylori*. The discrepancy between high in vitro and low in vitro antibiotic efficacy may be caused by degradation of the antibiotic in gastric acid, insufficient penetration through gastric mucus, or microbial resistance. *H. pylori* resistance to metronidazole is most common (10–50%) and appears to be higher in women. Resistance to clarithromycin is less than 10%; resistance to tetracycline and amoxicillin has been reported, but is uncommon.

Although the optimal regimen to eradicate *H. pylori* and cure peptic ulcer disease has not been established, a number of combinations are effective. The two-drug amoxicillin plus a proton pump inhibitor (PPI) regimen is associated with a wide variability in eradication rates (0–90%). More favorable and consistent eradication rates can be obtained with two-drug regimens that combine clarithromycin with a PPI or ranitidine bismuth citrate (RBC). Three-drug regimens that contain a PPI plus two antibiotics may be taken for 7 or 10 days rather than 14 days to minimize adverse effects and enhance compliance; however, eradication rates may be lower, especially with the 1-week regimen. The ideal duration of therapy and the optimal dose of clarithromycin when used in the three-drug regimen is under investigation. Three-drug regimens that contain either an H_2-receptor antagonist, sucralfate, or RBC (instead of a PPI) or azithromycin (instead of clarithromycin) are under investigation. Four-drug regimens of bismuth subsalicylate, metronidazole, and tetracycline or amoxicillin, and an antisecretory drug are effective and have lower drug costs, but are associated with a high frequency of adverse effects (up to 70%) and medication noncompliance. Frequent adverse effects include diarrhea, (up to 30%), nausea, and abnormal taste (with metronidazole and clarithromycin). An antisecretory drug should be included when the patient has an active ulcer in order to provide rapid relief of symptoms and enhance ulcer healing. Extending antisecretory drug therapy beyond the 7–14 days of antimicrobial therapy should be considered in ulcer patients with a history of ulcer complication who remain symptomatic upon cessation of the antimicrobial regimen.

The selection of an eradication regimen should be individualized and based on efficacy, tolerability, drug interaction potential, antibiotic resistance, cost, and the likelihood of compliance. Antibiotics should not be used for longer than 2 weeks. If treatment fails, a different antibiotic regimen should be considered. Until more information is available, ampicillin should not be substituted for amoxicillin, doxycycline should not be substituted for tetracycline, azithromycin should not be substituted for clarithromycin, an H_2-receptor antagonist should not be substituted for a PPI, and bismuth salts should not be interchanged. When eradicating *H. pylori*, omeprazole 20 mg and lansoprazole 30 mg are interchangeable. Patients should be instructed to take all of their medications (except PPIs) with meals and at bedtime (if necessary). PPIs should be taken prior to eating.[63–78]

DRUG TREATMENT REGIMENS USED TO ERADICATE *HELICOBACTER PYLORI*

DRUGS	DOSE	FREQUENCY	DURATION	EFFICACY[a]	ADVERSE EFFECTS[b]	COMPLIANCE[c]
Amoxicillin	1 g	bid–tid	14 days	Poor–fair	Low–medium	Likely
Omeprazole[d,e]	20 mg	bid–tid	14 days			
Clarithromycin	500 mg	tid	14 days	Fair–good	Low–medium	Likely
Omeprazole[d,e]	40 mg	qd	14 days			
Clarithromycin	500 mg	tid	14 days	Fair–good	Low–medium	Likely
RBC	400 mg	bid	28 days			
Clarithromycin	500 mg	bid	10–14 days	Good–excellent	Medium	Likely
Metronidazole	500 mg	bid	10–14 days			
Omeprazole[d,e]	20 mg	bid	10–14 days			
Clarithromycin	500 mg	bid	10–14 days	Good–excellent	Low–medium	Likely
Amoxicillin	1 g	bid	10–14 days			
Omeprazole[d,e]	20 mg	bid	10–14 days			
Amoxicillin	1 g	bid	14 days	Good	Medium	Likely
Metronidazole	500 mg	bid	14 days			
Omeprazole[d,e]	20 mg	bid	14 days			

(continued)

DRUG TREATMENT REGIMENS USED TO ERADICATE *HELICOBACTER PYLORI* (continued)

DRUGS	DOSE	FREQUENCY	DURATION	EFFICACY[a]	ADVERSE EFFECTS[b]	COMPLIANCE[c]
Tetracycline	500 mg	qid	14 days	Good	Medium	Unlikely
Metronidazole	500 mg	qid	14 days			
Sucralfate[e]	1 g	qid	14 days			
Clarithromycin	500 mg	bid	14 days	Good	Medium	Unlikely
Metronidazole	500 mg	bid	14 days			
RBC	400 mg	bid	14–28 days			
BSS	525 mg	qid	14 days	Good–excellent	Medium–high	Unlikely
Metronidazole	250 mg	qid	14 days			
Tetracycline	500 mg	qid	14 days			
H₂RA[f]	Conventional ulcer healing dosage regimen for 28 days					
BSS	525 mg	qid	14 days	Fair–good	Medium–high	Unlikely
Metronidazole	250 mg	qid	14 days			
Amoxicillin	500 mg	qid	14 days			
H₂RA[f]	Conventional ulcer healing dosage regimen for 28 days					

(continued)

515

DRUG TREATMENT REGIMENS USED TO ERADICATE *HELICOBACTER PYLORI* (continued)

DRUGS	DOSE	FREQUENCY	DURATION	EFFICACY[a]	ADVERSE EFFECTS[b]	COMPLIANCE[c]
BSS	525 mg	qid	7 days	Good–excellent	Medium–high	Unlikely
Metronidazole	500 mg	qid	7 days			
Tetracycline	500 mg	qid	7 days			
Omeprazole[d,e]	20 mg	bid	7 days			
BSS	525 mg	qid	7 days	Good–excellent	Medium–high	Unlikely
Metronidazole	500 mg	qid	7 days			
Clarithromycin	500 mg	bid	7 days			
Omeprazole[d,e]	20 mg	bid	7 days			

BSS = bismuth subsalicylate; H_2RA = H_2-receptor antagonist; PPI = proton pump inhibitor; RBC = ranitidine bismuth citrate.

[a] Efficacy (eradication rate): excellent >90%; good >80–90%; fair >70–80%; poor <70%.

[b] Adverse Effects = frequency of clinically important adverse effects.

[c] Compliance = estimate based on total number of tablets/capsules, frequency of administration, and clinically important adverse effects.

Antiemetics

DOLASETRON MESYLATE   Anzemet

Pharmacology. Dolasetron and its active metabolite, hydrodolasetron, are selective $5-HT_3$ antagonists. Dolasetron is approved for the prevention of chemotherapy-induced nausea and vomiting and for both the prevention and treatment of postoperative nausea and vomiting. Its use is similar to those of ondansetron and granisetron.[80–83] (*See* Antiemetic Drugs Comparison Chart.)

Adult Dosage. **PO or IV for chemotherapy-induced nausea and vomiting** 100 mg or 1.8 mg/kg. **IV for postoperative nausea and vomiting** 12.5 mg. **PO for postoperative nausea and vomiting** 100 mg. IV doses may be administered over a minimum of 30 sec or further diluted in 50 mL of NS or D5W and infused over a period of up to 15 min. In some dose-finding trials in adults, higher response rates were obtained with 200 mg PO and 2.4 mg IV than achieved with lower doses by the respective routes.[80,82]

Pediatric Dosage. **PO or IV for chemotherapy-induced nausea and vomiting** (2–16 yr) 1.8 mg/kg, to a maximum of 100 mg. **PO for postoperative nausea and vomiting** (2–16 yr) 0.35 mg/kg, to a maximum of 12.5 mg. **PO for postoperative nausea and vomiting** (2–16 yr) 1.2 mg/kg, to a maximum of 100 mg.

Dosage Forms. **Inj** 20 mg/mL; **Tab** 50, 100 mg.

Pharmacokinetics. Approximately 75% of dolasetron mesylate is dolasetron base. The apparent absolute bioavailability of oral dolasetron is approximately 75%. Little dolasetron is detected in the plasma, because of rapid conversion to hydrodolasetron by the ubiquitous enzyme, carbonyl reductase. Hydrodolasetron is partially metabolized in the liver and 61% is excreted unchanged in the urine. Hydrodolasetron has a V_d of 5.8 ± 1.5 L/kg and Cl of 0.56 ± 0.16 L/hr/kg. Its half-life is 7.3 ± 1.8 hr.

Adverse Reactions. Acute, reversible ECG changes (PR and QT_c prolongation, and QRS widening) have occurred in clinical trials and in healthy volunteers. Other adverse effects are similar to ondansetron and granisetron.

DRONABINOL   Marinol

Pharmacology. Dronabinol (delta-9-tetrahydrocannabinol [THC]) is an active antiemetic component of *Cannabis.* Its mechanism of action as an antiemetic is complex and poorly understood, but probably includes inhibition of the chemoreceptor trigger zone in the medulla.

Administration and Adult Dosage. **PO as an antiemetic** 5 mg/m^2 1–3 hr before chemotherapy, then q 2–4 hr after chemotherapy for a total of 4–6 doses/day. Dosage may be increased in 2.5 mg/m^2 increments, to a maximum of 15 mg/m^2/dose.[84–86] **PO for appetite stimulation** 2.5 mg before lunch and dinner or 2.5 mg at bedtime if unable to tolerate daytime administration. Dosage may be increased to a maximum of 20 mg/day.

Special Populations. *Pediatric Dosage.* **PO as an antiemetic during cancer chemotherapy** same as adult dosage in mg/m^2.

Geriatric Dosage. Same as adult dosage. (*See* Adverse Reactions.)

Dosage Forms. Cap 2.5, 5, 10 mg.

Patient Instructions. This drug may cause drowsiness. Until the extent of this effect is known, use caution when driving, operating machinery, or performing other tasks requiring mental alertness. Avoid excessive concurrent use of alcohol or other drugs that cause drowsiness. Store this medication in the refrigerator.

Missed Doses. Take this drug at regular intervals. If you miss a dose, take it as soon as you remember. If it is about time for the next dose, take that dose only. Do not double the dose or take extra.

Pharmacokinetics. *Onset and Duration.* Oral onset 30–60 min; peak 2–4 hr; duration is 4–6 hr, but may be longer in those who have not previously used the drug.[87,88] *Cannabis* smoking onset 15 sec–2 min; peak 8–16 min; duration 3–12 hr.[89]

Fate. Bioavailability is 4–12% orally, 2–50% by smoking. About 95% plasma protein bound. V_d is 8.9 ± 4.2 L/kg; Cl is 0.21 ± 0.054 L/hr/kg. Primarily metabolized by hydroxylation to active and inactive metabolites. Ultimately, 35% of metabolites are found in feces and 15% in urine, with <1% excreted unchanged in urine.[90–92]

$t_{1/2}$. Terminal phase 32 ± 12 hr, although time course of effects more closely parallels initial distribution phase.[90]

Adverse Reactions. Drowsiness occurs frequently. It may be accompanied by dizziness, ataxia, loss of balance, and disorientation to the point of being disabling. Other frequent side effects include dry mouth, orthostatic hypotension, and conjunctival injection.[93] The cannabis "high" experienced by some is not always well tolerated, especially by older patients.[94]

Contraindications. Allergy to dronabinol, marijuana, or sesame oil; mentally ill patients.

Precautions. Avoid during lactation. Use with caution in patients with hypertension or heart disease. Use with caution in patients with epilepsy.[84]

Drug Interactions. Not well studied, but some apparent interactions have been reported following *Cannabis* use. These include additive or supra-additive sedation with alcohol and other CNS depressants; additive hypertension and/or tachycardia with anticholinergics, antihistamines, sympathomimetics, or tricyclic antidepressants; and hypomania with disulfiram or fluoxetine.

Parameters to Monitor. Observe for frequency of emesis, drowsiness, or disorientation.

Notes. Dronabinol is at least as effective as **phenothiazines** for chemotherapy-induced nausea and vomiting,[86] but is not as effective as **serotonin antagonists** or IV **metoclopramide.**[95,96] It is not particularly effective for cisplatin-induced nausea and vomiting. It may not be as effective as smoking *Cannabis,* which is easier to titrate.[96] (*See* Antiemetic Drugs Comparison Chart.)

GRANISETRON   Kytril

Pharmacology. Granisetron is a selective antagonist at the 5-HT_3 (serotonin-S_3) receptor used for the prevention of nausea and vomiting associated with cancer chemotherapy. Its use in cancer chemotherapy is similar to that of ondansetron, and its efficacy and side effects are comparable to those of ondansetron.[97–99] (*See* Antiemetic Drugs Comparison Chart.)

Adult Dosage. IV for cancer chemotherapy-induced nausea and vomiting 10 μg/kg administered in 20–50 mL NS or D5W over 5 min, 30 min before the start of chemotherapy. **PO for cancer chemotherapy-induced nausea and vomiting** 1 mg up to 1 hr before chemotherapy and additional 1 mg doses at 12-hr intervals thereafter while receiving chemotherapy.

Pediatric Dosage. IV (>2 yr) same as adult dosage; however, this dosage may not be adequate for children.[98]

Dosage Forms. Inj 1 mg/mL; **Tab** 1 mg.

Pharmacokinetics. Oral absorption is approximately 60%. V_d is 30 ± 1.5 L/kg; Cl is 0.060 ± 0.54 L/hr/kg. Elimination is mostly by hepatic metabolism, with 16 ± 14% appearing in the urine as unchanged drug. The half-life is 5.3 ± 3.5 hr (may be longer in cancer patients than in normals). The metabolism of granisetron may be changed by inducers or inhibitors of the cytochrome P450 system, but dosage adjustment is not recommended.

Adverse Reactions. Similar to ondansetron.

ONDANSETRON HYDROCHLORIDE   Zofran

Pharmacology. Ondansetron is a selective antagonist at the 5-HT_3 (serotonin-S_3) receptor used for the prevention of nausea and vomiting associated with cancer chemotherapy, especially cisplatin, and for postoperative nausea and vomiting. It may also be useful for radiotherapy-induced nausea and vomiting. Ondansetron is thought to block these receptors at both peripheral sites in the GI tract as well as within the area postrema in the CNS.[100] It is not a dopamine receptor antagonist, so it has no extrapyramidal side effects. (*See* Notes.)

Administration and Adult Dosage. IV for chemotherapy-induced nausea or vomiting 0.15 mg/kg for 3 doses (30 min before chemotherapy, then 4 and 8 hr after) or 0.45 mg/kg, to a maximum of 32 mg as a single dose, or 8 mg IV as a single dose for cisplatin doses <100 mg/m^2.[99,101] (*See* Notes.) Infuse slowly over 15 min in 50 mL D5W or NS. **IV bolus for postoperative nausea or vomiting** 4 mg over 2–5 min before induction or postoperatively. **PO for chemotherapy- or radiotherapy-induced nausea or vomiting** 8 mg q 8 hr. **PO for postoperative nausea or vomiting** 16 mg 1 hr before surgery.

Special Populations. *Pediatric Dosage.* **IV for chemotherapy-induced nausea or vomiting** (<2 yr) safety and efficacy not established; (2–18 yr) same as adult dosage or 0.15 mg/kg for 2 doses for moderately emetogenic chemotherapy.[102–104] **IV for postoperative nausea or vomiting** 0.05–0.1 mg/kg, to a maximum of 4 mg as a single dose over 30 sec before the surgical incision.[105] **PO for chemotherapy-**

induced nausea and vomiting (4–12 yr) 4 mg q 8 hr. **PO for postoperative nausea or vomiting** 0.15 mg/kg 30–45 min prior to IV catheter placement.[106]

Geriatric Dosage. Same as adult dosage.

Other Conditions. In hepatic function impairment, do not exceed a single oral dose of 8 mg or a total daily IV dosage of 8 mg.

Dosage Forms. **Inj** 2 mg/mL; **Tab** 4, 8 mg; **Soln** 1.25 mg/mL.

Pharmacokinetics. *Fate.* Oral absorption is $62 \pm 15\%$.[90] V_d is 1.9 ± 0.5 L/kg; Cl is 0.35 ± 0.16 L/hr/kg in adults and may be higher in children.[90,97] The drug is extensively metabolized to glucuronide and sulfate conjugates.[97] About 5% appears in urine as unchanged ondansetron.[90]

$t_{1/2}$. 2.8 ± 0.6 hr in normal adults;[98] about 5 hr in the elderly.[96] However, the duration of activity is not related to the half-life.[99]

Adverse Reactions. Headache occurs frequently. Transient increased serum levels of hepatic enzymes also occur frequently, but these are probably caused by chemotherapy rather than by ondansetron.[99, 107–109]

Contraindications. None known.

Precautions. Pregnancy; lactation; suspected ileus. Patients who are hypersensitive to other 5-HT$_3$ antagonists may cross-react with ondansetron.[110]

Drug Interactions. The metabolism of ondansetron may be changed by inducers or inhibitors of the cytochrome P450 system, but dosage adjustment is not recommended.

Parameters to Monitor. Frequency of vomiting.

Notes. Protect vials from light; inspect for discoloration and particulate matter before using. **Dexamethasone** enhances the antiemetic effect of the 5-HT$_3$ antagonists[111,112]; the combination of ondansetron and dexamethasone is more effective than **metoclopramide** and dexamethasone for the acute component, but not for the delayed phase of severely emetogenic chemotherapy.[113,114] Several studies document the lack of additional efficacy beyond that achieved with a total daily ondansetron dosage of 0.45 mg/kg.[112,115] (*See* Antiemetic Drugs Comparison Chart.)

PROCHLORPERAZINE SALTS   Compazine, Various

Pharmacology. Prochlorperazine is a phenothiazine tranquilizer having antidopaminergic and weak anticholinergic activity. It suppresses the chemoreceptor trigger zone in the CNS and is used mainly for its antiemetic properties. It is not effective for the treatment of motion sickness or vertigo.

Administration and Adult Dosage. **PO as an antiemetic** 5–10 mg tid or qid; **PR as an antiemetic** 25 mg bid; **IM as an antiemetic** (deep in upper outer quadrant of buttock) 5–10 mg q 4–6 hr, to a maximum of 40 mg/day. **IM presurgically** (deep in upper outer quadrant of buttock) 5–10 mg 1–2 hr before induction, may repeat once before or after surgery; **IV presurgically** 2.5–10 mg 15–30 min before induction or as infusion (20 mg/L) started 15–30 min before induction. **SC** not recommended.

Special Populations. *Pediatric Dosage.* Not to be used in surgery, or in patients <9 kg or <2 yr. **PO or PR as an antiemetic** (9–13 kg) 2.5 mg daily–bid; (14–18 kg) 2.5 mg bid–tid; (19–39 kg) 2.5 mg tid–5 mg bid. (*See* Notes.) **IM as an antiemetic** (deep in upper outer quadrant of buttock) 0.13 mg/kg. **SC** not recommended.

Geriatric Dosage. Use the lower end of the recommended dosage range in elderly patients.

Dosage Forms. **Inj** 5 mg/mL; **Supp** 2.5, 5, 25 mg; **Syrup** 1 mg/mL; **Tab** 5, 10, 25 mg. Larger-dose tablets are available for psychiatric use. **SR Cap** not recommended.

Patient Instructions. This drug may cause drowsiness. Until the extent of this effect is known, use caution when driving, operating machinery, or performing other tasks requiring mental alertness. Avoid excessive concurrent use of alcohol or other drugs that cause drowsiness.

Missed Doses. Take this drug as prescribed. If you miss a dose, take it as soon as you remember. If it is about time for the next dose, take that dose only. Do not double the dose or take extra.

Pharmacokinetics. *Onset and Duration.* PO onset 30–40 min; PR onset 60 min; IM onset 10–20 min. Duration for all routes 3–4 hr.

Fate. The drug is well absorbed, but extensive and variable presystemic metabolism in the gut wall and liver limits bioavailability. Primarily eliminated by hepatic metabolism and biliary excretion.

$t_{1/2}$. 23 hr.[116]

Adverse Reactions. Extrapyramidal reactions, especially dystonias and dyskinesias, occur occasionally in adults and frequently in children (other extrapyramidal reactions are less likely because of the short duration of therapy when used as an antiemetic). Anticholinergic effects such as dry mouth, mydriasis, cycloplegia, urinary retention, decreased GI motility, and tachycardia occur occasionally. SC administration can cause local reactions at injection site.

Contraindications. Pediatric surgery; children <9 kg or <2 yr; coma or greatly depressed state caused by CNS depressants.

Precautions. Antiemetic action may mask signs and symptoms of overdose with other drugs and may mask the diagnosis and treatment of other conditions such as intestinal obstruction, brain tumor, or Reye's syndrome. Use with caution in conditions in which the drug's anticholinergic effects might be detrimental, in children with acute illnesses or dehydration, or in patients with a history of allergy to phenothiazine derivatives (eg, blood dyscrasias, jaundice). Avoid getting the concentrate or injectable solutions on hands or clothing because of the possibility of contact dermatitis.

Drug Interactions. Phenothiazines may decrease the efficacy of guanethidine or guanadrel or may have additive hypotensive effects with hypotensive drugs. Phenothiazines may inhibit the antiparkinson activity of levodopa.

Parameters to Monitor. Observe for extrapyramidal side effects and drug efficacy.

Notes. Protect the solution from light; a slight yellowish discoloration does not indicate altered potency, but markedly discolored solution should be discarded. Protect suppositories from heat. Prochlorperazine does not predictably reduce chemotherapy-induced nausea and vomiting in children and may even be associated with an increase in symptoms.[117] (*See* Antiemetic Drugs Comparison Chart.)

ANTIEMETIC DRUGS COMPARISON CHART

| | | INITIAL DOSE[a] | | INDICATIONS | | |
		Adult	Pediatric	Nausea and Vomiting[b]	Motion Sickness	Vertigo
ANTIHISTAMINES						
Buclizine Bucladin-S	Chew Tab 50 mg.	PO 50 mg.	—			X
Cyclizine Marezine	Tab 50 mg.	PO 50 mg.	PO (6–12 yr) 25 mg.		X	
Dimenhydrinate Dramamine Various	Cap 50 mg Tab 50 mg Chew Tab 50 mg Liquid 3.1 mg/mL Inj 50 mg/mL.	PO 50–100 mg IM, IV 50 mg.	PO (2–6 yr) 12.5–25 mg. (6–12 yr) 25–50 mg. IM, IV (>2 yr) 1.25 mg/kg.	X	X	X
Diphenhydra-mine Benadryl Various	Cap 25, 50 mg Tab 25, 50 mg Elxr 2.5 mg/mL Syrup 2.5 mg/mL Inj 10, 50 mg/mL.	PO 50 mg IM, IV 10–50 mg.	PO (2–6 yr) 6.25 mg or 1.25 mg/kg, (6–12 yr) 12.5 mg IM, IV (>9 kg) 1.25 mg/kg.	X	X	X
Meclizine Antivert Bonine Various	Cap 15, 25, 30 mg Tab 12.5, 25, 50 mg Chew Tab 25 mg.	PO 25–50 mg.	—	X	X	c

(continued)

523

ANTIEMETIC DRUGS COMPARISON CHART (continued)

DRUG	DOSAGE FORMS	INITIAL DOSE[a] Adult	INITIAL DOSE[a] Pediatric	INDICATIONS Nausea and Vomiting[b]	INDICATIONS Motion Sickness	INDICATIONS Vertigo
CANNABINOIDS						
***Dronabinol (C-II)*[d]** Marinol	Cap 2.5, 5, 10 mg.	PO 5 mg/m².	PO 5 mg/m².	X		
PHENOTHIAZINES						
Chlorpromazine Thorazine Various	Tab 10, 25, 50 mg Liquid 30, 100 mg/mL Syrup 2 mg/mL Supp 25, 100 mg Inj 25 mg/mL.	PO 10–25 mg PR 50–100 mg IM 25 mg.	PO, IM (>6 months) 0.55 mg/kg PR (>6 months) 1 mg/kg.	X		
Perphenazine Trilafon	Tab 2, 4, 8, 16 mg Liquid 3.2 mg/mL Inj 5 mg/mL.	PO 2–4 mg IM 5 mg.	—	X		
Prochlorperazine Compazine Various	Tab 5, 10, 25 mg Syrup 1 mg/mL Supp 2.5, 5, 25 mg Inj 5 mg/mL.	PO, IM 5–10 mg IV 2.5–10 mg PR 25 mg.	PO, PR (>9 kg or >2 yr) 2.5 mg IM (>9 kg or >2 yr) 0.13 mg/kg.	X		
Promethazine Phenergan Various	Syrup 1.25, 5 mg/mL Tab 12.5, 25, 50 mg Supp 12.5, 25, 50 mg Inj 25, 50 mg/mL.	PO, PR 25 mg IM, IV 12.5–25 mg.	PO, PR, IM (>2 yr) 0.25–0.5 mg/kg.	X	X	

(continued)

ANTIEMETIC DRUGS COMPARISON CHART (continued)

DRUG	DOSAGE FORMS	INITIAL DOSE[a] Adult	INITIAL DOSE[a] Pediatric	INDICATIONS Nausea and Vomiting[b]	INDICATIONS Motion Sickness	INDICATIONS Vertigo
Thiethylperazine Norzine Torecan	Tab 10 mg Supp 10 mg Inj 5 mg/mL.	PO, PR, IM 10 mg.	—	X		
Trifluopromazine Vesprin	Inj 10, 20 mg/mL.	IM 5–15 mg IM (elderly) 2.5 mg IV 1 mg.	IM (>2.5 yr) 0.2–0.25 mg/kg.	X		
SEROTONIN 5-HT$_3$ ANTAGONISTS						
Dolasetron Anzemet	Tab 50, 100 mg Inj 20 mg/mL.	PO 100 mg IV 1.8 mg/kg.	PO 1.8 mg/kg IV 1.8 mg/kg.	X		
Granisetron Kytril	Tab 1 mg Inj 1 mg/mL.	PO 1 mg IV 10 µg/kg.	IV (>2 yr) 10 µg/kg.	X		
Ondansetron Zofran	Tab 4, 8 mg Inj 2 mg/mL.	PO 8 or 16 mg IV 0.15–0.45 mg/kg (max 32 mg).	PO (>4 yr) 4 mg IV (>2 yr) 0.15 mg/kg.	X		
MISCELLANEOUS						
Dexamethazone Decadron Various	Tab 0.25, 0.5, 0.75, 1, 1.5, 2 mg Inj 4, 10, 20, 24 mg/mL.	PO, IV 10–20 mg.	PO, IV 8 mg/m².	e		

(continued)

525

ANTIEMETIC DRUGS COMPARISON CHART (continued)

		INITIAL DOSE[a]		INDICATIONS		
DRUG	DOSAGE FORMS	Adult	Pediatric	Nausea and Vomiting[b]	Motion Sickness	Vertigo
Droperidol Inapsine	Inj 2.5 mg/mL.	IM, IV 2.5 mg.	—	f		
Lorazepam (C-IV)[d] Ativan Various	Tab 0.5, 1, 2 mg Soln 2, 4 mg/mL.	PO 1–2 mg.	PO 0.05 mg/kg.	e		
Methylprednisolone Solu-Medrol Various	Inj 40, 125, 500 mg.	IV up to 100 mg.	IV 2–4 mg/kg.	e		
Metoclopramide Reglan	Inj 5 mg/mL.	IV 1–2 mg/kg.	IV 1–2 mg/kg.	X		
Trimethobenzamide Tigan Various	Cap 100, 250 mg Supp 100, 200 mg Inj 100 mg/mL.	PO 250 mg PR 200 mg IM 200 mg.	PO (14–40 kg) 100–200 mg PR (<14 kg) 100 mg, (14–40 kg) 100–200 mg.	X		

[a]Initial dose only; check prescribing information for subsequent dosage.
[b]Doses are for chemotherapy-induced nausea and vomiting. (*See* monograph for doses in postoperative nausea and vomiting.)
[c]Possibly effective.
[d]Controlled substance schedule designated in parentheses.
[e]Not labeled for this use; used as adjunctive for cancer chemotherapy-induced nausea and vomiting.
[f]Effective, but not labeled for this use.

Gastrointestinal Motility

BISACODYL
Dulcolax, Various

Pharmacology. Bisacodyl is a stimulant cathartic structurally similar to phenolphthalein that produces its effect by direct contact with colonic mucosa. It may stimulate water and electrolyte secretion in the colon.[118]

Administration and Adult Dosage. PO as a laxative/cathartic 10–30 mg; **PR** 10 mg. Adjust dosage based on response.

Special Populations. *Pediatric Dosage.* PO (>6 yr) 5–10 mg or 0.3 mg/kg hs or before breakfast; **PR** (<2 yr) 5 mg; (>2 yr) 10 mg.

Geriatric Dosage. Same as adult dosage.

Dosage Forms. EC Tab 5 mg; **Enema** (adult) 10 mg; **Supp** 10 mg.

Patient Instructions. Swallow tablets whole (not chewed or crushed) and do not take within 1 hour of antacids or dairy products. Do not use oral products in children <6 years of age.

Pharmacokinetics. *Onset and Duration.* Onset PO 6–12 hr; PR 15 min–1 hr.[119,120]

Fate. Absorption is less than 5% by oral or rectal route with subsequent conversion to the glucuronide salt and excretion in urine and bile. Rapidly converted in the gut by intestinal and bacterial enzymes to its active, but nonabsorbed, desacetyl metabolite.[121]

Adverse Reactions. Abdominal cramps occur frequently; with long-term use, metabolic acidosis or alkalosis, hypocalcemia, tetany, loss of enteric protein, and malabsorption occur occasionally; suppositories can cause proctitis and rectal inflammation.

Drug Interactions. Antacids or milk can dissolve the enteric coating of oral bisacodyl tablets, causing drug release in the stomach and gastric irritation.

Contraindications. Acute surgical abdomen; nausea, vomiting, or other symptoms of appendicitis; fecal impaction; intestinal or biliary tract obstruction; abdominal pain of unknown origin.

Notes. Useful for preoperative or preradiographic bowel preparation. Bisacodyl has been used in combination with **PEG electrolyte lavage solution** to decrease the amount of solution required.[118,122] (*See* PEG Electrolyte Lavage Solution.)

CISAPRIDE
Propulsid

Pharmacology. Cisapride is a prokinetic drug chemically related to metoclopramide. It acts primarily by facilitating the release of acetylcholine from postganglionic nerve endings of the myenteric plexus in GI smooth muscle attributed to serotonin 5-HT$_4$–receptor agonism and also appears to be a serotonin 5-HT$_3$–receptor antagonist. Unlike metoclopramide, cisapride does not have direct cholinergic or antiemetic effects and has no effect on serum prolactin or gastric secretion. Cisapride increases lower esophageal sphincter pressure and, unlike metoclopramide, it stimulates motility in all portions of the GI tract, including the esophagus and large intestine. It has no effect on normal gastric function and does not override normal homeostatic mechanisms.[123–125]

Administration and Adult Dosage. PO for the treatment of symptomatic nocturnal heartburn or esophagitis related to gastroesophageal reflux disease **(GERD)** 10 mg qid 15 min before meals and hs; may be increased to 20 mg qid if needed;[124,125] **PO for maintenance of healing of esophagitis related to GERD** 10–20 mg bid (before breakfast and hs) depending on initial severity of esophagitis or 20 mg hs;[124] **PO for functional dyspepsia or chronic constipation** 5–10 mg tid; **PO for symptomatic gastroparesis** 10 mg tid–qid, which appears to be more effective than 10 or 20 mg bid.[123–125]

Special Populations. *Pediatric Dosage.* (<18 yr) safety and efficacy not established. PO (Infants and children) 0.15–0.3 mg/kg tid or qid has been used.[123–125] (*See* Adverse Reactions.)

Geriatric Dosage. Same as adult dosage.

Other Conditions. In hepatic insufficiency, reduce the daily dosage by 50%. Dosage reduction in severe renal impairment does not appear necessary; however, some investigators recommend a 50% dosage reduction because of the accumulation of cisapride and/or norcisapride.[124,125] Administration of an extra dose after hemodialysis does not appear necessary.[126]

Dosage Forms. **Tab** 10, 20 mg; **Susp** 1 mg/mL.

Patient Instructions. Take this drug at least 15 minutes before meals. Cisapride may initially cause diarrhea or abdominal cramping, which usually disappears with continued use. Drowsiness may occur. Until the degree of drowsiness is known, use caution when driving, operating machinery, or performing other tasks that require mental alertness. Concomitant use of cisapride and alcohol has been shown to increase blood alcohol concentrations. Many drugs interact with cisapride. Ask your health care provider for a list of drugs to avoid. Do not exceed recommended doses. Seek medical attention if any of the following symptoms occur while taking cisapride: faintness, dizziness, irregular heartbeat or pulse, any other unusual symptom. Inform your physician of all concomitant medications and medical conditions.

Missed Doses. If you miss a dose, take it as soon as possible. If it is almost time for your next dose, skip the missed dose and return to your usual dosage schedule. Do not double doses.

Pharmacokinetics. *Onset and Duration.* PO onset 45 ± 15 min.

Fate. Oral bioavailability is $37.5 \pm 2.5\%$ because of first-pass metabolism in the liver and/or gut. Food increases the bioavailability, but not the rate of absorption.[125] Reduced gastric acidity decreases rate and extent of absorption of tablets. Cisapride is 98% plasma protein bound, primarily to albumin. V_d is about 2.4 L/kg;[124] Cl is 6 L/hr. Cisapride is extensively metabolized by CYP3A4, primarily to norcisapride, which is about one-sixth as active as the parent drug.[125,126] Less than 10% of cisapride is excreted unchanged in urine and feces. Norcisapride is eliminated renally and appears to accumulate in severe renal failure.[126] Steady-state serum concentrations are higher in the elderly because of a moderate prolongation of the half-life of cisapride and/or norcisapride.

$t_{1/2}$. 8.5 ± 1.5 hr in healthy subjects, prolonged in patients with severe hepatic failure, but not substantially increased in renal impairment.[123,124]

Adverse Reactions. Diarrhea, abdominal pain, constipation, flatulence, and rhinitis occur frequently and appear to be dose related. Diarrhea and abdominal cramping tend to subside after several days of continuous therapy.[125] Headache, fatigue, depression, and dizziness occur frequently and are not dose related. Urinary disorders, including incontinence, frequency, hesitancy, retention, and cystitis, are also reported frequently.[127] Although causality is not established, serious adverse reactions, including death, have occurred in infants and children, with several deaths from cardiovascular events. Seizures have been reported in patients with a prior history of seizures who were treated with cisapride, but a causal relationship has not been established. Pediatric deaths have been associated with seizures. Other postmarketing events in children include positive ANA, anemia, methemoglobinemia, hyper- and hypoglycemia, unexplained apnea, depression, apathy, visual changes accompanied by amnesia, and severe photosensitivity. Postmarketing events reported in adults include confusion, hallucinations, depression, suicide attempt, hyperprolactinemia, and galactorrhea. Extrapyramidal reactions and sinus tachycardia (with relapse upon rechallenge in some cases) occur rarely.

Contraindications. Concurrent use of CYP3A4 inhibitors; conditions that predispose to arrhythmias; respiratory failure; concurrent drugs that prolong the QT interval; GI hemorrhage or perforation or other situations where increased GI motility could be harmful. (Consult product information for details.)

Precautions. Pregnancy; lactation. Avoid in patients with second- or third-degree AV block. Weigh benefits and risks in patients who have or may develop prolongation of cardiac conduction intervals. (Consult product information for details.)

Drug Interactions. Sedative effects of benzodiazepines and of alcohol may be exaggerated by cisapride. Anticholinergics may decrease cisapride's efficacy. Acceleration of gastric emptying may affect the rate of absorption (increase or decrease) of other orally administered drugs. In some patients receiving oral anticoagulants, cisapride may result in prolonged coagulation times. Drugs that inhibit hepatic CYP3A4 (*see* Cytochrome P450 Interactions) may markedly increase the serum cisapride concentration and lead to a prolongation of the QT interval, resulting in ventricular arrhythmias, including torsades de pointes and even death; some patients had no pre-existing cardiac disease. (*See* Contraindications.)

Parameters to Monitor. Consider ECG prior to starting therapy. Monitor for symptomatic relief of GERD, dyspepsia, chronic constipation, or gastroparesis; discontinue cisapride if not effective. Monitor for adverse effects, especially diarrhea and abdominal cramping. Monitor for potential drug interactions. (*See* Contraindications.) Serum concentrations of drugs with a narrow therapeutic index may require reassessment after initiation and discontinuation of cisapride therapy. In patients receiving oral anticoagulants, measure the PT/INR within the first few days of the start or discontinuation of cisapride.

Notes. Cisapride has similar efficacy to standard doses of **H₂-receptor antagonists** when used to treat mild esophagitis, but is not effective in severe erosive esophagitis.[128] When combined with an H₂-receptor antagonist, some additional benefit may be achieved.[128] In some studies, cisapride remained an effective gastrokinetic for up to 3 yr of treatment.[124] When cisapride is used to treat constipation, optimal effects may require 2–3 months of therapy. Cisapride has fewer CNS side effects than **metoclopramide**.[124]

DIPHENOXYLATE HYDROCHLORIDE AND ATROPINE SULFATE
Lomotil, Various

Pharmacology. Diphenoxylate is a synthetic meperidine congener lacking analgesic activity that slows GI motility; atropine is added in subtherapeutic amounts to decrease abuse potential.

Administration and Adult Dosage. **PO for diarrhea** 2 tablets or 10 mL qid initially, then, if control is achieved (usually within 48 hr), decrease to a **maintenance dosage** as low as 2 tablets or 10 mL daily prn. If chronic diarrhea is not controlled in 10 days at the full dosage, then symptoms are unlikely to be controlled by further administration.

Special Populations. *Pediatric Dosage.* **Use liquid only.** (<2 yr) Not recommended. **PO for diarrhea** 0.3–0.4 mg/kg/day of diphenoxylate in 4 divided doses initially, not to exceed adult dosage. Reduce dosage once diarrhea is controlled.

Geriatric Dosage. Same as adult dosage.

Dosage Forms. **Syrup** 500 μg diphenoxylate and 5 μg atropine/mL; **Tab** 2.5 mg diphenoxylate and 25 μg atropine.

Patient Instructions. This drug may cause dry mouth, blurred vision, drowsiness, or dizziness; use caution while driving or performing other tasks requiring alertness, coordination, or physical dexterity. Avoid alcohol and other CNS depressants. Seek medical attention if diarrhea persists or if fever, palpitations, or abdominal distention occurs.

Missed Doses. If you miss a dose, take it as soon as possible. If it is almost time for your next dose, skip the missed dose and return to your usual dosage schedule. Do not double doses.

Pharmacokinetics. *Onset and Duration.* Onset 45–60 min; duration 3–4 hr.

Fate. Diphenoxylate is well absorbed from the GI tract and metabolized to an active metabolite, diphenoxylic acid. Both drug and metabolite attain peak serum levels in 2 hr. Diphenoxylate V_d is 3.8 ± 1.1 L/kg; Cl is 1.04 ± 0.14 L/hr/kg.[129] Conjugates of the drug and metabolite are excreted primarily in the urine.

$t_{1/2}$. (Diphenoxylate) 2.5 ± 0.6 hr; (diphenoxylic acid) 7.2 ± 0.7 hr.[130]

Adverse Reactions. Anticholinergic symptoms such as dry mouth, urinary retention, blurred vision, fever, or tachycardia may occur frequently with high daily dosages, or occasionally with usual dosages in children.[131] Drowsiness, dizziness, and headache occur occasionally.

Contraindications. Children <2 yr; obstructive jaundice; diarrhea associated with pseudomembranous enterocolitis or enterotoxin-producing bacteria. (*See* Notes.)

Precautions. Use with caution in children because of variable response and potential for toxicity (atropinism) with recommended dosages (particularly in Down syndrome patients), and in patients with acute ulcerative colitis, hepatic dysfunction, or cirrhosis. (*See* Notes.)

Drug Interactions. Because of its chemical similarity to meperidine, avoid diphenoxylate use with MAOIs. Use with caution in combination with CNS depressants.

Parameters to Monitor. Frequency and volume of bowel movements; body temperature. Observe for signs of atropine toxicity. Monitor for abdominal distention.

Notes. In chronic diarrhea, diphenoxylate 5 mg is about equipotent with **loperamide** 2 mg or **codeine** 30–45 mg. It may provide temporary symptomatic relief of infectious traveler's diarrhea if used cautiously with an antibiotic, but discontinue it if fever occurs, symptoms persist beyond 48 hr, or blood or mucus appears in the stool.[132,133]

DOCUSATE SALTS   Various

Pharmacology. Docusate is an anionic surfactant that lowers the surface tension of the oil–water interface of the stool, allowing fecal material to be penetrated by water and fat, thereby softening the stool. The emulsifying action also enhances the absorption of many fat-soluble drugs and mineral oil.[118,119,134]

Administration and Adult Dosage. **PO as a stool softener** (sodium salt) 50–500 mg/day in single or divided doses (give solution/syrup in milk or fruit juice to mask taste); begin therapy with up to 500 mg/day and adjust after maximal effects occur (about 3 days);[121] (calcium salt) 240 mg/day; (potassium salt) 100–300 mg/day. Use of 200 mg/day or less of the sodium salt in the hospital setting may be ineffective in altering the prevalence of constipation. **PR as enema** 50–100 mg in water.

Special Populations. *Pediatric Dosage.* **PO** (sodium salt) (<3 yr) 10–40 mg/day; (3–6 yr) 20–60 mg/day; (6–12 yr) 40–120 mg/day; (>12 yr) same as adult dosage; give solution/syrup in milk, fruit juice, or formula to mask taste; (calcium salt) (≥6 yr) 50–150 mg/day; (potassium salt) (≥6 yr) 100 mg/day.

Geriatric Dosage. Same as adult dosage. (*See* Notes.)

Dosage Forms. (Sodium salt: Colace, various) **Cap** 50, 100, 240, 250 mg; **Soln** 10, 50 mg/mL; **Syrup** 3.3, 4 mg/mL; **Tab** 100 mg. (Calcium salt: Surfak, various) **Cap** 50, 240 mg. (Potassium salt: Dialose, various) **Cap** 240 mg; **Tab** 100 mg.

Patient Instructions. Take this with a full glass of fluid; take the liquid or solution forms in milk, fruit juice, or infant formula to mask the bitter taste.

Missed Doses. If you miss a dose, take it as soon as possible. If it is almost time for your next dose, skip the missed dose and return to your usual dosage schedule.

Pharmacokinetics. *Onset and Duration.* Onset of effect on stools is 2–3 days after first dose with continuous use.

Fate. Drug action is local in the gut, but docusate may be partially absorbed in the duodenum and jejunum, and secreted in the bile.[131,134]

Adverse Reactions. Bitter taste, throat irritation, and nausea (more common with syrup and liquid) occur frequently, abdominal cramps occasionally. Docusate may change intestinal morphology and cellular function, and may cause fluid and electrolyte accumulation in the colon.[134]

Contraindications. Undiagnosed abdominal pain; intestinal obstruction; concomitant use with mineral oil.

Precautions. Rectal bleeding or failure to respond to therapy may indicate a serious condition and the need for medical attention.

Drug Interactions. Concomitant use with mineral oil may enhance mineral oil absorption.[118,119]

Parameters to Monitor. Frequency and consistency of stools; ease of defecation.

Notes. Surfactant stool softeners are useful for softening hard, dry stools, in painful anorectal conditions, and in cardiac and other conditions to lessen the strain of defecation. They are more useful in preventing constipation rather than treating it; however, they may not be effective for long-term prevention of constipation in institutionalized elderly patients.[118,135]

LACTULOSE
Cephulac, Chronulac

Pharmacology. Lactulose is a synthetic disaccharide analogue of lactose that contains galactose and fructose and is metabolized by colonic bacteria to lactic and small amounts of acetic and formic acids. These acids result in acidification of colonic contents, decreased ammonia absorption, diffusion of ammonia from plasma to GI tract, and an osmotic catharsis.[136]

Administration and Adult Dosage. **PO as a cathartic** 15–30 mL (10–20 g), to a maximum of 60 mL; **PO for hepatic encephalopathy** 30–45 mL (20–30 g) q 1 hr until laxation, then 30–45 mL tid or qid, titrated to produce about 2 or 3 soft stools/day. **PR for hepatic encephalopathy as an enema** 300 mL with 700 mL water or NS retained for 30–60 min, may repeat q 4–6 hr. Repeat immediately if evacuated too promptly.

Special Populations. *Pediatric Dosage.* **PO for hepatic encephalopathy** (infants) 2.5–10 mL/day in divided doses; (older children and adolescents) 40–90 mL/day in divided doses, titrated to produce 2 or 3 soft stools daily. If initial dose causes diarrhea, reduce dose immediately; if diarrhea persists, discontinue.

Geriatric Dosage. Same as adult dosage. (*See* Notes.)

Dosage Forms. **Syrup** 667 mg/mL.

Patient Instructions. This syrup may be mixed with fruit juice, water, or milk to improve its palatability. In the treatment of hepatic encephalopathy, 2–3 loose stools per day are common, but report any worsening of diarrhea. Report belching, flatulence, or abdominal cramps if they are bothersome.

Missed Doses. If you miss a dose, take it as soon as possible. If it is almost time for your next dose, skip the missed dose and return to your usual dosage schedule.

Pharmacokinetics. *Onset and Duration.* (Catharsis) onset 24–48 hr; duration 24–48 hr. (Hepatic encephalopathy) onset and duration variable; however, reversal of coma may occur within 2 hr of the first enema.

Fate. After oral administration, less than 3% is absorbed and most reaches the colon unabsorbed and unchanged. Unabsorbed drug is metabolized in the colon by bacteria to low-molecular-weight acids and carbon dioxide. The small amount of absorbed drug is excreted in the urine unchanged.[136]

Adverse Reactions. Flatulence, belching, and abdominal discomfort are frequent initially. Colonic dilation occurs occasionally. Excessive diarrhea and fecal water loss may result in hypernatremia.[137]

Contraindications. Patients who require a low-galactose diet.

Precautions. Use with caution in diabetics because of small amounts of free lactose and galactose in the drug. Rectal bleeding or failure to respond to therapy may indicate a serious condition and the need for medical attention.

Drug Interactions. Do not use other laxatives concomitantly, because their induction of loose stools may confound proper lactulose dosage titration for hepatic encephalopathy. Nonabsorbable antacids may interfere with the colonic acidification of lactulose. Theoretically, some antibacterials might interfere with the intestinal bacteria that metabolize lactulose; however, oral neomycin has been used concurrently in hepatic encephalopathy.[136]

Parameters to Monitor. (Hepatic encephalopathy) observe for changes in hepatic encephalopathy and number of stools per day. Periodically obtain serum sodium, chloride, potassium, and bicarbonate levels during prolonged use, especially in elderly or debilitated patients.

Notes. Lactulose is effective in hepatic encephalopathy, but as a general laxative it offers no advantage over less expensive drugs.[137,138] One study of constipation in the elderly found that up to 60 mL/day of 70% **sorbitol** was equivalent in laxative effects and caused less nausea than the same dosage of lactulose syrup.[139]

LOPERAMIDE   Imodium

Pharmacology. Loperamide is a synthetic antidiarrheal structurally similar to haloperidol and without appreciable opiate activity that causes a dose-related inhibition of colonic motility and affects water and electrolyte movement through the bowel. Tolerance has not been observed.

Administration and Adult Dosage. **PO for acute diarrhea (℞) or traveler's diarrhea** (over-the-counter [OTC]) 4 mg initially, then 2 mg after each unformed stool, to a maximum of 16 mg/day (8 mg/day for no more than 2 days OTC product). **PO for chronic diarrhea (℞)** initiate therapy as above, then individualize dosage; **usual maintenance dosage** is 4–8 mg/day in single or divided doses. If clinical improvement does not occur after treatment with 16 mg/day for a minimum of 10 days, symptoms are unlikely to be controlled by further use.

Special Populations. *Pediatric Dosage.* (<2 yr) not recommended. **PO for acute diarrhea (℞)** (2–5 yr) up to 1 mg tid as liquid; (6–8 yr) 2 mg bid; (8–12 yr) 2 mg tid. After first day of therapy, give 1 mg/10 kg after each loose stool, to a maximum daily dosage equal to the initial daily dosage. **PO for acute or traveler's diarrhea** (OTC) (2–5 yr) not recommended; (6–8 yr) 1 mg initially, then 1 mg after each loose stool, to a maximum of 4 mg/day for 2 days; (9–11 yr) 2 mg initially, then 1 mg after each loose stool, to a maximum of 6 mg/day for 2 days. **PO for chronic diarrhea** dosage not established.

Geriatric Dosage. Same as adult dosage.

Dosage Forms. **Cap** 2 mg; **Chew Tab** 2 mg; **Tab** 2 mg; **Liquid** 0.2, 1 mg/mL; **Chew Tab** 2 mg plus simethicone (Imodium Advanced).

Patient Instructions. This drug may cause drowsiness or dizziness. Until the severity of these reactions is known, use caution when performing tasks that require mental alertness. It may cause dry mouth. If diarrhea does not stop after a few days, or if abdominal pain, distention, or fever occurs, seek medical attention.

Missed Doses. If you miss a dose, take it as soon as possible. If it is almost time for your next dose, skip the missed dose and return to your usual dosage schedule.

Pharmacokinetics. *Onset and Duration.* Onset 45–60 min; duration 4–6 hr.

Fate. GI absorption is approximately 40%; 25% or more is excreted in the stool unchanged; less than 2% of a dose is recovered in the urine.[17,140]

$t_{\frac{1}{2}}$. 10.8 ± 1.7 hr.[17,140]

Adverse Reactions. Abdominal cramping, constipation, distention, headache, rash, tiredness, drowsiness, dizziness, and dry mouth occur frequently.[141]

Contraindications. (℞, OTC) patients who must avoid constipation; children <2 yr. (OTC) bloody diarrhea; body temperature over 38°C (101°F); diarrhea associated with pseudomembranous colitis; or enterotoxin-producing bacteria. (*See* Notes.)

Precautions. Use with caution in patients with ulcerative colitis. Discontinue if improvement is not observed in 48 hr. Use cautiously in patients with hepatic dysfunction.

Drug Interactions. Absorption of loperamide may be decreased by cholesterol-binding resins.

Parameters to Monitor. Frequency and volume of bowel movements; body temperature. Monitor for abdominal distention.

Notes. Adverse reactions may be less frequent and efficacy may be greater than with **diphenoxylate** with atropine.[141] Loperamide may provide temporary symptomatic relief of infectious traveler's diarrhea if used cautiously with an antibiotic, but discontinue if fever occurs or other symptoms persist beyond 48 hr, or blood or mucus in stool develops.[132,133,141]

MAGNESIUM SALTS   Various

Pharmacology. Magnesium salts act as saline cathartics that inhibit fluid and electrolyte absorption by increasing osmotic forces in the gut lumen. Part of the action may be caused by cholecystokinin release, which stimulates small bowel motility and inhibits fluid and electrolyte absorption from the small intestine.[118]

Administration and Adult Dosage. PO as a laxative/cathartic (citrate) 240 mL; (sulfate) 20–30 mL of 50% solution (10–15 g) in a full glass of water; (hydroxide; Milk of Magnesia) 30–60 mL with liquid; (concentrate) 10–30 mL. (*See* Notes.)

Special Populations. *Pediatric Dosage.* PO (citrate) one-half the adult dosage; (sulfate) (2–5 yr) 2.5–5 g, (≥6 yr) 5–10 g in one-half glass or more of water; (hydroxide; Milk of Magnesia) 0.5 mL/kg.[118]

Geriatric Dosage. Same as adult dosage.

Other Conditions. Avoid use in patients with impaired renal function.[118]

Dosage Forms. Soln (citrate) 77 mEq/dL magnesium, 300 mL; (sulfate) 50%; **Susp** (hydroxide; Milk of Magnesia) 7–8.5%, many sizes, (*see* Notes) (also available as concentrates with 10 mL equivalent to 20 or 30 mL of susp); **Tab** (hydroxide; Milk of Magnesia) 311 mg; **Pwdr** (sulfate) 150, 240, 454 g, 1.8 kg.

Patient Instructions. Take Milk of Magnesia or magnesium sulfate with at least one full glass of liquid. You may take magnesium sulfate with fruit juice to partially mask its bitter taste. Refrigerating magnesium citrate improves its palatability.

Pharmacokinetics. *Onset and Duration.* Onset is dose dependent: (high end of dosage range) 0.5–3 hr; (low end of dosage range) 6–8 hr.[121]

Fate. Slow absorption of 15–30% of a dose from the GI tract. Absorbed magnesium is rapidly excreted in the urine in normal renal function.[118,121]

Adverse Reactions. Abdominal cramping, excessive diuresis, nausea, vomiting, and diarrhea occur frequently. Excessive use can lead to electrolyte abnormalities; dehydration may occur if taken with insufficient fluids. Use in patients with renal impairment may lead to hypermagnesemia, CNS depression, and hypotension.[118]

Contraindications. Acute surgical abdomen; fecal impaction; intestinal obstruction; abdominal pain of unknown origin; nausea; vomiting.

Precautions. Rectal bleeding or failure to respond to therapy may indicate a serious condition and the need for medical attention. Avoid use in patients with impaired renal function.[118]

Drug Interactions. None known.

Parameters to Monitor. Periodic serum magnesium levels in patients with impaired renal function who are receiving long-term daily administration.

Notes. Magnesium salts are useful for preparing the bowel for radiologic examination and surgical procedures. The following amounts of various magnesium salts are approximately equivalent to 80 mEq of magnesium: 100 mL citrate; 2.4 g (30 mL) Milk of Magnesia; and 10 g sulfate. The sulfate salt is the most potent cathartic, but is the least palatable. (*See also* Magnesium Salts in the Renal and Electrolyte sections.)

METOCLOPRAMIDE   Reglan, Various

Pharmacology. Metoclopramide antagonizes central and peripheral dopamine (D) receptors, showing a higher affinity for D_1, D_4, and D_5 subtypes and a lesser affinity for D_2 and D_3 subtypes; it sensitizes receptors in the GI tract to acetylcholine (thought to be due to partial agonism at the serotonin 5-HT$_4$–receptor subtype) and exerts a direct effect on smooth muscle. At higher doses it has 5-HT$_3$–receptor blocking effects. It increases peristalsis of the gastric antrum, duodenum, and jejunum, relaxes the pyloric sphincter and duodenal bulb, and has little effect on the colon or gallbladder. In patients with gastroesophageal reflux disease (GERD), metoclopramide produces a dose-dependent increase and duration of action in lower esophageal sphincter (LES) pressure. Its antiemetic action results from a direct antidopaminergic effect on the chemoreceptor trigger zone and vomiting center, and 5-HT$_3$–receptor blocking effects. Metoclopramide increases prolactin secretion and serum prolactin. It also produces a transient increase in aldosterone secretion, thought to be related to direct stimulation of the adrenal gland via stimulation of the 5-HT$_4$–receptor.[142,143]

Administration and Adult Dosage. **PO for short-term treatment of symptomatic GERD in patients who fail to respond to conventional therapy** up to 15 mg qid 30 min before each meal and hs for 4–12 weeks or intermittent single doses of up to 20 mg; **PO for symptomatic diabetic gastroparesis** 10 mg qid 30 min before each meal and hs for 2–8 weeks; **IM or IV for severe symptoms associated with gastroparesis** 10 mg qid for up to 10 days; **IV to facilitate small bowel intubation or to aid in radiologic examination** 10 mg over 1–2 min; **PO to increase maternal milk supply** 10 mg tid for 10–14 days.[144] **PO, IM, or IV for treatment of hiccups, PO** 10 mg q 6 hr, or **IM, IV** 5–10 mg q 8 hr, continue treatment for 10 days after resolution;[145] **IV for prevention of cancer chemotherapy-induced emesis** (drugs with high emetic potential) 2 mg/kg 30 min before chemotherapy, then q 2 hr for 2 doses, and then q 3 hr for 3 more doses; (drugs with low emetic potential) 1 mg/kg may be adequate; **IM for prevention of postoperative nausea and vomiting** 10–20 mg near the end of surgery. Dilute IV doses over 10 mg to 50 mL and infuse over at least 15 min. (*See* Notes.)

Special Populations. *Pediatric Dosage.* **IV to facilitate small bowel intubation or to aid in radiologic examination** (<6 yr) 0.1 mg/kg; (6–14 yr) 2.5–5 mg; (>14 yr) same as adult dosage.

Geriatric Dosage. Begin at one-half the initial dose (usually 5 mg) and increase or decrease based on efficacy and side effects.

Other Conditions. With Cl_{cr} <40 mL/min, begin at one-half the initial dose (usually 5 mg) and increase or decrease based on efficacy and side effects.

Dosage Forms. **Tab** 5, 10 mg; **Soln** 10 mg/mL; **Syrup** 1 mg/mL; **Inj** 5 mg/mL.

Patient Instructions. Take each dose 30 minutes before meals and at bedtime. This drug may cause drowsiness. Until the degree of drowsiness is known, use caution when driving, operating machinery, or performing other tasks requiring mental alertness. Avoid excessive concurrent use of alcohol or other drugs that cause drowsiness. Report any involuntary movements (eg, muscle spasms and jerky movements of the head and face) that may occur, especially in children and the elderly.

Missed Doses. If you miss a dose, take it as soon as possible. If it is almost time for your next dose, skip the missed dose and return to your usual dosage schedule. Do not double doses.

Pharmacokinetics. *Onset and Duration.* (GI effects) PO onset 45 ± 15 min, IM 12.5 ± 2.5 min, IV 2 ± 1 min; duration 1–2 hr.

Fate. Bioavailability is PO 80 ± 15.5%, and IM 85 ± 11%. Peak serum concentration after a PO dose occurs in 1–2 hr, but may be delayed with impaired gastric emptying. The drug is about 30% plasma protein bound. V_d is 3.4 ± 1.3 L/kg, increased in uremia and in cirrhosis; Cl is 0.37 ± 0.08 L/hr/kg, decreased in uremia and in cirrhosis. About 85% of orally administered drug is recovered in the urine after 72 hr as unchanged and conjugated drug; 20% of an IV dose is excreted unchanged in urine.[90,146]

$t_{1/2}$. α phase 5 min; β phase 5.5 ± 0.5 hr, increasing to about 14 hr in severe renal failure. Half-life may also be prolonged in cirrhosis.[90,146]

Adverse Reactions. Most side effects are related to dosage and duration of use. Drowsiness, restlessness, fatigue, and lassitude occur in 10% of patients with a dosage of 10 mg qid, and in 70% with IV doses of 1–2 mg/kg. Acute dystonic reactions occur in 0.2% of patients receiving 30–40 mg/day, 2% in cancer chemotherapy-treated patients >35 yr receiving doses of 1–2 mg/kg, and 25% in cancer chemotherapy-treated children without prior diphenhydramine treatment. Parkinsonian symptoms, tardive dyskinesia, and akathisia occur less frequently. Rapid IV push produces transient, intense anxiety, and restlessness followed by drowsiness. Transient flushing of the face and/or diarrhea occur frequently following large IV doses. Hyperprolactinemia may occur, resulting in gynecomastia and impotence in males, and galactorrhea and amenorrhea in females. Fluid retention may result from transient elevation of aldosterone secretion that occurs after parenteral, but not oral administration.[142] Diarrhea, hypertension, and mental depression have been reported.

Contraindications. GI hemorrhage; mechanical obstruction or perforation; pheochromocytoma; epilepsy; concurrent use of drugs that cause extrapyramidal effects.

Precautions. Pregnancy; lactation. Use with caution in the elderly and in patients with hypertension, renal failure, or Parkinson's disease, a prior history of depression or attempted suicide, and following gut anastomosis. In patients with diabetic gastroparesis, insulin dosage or timing may require adjustment.

Drug Interactions. Absorption of drugs from the stomach or small bowel may be altered by metoclopramide (eg, digoxin and cimetidine absorption is decreased; cyclosporine absorption is increased). Anticholinergics and narcotics may antagonize GI effects of metoclopramide. Use with an MAOI may result in hypertension and the combination should be avoided. Additive sedation can occur with alcohol or other CNS depressants.

Parameters to Monitor. Monitor periodically for CNS effects, extrapyramidal reactions, and changes in Cr_s, blood glucose, or blood pressure. (GERD or diabetic gastroparesis) observe for symptomatic relief.

Notes. Tolerance to the drug's gastrokinetic effect may develop with long-term therapy;[147] however, this remains controversial.[146] Metoclopramide has been used in the treatment of neurogenic bladder, orthostatic hypotension, Tourette's syndrome, adynamic or chemotherapy-induced ileus, anorexia, and complications of scleroderma.[148] If extrapyramidal symptoms occur, administer **diphenhydramine** 50 mg IM or **benztropine** 1–2 mg IM.

Domperidone is a prokinetic agent expected to become available in the United States for the treatment of symptoms of diabetic gastroparesis. It selectively blocks peripheral D_2 receptors primarily in the gut, has antiemetic effects related to its action at the chemoreceptor trigger zone, and has no cholinergic activity. Domperidone does not readily cross the blood-brain barrier and therefore does not produce the CNS and extrapyramidal effects seen with metoclopramide. It increases the frequency and amplitude of antral and duodenal peristalsis, but has not shown consistent results in increasing LES pressure in GERD patients. Domperidone is metabolized by CYP3A4; drug interactions related to its inhibition are expected to occur. Cimetidine and antacids may interfere with domperidone's bioavailability and should not be coadministered. The dosage is 20 mg qid, before meals and at bedtime. The side effects associated with domperidone include headache, dry mouth, diarrhea, anxiety, and elevation in serum prolactin concentration.[149]

Erythromycin in low doses binds to motilin receptors in the GI tract to stimulate gastric emptying.[143,147] In gastroparesis, doses of 200 mg IV of the lactobionate salt, 250 mg PO of the ethylsuccinate salt, or 500 mg PO of the base 15–120 min before meals and at hs appear to be effective.[150] Differences in efficacy between the various salts of erythromycin have not been established.[150] Erythromycin has also been used in other GI motility disorders.[143,150,151]

PEG ELECTROLYTE LAVAGE SOLUTION   GoLYTELY, Various

Pharmacology. Polyethylene glycol (PEG) electrolyte lavage solution is an isoosmotic solution containing approximately 5.69 g/L sodium sulfate, 1.68 g/L sodium bicarbonate, 1.46 g/L sodium chloride, 745 mg/L potassium chloride, and 60 g/L PEG 3350 used for total bowel cleansing prior to GI examination. A solution lacking sodium sulfate, with a slight variation in other salts and PEG (NuLYTELY), and flavored solutions are available with improved palatability. PEG acts as an osmotic cathartic, and the electrolyte concentrations are such that there is little net fluid or electrolyte movement into or out of the bowel. This method of bowel cleansing is well suited for colonoscopy, but because of some residual lavage fluid retained in the colon, other cleansing methods may be preferred prior to barium enema. Colonic cleansing with **bisacodyl** 15 mg orally followed by 2 L of PEG lavage solution 8 hr later has been found to be equally effective and more acceptable to patients than 4 L of solution used alone. The drug may be useful as a GI evacuant in ingestions and overdoses with iron and some EC and SR drug products.[122,152-155]

Adult Dosage. PO or NG 200–300 mL orally q 10 min or by NG tube at a rate of 20–30 mL/min until about 4 L are consumed or the rectal effluent is clear. Give a 1-L trial before the full dosage in patients suspected of having bowel obstruction. Use the solution at least 4 hr before the examination, allowing the patient 3 hr for drinking and a 1-hr period to complete bowel evacuation. Another method is to give the solution the evening before the examination. Chilling the solution may improve its palatability, but do not add any additional ingredients. Withhold solid food for 2 hr and medication for 1 hr before the solution is administered.

Pediatric Dosage. PO or NG 25–40 mL/kg/hr for 4–10 hr appear safe and useful for bowel evacuation.

Dosage Forms. Available as powder for reconstitution and oral solution.

Pharmacokinetics. The first bowel movement usually occurs after 1 hr, with total bowel cleansing 3–4 hr after starting.

Adverse Reactions. Frequent side effects include nausea, abdominal fullness, bloating (in up to 50% of patients), cramps, anal irritation, and vomiting. Urticaria, rhinorrhea, and dermatitis occur occasionally. Do not use PEG electrolyte lavage solution in patients with GI obstruction, gastric retention, toxic colitis, toxic megacolon, ileus, or bowel perforation; however, the solution appears safe for patients with liver, kidney, or heart disease.

PSYLLIUM HUSK

Pharmacology. Psyllium is a bulk-forming cathartic that absorbs water and provides an emollient mass.

Administration and Adult Dosage. PO for constipation 2.5–12 g daily–tid, stirred in a full glass of fluid, followed by an additional glass of liquid. **PO for mild diarrhea** usual doses titrated to effect may be used to "firm up" effluent. **PO to lower cholesterol** 10–30 g/day in divided doses in combination with diet may decrease cholesterol in patients with mild to moderate hypercholesterolemia.[156,157]

Special Populations. *Pediatric Dosage.* **PO for constipation** (6–12 yr) 2.5–3 g (psyllium) daily–tid, with fluid as above.

Geriatric Dosage. Same as adult dosage.

Dosage Forms. Pwdr Metamucil, Sugar Free Orange Flavor (containing 65% or 92% psyllium), Konsyl (sugar-free, containing 100% psyllium) 3.7, 5.2 g packet, 111–621 g; **Pwdr** Metamucil Orange Flavor (containing 50% or 65% sucrose) 7, 11 g packet, 210, 420, 630, 960 g; **Pwdr** (effervescent, sugar-free, containing 63% psyllium) 5.4 g packet; **Wafer** Metamucil (containing 4.5 g fat) 1.7 g of psyllium per wafer, Fiberall (containing 78 kcal of carbohydrate) 3.4 g psyllium/wafer.

Patient Instructions. Mix with a full glass of fluid before taking and follow with another glass of liquid.

Pharmacokinetics. *Onset and Duration.* Onset 12–24 hr, but 2–3 days may be required for full effect.[118,158]

Fate. Not absorbed from GI tract.

Adverse Reactions. Flatulence occurs frequently. Serious side effects are rare, but esophageal, gastric, intestinal, and rectal obstruction have been reported. Allergic reactions and bronchospasm have occurred following inhalation of dry powder.[118,159]

Contraindications. Acute surgical abdomen; fecal impaction; intestinal obstruction; abdominal pain of unknown origin; nausea; vomiting.

Precautions. Rectal bleeding or failure to respond to therapy may indicate a serious condition and the need for medical attention. Use with caution in patients who require fluid restriction, because constipation may occur unless fluid intake is adequate. Psyllium may be hazardous in patients with intestinal ulcerations, stenosis, or disabling adhesions. Use effervescent Metamucil formulations (packet) with caution in patients who require potassium restriction (7.4 and 7.9 mEq potassium/packet). Use the noneffervescent formulations of Metamucil cautiously in diabetics, because they contain 50% or 65% sucrose. Sugar-free preparations include Konsyl and Metamucil Sugar Free.

Drug Interactions. None known.

Notes. Psyllium is useful in lessening the strain of defecation and for inpatients who are on low-residue diets or constipating medications. It is safe to use in pregnancy.[118]

Miscellaneous Gastrointestinal Drugs

ACTIVATED CHARCOAL
Various

Pharmacology. Activated charcoal is a nonspecific GI adsorbent with a surface area of 900–2000 m^2/g used primarily in the management of acute poisonings.[160]

Administration and Adult Dosage. **PO or via gastric tube** 50–120 g dispersed in liquid as soon as possible after ingestion of poison (the FDA suggests 240 mL diluent/30 g activated charcoal). Repeat administration of activated charcoal after gastric lavage. (*See* Notes.)

Special Populations. *Pediatric Dosage.* **PO or via gastric tube** (≤12 yr) 25–50 g or 1–2 g/kg dispersed in liquid; (>12 yr) same as adult dosage.[161]

Geriatric Dosage. Same as adult dosage.

Dosage Forms. **Pwdr** plain, or dispersed in water or sorbitol-water.

Patient Instructions. This drug causes the stools to turn black.

Pharmacokinetics. *Onset and Duration.* Onset is immediate; duration is continual while it remains in the GI tract.

Fate. Eliminated unchanged in the feces.

Adverse Reactions. Black stools; gritty consistency may cause emesis in some patients.

Precautions. Insufficient hydration or use in patients with decreased bowel motility may result in intestinal bezoars.

Drug Interactions. Activated charcoal may decrease the oral absorption and efficacy of many drugs. (*See* Notes.)

Parameters to Monitor. Passage of activated charcoal in the stools. If sorbitol or other cathartics are administered, limit their dosages to prevent excessive fluid and electrolyte losses.

Notes. A suspension of activated charcoal in 25–35% **sorbitol** may increase palatability of the drug; total dosage of sorbitol should not exceed 1 g/kg. Substances *not* adsorbed by activated charcoal include mineral acids, alkalis, iron, cyanide, lithium and other small ions, and alcohols. Repeated oral doses of activated charcoal (eg, 15–30 g q 4–6 hr) have been used to enhance the elimination of some drugs, most notably **carbamazepine, phenobarbital, salicylates,** and **theophylline.**

CHOLELITHOLYTIC DRUGS:

CHENODIOL
Chenix

URSODIOL
Actigall, Urso

Pharmacology. The oral bile acids chenodiol (chenodeoxycholic acid) and ursodiol (ursodeoxycholic acid) are used to dissolve small (<20 mm), radiolucent cholesterol gallstones in mildly symptomatic patients with a functioning gallbladder who are unable to undergo a cholecystectomy. The exact mechanism by which these drugs dissolve cholesterol gallstones is unclear. Chenodiol expands the bile acid pool, inhibits synthesis of cholesterol and bile acids, and reduces biliary cholesterol saturation, allowing solubilization of cholesterol. Ursodiol does not appear to inhibit the synthesis of bile acids, but it does suppress the synthesis, secretion, and intestinal absorption of cholesterol, and it promotes nonmicellar mechanisms of cholesterol solubilization. Stone fragmentation via extracorporeal shock-wave lithotripsy (ECSWL) with subsequent oral bile acid therapy is the norm; however, some clinicians begin oral therapy 2 weeks prior to ECSWL. Ursodiol may have effects on the immune system and has been studied in a variety of conditions. The use of ursodiol in primary biliary cirrhosis improves liver function tests and certain immune markers, relieves pruritus in some patients (after an initial 2-week exacerbation period), and in long-term (4-year) studies, extends the length of time before death or to liver transplantation. Ursodiol also appears to be effective in decreasing the number of patients experiencing multiple episodes of rejection and in improved 1-year survival rates following liver transplantation.[162–172]

Adult Dosage. PO for gallstone dissolution (chenodiol) 13–16 mg/kg/day; (ursodiol) 8–10 mg/kg/day. For both drugs, the dosage is given in 2–3 divided doses; higher dosages do not provide additional efficacy. Although studies conflict, a single bedtime dose may be more effective than multiple daily doses in reducing cholesterol saturation of bile. Complete gallstone dissolution usually requires 6–24 months of treatment and treatment should be continued for at least 3 months after stones or sludge are not apparent on ultrasonography, because of the possible presence of microscopic stones and/or crystals. Cessation of oral bile acid therapy results in gallstone recurrence in approximately 50% of patients within 5 yr. **Maintenance therapy** (ursodiol) 300 mg/day may decrease the recurrence rate by one-half, especially in patients <50 yr; maintenance therapy with chenodiol appears to be ineffective. **PO for prophylaxis against gallstone formation during weight loss** (ursodiol) 300 mg bid. **PO for biliary disorders associated with cystic fibrosis** (ursodiol) 15–20 mg/kg/day. **PO for primary biliary cirrhosis** (ursodiol) 12–15 mg/kg/day either divided or as a single bedtime dose. **PO as an adjunct to immunosuppressants following liver transplantation** (ursodiol) 10–15 mg/kg/day.

Dosage Forms. (Chenodiol) **Tab** 250 mg available from the manufacturer as an orphan drug. (Ursodiol) **Cap** 300 mg. Ursodial can be formulated into a suspension.[173]

Adverse Reactions. Chenodiol is not widely used because of its dose-related side effects: diarrhea (50%), increased AST and ALT (40%), usually reversible hepatitis (3%), and a 10% or greater increase in LDL cholesterol. Ursodiol has fewer and less severe adverse effects, but the safety of ursodiol beyond 24 months has not been established. Oral bile acids are not recommended during pregnancy. Combination therapy with the two drugs is no longer recommended.

MESALAMINE PREPARATIONS

Pharmacology. Mesalamine (5-aminosalicylic acid [5-ASA]) is thought to be the active moiety of sulfasalazine. Each molecule of olsalazine that reaches the colon is converted to 2 molecules of mesalamine. The mechanism of action of mesalamine in inflammatory bowel disease (IBD) is unknown, but appears to be topical rather than systemic. Mucosal production of arachidonic acid metabolites, through both the cyclo-oxygenase and lipoxygenase pathways, are increased in patients with chronic IBD. Mesalamine may block cyclo-oxygenase in the arachidonic cascade and downregulate production of inflammatory prostaglandins in the large bowel. Modulation of the lipoxygenase pathway may inhibit formation of chemotactically active leukotrienes and hydroxyeicosatetraenoic acids. Mesalamine inhibits macrophage and neutrophil chemotaxis, reduces intestinal mononuclear cell production of immunoglobulin (Ig) A and IgG antibodies, and is a scavenger of oxygen-derived free radicals, which are increased during active IBD.[174–177]

Administration and Adult Dosage.

INDICATION	ASACOL Mesalamine	DIPENTUM Olsalazine	PENTASA Mesalamine	ROWASA Mesalamine
Short-term treatment of active mild to moderate ulcerative colitis.	PO 800 mg tid, or 1.6 g tid[a] for 6 weeks.	PO 500 mg tid,[a] 1 g bid,[a] or 1 g tid[a] for 3–6 weeks.	PO 1 g qid for 6–8 weeks.	PR 2 g hs,[a,b] or 4 g hs[b] for 3–6 weeks (enema).
Maintenance of ulcerative colitis remission.	PO 800 mg bid.	PO 500 mg bid.[c]	PO 1 g bid[a] or 1 g qid.[a]	PR 1–2 g hs[a,b] (enema).
Short-term treatment of active mild to moderate Crohn's disease.	PO 800 mg tid[a] or 1.6 g tid[a] for 8–16 weeks.	a	PO 1 g qid[a] for 8–16 weeks.	a
Maintenance of Crohn's disease remission.	PO 800 mg– 1.6 g tid.[a]	a	PO 1 g bid or 1 g qid.[a]	a
Treatment of active proctitis.	PO 800 mg tid.	a	PO 1 g qid.	PR 1–2 g hs,[a,b] 4 g hs[b] (enema); 500 mg bid or tid[d] (suppository).

[a]Nonlabeled indication and dosage; optimal dosage regimen has not been determined.
[b]Retain enema for approximately 8 hr.
[c]Patients intolerant to sulfasalazine.
[d]Retain suppository for 1–3 hr or longer.
From references 174–181.

Special Populations. *Pediatric Dosage.* Safety and efficacy not established; however, pediatric use has been reported.[182,183]

Geriatric Dosage. No dosage reduction is necessary. However, older patients are more likely to have renal impairment. (*See* Precautions.)

Other Conditions. Dosage reduction may be considered in severe renal and/or hepatic impairment.[174] (*See* Precautions.)

Dosage Forms.

DRUG	ASACOL *Mesalamine*	DIPENTUM *Olsalazine*	PENTASA *Mesalamine*	ROWASA *Mesalamine*
Formulation.	Tablet enteric-coated pH dependent (pH 7), delayed release.	Capsule containing 5-ASA diamer; diazo bond is degraded by bacteria in colon.[a]	Capsule containing ethyl-cellulose-coated microgranules, controlled release.	Rectal suspension, suppository.
Site of action.	Distal ileum or colon.	Colon.	Proximal jejunum to colon.	Rectum or splenic flexure (enema); rectum (suppository).
Dosage forms.	EC Tab 400 mg.	Cap 250 mg.	SR Cap 250 mg.	Enema 4 g/60 mL; Supp 500 mg.

[a]Each molecule of olsalazine that reaches the colon is converted to 2 molecules of mesalamine.

Patient Instructions. (Oral) take mesalamine with food and a full glass of water. Swallow tablets or capsules whole without breaking or chewing. The tablet core (Asacol) or small beads (Pentasa) may appear in the stool after mesalamine is released, but this does not mean there was a lack of effect. Report intact or partially intact tablets in the stool (Asacol), because this may indicate that the expected amount of mesalamine was not released from the tablet. Report nausea, vomiting, abrupt change in character or volume of stools, or skin rashes. (Rectal) empty bowel immediately prior to insertion of enema or suppository. Use enema at bedtime and retain for 8 hours, if possible. Retain suppository for 1 to 3 hours or longer. Report signs of anal or rectal irritation.

Missed Doses. (Oral) if you miss a dose, take it as soon as possible. If it is almost time for your next dose, skip the missed dose and return to your usual dosage schedule. Do not double doses. (Rectal) if you miss a dose, use it as soon as possible if you remember it that same night. If you do not remember it until the next morning, skip the missed dose and return to your usual dosage schedule.

Pharmacokinetics. *Onset and Duration.* The onset of action of Asacol, Dipentum, and Pentasa is delayed because of the release characteristics of their dosage forms; duration of action varies depending on intestinal transit time.[174]

Fate. About $70 \pm 10\%$ of oral mesalamine is absorbed in the proximal small bowel when administered in an uncoated product or unbound to a carrier molecule; some absorption may occur in the distal small bowel, but mesalamine is poorly absorbed from the colon. Various oral dosage forms have been formulated to deliver mesalamine topically to the more distal sites of inflammation.[174,175,177] (*See* Dosage Forms and Notes.) After oral administration, about 50% of mesalamine from Pentasa is released in the small bowel and 50% is released in the colon, although the amount released may vary and is patient specific.[177] About $25 \pm 10\%$ of released mesalamine is absorbed following oral administration of Asacol or Pentasa; the remainder is excreted in the feces. About 98% of an oral olsalazine dose reaches the large bowel; less than 2% is absorbed. Mesalamine absorption from the enema is pH dependent; neutral solutions are better absorbed than acidic solutions.[174] Rowasa (at pH 4.5) is less than 15% rectally absorbed. Plasma protein binding: mesalamine ($55 \pm 15\%$); N-acetylmesalamine (80%); olsalazine and olsalazine-O-sulfate (greater than 99%).[174] Absorbed mesalamine is rapidly acetylated to N-acetyl-5-aminosalicylate (N-acetylmesalamine) in the intestinal mucosal wall and the liver. Absorbed olsalazine is conjugated in the liver to olsalazine-O-sulfate. N-acetylmesalamine is excreted in urine. Less than 1% of a dose of olsalazine is recovered unchanged in urine.

$t_{1/2}$. (Mesalamine) 1 ± 0.5 hr; (N-acetylmesalamine) 7.5 ± 1.5 hr; (olsalazine-O-sulfate) 7 days.[174]

Adverse Reactions. Adverse effects are usually less frequent than those reported with oral sulfasalazine. Headache, flatulence, abdominal pain, diarrhea, dizziness, and fatigue occur frequently with oral or rectal mesalamine. An acute intolerance syndrome develops in 3% of patients taking mesalamine; dose-dependent secretory diarrhea occurs in about 17% of patients receiving olsalazine 1 g/day, although it is sometimes difficult to distinguish these adverse effects from the underlying disease. Oral, esophageal, and duodenal ulceration as well as gastritis and GI bleeding have been reported. Dermatologic reactions, including acne, pruritus, urticaria, alopecia, and photosensitivity, occur occasionally. (*See* Contraindications.) Rarely, pericarditis, fatal myocarditis, hypersensitivity pneumonitis, pancreatitis, nephrotic syndrome, interstitial nephritis, and hepatitis occur. (*See* Precautions.) Anal irritation or a hypersensitivity reaction to mesalamine or the sulfite contained in the rectal suspension is rare; however, patients intolerant to sulfasalazine may also be sensitive to rectal mesalamine.

Contraindications. Pyloric stenosis; intestinal obstruction; salicylate hypersensitivity.

Precautions. Pregnancy, although recommended dosages do not appear to present a major teratogenic risk;[184,185] lactation. Renal tubular damage caused by absorbed mesalamine or its N-acetylated metabolite may occur, especially in patients with pre-existing renal impairment or those on concomitant 5-ASA-liberating medication. Use caution if mesalamine is used in patients with impaired hepatic function. Patients who experience rash or fever with sulfasalazine may have the same reaction to mesalamine or olsalazine, indicating possible cross-sensitivity to salicylates.

Drug Interactions. Increased PT in patients taking warfarin has been reported.

Parameters to Monitor. Improvement in abdominal cramping, diarrhea, and rectal bleeding. Monitor for adverse effects, including diarrhea (olsalazine), acute intolerance syndrome, and hypersensitivity reaction. Monitor BUN, Cr_s and urinalysis prior to and periodically during therapy. Monitor PT in patients taking concurrent warfarin.

Notes. The release characteristics of Pentasa are primarily time dependent, whereas those of Asacol are pH dependent; consequently, Asacol may not provide reliable site-specific release of 5-ASA if intestinal pH is inadequate. In 2–3% of patients taking Asacol, intact, or partially intact, tablets have been reported in the stool.

There appears to be no clinically important advantage of one oral mesalamine product over another, or over **sulfasalazine,** in treating or maintaining remission of mild to moderate ulcerative colitis.[174–176,178,180,186] A dose–response relationship exists when mesalamine is used to treat and maintain remission of mild to moderate ulcerative colitis.[178,186] A mesalamine preparation may be of benefit in the sulfasalazine-sensitive patient and in men who wish to have children because mesalamine does not alter sperm count, morphology, or motility.[175,186] The enema is as effective as oral sulfasalazine or **hydrocortisone** enema in patients with active mild to moderate left-sided ulcerative colitis and proctitis and is associated with a more rapid response and fewer and milder adverse effects.[175,178,180,187] A 1–2 g mesalamine enema may be as effective as the 4 g formulation in mild ulcerative colitis and proctitis.[180] Patients refractory to oral sulfasalazine and oral or rectal hydrocortisone may respond to rectal mesalamine. Rectal mesalamine combined with oral sulfasalazine or **corticosteroids** may enhance induction and maintenance of remission in patients with mild to moderate ulcerative colitis, but the risk of adverse effects is increased.[178,189]

In Crohn's disease with involvement of the ileum or proximal large bowel, oral formulations, which deliver mesalamine to the small bowel and colon, are preferable to sulfasalazine or olsalazine. Oral mesalamine preparations appear effective in treating active mild to moderate Crohn's disease (including ileal or ilealcolonic), maintaining remission, and preventing recurrence after curative surgery; however, optimal dosage regimens require further clarification.[177,179,188] Rectal mesalamine appears to be less effective in Crohn's disease, but efficacy is dependent on disease location and severity.[177,179] Mesalamine is reported to improve the quality of life in Crohn's patients, but assessment instruments require validation.[174,190] (*See also* Sulfasalazine.)

Balsalazide disodium (Colazide) is a mesalamine prodrug that releases mesalamine after colonic cleavage of the diazo bond that links it to the inactive carrier 4-aminobenzoyl-β-alanine in a fashion similar to that of olsalazine and sulfasalazine. It appears to be more effective and faster acting than delayed-release mesalamine in acute treatment of mild to moderate ulcerative colitis and may be better tolerated. Dosage used investigationally for ulcerative colitis is 2.25 g PO tid.[191] It is available in 2.25 g tablets (equivalent to 780 mg of mesalamine).

OCTREOTIDE   Sandostatin

Pharmacology. Octreotide is a synthetic octapeptide with pharmacologic actions similar to somatostatin. The actions of somatostatin are regulated by somatostatin receptors (5 known subtypes) located in regions of the brain, leptomeninges, anterior pituitary, endocrine and exocrine pancreas, GI mucosa, and cells of the immune system. Octreotide binds to somatostatin-receptor subtypes 2 and 5 and, to a lesser extent, subtype 3, but not to subtypes 1 and 4. It suppresses the secretion of numerous substances, including serotonin, gastrin, vasoactive intestinal peptide (VIP), insulin, glucagon, secretin, motilin, pancreatic polypeptide, and growth hormone (GH). It suppresses the luteinizing hormone response to gonadotropin-releasing hormone, and the secretion of thyroid-stimulating hormone (TSH). It also decreases splanchnic blood flow.[192,193]

Administration and Adult Dosage. Deep SC administration is recommended for symptom control. **SC for symptomatic treatment of severe diarrhea and facial flushing associated with metastatic carcinoid tumors** 100–600 μg/day in 2–4 divided doses during the first 2 weeks of therapy; **maintenance dosages** of 50–1500 μg/day (median about 450 μg/day) have been used. **SC for symptomatic treatment of profuse watery diarrhea associated with VIP-secreting tumors (VIPomas)** 200–300 μg/day in 2–4 divided doses for the first 2 weeks (range 150–750 μg/day) to control symptoms, then adjust dosage based on therapeutic response; dosages over 450 μg/day are usually not required. **SC to reduce GH and/or IGF-I (insulin-like growth factor I, somatomedin C) in patients with acromegaly** 50 μg tid initially, increase dosage q 2 weeks based on IGF-I concentration. The most common dosage is 100 μg tid, with some patients requiring 500 μg tid although doses >600 μg/day are rarely of additional benefit.[193] A more rapid titration can be obtained by drawing multiple GH concentrations from 0 to 8 hr after the octreotide dose. The goal is to achieve GH <5 μg/L (or IGF-I concentration <1.9 units/mL in men and <2.2 units/mL in women). Discontinue octreotide for about 4 weeks each year in acromegalics who have received irradiation; if clinical symptoms or abnormal laboratory results recur, resume therapy. **IV** same dosage as SC, diluted in 50–200 mL of NS or D5W and infused over 15–30 min, or given by IV push over 3 min. In emergency situations (eg, carcinoid crisis), give by rapid IV bolus. (*See* Notes.)

Special Populations. *Pediatric Dosage.* SC 1–10 μg/kg are well tolerated in patients ≥1 month. Studies of various GI disorders used widely varying dosages in children 3 days–16 yr.[194] Octreotide has been studied in the treatment of hyperinsulinemic hypoglycemia in neonates in varying dosages.[194,195] **SC for anti-VIP effects** 3.5 μg/kg/day divided q 8 hr has been used.[196]

Geriatric Dosage. Dosage reduction is recommended because of decreased renal clearance.

Other Conditions. The effect of hepatic disease on the disposition of octreotide is unknown. Reduction of maintenance dosages may be required in patients with renal impairment and those undergoing dialysis.[197]

Dosage Forms. **Inj** 50, 100, 200, 500, 1000 μg/mL.

Patient Instructions. Instruct patient in sterile SC injection technique. Avoid multiple SC injections at the same site within a short period of time. Systematically rotate injection sites. Do not use solution if particulates and/or discoloration are present. Store medication in refrigerator, but do not allow it to freeze; individual ampules can remain at room temperature for up to 24 hours. Sandostatin is stable at room temperature for 14 days if protected from light. Pain at injection site can be minimized by using the smallest volume necessary to obtain the desired dose and by bringing the solution to room temperature prior to injection, but do not warm artificially. Stop medication and report if symptoms of high or low blood sugar occur.

Missed Doses. If you miss a dose, take it as soon as possible. If it is almost time for your next dose, skip the missed dose and return to your usual dosage schedule.

Do not double doses. Although you will not be harmed by forgetting a dose, the symptoms that you are trying to control may reappear. To be able to control your symptoms, your doses should be evenly spaced over a period of 24 hours.

Pharmacokinetics. *Onset and Duration.* SC peak concentrations occur in 0.4 hr (0.7 hr in acromegaly). Duration is up to 12 hr, depending on tumor type.

Fate. Oral absorption is poor; SC and IV routes are bioequivalent. The drug is 65% protein bound (41% in acromegaly), primarily to lipoprotein and, to a lesser extent, albumin. V_d is 0.35 ± 0.22 L/kg; Cl is 0.16 ± 0.08 L/hr/kg. V_d and Cl are both increased in acromegaly; Cl is decreased in the elderly by 26% and in those with renal impairment. Octreotide exhibits nonlinear pharmacokinetics at dosages of 600 µg/day or greater. About 32% is excreted unchanged in urine.

$t_{1/2}$. 1.5 ± 0.4 hr; increased by 46% in the elderly.

Adverse Reactions. Single doses of octreotide can inhibit gallbladder contractility and decrease bile secretion. About one-half of patients on octreotide for 12 months or longer experience cholesterol gallstones or sludge, unrelated to age, gender, or dosage. About 5–10% of nonacromegalic patients and 34–61% of acromegalics experience diarrhea, loose stools, nausea, and abdominal discomfort. The severity, but not the frequency, is dose dependent; symptoms spontaneously subside in about 14 days.[193] Diabetics appear to be especially susceptible to nausea and abdominal cramping.[192] Hypoglycemia (in 3%) and hyperglycemia (in 16%) is more common in acromegalics than nonacromegalics (1.5%). Octreotide suppresses the secretion of TSH, alters the balance between insulin, glucagon, and GH, and may be responsible for cardiac conduction abnormalities, which are particularly frequent in acromegaly: bradycardia (21%), conduction abnormalities (10%), and arrhythmias (9%). Adverse reactions that occur in 1–10% of patients include vomiting, flatulence, constipation, and headache. Adverse GI effects often diminish with time.[198] Pain on injection occurs frequently and can be minimized by warming the solution prior to injection and using the smallest possible drug volume to obtain the appropriate dose. Several cases of pancreatitis have been reported. Abnormal Schilling's tests and decreased vitamin B_{12} levels have been reported.

Precautions. Pregnancy; lactation. Use with caution in patients with diabetic gastroparesis because octreotide slows GI transit time;[192] insulin-dependent diabetics may require a reduction in insulin dosage.

Drug Interactions. In acromegaly, reduction of dosage of medications causing bradycardia (eg, β-blockers) may be required. In all patients, the dosage of calcium-channel blocking drugs, diuretics, insulin, or oral hypoglycemics may require an adjustment with concurrent octreotide. Octreotide may decrease the absorption of some orally administered nutrients and drugs (eg, fat, cyclosporine).

Parameters to Monitor. Perform ultrasound of the gallbladder periodically during extended therapy. Obtain baseline and periodic total and/or free T_4 during long-term therapy. Monitor closely for hyper- or hypoglycemia, especially in diabetics. Periodically monitor vitamin B_{12} during long-term therapy. Evaluate cardiac function both at baseline and periodically during therapy, especially in acromegalics. Monitor serum concentrations of drugs whose absorption may be affected by octreotide (eg, cyclosporine). In acromegaly, evaluate GH or IGF-I concentrations q 6 months. However, symptomatic benefit (eg, relief of headaches, joint pain, excessive perspiration) may be greater than actual decreases in laboratory values.[193] In carcinoid, measurement of urinary 5-hydroxyindole acetic acid, serum serotonin, and serum substance P may be useful in monitoring the usefulness of octreotide therapy.

Notes. Octreotide has been investigated for a variety of conditions, including GH-secreting pituitary tumors; insulinomas; thyrotropinomas (dosage: 100–300 µg/day); hypotension caused by carcinoid crisis or autonomic neuropathy; Zollinger-Ellison syndrome; glucagonomas; diabetes mellitus; AIDS-related diarrhea (dosage: 150–1500 µg/day for 14 days based on stool volume); secretory diarrhea (dosage: 50–500 µg/day) due to ileostomy, short-bowel syndrome, intestinal graft-versus-host disease, radiation colitis, and intestinal fistulas; pancreatic or liver transplantation; colon cancer; dumping syndrome; psoriasis; resistant hypercalcemia; and intrathecally and intraventricularly for pain management.[192,193,198–200] Octreotide is reportedly ineffective in bleeding due to peptic ulcers, although this is controversial; however, it is effective in treating bleeding due to esophageal varices (dosage: 50 µg IV bolus then 50 µg/hr continuous infusion for 48 hours).[193,200] Octreotide's effectiveness in treating acute pancreatitis remains uncertain.[193] Octreotide is not compatible in PN solutions. Octreotide 200 µg/mL is stable for up to 60 days in polypropylene syringes under refrigeration and protected from light.[201]

SULFASALAZINE   Azulfidine, Various

Pharmacology. Sulfasalazine is a conjugate of sulfapyridine and mesalamine that is thought to be the primary active moiety. (*See* Mesalamine Preparations.)

Administration and Adult Dosage. **PO for short-term treatment of active mild to moderate ulcerative colitis or Crohn's disease** 4–6 g/day in equally divided doses; do not exceed an interval of 8 hr between nighttime and morning doses; administer after meals when feasible.[177,179,180] A lower initial dosage may decrease adverse GI effects. **PO for maintenance of remission of ulcerative colitis** 1–2 g/day in divided doses.[180] Dosages up to 12 g/day have been used; however, dosages >4 g/day are associated with an increased frequency of adverse effects. Low-dose therapy is not effective in maintaining remission in Crohn's disease.[177,179] **PO for desensitization of allergic patients** reinstitute sulfasalazine at a total daily dosage of 50–250 mg; thereafter, double the daily dosage q 4–7 days until the desired therapeutic effect is achieved. If symptoms of sensitivity recur, discontinue sulfasalazine. Do not attempt desensitization in patients who have a history of agranulocytosis or an anaphylactic reaction during previous sulfasalazine therapy. Consider **mesalamine** instead of desensitization in sulfasalazine-sensitive patients.

Special Populations. *Pediatric Dosage.* (<2 yr) contraindicated; (≥2 yr) **PO for short-term treatment of active mild to moderate ulcerative colitis or Crohn's disease** 40–60 mg/kg/day in 3–6 equally divided doses. Additional age-related information is available.[182] **PO for maintenance of remission of ulcerative colitis** 30 mg/kg/day in 4 equally divided doses.

Geriatric Dosage. No dosage reduction is necessary. However, older patients may have renal impairment.

Other Conditions. Consider dosage reduction in severe renal or hepatic impairment.[174]

Dosage Forms. **Tab** 500 mg; **EC Tab** 500 mg; **Susp** 50 mg/mL.

Patient Instructions. Take each dose after meals or with food, and drink at least 1 full glass of water with each dose; drink several additional glasses of water daily. This medication must be taken continually to be effective. It is often necessary to continue medication even when symptoms such as diarrhea and abdominal cramping have been controlled. Report any nausea, vomiting, abrupt change in character or volume of stools, or skin rashes. Sulfasalazine may cause an orange-yellow discoloration of the urine or skin. Reversible infertility may occur in males.

Missed Doses. If you miss a dose, take it as soon as possible. If it is almost time for your next dose, skip the missed dose and return to your usual dosage schedule. Do not double doses.

Pharmacokinetics. ***Onset and Duration.*** Maximum effect is in 1–2 weeks; duration is 10 ± 2 hr following an oral dose.[17]

Serum Levels. (Sulfapyridine) levels >50 mg/L (200 μmol/L) are associated with increased toxicity.[17] Therapeutic effect appears to be related to topical mesalamine levels in the bowel.[174,175,177]

Fate. Sulfasalazine is about 30% absorbed from the small intestine, but the absorbed drug is almost completely secreted unchanged in the bile. It is then metabolized in the large bowel, probably by intestinal bacteria, to **sulfapyridine** and mesalamine. Most of the sulfapyridine is absorbed from the bowel. Plasma protein binding: sulfasalazine (>99%); sulfapyridine (50%); mesalamine ($55 \pm 15\%$); N-acetylmesalamine (80%). Sulfapyridine is metabolized by the liver and excreted in the urine; slow acetylators have higher serum sulfapyridine concentrations. After an oral dose of sulfasalazine, about 91% of sulfapyridine is recovered in the urine in 3 days as sulfapyridine, its metabolites, and small amounts of sulfasalazine. Mesalamine is eliminated primarily in the feces; only a small portion is absorbed, metabolized, and excreted in the urine as N-acetylmesalamine.[17]

$t_{\frac{1}{2}}$. (Sulfapyridine) 9 ± 4 hr, depending on acetylator phenotype.[17] (*See also* Mesalamine Preparations.)

Adverse Reactions. Anorexia, nausea, vomiting, dyspepsia, and headache occur in about one-third of patients and are related to serum sulfapyridine concentrations. Leukopenia occurs frequently. Mild allergic reactions, including rash, pruritus, and fever, are common.[177] Rare toxic hypersensitivity reactions (caused by sulfapyridine) include neutropenia, agranulocytosis, hepatitis, pancreatitis, pericarditis, pneumonitis, peripheral neuropathy, and severe hemolytic anemia.[175,177,202] Sulfasalazine may cause an orange-yellow discoloration of the urine or skin and may precipitate acute attacks of porphyria. In men, sulfasalazine frequently leads to a reversible decrease in sperm count and abnormal sperm morphology and motility.[177]

Contraindications. Intestinal or urinary obstruction; porphyria; infants <2 yr; hypersensitivity to sulfasalazine, its metabolites, sulfonamides, or salicylates.

Precautions. Pregnancy, despite reports of safety; lactation. Use with caution in patients with renal or hepatic impairment, blood dyscrasias, slow acetylators, bronchial asthma, G-6-PD deficiency, or severe allergies.

Drug Interactions. Reduced metabolism of dietary folate has been reported in sulfasalazine-treated patients.[177] Consider folic acid supplementation in patients on long-term therapy. Decreased digoxin bioavailability has been reported when sulfasalazine is concurrently administered.

Parameters to Monitor. Monitor therapeutic response (decrease in degree and frequency of diarrhea, rectal bleeding, abdominal cramping) and adverse effects (headache, anorexia, dyspepsia, nausea, hypersensitivity reactions). Obtain baseline and periodic CBC, reticulocyte counts, and urinalysis. Monitor serum folate periodically in patients on long-term therapy.[17] Monitor serum digoxin levels during initiation and after discontinuation of sulfasalazine.

Notes. There appears to be no important therapeutic advantage of sulfasalazine over oral **mesalamine** when used to treat or maintain remission of ulcerative colitis; however, the higher sulfasalazine dosages used to treat active disease are associated with an increased frequency of adverse effects.[180,186] Crohn's disease patients with involvement of the ileum do not respond as well to sulfasalazine as those with only large bowel disease.[177,179] Combining sulfasalazine with an oral or rectal **corticosteroid** or with rectal mesalamine may be of benefit in patients with ulcerative colitis who do not respond to single-drug therapy.[180,187] In ulcerative colitis patients receiving maintenance therapy, there was less absorption and greater acetylation of 5-ASA with sulfasalazine or olsalazine than with mesalamine (Asacol).[203] Sulfasalazine has also been used to treat ankylosing spondylitis and rheumatoid arthritis.[186] Occasionally, the EC tablet may appear whole in the stool; if this occurs, switch the patient to the uncoated form. (*See also* Mesalamine Preparations.)

■ REFERENCES

1. Pinson JB, Weart CW. Antacid products, H₂-receptor antagonists, antireflux and anti-flatulence products. In, Covington TR et al., eds. *Handbook of nonprescription drugs.* 11th ed. Washington, DC: American Pharmaceutical Association; 1996.
2. Soll AH. Peptic ulcer and its complications. In, Feldman M et al., eds. *Sleisenger and Fordtran's gastrointestinal and liver disease: pathophysiology/diagnosis/management.* 6th ed. Philadelphia: WB Saunders; 1998:620–78.
3. Smythe MA, Zarowitz BJ. Changing perspectives of stress gastritis prophylaxis. *Ann Pharmacother* 1994;28:1073–85.
4. Lambert JR, Midolo P. The actions of bismuth in the treatment of *Helicobacter pylori* infection. *Aliment Pharmacol Ther* 1997;11(suppl 1):27–33.
5. Tillman LA et al. Review article: safety of bismuth in the treatment of gastrointestinal diseases. *Aliment Pharmacol Ther* 1996;10:459–67.
6. McColm AA et al. Ranitidine bismuth citrate: a novel anti-ulcer agent with different physiochemical characteristics and improved biological activity to a bismuth-citrate-ranitidine admixture. *Aliment Pharmacol Ther* 1996;10:241–50.
7. Feldman M, Burton ME. Histamine₂-receptor antagonists. Standard therapy for acid-peptic diseases (Part I). *N Engl J Med* 1990;323:1672–80.

8. Feldman M, Burton ME. Histamine$_2$-receptor antagonists. Standard therapy for acid-peptic diseases (Part II). *N Engl J Med* 1990;323:1749–55.

9. Lipsy RJ et al. Clinical review of histamine$_2$-receptor antagonists. *Arch Intern Med* 1990;150:745–51.

10. Navab F, Steingrub J. Stress ulcer: is routine prophylaxis necessary? *Am J Gastroenterol* 1995;90:708–12.

11. Amsden GW et al. Pharmacodynamics of bolus famotidine versus infused cimetidine, ranitidine, and famotidine. *J Clin Pharmacol* 1994;34:1191–8.

12. O'Keefe G, Maier RV. Current management of patients with stress ulceration. *Adv Surg* 1996;30:155–77.

13. Chhattriwalla Y et al. The use of cimetidine in the newborn. *Pediatrics* 1980;65:301–2.

14. Dimand RJ. Use of H$_2$-receptor antagonists in children. *DICP* 1990;24(suppl):S42–6.

15. Buck ML. Use of famotidine in infants and children. *Pediatr Pharmacother* 1998;4(2):1–6.

16. Gladziwa U, Klotz U. Pharmacokinetic optimisation of the treatment of peptic ulcer in patients with renal failure. *Clin Pharmacokinet* 1994;27:393–408.

17. Lauritsen K et al. Clinical pharmacokinetics of drugs used in the treatment of gastrointestinal disease (Part II). *Clin Pharmacokinet* 1990;19:94–125.

18. Wagner BKJ et al. Famotidine pharmacokinetics in patients undergoing cardiac surgery. *Drug Invest* 1994; 8:271–7.

19. Freston JW. Long-term acid control and proton pump inhibitors: interactions and safety issues in perspective. *Am J Gastroenterol* 1997;92(4 suppl):51S–57S.

20. Smallwood RA. Safety of acid suppressing drugs. *Dig Dis Sci* 1995;40(suppl):63S–80S.

21. Welage LS, Berardi RR. Drug interactions with antiulcer agents: considerations in the treatment of acid-peptic disease. *J Pharm Pract* 1994;7:177–95.

22. Bianchi Porro G et al. Double-blind, double-dummy endoscopic comparison of the mucosal protective effects of misoprostol vs ranitidine on naproxen-induced mucosal injury to the stomach and duodenum in rheumatic patients. *Am J Gastroenterol* 1997;92:663–7.

23. Yeomans ND et al. A comparison of omeprazole with ranitidine for ulcers associated with nonsteroidal anti-inflammatory drugs. *N Engl J Med* 1998;338:719–26.

24. Taha AS et al. Famotidine for the prevention of gastric and duodenal ulcers caused by nonsteroidal anti-inflammatory drugs. *N Engl J Med* 1996;334:1435–9.

25. Hudson N et al. Famotidine for healing and maintenance in nonsteroidal anti-inflammatory drug–associated gastroduodenal ulceration. *Gastroenterology* 1997;112:1817–22.

26. Wallace JL. Nonsteroidal anti-inflammatory drugs and gastroenteropathy; the second hundred years. *Gastroenterology* 1997;112:1000–16.

27. Berardi RR. Therapeutic approaches to gastroesophageal reflux disease. *J Pharm Care Pain & Sympt Control* 1998;6:37–63.

28. Burnakis TG. The histamine receptor antagonist cimetidine in the treatment of herpes zoster. *Hosp Pharm* 1997;32:1162–7.

29. Raskin JB et al. Misoprostol dosage in the prevention of nonsteroidal anti-inflammatory drug–induced gastric and duodenal ulcers: a comparison of three regimens. *Ann Intern Med* 1995;123:344–350.

30. Silverstein FE et al. Misoprostol reduces serious gastrointestinal complications in patients with rheumatoid arthritis receiving nonsteroidal anti-inflammatory drugs. *Ann Intern Med* 1995;123:241–9.

31. Philips AC et al. NSAIDs and the elderly: toxicity and economic implications. *Drugs Aging* 1997;10:119–30.

32. Koch M et al. Prevention of nonsteroidal anti-inflammatory drug–induced gastrointestinal mucosal injury; a meta-analysis of randomized controlled clinical trials. *Arch Intern Med* 1996;156:3421–32.

33. Hawkey CJ et al. Omeprazole compared with misoprostol for ulcers associated with nonsteroidal anti-inflammatory drugs. *N Engl J Med* 1998;338:727–34.

34. Isdale A, Wright V. Misoprostol/NSAID fixed combinations: help or hindrance in clinical practice? *Drug Safety* 1995;12:291–8.

35. Younossi ZM et al. Effect of combined anticoagulation and low-dose ASA treatment on upper gastrointestinal bleeding. *Dig Dis Sci* 1997;42:79–82.

36. Balaban DH et al. Nasogastric omeprazole: effects on gastric pH in critically ill patients. *Am J Gastroenterol* 1997;92:79–83.

37. Phillips JO et al. A prospective study of simplified omeprazole suspension for the prophylaxis of stress-related mucosal damage. *Crit Care Med* 1996;24:1793–800.

38. Blum RA. Lansoprazole and omeprazole in the treatment of acid peptic disorders. *Am J Health-Syst Pharm* 1996;53:1401–15.

39. Langtry HD, Wilde MI. Lansoprazole. *Drugs* 1997;54:473–500.

40. Zimmermann AE, Katona BG. Lansoprazole: a comprehensive review. *Pharmacotherapy* 1997;17:308–26.

41. Hirschowitz BI. Zollinger-Ellison syndrome: pathogenesis, diagnosis, and management. *Am J Gastroenterol* 1997;92(4 suppl):44S–50S.

42. Berardi RR, Welage LS. Proton pump inhibitors in acid-related disease. *Am J Health-Syst Pharm* 1998; 55: 2289–98.

43. Walters JK et al. The use of omeprazole in the pediatric population. *Ann Pharmacother* 1998;32:478–81.

44. Freston JW. Long-term acid control and proton pump inhibitors: interactions and safety issues in perspective. *Am J Gastroenterol* 1997;92(4 suppl):51S–7S.

45. Kuipers EJ et al. Atrophic gastritis and *Helicobacter pylori* infection in patients with reflux esophagitis treatment with omeprazole or fundoplication. *N Engl J Med* 1996;334:1018–22.

46. Kuipers EJ. *Helicobacter pylori* and the risk and management of associated diseases: gastritis, ulcer disease, atrophic gastritis, and gastric cancer. *Aliment Pharmacol Ther* 1997;11(suppl 1):71–88.

47. Andersson T. Pharmacokinetics, metabolism and interactions of acid pump inhibitors. Focus on omeprazole, lansoprazole, and pantoprazole. *Clin Pharmacokinet* 1996;31:9–28.

48. Collen D et al. Primary gastroduodenal prophylaxis with omeprazole for NSAID users. *Gastroenterology* 1996;110:A86. Abstract.

49. Mohiuddin MA et al. Effective gastric acid suppression after oral administration of enteric-coated omeprazole granules. *Dig Dis Sci* 1997;42:715–9.

50. Sharma VK et al. Nonencapsulated, intact omeprazole granules effectively suppress intragastric acidity when administered via a gastrostomy. *Am J Gastroenterol* 1997;92:848–51.

51. Zagari M et al. Proton pump inhibitors versus H2-receptor antagonists for the treatment of erosive gastroesophageal disease: a cost-comparative study. *Am J Manag Care* 1995;1:247–55.

52. Fitton A et al. Pantoprazole: a review of its pharmacological properties and therapeutic use in acid-related disorders. *Drugs* 1996;51:460–82.

53. Mossner J et al. One-year prophylactic efficacy and safety of pantoprazole in controlling gastroesophageal reflux symptoms in patients with healed reflux oesophagitis. *Ailment Pharmacol Ther* 1997;11:1087–92.

54. Bardhan KD et al. Pantoprazole-based 10 day triple therapy is effective in *Helicobacter pylori* eradication. *Aliment Pharmacol Ther* 1998;12:185–9.

55. Prakash A et al. Rabeprazole. *Drugs* 1998;55:261–7.

56. Cloud ML et al. Rabeprazole in the treatment of acid-peptic diseases: results of three placebo-controlled dose–response clinical trials in duodenal ulcer, gastric ulcer, and gastroesophageal reflux disease (GERD). *Dig Dis Sci* 1998;43:993–1000.

57. McCarthy DM. Sucralfate. *N Engl J Med* 1991;325:1017–25.

58. Jensen SL, Jensen PF. Role of sucralfate in peptic disease. *Dig Dis* 1992;10:153–61.

59. Ben-Menachem T et al. Prophylaxis for stress-related gastric hemorrhage in the medical intensive care unit. A randomized, controlled, single-blind study. *Ann Intern Med* 1994;121:568–75.

60. *USP-DI*, Vol. I. Rockville, MD. The United States Pharmacopoeal Convention, 1998.

61. Ben-Menachem T et al. Prophylaxis for stress-related gastrointestinal hemorrhage: a cost-effectiveness analysis. *Crit Care Med* 1996;24:338–45.

62. Cook DJ et al. Stress ulcer prophylaxis in critically ill patients; resolving discordant meta-analyses. *JAMA* 1996;275:308–14.

63. The Report of the Digestive Health Initiative International Update Conference on *Helicobacter pylori*. *Gastroenterology* 1997;113(suppl):S4–8.

64. Soll AH. Medical treatment of peptic ulcer disease: practice guidelines. *JAMA* 1996;275:622–9.

65. Graham KS et al. Variability with omeprazole-amoxicillin combinations for treatment of *Helicobacter pylori* infection. *Am J Gastroenterol* 1995;90:1415–7.

66. Markaham A, McTavish D. Clarithromycin and omeprazole: as *Helicobacter pylori* eradication therapy in patients with *H. pylori*–associated gastric disorders. *Drugs* 1996;51:161–78.

67. Al-Assi MT et al. Azithromycin triple therapy for *Helicobacter pylori* infection: azithromycin, tetracycline, and bismuth. *Am J Gastroenterol* 1995;90:403–5.

68. Pounder RE, Williams MP. The treatment of *Helicobacter pylori* infection. *Aliment Pharmacol Ther* 1997; 11(suppl 1):35–41.

69. Hunt RH. Peptic ulcer disease: defining the treatment strategies in the era of *Helicobacter pylori*. *Am J Gastroenterol* 1997;92(suppl):36S–43S.

70. Hopkins RJ. Current FDA-approved treatments for *Helicobacter pylori* and the FDA approval process. *Gastroenterology* 1997;113(suppl):S126–30.

71. Unge P. What other regimens are under investigation to treat *Helicobacter pylori* infection? *Gastroenterology* 1997;113(suppl):S131–48.

72. Laine L et al. Randomized comparison of differing periods of twice-a-day triple therapy for the eradication of *Helicobacter pylori*. *Aliment Pharmacol Ther* 1996;10:1029–33.

73. Peterson WL. The role of antisecretory drugs in the treatment of *Helicobacter pylori* infection. *Aliment Pharmacol Ther* 1997;11(suppl 1):21–5.

74. Mégraud F. Resistance of *Helicobacter pylori* to antibiotics. *Aliment Pharmacol Ther* 1997;11(suppl 1):43–53.

75. Fennerty MB. What are the treatment goals for *Helicobacter pylori* infection? *Gastroenterology* 1997;113 (suppl 6):S120–5.

76. Hackelsberger A, Malfertheiner P. A risk-benefit assessment of drugs used in the eradication of *Helicobacter pylori* infection. *Drug Safety* 1996;11:30–52.

77. Robinson DM et al. Guidelines for the treatment of *Helicobacter pylori* in the pediatric population. *Ann Pharmacother* 1997;31:1247–9.

78. Bodger K et al. Clinical economics review: *Helicobacter pylori*–associated peptic ulcer disease. *Aliment Pharmacol Ther* 1997;11:273–82.

79. Berardi RR. Peptic ulcer disease. In, DiPiro JT et al., eds. *Pharmacotherapy: a pathophysiologic approach.* 4th ed. Stamford, CT: Appleton & Lange; in press.

80. Kris MG et al. Dose-ranging evaluation of the serotonin antagonist dolasetron mesylate in patients receiving high-dose cisplatin. *J Clin Oncol* 1994;12:1045–9.

81. Hesketh P et al. Double-blind, randomized comparison of the antiemetic efficacy of intravenous dolasetron mesylate and intravenous ondansetron in the prevention of acute cisplatin-induced emesis in patients with cancer. *J Clin Oncol* 1996;14:2242–9.

82. Fauser AA et al. Therapeutic equivalence of single oral doses of dolasetron mesilate and multiple doses of ondansetron for the prevention of emesis after moderately emetogenic chemotherapy. *Eur J Cancer* 1996;32A: 1523–9.

83. Rubenstein EB et al. Randomized, double blind, dose-response trial across four oral doses of dolasetron for the prevention of acute emesis after moderately emetogenic chemotherapy. *Cancer* 1997;79:1216–24.

84. Poster DS et al. Δ^9-tetrahydrocannabinol in clinical oncology. *JAMA* 1981;245:2047–51.

85. Cocchetto DM et al. A critical review of the safety and antiemetic efficacy of delta-9-tetrahydrocannabinol. *Drug Intell Clin Pharm* 1981;15:867–75.

86. Voth EA, Schwartz RH. Medicinal applications of delta-9-tetrahydrocannabinol and marijuana. *Ann Intern Med* 1997;126:791–8.

87. Lemberger L et al. Delta-9-tetrahydrocannabinol. Temporal correlation of the psychologic effects and blood levels after various routes of administration. *N Engl J Med* 1972;286:685–8.

88. Hollister LE et al. Do plasma concentrations of Δ^9-tetrahydrocannabinol reflect the degree of intoxication? *J Clin Pharmacol* 1981;21(suppl 8–9):171S–7S.

89. Huestis MA et al. Characterization of the absorption phase of marijuana smoking. *Clin Pharmacol Ther* 1992;52:31–41.

90. Benet LZ et al. Design and optimization of dosage regimens; pharmacokinetic data. In, Hardman JG et al., eds. *Goodman and Gilman's the pharmacological basis of therapeutics.* 9th ed. New York: McGraw-Hill; 1996:1707–92.

91. Wall ME et al. Metabolism, disposition, and kinetics of delta-9-tetrahydrocannabinol in men and women. *Clin Pharmacol Ther* 1983;34:352–63.

92. Agurell S et al. Pharmacokinetics and metabolism of Δ^1-tetrahydrocannabinol and other cannabinoids with emphasis in man. *Pharmacol Rev* 1986;38:21–43.

93. Devine ML et al. Adverse reactions to delta-9-tetrahydrocannabinol given as an antiemetic in a multicenter study. *Clin Pharm* 1987;6:319–22.

94. Anon. Synthetic marijuana for nausea and vomiting due to cancer chemotherapy. *Med Lett Drugs Ther* 1985; 27:97–8.

95. Gralla RJ et al. Antiemetic therapy: a review of recent studies and a report of a random assignment trial comparing metoclopramide with delta-9-tetrahydrocannabinol. *Cancer Treat Rep* 1984;68:163–72.

96. Doblin RE, Kleiman MAR. Marijuana as antiemetic medicine: a survey of oncologists' experiences and attitudes. *J Clin Oncol* 1991;9:1314–9.

97. Colthup PV, Palmer JL. The determination in plasma and pharmacokinetics of ondansetron. *Eur J Cancer Clin Oncol* 1989;25(suppl 1):S71–4.

98. Adams VR, Valley AW. Granisetron: the second serotonin-receptor antagonist. *Ann Pharmacother* 1995;29:1240–51.

99. Beck TM et al. Stratified, randomized, double-blind comparison of intravenous ondansetron administered as a multiple-dose regimen versus two single-dose regimens in the prevention of cisplatin-induced nausea and vomiting. *J Clin Oncol* 1992;10:1969–75.

100. Freeman AJ et al. Selectivity of 5-HT$_3$ receptor antagonists and anti-emetic mechanisms of action. *Anticancer Drugs* 1992;3:79–85.

101. Brown GW et al. The effectiveness of a single intravenous dose of ondansetron. *Oncology* 1992;49:273–8.

102. Holdsworth MT et al. Assessment of chemotherapy-induced emesis and evaluation of a reduced-dose intravenous ondansetron regimen in pediatric outpatients with leukemia. *Ann Pharmacother* 1995;29:16–21.

103. Billett AL, Sallan SE. Antiemetics in children receiving cancer chemotherapy. *Support Care Cancer* 1994;2:279–85.

104. Foot ABM, Hayes C. Audit of guidelines for effective control of chemotherapy and radiotherapy induced emesis. *Arch Dis Child* 1994;71:475–80.

105. Watcha MF et al. The dose-response relationship of ondansetron in preventing postoperative emesis in pediatric patients undergoing ambulatory surgery. *Anesthesiology* 1995;82:47–52.

106. Rose JB et al. Preoperative oral ondansetron for pediatric tonsillectomy. *Anesth Analg* 1996;82:558–62.

107. Blackwell CP, Harding SM. The clinical pharmacology of ondansetron. *Eur J Cancer Clin Oncol* 1989;25(suppl 1):S21–4.

108. Hesketh PJ et al. GR 38032F (GR-C507/75): a novel compound effective in the prevention of acute cisplatin-induced emesis. *J Clin Oncol* 1989;7:700–5.

109. Grunberg SM et al. Dose ranging phase I study of the serotonin antagonist GR38032F for prevention of cisplatin-induced nausea and vomiting. *J Clin Oncol* 1989;7:1137–41.

110. Kataja V, de Bruijn KM. Hypersensitivity reactions associated with 5-hydroxytryptamine$_3$-receptor antagonists: a class effect? *Lancet* 1996;347:584–5.

111. Italian Group for Antiemetic Research. Persistence of efficacy of three antiemetic regimens and prognostic factors in patients undergoing moderately emetogenic chemotherapy. *J Clin Oncol* 1995;13:2417–26.

112. Chaffee BJ, Tankanow RM. Ondansetron—the first of a new class of antiemetic agents. *Clin Pharm* 1991;10:430–46.

113. Roila F. Control of acute cisplatin-induced emesis over repeat courses of chemotherapy. *Oncology* 1996;53(suppl 1):65–72.

114. Italian Group for Antiemetic Research. Ondansetron versus metoclopramide, both combined with dexamethasone, in the prevention of cisplatin-induced delayed emesis. *J Clin Oncol* 1997;15:124–30.

115. Grunberg SM et al. Randomized double-blind comparison of three dose levels of intravenous ondansetron in the prevention of cisplatin-induced emesis. *Cancer Chemother Pharmacol* 1993;32:268–72.

116. Vozeh S et al. Pharmacokinetic drug data. *Clin Pharmacokinet* 1988;15:254–82.

117. Zeltzer L et al. Paradoxical effects of prophylactic phenothiazine antiemetics in children receiving chemotherapy. *J Clin Oncol* 1984;2:930–6.

118. Covington TR et al., eds. *Handbook of nonprescription drugs.* 11th ed. Washington, DC: American Pharmaceutical Association; 1996.

119. Jinks MJ, Fuerst RH. Geriatric therapy. In, Koda-Kimble MA, Young LY, eds. *Applied therapeutics: the clinical use of drugs.* 5th ed. Vancouver, WA: Applied Therapeutics; 1992:7-1–19.

120. Anon. Laxative drug products for over-the-counter human use; tentative final monograph. *Fed Regist* 1985;50:2124–58.

121. Brunton LL. Agents affecting gastrointestinal water flux and motility; emesis and antiemetics; bile acids and pancreatic enzymes. In, Hardman JG et al., eds. *Goodman and Gilman's the pharmacological basis of therapeutics.* 9th ed. New York: McGraw-Hill; 1996:917–36.

122. Adams WJ et al. Bisacodyl reduces the volume of polyethylene glycol solution required for bowel preparation. *Dis Colon Rectum* 1994;37:229–33.

123. Hatlebakk JG, Berstad A. Pharmacokinetic optimisation in the treatment of gastroesophageal reflux disease. *Clin Pharmacokinet* 1996;31:386–406.

124. Wiseman LR, Faulds D. Cisapride. An updated review of its pharmacology and therapeutic efficacy as a prokinetic agent in gastrointestinal motility disorders. *Drugs* 1994;47:116–52.

125. Barone JA et al. Cisapride: a gastrointestinal prokinetic drug. *Ann Pharmacother* 1994;28:488–500.

126. Gladziwa U et al. Pharmacokinetics and pharmacodynamics of cisapride in patients undergoing hemodialysis. *Clin Pharmacol Ther* 1991;50:673–81.

127. Boyd IW, Rohan AP. Urinary disorders associated with cisapride. *Med J Aust* 1994;160:579–80.

128. Kahrilas PJ. Gastroesophageal reflux disease. *JAMA* 1996;276:983–8.

129. Karim A et al. Pharmacokinetics and metabolism of diphenoxylate in man. *Clin Pharmacol Ther* 1972;13:407–19.

130. Jackson LS, Stafford JE. The evaluation and application of a radioimmunoassay for the measurement of diphenoxylic acid, the major metabolite of diphenoxylate hydrochloride (Lomotil), in human plasma. *J Pharmacol Methods* 1987;18:189–97.

131. Gattuso JM, Kamm MA. Adverse effects of drugs used in the management of constipation and diarrhoea. *Drug Safety* 1994;10:47–65.

132. Wolfe MS. Acute diarrhea associated with travel. *Am J Med* 1990;88(suppl 6A):34–7.

133. DuPont HL. Travellers' diarrhoea. Which antimicrobial? *Drugs* 1993;45:910–7.

134. Anon. The safety of stool softeners. *Med Lett Drugs Ther* 1997;19:45–6.

135. Castle SC et al. Constipation prevention: empiric use of stool softeners questioned. *Geriatrics* 1991;46:84–6.

136. Crossley IR, Williams R. Progress in the treatment of chronic portasystemic encephalopathy. *Gut* 1984;25:85–98.

137. Kot TV, Pettit-Young NA. Lactulose in the management of constipation: a current review. *Ann Pharmacother* 1992;26:1277–82.

138. Anon. Lactulose (Chronulac) for constipation. *Med Lett Drugs Ther* 1980;22:2–4.

139. Lederle FA et al. Cost-effective treatment of constipation in the elderly: a randomized double-blind comparison of sorbitol and lactulose. *Am J Med* 1990;89:597–601.

140. Killinger JM et al. Human pharmacokinetics and comparative bioavailability of loperamide hydrochloride. *J Clin Pharmacol* 1979;19:211–8.

141. Ericcson CD, Johnson PC. Safety and efficacy of loperamide. *Am J Med* 1990;88(suppl 6A):10–4.

142. Rizzi CA et al. Regulation of plasma aldosterone levels by metoclopramide: a reappraisal of its mechanism from dopaminergic antagonism to serotonergic agonism. *Neuropharmacology* 1997;36:763–8.

143. Scarpignato C. Pharmacological stimulation of gastrointestinal motility: where we are and where are we going? *Dig Dis* 1997;15(suppl 1):112–36.

144. Anderson PO, Valdés V. Increasing breast milk supply. *Clin Pharm* 1993;12:479–80.

145. Lewis JH. Hiccups: reasons and remedies. In, Lewis JH, ed. *A pharmacologic approach to gastrointestinal disorders.* Baltimore: Williams & Wilkins; 1994:209–27.

146. Brown CK, Khanderia U. Use of metoclopramide, domperidone, and cisapride in the management of diabetic gastroparesis. *Clin Pharm* 1990;9:357–65.

147. Drenth JPH, Engels LGJB. Diabetic gastroparesis. A critical reappraisal of new treatment strategies. *Drugs* 1992;44:537–53.

148. Stewart RB et al. Metoclopramide: an analysis of inappropriate long-term use in the elderly. *Ann Pharmacother* 1992;26:977–9.

149. Barone J. Domperidone: mechanism of action and clinical use. *Hosp Pharm* 1998;33:191–7.

150. Weber FH, et al. Erythromycin: a motilin agonist and gastrointestinal prokinetic agent. *Am J Gastroenterol* 1993;88:485–90.

151. Lartey PA et al. New developments in macrolides: structures and antibacterial and prokinetic activities. *Adv Pharmacol* 1994;28:307–43.

152. DiPalma JA, Brady CE. Colon cleansing for diagnostic and surgical procedures: polyethylene glycol-electrolyte lavage solution. *Am J Gastroenterol* 1989;84:1008–16.

153. Goodale EP, Noble TA. Pediatric bowel evacuation with a polyethylene glycol and iso-osmolar electrolyte solution. *DICP* 1990;23:1008–9.

154. Fordtran JS et al. A low-sodium solution for gastrointestinal lavage. *Gastroenterology* 1990;98:11–6.

155. Tenenbein M. Whole bowel irrigation as a gastrointestinal decontamination procedure after acute poisoning. *Med Toxicol Adv Drug Exp* 1988;3:77–84.

156. Glore SR et al. Soluble fiber and serum lipids: a literature review. *J Am Diet Assoc* 1994;94:425–36.

157. Chan EK, Schroeder DJ. Psyllium in hypercholesterolemia. *Ann Pharmacother* 1995;29:625–6.

158. Tedesko FJ et al. Laxative use in constipation. *Am J Gastroenterol* 1985;80:303–9.

159. Freeman GL. Psyllium hypersensitivity. *Ann Allergy* 1994;73:490–2.

160. Cooney DO. *Activated charcoal in medical applications.* New York: Marcel Dekker; 1995.

161. Palatnick W, Tennenbein M. Activated charcoal in the treatment of drug overdose. *Drug Safety* 1992;7:3–7.

162. Paumgartner G et al. Ursodeoxycholic acid treatment of cholesterol gallstone disease. *Scand J Gastroenterol* 1994;29(suppl 204):27–31.

163. Strandvik B, Lindblad A. Cystic fibrosis. Is treatment with ursodeoxycholic acid of value? *Scand J Gastroenterol* 1994;29(suppl 204):65–7.

164. Krasman ML et al. Biliary tract disease in the aged. *Clin Geriatr Med* 1991;7:347–70.

165. Rubin RA et al. Ursodiol for hepatobiliary disorders. *Ann Intern Med* 1994;121:207–18.

166. Plaisier PW et al. Dissolution of gallstones. *Dig Dis* 1993;11:181–8.

167. Broughton G II. Chenodeoxycholate: the bile acid. The drug. A review. *Am J Med Sci* 1994;307:54–63.

168. Kaplan MM. Primary biliary cirrhosis. *N Engl J Med* 1996;335:1570–80.

169. Barnes D et al. A randomized clinical trial of ursodeoxycholic acid as adjuvant treatment to prevent liver transplant rejection. *Hepatology* 1997;26:853–7.

170. Clavien PA et al. Evidence that ursodeoxycholic acid prevents steroid-resistant rejection in adult liver transplantation. *Clin Transplant* 1996;10:658–62.

171. Neuberger J. Primary biliary cirrhosis. *Lancet* 1997;350:875–9.

172. Poupon RE et al. Combined analysis of randomized controlled trials of ursodeoxycholic acid in primary biliary cirrhosis. *Gastroenterology* 1997;113:884–90.

173. Mallett MS et al. Stability of ursodiol 25 mg/ml in an extemporaneously prepared oral liquid. *Am J Health-Syst Pharm* 1997;54:1401–4.

174. Small RE, Schraa CC. Chemistry, pharmacology, pharmacokinetics, and clinical applications of mesalamine for the treatment of inflammatory bowel disease. *Pharmacotherapy* 1994;14:385–98.

175. Goldenberg MM. Critical drug appraisal: mesalamine in the treatment of inflammatory bowel disease. *P & T* 1997;(October):498–510.

176. Bonapace CR, Mays DA. The effect of mesalamine and nicotine in the treatment of inflammatory bowel disease. *Ann Pharmacother* 1997;31:907–13.

177. Elton E, Hanauer SB. Review article: the medical management of Crohn's disease. *Aliment Pharmacol Ther* 1996;10:1–22.

178. Robinson M. Optimizing therapy for inflammatory bowel disease. *Am J Gastroenterol* 1997;92(suppl 12): 12S–7S.

179. Hanauer SB, Meyers S. Management of Crohn's disease in adults. *Am J Gastroenterol* 1997;92:559–66.

180. Kornbluth A, Sachar DB. Ulcerative colitis practice guidelines for adults. *Am J Gastroenterol* 1997; 92:204–11.

181. Bitton A, Peppercorn MA. Medical therapy of ulcerative proctitis and protosigmoiditis, including refractory disease. *Inflam Bowel Dis* 1995;1:207–19.

182. Winter H, Grand R. Medical therapy for children with inflammatory bowel disease. *Inflam Bowel Dis* 1996; 2:269–75.

183. D'Agata ID et al. Mesalamine in pediatric inflammatory bowel disease: a 10-year experience. *Inflam Bowel Dis* 1996;2:229–35.

184. Bell CM, Habal FM. Safety of topical 5-aminosalicylic acid in pregnancy. *Am J Gastroenterol* 1997;92: 2201–2.

185. Diav-citrin O et al. The safety of mesalamine in human pregnancy: a prospective controlled cohort study. *Gastroenterology* 1998;114:23–8.

186. Sutherland LR et al. Alternatives to sulfasalazine: a meta-analysis of 5-ASA in the treatment of ulcerative colitis. *Inflam Bowel Dis* 1997;3:65–78.

187. Kam L et al. A comparison of mesalamine suspension enema and oral sulfasalazine for treatment of active distal ulcerative colitis in adults. *Am J Gastroenterol* 1996;91:1338–42.

188. Camma C et al. Mesalamine in the maintenance treatment of Crohn's disease: a meta-analysis adjusted for confounding variables. *Gastroenterology* 1997;113:1465–73.

189. d'Albasio G et al. Combined therapy with 5-aminosalicylic acid tablets and enemas for maintaining remission in ulcerative colitis: a double-blind study. *Am J Gastroenterol* 1997;97:1143–7.

190. Irvine EJ. Quality of life issues in patients with inflammatory bowel disease. *Am J Gastroenterol* 1997;92 (12 suppl):18S–24S.

191. Green, JRB and the Abacus Investigator Group. Balsalazide is more effective and better tolerated than mesalamine in the treatment of acute ulcerative colitis. *Gastroenterology* 1998;114:15–22.

192. Mosdell KW, Visconti JA. Emerging indications for octreotide therapy (part 1). *Am J Hosp Pharm* 1994; 51:1184–92.

193. Lamberts SWJ et al. Octreotide. *N Engl J Med* 1996;334:246–54.

194. Tauber MT et al. Clinical use of the long acting somatostatin analogue octreotide in pediatrics. *Eur J Pediatr* 1994;153:304–10.

195. Barrons RW. Octreotide in hyperinsulinism. *Ann Pharmacother* 1997;31:239–41.

196. Colon AR. Drug therapy in pediatric gastrointestinal disease. In, Lewis JH, ed. *A pharmacologic approach to gastrointestinal disorders.* Baltimore: Williams & Wilkins; 1994:519–34.

197. Harris AG. Somatostatin and somatostatin analogues: pharmacokinetics and pharmacodynamic effects. *Gut* 1994;35(suppl 3):S1–4.

198. Mosdell KW, Visconti JA. Emerging indications for octreotide therapy (part 2). *Am J Hosp Pharm* 1994; 51:1317–30.

199. Cascinu S et al. Inhibition of tumor cell kinetics and serum insulin growth factor I levels by octreotide in colorectal cancer patients. *Gastroenterology* 1997;113:767–72.

200. Imperiale TF, Birgisson S. Somatostatin or octreotide compared with H_2 antagonists and placebo in the management of acute nonvariceal upper gastrointestinal hemorrhage: a meta-analysis. *Ann Intern Med* 1997;127: 1062–71.

201. Ripley RG et al. Stability of octreotide acetate in polypropylene syringes at 5 and 20°C. *Am J Health-Syst Pharm* 1995;52:1910–1.

202. Laasila K, Leirisalo-Repo M. Side effects of sulphasalazine in patients with rheumatic diseases or inflammatory bowel disease. *Scand J Rheumatol* 1994;23:338–400.

203. Stretch GL et al. 5-amino salicylic acid absorption and metabolism in ulcerative colitis patients receiving maintenance sulfphasalazine, olsalazine or mesalazine. *Aliment Pharmacol Ther* 1996;10:941–7.

Hematologic Drugs

Coagulants and Anticoagulants

ALTEPLASE
Activase

Pharmacology. Alteplase (recombinant tissue-type plasminogen activator [rt-PA]) is a 1-chain tissue plasminogen activator (fibrinolytic) produced by recombinant DNA technology. It has a high affinity for fibrin-bound plasminogen, allowing activation on the fibrin surface. Most plasmin formed remains bound to the fibrin clot, minimizing systemic effects.[1–3]

Administration and Adult Dosage. **Accelerated IV infusion for post-MI clot lysis** (preferred) 15 mg as a bolus, followed by 0.75 mg/kg (up to 50 mg) over 30 min, then 0.5 mg/kg (up to 35 mg) over the next 60 min. Start heparin infusion (to an aPTT of 1.5–2.0 times control) with or upon completion of the alteplase infusion and continue for at least 48 hr. (*See* Notes.) **Alternatively, IV infusion for post-MI clot lysis** 60 mg over 1 hr (6–10 mg in the first 1–2 min), then 20 mg/hr for 2 hr to a total of 100 mg (for patients <65 kg, administer a dose of 1.25 mg/kg over 3 hr). Begin as soon as possible after acute MI symptoms. Adjunctive heparin is also recommended.[2,4,5] **IV infusion for pulmonary embolism** 100 mg over 2 hr. Institute heparin infusion immediately following alteplase infusion when the aPTT or thrombin time returns to 2 times normal. Alternatively, 0.6 mg/kg as a single dose over 2 min in addition to heparin infusion has been used successfully.[6] **IV infusion for acute ischemic stroke** 0.9 mg/kg, to a maximum of 90 mg; give 10% initially as a bolus, with the remainder given over the next 60 min. Avoid anticoagulants or antiplatelet drugs for 24 hr after treatment.[7,8]

Special Populations. *Pediatric Dosage.* Safety and efficacy not established.

Geriatric Dosage. Same as adult dosage.

Dosage Forms. Inj 50, 100 mg.

Pharmacokinetics. *Onset and Duration.* Duration is several hours because of binding with fibrin. However, rethrombosis after reperfusion appears to be inversely proportional to serum half-life.[2]

Fate. There is rapid uptake by hepatocytes and fibrin binding. V_c is 3.8–6.6 L and $V_{d\beta}$ is 0.1 ± 0.01 L/kg; Cl is 0.6 ± 0.24 L/hr/kg.[2,9]

$t_{1/2}$. α phase 4.8 ± 2.4 min; β phase 26 ± 10 min.[9]

Adverse Reactions. Bleeding from GI and GU tracts and ecchymoses occur frequently. Retroperitoneal or gingival bleeding or epistaxis occur occasionally. Superficial bleeding from trauma sites may also occur. The overall risk of intracranial hemorrhage is 0.1–0.75%.[7] In ISIS-3 the rates for definite or possible cerebral bleed were as follows: rt-PA (**deuteplase,** a two-chain form of alteplase), 0.5%; **streptokinase,** 0.2%; **anistreplase,** 0.7%.[10] Independent risk factors for thrombolytic-induced intracranial hemorrhage with alteplase include age >65 yr, body weight <70 kg, and hypertension on hospitalization.[4]

Contraindications. Active internal bleeding; history of CVA; recent (within 2 months) intracranial or intraspinal surgery or trauma; intracranial neoplasm, AV malformation, or aneurysm; bleeding diathesis; severe uncontrolled hypertension.

Precautions. Use with caution in the following: pregnancy; recent (within 10 days) major surgery, trauma, GI or GU bleeding; cerebrovascular disease; systolic blood pressure of 180 mm Hg or above, diastolic of 110 mm Hg or above; high likelihood of left heart thrombus; acute pericarditis; subacute bacterial endocarditis; hemostatic defects; significant liver dysfunction; septic thrombophlebitis; age >75 yr; concurrent oral anticoagulants. Avoid IM injections and noncompressible arterial punctures; minimize arterial and venous punctures and excessive patient handling. Stop immediately if severe bleeding or anaphylactoid reaction occurs.

Drug Interactions. Preliminary data from a nonrandomized study suggest that concurrent IV nitroglycerin therapy may impair the thrombolytic effect of alteplase in acute MI.[11] Anticoagulants or antiplatelet drugs may increase the risk of bleeding.

Parameters to Monitor. For short-term thrombolytic therapy of MI, laboratory monitoring is of little value. No correlation has been made between clotting test results and likelihood of hemorrhage or efficacy.[2]

Notes. Other than cerebral hemorrhage, no clear differences in bleeding risk have been observed with the various thrombolytics.[2,4] Data from the ISIS-3 trial show the 5-week mortality for **duteplase, streptokinase,** and **anistreplase** to be virtually identical.[10] Based on the GUSTO trial, some investigators suggest that the accelerated alteplase regimen be used for patients <75 yr with anterior or large infarctions presenting within 4 hr of symptoms. The absolute survival advantage over streptokinase was 0.9%, representing a 14% risk reduction.[5,12] Double-bolus alteplase (50 mg IV over 1–3 min followed by 40–50 mg IV 30 min later) was compared to accelerated infusion alteplase in an attempt to shorten and simplify administration. However, the double-bolus method was associated with a slightly higher rate of intracranial hemorrhage and is not recommended.[13]

ANISTREPLASE   Eminase

Pharmacology. Anistreplase (anisoylated plasminogen-streptokinase activator complex [APSAC]) is an acylated form of the streptokinase-plasminogen complex that is temporarily inactive. After deacylation, the streptokinase-plasminogen complex promotes thrombolysis by converting plasminogen to the proteolytic enzyme plasmin. Thrombolysis occurs through the action of plasmin on fibrin.[4,7,9,14,15]

Adult Dosage. IV for post-MI clot lysis 30 units over 2–5 min as a single injection. Adjunctive IV heparin is associated with higher bleeding rates than aspirin alone in anistreplase-treated patients and offers no additional improvement in outcome.

Dosage Forms. Inj 30 units.

Pharmacokinetics. Deacylation and thrombolysis begin immediately after injection. Duration of fibrinolytic activity is 4–6 hr. Anistreplase undergoes deacylation and local inactivation in the circulation by inhibitor complex formation and proteolysis, and to a lesser extent is metabolized rapidly by the liver. V_d is 0.084 ± 0.027 L/kg, with a Cl of 0.055 ± 0.02 L/hr/kg and half-life of 1.2 ± 0.4 hr.

Adverse Reactions. Data from ISIS-3 indicate that bleeding was slightly more common with anistreplase than with streptokinase or rt-PA; however, major bleeding rates were similar. In ISIS-3 the rates for definite or possible cerebral bleeding were as follows: **anistreplase,** 0.7%; **streptokinase,** 0.2%; rt-PA (**duteplase,** a two-chain form of alteplase), 0.5%.[10] Allergic reactions similar to those reported with streptokinase include rash, erythema, bronchoconstriction, and, rarely, anaphylaxis. Precautions and monitoring parameters are the same as for streptokinase.

Notes. Ease of administration (30 units given over 2–5 min as a single IV injection) is a potential advantage of anistreplase for the emergent treatment of acute MI in some settings (eg, in the field). However, anistreplase is more expensive than streptokinase, has the same allergy profile, offers no efficacy advantage, and is potentially associated with a slightly higher bleeding risk.

CLOPIDOGREL BISULFATE   Plavix

Pharmacology. Clopidogrel is an antiplatelet agent that prevents platelet aggregation by direct inhibition of ADP binding to receptor sites and subsequent activation of the glycoprotein IIb/IIIa complex. This action is irreversible and consequently platelets exposed to clopidogrel are inhibited for their life span.

Adult Dosage. **PO for reduction of stroke, MI, or vascular death** 75 mg once daily.

Dosage Forms. **Tab** 75 mg.

Pharmacokinetics. Clopidogrel is rapidly absorbed; bioavailability is about 50%; 98% is bound to plasma proteins. The parent compound has no platelet-inhibiting activity and undergoes extensive hepatic metabolism to a carboxylic acid derivative (main metabolite) and an unidentified active metabolite. The half-life of the carboxylic acid metabolite is about 8 hr.

Adverse Reactions. The most frequent side effects are diarrhea in 4.5%, rash in 4.2%, GI hemorrhage in 2%, and GI ulcers in 0.7% of patients. Serious, but less frequent, side effects include intracranial hemorrhage in 0.4%, and severe neutropenia in 0.04%. The drug is contraindicated in active bleeding, such as in patients with peptic ulcer or intracranial hemorrhage. Use with caution in patients at increased risk of bleeding from trauma, surgery, or other conditions. Clopidogrel should be discontinued 7 days prior to elective surgery if an antiplatelet effect is not desired.

Drug Interactions. Use with caution in patients receiving anticoagulants, or drugs that inhibit platelet function, including NSAIDs.

Notes. The overall risk reduction for clopidogrel was 8.7% greater than **aspirin** in the CAPRIE study in patients at risk for an ischemic event.[16]

DALTEPARIN   Fragmin

Pharmacology. Dalteparin is a low-molecular-weight heparin (average mass 3000–8000 daltons) prepared by depolymerization and chromatographic purification of unfractionated porcine intestinal mucosa heparin. Other pharmacological properties are similar to enoxaparin.[17] (*See* Low-Molecular-Weight Heparins Comparison Chart.)

Adult Dosage. **SC for prevention of DVT and pulmonary embolus (PE) following abdominal surgery** 2500 IU 1–2 hr before surgery and once daily for 5–10 days. **SC for prevention of DVT and PE following abdominal surgery in high-risk patients (eg, with malignancy)** 2500 IU 1–2 hr before surgery, 2500 IU 12 hr later, then 5000 IU once daily for 5–10 days. **SC for prevention of DVT and PE following hip replacement surgery** 2500 IU 2 hr before and 12 hr after surgery and then 5000 IU once daily for 6–13 days.

Dosage Forms. **Inj** 2500 IU/0.2 mL, 5000 IU/0.2 mL; 95,000 IU.

Pharmacokinetics. Bioavailability following SC injection is about 87 ± 6%. Following SC doses V_d is 0.04–0.06 L/kg; following a single IV dose Cl is 0.025 ± 0.0054 L/hr/kg and the terminal half-life is 2.1 ± 0.3 hr; after SC administration the apparent half-life is 3–5 hr. Dalteparin is eliminated primarily by the kidney.

Adverse Reactions. Overall, rates of major and minor bleeding complications are similar to unfractionated **heparin.** Hematoma or pain at the injection site occurs frequently. Thrombocytopenia occurs in less than 1% of patients; however, dalteparin should be used with extreme caution in patients with a history of heparin-induced thrombocytopenia (in vitro platelet testing is recommended before considering use). Rash, fever, skin necrosis, and anaphylactoid reactions occur rarely. Contraindications, precautions, drug interactions, and monitoring parameters are the same as for enoxaparin.

ENOXAPARIN SODIUM   Lovenox

Pharmacology. Enoxaparin is a low-molecular-weight heparin (average mass 3500–5500 daltons) prepared by depolymerization of unfractionated porcine intestinal mucosa heparin. Like unfractionated **heparin,** enoxaparin binds with antithrombin III, accelerating the rate at which antithrombin III neutralizes several activated clotting factors. However, enoxaparin has many biological properties that differ from those of unfractionated heparin. Enoxaparin possesses a higher ratio of antifactor Xa to antifactor IIa activity, reduced interactions with platelets, and less lipoprotein lipase–releasing activity. It also has a lower affinity for platelet factor 4, von Willebrand factor (VIIIR), and vascular endothelium. At recommended dosages, single injections do not markedly affect platelet aggregation, prothrombin time, or aPTT.[18–23] (*See* Low-Molecular-Weight Heparins Comparison Chart.)

Administration and Adult Dosage. **SC for prevention of DVT and pulmonary embolus (PE) following hip or knee replacement surgery** 30 mg bid for 7–10 days started 12–24 hr postoperatively. **SC for prevention of DVT and PE following abdominal surgery** 40 mg once daily for 7–10 days started 2 hr prior to surgery.[18] **SC for active DVT treatment** 1 mg/kg q 12 hr initiated with warfarin therapy; continue for a minimum of 5 days and until a warfarin target INR of 2.0 is achieved on 2 consecutive days. **SC for unstable angina or non–Q-wave MI** 1 mg/kg q 12 hr results in a 16.2% risk reduction for the combined end point of death, MI, and recurrent angina at 14 days over therapy with a standard IV heparin infusion.[19] **SC for active PE treatment** 0.5–3.5 mg/kg/day in divided doses (usually 1 mg/kg bid), initiated with warfarin. Enoxaparin (and other low-molecular-weight heparins) may be safe and effective in the treatment of pulmonary embolus; however, confirmative studies are necessary before they can be routinely recommended as an alternative to standard heparin infusions.

Special Populations. *Pediatric Dosage.* **SC for treatment** (neonates) 1.6 mg/kg bid; (older infants and children) 1 mg/kg bid dosages have been used.

Geriatric Dosage. Elderly patients may have reduced elimination; use with caution in these patients.

Other Conditions. Elimination may be delayed in renal insufficiency; use with caution in these patients.

Dosage Forms. **Inj** 30 mg/0.3 mL, 40 mg/0.4 mL.

Pharmacokinetics. *Onset and Duration.* Peak antifactor Xa occurs 3–5 hr after SC injection and persists for about 12 hr following a 40 mg SC injection.

Fate. Mean absolute bioavailability following SC injection is about 92%. V_d is about 6 L and Cl is about 1.5 L/hr after IV administration. Some hepatic desulfation and depolymerization occurs, but most of the drug is eliminated renally.

$t_{1/2}$. The apparent half-life after SC administration is 4.5 hr.

Adverse Reactions. Overall, rates of major and minor bleeding complications in comparative studies with unfractionated heparin are similar. In clinical trials of enoxaparin in hip replacement surgery, major bleeding occurred in 4% of patients compared with 6% of unfractionated heparin-treated patients. Thrombocytopenia, fever, pain on injection, asymptomatic increases in transaminase levels, hypochromic anemia, and edema occur frequently. Skin necrosis occurs occasionally.

Contraindications. Hypersensitivity to heparin or pork-derived products; active major bleeding; thrombocytopenia associated with positive in vitro testing for antiplatelet antibody in the presence of a low-molecular-weight heparin.

Precautions. If epidural or spinal anesthesia or spinal puncture is employed, patients receiving low-molecular-weight heparins for prevention of thromboembolic complications are at risk for developing epidural or spinal hematoma which can result in permanent paralysis. The risk of these events may be higher when postoperative indwelling epidural catheters are used. Use with caution in patients with renal impairment.

Drug Interactions. Use with caution in patients receiving oral anticoagulants or drugs that inhibit platelet function, including NSAIDs.

Parameters to Monitor. Monitor CBC, including platelet count and stool for occult blood periodically; aPTT monitoring is not required.

LOW-MOLECULAR-WEIGHT HEPARINS COMPARISON CHART

DRUG	DOSAGE FORMS	ADULT DOSAGE	AVERAGE MASS (DALTONS)	AF-Xa[a] (IU/MG)	AF-Xa/AF-IIa[b] RATIO	HALF-LIFE (HR)
Ardeparin Normiflo	Inj 5000, 10,000 units.	SC for DVT prophylaxis 50 units/kg q 12 hr.	5500–6500	100	—	3.3
Dalteparin Fragmin	Inj 2500, 5000 IU/0.2 mL.	SC for DVT prophylaxis 2500–5000 IU/day SC for DVT treatment 120 IU/kg bid.	3000–8000	160	4:1	2.8–4
Danaparoid[c] Orgaran	Inj 750 units/ 0.6 mL.	SC for DVT prophylaxis 750 units bid SC for DVT treatment 2000 units q 12 hr.	6500	—	3.35:1	18.3
Enoxaparin Lovenox	Inj 30 mg/0.3 mL, 40 mg/0.4 mL.	SC for DVT prophylaxis 30 mg bid; SC post-abdominal surgery 40 mg/day SC for DVT treatment 1 mg/kg q 12 hr.	3500–5500	100	2.7:1	3.5–5.9

(continued)

DRUG	DOSAGE FORMS	ADULT DOSAGE	AVERAGE MASS (DALTONS)	AF-Xa[a] (IU/MG)	AF-Xa/AF-IIa[b] RATIO	HALF-LIFE (HR)
Nadroparin Fraxiparin (Investigational, Sanofi)	—	SC for DVT prophylaxis 4400 IU once daily SC for DVT treatment 90–92 IU/kg bid.	4500	85	3.2:1	2.3–5.6
Tinzaparin Innohep Logiparin (Investigational, Novo)	—	SC for DVT prophylaxis 50–75 IU/kg once daily SC for DVT treatment 175 IU/kg once daily.	4900	86	1.9:1	1.85

[a]Antifactor Xa activity.

[b]Antifactor Xa:antifactor IIa ratio. The ratio for unfractionated heparin is 1.

[c]A heparinoid; mixture of low-molecular-weight sulfated nonheparin glycosaminoglycans: heparan sulfate (84%), dermatan sulfate (12%), and chondroitin sulfate (4%).

From references 2, 17, 20, 22, 24, and 25.

HEPARIN SODIUM   Various

Pharmacology. A heterogeneous, unfractionated group of mucopolysaccharides derived from the mast cells of animal tissues. It binds with antithrombin III, accelerating the rate at which antithrombin III neutralizes *activated forms* of factors XII, XI, IX, X, VII, and II. It is active in vitro and in vivo.

Administration and Adult Dosage. Express dosage in units only; dosage must be individually titrated to desired effect (usually 1.5–2.5 times aPTT).[1,5,26] Weight-based nomogram and computer-assisted dosage of heparin are effective, safe, and superior to "standard care" or empiric approaches.[27–29] **IV for thrombophlebitis or pulmonary embolus (PE)** (continuous infusion) 50–100 units/kg initially, then 15–25 units/hr/kg; alternatively, 5000 units initially, then 1000 units/hr; (intermittent) 75–125 units/kg q 4 hr.[1,5,26,30] Duration of therapy for thrombophlebitis or PE is 7–10 days, followed by oral anticoagulation (preferably initiated during the first 24 hr of heparin therapy).[26,31] A 5-day course of heparin has been shown to be as effective as a 10-day course in treating deep vein thrombosis.[32] **SC for thrombophlebitis or PE** 10,000–20,000 units initially (preceded by a 5000-unit IV loading dose), then 8000–10,000 units q 8 hr or 15,000–20,000 units q 12 hr. **SC for prophylaxis of deep vein thrombosis (low-dose)** 5000 units 2 hr before surgery, repeated q 8–12 hr for 5–7 days or until patient is ambulatory.[33] **IV for heparin lock flush** inject sufficient solution (of 10 or 100 units/mL) into injection hub to fill the entire set after each heparin lock use. Some institutions reserve the 100 units/mL solution for flushing triple-lumen central catheters and use NS for all other catheters.

Special Populations. *Pediatric Dosage.* Same as adult dosage in units/kg.

Geriatric Dosage. Same as adult dosage.

Other Conditions. Patients with PE may require larger heparin doses than patients with thrombophlebitis.[30] (*See* Administration and Adult Dosage.) Patients with severe renal dysfunction may require lower dosages.[2] There is no good evidence that liver disease markedly affects dosage requirements.

Dosage Forms. Inj 1000, 2500, 5000, 7500, 10,000, 15,000, 20,000, 40,000 units/mL; 2, 40, 50, 100 units/mL (prediluted); **Heparin Lock Flush** 10, 100 units/mL.

Patient Instructions. This drug is potentially harmful when taken with nonprescription or prescription drugs. Consult your physician or pharmacist when considering the use of other medications, particularly aspirin-containing products.

Pharmacokinetics. *Onset and Duration.* Onset immediate after IV administration.

Serum Levels. The relationship between heparin serum concentrations and aPTT response may vary between reagents and reagent lots. It is recommended that each laboratory establish a therapeutic aPTT range corresponding to heparin serum concentrations of 0.2–0.4 unit/mL using protamine titration.[2] Circadian variation in heparin activity may occur, and aPTT response may vary during the day at a given infusion rate.[34]

Fate. SC bioavailability is 20–40% and is dose dependent.[2] There is no biotransformation in plasma or liver; transfer and storage in reticuloendothelial cells has been suggested.[26,35] V_d is 0.058 ± 0.011 L/kg (approximates plasma volume).[9] Cl is dose dependent; Cl may be increased in PE, but this has not been a consistent finding.[26]

$t_{\frac{1}{2}}$. (Pharmacologic) 90 ± 60 min, dose related; higher doses lead to increased half-life; half-life may be decreased in pulmonary embolus, but this has not been a consistent finding.[26,30,35,36] Shorter half-life is also reported in smokers than in nonsmokers.[2]

Adverse Reactions. Bleeding occurs in 3–20% of patients receiving short-term, high-dose therapy.[26,37] Bleeding risk is increased by 3-fold when the aPTT is 2.0–2.9 and by 8-fold when the aPTT is >3.0 times control.[26] Heparin administration by continuous IV infusion may cause a lower frequency of bleeding complications than intermittent IV administration.[26] Renal dysfunction, liver disease, and other factors (serious cardiac illness, malignancy, age >60 yr, and maximum aPTT greater than 2.2 times control) may increase bleeding risk.[2,35,37] (*See* Precautions.) Thrombocytopenia occurs frequently (usually 1–5%) and may be more common with heparin derived from bovine lung. (*See* Notes.) However, recent studies suggest little difference and an overall decline in prevalence.[26,38,39] The decline may be related to improved manufacturing techniques and reduced therapy duration.[38] Osteoporosis and bone fractures occur rarely with doses of 15,000 units/day or more for longer than 5 months.[26] Rarely patients receiving prolonged therapy or with diabetes or renal dysfunction may develop marked hyperkalemia.[40]

Contraindications. Active bleeding; thrombocytopenia; threatened abortion; subacute bacterial endocarditis; suspected intracranial hemorrhage; regional or lumbar block anesthesia; severe hypotension; shock; and after eye, brain, or spinal cord surgery.

Precautions. Risk factors for hemorrhage may include IM injections, trauma, recent surgery, age >60 yr, malignancy, peptic ulcer disease, potential bleeding sites, and acquired or congenital hemostatic defects.[26]

Drug Interactions. Anticoagulants or antiplatelet drugs including aspirin and other NSAIDs may increase risk of bleeding.

Parameters to Monitor. Baseline aPTT, PT/INR, hematocrit, and platelet count. Obtain aPTT (therapeutic range 1.5–2.5 times control) 3 or 4 times (or until therapeutic range is achieved) on day 1, and at least daily thereafter. Monitor platelets and hematocrit every other day and signs of bleeding (melena, hematuria, ecchymoses, hematemesis, epistaxis) daily.[1,5,26]

Notes. Heparin-induced thrombocytopenia is a potentially serious, and sometimes fatal, complication of heparin therapy. **Lepirudin** (Refludan) 0.4 mg/kg IV as a bolus followed by a 0.15 mg/kg/hr IV infusion for 2–10 days is approved for management of heparin-induced thrombocytopenia; it may reduce death, amputation, and other thromboembolic complications. Other agents including **danaparoid** (Orgaran), **ancrod** (Venacil, compassionate use-Knoll), **dextran**, and **argatroban** (Novastan, investigational—Mitsubishi Chemical) have also been used successfully in these patients.[41]

PHYTONADIONE   AquaMephyton, Konakion, Mephyton

Pharmacology. Vitamin K is a required cofactor for the hepatic microsomal enzyme system that carboxylates glutamyl residues in precursor proteins to γ-carboxyglutamyl residues. These proteins are present in vitamin K–dependent clotting factors (II, VII, IX, and X) and anticoagulation proteins (protein C and protein S), as well as bone (osteocalin), and some plasma proteins (protein Z), and the protein of several organs (kidney, lung, and testicular tissue).[42-44]

Administration and Adult Dosage. The normal daily nutritional requirement is about 0.03–1.5 μg/kg.[43,45,46] The adult RDA is 70 μg/day for men 19–24 yr and 80 μg/day for men >25 yr; it is 60 μg/day for women 19–24 yr and 65 μg/day for women >25 yr.[47] **PO, SC, or IM to reverse bleeding** (Konakion may only be given IM) 2.5–10 mg up to 25 mg initially. A single dose of 1–5 mg is usually sufficient to normalize PT during anticoagulant therapy, but in the presence of severe bleeding, 20–50 mg may be needed.[43,47] The initial dose may be repeated, based on PT and clinical response, after 12–48 hr if given PO and 6–8 hr if given parenterally. Use the smallest dosage possible to reverse anticoagulants, to obviate possible refractoriness to further anticoagulant therapy.[43,48] Do not give AquaMephyton intravenously unless it is absolutely essential, and do not exceed an infusion rate of 1 mg/min. The drug may be diluted in preservative-free dextrose or saline solution just prior to use. **PO for antenatal use in pregnant women receiving anticonvulsants** 20 mg/day throughout the last 4 weeks of pregnancy.[44]

Special Populations. *Pediatric Dosage.* RDAs are (<6 months) 5 μg/day; (6 months–1 yr) 10 μg/day; (1–3 yr) 15 μg/day; (4–6 yr) 20 μg/day; (7–10 yr) 30 μg/day; (11–14 yr) 45 μg/day; (15–18 yr) 55 μg/day for females, 65 μg/day for males.[47] **IM for prophylaxis of hemorrhagic disease of the newborn** 0.5–1 mg within 1 hr of birth. **SC or IM for treatment of hemorrhagic disease of the newborn** 1 mg; more if mother has been receiving an oral anticoagulant.

Geriatric Dosage. (>55 yr) the RDA is 65 μg/day for women and 80 μg/day for men.[47]

Dosage Forms. Tab (Mephyton) 5 mg; **Inj** (AquaMephyton, Konakion) 2, 10 mg/mL.

Pharmacokinectics. *Onset and Duration.* Reversal of anticoagulant effect is variable among individuals; parenteral onset is often within 6 hr; peak and duration is variable among individuals and with dose. A 5 mg IV dose usually returns PT to normal in 24–48 hr.[49] Large doses may cause prolonged refractoriness to oral anticoagulants.[43,48]

Fate. Absorbed from the GI tract via intestinal lymphatics only in the presence of bile; well absorbed after parenteral administration. Metabolized in the liver to hydroquinone form and epoxide form which are interconvertible with the quinone.[42] Little storage occurs in the body. In the absence of bile, hypoprothrombinemia develops over a period of several weeks.[43,48,50]

Adverse Reactions. The drug itself appears to be nontoxic; however, severe reactions (eg, flushing, dyspnea, chest pain) and occasionally deaths have occurred after IV administration of AquaMephyton, possibly caused by the emulsifying agents.[43,46,51] This product should rarely be used IV, and only when other routes of administration are not feasible. A transient flushing sensation, peculiar taste, and pain and swelling at the injection site may occur. Large parenteral doses in neonates have caused hyperbilirubinemia.

Contraindications. Konakion is contraindicated for other than IM use.

Precautions. Temporary refractoriness to oral anticoagulants may occur, especially with large doses of vitamin K. Reversal of anticoagulant activity may restore previous thromboembolic conditions. Either no effect or worsening of hypoprothrombinemia may occur in severe liver disease, and repeated doses are not warranted if response to the initial dose is unsatisfactory.[43,51]

Drug Interactions. Mineral oil and cholesterol-binding resins may impair phytonadione absorption.

Parameters to Monitor. Monitor PT before, and at intervals after, administration of the drug; the interval depends on the route of administration, the condition being treated, and the patient's status. (*See* Administration and Adult Dosage.)

Notes. Protect drug from the light at all times. Phytonadione reverses the effects of oral anticoagulant therapy, but has no antagonist activity against heparin.

RETEPLASE   Retavase

Pharmacology. Reteplase (recombinant plasminogen activator [r-PA]) is a nonglycosylated mutant of wild-type tissue plasminogen activator. In animals, this modification results in less high-affinity fibrin binding, longer half-life, and greater thrombolytic potency than **alteplase** (r-tPA).

Adult Dosage. **IV for post-MI clot lysis** two 10 IU boluses 30 min apart, with adjunctive IV heparin given as a 5000-unit bolus followed by 1000 units/hr (aPTT target 1.5–2.0 times control) for at least 24 hr.

Dosage Forms. **Inj** 10.8 IU.

Adverse Reactions. (*See* Alteplase.)

Notes. In the Reteplase Angiographic Phase II International Dose-finding study (RAPID) open-label MI trial, reteplase achieved more rapid, complete, and sustained thrombolysis than standard-dose rt-PA with comparable bleeding risk.[52] The RAPID trial did not, however, have sufficient power to detect differences in mortality between the groups. The GUSTO-III trial found reteplase equivalent to accelerated-infusion **alteplase** in MI for the combined end points of death or nonfatal, disabling stroke.[53] The International Joint Efficacy Comparison of Thrombolytics (INJECT) trial suggests that reteplase mortality rates are similar to those observed with streptokinase.[54]

STREPTOKINASE   Kabikinase, Streptase

Pharmacology. A bacterial protein derived from group C β-hemolytic streptococci. It acts indirectly, forming a streptokinase–plasminogen activator complex that activates other plasminogen, converting it to the proteolytic enzyme plasmin. Plasmin then hydrolyzes fibrin, fibrinogen, factors V, VIII, II, complement, and kallikreinogen.

Administration and Adult Dosage. IV for post-MI clot lysis 1.5 million IU over 60 min. **IV for pulmonary embolism, DVT, arterial thrombosis, or embolism** 250,000 IU over 30 min, followed by 100,000 IU/hr for 24–72 hr (72 hr if DVT suspected).[55] Institute heparin therapy. (*See* Notes and Parameters to Monitor.) **For arteriovenous cannula occlusion** slowly instill 250,000 IU in 2-mL solution into each occluded limb of cannula; clamp for 2 hr, aspirate contents, and flush with NS. **Selective intra-arterial infusion** (investigational) 5000 IU/hr for 5–48 hr.[56,57] (*See* Notes.)

Special Populations. *Pediatric Dosage.* Safety and efficacy not established.

Geriatric Dosage. Same as adult dosage.

Dosage Forms. Inj 250,000, 600,000, 750,000, 1.5 million IU.

Pharmacokinetics. *Onset and Duration.* Onset of fibrinolytic activity immediately following IV administration; duration 8–24 hr following discontinuation of the infusion.[58]

Fate. V_d is 0.08 ± 0.04 L/kg; Cl is 0.1 ± 0.04 L/hr/kg.[9] Clearance results, in part, from formation of an antigen-antibody complex that remains soluble and is rapidly removed.[2] Local inactivation in the circulation by inhibitor complex formation and proteolysis occurs. It is postulated that the reticuloendothelial system also contributes to clearance.[59]

$t_{1/2}$. α phase averages 18–23 min and is related to antigen-antibody formation; β phase averages 83 min and appears to be related to clearance by the reticuloendothelial system.[2,59]

Adverse Reactions. Surface bleeding complications occur frequently and are primarily related to invasive procedures (eg, venous cutdowns, arterial punctures, and sites of surgical intervention). Severe internal bleeding is reported occasionally; however, its prevalence is no greater than with other thrombolytics or standard anticoagulant therapy. Transient hypotension occurs occasionally. In ISIS-3 the rates for definite or possible cerebral bleeding were as follows: streptokinase, 0.2%; rt-PA (**duteplase,** a two-chain form of alteplase), 0.5%; **anistreplase,** 0.7%.[10] Occasional allergic reactions include fever, urticaria, itching, flushing, and musculoskeletal pain. Anaphylactoid reactions occur rarely with preparations now in use.[2,60]

Contraindications. (*See* Alteplase.)

Precautions. (*See* Alteplase.) Prior exposure to anistreplase or streptokinase within the last 12 months.

Drug Interactions. Anticoagulants or antiplatelet drugs may increase risk of bleeding.

Parameters to Monitor. For short-term thrombolytic therapy of MI, laboratory monitoring is of little value. For IV continuous infusion, monitor thrombin time, aPTT, or PT to detect activation of the fibrinolytic system, performed 3–4 hr after initiating therapy and q 12 hr throughout treatment.[60] No correlation has been made between clotting test results and likelihood of hemorrhage or efficacy; however, prolongation of the thrombin time to 2–5 times normal control value has been recommended.

Notes. In addition to post-MI clot lysis, streptokinase is recommended only for treatment of thrombosis involving the axillary-subclavian system or the popliteal vein or deep veins of the thigh and pelvis, and for patients in whom massive pulmonary emboli have caused obstruction of blood flow to one or more lung segments or when clinical shock is present.[60] The risk of stroke and intracranial bleeding appears to be less with streptokinase (by a difference of ≤0.5%) than with other thrombolytic agents.[61] Thrombolytic therapy may help prevent venous valvular damage and the development of venous or pulmonary hypertension.[62] The recommended fixed dosage schedule results in sufficient activation of plasminogen in 95% of patients.[63] However, consider using **alteplase** in those patients with exposure to streptokinase or anistreplase in the last 12 months.[4] The benefits of instituting anticoagulant therapy with heparin after completion of the thrombolytic infusion are not clear. However, it is recommended that heparin infusion (to an aPTT of 1.5–2.0 times control) be given only in the presence of high risk for systemic or venous thromboembolism (eg, anterior MI, CHF, previous embolus, atrial fibrillation). Heparin is initiated without a bolus 4 hr after the start of streptokinase infusion (or when aPTT is less than twice control) and continued for at least 48 hr.[4,7]

TICLOPIDINE   Ticlid

Pharmacology. Ticlopidine is an antiplatelet agent that inhibits most known stimuli (eg, ADP, collagen, epinephrine) for platelet aggregation. It prolongs bleeding time, normalizes shortened platelet survival, suppresses platelet growth factor release, and may block von Willebrand factor and fibrinogen interactions with platelets.[64–66]

Adult Dosage. PO for thrombotic stroke reduction in patients with stroke, or stroke precursors, patients with unstable angina, or those undergoing coronary artery bypass graft, or coronary angioplasty 250 mg bid.

Dosage Forms. Tab 250 mg.

Pharmacokinetics. The onset of clinical effect is delayed, with maximum efficacy being achieved in 3–8 days. Approximately 80% of the drug is absorbed orally, with peak serum concentrations occurring in about 2 hr. Ticlopidine undergoes extensive liver metabolism to possibly active metabolites, with only 2% excreted unchanged in urine. Half-life is 4–5 days with repeated dosage.

Adverse Reactions. Diarrhea and rash occurs frequently. Minor bleeding such as bruising, petechiae, epistaxis, and hematuria occurs occasionally. Severe neutropenia occurs in about 0.8% of patients and mild to moderate neutropenia in about 1.6% of patients during the first 3 months of therapy; neutropenia usually resolves within 3 weeks of discontinuation, although sepsis and death have been reported. Thrombocytopenia, thrombotic thrombcytopenic purpura (TTP), and cholestasis occur rarely.[66,67] Obtain CBC and differential counts q 2 weeks during the first 3 months of therapy; more frequent monitoring is recommended if the absolute neutrophil count is consistently declining or is less than 30% of the baseline value or if patients demonstrate signs and symptoms of TTP (weakness, pallor, petechiae or purpura), dark urine, jaundice, or neurologic changes.

Notes. The Ticlopidine Aspirin Stroke Study (TASS) trial found a 12% risk reduction in nonfatal stroke or cardiovascular death with ticlopidine compared to aspirin in high-risk (previous TIA or minor stroke) men and women. For secondary stroke prevention, the Canadian American Ticlopidine Study (CATS) trial found that the risk of stroke, MI, or cardiovascular death was reduced by 23% with ticlopidine over placebo. Ticlopidine has also been shown to markedly reduce MI, cardiovascular death, and ECG evidence of ischemia in patients with unstable angina.[68,69] Reserve ticlopidine for patients intolerant to aspirin. **Clopidogrel** (Plavix) is a safer alternative with similar efficacy that should replace ticlopidine.

UROKINASE   Abbokinase

Pharmacology. Urokinase is a proteolytic enzyme produced by renal parenchymal cells that acts to directly convert plasminogen to plasmin with effects similar to streptokinase.[2]

Adult Dosage. **IV for pulmonary emboli** 4400 IU/kg loading dose over 10 min, followed by 4400 IU/kg/hr for 12 hr. Heparin therapy is initiated without a loading dose after discontinuation of the thrombolytic when the thrombin time, or other coagulation test, no longer exceeds 2 times normal control. **Selective intracoronary infusion** 6000 IU/min for up to 2 hr. **IV for catheter clearance** attach a 1-mL tuberculin syringe filled with 5000 IU reconstituted solution (Open-Cath) and slowly inject an amount equal to the catheter volume; aspirate and repeat q 5 min as necessary. If not successful, allow urokinase to remain in the catheter for 30–60 min before attempting to aspirate. For central venous catheters whose function has not been restored by the bolus method, a 6- or 12-hr infusion of 40,000 IU/hr (5000 IU/mL at 8 mL/hr) in adults may be useful.[70]

Dosage Forms. **Inj** 5000, 9000, 250,000 IU.

Pharmacokinetics. The drug's half-life is about 10–20 min.

Adverse Reactions. Side effects, contraindications, and precautions are similar to streptokinase, although allergic reactions occur much less frequently.

WARFARIN SODIUM   Coumadin, Panwarfin, Various

Pharmacology. Warfarin prevents the conversion of vitamin K back to its active form from vitamin K epoxide. This impairs formation of the vitamin K–dependent clotting factors VII, IX, X, II (prothrombin) and proteins C and S (physiologic anticoagulants). The (S)-warfarin enantiomer is approximately 4-fold more potent an anticoagulant than (R)-warfarin.[2,71]

Administration and Adult Dosage. **PO or IV** 5–7.5 mg/day (range, 2–10 mg/day), titrating dosage to an INR of 2.0–3.0 for treatment or prophylaxis of venous thrombosis, pulmonary embolism, systemic embolism, tissue heart valves, valvular heart disease, atrial fibrillation (AF) (except patients <60 yr with "lone AF"), and recurrent systemic embolism. Adjust dosage to an INR of 2.5–3.5 for management of mechanical prosthetic valves (upper end of range for caged-ball, tilting-disk, and mitral position valves);[72] adding **aspirin** 100 mg/day offers additional protection, but increases the risk of mild bleeding.[4,26] For post-MI patients who are at increased risk of systemic or pulmonary embolism, maintain a warfarin dosage that achieves an INR of 2.5–3.5 for up to 3 months. Low-dose warfarin

(1 mg/day) without measurable changes in PT/INR begun 3 days before central venous catheter placement and continued while the catheter remains in place is recommended to reduce the risk of axillary-subclavian venous thrombosis.[5,73] (*See* Notes.)

Special Populations. *Pediatric Dosage.* (<18 yr) safety and efficacy not established. However, when used, dosage is titrated based on INR as in adult dosage.

Geriatric Dosage. Same as adult dosage. (*See also* Precautions.)

Other Conditions. Large variability in response requires that dosage be carefully individualized in all patients. Patients with liver disease, CHF, hyperthyroidism, or fever may be particularly sensitive to warfarin. Renal failure does not enhance the hypoprothrombinemic response to warfarin; however, these patients may have compromised hemostatic mechanisms that predispose to bleeding.[74]

Dosage Forms. **Tab** 1, 2, 2.5, 4, 5, 7.5, 10 mg.

Patient Instructions. This drug is potentially harmful when taken with nonprescription or prescription drugs. Consult your physician or pharmacist when considering the use of other medications, particularly aspirin-containing products.

Missed Doses. Take this drug at the same time each day. It is important that you try not to miss any doses. If you do miss a dose, take it as soon as you remember. If it is about time for the next dose, take that dose only. Do not double the dose or take extra.

Pharmacokinetics. *Onset and Duration.* Peak PT effect is in 36–72 hr;[75] at least 4–6 days of warfarin therapy are required before full therapeutic effect is achieved.[1,26] Duration after discontinuation depends on resynthesis of vitamin K–dependent clotting factors II, VII, IX, and X (which requires about 4–5 days).

Fate. Completely absorbed orally; well absorbed following small bowel resection;[76] 99 ± 1% is plasma protein bound.[9] V_d (racemic) is 0.14 ± 0.06 L/kg; Cl (racemic) is 0.0027 ± 0.0014 L/hr/kg.[9] It undergoes oxidative P450 enzyme biotransformation in the liver: (R)-warfarin, CYP1A2; (S)-warfarin, CYP2C subfamily,[77] producing warfarin alcohols, which have minor anticoagulant activity.[78,79] Less than 2% is excreted unchanged in urine.[9]

$t_{1/2}$. 37 ± 15 hr,[9,80] unchanged in acute hepatic disease.[81] Enantiomer half-lives: (R)-warfarin 43 ± 14 hr; (S)-warfarin 32 ± 12 hr.[9]

Adverse Reactions. Bleeding (major and minor) occurs frequently (6–29%); fatal or life-threatening hemorrhage has been reported in 1–8%. Risk factors for increased bleeding include PT ratio greater than 2.0, age >60 yr, and other co-morbid conditions. Rarely, skin necrosis (occurring early in therapy and involving the breast, buttocks, thigh, or penis), purple-toe syndrome (occurring after 3–8 weeks of therapy), and alopecia may occur.[1,26,37,82,83]

Contraindications. Pregnancy; threatened abortion; blood dyscrasias; bleeding tendencies; unsupervised patients with senility, alcoholism, psychosis, or lack of cooperation; anticipated spinal puncture procedure; regional or lumbar anesthesia.

Precautions. Avoid all IM injections because of the risk of hematoma. Several other factors may influence response: diet, travel, and environment. Monitor patients with liver disease, CHF, atrial fibrillation, hyperthyroidism, or fever especially carefully. The elderly have a higher risk of major trauma (eg, hip fractures) and physiologic changes in subcutaneous tissues and joint spaces, which may allow bleeding to expand unchecked.[83]

Drug Interactions. There are many important interactions that have potential clinical importance. Careful monitoring and appropriate dosage adjustment is recommended when any potential interacting drug is added or discontinued. Some agents commonly associated with increased warfarin effect include amiodarone, cimetidine, ciprofloxacin, clofibrate, erythromycin, fluconazole, fluvoxamine, lovastatin, metronidazole, quinidine, and trimethoprim-sulfamethoxazole. Some agents commonly associated with decreased warfarin effect include barbiturates, carbamazepine, cholestyramine, griseofulvin, and rifampin. (*See* references 84 and 85 for more comprehensive information regarding warfarin drug interactions.)

Parameters to Monitor. PT/INR daily while hospitalized, then weekly to monthly to monitor therapeutic effect; hematocrit; stool guaiac; urinalysis (for hematuria) for toxicity. Also observe for ecchymoses, hemoptysis, and epistaxis.

Notes. Loading dose has no therapeutic advantage and may be unsafe because of excessive depression of factor VII.[26] Predictive techniques using small loading doses (eg, 10 mg/day for 2–3 days) were developed using a therapeutic range target much higher than current recommendations. With the current narrow and lower therapeutic target, the predictive error of these techniques may be unacceptable.[26] **Phytonadione** begins to restore the PT toward normal within 4–8 hr, although large doses may induce a subsequent resistance to anticoagulant effect lasting one or more weeks.[86] A small oral dose (eg, 2.5 mg) or small slow IV injection (0.5–1 mg) of phytonadione may be used to bring an elevated PT/INR back into target range without resulting resistance.[4] Treat the first episode of venous thrombosis for 6 weeks in patients with reversible risk factors and 6 months in others. Consider continuing warfarin for an indefinite period in patients with active cancer or recurrent venous thrombosis.[87]

Hematopoietics

EPOETIN ALFA   Epogen, Procrit

Pharmacology. Epoetin alfa (erythropoietin [EPO]) is a recombinant human glycoprotein produced from mammalian cells that stimulates RBC production. The product contains the identical amino acid sequence and produces the same biologic effects as natural erythropoietin.[88–91]

Administration and Adult Dosage. **IV or SC for dialysis or nondialysis chronic renal failure patients** 50–100 units/kg 3 times/week initially, increased or decreased by 25 units/kg to maintain a target hematocrit of 30–36%. When the target hematocrit is reached (or when there is an increase >4 points in any 2-week period), reduce the dosage to 25 units/kg 3 times/week. If at any time the hematocrit exceeds 36%, discontinue epoetin until the target hematocrit is achieved and then resume at a lower dosage. Individualize the maintenance dosage to maintain the target hematocrit. **IV or SC for zidovudine-treated or HIV-infected patients** 100 units/kg 3 times/week for 8 weeks initially, increased or decreased by 50–100 units/kg based on response; maximum effective dosage is 300 units/kg 3 times/week. If hematocrit exceeds 40%, discontinue epoetin until the hematocrit returns to 36%, then reduce dosage by 25%; adjust dosage to maintain desired hematocrit target. Patients with initial erythropoietin levels >500 units/L are unlikely to respond to epoetin. **SC for chemotherapy-treated cancer patients** 150 units/kg 3 times/week for 8 weeks initially, increasing to 300 units/kg 3 times/week if there is an unsatisfactory reduction in transfusion requirement or an unsatisfactory increase in hematocrit. If hematocrit exceeds 40%, discontinue epoetin until the hematocrit returns to 36%, then reduce dosage by 25%; adjust dosage to maintain desired hematocrit target.

Special Populations. *Pediatric Dosage.* Safety and efficacy not established. **SC for anemia of prematurity** (preterm neonates) 200 units (140 units/kg) every other day for 10 doses;[92] alternatively, 250 units/kg 3 times/week.[91] **SC or IV for anemia of end-stage renal disease** (newborn–18 yr) 50 units/kg 3 times/week has been used.[93,94]

Geriatric Dosage. Same as adult dosage.

Dosage Forms. Inj 2000, 3000, 4000, 10,000 units/mL.

Pharmacokinetics. *Onset and Duration.* In response to administration 3 times/week, reticulocyte count increases within 10 days followed by increases in RBC count, hematocrit, and hemoglobin in about 2–6 weeks.

Fate. Not orally bioavailable. Peak serum levels occur 5–24 hr after SC administration. V_d is 0.033–0.055 L/kg; Cl is about 0.00282 L/hr/kg.[88]

$t_{1/2}$. 9.3 ± 3.3 hr initially; 6.2 ± 1.8 hr during long-term therapy.[88]

Adverse Reactions. Hypertension, headache, tachycardia, nausea, vomiting, clotted vascular access, shortness of breath, hyperkalemia, and diarrhea occur frequently. Occasionally seizures and rarely CVA, TIA, or MI occur.[88–91]

Contraindications. Uncontrolled hypertension. Hypersensitivity to mammalian cell-derived products or albumin.

Precautions. Pregnancy. Use cautiously with a known history of seizure or underlying hematologic disease including sickle cell anemia, myelodysplastic syndromes, or hypercoagulable states.

Drug Interactions. None known.

Parameters to Monitor. Evaluate iron stores prior to and during therapy. Supplemental iron may be required to maintain a transferrin saturation of at least 20% and ferritin levels of at least 100 μg/L. Determine hematocrit twice a week for 2–6 weeks or until stabilized in the target range; monitor at regular intervals thereafter. Monitor CBC with differential, platelet count, BUN, Cr_s, serum uric acid, serum phosphorus, and serum potassium at regular intervals.

FERROUS SALTS
Various

Pharmacology. Ferrous salts are soluble forms of iron, an essential nutrient that functions primarily as the oxygen-binding core of heme in RBCs (as hemoglobin), muscles (as myoglobin), and in the respiratory enzyme cytochrome C.

Administration and Adult Dosage. **PO as a dietary supplement** RDA for adult males is 10 mg/day, and for adult females (19–51 yr) is 15 mg/day.[47] **PO for treatment of iron deficiency** 2–3 mg/kg/day of elemental iron in divided doses. (*See* Ferrous Salts Comparison Chart for usual dosage ranges for individual salts.) Dose-related adverse effects may be decreased by using suboptimal dosages, by increasing the daily dosage gradually, or by administering with a small amount of food (although this latter method reduces absorption). After hemoglobin is normalized, continue oral therapy for 3–6 months to replenish iron stores.

Special Populations. *Pediatric Dosage.* **PO for prophylaxis** RDA (infants) 6 mg/day; (1–10 yr) 10 mg/day; (11–18 yr, males) 12 mg/day; (11–18 yr, females) 15 mg/day.[47] **PO for treatment** (infants) 10–25 mg of elemental iron in 3–4 divided doses; (6 months–2 yr) up to 6 mg/kg/day of elemental iron in 3–4 divided doses; (2–12 yr) 3 mg/kg/day of elemental iron in 3–4 divided doses.

Geriatric Dosage. Same as adult dosage, except dosage in women >51 yr is 10 mg/day of elemental iron.

Other Conditions. Iron requirement during pregnancy is approximately twice that of the normal, nonpregnant woman because of an expanding blood volume and the demands of the fetus and placenta. The RDA in pregnancy is 30 mg/day, and a prophylactic dose of 15–30 mg/day of elemental iron during the second and third trimesters has been recommended to prevent depletion of maternal iron stores. Iron-deficient patients may need higher doses.

Dosage Forms. (*See* Ferrous Salts Comparison Chart.)

Patient Instructions. Take this drug with a full glass of water on an empty stomach (1 hour before or 2 hours after meals) for best absorption. Take liquid preparations in water or juice, and drink with a straw to minimize tooth staining. If gastric distress or nausea occurs, a small quantity of food may be taken with the drug, but do not take with antacids because absorption is decreased. Iron preparations may cause constipation and black stools. Keep all iron products out of the reach of children.

Missed Doses. Take this drug at regular intervals. If you miss a dose, take it as soon as you remember. If it is about time for the next dose, take that dose only. Do not double the dose or take extra.

Pharmacokinetics. *Onset and Duration.* Response to equivalent amounts of oral or parenteral therapy is essentially the same. Reticulocytes increase within 4–7 days and reach a peak about the tenth day. An increase in hemoglobin of 2 g/dL or more and a 6% increase in hematocrit should occur in about 3–4 weeks. Three to 6 months of therapy are generally required for restoration of iron stores.[95,96]

Serum Levels. Normal is 65–170 μg/dL (12–30 μmol/L) in adult males, 50–170 μg/dL (9–30 μmol/L) in adult females, and 50–120 μg/dL (9–21 μmol/L) in children. A decrease in the transferrin saturation (serum iron ÷ total iron–binding capacity × 100) is an indication of preanemic iron deficiency. A transferrin saturation <16% or plasma ferritin concentration <12 μg/L indicates probable iron deficiency.[95,96] In overdosage, toxicity may occur at iron levels >350 μg/dL (63 μmol/L). Chelation therapy is indicated at these levels, especially if the patient is symptomatic.[95]

Fate. Iron is absorbed primarily from the duodenum at a rate dependent on the amount of iron in storage sites. About 10% of dietary iron is absorbed in normal subjects, 20% in iron-deficient patients, and as much as 70% of medicinal iron is absorbed during marked iron deficiency or increased erythropoiesis. In the plasma, iron is oxidized to the ferric state, combined with transferrin, and either used or stored as ferritin (mostly in the reticuloendothelial system and hepatocytes). The average loss in the healthy adult male is about 1 mg/day. GI loss of extravasated red cells, iron in bile, and exfoliated mucosal cells accounts for two-thirds of this iron. The other one-third is lost in the skin and urine. Menstruating women have an additional loss of about 0.5 mg/day.

Adverse Reactions. Side effects are primarily related to the dose of elemental iron. Frequent GI irritation, constipation, and stained teeth (liquid preparations only—dilute and use a drinking straw). An increased risk of cancer associated with excessive iron stores has been reported.[97]

Contraindications. Hemochromatosis; hemosiderosis; hemolytic anemias in which no true iron deficiency exists.

Precautions. Use with caution in patients with peptic ulcer, regional enteritis, or ulcerative colitis. Serious acute poisoning (which can be fatal) occurs frequently in children: doses as low as 20 mg/kg of elemental iron can cause toxicity; 40 mg/kg is considered serious; and greater than 60 mg/kg is potentially lethal.[98]

Drug Interactions. Food, calcium carbonate, sodium bicarbonate, and possibly magnesium trisilicate can reduce iron absorption. Vitamin E can reduce utilization of iron in iron deficiency anemia. Iron salts can reduce oral absorption of carbidopa/levodopa, methyldopa, penicillamine, quinolones, tetracyclines, and thyroid hormones.

Parameters to Monitor. Periodic reticulocyte count, hemoglobin, and hematocrit. (*See* Onset and Duration.)

Notes. Ferrous salts are used in prevention and treatment of iron deficiency anemias. Such anemias occur most frequently with exceptional blood losses (eg, pathologic bleeding, menstruation) and during periods of rapid growth (eg, infancy, adolescence, pregnancy). Iron is ineffective in hemoglobin disturbances not caused by iron deficiency. Concurrent administration of high doses of **vitamin C** may enhance absorption (particularly when given with SR formulations), but cost/benefit may not warrant its use. Wide variation in dissolution and absorption exists among SR and EC products, and the frequency of adverse effects, although negligible, probably reflects the small amount of ionic iron available for absorption because of transport of the iron past the duodenum and proximal jejunum.[99]

FERROUS SALTS COMPARISON CHART

DRUG	SOLID DOSAGE FORMS[a]	ADULT DOSAGE (CAP OR TAB/DAY)	ELEMENTAL IRON/CAP OR TAB (%)	(mg Fe)	OTHER DOSAGE FORMS[a]
Carbonyl Iron	Cap 50 mg iron.	3	100	50	
Ferrous Fumarate	Chew Tab 100 mg	1–4	33	33	Drp 75 mg/mL
	Tab 63, 200, 324, 325, 350 mg.	1–4	33	20, 66	Susp 20 mg/mL.
		1–2	33	106, 106, 115	
Ferrous Gluconate	Tab 240, 325 mg.	3–6	11	27, 36	Elxr 60 mg/mL.
Ferrous Sulfate Exsiccated	SR Tab 160 mg	1–2	30	50	
	Tab 187, 200 mg.	3–4	30	60, 65	
Ferrous Sulfate Hydrous	SR Cap/Tab various	—	20	—	Drp 125 mg/mL
	Cap 250 mg	3	20	50	Elxr 44 mg/mL
	Tab 195, 300, 324 mg.	3–6	20	39	Syrup 18 mg/mL.
		3	20	60, 65	
Polysaccharide-Iron Complex	Cap 150 mg iron	1–2	—	150	Elxr 20 mg/mL iron.
	Tab 50 mg iron.	2–4	—	50	

[a]Doses listed represent total iron salt, not elemental iron, except for carbonyl iron and polysaccharide-iron complex.

FILGRASTIM
Neupogen

Pharmacology. Filgrastim is an *Escherichia coli*–derived (nonglycosylated) recombinant human granulocyte colony–stimulating factor (G-CSF). G-CSF is one of many glycoprotein hormones that regulate the proliferation and differentiation of hematopoietic progenitor cells and the function of mature blood cells. Specifically, G-CSF promotes proliferation and maturation, and enhances the function and migration of neutrophil granulocytes. G-CSF also promotes pre–B-cell activation and growth, and acts in synergy with interleukin-3 to support megakaryocyte and platelet production.[89,100]

Administration and Adult Dosage. **SC or IV for myelosuppressive cancer chemotherapy** 5 μg/kg/day as a single injection. The drug is usually discontinued once the post-nadir ANC reaches 1500–2000/μL. Based on severity of ANC nadir, dosage may be increased in 5 μg/kg/day increments for each chemotherapy cycle. **SC continuous infusion for chemotherapy-induced febrile neutropenia** 12 μg/kg/day beginning within 12 hr of empiric antibiotic therapy and continued until neutrophil count is greater than 5000/μL and the patient is afebrile for 4 days.[101] **IV or SC for bone marrow transplant patients** 10 μg/kg/day infused IV over 4 or 24 hr or as a continuous SC infusion, decreasing to 5 μg/kg/day when ANC is greater than 1000/μL for 3 consecutive days. Discontinue therapy if the ANC remains >1000/μL for 3 more consecutive days; resume at a dosage of 5 μg/kg/day when ANC becomes less than 1000/μL. **SC for severe chronic neutropenia** (congenital) 6 μg/kg bid; (idiopathic or cyclic) 5 μg/kg/day. Target ANC range is 1500–10,000/μL; decrease dosage if ANC is persistently >10,000/μL. **SC with erythropoietin to decrease hematologic toxicity from zidovudine** 3.6 μg/kg/day initially, increasing or decreasing weekly by 1 μg/kg/day to maintain a target ANC of 1500–5000/μL.[102]

Special Populations. *Pediatric Dosage.* Safety and efficacy not established. **IV or SC** adult dosages in μg/kg are well tolerated.

Geriatric Dosage. Same as adult dosage.

Dosage Forms. Inj 300 μg/mL.

Patient Instructions. Your pharmacist or physician should instruct you on proper dosage, administration, and disposal. Store vials in the refrigerator, but do not freeze. Vials are designed for single use only; discard any unused portion. Bring vial to room temperature before administration; do not shake.

Pharmacokinetics. *Onset and Duration.* Increase in neutrophilic band forms occurs within about 60 min following administration. With discontinuation of therapy, neutrophil counts return to baseline values in about 4 days.[100]

Fate. Not orally bioavailable. V_d is about 0.15 L/kg; Cl is 0.03–0.042 L/hr/kg.

$t_{1/2}$. 3.5–3.85 hr.

Adverse Reactions. Mild to moderate bone pain responsive to nonnarcotic analgesics is reported frequently. Transient decreases in blood pressure occur occasionally. During long-term therapy, splenomegaly occurs frequently; occasional exacerbation of skin disorders, alopecia, hematuria, proteinuria, thrombocytopenia, and osteoporosis were also reported. Other adverse effects occur during administration of filgrastim that are likely the consequence of the underlying malignancy or cytotoxic chemotherapy. Acute reactions to sargramostim (eg, febrile episodes, flushing, hypotension, tachycardia, and hypoxia) appear to be more common than with filgrastim.[89,100,102,103]

Contraindications. History of hypersensitivity to *E. coli*–derived proteins. Do not use within the period of 24 hr before and 24 hr after administration of cytotoxic chemotherapy.

Precautions. Use with caution in any malignancy with myeloid characteristics because of the possibility of tumor growth. The efficacy of filgrastim has not been established in patients receiving nitrosoureas, mitomycin, fluorouracil, or cytarabine.

Drug Interactions. None known.

Parameters to Monitor. Perform a CBC and platelet count prior to chemotherapy and twice a week during filgrastim therapy. Regular monitoring of WBC counts at the time of recovery from the postchemotherapy nadir is recommended to avoid excessive leukocytosis.

Notes. Other potential uses for filgrastim include AIDS-related neutropenia, myelodysplastic syndromes, and drug-induced neutropenia or aplastic anemia. Further clinical trials are needed to prove that use for these and other indications is beneficial, safe, and cost effective.

IRON DEXTRAN   DexFerrum, InFeD, Various

Pharmacology. (*See* Ferrous Salts.) The overall response to parenteral iron is no more rapid or complete than the response to orally administered iron, so iron dextran is indicated only when oral iron therapy is determined to be ineffective or impossible.

Administration and Adult Dosage. The total cumulative amount required for restoration of hemoglobin (Hb) in g/dL and body stores of iron can be approximated using lean body weight (LBW) in kg (or actual body weight if less than LBW) from the formula:

$$\text{Total mg Iron} = [0.0442 \times (\text{Desired Hb} - \text{Observed Hb}) \times \text{LBW} + (0.26 \times \text{LBW})] \times 50$$

To calculate dose in mL, divide the result by 50. Usual Hb target for adults is 14.8 g/dL. The dose of iron required secondary to blood loss can be estimated from the formula:

$$\text{Total mg Iron} = \text{Blood Loss (mL)} \times \text{Hematocrit (observed, as decimal fraction)}$$

Deep IM (in upper outer quadrant of buttock only, using Z-track technique) 25 mg (0.5-mL) test dose the first day, then, if no adverse reaction occurs, administer a maximum daily dose of 100 mg (2 mL) until the total calculated amount is reached. **Slow IV** test dose of 25 mg (0.5 mL) over at least 30 sec the first day; if no adverse reaction occurs after a minimum of 1 hr, proceed (until the total calculated amount is reached) by daily increments over 2–3 days, to a maximum dose of 100 mg/day at a rate not to exceed 50 mg/min.[102] **IV in erythropoietin-treated dialysis patients** 100–200 mg/week after dialysis. **Total dose IV infusion** is an off-label use and is discouraged by the FDA, but is widely used. The total calculated dose of iron dextran is diluted in 500 mL of NS (dextrose solutions cause increased local phlebitis) and infused at a rate of 6 mg/min after a 30 mL test dose is delivered over 2 min.[104]

Special Populations. *Pediatric Dosage.* (<4 months) safety and efficacy not established; (5–15 kg) total cumulative amount required for restoration of Hb (in g/dL) and body stores of iron can be estimated using body weight (W) in kg from the formula:

$$\text{Total mg Iron} = [0.0442 \times (\text{Desired Hb} - \text{Observed Hb}) \times W + (0.26 \times W)] \times 50$$

To calculate dose in mL, divide the result by 50. Usual Hb target for children ≤15 kg is 12 g/dL. Maximum daily dose is (infants <5 kg) 25 mg (0.5 mL), (children <10 kg) 50 mg (1 mL), (children >15 kg) same as adult dosage.

Geriatric Dosage. Same as adult dosage.

Dosage Forms. **Inj** 50 mg elemental iron/mL.

Pharmacokinetics. *Onset and Duration.* Hematologic response is the same as with oral therapy, although total body stores of iron are replaced when the above dosage regimens are used.

Serum Levels. (*See* Ferrous Salts.)

Fate. Following IV administration, the inert complex is gradually cleared from the plasma by the reticuloendothelial cells of the liver, spleen, and bone marrow. With doses >500 mg, the rate of uptake is 10–20 mg/hr. Iron dextran is then dissociated and released as free ferric iron (at a rate controlled by the serum iron level), which combines with transferrin and is incorporated into hemoglobin within the bone marrow.[104–106] Although all iron is eventually released in this manner, many months are often required for this process to be completed.[95]

Adverse Reactions. Hypotension and peripheral vascular flushing occur with too rapid IV administration. Mild, transient reactions including flushing, fever, myalgia, arthralgia, and lymphadenopathy usually occur only occasionally, although they occur in 80–90% of patients with active rheumatoid arthritis or active SLE. Immediate anaphylactoid reactions, which may be life threatening, occur in 0.1–0.6% of patients.[107] A predictive test for predisposition to anaphylaxis is not available. IM administration has been associated with variable degrees of soreness, sterile abscess formation, tissue staining, and sarcoma formation.[105] Total dose infusion appears to be tolerated as well as divided doses.[104]

Contraindications. Anemias other than iron deficiency anemia; hemochromatosis; hemosiderosis; SC administration.

Precautions. Pregnancy. Use with extreme caution in the presence of serious liver impairment. Patients with rheumatoid arthritis may have an acute exacerbation or reactivation of joint pain and swelling following administration. History of allergies and/or asthma. Because of the potential for anaphylactoid reactions, have epinephrine, diphenhydramine, and methylprednisolone immediately available during iron dextran administration. Use parenteral iron only in patients in whom an iron-deficient state has been clearly established and who are not amenable to oral therapy.

Drug Interactions. None known.

Parameters to Monitor. (*See* Ferrous Salts.)

MACROPHAGE COLONY-STIMULATING FACTOR   (Investigational)

Pharmacology. Macrophage colony-stimulating factor (M-CSF) is a cytokine that promotes proliferation of macrophages and monocytes, enhances macrophage antitumor and antimicrobial activity, and stimulates the release of G-CSF, GM-CSF, interferon, interleukin-1, and tumor necrosis factor. Antitumor response has been observed in a limited number of patients. M-CSF is also being evaluated in the treatment of fungal infections following bone marrow transplant, where macrophage activation may be critical for host defense response. Complete or partial clinical improvement has been observed in some patients.[89] M-CSF is being used investigationally in 3 forms: native protein from urine, a glycosylated recombinant form, and a truncated nonglycosylated form.

Adult Dosage. Most clinical trials evaluated the antitumor and antimicrobial activities of M-CSF. Phase I dose escalation studies using 10–160 μg/kg/day show increased circulating monocytes (at greater than 30 μg/kg/day) and increased antibody-dependent, monocyte-mediated cytotoxicity (at 50–80 μg/kg/day).

Adverse Reactions. Adverse reactions to M-CSF include fever and ophthalmologic toxicity (conjunctivitis, iritis).

SARGRAMOSTIM   Leukine

Pharmacology. Sargramostim is a yeast-derived (glycosylated) recombinant human granulocyte-macrophage colony-stimulating factor (GM-CSF). GM-CSF is one of many glycoprotein hormones that regulate the proliferation and differentiation of hematopoietic progenitor cells and the function of mature blood cells. Specifically, GM-CSF promotes proliferation, maturation, and function of neutrophils, eosinophils, monocytes, and macrophages. GM-CSF also stimulates production of cytokines including interleukin-1 and tumor necrosis factor.[100,103,108]

Adult Dosage. **IV following autologous bone marrow infusion** 250 μg/m^2/day given as a 2-hr infusion beginning 2–4 hr after the autologous bone marrow infusion. Give the first dose no sooner than 24 hr after the last chemotherapy dose or before 12 hr following the last dose of radiotherapy. Continue sargramostim until the ANC is >1500/μL for 3 consecutive days. **IV for bone marrow transplantation failure or delay in engraftment** 250 μg/m^2/day for 14 days as a 2-hr infusion, repeated in 7 days if engraftment has not occurred. If there is no improvement, a third course with 500 μg/m^2/day given for 14 days may be tried. **SC for AIDS patients receiving ganciclovir** 1–15 μg/kg/day has been used investigationally.

Dosage Forms. **Inj** 250, 500 mg.

Adverse Reactions. Acute reactions (eg, febrile episodes, flushing, hypotension, tachycardia, and hypoxia) appear to be more common than with filgrastim. Other adverse reactions that occur frequently with GM-CSF are bone pain, lethargy, rash, and fluid retention.

Notes. Sargramostim is indicated for myeloid reconstitution after autologous bone marrow transplantation. It has also been used with some success to maintain normal neutrophil counts in AIDS patients receiving **ganciclovir.** Other potential uses for GM-CSF include AIDS-related neutropenia, myelodysplastic syndromes, and congenital, chronic, or drug-induced neutropenia and aplastic anemia. Controlled clinical trials are needed to prove that use for these and other indications is beneficial, safe, and cost effective. Clinical and laboratory evidence appears to suggest GM-CSF enhances the effect of **zidovudine** against HIV.[89,100,103,108–110]

■ REFERENCES

1. Hyers TM et al. Antithrombotic therapy for venous thromboembolic disease. *Chest* 1995;108:335S–51S.
2. Lutomski DM et al. Pharmacokinetic optimisation of the treatment of embolic disorders. *Clin Pharmacokinet* 1995;28:67–92.
3. International Society and Federation of Cardiology and World Health Organization Task Force on Myocardial Reperfusion. Reperfusion in acute myocardial infarction. *Circulation* 1994;90:2091–102.
4. Becker RC, Ansell J. Antithrombotic therapy: an abbreviated reference for clinicians. *Arch Intern Med* 1995;155:149–61.
5. The GUSTO Investigators. An international randomized trial comparing four thrombolytic strategies for acute myocardial infarction. *N Engl J Med* 1993;329:673–82.
6. Levine M et al. A randomized trial of a single bolus dosage regimen of recombinant tissue plasminogen activator in patients with acute pulmonary embolism. *Chest* 1990;98:1473–9.
7. Cairns JA et al. Coronary thrombolysis. *Chest* 1995;108:401S–23S.
8. The National Institute of Neurological Disorders rt-PA Stroke Study Group. Tissue plasminogen activator for acute ischemic stroke. *N Engl J Med* 1995;333:1581–7.
9. Benet LZ et al. Design and optimization of dosage regimens; pharmacokinetic data. In, Hardman JG et al., eds. *Goodman and Gilman's the pharmacological basis of therapeutics.* 9th ed. New York: McGraw-Hill; 1996:1707–92.
10. Third International Study of Infarct Survival Collaborative Study. ISIS-3: a randomized comparison of streptokinase vs tissue plasminogen activator vs anistreplase and of aspirin plus heparin vs aspirin alone among 41,299 cases of suspected acute myocardial infarct. *Lancet* 1992;339:753–70.
11. Nicolini FA et al. Concurrent nitroglycerin therapy impairs tissue-type plasminogen activator-induced thrombolysis in patients with acute myocardial infarction. *Am J Cardiol* 1994;74:662–6.
12. Fuster V. Coronary thrombolysis—a perspective for the practicing physician. *N Engl J Med* 1993;329:723–4.
13. The Continuous Infusion Versus Double-Bolus Administration of Alteplase (COBALT) Investigators. A comparison of continuous infusion of alteplase with double-bolus administration for acute myocardial infarction. *N Engl J Med* 1997;337:1124–30.
14. Munger MA, Forrence EA. Anistreplase: a new thrombolytic for the treatment of acute myocardial infarction. *Clin Pharm* 1990;9:530–40.
15. O'Connor CM et al. A randomized trial of intravenous heparin in conjunction with anistreplase (anisoylated plasminogen streptokinase activator complex) in acute myocardial infarction: the Duke University Clinical Cardiology Study (DUCCS) 1. *J Am Coll Cardiol* 1994;23:11–8.
16. CAPRIE Steering Committee. A randomized, blinded, trial of clopidogrel versus aspirin in patients at risk for ischaemic events (CAPRIE). *Lancet* 1996;348:1329–39.
17. Howard PA. Dalteparin: a low-molecular-weight heparin. *Ann Pharmacother* 1997;31:192–203.
18. Charland SL, Klinter DEJ. Low-molecular-weight heparins in the treatment of pulmonary embolism. *Ann Pharmacother* 1998;32:258–64.
19. Spinler SA, Nawarskas JJ. Low-molecular-weight heparins for acute coronary syndromes. *Ann Pharmacother* 1998;32:103–10.
20. Green D et al. Low molecular weight heparin: a critical analysis of clinical trials. *Pharmacol Rev* 1994;46:89–109.

21. Noble S et al. Enoxaparin. A reappraisal of its pharmacology and clinical applications in the prevention and treatment of thromboembolic disease. *Drugs* 1995;49:388–410.

22. Levine M et al. A comparison of low-molecular-weight heparin administered primarily at home with unfractionated heparin administered in the hospital for proximal deep-vein thrombosis. *N Engl J Med* 1996;334: 677–81.

23. Lensing AWA et al. Treatment of deep venous thrombosis with low-molecular-weight heparins. A meta-analysis. *Arch Intern Med* 1995;155:601–7.

24. Verstraete M. Pharmacotherapeutic aspects of unfractionated and low molecular weight heparins. *Drugs* 1990;40:498–530.

25. de Valk HW et al. Comparing subcutaneous danaparoid with intravenous unfractionated heparin for the treatment of venous thromboembolism. A randomized controlled trial. *Ann Intern Med* 1995;123:1–9.

26. Carter BL. Therapy of acute thromboembolism with heparin and warfarin. *Clin Pharm* 1991;10:503–18.

27. Raschke RA et al. The weight-based heparin dosing nomogram compared with a "standard care" nomogram. A randomized controlled trial. *Ann Intern Med* 1993;119:874–81.

28. Kershaw B et al. Computer-assisted dosing of heparin. Management with pharmacy-based anticoagulation service. *Arch Intern Med* 1994;154:1005–11.

29. Gunnarsson PS et al. Appropriate use of heparin. Empiric vs nomogram-based dosing. *Arch Intern Med* 1995; 155:526–32.

30. Simon TL et al. Heparin pharmacokinetics: increased requirements in pulmonary embolism. *Br J Haematol* 1978;39:111–20.

31. Kruchoski ME, Emory CE. Initiating heparin and warfarin therapy concurrently. *Hosp Pharm* 1986;21:174.

32. Hull RD et al. Heparin for 5 days as compared with 10 days in the initial treatment of proximal venous thrombosis. *N Engl J Med* 1990;322:1260–4.

33. Melamed AJ, Suarez J. Detection and prevention of deep venous thrombosis. *Drug Intell Clin Pharm* 1988; 22:107–14.

34. Cooke HM, Lynch A. Biorhythms and chronotherapy in cardiovascular disease. *Am J Hosp Pharm* 1994;51: 2569–80.

35. Estes JW. Clinical pharmacokinetics of heparin. *Clin Pharmacokinet* 1980;5:204–20.

36. Hirsh J et al. Heparin kinetics in venous thrombosis and pulmonary embolism. *Circulation* 1976;53:691–5.

37. Landefeld CS et al. A bleeding risk index for estimating the probability of major bleeding in hospitalized patients starting anticoagulant therapy. *Am J Med* 1990;89:569–78.

38. Bailey RT et al. Heparin-associated thrombocytopenia: a prospective comparison of bovine lung heparin, manufactured by a new process, and porcine intestinal heparin. *Drug Intell Clin Pharm* 1986;20:374–8.

39. Becker PS, Miller VT. Heparin-induced thrombocytopenia. *Stroke* 1989;20:1449–59.

40. Oster JR et al. Heparin-induced aldosterone suppression and hyperkalemia. *Am J Med* 1995;98:575–86.

41. Gupta AK et al. Heparin-induced thrombocytopenia. *Ann Pharmacother* 1998;32:55–9.

42. Uotila L. The metabolic functions and mechanism of action of vitamin K. *Scand J Clin Lab Invest* 1990; 201(suppl):109–17.

43. Hardman JG et al., eds. *Goodman and Gilman's the pharmacological basis of therapeutics.* 9th ed. New York: McGraw-Hill; 1996:1583–5.

44. Thorp JA et al. Current concepts and controversies in the use of vitamin K. *Drugs* 1995;49:376–87.

45. Frick PG et al. Dose response and minimal daily requirement for vitamin K in man. *J Appl Physiol* 1967;23:387–9.

46. Mattea EJ, Quinn K. Adverse reactions after intravenous phytonadione administration. *Hosp Pharm* 1981;16:224–35.

47. Food and Nutrition Board, NRC. *Recommended dietary allowances.* 10th ed. Washington, DC: National Academy Press; 1989.

48. Koch-Weser J, Sellers EM. Drug interactions with coumarin anticoagulants (2 parts). *N Engl J Med* 1971; 285:487–9, 547–58.

49. Zieve PD, Solomon HM. Variation in the response of human beings to vitamin K. *J Lab Clin Med* 1969; 73:103–10.

50. Woolf IL, Babior BM. Vitamin K and warfarin. *Am J Med* 1972;53:261–7.

51. O'Reilly RA et al. Intravenous vitamin K1 injections: dangerous prophylaxis. *Arch Intern Med* 1995;155:2127.

52. Lopez LM. Clinical trials in thrombolytic therapy, Part 2: The open-artery hypothesis and RAPID-1 and RAPID-2. *Am J Health-Syst Pharm* 1997;54(suppl):S27–30.

53. The Global Use of Strategies To Open Occluded Coronary Ateries (GUSTO III) Investigators. A comparison of reteplase with alteplase for acute myocardial infarction. *New Engl J Med* 1997;337:1118–23.

54. Randomised, double-blind comparison of reteplase double-bolus administration with streptokinase in acute

myocardial infarction: trial to investigate equivalence. International Joint Efficacy Comparison of Thrombolytics (INJECT). *Lancet* 1995;346:329–36.

55. Rogers LQ, Lutcher CL. Streptokinase therapy for deep vein thrombosis: a comprehensive review of the English literature. *Am J Med* 1990;88:389–95.

56. Katzen BT, van Breda A. Low dose streptokinase in the treatment of arterial occlusion. *AJR* 1981;136:1171–8.

57. Belkin M et al. Intra-arterial fibrinolytic therapy. *Arch Surg* 1986;121:769–73.

58. Fletcher AP et al. The maintenance of a sustained thrombolytic state in man. I. Induction and effects. *J Clin Invest* 1959;38:1096–110.

59. Fletcher AP et al. The clearance of heterologous protein from the circulation of normal and immunized man. *J Clin Invest* 1958;37:1306–15.

60. Sherry S et al. Thrombolytic therapy in thrombosis: a National Institutes of Health consensus development conference. *Ann Intern Med* 1980;93:141–4.

61. Levine MN et al. Hemorrhagic complications of thrombolytic therapy in the treatment of myocardial infarction and venous embolism. *Chest* 1995;108:291S–301S.

62. Goldhaber SZ. Contemporary pulmonary embolism thrombolysis. *Chest* 1995;107(suppl):45S–51S.

63. Marder VJ. The use of thrombolytic agents: choice of patient, drug administration, laboratory monitoring. *Ann Intern Med* 1979;90:802–8.

64. Haynes RB et al. A critical appraisal of ticlopidine, a new antiplatelet agent. Effectiveness and clinical indications for prophylaxis of atherosclerotic events. *Arch Intern Med* 1992;152:1376–80.

65. Matchar DB et al. Medical treatment for stroke prevention. *Ann Intern Med* 1994;121:41–53.

66. Carlson JA, Maesner JE. Fatal neutropenia and thrombocytopenia associated with ticlopidine. *Ann Pharmacother* 1994;28:1236–8.

67. Cassidy LJ et al. Probable ticlopidine-induced cholestatic hepatitis. *Ann Pharmacother* 1995;29:30–2.

68. Hass WK et al. A randomized trial comparing ticlopidine hydrochloride with aspirin for the prevention of stroke in high-risk patients. *N Engl J Med* 1989;321:501–7.

69. Gent M et al. The Canadian American Ticlopidine Study (CATS) in thromboembolic stroke. *Lancet* 1989; 1:1215–20.

70. Haire WD, Lieberman RP. Thrombosed central venous catheters: restoring function with 6-hour urokinase infusion after failure of bolus urokinase. *J Parenter Enteral Nutr* 1992;16:129–32.

71. Breckenridge A et al. Pharmacokinetics and pharmacodynamics of the enantiomers of warfarin in man. *Clin Pharmacol Ther* 1974;15:424–30.

72. Fihn SD. Aiming for safe anticoagulation. *N Engl J Med* 1995;333:54–5. Editorial.

73. Bern MM et al. Very low doses of warfarin can prevent thrombosis in central venous catheters. *Ann Intern Med* 1990;112:423–8.

74. O'Reilly RA, Aggeler PM. Determinants of the response to oral anticoagulant drugs in man. *Pharmacol Rev* 1970;22:35–96.

75. Nagashima R et al. Kinetics of pharmacologic effects in man: the anticoagulant action of warfarin. *Clin Pharmacol Ther* 1969;10:22–35.

76. Lutomski DM et al. Warfarin absorption after massive small bowel resection. *Am J Gastroenterol* 1985;80:99–102.

77. Slaughter RL, Edwards DJ. Recent advances: the cytochrome P450 enzymes. *Ann Pharmacother* 1995;29:619–24.

78. Yacobi A et al. Serum protein binding as a determinant of warfarin body clearance and anticoagulant effect. *Clin Pharmacol Ther* 1976;19:552–8.

79. Lewis RJ et al. Warfarin metabolites: the anticoagulant activity and pharmacology of warfarin alcohols. *J Lab Clin Med* 1973;81:925–31.

80. O'Reilly RA et al. Studies on the coumarin anticoagulant drugs: the pharmacodynamics of warfarin in man. *J Clin Invest* 1963;42:1542–51.

81. Williams RL et al. Influence of acute viral hepatitis on disposition and pharmacologic effect of warfarin. *Clin Pharmacol Ther* 1976;20:90–7.

82. Hirsh J. Drug therapy: oral anticoagulant drugs. *N Engl J Med* 1991;324:1865–75.

83. Landefeld CS, Goldman L. Major bleeding in outpatients treated with warfarin: incidence and prediction by factors known at the start of outpatient therapy. *Am J Med* 1989;87:144–52.

84. Hansten PD, Horn JR. *Drug interactions and updates quarterly.* Vancouver, WA: Applied Therapeutics; 1998 (updated quarterly).

85. Tatro DS, ed. *Drug interaction facts.* St. Louis: JB Lippincott; 1998 (updated quarterly).

86. Deykin D. Warfarin therapy (second of two parts). *N Engl J Med* 1970;283:801–3.

87. Hirsh J. The optimal duration of anticoagulant therapy for venous thrombosis. *N Engl J Med* 1995;332: 1710–1. Editorial.

88. Schwenk MH, Halstenson CE. Recombinant human erythropoietin. *DICP* 1989;23:528–36.
89. Petersdorf SH, Dale DC. The biology and clinical applications of erythropoietin and the colony-stimulating factors. *Adv Intern Med* 1995;40:395–428.
90. Erslev AJ. Erythropoietin. *N Engl J Med* 1991;324:1339–44.
91. Zachée P. Controversies in selection of epoetin dosages. Issues and answers. *Drugs* 1995;49:536–47.
92. Ohis RK, Christensen RD. Recombinant erythropoietin compared with erythrocyte transfusion in the treatment of anemia of prematurity. *J Pediatr* 1991;119:781–8.
93. Ongkingco JR et al. Use of low-dose subcutaneous recombinant human erythropoietin in end-stage renal disease: experience with children receiving continuous cycling peritoneal dialysis. *Am J Kidney Dis* 1991;18:446–50.
94. Rigden SP et al. Recombinant human erythropoietin therapy in children maintained by haemodialysis. *Pediatr Nephrol* 1990;4:618–22.
95. Hardman JG et al., eds. *Goodman and Gilman's the pharmacological basis of therapeutics.* 9th ed. New York: McGraw-Hill; 1996.
96. Koeller JM, Van Den Berg C. Anemias. In, Koda-Kimble MA, Young LY, eds. *Applied therapeutics: the clinical use of drugs.* 6th ed. Vancouver, WA: Applied Therapeutics; 1995:88.3–88.17.
97. Stevens RG. Iron and the risk of cancer. *Med Oncol Tumor Pharmacother* 1990;7:177–81.
98. Olson KR, ed. *Poisoning and drug overdose.* Norwalk, CT: Appleton & Lange; 1990.
99. Middleton EJ et al. Studies on the absorption of orally administered iron from sustained-release preparations. *N Engl J Med* 1966;274:136–9.
100. Anon. G-CSF and GM-CSF: white blood cell growth factors. *Hosp Pharm* 1990;25:881–2.
101. Maher DW et al. Filgrastim in patients with chemotherapy-induced febrile neutropenia. *Ann Intern Med* 1994;121:492–501.
102. Miles SA et al. Combined therapy with recombinant granulocyte colony-stimulating factor and erythropoietin decreases hematologic toxicity zidovudine. *Blood* 1991;77:2109–17.
103. Demuynck H et al. Comparative study of peripheral blood progenitor cell collection in patients with multiple myeloma after single-dose cyclophosphamide combined with rhGM-CSF or rhG-CSF. *Br J Haematol* 1995;90:384–92.
104. Auerbach M et al. A randomized trial of three iron dextran infusion methods for anemia in EPO-treated dialysis patients. *Am J Kidney Dis* 1998;31:81–6.
105. Kumpf VJ, Holland EG. Parenteral iron dextran therapy. *DICP* 1990;24:162–6.
106. Wood JK et al. The metabolism of iron-dextran given as a total-dose infusion to iron deficient Jamaican subjects. *Br J Haematol* 1968;14:119–29.
107. Novey HS et al. Immunologic studies of anaphylaxis to iron dextran in patients on renal dialysis. *Ann Allergy* 1994;72:224–8.
108. Hogan KR, Peters MD. Granulocyte-macrophage colony-stimulating factor in neutropenia. *DICP* 1991;25:32–5.
109. Grossberg HS, Bonnem EM. GM-CSF with ganciclovir for the treatment of CMV retinitis in AIDS. *N Engl J Med* 1989;320:1560. Letter.
110. Groopman JE. Granulocyte-macrophage colony-stimulating factor in human immunodeficiency virus disease. *Semin Hematol* 1990;27(suppl 3):8–14.

Hormonal Drugs

Adrenal Hormones

Class Instructions: Corticosteroids. (Systemic use) these drugs may be taken with food, milk, or an antacid to minimize stomach upset. Take single daily doses or alternate-day doses in the morning prior to 9 AM. Take multiple daily doses at evenly spaced intervals during the day. Report unusual weight gain, lower extremity swelling, muscle weakness, black tarry stools, vomiting of blood, facial swelling, menstrual irregularities, prolonged sore throat, fever, cold, infection, serious injury, fatigue, anorexia, nausea, vomiting, diarrhea, weight loss, dizziness, or low blood sugar. Consult physician during periods of increased stress. If you are diabetic, you may have increased requirements for insulin or oral hypoglycemics. Carry appropriate identification if you are taking long-term corticosteroid therapy. Do not discontinue this medication without medical approval; tell any new health care provider that you are taking a corticosteroid. Avoid immunizations with live vaccines.

Missed Doses. If a dose is missed and the proper schedule is *every other day,* take it as soon as possible and resume the schedule unless it is past noon. In that case, wait until the next morning and resume every-other-day administration. If the proper schedule is *once a day,* take the dose as soon as possible. If you do not remember until the next day, do not double that day's dose; skip the missed dose. If the proper schedule is *several times a day,* take the dose as soon as possible and resume the normal schedule. If you do not remember until the next dose is due, then take both the regular dose and the missed dose, and resume the normal dosage schedule.

COSYNTROPIN   Cortrosyn

Pharmacology. Cosyntropin is a synthetic polypeptide containing the first 24 of the 39 amino acids of natural **corticotropin (adrenocorticotropic hormone [ACTH])** and retaining the full activity of corticotropin with decreased antigenicity. Cosyntropin 250 μg is equivalent to corticotropin 25 units. Cosyntropin stimulates the adrenal cortex to produce and secrete gluco- and mineralocorticoids and androgens similar to corticotropin. Cosyntropin is used as a diagnostic agent to detect adrenocortical insufficiency, but can also be used therapeutically as a substitute for corticotropin.[1–4]

Adult Dosage. **IM or IV for diagnostic use** hold exogenous cortisone or hydrocortisone on the test day and, if the patient is not taking spironolactone or an estrogen, a baseline cortisol level (which should exceed 5 μg/dL) is drawn in the morning just before the dose. Then, cosyntropin 250 μg in 1 mL of NS is given IM, or 250 μg in 2–5 mL NS is given IV push over 2 min. Normal cortisol levels are >18 μg/dL (500 nmol/L) 30 min after the injection and ≥7 μg/dL (190 nmol/L) above baseline. If the cortisol level is drawn 60 min postadministration, then an approximate doubling of the baseline cortisol value indicates a normal response. Alternatively, give an infusion of 250 μg in D5W or NS over 6 hr in the morning with serum cortisol levels drawn before and after. The second cortisol level should be >18 μg/dL (500 nmol/L) and ≥7 μg/dL (190 nmol/L) above baseline. **IV for therapeutic use** 250 μg infused IV over 8 hr elicits maximal adrenocortical secretion.

Pediatric Dosage. IM or IV as a diagnostic agent (≤2 yr) 125 μg given as above.

Dosage Forms. Inj 250 μg.

Adverse Reactions. (Diagnostic use) rare reports of hypersensitivity. (Therapeutic use) salt and water retention, and virilization occur.

DEXAMETHASONE   Decadron, Hexadrol, Various

Pharmacology. Dexamethasone is a potent, long-acting glucocorticoid lacking sodium-retaining activity with low to moderate doses. (*See* Prednisone and the Oral Corticosteroids Comparison Chart.)

Administration and Adult Dosage. Total daily dosage is variable depending on the clinical disorder and patient response. **PO for acute, self-limited allergic disorders or exacerbation of chronic allergic disorders** 0.75–9 mg/day in 2 divided doses on the first day, then tapered over 7 days and discontinued. **IV for cerebral edema** 10 mg (as the sodium phosphate) initially, followed by 4 mg IM or IV q 6 hr for several days until maximal response occurs; then decrease the dosage over 5–7 days and discontinue. **PO or IV as an antiemetic with cancer chemotherapy** (usually in combination with other antiemetics) 10–20 mg immediately prior to therapy; optionally, up to 40 mg may be given after chemotherapy.[5–8] **PO or IV for acute exacerbations of multiple sclerosis** (after 200 mg/day prednisolone given for 1 week) 4–8 mg dexamethasone every other day for 1 month. **PO as the dexamethasone suppression test to screen for Cushing's disease** 1 mg at 11 PM; a measured serum cortisol at 8 AM the next morning <5 μg/dL (140 nmol/L) indicates a normal response.[9] Alternatively, PO 0.5 mg q 6 hr for 48 hr (8 doses), with a 24-hr urine collected for 17-hydroxycorticosteroids (17-OHCs) during the second 24-hr period. A normal response is 2.5 mg (6.9 μmol) or less of 17-OHCs during the second 24-hr period.[9] **PO as a Cushing's syndrome test to distinguish pituitary origin from other causes** 2 mg q 6 hr for 48 hr (8 doses). A normal response is a 24-hr urine concentration of less than 2.5 mg (6.9 μmol) of 17-OHCs.[9] (*See* Notes.) **IM (aqueous) in the mother for antenatal prevention of neonatal distress syndrome** starting 24 hr or more before premature delivery, give 5 mg q 12 hr for 4 doses, or 12 or 16 mg q 24 hr for 2 doses.[10] **IV for septic shock** not recommended because of a lack of efficacy and a possible increase in mortality.[11,12] **IM (depot) for prolonged systemic effect** 8–16 mg q 1–3 weeks. (*See also* Inhaled Corticosteroids Comparison Chart in the Respiratory Drugs section.)

Special Populations. *Pediatric Dosage.* **PO, IM, or IV for airway edema** 0.25–0.5 mg/kg/dose q 6 hr prn for croup or beginning 24 hr before planned extubation, then for 4–6 doses; **PO, IM, or IV as an anti-inflammatory or immuno-**

suppressive 0.03–0.15 mg/kg/day divided q 6–12 hr; **PO, IM, or IV for cerebral edema** 1.5 mg/kg once, then 1.5 mg/kg/day divided q 4–6 hr for 5 days, then taper over the next 5 days and discontinue. **IV to prevent hearing loss and other neurologic sequelae in *Haemophilus influenzae* bacterial meningitis** (>2 months) 0.15 mg/kg q 6 hr, beginning no sooner than 20 min before (or with) the first dose of antibiotics and continued for 4 days.[12–15]

Geriatric Dosage. Consider using a lower dosage for decreased body size.

Patient Instructions. (*See* Class Instructions: Corticosteroids.)

Dosage Forms. Elxr 0.1 mg/mL; **Soln** 0.1, 1 mg/mL; **Tab** 0.25, 0.5, 0.75, 1, 1.5, 2, 4, 6 mg; **Inj** 4, 10, 20, 24 mg/mL; **Depot Inj** 8, 16 mg/mL (as acetate).

Pharmacokinetics. *Onset and Duration.* (*See* Oral Corticosteroids Comparison Chart.)

Serum Levels. Serum concentration is not directly correlated with therapeutic effect.[2,16]

Fate. After oral administration, 78 ± 14% is absorbed; 68% is plasma protein bound. V_d is 0.82 ± 0.22 L/kg. The drug is eliminated primarily by hepatic metabolism, with about 2.6 ± 0.6% excreted unchanged in urine.[3,17,18]

$t_{1/2}$. (Males) 3.5 ± 0.87 hr; (females) 2.4 ± 0.16 hr.[3,17,18]

Adverse Reactions. (*See* Prednisone Adverse Reactions.) Perineal itching or burning may occur after IV administration.[19]

Contraindications. Systemic fungal infections (except as maintenance therapy in adrenal insufficiency); administration of live virus vaccines to patients receiving an immunosuppressive dosage of dexamethasone; IM use in idiopathic thrombocytopenic purpura.

Precautions. (*See* Prednisone.)

Parameters to Monitor. (*See* Prednisone.)

Notes. The dexamethasone suppression test for diagnosis of depression is of unproven value.[20,21] Variations of the dexamethasone suppression test (for Cushing's disease screening) have been used.[1,9]

METHYLPREDNISOLONE SODIUM SUCCINATE   Solu-Medrol, Various

Pharmacology. Methylprednisolone sodium succinate is an injectable glucocorticoid that has about 1.25 times greater anti-inflammatory potency than prednisone or prednisolone and a similar duration of biologic activity. (*See* Oral Corticosteroids Comparison Chart.) It is commonly used when oral therapy is not possible and in situations in which large parenteral doses are necessary. Evidence of efficacy in improving the outcome of septic shock is lacking, and, because of increased mortality in some patient groups, the use of methylprednisolone in septic shock is not recommended. Patients with acute spinal cord injury treated with high-dose methylprednisolone within 8 hr may have improved neurologic recovery.[3,11–13,18,22–24]

Adult Dosage. IV initial dosage 10–40 mg given over one to several minutes; dosages up to 30 mg/kg q 4–6 hr (high-dose therapy) for up to 48–72 hr are used for severe, acute conditions. Infuse large doses (≥250 mg) slowly (eg, over 1–2 hr), because arrhythmias and sudden death have occurred with rapid infusions. **IV for acute spinal cord injury** 30 mg/kg over 15 min, begun within 8 hr of injury, followed 45 min later by a continuous IV infusion of 5.4 mg/kg/hr for 23 hr.

Pediatric Dosage. IV as an anti-inflammatory or immunosuppressive 0.16–0.8 mg/kg/day in 2–4 divided doses.

Dosage Forms. Inj 40, 125, 500 mg, 1, 2 g; **Depot Inj** (as acetate) 20, 40, 80 mg/mL. (*See also* Oral Corticosteroids Comparison Chart.)

Pharmacokinetics. Plasma protein binding is 78 ± 3%. V_d is 1.2 ± 0.2 L/kg; Cl is 0.37 ± 0.054 L/hr/kg. The drug is extensively metabolized, with 4.9 ± 2.3% excreted unchanged in urine. The serum half-life is 2.2 ± 0.5 hr and is not affected by renal function.

Adverse Reactions. Side effects are similar to prednisone in equivalent dosages. Ketoconazole reduces methylprednisolone elimination, possibly leading to excessive corticosteroid effect. (*See also* Prednisone Drug Interactions.)

PREDNISONE   Deltasone, Orasone, Various

Pharmacology. Prednisone is a synthetic glucocorticoid with less sodium-retaining activity than hydrocortisone. Prednisone is inactive until converted into **prednisolone.** At the cellular level, glucocorticoids appear to act by controlling the rate of protein synthesis. Clinically, these drugs are used primarily for their anti-inflammatory and immunosuppressant effects.

Administration and Adult Dosage. Total daily dosage is variable, depending on the clinical disorder and patient response.[16,25] Daily divided high-dose therapy for initial control of more severe disease states may be necessary until satisfactory control is obtained, usually 4–10 days for many allergic and collagen diseases. Administration of a short- or intermediate-acting preparation given as a single dose in the morning (prior to 9 AM) is likely to produce fewer side effects and less pituitary-adrenal suppression than either a divided dosage regimen with the same agent or an equivalent dosage of a long-acting agent.[16] Alternate-day therapy (ie, total 48-hr dosage administered every other morning) with intermediate-acting agents (eg, prednisone) further reduces the prevalence and degree of side effects. However, it may not be uniformly effective in treating all disease states, unless large doses are used (eg, 40–60 mg every other day for adults requiring long-term corticosteroid therapy for asthma).[16,26,27] Complete adrenal suppression may not occur with single daily doses given either in the morning or evening if the prednisone dose is 15 mg or less, but Cushing's syndrome may still occur and patients should receive supplemental corticosteroids during periods of unusual stress. **In times of stress** (eg, surgery, severe trauma, serious illness), patients on long-term corticosteroid therapy (>5 mg/day prednisone or equivalent) should receive supplemental IV **hydrocortisone** 100–300 mg/day or PO prednisone 25–75 mg/day in divided doses.[2,3,16,25,28] Guidelines for withdrawal from glucocorticoid therapy have been published.[2,9]

Common initial doses are: **PO for acute asthma exacerbations in adults and adolescents** 40 mg 2–4 times/day for 3–5 days; hospitalized patients may require a parenteral preparation. Reduce dosage to minimum effective maintenance dosage as soon as possible; **PO as an adjunct therapy for *Pneumocystis carinii* pneumonia** (with an arterial PO$_2$ of 70 mm Hg or less, or an arterial-alveolar gradient ≥35 mm Hg) 40 mg bid for 5 days begun with antimicrobial therapy, then 20 mg bid for 5 days, then 20 mg/day for the duration of antimicrobial therapy; **PO for arthritis** 10 mg/day; **PO for collagen diseases** 1 mg/kg/day; **PO for acute gout** 30–50 mg/day, gradually decreased over 10 days; **PO for rheumatic carditis** 40 mg/day; **PO for nephrotic syndrome** 60 mg/day; **PO for skin disorders** 40 mg/day, up to 240 mg/day in pemphigus; **PO for ulcerative colitis** 10–30 mg/day or, if severe, 60–120 mg/day; **PO for thrombocytopenia** 0.5 mg/kg/day; **PO for organ transplantation** (in combination with cyclosporine) 200 mg once, then taper dosage in 40 mg increments daily until reaching a dose of 20 mg/day; continue at 20 mg/day for 60 days, then reduce dosage to 10 mg/day and make further dosage adjustments based on the clinical situation; **PO for acute exacerbations of multiple sclerosis** 200 mg/day for 1 week, then 80 mg every other day for 1 month.[3,12,26–33]

Special Populations. *Pediatric Dosage.* Dosage depends on disease state and patient response. *Common initial doses are:* **PO for acute asthma** 1–2 mg/kg/day in 1–2 divided doses; **PO for inflammation or immunosuppression** 0.2–1 mg/kg/day in 2–4 divided doses.[13]

Dosage Forms. **Soln** 1, 5 mg/mL; **Syrup** 1 mg/mL; **Tab** 1, 2.5, 5, 10, 20, 50 mg.

Patient Instructions. (*See* Class Instructions: Corticosteroids.)

Pharmacokinetics. *Onset and Duration.* (*See* Oral Corticosteroids Comparison Chart.)

Serum Levels. Serum concentration is not directly correlated with therapeutic effect.[2,16] A timed prednisolone serum drug level may be useful in estimating clearance and identifying abnormalities in absorption, elimination, or patient compliance.[34]

Fate. Bioavailability is 77–99%, with peak levels occurring 1–4 hr postingestion;[18] 90–95% is plasma protein bound, depending on serum concentration. Prednisone is metabolized in the liver to its active form, prednisolone.[2,16] Liver disease does not impair conversion to active metabolite. In fact, patients with liver disease and hypoalbuminemia are more likely to suffer major side effects of prednisone as a result of decreased protein binding and reduced prednisolone clearance.[2,16,35,36] V_d of prednisolone is 1.5 ± 0.2 L/kg. Over 90% of metabolites are excreted in urine; $3 \pm 2\%$ of a dose of prednisone is excreted unchanged in urine with an additional $15 \pm 5\%$ excreted as prednisolone.[3,18,35]

t$_½$. (Prednisone) 3.4 hr; (prednisolone) 2–5 hr.[18,35] Biologic half-life exceeds serum half-life. (*See* Oral Corticosteroids Comparison Chart.)

Adverse Reactions. Dose- and duration-related side effects include fluid and electrolyte disturbances (with possible edema and hypertension), hyperglycemia and glycosuria, spread of herpes conjunctivitis, activation of tuberculosis, peptic ulcers (possibly), osteoporosis, bone fractures,[37] myopathy, menstrual irregularities, behavioral disturbances (increasing with dosages >40 mg/day),[38] poor wound healing, ocular cataracts, glaucoma, arrest of growth (in children), hirsutism, pseudotumor cerebri (primarily in children), and Cushing's syndrome (moon face, buffalo hump, central obesity, easy bruising, acne, hirsutism, and striae).[2,16,25] Prolonged therapy may lead to suppression of pituitary-adrenal function. Too rapid withdrawal of long-term therapy can cause acute adrenal insufficiency (eg, fever, myalgia, arthralgia, and malaise); adrenally suppressed patients are also unable to respond to stress.

Contraindications. Systemic fungal infections (except as maintenance therapy in adrenal insufficiency); administration of live virus vaccines in patients receiving immunosuppressive doses of corticosteroids.

Precautions. Pregnancy. Use with caution in diabetes mellitus; osteoporosis; peptic ulcer; esophagitis; tuberculosis; and other acute and chronic bacterial, viral, and fungal infections; hypertension or other cardiovascular diseases; hypothyroidism; immunizations; hypoalbuminemia; psychosis; and liver disease. Suppression of PPD and other skin test reactions may occur.

Drug Interactions. Corticosteroids may increase serum glucose levels, and an increase in the dosage of antidiabetic drugs may be required. Corticosteroids may decrease salicylate serum levels. Amphotericin B and loop and thiazide diuretics may enhance corticosteroid-induced potassium depletion. Carbamazepine, phenobarbital (and possibly other barbiturates), phenytoin (best documented with dexamethasone), rifampin, and possibly aminoglutethimide increase the metabolism of corticosteroids. Ketoconazole reduces methylprednisolone elimination, but its effect on other corticosteroids is not well established.

Parameters to Monitor. Observe for behavioral disturbances and signs or symptoms of Cushing's syndrome. With short-term, high-dose therapy, frequently monitor serum potassium and glucose, and blood pressure. With long-term therapy, monitor these parameters occasionally and perform periodic eye examinations and possibly stool guaiac. Monitor growth in infants and children on prolonged therapy.

Notes. Other, more expensive glucocorticoids offer minimal advantages over prednisone in most clinical situations.[3,39] Dosage ranges for **prednisolone** are the same as those for prednisone. Patients who have received daily glucocorticoid therapy for asthma for less than 2 weeks *do not* require dosage tapering to prevent acute adrenal insufficiency; however, dosage tapering may be required to maintain an adequate clinical response.[25,29] Efficacy in patients with stable COPD is controversial.[40,41]

ORAL CORTICOSTEORIDS COMPARISON CHART

DURATION AND DRUG	DOSAGE FORMS	EQUIVALENT ANTI-INFLAMMATORY DOSE (MG)[a]	RELATIVE ANTI-INFLAMMATORY POTENCY[a]	RELATIVE MINERALO-CORTICOID ACTIVITY	SERUM HALF-LIFE (HR)	COMMENTS
SHORT-ACTING GLUCOCORTICOIDS (BIOLOGIC ACTIVITY 8–12 HR)						
Cortisone Various	Tab 5, 10, 25 mg.	25	0.8	0.8	0.5	Must be metabolized to active form (hydrocortisone).
Hydrocortisone Various	Tab 5, 10, 20 mg Susp (as cypionate) 2 mg/mL.	20	1	1	1.5	Daily secretion in man is 20 mg.
INTERMEDIATE-ACTING GLUCOCORTICOIDS (BIOLOGIC ACTIVITY 12–36 HR)						
Methylprednisolone Medrol Various	Tab 2, 4, 8, 16, 24, 32 mg.	4	5	0.5	2.3	Minimal sodium-retaining activity.
Prednisolone Various	Tab 5 mg Syrup 1, 3 mg/mL.	5	4	0.8	2–5	Minimal sodium-retaining activity.
Prednisone Various	Tab 1, 2.5, 5, 10, 20, 50 mg Soln 1, 5 mg/mL Syrup 1 mg/mL.	5	4	0.8	3.4	Must be metabolized to active form (prednisolone).
Triamcinolone Aristocort Kenacort Various	Tab 1, 2, 4, 8 mg Syrup 0.8 mg/mL.	4	5	0	2.6	

(continued)

ORAL CORTICOSTEOIDS COMPARISON CHART (continued)

DURATION AND DRUG	DOSAGE FORMS	EQUIVALENT ANTI-INFLAMMATORY DOSE (MG)[a]	RELATIVE ANTI-INFLAMMATORY POTENCY[a]	RELATIVE MINERALO-CORTICOID ACTIVITY	SERUM HALF-LIFE (HR)	COMMENTS
LONG-ACTING GLUCOCORTICOIDS (BIOLOGIC ACTIVITY 36–54 HR)						
Betamethasone Celestone	Tab 0.6 mg	0.6	25	0	5+	Minimal sodium-retaining activity, but with high doses, retention may occur.
Dexamethasone Decadron Hexadrol Various	Tab 0.25, 0.5, 0.75, 1, 1.5, 2, 4, 6 mg Elxr 0.1 mg/mL Soln 0.1, 1 mg/mL.	0.75	30	0	Males 3.5 Females 2.4	No sodium-retaining activity with low to moderate doses.
MINERALOCORTICOID (BIOLOGIC ACTIVITY 18–36 HR)						
Fludrocortisone Florinef	Tab 100 μg	—	10	125	3.5+	Mineralocorticoid used in Addison's disease.

[a]Anti-inflammatory potency does not correlate with immunosuppressive effects.[42]
From references 2, 3, 17, 18, 25, 35, and 43.

TOPICAL CORTICOSTEROIDS

Pharmacology. Topical corticosteroids have nonspecific, local anti-inflammatory effects in the dermal and epidermal skin layers which probably occur by inhibiting mediators in the arachidonic acid pathway in cells, by suppressing DNA synthesis at the cellular level, and by decreasing the influx of white blood cells into the local area. Potency is dependent on the characteristics and concentration of the drug and the vehicle used and is usually measured by the assessment of the relative degree of skin blanching (vasoconstrictor assay).[44-48]

Adult Dosage. Uses for the nonprescription hydrocortisone preparations include relief of itching, inflammation, and rashes caused by eczema; insect bites; poison oak, ivy, or sumac; soaps, detergents, or cosmetics; jewelry; seborrheic dermatitis, psoriasis; and external genital or anal itching. Prescription indications include relief of inflammatory and pruritic manifestations of corticosteroid-responsive dermatoses including contact or atopic dermatitis; nummular, stasis, or asteatotic eczema; lichen planus; lichen simplex chronicus; insect and arthropod bite reactions; and first- and second-degree localized burns and sunburns. These products are usually applied sparingly in a light film, 2–4 times/day; however, with continuous use, a repository effect may make 1–2 applications/day as effective. High-potency agents should be reserved for short-term or intermittent use only, but may be more effective and cause fewer adverse effects than continuous therapy with lower potency products. Treatment with very high-potency agents should not exceed 2 consecutive weeks and the total dosage should not exceed 50 g/week, because of the hypothalmic-pituitary-adrenal (HPA) axis suppressing potential.[44-48]

Dosage Forms. (*See* Topical Corticosteroids Comparison Chart.)

Patient Instructions. Avoid prolonged use around the eyes (or contact with the eyes); in the genital and rectal areas; on the face, armpits, and in skin creases; or use with occlusive dressings unless directed.

Missed Doses. Apply a missed dose as soon as you remember unless it is almost time for the regular schedule. If it is almost time for the regular application, then continue on the regular schedule. Do not apply a double dose.

Pharmacokinetics. The absorption of these drugs is dependent on the physical properties of the drug itself, the surface area of use, the thickness of the skin (greater absorption from the face, in skin folds, in the perineum, and on denuded skin; lesser absorption from the palms and soles), skin temperature or hydrational state (greater with increased skin temperature, or increased hydration), the age of the patient (children have a greater surface area:mass ratio and increased systemic effects), the use of occlusive dressings, the vehicle, application frequency, and length of treatment. Approximately 12–30 g is sufficient to cover the adult body one time. (*See* Topical Corticosteroids Comparison Chart.)

Adverse Reactions. Adverse reactions occur more frequently with increasing product potency and include local burning, itching, irritation, erythema, dryness, folliculitis, hypertrichosis, acneiform eruptions, hypopigmentation, rosacea, skin atrophy, striae, telangiectasias, purpura, perioral dermatitis, overgrowth of skin bacteria and fungi, allergic contact dermatitis, and cataracts or glaucoma with prolonged application around the eye. Systemically, there may be enough absorption of potent steroids to cause suppression of the HPA axis, causing symptoms of Cushing's syndrome, and growth retardation, particularly in young children.

TOPICAL CORTICOSTEROIDS COMPARISON CHART

CLASS AND DRUG	BRAND NAMES	DOSAGE FORMS	STRENGTHS
LOW-POTENCY AGENTS (Modest anti-inflammatory effects. Safest for chronic application, face and intertriginous areas, use under occlusion, and use on young children and infants.)			
Aclometasone Dipropionate	Aclovate	Cream, Ointment	0.05%
Desonide	Tridesilon, Various	Ointment	0.05%
Fluocinolone Acetonide	Various	Cream	0.01%
Hydrocortisone	Hytone, Various	Cream, Lotion, Ointment, Solution, Foam	0.5–2.5%
Hydrocortisone Acetate	Various	Cream, Ointment	0.5, 1%
MEDIUM-POTENCY AGENTS (Effective for moderate inflammatory dermatoses [eg, chronic eczematous dermatoses]. May be used for a limited duration of time on the face and intertriginous areas.)			
Betamethasone Valerate	Valisone, Various	Cream Lotion Ointment	0.01–0.1% 0.1% 0.1%
Desoximetasone	Topicort, Various	Cream	0.05%
Fluocinolone Acetonide	Synalar, Various	Cream, Ointment, Solution	0.01, 0.025% 0.01%
Hydrocortisone Valerate	Westcort	Cream, Ointment	0.2%
Mometasone Furoate	Elocon	Cream, Lotion, Ointment	0.1%
Triamcinolone Acetonide	Aristocort, Kenalog	Cream, Lotion, Ointment	0.025%, 0.1%
HIGH-POTENCY AGENTS (May be used for more severe eczematous dermatoses [eg, lichen simplex chronicus, psoriasis]. May be used for intermediate duration, with the exception of areas of thickened skin and chronic conditions. May be used on the face or in intertriginous areas for short periods of time.)			
Amcinonide	Cyclocort	Ointment	0.1%
Betamethasone Dipropionate	Diprosone, Various	Cream, Ointment	0.05%
Desoximetasone	Topicort	Cream	0.25%
Diflorasone Diacetate	Psorcon, Various	Ointment	0.05%
Fluocinolone Acetonide	Synalar-HP	Cream	0.2%

(*continued*)

TOPICAL CORTICOSTEROIDS COMPARISON CHART (continued)

CLASS AND DRUG	BRAND NAMES	DOSAGE FORMS	STRENGTHS
Fluocinonide	Lidex, Various	Cream, Gel, Ointment	0.05%
Halcinonide	Halog	Cream, Ointment	0.1%
Triamcinolone Acetonide	Aristocort, Kenalog	Cream, Ointment	0.5%

VERY–HIGH-POTENCY AGENTS (Used primarily as an alternative to systemic corticosteroids when local areas are involved. Used on thick, chronic lesions of psoriasis, lichen simplex chronicus, or discoid lupus erythematosus. Skin atrophy is likely. Use for short duration on small areas. Do not use with occlusive dressings.)

Betamethasone Dipropionate, Augmented	Diprolene	Cream	0.05%
Clobetasol Propionate	Temovate	Cream	0.05%
Diflorasone Diacetate	Psorcon	Ointment	0.05%
Halobetasol Propionate	Ultravate	Cream, Ointment	0.05%

From references 44–48.

Antidiabetic Drugs

ACARBOSE
Precose

Pharmacology. Acarbose is an oral α-glucosidase inhibitor indicated for the management of hyperglycemia caused by type 2 diabetes mellitus. Inhibition of this gut enzyme system effectively reduces the rate of complex carbohydrate digestion and the subsequent absorption of glucose, lowering postprandial glucose excursions in type 2 diabetes. In obese and nonobese patients with type 2 diabetes, acarbose monotherapy is associated with a 0.5–1% decrease in hemoglobin A_{1c}.[49] **Miglitol** (Glyset, Bayer) is an α-glucosidase inhibitor that has similar indications, uses, side effects, and dosage as acarbose. The clinical benefits, if any, of miglitol over acarbose have not been determined.

Adult Dosage. **PO for type 2 diabetes** 25 mg, tid initially, just prior to meals. Increase to 50 mg tid after 4–8 weeks, and again to 100 mg tid after 4–8 additional weeks, if necessary. Dosages >100 mg tid are not recommended because of increased risk of hepatotoxicity.

Dosage Forms. Tab 50, 100 mg.

Pharmacokinetics. The drug is poorly absorbed from the GI tract (<2%) and undergoes extensive metabolism in the GI tract via intestinal flora and digestive enzymes. All metabolites and absorbed acarbose are excreted via the kidneys. The half-life with normal renal function is about 2 hr.

Adverse Reactions. The major side effect of acarbose is flatulence. Acarbose monotherapy is not associated with hypoglycemia; however, patients managed with combination therapy (acarbose plus a sulfonylurea or insulin) may have hypoglycemia secondary to the other drug. In this setting, do not manage hypoglycemia with a complex carbohydrate (eg, sucrose), but rather with oral glucose (if the patient is conscious) or IV glucose or glucagon (if the patient is unconscious). Attempting to manage hypoglycemia with oral sugar sources other than glucose is not effective in acarbose-treated patients and may have grave consequences. Acarbose is contraindicated in patients with inflammatory bowel disease, colonic ulceration, obstructive bowel disorders, type 1 diabetes, or in those with a history of diabetic ketoacidosis. Acarbose is not recommended in patients with a Cr_s >2 mg/dL, because it may accumulate in serum and long-term studies have not been performed in this population. Use the drug with caution in patients with disorders of digestion or absorption or those with a medical condition that might deteriorate with increased intestinal gas formation.

ALDOSE REDUCTASE INHIBITORS

Prolonged hyperglycemia causes excess flux of glucose into tissues, and glucose is shunted to the polyol pathway, resulting in excess sorbitol production. Excess intracellular sorbitol causes a reduction in the uptake of myoinositol and ultimately a downregulation in the Na^+/K^+-ATPase system. This process is thought to be one of the biochemical mechanisms leading to the development of neuropathy, collagen disorders, cataracts, and possibly retinopathy in diabetics. Because aldose reductase is the rate-limiting enzyme in this pathway, aldose reductase inhibitors are being studied as a possible means of decreasing the sorbitol-linked sequelae of diabetes.[50] Although this is a promising class of drugs, the side effects, dosage regimens, and long-term benefits are yet to be determined. **Tolrestat** (Alredase, Ayerst) has a serum half-life of 10–13 hr and has been used investigationally in doses of 100 mg bid. In one study, tolrestat was shown to reduce the rate of progression of neuropathy compared to placebo.[49] Other aldose reductase inhibitors, **epalrestat, minalrestat** (Wyeth-Ayerst), **ponalrestat** (Prodiax, Merck), **zenarestat** (Warner, Lambert), and **zopolrestat** (Alond, Pfizer), are also currently under investigation.[50,51]

BECAPLERMIN   Regranex

Pharmacology. Becaplermin is a recombinant human platelet–derived growth factor (rhPDGF-BB). Endogenous platelet–derived growth factor (PDGF) stimulates proliferation and migration of cells important to the healing process and rhPDGF-BB has similar activity to the natural compound. Becaplermin gel is indicated for the treatment of diabetic neuropathic ulcers of the lower extremities that involve the subcutaneous tissue or beyond that have an adequate blood supply.[52]

Administration and Adult Dosage. **Top for ulcer healing** the area of the ulcer determines the amount of gel to apply. (*See* chart, p. 597.) Squeeze the calculated length of gel onto the waxed paper device included in the package. Spread a thin layer (1/16 inch) over the ulcer using a tongue depressor or cotton-tipped applicator. Cover ulcer with saline-moistened dressing for 12 hr. After 12 hr, remove dressing and rinse the ulcer with saline or water to remove residual gel. Cover the ulcer with a moistened dressing (without becaplermin gel) until the next application 12 hr later. Measure ulcer size weekly or biweekly and adjust the amount of gel applied accordingly. Apply gel until the ulcer is completely healed. Reassess continued therapy for ulcers that do not decrease in size by 30% after 10 weeks of treatment or those that do not completely heal in 20 weeks. (*See* Notes.)

Special Populations. *Pediatric Dosage.* (<16 yr) safety and efficacy not established; (≥16 yr) same as adult dosage.

Geriatric Dosage. Same as adult dosage.

DOSAGE GUIDELINES IN INCHES

Tube Size	Formula[a]
2 g	Length × Width × 1.3
7.5 or 15 g	Length × Width × 0.6

Example: If the ulcer measures 1 inch by 2 inches, then apply a 2.6-inch length of gel if the 2-g tube is used (1 × 2 × 1.3 = 2.6), or 1.2 inch if the 7.5- or 15-g tube is used (1 × 2 × 0.6 = 1.2).

DOSAGE GUIDELINES IN CENTIMETERS

Tube Size	Formula[a]
2 g	Length × Width ÷ 2
7.5 or 15 g	Length × Width ÷ 4

Example: If the ulcer measures 4 cm by 2 cm, then apply a 4-cm length of gel if the 2-g tube is used ([4 × 2] ÷ 2 = 4), or 2 cm if the 7.5- or 15-g tube is used ([4 × 2] ÷ 4 = 2).

---

[a]Measure the greatest length and width of the ulcer for all calculations.

Dosage Forms. Gel 100 μg/g.

Patient Instructions. Wash hands thoroughly. Do not touch tip of tube to the ulcer or other surface. Squeeze the calculated length of gel onto a clean surface such as waxed paper. Apply a thin layer (thickness of a dime) once daily with an application aid such as a tongue depressor or cotton swab. Cover the ulcer with a moistened dressing for 12 hours. After 12 hours remove dressing and rinse ulcer site. Place moistened dressing over ulcer for an additional 12 hours (no gel applied). Store the tube of gel in refrigerator.

Missed Doses. If you miss a dose, apply it as soon as you remember. If it is almost time for the next application, apply that dose only. Do not double the dose or apply extra.

Pharmacokinetics. *Fate.* Systemic absorption is erratic with some patients having nonquantifiable levels, while others have baseline levels that may or may not vary during the treatment period. In rats, systemic bioavailability is less than 3%.

Adverse Reactions. Erythematous rash occurs in 2% of patients, possibly caused by preservatives. No increase of infections, cellulitis, or osteomyelitis has occurred.

Contraindications. Known neoplasm at application site.

Precautions. For external use only. Use with caution in patients allergic to parabens or m-cresol.

Parameters to Monitor. Measure ulcer size weekly or biweekly.

Notes. Good ulcer care including sharp debridement, pressure relief, and infection control should accompany the use of becaplermin gel.[52]

GLUCAGON   Gluca Gen, Various

Pharmacology. Glucagon is a counter-regulatory hormone that increases blood glucose levels by induction of glycogenolysis. It is indicated for the treatment of the unconscious hypoglycemic patient, but it is effective only in patients with adequate hepatic glycogen stores. Glucagon has also been used as a bowel relaxant during diagnostic procedures and in overdosage with β-blockers or calcium-channel blockers.

Adult Dosage. IM, SC, or IV for hypoglycemia 0.5–1 mg. Response is usually observed in 10–20 min.

Dosage Forms. Inj 1, 10 mg.

Adverse Reactions. Glucagon occasionally causes nausea and vomiting, so position patients to prevent aspiration. Administration of glucagon may occasionally result in generalized allergic reactions such as urticaria, respiratory distress, and hypotension. Glucagon may also precipitate hypertensive crisis in the patient with underlying pheochromocytoma (secondary to release of catecholamines).

INSULINS

Pharmacology. Insulin promotes cellular uptake of glucose, fatty acids, and amino acids, and their conversion to glycogen, triglycerides, and proteins. Beef and pork insulins are extracted and purified from the animal's pancreas. Human insulin is produced either by recombinant DNA technology or by enzymatic conversion of pork insulin to human. No differences in side effects or long-term control of diabetes have been observed between human insulin and highly purified pork insulin.

Administration and Adult Dosage. SC for type 1 diabetes usual initial dosage ranges from 0.6–0.75 unit/kg/day in divided doses.[53] During the first week of therapy, the dosage requirement may escalate to 1 unit/kg/day in divided doses because of insulin resistance and the usual age group (adolescents) being treated. The dosage requirement may temporarily decrease to 0.1–0.5 unit/kg/day if the patient experiences a "honeymoon phase." Dosage adjustments are made on the basis of clinical symptoms, blood glucose levels, and hemoglobin A_{1c} values. Insulin may be administered by various methods depending on a number of factors. Single daily SC injections of intermediate-acting insulin are often used, but should not usually be used in the type 1 patient, because although single daily injections may offer protection from diabetic ketoacidosis, they are not sufficient to prevent long-term complications. Intensive forms of insulin therapy, which may provide better glycemic control, include the split-and-mixed regimen (2 SC injections daily of mixed short- and long-acting insulin), multiple daily SC doses of short-acting insulin in combination with a single injection of long-acting insulin, and insulin pump therapy. **IV, SC, or IM for diabetic ketoacidosis (IV preferred for**

patients in shock) 0.1 unit/kg, followed by a continuous infusion of 0.1–0.2 unit/hr/kg. If the serum glucose does not change in the first hour, double the insulin rate, with further adjustments in insulin dosage based on glucose levels.[54] Fluid and electrolyte repletion must accompany insulin therapy. **SC for type 2 diabetes** those who require insulin (patients unresponsive to oral agent therapy or patients with extreme hyperglycemia [fasting serum glucose >200–225 mg/dL]) may need as little as 5–10 units/day or more than 100 units/day.[54] Patients who require <30 units/day may be well controlled with 1 injection/day of intermediate-acting insulin; patients who require more than 30 units/day should be treated with 2 or more injections per day. Insulin resistance in the type 2 population is usually associated with obesity. Weight reduction and improved glycemic control usually improve insulin response.

Special Populations. *Pediatric Dosage.* (*See* Administration and Adult Dosage.) **Common maintenance dosages** are 0.6–0.9 unit/kg/day in divided doses in prepubertal children, up to 1.5 units/kg/day during puberty, and <1 unit/kg/day after puberty. Requirements may occasionally be as high as 200 units/day during growth spurts.

Geriatric Dosage. Same as adult dosage.

Other Conditions. Insulin requirements may be decreased in patients with renal or hepatic impairment, or hypothyroidism. Requirements may be increased during pregnancy (especially in the second and third trimesters), in patients with high fever, hyperthyroidism, or severe infections; and following trauma or surgery.

Dosage Forms. (*See* Insulins Comparison Chart.)

Patient Instructions. Instruct patients in the following areas: use of insulin syringes and needles; storage, mixing, and handling of insulin; urine ketone testing; blood glucose testing; adherence to proper diet and regular meals; personal hygiene (especially the feet); and recognition and treatment of hypoglycemia and hyperglycemia. (*See* Sulfonylurea Agents.)

Pharmacokinetics. *Onset and Duration.* Human insulin is more soluble than animal source insulins and may have a shorter onset and duration of action. (*See* Insulins Comparison Chart.)

Serum Levels. Diabetics vary widely in their response to insulin, and serum levels are not normally monitored clinically.

Fate. The rate of absorption depends on the insulin type. (*See* Insulins Comparison Chart.) Serum levels are affected by obesity, diet, degree of activity, pancreatic β-cell activity, growth hormone, and circulating antibodies. Insulin is primarily metabolized in the liver, although the kidneys are responsible for the metabolism of up to 50% of the daily insulin output.[55]

$t_{1/2}$. (Regular insulin) 4–5 min after IV administration.

Adverse Reactions. Hypoglycemia is dose related. Patients being treated with intensive insulin regimens of 3 or more injections/day are more prone to hypoglycemic episodes than are patients treated with the conventional 1–2 injections/day.[56] Local allergic reactions, with an onset of 15 min–4 hr, are usually caused by insulin impurities, and 70% of these patients have a history of interrupted treatment. Immune or nonimmune insulin resistance occurs occasionally. Lipohypertrophy at the injection site may occur, especially with repeated use of the same site. Lipoatrophy may also occur at the injection site and may be less frequent with the highly purified animal or human insulins. Allergy, resistance, and lipoatrophy may be overcome by switching to a more highly purified product (eg, human insulin). In general, pork insulin is less antigenic than beef-pork or pure beef insulin (neither is available in the United States) because it is more structurally similar to human insulin, which is the least immunogenic.[57]

Contraindications. Hypoglycemic episodes.

Precautions. Use with caution in patients with renal or hepatic disease, or hypothyroidism. Insulin requirements may change with exercise or infection, or when switching animal sources or to more purified products.

Drug Interactions. Alcohol may produce hypoglycemia, especially in fasting patients; moderate increases in blood glucose may occur in nonfasting patients. Oral contraceptives, corticosteroids, furosemide, niacin (large doses), diazoxide, thiazide diuretics, and thyroid hormones (large doses) may increase insulin requirements. Anabolic steroids may decrease the insulin requirement. Avoid MAOIs in diabetics because they may interfere with the normal adrenergic response to hypoglycemia, prolonging the action of antidiabetic agents. β-Blockers prolong hypoglycemic episodes and inhibit tachycardia and tremors, which are signs of hypoglycemia (sweating is not inhibited); hypertension may occur during hypoglycemia; cardioselective β-blockers (eg, atenolol, metoprolol) are less likely to cause problems than nonselective types (eg, nadolol, propranolol).

Parameters to Monitor. Monitor blood glucose routinely. (*See* Blood Glucose Monitors Comparison Chart.) Long-term diabetic control is best monitored using hemoglobin A_{1c}.[53] The patient should continually watch for subjective symptoms of hypoglycemia and hyperglycemia. Observe for signs of lipoatrophy, lipohypertrophy, and allergic reactions.

Notes. Insulin is stable for 1–2 months at constant room temperature and up to 24 months under refrigeration. Insulin is adsorbed by glass and plastic IV infusion equipment, with little difference between glass and plastic; maximal adsorption occurs within 15 sec. Adsorption may be minimized by the addition of small amounts (1–2%) of **albumin** to the infusion container; however, this may be costly and unnecessary because patient response is generally adequate without addition of albumin. Variation can be minimized by flushing all new IV administration equipment with 50 mL of the insulin-containing solution (thereby saturating "binding sites") before it is used.[58]

Pump devices are available to deliver insulin depending on or independent of a measured serum glucose level. "Open-loop" devices can deliver insulin at a constant rate and can be manually controlled. "Closed-loop" devices (the "artificial pancreas") can deliver insulin at variable rates in response to serum glucose, but are used only in the experimental setting.

Novel forms of insulin delivery are currently under investigation, with inhaled insulin showing the most promise. Pulmonary tissue provides a large absorptive surface for insulin. Insulin can effectively be delivered as an inhaled aerosol and in one study had an onset of action that was 23 min earlier than SC regular insulin, and sustained its action for >3 hr. Ninety-nine units of inhaled insulin were metabolically equivalent to 10 units of SC insulin.[59]

Human insulin is the insulin of choice for patients with insulin resistance, pregnancy, or allergy, new insulin-dependent patients, or any patient taking insulin intermittently.

INSULIN ANALOGUES

Insulin injected SC does not result in serum insulin concentrations that mimic normal physiologic insulin response. Over 30 human insulin analogues with differing pharmacokinetic profiles have been produced using recombinant DNA technology. The goal of insulin analogue research is to produce a human insulin analogue with a rapid action (to provide bolus postprandial insulin) and a human insulin analogue with a slow, extended release pattern (to provide basal insulin). **Insulin lispro** (Humalog) is a rapid-acting analogue with a pharmacokinetic profile between that of IV and SC regular human insulin. It has an onset in 15 min or less, a peak at 1–2 hr and a duration of 2–4 hr. Humalog offers a pharmacokinetic profile that is superior to regular human insulin when used to cover postprandial glycemic excursions. Long-acting analogues (eg, **insulin glargine**—Hoechst Marion Roussel) are also being evaluated.[60] Humalog is available as injection 100 units/mL.

INSULINS COMPARISON CHART[a]

PRODUCT	MANUFACTURER	STRENGTH
SHORT-ACTING (ONSET, 0.5–2 HR; PEAK, 3–4 HR; DURATION, 4–8 HR)		
Pork		
Iletin II Regular	Lilly	U-100, U-500
Purified Pork Regular	Novo/Nordisk	U-100
Human		
Humalog[b]	Lilly	U-100
Humulin Regular	Lilly	U-100
Novolin R	Novo/Nordisk	U-100
Velosulin	Novo/Nordisk	U-100
INTERMEDIATE-ACTING (ONSET, 2–4 HR; PEAK, 8–14 HR; DURATION, 14–24 HR)		
Pork		
Iletin II Lente	Lilly	U-100
Iletin II NPH	Lilly	U-100
Purified Pork Lente	Novo/Nordisk	U-100
Purified Pork NPH	Novo/Nordisk	U-100
Human		
Humulin L (Lente)	Lilly	U-100
Humulin N (NPH)	Lilly	U-100
Novolin L (Lente)	Novo/Nordisk	U-100
Novolin N (NPH)	Novo/Nordisk	U-100

(*continued*)

INSULINS COMPARISON CHART[a] (continued)

PRODUCT	MANUFACTURER	STRENGTH
LONG ACTING (ONSET, 6–14 HR; PEAK, NONE; DURATION, 20–30 HR)		
Human		
Humulin U (Ultralente)	Lilly	U-100
FIXED COMBINATIONS[c] (ONSET, 0.5–1 HR; PEAK, 3–10 HR; DURATION, 14–18 HR)		
Human		
Humulin 70/30[c]	Lilly	U-100
Novolin 70/30[c]	Novo/Nordisk	U-100
Humulin 50/50[c]	Lilly	U-100

[a]There may be variations within the ranges of onset, peak, and duration among manufacturers. Onset and duration may be prolonged in long-standing diabetes, and large doses may have prolonged durations of action. Site of injection, depth of injection, and whether site is exercised, massaged, or has heat applied to it also affect rate of insulin absorption. Human insulins have a slightly more rapid onset and a shorter duration of action than animal-derived insulins.

[b]SC Humalog is more rapidly absorbed and has a shorter duration than other human insulins (onset, 0–0.25 hr; peak, 1–2 hr; duration, 2–4 hr).

[c]These products contain isophane and regular insulin in the specified proportions; the first number designates the percentage of isophane insulin and the second designates the percentage of regular insulin.

From references 53, 56, and product information.

METFORMIN   Glucophage

Pharmacology. Metformin is a biguanide antihyperglycemic agent used in the management of type 2 diabetes mellitus. It does not affect insulin secretion, but rather reduces hepatic glucose production and enhances glucose utilization by muscle. Reported increases in glucose utilization in muscle are 7–35%. In addition to blood glucose reductions (mean 53 mg/dL), metformin may also have beneficial effects on serum lipids.[61] (*See* Notes.)

Administration and Adult Dosage. **PO for type 2 diabetes** initiate 500 mg tablets with a dosage of 1 tablet bid with the morning and evening meals. Increase dosage in 500 mg/day increments at weekly intervals, to a maximum of 2.5 g/day. Initiate 850 mg tablets with 1 tablet/day before the morning meal. Increase dosage in 850 mg/day increments q 2 weeks, to a maximum of 850 mg tid. Individualize maintenance dosage based on glycemic response. Give all dosages up to 2 g/day in 2 divided doses; larger dosages require a tid regimen to reduce GI discomfort.

Special Populations. *Pediatric Dosage.* Safety and efficacy not established.

Geriatric Dosage. Initial and maintenance dosages should be lower in the elderly. Avoid usual maximum adult dosage. Metformin should not be started in patients ≥80 years of age unless renal function is normal.

Dosage Forms. **Tab** 500, 850 mg.

Patient Instructions. Take metformin just prior to meals in order to reduce gastrointestinal side effects (diarrhea, nausea, and heartburn). Contact your physician if gastrointestinal side effects persist. Do not take metformin if you develop a serious medical condition such as myocardial infarction, stroke, or serious infection; require surgery; consume excessive amounts of alcohol; or require x-ray procedures with contrast dyes. Discontinue metformin and contact your health care provider immediately if hyperventilation, muscle pain, malaise, or unexplained drowsiness, or other unusual symptoms occur that may indicate the development of lactic acidosis.

Missed Doses. Take as soon as possible, unless near time of next dose. Do not double doses.

Pharmacokinetics. *Serum Levels.* Not monitored clinically.

Fate. Absorption half-life is 0.9–2.6 hr; absolute bioavailability is 50–60%. Peak serum levels are 1–2 mg/L in patients with type 2 diabetes. Plasma protein binding is negligible; V_d is 654 ± 358 L after a single 850 mg oral dose; Cl is proportional to renal function. Metformin is excreted in the urine unchanged.[61]

$t_{½}$. 1.7–4.5 hr in patients with normal renal function.[61]

Adverse Reactions. Acute side effects may occur in as many as 30% of patients treated with metformin. The side effects include primarily GI complaints, such as diarrhea, abdominal discomfort, nausea, anorexia, and metallic taste. GI side effects are usually transient and dose related, and can be mitigated by giving the drug just prior to meals, initiating therapy with small doses, and increasing the dosage slowly. Metformin reduces serum **vitamin B_{12}** levels in approximately 7% of patients, but is rarely associated with anemia. If vitamin B_{12} deficiency anemia occurs, it may be treated with vitamin B_{12} supplementation or by discontinuing metformin. Lactic acidosis has been reported; however, almost all cases occur in patients in whom metformin was contraindicated or in patients who attempted suicide by overdose. Lactic acidosis occurs in 0.03 case/1000 patient-yr, with fatalities in about 50% of cases.[61]

Contraindications. Patients with acute or chronic metabolic acidosis; patients undergoing radiographic studies requiring contrast media (withhold metformin for 48 hr after contrast media administration); abnormal Cl_{cr} or Cr_s >1.5 mg/dL in males or >1.4 mg/dL in females; any disease that can cause hypoxia and could result in accumulation of lactate (eg, CHF requiring pharmacologic treatment, myocardial infarction, severe infections, stroke); or hepatic dysfunction.

Precautions. Avoid in pregnancy and lactation.

Drug Interactions. Furosemide and nifedipine increase serum levels of metformin, the clinical relevance of which is unknown. Cimetidine reduces the tubular secretion of metformin and may increase peak serum concentrations by as much as 60%.[62] (*See also* Insulin Drug Interactions.)

Parameters to Monitor. Monitor renal function, hepatic function, and CBC prior to initiation of therapy and at least annually thereafter. Monitor renal function more closely in the elderly because of the age-related changes in renal function and greater risk for acute renal failure. (*See* Contraindications.) The goal of therapy is to reduce fasting blood glucose and glycosylated hemoglobin levels to normal or near normal using the lowest effective dosage of the drug.

Notes. Because of its effect on weight and lipids, metformin is an appropriate choice for initial monotherapy in obese, new-onset type 2 diabetic patients, whereas **sulfonylureas** are usually a better choice for nonobese patients. In patients who do not respond to metformin monotherapy, combination therapy with a sulfonylurea may be effective. Weight loss has been associated with metformin therapy (mean 0.8 kg); weight gain (mean 2.8 kg) has been found in patients treated with sulfonylureas.[63] Reductions in total cholesterol, LDL cholesterol, and triglycerides of 5, 8, and 16%, respectively, and an increase of 2% in HDL cholesterol have been reported.

REPAGLINIDE
Prandin

Pharmacology. Repaglinide is a meglitinide agent that stimulates insulin release from the pancreas, although it is structurally unrelated to sulfonylureas. Compared to the sulfonylureas, repaglinide has a quicker onset of action and a shorter duration of action, thereby resulting in a lower risk of prolonged hypoglycemia.[64]

Administration and Adult Dosage. **PO for type 2 diabetes** newly treated patients with HbA_{1c} <8% should start with 0.5 mg within 30 min before each meal. Patients previously treated with antidiabetic agents should start with 1 or 2 mg within 30 min before each meal. Increase dosage based on glycemic response, to a maximum of 4 mg/dose or 16 mg/day. Starting doses of repaglinide are unchanged when taken concurrently with metformin.

Special Populations. *Pediatric Dosage.* Safety and efficacy not established.

Geriatric Dosage. Dosage adjustment is not needed unless renal function is compromised. However, the elderly are more sensitive to hypoglycemia and should be monitored closely with initiation of therapy.

Other Conditions. No adjustment of the initial dosage is required in renal impairment, but use caution with subsequent dosage increases. In patients with hepatic abnormalities, wait longer before increasing the dosage.

Dosage Forms. **Tab** 0.5, 1, 2 mg.

Patient Instructions. Take each dose 0 to 30 minutes before each meal, usually 15 minutes. Recognize signs and symptoms of hypoglycemia and treat accordingly. Skip your dose if you will miss a meal. Add a dose when you eat an extra meal.

Missed Doses. If you miss a dose, take your regular dose at your next scheduled meal. Do not double the dose.

Pharmacokinetics. *Fate.* Oral bioavailability is 56%. Peak plasma concentrations occur within 1 hr; food reduces mean peak concentration by 20%, although time to peak concentration is not altered. Serum concentrations are higher and prolonged in those with liver impairment. Plasma protein binding is >98%. V_d is 31 L; Cl is 38 L/hr. The drug is primarily metabolized in the liver by CYP3A4 to inactive metabolites excreted in the feces.

$t_{1/2}$. About 1 hr.

Adverse Reactions. The most frequent side effect is hypoglycemia. Upper respiratory infections, sinusitis, nausea, diarrhea, constipation, arthralgia, and headache have also been reported, but their frequency is equal to or only slightly higher than placebo.

Contraindications. Diabetic ketoacidosis; type 1 diabetes.

Precautions. Pregnancy; lactation. Use cautiously in patients with renal impairment and in those at increased risk of hypoglycemia, including those with hepatic or adrenal insufficiency and in debilitated, elderly, or malnourished patients. Hypoglycemia is more frequent in treatment of previously untreated patients and in those with HbA$_{lc}$ <8%.[65]

Drug Interactions. Inhibitors of CYP3A4 (eg, ketoconazole, miconazole, erythromycin) inhibit the metabolism of repaglinide. CYP3A4 inducers (eg, troglitazone, rifampin, barbiturates, carbamazepine) may reduce serum levels of repaglinide.

Parameters to Monitor. Monitor fasting blood glucose and HbA$_{lc}$ periodically.

SULFONYLUREA AGENTS

Pharmacology. Sulfonylureas acutely enhance insulin secretion from pancreatic β cells and potentiate insulin action on several extrahepatic tissues. Long-term, sulfonylureas increase peripheral utilization of glucose, suppress hepatic gluconeogenesis, and possibly increase the sensitivity and/or number of peripheral insulin receptors. Second-generation sulfonylureas (eg, **glyburide, glipizide**) are more potent than first-generation agents and are used in much smaller dosages, with lower resultant blood levels. These lower serum concentrations decrease the likelihood of protein-binding displacement and hepatic metabolic interference.

Administration and Adult Dosage. (*See* Sulfonylurea Agents Comparison Chart.)

Special Populations. *Pediatric Dosage.* Not used in children.

Geriatric Dosage. Start at lower end of dosage range and slowly titrate upward if needed. Observe precautions with renal or hepatic impairment.

Other Conditions. Dosage alterations may be necessary with all sulfonylureas in patients with severe hepatic dysfunction. With renal disease, especially in geriatric patients, there is an increased duration of action with **chlorpropamide, acetohexamide,** and possibly **glyburide.**[66]

Dosage Forms. (*See* Sulfonylurea Agents Comparison Chart.)

Patient Instructions. Eat an approved diet consistently on a day-to-day basis. Take this medication at the same time each day (in the morning for once-daily medications). Report factors that might alter blood glucose levels (eg, infection, fasting states) as well as any side effects.

Missed Doses. Take a missed dose as soon as you remember unless it is near time of the next dose. Do not double doses.

Pharmacokinetics. (*See* Sulfonylurea Agents Comparison Chart.)

Adverse Reactions. Hypoglycemic reactions (especially with **chlorpropamide**), anorexia, nausea, vomiting, diarrhea, allergic skin reactions, and cholestatic jaundice occur occasionally. Hematologic disorders, mild disulfiram-like reaction to alcohol, hyponatremia (most common with **chlorpropamide,** but may occur with **tolbutamide**), and bone marrow suppression occur rarely.[67]

Contraindications. Pregnancy; type 1 diabetes; juvenile, unstable, or brittle diabetes; diabetes complicated by acidosis, ketosis, diabetic coma, major surgery, severe infection, or severe trauma.

Precautions. Chlorpropamide may cause hyponatremia, particularly in elderly women taking diuretics.[68]

Drug Interactions. Drugs that have been reported to enhance sulfonylurea effects include chloramphenicol (chlorpropamide and tolbutamide), dicumarol, fluconazole (glipizide, glyburide, tolbutamide, and possibly others), sulfonamides, and high-dose salicylates. Rifampin stimulates the metabolism of tolbutamide and possible other sulfonylureas. Drugs that impair glucose tolerance include oral contraceptives, corticosteroids, thiazide diuretics, furosemide, thyroid hormones (large doses), and niacin.[69] Acute ingestion of alcohol in combination with sulfonylureas can produce severe hypoglycemia. (*See also* Insulin Drug Interactions.)

Parameters to Monitor. Monitor clinical symptoms of hyperglycemia (mainly polyphagia, polyuria, polydipsia, or numbing or tingling of feet) or hypoglycemia (hunger, nervousness, warmth, sweating, palpitations, headaches, confusion, drowsiness, anxiety, blurred vision, or paresthesias of lips). Monitor fasting serum glucose levels frequently at the initiation of therapy to gauge the adequacy of the dosage. Self-monitoring of fasting and selected postprandial blood glucose levels by the patient is also helpful. (*See* Blood Glucose Monitors Comparison Chart.) Long-term diabetic control may best be monitored using hemoglobin A_{1c}.

Notes. Sulfonylureas are usually an appropriate choice for nonobese, new-onset type 2 diabetic patients, whereas **metformin** may be more appropraite for obese type 2 patients.[70] Individualize the choice of sulfonylurea based on the patient's characteristics (eg, renal function, hepatic function, likelihood of hypoglycemia) and the pharmacokinetics of the drugs. Glyburide, glipizide, glimepiride, and chlorpropamide are more effective at lowering blood glucose than acetohexamide, tolazamide, or tolbutamide.[57] Acetohexamide, tolazamide, and tolbutamide should probably be reserved for mild hyperglycemia or in those likely to develop hypoglycemia (eg, the elderly). In patients who do not respond to sulfonylurea monotherapy, combination therapy with **insulin, metformin, troglitazone,** or **acarbose** may be effective.[70]

SULFONYLUREA AGENTS COMPARISON CHART

DRUG	DOSAGE FORMS	DAILY DOSAGE	FATE	DURATION (HR)	COMMENTS
FIRST GENERATION					
Acetohexamide Dymelor Various	Tab 250, 500 mg.	250 mg–1.5 g in 2 divided doses.	65% converted to an active metabolite (hydroxyhexamide).	12–18	May be useful in the elderly and others prone to hypoglycemia, but avoid in patients with renal dysfunction.
Chlorpropamide Diabinese Various	Tab 100, 250 mg.	100–500 mg in a single dose.	Metabolized, and 20% excreted unchanged.	24–72	Avoid in elderly and in patients with renal dysfunction. Causes disulfiram-like reaction in 30% of patients.
Tolazamide Tolinase Various	Tab 100, 250, 500 mg.	100 mg–1 g in 1–2 divided doses.	Converted to weakly active metabolites.	16–24	Delayed onset of action (3–4 hr). May be useful in the elderly and others prone to hypoglycemia.
Tolbutamide Orinase Various	Tab 500 mg.	500 mg–3 g in 2–3 divided doses.	Converted to inactive compounds.	6–12	May be useful in the elderly and others prone to hypoglycemia.

(continued)

SULFONYLUREA AGENTS COMPARISON CHART (continued)

DRUG	DOSAGE FORMS	DAILY DOSAGE	FATE	DURATION (HR)	COMMENTS
SECOND GENERATION					
Glimepiride Amaryl	Tab 1, 2, 4 mg.	1–8 mg in a single dose.	Converted to inactive and active metabolites.	24	Similar to glyburide.
Glipizide Glucotrol	Tab 5, 10 mg SR Tab 5, 10 mg.	Non-SR 5–40 mg in 1–2 divided doses. SR 5–20 mg in a single dose.	Converted to inactive metabolites.	10–24 (non-SR) 18–24 (SR)	Take non-SR product on an empty stomach.
Glyburide DiaBeta Glynase Micronase Various	Tab 1.25, 2.5, 5 mg Tab (micronized) 1.5, 3, 6 mg.	Nonmicronized 1.25–20 mg in 1–2 divided doses Micronized 0.75–12 mg in 1–2 divided doses.	Converted to inactive and active metabolites.	18–24	The micronized product (Glynase, various) offers no advantage over the nonmicronized products.

From references 67, 68 and product information.

TROGLITAZONE   Rezulin

Pharmacology. Troglitazone is a thiazolidinedione antihyperglycemic agent used to improve insulin sensitivity in patients with type 2 diabetes. Insulin-dependent glucose disposal in skeletal muscle is improved while hepatic glucose production is decreased, both contributing to troglitazone's glucose-lowering effects. Troglitazone is only effective in the presence of insulin; by itself it does not lead to hypoglycemia and does not increase insulin secretion. Because insulin is required for its action, troglitazone should not be used in patients with type 1 diabetes.[71] (*See* Notes.)

Administration and Adult Dosage. **PO for type 2 diabetes (monotherapy)** 400 or 600 mg once daily with food; after a 6–8 week trial of 400 mg/day, dosage can be increased to 600 mg/day. If no response occurs at the maximum dose of 600 mg/day other therapeutic options should be considered; **(combination therapy with insulin or a sulfonylurea)** 200 mg once daily initially, increasing q 2–4 weeks to a maximum of 600 mg/day. Dosages of insulin or sulfonylurea may need to be decreased based on the glucose-lowering response of achieved. For those on **insulin,** decrease the insulin dosage by 10–25% when fasting plasma glucose levels are <120 mg/dL.

Special Populations. *Pediatric Dosage.* Safety and efficacy not established.

Geriatric Dosage. (>65 yr) no differences in efficacy or safety; dosage adjustments are not required.

Other Conditions. No dosage adjustment is required in renal impairment.

Dosage Forms. **Tab** 200, 300, 400 mg.

Patient Instructions. Take once daily with a meal. If you are taking insulin or a sulfonylurea, you should understand the signs and symptoms of hypoglycemia and its appropriate treatment. Report any nausea, vomiting, abdominal pain, loss of appetite, or dark urine immediately to your health care provider. Because troglitazone may decrease the effectiveness of oral contraceptives, a higher contraceptive dose or alternative method may be required.

Missed Doses. If you miss a dose at the regular meal, take at the next meal. If you forget to take a dose one day, take your regular dose the next day. Do not double the dose on the next day.

Pharmacokinetics. *Fate.* Maximum plasma concentration occurs in 2–3 hr; food increases the extent of absorption by 30–85%. Steady-state serum levels are achieved in 3–5 days. Extensively bound to serum albumin (>99%). V_d is 10.5–26.5 L/kg. Metabolized in the liver to inactive compounds. Troglitazone is primarily excreted in the feces (85%).

$t_{1/2}$. 16–34 hr.

Adverse Reactions. Side effects from troglitazone are rare. Abnormal liver function tests (AST, ALT) are reported in about 2% of patients and are generally reversible on drug discontinuation. Severe hepatotoxicity requiring liver transplant or causing death is estimated to occur in 1 in 60,000 patients.

Contraindications. Troglitazone should be used cautiously in patients with hepatic disease.

Precautions. Premenopausal anovulatory individuals may resume ovulation, placing them at risk for pregnancy. Use cautiously in patients with hepatic abnormalities.

Drug Interactions. Ethinyl estradiol and norethindrone plasma concentrations are reduced by 30%, resulting in possible loss of contraceptive efficacy. Absorption of troglitazone is reduced when administered with cholestyramine.

Parameters to Monitor. Monitor serum ALT levels at the start of therapy, monthly for the first 8 months, q 2 months for the remainder of the first year, and periodically thereafter. Perform liver function tests at the first sign of hepatic dysfunction. If ALT levels are over 1.5–2 times the upper limit of normal, repeat liver function tests within 1 week, then weekly until levels return to normal or rise to 3 times the upper limit of normal, at which point discontinue troglitazone.

Notes. In type 2 diabetics on insulin therapy, troglitazone often results in a decreased requirement for **insulin.** Some patients have been able to discontinue their exogenous insulin.[71] Patients on concomitant therapy with insulin or **sulfonylureas** should not alter the doses of the latter medications until positive changes in fasting plasma glucose levels are obtained (fasting blood sugars <120 mg/dL). Troglitazone may also lower blood pressure (BP) in patients with essential hypertension. In one 8-week study, the average BP decreased from 164/94 to 146/82 in patients taking troglitazone 200 mg bid.[72]

BLOOD GLUCOSE MONITORS COMPARISON CHART

NAME AND MANUFACTURER	TEST STRIP USED	RANGE (MG/DL)	TEST TIME	FEATURES
Accu-Chek Advantage (Boehringer Mannheim)	Advantage	10–600	40 sec	No cleaning, wiping, or timing; touchable test strips; time and date; 100-value memory.
Accu-Chek Easy (Boehringer Mannheim)	Easy Test Strips	20–500	15–60 sec	Large display; 30-value memory.
Accu-Chek Instant (Boehringer Mannheim)	Instant Glucose	20–500	12 sec	No wiping or timing; 9-value memory.
Accu-Chek III (Boehringer Mannheim)	Chemstrip bG	20–500	2 min	Time and date; 20-value memory; icons to guide tester; test strips may be visually read.
CheckMate Plus (Cascade Medical)	CheckMate Plus	25–500	15–70 sec	Display provides words for guidance; no wiping or timing; data port allows downloading to a PC.
Companion 2 Sensor (Medisense)	Pen 2/Companion 2	20–600	20 sec	Same as for Pen 2 Sensor; credit-card size; large display widow.
Diascan-S (Home Diagnostics)	Diascan	10–600	90 sec	10-value memory; technique error notification.
ExacTech (Medisense)	ExacTech	40–450	30 sec	Credit-card size and shape; no wiping, timing, or cleaning; last reading recall.
ExacTech RSG (Medisense)	ExacTech RSG	40–450	30 sec	No calibration required.
Glucometer Elite Diabetes Care System (Bayer)	Glucometer Elite	20–500	30 sec	No buttons; turns on when test strip inserted; blood touched to tip of test strip is automatically drawn.
Glucometer Encore Diabetes Care System (Bayer)	Glucometer Encore	10–600	15–60 sec	10-value memory.

(continued)

611

BLOOD GLUCOSE MONITORS COMPARISON CHART (continued)

NAME AND MANUFACTURER	TEST STRIP USED	RANGE (MG/DL)	TEST TIME	FEATURES
MediSense 2 Card (Medisense)	MediSense 2 or Precision Q.I.D.	20–600	20 sec	Credit-card size, extra large display window.
MediSense 2 Pen (Medisense)	MediSense 2 or Precision Q.I.D.	20–600	20 sec	No cleaning, wiping, timing; pen size; individually wrapped test strips.
One Touch Basic (LifeScan)	Genuine One Touch	0–600	45 sec	No timing or wiping; large display.
One Touch Profile (LifeScan)	One Touch	0–600	45 sec	No timing or wiping; large display; time and date; 250-result memory; 14- and 30-day test average.
Precision Q.I.D. (MediSense)	Precision Q.I.D.	20–600	20 sec	Automatic start when small blood sample applied; OK to touch strip; large display; data-downloading capacity.
Prestige (Home Diagnostics)	Prestige	25–600	20–50 sec	Blood application outside or inside the monitor; large digital display.
Select GT (Chronimed)	Select GT	30–600	50 sec	Large display; blood application inside or outside the meter, 100-test memory.
Supreme II (Chronimed)	Supreme	30–600	50 sec	Large display; blood application inside or outside the meter; 100-test memory.
SureStep (LifeScan)	SureStep	0–500	15–30 sec	Large display; touchable test strip; 10-test memory.
ULTRA+ (Home Diagnostics)	ULTRA+	30–600	45 sec	Large digital display; test strip absorbs entire blood sample to prevent splashing.

Adapted from reference 73.

BLOOD GLUCOSE TEST STRIPS COMPARISON CHART

NAME AND MANUFACTURER	COLOR CHART INCREMENTS (MG/DL)	PROCEDURE
Chemstrip bG (Boehringer Mannheim)	20, 40, 80, 120, 180, 240, 400, 800.	Wipe after 1 min, read after 2 min.
Diascan (Home Diagnostics)	20, 40, 80, 120, 180, 300, 500, 800.	Wipe after 30 sec, read 60 sec later.
Glucostix Reagent Strips (Miles)	20, 40, 70, 110, 140, 180, 250, 400, 800.	Blot after 30 sec, read 90 sec later.
Select GT Strips (Chronimed)	Low, 20, 40, 70, 120, 180, 240, 400, high.	Wait 60 sec, turn strip over and read.
Supreme Strips (Chronimed)	Low, 20, 40, 70, 120, 180, 240, 400, high.	Wait 60 sec, turn strip over and read.

Adapted from reference 73.

613

Contraceptives

Class Instructions: Oral Contraceptives. Take drug at approximately the same time each day for maximum efficacy. This drug may be taken at bedtime or with food, milk, or an antacid if stomach upset occurs. Use an additional form of contraception concurrently during the first 7 days of the oral progestin-only products or if you do not start your oral contraceptives on day 1 of menses. If spotting occurs and no oral doses have been missed, continue to take tablets even if spotting continues. Report immediately if any of the following occur: new severe or persistent headache; blurred or loss of vision; shortness of breath; severe leg, chest, or abdominal pain; or any abnormal vaginal bleeding. Hormonal contraceptives do not protect against HIV infection or other sexually transmitted diseases.

COMBINATION ORAL CONTRACEPTIVES

Pharmacology. These products contain an estrogen, either ethinyl estradiol or mestranol, and one of several 19-nortestosterone progestins, which are taken in a cyclic fashion, usually 21 of 28 days. As contraceptives, estrogens suppress follicle-stimulating hormone and luteinizing hormone (LH) to inhibit ovulation, cause edematous endometrial changes that are hostile to implantation of the fertilized ovum, accelerate ovum transport, and produce degeneration of the corpus luteum (luteolysis). Progestins inhibit ovulation by suppression of LH, inhibit sperm capacitation, slow ovum transport, produce a thinning endometrium that hampers implantation, and cause cervical mucus changes that are hostile to sperm migration. Induction of a pseudopregnancy state and anovulation improves symptoms of endometriosis. Anovulatory dysfunctional uterine bleeding caused by unopposed estrogen or estrogen withdrawal responds to progestins. (*See* Contraception Efficacy, and Risks and Benefits of Oral Contraceptives Comparison Charts.)

Administration and Adult Dosage. PO for contraception (monophasic combinations) 1 tablet daily beginning on the first day of menses and continued for 21 days; stop for 7 days and start the next cycle of 21 tablets. Combination 28-day products (7 inert or iron tablets) are taken 1 tablet daily continuously; (multiphasic combinations) 1 tablet daily beginning on the first day of menses (Triphasil only) or manufacturer states first Sunday following the beginning of menstruation (if menstruation begins on Sunday, take first tablet on that day), although day-1 start is most effective, then 1 tablet daily for 21 or 28 days as above. **PO for contraception postpartum** start 6 weeks postpartum if not breastfeeding; lactation may prolong period of infertility. **PO for contraception postabortion** start immediately if gestation is terminated at 12 weeks or earlier; start in 1 week if gestation is terminated at 13–28 weeks. **PO for emergency postcoital contraception** (Ovral, Preven) 2 tablets taken as soon as possible after coitus, and 2 more tablets taken 12 hr later, but within 72 hr after coitus; or (Lo-Ovral) 4 tablets taken as soon as possible after coitus and 4 more taken 12 hr later, but within 72 hr after coitus.[74–76] (*See* Notes.) **PO for dysfunctional uterine bleeding (anovulatory cycles)** (any combination agent) 1 tablet daily to qid for 5–7 days for acute bleeding, then 1 tablet daily cyclically as for contraception for 3 months to prevent further bleeding.[77] **PO for dysmenorrhea or endometriosis** (any combination tablet) 1 tablet daily continuously for 15 weeks, followed by 1 drug-free week; repeat 16-week cycle for 6–12 months to induce a pseudopregnant state.[78]

Special Populations. *Geriatric Dosage.* Same as adult dosage.

Other Conditions. Discontinue oral contraceptives at least 2 weeks before elective major surgery and do not reinstitute until at least 2 weeks afterward. Stop immediately in patients undergoing emergency surgery or immobilization for long time periods; institute low-dose SC heparin or other appropriate thromboembolytic prophylaxis in the postoperative period and restart cycle 4 weeks after return to normal activities.[76] Start with an agent containing at least 50 μg estrogen in women receiving rifampin, or any cytochrome P450-inducing anticonvulsant.[74–76]

Dosage Forms. (*See* Oral Contraceptive Agents Comparison Chart.)

Patient Instructions. (*See* Class Instructions: Oral Contraceptives.) (Contraception) any menstrual irregularities and bothersome side effects should diminish after the first 3–4 cycles. Report if no menses occur for 2 months. (Acute anovulatory bleeding) expect heavy and severely cramping flow 2–4 days after stopping therapy, with normal periods thereafter.

Missed Doses. If you miss 1 active dose, take it as soon as you remember it and take the next tablet at the correct time even if you take 2 tablets on the same day or at the same time. If you miss 2 active doses in week 1 or 2, take 2 tablets on the day you remember and 2 tablets the next day. If you miss 2 active doses in week 3 or miss 3 or more active tablets, then either (if you start on day 1) start a new pack the same day, or (if you start on Sunday) take 1 tablet daily until Sunday, then start a new pack that day. Use an alternative form of contraception for the next 7 days after you miss 2 or more active doses in weeks 1, 2, or 3, or abstain from sex for the next 7 days.

Pharmacokinetics. *Onset and Duration.* Onset of contraception after 1 week of oral regimen. Dysfunctional uterine bleeding should decrease within 12–24 hr of starting regimen.[77]

Serum Levels. No correlation of estradiol or mestranol serum levels with pharmacologic activity.

Fate. There is marked intra- and interpatient variability in the pharmacokinetics of all these agents. All are concentrated in body fat and endometrium, and penetrate poorly into breast milk.[79–88] **Desogestrel** is a prodrug that undergoes extensive first-pass and possibly gut-wall metabolism to its active form, 3-ketodesogestrel. Bioavailability is $62.7 \pm 7\%$; 65% bound to albumin and 35% to sex hormone–binding globulin (SHBG); SHBG increases by about 200% during long-term use. V_d is 2.4 ± 1.1 L/kg; Cl is 0.2 ± 0.1 L/hr/kg. About 45% is recovered in urine as glucuronides (38–61%), sulfates (23–29%), and unconjugated forms (14–28%); 30.9% is recovered in feces.[79,80,89–91]

Ethinyl estradiol is rapidly absorbed, with peak concentrations in 60 ± 30 min; bioavailability is $59 \pm 13\%$.[79,84,85] It undergoes extensive small intestine and hepatic first-pass metabolism and conjugation to sulfates, and hydroxylation to active 2-hydroxylethinyl estradiol and other hydroxylated metabolites. Ethinyl estradiol is 98.5% bound to albumin and is not bound to SHBG. V_d is 5 ± 2 L/kg; reported Cl has ranged from 0.4 ± 0.2 to 1 ± 0.3 L/hr/kg. About 23–59% is excreted in urine, 30–53% in feces as glucuronides and sulfates, and 28–43% undergoes enterohepatic circulation with a rebound in estradiol levels 10–14 hr after administration.[76,79,81–85,89,91] (*See* Estradiol and Its Esters monograph for estrogen replacement.)

Ethynodiol diacetate undergoes rapid absorption and hydrolysis to norethindrone and its metabolites in vivo. (*See* Progestin-only contraceptives.) **Mestranol** approximately 54% is demethylated to ethinyl estradiol; serum levels of ethinyl estradiol after oral administration of 50 μg of mestranol are equivalent to those after 35 μg of ethinyl estradiol.[85,88] **Norgestrel/levonorgestrel, norethindrone and norethindrone acetate** (*See* Progestin-only contraceptives.) **Norethynodrel** is rapidly converted to norethindrone in vito.[81,88] (*See* Progestin-only contraceptives.) **Norgestimate** undergoes hepatic and gut metabolism to levonorgestrel ($15.4 \pm 5.4\%$), norgestrel acetate ($9.5 \pm 1.7\%$), norgestrel oxime ($10.6 \pm 1.8\%$), and $8.1 \pm 4.5\%$ as other conjugated metabolites.[82] It is not bound to SHBG. From 35 to 49% is excreted in urine (57% conjugated sulfates and glucuronides and 12% unconjugated) and 16–49% in feces.

$t_{1/2}$. (Desogestrel) α phase 1.6 hr, β phase 24 ± 5 hr;[89,90] (ethinyl estradiol) α phase 50 ± 7 min, β phase 15 ± 3 to 33 ± 10 hr;[79,89] (levonorgestrel) α phase 0.3 ± 0.2 hr, β phase 31.4 ± 18.5 hr;[78–84,87,88] (norgestimate) 16 hr, (norethindrone) α phase 0.7 ± 0.3 hr, β phase 7.6 ± 1.9 hr.[79–83,88,92]

Adverse Reactions. The risk of major congenital malformations is not increased if oral contraceptives are taken during pregnancy.[93,94] Most of the risks of oral contraceptives are minimal with the lower dosages of estrogens and newer progestins currently available.[76,94–98] (*See* Risks and Benefits of Oral Contraceptives, and Hormone Excess and Deficiency Symptomatology Comparison Charts.)

Contraindications. Known or suspected pregnancy; presence or history of thrombophlebitis or thromboembolic disorders; presence or history of carcinoma of breast or genitals, or other estrogen-dependent tumors; cerebral vascular or coronary artery disease; uncontrolled hypertension; focal migraine; markedly impaired liver function; hepatic adenoma or carcinoma; cholestatic jaundice of pregnancy or jaundice with prior pill use; undiagnosed abnormal genital bleeding; malabsorption syndrome, heavy smoking (>15 cigarettes/day) in women ≥35 yr;[76,96] polycythemia vera because of greater tendency for deep vein thrombosis. (*See* Notes.)

Precautions. Use with caution in patients with hyperlipidemia, diabetes, conditions that may be aggravated by fluid retention (eg, hypertension, convulsions, migraine, and cardiac or renal dysfunction), or severe varicosities, in adolescents in whom regular menses are not established, and during lactation.

Drug Interactions. Oral contraceptives may be less effective, resulting in increased breakthrough bleeding or pregnancy, when given with some antibiotics (eg, ampicillin, griseofulvin, metronidazole, nitrofurantoin, neomycin, penicillin, rifampin, tetracycline), or anticonvulsants (eg, barbiturates, carbamazepine, phenytoin). Administer doses of vitamin C ≥1 g/day at least 4 hr before or after oral contraceptives to avoid increasing the bioavailability of ethinyl estradiol; use caution if long-term vitamin C intake is discontinued.[76,99]

Parameters to Monitor. Complete pretreatment physical examination with special reference to blood pressure, breasts, abdomen, pelvic organs, and Pap smear at least q 1–2 yr.

Notes. The initial oral contraceptive prescribed should be a combined product (eg, Ovcon-35, Ortho-Cept, Desogen, Ortho-Novum 7/7/7, Tri-Norinyl, Ortho-Cyclen) containing the smallest effective dose of estrogen (≤35 μg ethinyl estradiol) and progestin (≤0.15 mg desogestrel or levonorgestrel, ≤1 mg norethindrone, or ≤0.25 mg norgestimate) that provides an acceptable pregnancy rate and minimizes side effects.[74,76] Prescribing oral contraceptives to smokers >35 yr requires adequate informed consent because of a doubled risk of carciovascular disease.[95,97] The health risks of pregnancy in healthy, nonsmoking women in their forties is greater than the risks of taking sub-50 μg estrogen or progestin-only contraceptives.[94,97] (*See* Risks and Benefits of Oral Contraceptives Comparison Chart.) For emergency postcoital contraception, 2 doses of Ovral is the standard of care, but might be somewhat less effective than high-dose estrogens.[100]

PROGESTIN-ONLY CONTRACEPTIVES:	
LEVONORGESTREL/NORGESTREL	Norplant, Ovrette
MEDROXYPROGESTERONE ACETATE	Depo-Provera
NORETHINDRONE	Micronor, Nor-Q.D.

Pharmacology. Norgestrel and norethindrone are 19-nortestosterone derivatives; only the 1-isomer of norgestrel (levonorgestrel) is active. Medroxyprogesterone acetate is a 17α-acetoxyprogesterone derivative with greater progestational activity and oral efficacy than native progesterone. These compounds share the actions of progestins, although progestin-only contraceptives suppress ovulation in only about 50% of cycles. (*See* Combination Oral Contraceptives.)

Administration and Adult Dosage. PO (norethindrone) 0.35 mg/day, or (norgestrel) 0.075 mg/day continuously at the same time each day, starting on the first day of menses or immediately postpartum. IM (medroxyprogesterone acetate) 150 mg q 3 months, starting within 5 days of menses or immediately postabortion or postpartum (within 5 days to 6 weeks of delivery). In breastfeeding mothers, the first dose is recommended at 6 weeks postpartum, although some clinicians give it between 3 and 6 weeks postpartum.[74,101–105] Subdermal (levonorgestrel) 216 mg (6 Norplant implants) q 5 yr; insert within 7 days of onset of menstruation, immediately postabortion, or no earlier than 6 weeks postpartum if breastfeeding; insertion and removal requires a simple surgical procedure performed by trained personnel.[106] (*See also* Progesterone.)

Dosage Forms. Tab (norethindrone) 0.35 mg (Micronor, Nor-Q.D.); (norgestrel) 0.075 mg (Ovrette). **Implant Pellet** (levonorgestrel) kit of 6 capsules each containing 36 mg (Norplant). **Inj** (medroxyprogesterone acetate) use only the 150 mg/mL dosage form of Depo-Provera for contraception.

Patient Instructions. (*See* Class Instructions: Oral Contraceptives.) Spotting and breakthrough bleeding occur more frequently than with the combination oral contraceptives during the first few months of use; notify prescriber if this persists through the third month.[74,94,106] (Depo-Provera) use an alternative form of contraception for the first 2 weeks if your first injection is more than 5 days after the start of menses. Cessation of menses is common after 1–2 years. (Norplant) use an alternative form of contraception for the first 24 hours if inserted more than 7 days after the start of menses. Irregular bleeding patterns should become more regular 9–12 months after insertion. The implants may be visible under the skin. Removal at 5 years must be done by trained personnel.

Missed Doses. (Oral) If you miss a dose, even if it is taken only 3 hours late, use an additional backup method for the next 48 hours. Take the missed dose as soon as you remember. If menses do not occur within 45 days, discontinue the contraceptive, use an alternate nonhormonal method of contraception, and make sure you are not pregnant. Because of the higher risk of failure if 1 tablet is missed every 1–2 cycles, consider changing the time of tablet taking or using a different contraceptive.

Pharmacokinetics. *Onset and Duration.* (Oral) onset after 1 week; duration 24 hr. (Depo-Provera) onset is within 24 hr if given within 5 days of menses; the drug prevents ovulation the first month of use; ovulation is inhibited for at least 14 weeks after 150 mg IM; mean interval before return of ovulation after last injection is 9 months; 70% of former users conceive within first 12 months after stopping.[80,101,102] (Norplant) onset is within 24 hr after subdermal implantation if inserted within 7 days of menses; immediately reversible once removed, normal ovulatory cycles return during first month after removal.

Serum Levels. (Ovulation inhibition) levonorgestrel 0.2 µg/L (0.64 nmol/L); medroxyprogesterone over 0.1 µg/L (0.25 nmol/L);[99–102] norethindrone 0.4 µg/L (1.34 nmol/L).[106]

Fate. **Levonorgestrel** is 99.7 ± 16% absorbed orally with no first-pass metabolism.[79–84,87] Peak serum levels occur in 1.1 ± 0.4 hr, are dose dependent, and exhibit considerable interindividual variation. Oral administration of 30 µg yields peak levels of 0.9 ± 0.7 µg/L (2.9 ± 2.2 nmol/L); 150 µg yields 3.6 ± 0.5 µg/L (11.5 ± 1.6 nmol/L); 250 µg yields 5 ± 0.5 µg/L (16 ± 1.6 nmol/L). Within 24 hr after implantation of Norplant, levonorgestrel produces serum levels greater than 0.3 µg/L (0.96 nmol/L). Release of 80 µg/day of levonorgestrel during the first 6–12 months yields levels of 0.4 ± 0.1 µg/L (1.1 ± 0.4 nmol/L); thereafter, release of 25–35 µg/day yields levels that remain above 0.28 ± 0.16 µg/L (0.9 ± 0.5 nmol/L) for the remainder of the 5 yr. Levels are unmeasurable within 48 hr after removal of the implant.[106] Levonorgestrel is concentrated in body fat and endometrium, but penetrates poorly into breast milk (approximately 10% of serum levels); it is bound 69.4% to sex hormone–binding globulin and 30% to albumin. V_d is 1.5 ± 0.4 L/kg; Cl is 0.05 ± 0.01 L/hr/kg. Conjugated glucuronides, sulfates, and unconjugated levonorgestrel and its metabolites are excreted 45% in urine and 32% in feces.[82,87] (*See* Medroxyprogesterone Acetate and Norethindrone.)

$t_{1/2}$. (Levonorgestrel) α phase 0.3 $\pm$ 0.2 hr, β phase 31.4 $\pm$ 18.5 hr;[79–84,87,88] (medroxyprogesterone acetate) about 50 days, reflecting slow IM absorption from depot; (norethindrone) α phase 0.7 $\pm$ 0.3 hr, β phase 6.4 $\pm$ 3 hr.[79–83,88,92]

Adverse Reactions. Menstrual irregularities, including spotting, breakthrough bleeding, prolonged cycles, and amenorrhea are frequent. Because ovulation is suppressed in only about 50% of cycles, functional ovarian cysts may occur. Most resolve spontaneously within 4 weeks, and surgical intervention is usually not necessary. Ectopic pregnancy occurs in 6% of all pregnancies. Low doses of progestins have minimal impact on serum glucose, insulin or lipid levels; coagulation; liver, or thyroid function; blood pressure; or cardiovascular complications.[74,94,101,102,106] (Depo-Provera) menstrual irregularities, spotting, and breakthrough bleeding are frequent in the first 12 months after IM injection; amenorrhea (after 1 yr), infertility (up to 18 months), and weight gain of 1–1.5 kg also occur. Reversible reduced bone density changes occur with over 5 yr of use as contraceptive, but there is no clinical evidence of fractures. Long-term use (>5 yr) does not increase the overall risk of ovarian, liver, breast, or cervical cancer, but reduces the risk of endometrial cancer for at least 8 yr after stopping.[94,101,102,107] (Norplant) the most frequent adverse effects include irregular menstrual bleeding, headaches, weight gain, mood changes and depression, premenstrual bilateral mastalgia, galactorrhea (especially upon discontinuation of lactation), acne, outbreaks of genital herpes in patients with a previous history. Rarely, rash, implant expulsions, and local complications (eg, infection, hematoma formation, irritation, allergic reactions to adhesives) occur.[106–109]

Contraindications. Thrombophlebitis or history of deep vein thrombophlebitis or thromboembolic disorders; known or suspected carcinoma of the breast or endometrium, or other estrogen-dependent tumors; undiagnosed abnormal genital bleeding. Known or suspected pregnancy is a contraindication, but the risk of congenital malformations is not increased when progestin-only contraceptives are taken during pregnancy.[94,103] Although acute liver disease, benign or malignant liver tumors, history of cholestatic jaundice of pregnancy, or jaundice with prior hormonal contraceptive use are listed as contraindications by manufacturers, liver disease is not considered by others to be a contraindication to progestin-only contraceptives.[94]

Precautions. Use with caution in patients with a history of depression, diabetes, gestational diabetes, coronary artery disease, cerebrovascular disease, hyperlipidemia, liver disease, or hypertension. Although progestins are not harmful to the fetus during the first 4 months of pregnancy, confirm a negative pregnancy test before reinjecting women >2 weeks late for their IM injection.[94,103] Progestin-only contraceptives used during breastfeeding are unlikely to pose any risk to the infant,[94,101–105] and they usually do not decrease breast milk production if begun after 6 weeks postpartum.

Drug Interactions. Rifampin and cytochrome P450–inducing anticonvulsants can decrease efficacy. Long-term use of griseofulvin can increase menstrual irregularities.[74,94,101,102,106]

Parameters to Monitor. Complete pretreatment physical examination with special reference to blood pressure, breasts, abdomen, pelvic organs, and Pap smear at least q 1–2 yr.

Notes. Progestin-only contraceptives are the hormonal contraceptives of choice during breastfeeding or in patients with contraindications to estrogen therapy (eg, hypertension, diabetes, hyperlipidemia, smokers).[74,94,101,102] Long-term noncontraceptive benefits of IM medroxyprogesterone acetate include decreases in menstrual blood loss, anemia, candidal vulvovaginitis, pelvic inflammatory disease, and endometrial cancer. A 30% reduction in seizure frequency was observed in a small group of women with uncontrolled seizures who became amenorrheic with medroxyprogesterone.[101,102]

CONTRACEPTION EFFICACY COMPARISON CHART

METHOD	AVERAGE PREGNANCY RATES PER 100 WOMAN-YR
Oral Monophasic Combination	
<30 µg ethinyl estradiol (EE)[a]	0.75
35–49 µg EE	0.27
50 µg EE	0.16
Oral Multiphasic Combination	0.33
Oral Progestin Only[a]	
Age 25–30 yr	3.1
Age 30–34 yr	2.0
Age 35–39	1.0
Age >40 yr	0.3
Lactating	0.3
Subdermal Progestin Implant	0.2
Injectable Depot Progestin	0.3
Emergency Postcoital (within 72 hr of intercourse)	
Ovral 2 tablets q 12 hr for 2 doses	0.2–2.5[b]
Ethinyl estradiol 5 mg/day for 5 days	0.5–1.6[b]
Intrauterine Device	
Copper T 380	0.5
Progestasert	2.9
Barrier Method	
Diaphragm	1.9
Condom[c]	3.6
Vaginal Sponge	10
Cervical Cap	13
Vaginal Spermicide (cream, foam, jelly)	11.9
Other	
Tubal Sterilization	<1
Coitus Interruptus	6.7
Rhythm	15.5
Abstinence Method	70

[a]Mestranol 50 µg is approximately equal to 35 µg of ethinyl estradiol.
[b]Postcoital contraception numbers represent the percentage of women in whom pregnancies occur.
[c]Protects against most sexually transmitted diseases.
From references 74, 75, 93, 94, 102, 106, and 110–112.

ORAL CONTRACEPTIVE AGENTS COMPARISON CHART

| | | | | POTENCY[d] | | | BREAKTHROUGH |
PRODUCT	CYCLE[a]	ESTROGEN[b]	PROGESTIN[c]	Estrogenic[e]	Progestational[f]	Androgenic[g]	BLEEDING AND SPOTTING (%)[h]
MONOPHASIC COMBINATION AGENTS CONTAINING <50 µg OF ESTROGEN							
Alesse, Levlite	21, 28	Ethinyl estradiol 20 µg.	Levonorgestrel 0.1 mg.	+	+	+	8
Loestrin 1/20	21, 28	Ethinyl estradiol 20 µg.	Norethindrone acetate 1 mg.	+	++	++	25
Desogen, Ortho-Cept	21, 28	Ethinyl estradiol 30 µg.	Desogestrel 0.15 mg.	+	+	±	4
Loestrin 1.5/30	21, 28	Ethinyl estradiol 30 µg.	Norethindrone acetate 1.5 mg.	+	+++	+++	31
Levlen, Levora, Nordette	21, 28	Ethinyl estradiol 30 µg.	Levonorgestrel 0.15 mg.	+	+	++	14
Lo-Ovral	21, 28	Ethinyl estradiol 30 µg.	Norgestrel 0.3 mg.	+	+	++	10
Brevicon, ModiCon, Various	21, 28	Ethinyl estradiol 35 µg.	Norethindrone 0.5 mg.	++	+	+	15
Ovcon-35	21, 28	Ethinyl estradiol 35 µg.	Norethindrone 0.4 mg.	++	+	+	19
Demulen 1/35, Zovia	21, 28	Ethinyl estradiol 35 µg.	Ethynodiol diacetate 1 mg.	+	++	+	38

(continued)

ORAL CONTRACEPTIVE AGENTS COMPARISON CHART (continued)

PRODUCT	CYCLE[a]	ESTROGEN[b]	PROGESTIN[c]	Estrogenic[e]	Progestational[f]	Androgenic[g]	BREAKTHROUGH BLEEDING AND SPOTTING (%)[h]
Norinyl 1+35, Ortho-Novum 1/35, Various	21, 28	Ethinyl estradiol 35 µg.	Norethindrone 1 mg.	++	++	+	15
Ortho-Cyclen	21, 28	Ethinyl estradiol 35 µg.	Norgestimate 0.25 mg.	++	++	+	11
BIPHASIC[i] COMBINATION PRODUCTS CONTAINING <50 µg OF ESTROGEN							
Jenest-28	28	Ethinyl estradiol 35 µg (days 1–21).	Norethindrone 0.5 mg (days 1–7); 1 mg (days 8–21).	++	+	+	7
Mircette	28	Ethinyl estradiol 20 µg (days 1–21); 10 µg (days 24–28).	Desogestrel 0.15 mg (days 1–21).	+	+	±	12
Ortho-Novum 10/11, Various	21, 28	Ethinyl estradiol 35 µg (days 1–21).	Norethindrone 0.5 mg (days 1–10); 1 mg (days 11–21).	++	+	+	20

(continued)

ORAL CONTRACEPTIVE AGENTS COMPARISON CHART (continued)

PRODUCT	CYCLE[a]	ESTROGEN[b]	PROGESTIN[c]	Estrogenic[e]	POTENCY[d] Progestational[f]	Androgenic[g]	BREAKTHROUGH BLEEDING AND SPOTTING (%)[h]
TRIPHASIC[c] COMBINATION PRODUCTS CONTAINING <50 μg OF ESTROGEN							
Estrostep	21, 28	Ethinyl estradiol 20 μg (days 1–5); 30 μg (days 6–12); 35 μg (days 13–21).	Norethindrone acetate 1 mg (days 1–21).	+	+	+	—
Ortho-Novum 7/7/7	21, 28	Ethinyl estradiol 35 μg (days 1–21).	Norethindrone 0.5 mg (days 1–7); 0.75 mg (days 8–14); 1 mg (days 15–21).	++	+	+	12
Ortho Tri-Cyclen	21, 28	Ethinyl estradiol 35 μg (days 1–21).	Norgestimate 0.18 mg (days 1–7); 0.215 mg (days 8–14); 0.25 mg (days 15–21).	++	+	±	9

(continued)

PRODUCT	CYCLE[a]	ESTROGEN[b]	PROGESTIN[c]	Estrogenic[e]	Progestational[f]	Androgenic[g]	BREAKTHROUGH BLEEDING AND SPOTTING (%)[h]
Tri-Norinyl	21, 28	Ethinyl estradiol 35 μg (days 1–21).	Norethindrone 0.5 mg (days 1–7); 1 mg (days 8–16); 0.5 mg (days 17–21).	++	+	+	15
Tri-Levlen, Triphasil	21, 28	Ethinyl estradiol 30 μg (days 1–6); 40 μg (days 7–11); 30 μg (days 12–21).	Levonorgestrel 0.05 mg (days 1–6); 0.075 mg (days 7–11); 0.125 mg (days 12–21).	+	+	+	15

MONOPHASIC COMBINATION AGENTS CONTAINING 50 μg OF ESTROGEN

PRODUCT	CYCLE[a]	ESTROGEN[b]	PROGESTIN[c]	Estrogenic[e]	Progestational[f]	Androgenic[g]	BREAKTHROUGH BLEEDING AND SPOTTING (%)[h]
Norinyl 1 + 50, Ortho-Novum 1/50, Various	21, 28	Mestranol 50 μg.	Norethindrone 1 mg.	++	++	+	11
Demulen 1/50, Zovia	21, 28	Ethinyl estradiol 50 μg.	Ethynodiol diacetate 1 mg.	+	++	+	13

(continued)

ORAL CONTRACEPTIVE AGENTS COMPARISON CHART (continued)

PRODUCT	CYCLE[a]	ESTROGEN[b]	PROGESTIN[c]	POTENCY[d] Estrogenic[e]	POTENCY[d] Progestational[f]	POTENCY[d] Androgenic[g]	BREAKTHROUGH BLEEDING AND SPOTTING (%)[h]
Ovcon-50	21, 28	Ethinyl estradiol 50 μg.	Norethindrone 1 mg.	++	++	++	12
Ovral	21, 28	Ethinyl estradiol 50 μg.	Norgestrel 0.5 mg.	++	+++	+++	5
PROGESTIN ONLY							
Micronor, Nor-Q.D.	Continuous	None	Norethindrone 0.35 mg.	0	+++	+	42
Ovrette	Continuous	None	Norgestrel 0.075 mg.	0	+	+	35
POSTCOITAL							
Preven	2 doses of 2 tablets each (*See* monograph)	Ethinyl estradiol 50 μg.	Levonorgestrel 0.25 mg.	—	—	—	—

+++ = High; ++ = moderate; + = Low; ± = Very low.

[a] 28-day cycles contain 7 inert or iron tablets to complete the 28-day cycle.

[b] Estrogen equivalent potency: ethinyl estradiol is about 1.5 times as potent as mestranol. Inhibition of ovulation requires 50 μg of ethinyl estradiol or 80 μg of mestranol.

(continued)

ORAL CONTRACEPTIVE AGENTS COMPARISON CHART (continued)

[c] Most products contain either norethindrone or norgestrel. Norethindrone may be preferred over norgestrel, which has a marked adverse effect on lipid profile (decreased HDL, increased LDL). Only levonorgestrel is biologically active and exists in newer preparations. Older preparations contain norgestrel, which also has an inactive d-isomer. Desogestrel and norgestimate have positive effects on lipids.

[d] Potency designations are based on laboratory tests of individual components. Applicability of these methods for combination products used clinically has been questioned.

[e] Overall estrogenic effect as modified by antiestrogenic or estrogenic effect of progestational component. Relative estrogenic potency as measured by affinity for estrogen receptor (all are relatively weak); norethynodrel > ethynodiol diacetate > norethindrone acetate > norethindrone > levonorgestrel/norgestimate/desogestrel. Antiestrogenic potency: norethindrone acetate > levonorgestrel > ethynodiol diacetate > norethynodrel > norgestimate > desogestrel.

[f] Progestational potency as measured by delay of menses test. Relative progestogenic potency: norgestimate > desogestrel > levonorgestrel > norethindrone > norethindrone acetate > ethynodiol diacetate > norethynodrel.

[g] Relative androgenic potency (prostate growth in rats): levonorgestrel > norethindrone > norethindrone acetate > ethynodiol diacetate > norethynodrel > norgestimate > desogestrel.

[h] Prevalence of breakthrough bleeding (BTB) decreases from the first cycle to third cycle by 50–66% per cycle; these figures represent data submitted to FDA on prevalence of BTB in the third cycle of use. BTB can result from either estrogen or progestin deficiency. Bleeding decreases after the first 6 months of use regardless of the formulation used.

[i] Bi- and triphasic compounds are overall estrogen dominant.

From references 74, 76, 83, and 95.

RISKS AND BENEFITS OF ORAL CONTRACEPTIVES COMPARISON CHART

CONDITION	CLINICAL INFORMATION	COMMENTS
RISKS		
Breast Cancer	Controversial. Overall, lifetime risk is not increased. A meta-analysis of 27 studies indicates a relative risk of 1.16 after 4–12 yr of use. The relative risk is increased to 3 if started in teenage years and duration is >10 yr.	Further information required regarding risk with progestin-only contraceptives.
Cerebrovascular Accidents	Risk of hemorrhagic stroke is increased 2.5-fold compared to nonusers; ever-users have a 1.5-fold risk compared to never-users. Risk is mostly in heavy smokers >35 yr and with predisposing risk factors (eg, hypertension, diabetes, hyperlipidemia). Odds ratio is 2.9 with combined oral contraceptives (OCs) containing 50 μg of estrogen, 1.8 for combined OCs with 30–40 μg estrogen, and 0.9 for progestin-only products.	Related to both the estrogen and progestin components. Minimal risk with 35 μg/day and progestin-only preparations.
Cervical Cancer	Increased risk of cervical erosions, eversions, dysplasias, and conversion to cancer in situ. Relative risk is 1.8–2.1 times that of nonusers and increased with duration of use over 5 yr; other risk factors include multiple sexual partners and early sexual activity.	May increase risk of herpes or papillomavirus infection, which accelerate progression of preinvasive lesions.
Gallbladder Disease	Relative risk of 1.36 for gallstones in users compared to nonusers only during the first 4 yr of use, then risk returns to baseline.	Estrogens increase cholesterol saturation.
Hepatic Tumors	Both benign and malignant tumors reported. Relative risk is 2.6 for users; 9.6 with duration of use over 5 yr. Shock can result from rupture of mass. Surgical intervention may be needed, because tumors are not always reversible after discontinuation. Risk is greater in smokers and those with a history of hepatitis B infection or diabetes.	Unknown, although mestranol and higher-dosage formulations are implicated. Progestin-only contraceptives not implicated.

(continued)

CONDITION	CLINICAL INFORMATION	COMMENTS
Hyperglycemia	Abnormal glucose tolerance found in predisposed individuals (eg, subclinical or gestational diabetes) and rare cases of diabetic ketoacidosis reported. These effects are minimal with combinations containing ≤35 µg/day of ethinyl estradiol or newer progestins. Norgestrel has greatest insulin-antagonizing activity.	Hyperinsulinemia with relative insulin resistance caused by progestins with minimal effect from estrogens.
Hyperlipidemia	Elevated triglycerides; may precipitate pancreatitis in patients with underlying hyperlipidemia; adverse effects on lipids are greatest with progestin-dominant products, especially levonorgestrel and ethynodiol diacetate, and lowest with norgestimate and desogestrel.	Estrogens increase triglycerides and HDL; progestins increase LDL and decrease HDL. Minimal effect with progestin-only products.
Hypertension	Mild BP elevations of 4 mm Hg systolic and 1 mm Hg diastolic, usually reversible upon drug discontinuation, occur in 1–5% of users. Rare with low-dose products. More common in older women and in those with a family history of hypertension.	Related to both estrogen and progestin components. Consider progestin-only contraceptives.
Infertility	Little risk of permanent sterility. Conception rate after discontinuation may temporarily lag behind that of nonusers for a few months.	Risk concentrated in older women with a long history of contraceptive use.
Myocardial Infarction	No increased risk in healthy nonsmokers; risk is increased 2.8 times that of nonusers in smokers >35 yr with presence of other predisposing factors (eg, hyperlipidemia, diabetes, hypertension). Relative risk of 1.9 for current and past users of low-dose products.	Questionably thromboembolic because risk reverses after drug discontinuation.

(continued)

RISKS AND BENEFITS OF ORAL CONTRACEPTIVES COMPARISON CHART (continued)

CONDITION	CLINICAL INFORMATION	COMMENTS
Postpill Amenorrhea	Prevalence is 0.2–2.6% after use; check for pituitary tumor in presence of galactorrhea.	Risk is increased if menses were irregular prior to starting. Unrelated to duration or dose.
Thromboembolism and Thrombophlebitis	Risk is increased 2.8-fold that of nonuser; risk is concentrated in smokers, sedentary females >50 yr, and duration of use >5 yr. Desogestrel-containing products have a 2-fold risk compared with other progestins and 4- to 5-fold that of nonusers. Minimal risk with progestin-only products.	Related to desogestrel and to estrogen dose. Estrogens decrease antithrombin III and increase coagulation factors and platelet aggregation.
Teratogenesis	No increased risk of congenital cardiac, limb, or other malformations if oral or progestin-only contraceptives taken during pregnancy. Reports of masculinization of female genitalia reported when high doses of progestin were used for threatened abortion.	Exhaustive review of 18 prospective studies and meta-analysis of 12 prospective cohorts show relative risk of 0.99–1.04.
BENEFITS[a]		
Breast Disease	A 50–75% reduction in fibrocystic disease and fibroadenoma with >2 yr of use.	Protection greatest with progestin-dominant products. Does not prevent breast cancer.
Endometrial Cancer	A 54–72% reduction in endometrial cancer with ≥2 yr of continuous use. Benefit persists for as long as 15 yr after drug discontinuation. Greatest effects in nulliparous women.	Progestin component protective against endometrial adenomatous hyperplasia (precursor to adeno cancer) by opposing estrogen effect.
Ovarian Cancer	A 30% risk reduction with duration of use ≤4 yr, 60% risk reduction with >5 yr, 80% risk reduction with >12 yr of use compared to nonusers. Protection persists for 10 yr after drug discontinuation.	Mechanism unknown.

(continued)

RISKS AND BENEFITS OF ORAL CONTRACEPTIVES COMPARISON CHART (continued)

CONDITION	CLINICAL INFORMATION	COMMENTS
Ovarian Cysts	An 80–90% risk reduction.	Less protection with triphasics and low-dose products.
Pelvic Inflammatory Disease/Ectopic Pregnancy	Risk reduction of 50–70% with >1 yr of use and beneficial reduction of ectopic pregnancy rate.	Does not protect against gonorrhea or chlamydial cervicitis.
Menstrual Cycle Effects	A 90% improvement in dysmenorrhea and 50% reduced risk of iron deficiency anemia. Reduction in premenstrual symptoms (eg, anxiety, depression, and headache).	Decrease in menstrual flow and menstrual fluid prostaglandins.
Acne	Combined oral contraceptives lower serum testosterone levels with improvement of acne.	Use least androgenic progestins (eg, desogestrel, norgestimate) for greatest effect.
Rheumatoid Arthritis	A 50% reduction in frequency.	Progesterone attenuates immune response.

aMost risks and benefits have been documented with the higher-dose estrogen products (>50 µg/day).
From references 74, 76, 93–98, and 110–115.

HORMONE EXCESS AND DEFICIENCY SYMPTOMATOLOGY COMPARISON CHART

CONDITION	SYMPTOMATOLOGY
Estrogen Excess[a]	Estrogen excess may also be a result of progestin deficiency. Symptoms include nausea, vomiting, vertigo, leukorrhea, increase in leiomyoma size, uterine cramps, breast tenderness with fluid retention, cystic breast changes, cholasma, edema, and fluid retention resulting in abdominal or leg pain with cyclic weight gain, headaches on pill days, and hypertension.
Estrogen Deficiency	Estrogen deficiency may also be a result of progestin excess. Symptoms include irritability, nervousness, decreased libido, hot flashes, early and midcycle breakthrough bleeding and spotting (days 1–7), atrophic vaginitis, dyspareunia, no withdrawal bleeding with continued contraceptive use, and decreased amount of withdrawal bleeding.
Progestin Excess	Progestin excess may also be a result of estrogen deficiency. Symptoms include increased appetite and weight gain on nonpill days, tiredness, fatigue, weakness, depression, decreased libido, decreased length of menstrual flow, *Candida* vaginitis, headaches on nonpill days, and breast tenderness on nonpill days.
Progestin Deficiency	Progestin deficiency may also be a result of estrogen excess. Symptoms include late breakthrough bleeding (days 8–21), heavy menstrual flow and clots, dysmenorrhea, and delayed onset of menses following last pill.
Androgen Excess	Symptoms include increased appetite and weight gain, oily scalp, acne, and hirsutism.

[a]Less likely with preparations containing <50 µg/day ethinyl estradiol.

From references 74 and 94–96.

Female Sex Hormones

ESTRADIOL AND ITS ESTERS   Alora, Climara, Combi Patch, Delestrogen,
                                      Estinyl, Estrace, Estraderm, Estring, Vivelle, Various

Pharmacology. Estradiol (17β-estradiol; E_2) is the most potent of the naturally occurring estrogens and is the major estrogen secreted during the reproductive years. Estradiol and other estrogens produce characteristic effects on specific tissues (such as breast), cause proliferation of vaginal and uterine mucosa, increase calcium deposition in bone, and accelerate epiphyseal closure following initial growth stimulation. Addition of the ethinyl radical results in an orally active compound that is 200 times more potent than estradiol. (*See* Notes.)

Administration and Adult Dosage. For patients with an intact uterus, either continuous daily or monthly (minimum of 10–12 days) administration of a progestin is recommended to induce endometrial sloughing and decrease the risk of endometrial cancer; administration of progestin quarterly (14 days of progestin q 3 months) might also be effective.[116–118] **PO for postmenopausal symptoms and atrophic vaginitis** administer daily or, if uterus is present, continuous daily or in cyclic regimen of 3 weeks on followed by 1 week off, using the smallest effective dosage (micronized estradiol) 0.5–2 mg/day initially, adjusted as necessary to control symptoms; (ethinyl estradiol) 0.02 mg/day or every other day, to a maximum of 0.05 mg/day; severe cases may require 0.05 mg tid initially until improvement, then decrease to 0.05 mg/day; administer as with micronized estradiol. **Top patch for postmenopausal symptoms or osteoporosis** initiate with 50 μg/day patch; patch is changed once (Climara) or twice (Estraderm, Vivelle) weekly and is administered continuously or cyclically (eg, for 3 weeks followed by 1 week without patch). Dosage may be increased to a 75 or 100 μg/day patch if symptoms are not controlled. Combi Patch can be used continuously or sequentially, in which a 50 μg/day estradiol-only patch is used for the first 14 days and Combi Patch is used for the second 14 days of a 28-day cycle. Start either method with the 0.14 mg norethindrone patch and change the patch twice weekly. (*See* Notes.) **Vag for postmenopausal vasomotor symptoms and atrophic vaginitis** 200–400 μg/day as micronized estradiol cream for 1–2 weeks, then reduce to 100–200 μg/day for 1–2 weeks, then to maintenance of 100 μg 1–3 times/week. **Vag for symptoms of urogenital atrophy** (Estring) insert one 2 mg ring into the upper vagina every 3 months. **PO for prevention of osteoporosis** use minimum effective dosage of 2 mg/day micronized estradiol or 20 μg/day of ethinyl estradiol, or equivalent. **PO for dysfunctional uterine bleeding** 0.05–0.1 mg/day of micronized estradiol or 10–20 μg/day of ethinyl estradiol for 10–20 days with addition of progestin the third week.[77] **PO for palliation of breast cancer in postmenopausal women** (ethinyl estradiol) 1 mg tid, or (micronized estradiol) 10 mg tid for at least 3 months. **PO for palliation of advanced inoperable prostatic cancer** (ethinyl estradiol) 0.15–2 mg/day, or (micronized estradiol) 1–2 mg tid. **IM for postmenopausal symptoms and prevention of osteoporosis** when oral or vaginal therapy does not provide expected response, is poorly tolerated, or when noncompliance occurs (estradiol cypionate) 1–5 mg q 3–4 weeks; (estradiol valerate) 10–20 mg q 4 weeks. **IM for dysfunctional uterine bleeding** (estradiol valerate) 20 mg initially, then 5 mg q 2 weeks with addition of progestin. **IM for palliation of advanced inoperable prostatic cancer** (polyestradiol phosphate) 40 mg q 2–4 weeks; (estradiol valerate) 30 mg or more q 1–2 weeks depending on patient response.

Special Populations. *Geriatric Dosage.* Same as adult dosage.

Other Conditions. Because estrogens can increase the risk of postsurgery thromboembolic complications, discontinue estrogens at least 4 weeks before surgery if feasible.

Dosage Forms. **Tab** (micronized estradiol) 0.5, 1, 2 mg; (ethinyl estradiol) 0.02, 0.05, 0.5 mg; **SR Patch** (estradiol) 25, 37.5, 50, 75, 100 μg/day; **SR Patch** (estriol) 50 μg/day plus norethindrone acetate 140 or 250 μg/day (Combi Patch). (*See* Notes.) **Vag Crm** (estradiol) 100 μg/g; **Vag Ring** (estradiol) 2 mg (Estring); **Inj** (estradiol cypionate in oil) 5 mg/mL; 2 mg/mL with testosterone cypionate 50 mg/mL (DepoTestadiol, various); (estradiol valerate in oil) 10, 20, 40 mg/mL; 2 mg/mL with testosterone enanthate 90 mg/mL (Androgyn LA, various); (polyestradiol phosphate) 40 mg/mL.

Patient Instructions. Report immediately if any of the following occur: new severe or persistent headache or vomiting; blurred or lost vision; speech impairment; calf, chest, or abdominal pain; weakness or numbness of extremities; or any abnormal vaginal bleeding. This (oral) drug may be taken with food, milk, or an antacid to minimize stomach upset. (Patch) discard the protective liner and apply the patch to a clean, dry, and intact area of skin, preferably on the abdomen. Avoid excessively hairy, oily, or irritated areas. Apply immediately after opening and press the patch firmly in place with the palm of your hand for about 10 seconds to ensure good contact, particularly around the edges. Do not apply to the breasts or the waistline. To minimize irritation, rotate sites with an interval of at least 1 week between applications to a particular site.

Pharmacokinetics. *Onset and Duration.* (Menopausal symptoms) onset of therapeutic E_2 levels after oral or vaginal administration is 0.5–1 hr, with peak levels at 5 hr and progressive decline toward baseline by 12–24 hr. Onset of relief of menopausal symptoms occurs within days of first cycle of therapy. Reductions of luteinizing hormone (LH) and follicle-stimulating hormone (FSH) levels occur within 3 hr and 6 hr, respectively, with a duration of 24 hr.[89,119] Peak E_2 levels after IM products are (valerate) 2.2 days, (cypionate) 4 days. Duration of depot products is variable following IM injection; (valerate) 14–21 days, (cypionate) 14–28 days, (polyestradiol phosphate) 14–28 days.[119,120] (Cancer) response to estradiol therapy should be apparent within 3 months after initiation of oral therapy.

Serum Levels. (Relief of menopausal symptoms) E_2 levels: apparent over 40 ng/L (147 pmol/L); 80% relief with 68 ng/L (250 pmol/L); 100% relief with 112 ng/L (411 pmol/L).[80,100,116,117,119,121,122] (Prevention of osteoporosis) 60 ng/L (220 pmol/L).

Fate. (Ethinyl estradiol) PO administration of 20 μg yields ethinyl estradiol levels of 25 ng/L (84 pmol/L); 30 μg yields 60 ng/L (202 pmol/L). (*See* Combination Oral Contraceptives.)

(Estradiol) oral bioavailability of micronized estradiol (E_2) is 4.9 ± 5% because of extensive and rapid first-pass metabolism.[123] Topical absorption may be affected by skin thickness and site of patch application: 100% (abdomen) and 85% (thigh).[100,122] Oral or vaginal administration results in unphysiologic levels of estrone ($E_1 > E_2$; E_1 is less after Vaginal than PO administration).[80,100,116,119–123] Patch yields levels of $E_2 > E_1$ (minor E_1 elevations).[100,116,119–123] Steady-state E_2 level after PO administration of 1 mg estradiol is 35 ± 5 ng/L (128 ± 18 pmol/L) or an increase of 25 ng/L (92 pmol/L) over baseline; after 2 mg, 63 ± 11 ng/L (231 ± 40 pmol/L) or 40 ng/L (147 pmol/L) over baseline; after 4 mg, 121 ± 15 ng/L (444 ± 55 pmol/L) or 50 ng/L (183 pmol/L) over baseline; after 6 mg, 207 ± 200 ng/L (760 ± 734 pmol/L).[80,119] Vaginal 0.2 mg estradiol yields 80 ± 19 ng/L (293 ± 7 pmol/L) of E_2.[119] Patch 25 μg yields 25 ng/L (92 pmol/L); 50 μg yields 38 ± 10 ng/L (138 ± 36 pmol/L); 100 μg yields 89 ± 82 ng/L (327 ± 302 pmol/L) of E_2.[100,122] (*See* Notes.)

Estradiol is about 60% bound to albumin and 38% to sex hormone–binding globulin, 3% unbound. It is widely distributed and concentrated in fat. V_d is 10.9 ± 2.9 L; Cl is 24.2 ± 7 L/hr/m^2 or 0.77 L/hr/kg.[80,119,120] Estradiol and its esters are converted in the liver, endometrium, and intestine, 15% to estrone (active), 65% to estrone sulfate and its conjugates (primarily sulfates and glucuronides with reconversion of 5% estrone and 1.4% estrone sulfate back to E_2). E_2 is excreted 50% in urine and 10% in feces, with some enterohepatic circulation. Less than 1% is excreted unchanged in urine and 50–80% as conjugates: estrone 20%, estriol 20%, estradiol glucuronide 7%.[80,119,120] (Estradiol valerate and cypionate) these are slowly hydrolyzed to E_2 and their respective free acids. (Polyestradiol phosphate) slowly hydrolyzed to E_2.

$t_{1/2}$. (Estradiol) 1 hr;[80,119,120] (ethinyl estradiol) α phase 50 ± 7 min; β phase 15 ± 3 to 33 ± 10 hr.[79–89]

Adverse Reactions. (*See* Postmenopausal Hormone Replacement Risks and Benefits Comparison Chart.) Nausea, vomiting, bloating, breast tenderness, and spotting occur frequently. (*See* Hormone Excess and Deficiency Symptomatology Comparison Chart.) Hypercalcemia occurs occasionally in patients with breast cancer. Thromboembolism, thrombophlebitis, diabetes, hypertension, and gallbladder disease are less likely to occur with hormone replacement dosages than with oral contraceptive dosages. Pain at injection site occurs frequently. Occasional redness and irritation at application site with patch; rash rarely.

Contraindications. Pregnancy; history or presence of estrogen-dependent cancer (except in appropriate patients treated for metastatic disease); undiagnosed abnormal genital bleeding; history or presence of thromboembolism or severe thrombophlebitis. A history of breast cancer may not be an absolute contraindication to estrogen therapy in women with severe menopausal symptoms.[116,124] Active or severe chronic liver disease is a contraindication for combinations with testosterone.

Precautions. Use with caution in patients with disease states that may be exacerbated by increased fluid retention (eg, asthma; epilepsy; migraine; and cardiac, hepatic, or renal dysfunction); in women with a strong family history of breast cancer or presence of fibrocystic disease, fibroadenoma, or abnormal mammogram; in women with fibromyomata, cardiovascular disease, diabetes, hypertriglyceridemia, severe liver disease, or history of jaundice during pregnancy; and in young patients in whom bone growth is not complete. Oral estrogen can increase thyroid-binding globulin and cause false elevations in total T_4 and T_3 and false depression of resin T_3 uptake while the thyroid index, thyroid-stimulating hormone, and the patient remain euthyroid. Estrace 2 mg and Estinyl 0.02 mg both contain tartrazine, which may cause allergic reactions, including bronchospasm, in susceptible individuals.

Drug Interactions. Estrogens may reduce the effects of tricyclic antidepressants and of warfarin, and may increase the effects of corticosteroids by increasing their half-lives. Barbiturates, rifampin, and other cytochrome P450 inducers may decrease estrogen levels.

Parameters to Monitor. Signs and symptoms of side effects, especially abnormal bleeding. Pretreatment and physical examination with reference to blood pressure, breasts, abdomen, pelvic organs, and Pap smear. Baseline laboratory tests should include glucose, triglycerides, cholesterol, liver function tests, and calcium. Repeat physical examination annually; repeat laboratory tests only if abnormal at baseline.

Notes. Estradiol has been advocated as the estrogen replacement of choice because it is the principal estrogen of the reproductive years; however, advantages over other estrogens have not been established. Synthetic 17α-alkylated estrogens (eg, ethinyl estradiol) are generally not recommended in menopausal replacement therapy because of their potent hepatic effects. The combination of an **androgen** with estrogen is indicated for moderate to severe vasomotor symptoms in patients not improved by estrogen alone. Potential benefits include increased libido and psychological well-being. An alternative to estrogens for hot flashes is **megestrol acetate** 20 mg bid, which reduced hot flashes by 50% during 4 weeks of use in one study.[125] The combination of **norethindrone acetate** and estradiol in a single patch (Combi Patch) results in less endometrial hyperplasia than an estradiol-only patch.

Nonoral estradiol administration (eg, patch, vaginal, implant, injection), avoids first-pass effect and theoretically results in a preferable premenopausal physiologic serum level ratio of $E_2 > E_1$. Oral administration results in an unphysiologic ratio of $E_2 < E_1$ (E_1 levels are not directly related to efficacy).[80,100,119,120,122,126] Avoiding the first-pass effect allows a smaller dosage to be used and prevents undesirable changes from liver stimulation (ie, increases in renin substrate, sex hormone–binding globulin, thyroxine-binding globulin, coagulation factors, transferrin, growth hormone levels, and cortisol-binding globulin, and a reduction in insulin-like growth factor) and their subsequent sequelae (ie, gallbladder disease, hypertension, and hypercoagulable states in some women).[100,122,126,127] Hepatic stimulation varies with oral preparations, with ethinyl estradiol > conjugated estrogens > E_2. Enhanced liver action is also responsible for the cardioprotective effects on lipids, and occurs even with vaginal estrogens.[128] Transdermal administration appears to exert favorable effects on serum lipoproteins (ie, elevation of high-density lipoproteins and depression of low-density lipoproteins) after more than 4 months of use, and protects against bone loss and fractures similarly to oral estrogens.[100,122,126,127] However, one study found no effect on lipid profile,[100] and there are no studies that evaluate long-term estradiol patch use as protection against cardiovascular disease.

Postmenopausal women most likely to develop osteoporosis are whites and Asians, whereas blacks are at less risk.[116,126,129] In women in whom estrogen replacement therapy is intolerable or contraindicated, **alendronate sodium** (Fosamax) 10 mg/day PO has increased bone mass and reduced vertebral fractures, vertebral deformities, and loss of height. It must be taken at least 30 min before the first food, beverage, or medications of the day with a full glass of plain tap water only, and the person must remain in an upright position after taking the tablet because erosive esophagitis has occurred.[130,131] A trend toward reduction in the incidence of nonvertebral fractures also occurs. Concomitant estrogen replacement and alendronate in the treatment of osteoporosis in postmenopausal women is not recommended because of limited clinical experience. **Calcitonin salmon** (Miacalcin) 200 IU/day intranasally has increased bone mass in women >5 yr postmenopausal with low bone mass who cannot take estrogens.[132] Intermittent administration of **etidronate disodium** (Didronel) 400 mg/day PO 2 hr before or after a meal for 14 days, given q 3–3.5 months, can increase bone mass and offers an effective alternative for patients unable to take estrogens. Further studies are required to determine its safety because abnormal mineralization, microfractures, increased bone pain, and increased frequency of nonvertebral fractures have been reported occasionally.[129,133] Slow-release **fluoride** (Slow Fluoride) appears to be useful in a dosage of 25 mg/day for up to 4 years, but immediate-release products are not useful because the drug is irritating to the GI tract and the new bone formed is brittle and subject to fracture.[134]

ESTROGENS, CONJUGATED	Premarin, Premphase, Prempro, Various
ESTROGENS, ESTERIFIED	Estratab, Menest, Various

Pharmacology. Conjugated estrogens contain a mixture of 50–65% sodium estrone sulfate, 20–35% sodium equilin sulfate, and other estrogenic substances obtained from the urine of pregnant mares. Esterified estrogens are a combination of 75–85% sodium estrone sulfate and 6.5–15% sodium equilin sulfate prepared from Mexican yams. (*See* Estradiol and Its Esters.)

Administration and Adult Dosage. For patients with an intact uterus, continuous daily or monthly (for a minimum of 10–12 days) administration of a progestin is recommended to induce endometrial sloughing and decrease the risk of endometrial cancer; administration of progestin quarterly (14 days of progestin q 3 months) might also be effective.[116–118] **PO for postmenopausal symptoms and atrophic vaginitis** use smallest effective dosage in the range of 0.3–1.25 mg/day continuously or, if uterus is present, in cycles of 21–25 days/month. **PO for prevention of postmenopausal osteoporosis** use minimum effective dosage of 0.625 mg/day continuously, or cyclically if uterus is present, or 0.3 mg/day if 1.5 g/day of elemental calcium is also used; higher dosages of 1.25 mg/day may be necessary following fractures caused by osteoporosis.[116] For women experiencing migraine or other symptoms during the withdrawal period, a 5-day/week regimen or a shorter withdrawal period may be used. **Vag for postmenopausal symptoms and/or atrophic vaginitis** 1.25–2.5 mg/day; (atrophic vaginitis) 0.3 mg 3 times/ week might be effective.[121] **PO for dysfunctional uterine bleeding** 1.25–2.5 mg/day for 10 days.[77] **IV (preferred) or IM for rapid cessation of dysfunctional uterine bleeding** 25 mg of conjugated estrogens, may repeat in 6–12 hr prn, to a maximum of 3 doses.[77] **IV for bleeding from uremia** 0.6 mg/kg/day diluted in 50 mL of NS and infused over 30–40 min for 5 days; dosages as high as 60 mg/day IV have been used.[135,136] **PO for palliation of breast cancer** (patients should be ≥5 yr postmenopausal) 10 mg tid. **PO for palliation of prostatic cancer** 1.25–2.5 mg tid.

Special Populations. *Geriatric Dosage.* Same as adult dosage.

Dosage Forms. Tab (conjugated) 0.3, 0.625, 0.9, 1.25, 2.5 mg; 0.625 mg with medroxyprogesterone acetate 2.5 mg (Prempro); 0.625 mg with medroxyprogesterone acetate 5 mg (Premphase); 0.625 mg with methyltestosterone 5 mg; 1.25 mg with methyltestosterone 10 mg (Premarin with methyltestosterone); (esterified) 0.3, 0.625, 1.25, 2.5 mg; 0.625 mg with testosterone 1.25 mg (Estratest H.S., Menogen H.S.); 1.25 mg with testosterone 2.5 mg (Estratest, Menogen); **Inj** (conjugated) 25 mg; **Vag Crm** (conjugated) 0.625 mg/g.

Patient Instructions. Report immediately if any of the following occur: new severe or persistent headache or vomiting; blurred or loss of vision; speech impairment; calf, chest, or abdominal pain; weakness or numbness of extremities; or any abnormal vaginal bleeding. This (oral) drug may be taken with food, milk, or an antacid to minimize stomach upset.

Pharmacokinetics. *Onset and Duration.* (Menopausal symptoms) PO peak onset of equilin sulfate is 4 hr; onset of estrone is 3 hr, with a peak of 5 hr; duration is >24 hr. After vaginal administration, onset of therapeutic estradiol levels is 3 hr and peak occurs in 6 hr, with decline over 24 hr to baseline values. Gonadotropin suppression occurs within 1 month of therapy, although suppression to premenopausal levels may not occur.[122] (Uremia) improvement in bleeding time occurs within 6 hr after starting estrogens; maximum improvement occurs within 2–5 days after initiation of estrogens; effects last 3–10 days after drug discontinuation.[135,136]

Serum Levels. (*See* Estradiol and Its Esters.)

Fate. Both conjugated equilin and estrone sulfate are rapidly absorbed and hydrolyzed to unconjugated forms when given orally or vaginally. Oral administration of 0.3 mg yields steady-state estradiol (E_2) levels of 48 ± 12 ng/L (175 ± 45 pmol/L) or an increase of 20 ng/L (73 pmol/L) over baseline; 0.625 mg yields 103 ± 33 ng/L (378 ± 120 pmol/L) or 50 ng/L (184 pmol/L) over baseline; 1.25 mg yields 125 ± 66 ng/L (460 ± 243 pmol/L) or 70 ng/L (257 pmol/L) over baseline. Vaginal administration of 0.3 mg yields steady-state E_2 levels of −7 ± 22 ng/L (−26 ± 81 pmol/L); 0.625 mg yields 36 ± 16 ng/L (131 ± 57 pmol/L); 1.25 mg yields 94 ± 44 ng/L (344 ± 161 pmol/L).[80,119,120] (Estrone sulfate) V_d is 38 ± 13 L; Cl is 3.9 ± 1.2 L/hr/m^2.[137,138] Estrone sulfate is rapidly converted to estrone and estradiol. (Equilin sulfate) Cl is 7.3 ± 4 L/hr/m^2. Approximately 30% of equilin sulfate is metabolized to active 17β-dihydroequilin sulfate and 2% to active 17β-dihydroequilin.[137] Inactivation of estrogens occurs mainly in the liver, with degradation to less active estrogenic products (eg, estrone). Metabolites are conjugated with sulfate and glucuronic acid; urinary recovery is 70–88% within 5 days after oral administration. (*See* Estradiol and Its Esters.)

$t_{1/2}$. (Estrone sulfate) α phase 3.2 ± 0.5 min; β phase 4–5 hr. (Equilin) 19–27 min. (Equilin sulfate) 190 min. (17β-dihydroequilin) α phase 5.5 ± 2 min; β phase 45 ± 5 min. (17β-dihydroequilin sulfate) α phase 5 ± 0.5 min; β phase 2.5 ± 0.6 hr.[137]

Adverse Reactions. (*See* Estradiol and Its Esters.)

Contraindications. (*See* Estradiol and Its Esters.)

Precautions. (*See* Estradiol and Its Esters.)

Drug Interactions. (*See* Estradiol and Its Esters.)

Parameters to Monitor. (*See* Estradiol and Its Esters.)

Notes. Both oral and vaginal administration result in an unphysiologic $E_1 > E_2$ ratio, although higher E_2 levels occur orally than vaginally.[119–122] (*See* Estradiol Notes, and Postmenopausal Hormone Replacement Risks and Benefits Comparison Chart.)

ESTRONE AND ITS ESTERS	Various
ESTROPIPATE	Ogen, Various

Pharmacology. Estrone (E_1) is the major estrogen produced in the post-menopausal period. It is one-half as potent as estradiol (E_2) and shares the actions of other estrogens. Estropipate is estrone sulfate stabilized with inert piperazine. (*See* Estradiol and Its Esters.)

Administration and Adult Dosage. For patients with intact uterus, either continuous daily or monthly administration (minimum of 10–12 days) of progestin is recommended to induce endometrial sloughing and decrease the risk of endometrial cancer; administration of progestin quarterly (14 days of progestin q 3 months) might also be effective.[116–118] **PO for postmenopausal symptoms and prevention of osteoporosis** (estropipate) use smallest effective dosage in the range of 0.625–5 mg/day continuously or in cycles of 21–25 days/month; administer as with conjugated estrogens. **Vag for postmenopausal symptoms and/or atrophic vaginitis** (estropipate) 3–6 mg/day. **IM for postmenopausal symptoms and prevention of osteoporosis** when oral or vaginal therapy does not provide expected response or is poorly tolerated, or when noncompliance occurs (estrone) 0.1–0.5 mg 2–3 times/week. **IM for dysfunctional uterine bleeding** (estrone) 2–5 mg/day for several days. **IM for breast cancer in postmenopausal women** (estrone) 5 mg 3 times/week. **PO for palliation of inoperable advanced prostatic cancer** (estropipate) 3–6 mg tid. **IM for inoperable advanced prostatic cancer** (estrone) 2–4 mg 2–3 times/week.

Special Populations. *Geriatric Dosage.* Same as adult dosage.

Dosage Forms. **Tab** (estropipate, as conjugated estrogens equivalent) 0.625, 1.25, 2.5, 5 mg; **Vag Crm** (estropipate) 1.5 mg/g; **Inj** (estrone) 2, 5 mg/mL.

Patient Instructions. Report immediately if any of the following occur: new severe or persistent headache or vomiting; blurred or loss of vision; speech impairment; calf, chest, or abdominal pain; weakness or numbness of extremities; or any abnormal vaginal bleeding. This (oral) drug may be taken with food, milk, or an antacid to minimize stomach upset.

Pharmacokinetics. *Fate.* Estrone is not orally active because of enzymatic degradation in the gut and liver. Addition of a piperazine moiety increases oral absorption such that E_2 levels are similar to those after administration of estradiol. Oral administration of 0.6 mg estropipate yields E_2 serum levels of 34 ng/L (124 pmol/L); 1.2 mg yields 42 ng/L (154 pmol/L).[80,119,120] Estrone is hydroxylated to α-hydroxyestrone, estriol, and 2-hydroxyestrone.[80,123] (*See* Estradiol and Its Esters.)

$t_{1/2}$. (Estrone) estimated to be 12 hr in serum; however, this does not reflect events in peripheral tissues; (estrone sulfate) 4–5 hr.[80,119,120,123]

Adverse Reactions. (*See* Estradiol and Its Esters.)

Contraindications. (*See* Estradiol and Its Esters.)

Precautions. (*See* Estradiol and Its Esters.)

Drug Interactions. (*See* Estradiol and Its Esters.)

Parameters to Monitor. (*See* Estradiol and Its Esters.)

Notes. (*See* Estradiol and Its Esters.)

RALOXIFENE   Evista

Pharmacology. Raloxifene is a selective estrogen receptor modulator similar to tamoxifen. It acts like an estrogen in the bone and like an estrogen antagonist on the breast and uterus. Raloxifene increases bone mineral density, but its effects on fracture rate is not yet known; it decreases serum LDL cholesterol levels, but does not stimulate endometrial growth.[139,140] It is also being studied for use in prevention of breast cancer.

Adult Dosage. **PO for prevention of postmenopausal osteoporosis** 60 mg once daily with supplemental calcium.

Dosage Forms. **Tab** 60 mg.

Pharmacokinetics. Oral bioavailability is 2% because of an extensive first-pass effect. It is highly bound to albumin and α_1-acid glycoprotein and has a V_d of 2348 L/kg. Cl is 40–60 L/hr/kg. The drug is metabolized to glucuronide metabolites, some of which undergo enterohepatic recycling and can be converted back to the parent drug. Metabolites are excreted primarily in feces. The half-life is about 28 hr.

Adverse Reactions. Hot flashes occur in 25–30% of women; leg cramps are also frequent. It increases the risk of venous thrombosis and is a teratogen. Raloxifene is contraindicated in women who may become pregnant, or who have a history of venous thrombotic events.

Drug Interactions. Cholestyramine (and presumably colestipol) binds raloxifene and reduces its absorption and enterohepatic recirculation. The drugs should not be coadministered. Raloxifene decreases the effect of warfarin, and PT should be monitored carefully when they are given together.

ESTROGENS COMPARISON CHART

DRUG	DOSAGE FORMS	EQUIPOTENT PHYSIOLOGIC DOSE[a,b]	COMMENTS
STEROIDAL AGENTS			
Conjugated Estrogens Premarin Various	Tab 0.3, 0.625, 0.9, 1.25, 2.5 mg Vag Crm 0.625 mg/g Inj 25 mg.	0.625 mg.	Mixture of 50–65% sodium estrone sulfate, 20–35% equilin sulfate, and other estrogenic substances from the urine of pregnant mares. Expensive; nausea is rare.
Esterified Estrogens Estratab Menest Various	Tab 0.3, 0.625, 1.25, 2.5 mg.	0.625 mg.	Similar to conjugated estrogens. Mixture of 75–85% sodium estrone sulfate and 6.5–15% sodium equilin sulfate obtained from Mexican yams.
Estradiol, Micronized Estrace	Tab 0.5, 1, 2 mg Vag Crm 100 µg/g.	1 mg.	Moderate cost; some nausea with oral; estradiol is the major estrogen secreted during the reproductive years.
Estradiol Climara Estraderm Vivelle	SR Patch 25, 37.5, 50, 75, 100 µg/day.	50 µg/day.	Estraderm contains alcohol; Climara and Vivelle do not contain alcohol and may be less irritating to the skin.
Estradiol Cypionate Depo-Estradiol Various	Inj (in oil) 5 mg/mL.	—	Pain at injection site; variable onset with a duration of 14–28 days.

(continued)

ESTROGENS COMPARISON CHART (continued)

DRUG	DOSAGE FORMS	EQUIPOTENT PHYSIOLOGIC DOSE[a,b]	COMMENTS
Estradiol Valerate Delestrogen Various	Inj (in oil) 10, 20, 40 mg/mL.	1 mg.	Pain at injection site; variable onset with a duration of 14–21 days.
Ethinyl Estradiol Estinyl Feminone	Tab 0.02, 0.05, 0.5 mg.	5 μg.	Not recommended for estrogen replacement because of its potent hepatic effects. (*See* Estradiol Notes.)
Estrone Various	Inj 2, 5 mg/mL.	0.9 mg.	No advantage over conjugated/esterified estrogens; estrone is the major estrogen of the postmenopausal years.
Estropipate Ogen Various	Tab 0.625, 1.25, 2.5, 5 mg Vag Crm 1.5 mg/g.	0.625 mg.	Ogen 0.625 mg = 0.75 mg estropipate. Ogen 1.25 mg = 1.5 mg estropipate. Ogen 2.5 mg = 3 mg estropipate. Ogen 5 mg = 6 mg estropipate.
Quinestrol Estrovis	Tab 100 mg.	—	Promoted for once-a-week estrogen therapy because it is stored in fat and gradually released.
NONSTEROIDAL AGENTS			
Chlorotrianisene Tace	Cap 12, 25 mg.	12 mg.	Expensive; weak estrogenic activity, metabolized by liver to a more active compound. Infrequently used because of long duration of action because of storage in adipose tissue.

(continued)

ESTROGENS COMPARISON CHART (continued)

DRUG	DOSAGE FORMS	EQUIPOTENT PHYSIOLOGIC DOSE[a,b]	COMMENTS
Dienestrol Various	Vag Crm 0.01%.	—	
Diethylstilbestrol Various	Tab 1, 5 mg.	0.25 mg.	Antineoplastic agent no longer indicated for estrogen replacement therapy. Inexpensive; frequent nausea.
Diethylstilbestrol Diphosphate Stilphostrol	Tab 50 mg Inj 50 mg/mL.	0.4 mg.	

[a]Potency of estrogens: estradiol > estrone > estriol. Potency is based on the effects on the liver.
[b]*See* monographs or product information for exact dosage regimens for various uses.

POSTMENOPAUSAL HORMONE REPLACEMENT RISKS AND BENEFITS COMPARISON CHART

RISKS/BENEFITS	CLINICAL INFORMATION	COMMENTS
Cancer, Breast	Controversial; no association with <5 yr duration of use to relative risk of 1.25–1.45 among current users with >5 yr duration of use; highest risk of 1.7 reported among long-term users >60 yr. No risk found in past users, regardless of duration of use. Two meta-analyses show minimal risk with >15 yr of use.	Addition of progestin does not reduce risk. Regular mammography is recommended. Consider limiting duration of treatment to <5 yr if risks of cancer outweigh cardioprotective benefits.
Cancer, Colon	A 46% decrease in colon cancer risk; no effect on rectal cancer.	In slender women, risk is reduced by up to 75%.
Cancer, Endometrial	Relative risk of 8.2 with unopposed estrogen use; risk increases with higher dosage and duration >5 yr; 34% risk after 3 yr; 20% lifetime probability of needing a hysterectomy with unopposed estrogen therapy.	Relative risk of 1 with the concurrent addition of a minimum of 10–14 days of progestin. No increased risk of estrogen hyperplasia or need for hysterectomy with concurrent progestin therapy.
Cardiovascular Disease	Three meta-analyses and a cohort study suggest a 40–50% reduction in the risk of coronary and fatal heart disease with unopposed estrogens; benefits may be greater in those with heart disease and >15 yr duration of use. Decreased lifetime probability of developing coronary artery disease. Unknown protection against stroke.	Combination with progestin may be protective, but data are insufficient. May be related to estrogen's effects on lipids or direct effect of relaxing blood vessel walls.
Hypertension	Estrogens can reduce BP.	Hormone replacement is not contraindicated in hypertension.
Lipids	Unopposed oral estrogens reduce LDL and increase HDL by 10–15%; however, estrogens can increase triglyceride levels.	Progesterone antagonizes beneficial estrogen lipid effects less than medroxyprogesterone. Most favorable effects on lipids occur with estrogen alone. Nonoral estrogens (eg, patch, vaginal) produce less HDL beneficial effects.

(continued)

POSTMENOPAUSAL HORMONE REPLACEMENT RISKS AND BENEFITS COMPARISON CHART (continued)

RISKS/BENEFITS	CLINICAL INFORMATION	COMMENTS
Gallbladder Disease	Estrogen treatment is associated with a 2.1 relative risk (RR). RR of 2.6 with >10 yr of use; RR of 2.4 for users of 1.25 mg or more of conjugated/estrified estrogen.	Mortality unaffected; may require cholecystectomy.
Osteoporosis	Inhibits bone resorption and prevents bone loss; 15–50% increase in bone density if begun within 3 yr of menopause. Osteoporosis risk increased in Caucasian and Asian ethnic groups, in sedentary lifestyle, in smokers, with low calcium and vitamin D intake, and excessive alcohol or thyroxine intake.	Alendronate (Fosamax) orally, intranasal calcitonin (Miacalcin), etidronate (Didronel), and slow-release fluoride may also be effective. (*See* Estradiol Notes.)
Fractures	One-half as many fractures of spinal and hip bones with >5 yr of use; 28% reduction with 10 yr use; 40% with 15 yr use; and 55% with 20 yr. Risk returns near baseline 6 yr or more after cessation of therapy. Decreased lifetime probability of osteoporotic fracture. Risk increases 4-fold for each 1 SD decrease in bone density at the hip; 66% of femoral neck fractures occur when bone density is below the lowest quartile.	Bone densitometry can identify women at highest risk.
Vaginal Bleeding	Unpredictable bleeding occurs in 35–40% of women with uteruses yearly.	Amenorrhea usually occurs after 6–8 months of combination estrogen/progestin therapy.

From references 116, 118, 124, 127, 129, 138, and 141–147.

MEDROXYPROGESTERONE ACETATE Depo-Provera, Provera, Various

Pharmacology. Medroxyprogesterone is a 17α-acetoxyprogesterone derivative with greater progestational effects and oral efficacy than progesterone. Progesterone transforms an estrogen-primed proliferative endometrium into a secretory endometrium.

Administration and Adult Dosage. PO for secondary amenorrhea and dysfunctional uterine bleeding, and to induce withdrawal bleeding following postmenopausal estrogen replacement therapy 5–10 mg/day for 5–10 days, depending on degree of endometrial stimulation desired, beginning on the presumed day 1–12 of the cycle (during the first week of estrogen administration). In cases of secondary amenorrhea, therapy can be started at any time. **PO for postmenopausal symptoms and osteoporosis** (combined with continuous estrogen) 2.5–5 mg/day.[148,149] (*See* Notes.) **PO for relief of vasomotor symptoms** 20 mg/day; **IM for relief of vasomotor symptoms** 150 mg/day.[150] (*See* Notes.) **IM for endometrial or renal carcinoma** 400 mg–1 g/week initially for a few weeks, then, if improvement occurs, reduce to maintenance dosage of 400 mg/month. (*See also* Progestin-Only Contraceptives.)

Special Populations. *Geriatric Dosage.* Same as adult dosage.

Dosage Forms. Tab 2.5, 5, 10 mg; **Inj** 150, 400 mg/mL.

Patient Instructions. Report immediately if any of the following occur: new severe or persistent headache; blurred vision; calf, chest, or abdominal pain; or any abnormal vaginal bleeding. This (oral) drug may be taken with food, milk, or an antacid to minimize stomach upset. (Dysfunctional uterine bleeding) expect heavy and severely cramping flow 2–4 days after stopping therapy; expect a normal period after a few days.

Pharmacokinetics. *Onset and Duration.* Withdrawal bleeding (in estrogen-primed endometrium) occurs 3–7 days after last dose.[101,102] Onset of symptomatic relief of hot flashes within 4–7 days; maximum relief after 1 month; duration 8–20 weeks after discontinuation.[150]

Serum Levels. Inhibition of ovulation and tumor response occurs with medroxyprogesterone levels >0.1 μg/L (0.25 nmol/L).[99,101,102,151]

Fate. Medroxyprogesterone acetate (MPA) is rapidly absorbed orally with no first-pass metabolism; oral bioavailability is 5.7 ± 3.8%; IM bioavailability is 2.5 ± 1.7%, with a large interpatient variation in serum levels after oral or IM administration.[80,151] Higher concentration depot formulation is associated with lower serum concentrations, but equivalent bioavailability.[152] Peak concentrations occur in 2–7 hr and are 2–10 times higher after oral than after IM depot injection. PO 10 mg yields peak levels of 3–4 μg/L (7.5–10 nmol/L), declining to 0.3–0.6 μg/L (0.8–1.5 nmol/L) by 24 hr; PO 100 mg yields 13 ± 7 μg/L (34 ± 18 nmol/L), declining to 2 μg/L (5 nmol/L) by 24 hr; PO 500 mg yields 13 ± 8 μg/L (34 ± 21 nmol/L). After 150 mg IM of the 150 mg/mL formulation, peak levels of 8.3 ± 3.2 μg/L (21 ± 8 nmol/L) occur within a few days, declining to levels of 0.8 ± 0.7 μg/L (2 ± 1.8 nmol/L) for 92 ± 44 days. After 400 mg IM of the 400 mg/mL formulation, peak serum levels of 6.2 ± 2.3 μg/L (16 ± 6 nmol/L) are achieved after 16.3 ± 15.6 days.[80,92,101,102,152] The drug is stored in fat; over 90% is protein bound to albumin; 83% of a dose is present in serum as the parent drug and conjugated medroxyprogesterone; it is hydroxylated to 6-β-hydroxy-MPA, and 21-hydroxy-MPA, which have unknown activity. From 15 to 20% of a dose is excreted in urine as glucuronide and sulfate conjugates; 45–80% is excreted in feces.[92]

$t_{1/2}$. 50 days, reflecting slow IM absorption from depot.

Adverse Reactions. Frequent breast tenderness, weight gain, and depression occur. Adverse lipid effects (increased low-density lipoproteins, decreased high-density lipoproteins) occur with dosages ≥10 mg/day; dosages of 2.5–5 mg/day have negligible effects.[118,148,152] (*See also* Progestin-Only Contraceptives, Postmenopausal Hormone Replacement Risks and Benefits Comparison Chart, and Hormone Excess and Deficiency Symptomatology Comparison Chart.)

Contraindications. Known or suspected pregnancy or as a diagnostic test for pregnancy. Thrombophlebitis, history of deep vein thrombophlebitis, or thromboembolic disorders; known or suspected carcinoma of the breast or endometrium, or other estrogen-dependent tumors; undiagnosed abnormal genital bleeding. Although acute liver disease, benign or malignant liver tumors, and history of cholestatic jaundice of pregnancy or jaundice with prior hormonal contraceptive use are listed as contraindications by manufacturers, liver disease is not considered by others to be a contraindication to progestin-only contraceptives.[94]

Precautions. Use with caution in patients with a history of depression, diabetes, gestational diabetes, coronary artery disease, cerebrovascular disease, hyperlipidemia, liver disease, or hypertension. Although progestins are not harmful to the fetus during the first 4 months of pregnancy; confirm a negative pregnancy test before reinjecting women more than 2 weeks late for their IM injection.[94,103] Progestin-only contraceptives used during breastfeeding are unlikely to pose any risk to the infant,[94,101–105] and they usually do not decrease breast milk production if begun after 6 weeks postpartum.

Drug Interactions. Rifampin and cytochrome P450-inducing anticonvulsants can increase progestin metabolism. Long-term use of griseofulvin can increase menstrual irregularities.[74,94,101,102,106]

Parameters to Monitor. Complete pretreatment physical examination with special reference to blood pressure, breasts, abdomen, pelvic organs, and Pap smear yearly.

Notes. Continuous administration of low-dose progestin and estrogen combinations in postmenopausal syndrome causes amenorrhea in more than 50% of women and does not appear to negatively influence blood lipids when compared to cyclic therapy.[118,148,149,153] Concurrent administration of estrogen with progestin for amenorrhea may be associated with less breakthrough bleeding than with progestin alone. There is no evidence that progestins are effective in preventing habitual abortion or treating threatened abortion.

NORETHINDRONE	Norlutin
NORETHINDRONE ACETATE	Aygestin, Norlutate

Pharmacology. Norethindrone and norethindrone acetate are 19-nortestosterone derivatives that share the actions of progestins. They have oral efficacy, increased progestational activity compared to progesterone, and reduced androgenic activity compared to androgens. Norethindrone acetate differs from norethindrone only in potency; the acetate is twice as potent. (*See also* Medroxyprogesterone Acetate, and Progesterone.)

Administration and Adult Dosage. PO for withdrawal bleeding following post-menopausal estrogen replacement therapy or combined for estrogen replacement therapy (norethindrone) 5–20 mg/day or (norethindrone acetate) 2.5–10 mg/day starting on day 15–20 of the cycle and continuing for 5–10 days; or (norethindrone) 1–2.5 mg/day or (norethindrone acetate) 0.5–1 mg/day continuously combined with estrogen.[148,149,153] (*See* Medroxyprogesterone Acetate Notes.) **PO for amenorrhea or abnormal uterine bleeding** (norethindrone) 5–20 mg/day, or (norethindrone acetate) 2.5–10 mg/day starting on day 5 and ending on day 25 of menses. In cases of secondary amenorrhea, therapy can be started at any time.[77] **PO for endometriosis** (norethindrone) 10 mg/day, or (norethindrone acetate) 5 mg/day for 2 weeks, increasing in (norethindrone) 5 mg/day or (norethindrone acetate) 2.5 mg/day increments q 2 weeks until a maintenance dosage of (norethindrone) 30 mg/day or (norethindrone acetate) 15 mg/day is reached.[78]

Special Populations. *Geriatric Dosage.* Same as adult dosage.

Dosage Forms. Tab (norethindrone) 5 mg (Norlutin); (norethindrone acetate) 5 mg (Aygestin, Norlutate).

Patient Instructions. Report immediately if any of the following occur: new severe or persistent headache; blurred vision; calf, chest, or abdominal pain; or any abnormal vaginal bleeding. This (oral) drug may be taken with food, milk, or an antacid to minimize stomach upset. (Dysfunctional uterine bleeding) expect heavy and severely cramping flow 2–4 days after stopping therapy; expect a normal period after a few days.

Pharmacokinetics. *Onset and Duration.* (Uterine bleeding) after oral administration, acute bleeding should decrease in 1–2 days and stop in 3–4 days. (Withdrawal bleeding) onset 3–7 days after last oral dose.[79]

Fate. (Norethindrone) marked intra- and interpatient variability in pharmacokinetics. Norethindrone and its acetate are rapidly and completely absorbed with mean bioavailability of 64 ± 16% because of first-pass metabolism.[79–83,92] Norethindrone acetate is rapidly converted to norethindrone in vivo.[79,83,85,88] Oral administration of 1 mg of norethindrone yields peak levels of 4.8 ± 0.3 to 17 ± 8 μg/L (16 ± 0.9 to 57 ± 26 nmol/L), declining to 0.4 μg/L (1.3 nmol/L) after 24 hr; 3 mg yields peak levels of 8.3 ± 0.8 μg/L (27.8 ± 2.5 nmol/L). The drug is 35.5% bound to sex hormone–binding globulin and 61% bound to albumin. It is concentrated in body fat and endometrium; breast milk levels are 10% of maternal serum levels. V_d is 4.3 ± 9 L/kg; Cl is 0.5 ± 1.5 L/hr/kg. Over 50% is eliminated in urine and

20–40% in feces as conjugated glucuronides and sulfates; less than 5% of norethindrone and its acetate are excreted as unchanged norethindrone.[79–83,88,92]

$t_{1/2}$. (Norethindrone) 6.4 ± 3 hr.[79–83,88,92]

Adverse Reactions. (*See* Medroxyprogesterone Acetate, Postmenopausal Hormone Replacement Risks and Benefits Comparison Chart, and Hormone Excess and Deficiency Symptomatology Comparison Chart.)

Contraindications. (*See* Medroxyprogesterone Acetate, and Postmenopausal Hormone Replacement Risks and Benefits Comparison Chart.)

Precautions. (*See* Medroxyprogesterone Acetate, Postmenopausal Hormone Replacement Risks and Benefits Comparison Chart, and Hormone Excess and Deficiency Symptomatology Comparison Chart.)

Drug Interactions. (*See* Medroxyprogesterone Acetate.)

Parameters to Monitor. (*See* Medroxyprogesterone Acetate.)

Notes. (*See* Medroxyprogesterone Acetate.)

PROGESTERONE	Crinone, Progestasert, Various
HYDROXYPROGESTERONE CAPROATE	Duralutin, Various

Pharmacology. Progesterone is the natural hormone that induces secretory changes in the endometrium, relaxes uterine smooth muscle, and maintains pregnancy. Hydroxyprogesterone is a natural progestin with minimal progestational activity; esterification with caproic acid produces a progestational compound more potent than progesterone with a prolonged duration of activity.

Administration and Adult Dosage. **IM for secondary amenorrhea or dysfunctional uterine bleeding** (progesterone) 5–10 mg/day for 6–8 days or (only for amenorrhea) 100–150 mg as a single dose; (hydroxyprogesterone caproate) 375 mg, may repeat in 4 weeks prn. **IM for palliation of metastatic endometrial cancer** (hydroxyprogesterone caproate) 500 mg–1 g 2–3 times/week. **Intrauterine for contraception** (progesterone) 38 mg q 12 months, releases 68 μg/day; insert at any time during menstrual cycle or within 7 days of onset of menses, immediately postabortion, or no earlier than 6 weeks postpartum if breastfeeding; insertion and removal are done by trained personnel. **Vag for progesterone supplementation** (progesterone) 90 mg daily. **PO to induce withdrawal bleeding following postmenopausal estrogen replacement therapy** (micronized progesterone) 200 mg/day for first 12 days of cycle.[118] (*See* Notes.)

Special Populations. *Geriatric Dosage.* Same as adult dosage.

Dosage Forms. **Inj** (progesterone in oil) 50 mg/mL; (hydroxyprogesterone caproate in oil) 125, 250 mg/mL; **Intrauterine** (progesterone) 38 mg (Progestasert); **Vag Gel** (progesterone 8%) 90 mg/applicatorful (Crinone).

Patient Instructions. Report immediately if any of the following occur: new severe or persistent headache; blurred vision; calf, chest, or abdominal pain; or any abnormal vaginal bleeding. (Dysfunctional uterine bleeding) expect heavy flow and severe cramping 2–4 days after injection; expect a normal period after a few days. (Progestasert only) you may experience increased menstrual flow, cramping, and spotting. Check the position of the strings monthly after each period or after abnormal cramping to ensure proper placement of the IUD. Contact your prescriber immediately if the strings are missing, if you miss a menstrual period or if you have fever, pelvic pain, severe cramping, unusual vaginal bleeding, or any signs of infection.

Pharmacokinetics. *Onset and Duration.* (Amenorrhea) onset of withdrawal bleeding occurs 48–72 hr after last dose of IM progesterone and 2 weeks after IM hydroxyprogesterone caproate; (dysfunctional uterine bleeding) onset within 6 days of IM progesterone.[77] Duration is 12–24 hr with oral progesterone, 9–17 days with IM hydroxyprogesterone caproate. (Contraception) onset within 24 hr after insertion of Progestasert.

Serum Levels. (Endometrial progestational activity [luteal phase]) 15 μg/L (48 nmol/L) or greater of progesterone.

Fate. (Progesterone) bioavailability of oral progesterone is incomplete because of first-pass metabolism with wide interpatient variation; micronized forms are somewhat better absorbed.[80,118,153,154] Higher levels of progesterone and active metabolites occur after IM, vaginal, or rectal administration, because first-pass effect is avoided. Serum levels of progesterone after oral and IM increase rapidly to reach luteal phase values within 2.4 ± 1.1 hr and remain elevated for <12 hr after oral administration and for 48 hr after IM administration. PO 100 mg micronized progesterone yields peak progesterone levels of 7 ± 3.4 μg/L (23 ± 11 nmol/L); 200 mg yields 28 ± 19 μg/L (89 ± 59 nmol/L); IM 100 mg yields 60 μg/L (192 nmol/L); Vag 200 mg bid yields 19 ± 2 μg/L (61 ± 7 nmol/L); Vag 400 mg once daily yields 29 ± 53 μg/L (93 ± 188 nmol/L).[80,153,155] Oral progesterone V_d is 850 ± 265 L/kg; Cl is 18.7 ± 38 L/hr/kg.[153] Progesterone circulates 80% bound to albumin and 17% to corticosteroid-binding globulin, and distributes into fat. It undergoes rapid gut and hepatic metabolism, with formation of active metabolites: 20α-dihydroprogesterone (25–50% of the progestational activity of progesterone), 17-hydroxyprogesterone, and 11-deoxycorticosterone (a potent mineralocorticoid).[80,156,157] Hydroxyprogesterone caproate is cleaved to form 17-hydroxyprogesterone in the body; 17-hydroxyprogesterone, whether formed from progesterone or exogenously administered, is further metabolized to 11-deoxycortisol and then cortisol. Urinary excretion of progesterone is 50–60% as 5β-pregnanediol glucuronide and other conjugated glucuronic acid or sulfate metabolites; 5–10% excreted in feces.

$t_{1/2}$. (Progesterone) α phase 5 min; β phase 32.6 ± 9.3 hr.[153]

Adverse Reactions. Local reactions and swelling at the site of progesterone injection. The beneficial effects of estrogen-increased high-density lipoprotein levels are not reversed by progesterone.[118] (*See* Postmenopausal Hormone Replacement Risks and Benefits Comparison Chart, and Hormone Excess and Deficiency Symptomatology Comparison Chart.) (Progestasert) intermenstrual spotting and menstrual bleeding irregularities, expulsion, ectopic pregnancy, uterine perforation, pelvic inflammatory disease, cramping, and pain. Intrauterine administration of contraceptive doses of progesterone has no systemic effects.[74]

Contraindications. (*See* Medroxyprogesterone Acetate.) **Progestasert** pregnancy; active, recent, or recurrent pelvic infections, including gonorrhea or *Chlamydia* infection.

Precautions. (*See* Medroxyprogesterone Acetate, and Postmenopausal Hormone Replacement Risks and Benefits Comparison Chart, and Hormone Excess and Deficiency Symptomatology Comparison Chart.)

Drug Interactions. (*See* Medroxyprogesterone Acetate.)

Parameters to Monitor. Complete pretreatment and annual physical examination with special reference to blood pressure, breasts, abdomen, pelvic organs, and Pap smear.

Notes. Progesterone is widely used in the treatment of premenstrual syndrome; however, in double-blind, controlled trials, oral micronized and vaginal progesterone were no better than placebo.[158,159]

Thyroid and Antithyroid Drugs

IODIDES   Various

Pharmacology. Iodide inhibits the synthesis and release of thyroid hormone and preoperatively decreases the size and vascularity of the hyperplastic thyroid gland. Large doses block the uptake of radioactive iodine by the thyroid gland.

Administration and Adult Dosage. PO for hyperthyroidism, as an adjunct to antithyroid agents or for preoperative thyroidectomy preparation 50–100 mg q 8 hr diluted in a glass of water, milk or juice; dosages as high as 500 mg/day have been used. Use for 7–10 days before surgery. **PO for thyroid storm** 200 mg q 6 hr. **PO for prophylaxis in radiation emergency** 100 mg iodine immediately before or within 1–2 hr after exposure and daily for 3–7 days, to a maximum of 10 days after exposure. However, administration of smaller doses of 30–50 mg iodine and continued suppression with doses of 15–50 mg/day may also be effective.[160]

Special Populations. *Pediatric Dosage.* **PO for thyrotoxicosis** 300 mg (6 drops SSKI) q 8 hr diluted as above. **PO for prophylaxis in a radiation emergency** (<1 yr) 50 mg iodine immediately before or after exposure and daily for 3–7 days, to a maximum of 10 days after exposure; (>1 yr) same as adult dosage.

Geriatric Dosage. Same as adult dosage.

Dosage Forms. Soln (SSKI) 50 mg/drop iodide (1 g/mL); (Lugol's or strong iodine) 8 mg/drop iodide (50 mg/mL iodine plus 100 mg/mL potassium iodide); (potassium iodide) 21 mg/drop iodide; **Tab** 100 mg iodide (130 mg potassium iodide); **EC Tab** not recommended.

Patient Instructions. Dilute solution in 240 mL (8 fl oz) of liquid before taking; it may be taken with food, milk, or an antacid to minimize stomach upset. Do not use if solution turns brownish-yellow. If crystals form in the solution, they may be dissolved by warming the closed container in warm water. Dissolve tablets in one-half glass of water or milk before taking. Do not use if you are breastfeeding; advise your physician if you are pregnant. Discontinue use and report if fever, skin rash, epigastric pain, or joint swelling occur.

Pharmacokinetics. *Onset and Duration.* Onset is in 24–48 hr in hyperthyroidism, with maximum effect in 10–15 days. (*See* Notes.)

Serum Levels. Iodide levels >50 μg/L (0.4 mmol/L) inhibit iodide binding by thyroid in hyperthyroidism; levels >200 μg/L (1.6 mmol/L) inhibit iodide uptake by normal thyroid.[161]

Fate. Iodide is well absorbed throughout the GI tract and concentrated in the thyroid, stomach, and salivary glands. Renal clearance is 1.8 L/hr/kg; approximately 100 μg of iodine is excreted in urine daily; fecal excretion of iodine is negligible.[161]

Adverse Reactions. Any adverse reaction warrants drug discontinuation. Goiter, hypothyroidism, and hyperthyroidism occur frequently in euthyroid patients with a history of a thyroid disorder.[162–166] Iodism occurs with prolonged use and is indicated by metallic taste, GI upset, soreness of teeth and gums, coryza, frontal headaches, painful swelling of salivary glands, diarrhea, acneiform skin eruptions, and erythema of face and chest. Rarely, hypersensitivity occurs and is manifested by angioedema, cutaneous hemorrhages, and symptoms resembling serum sickness. (*See* Precautions.)

Contraindications. Pulmonary tuberculosis; pulmonary edema.

Precautions. Pregnancy, because fetal goiter, asphyxiation, and death may occur;[166] lactation. Use iodides or iodine-containing drugs (eg, amiodarone) with caution in patients with untreated Hashimoto's thyroiditis, in iodide-deficient patients, in children with cystic fibrosis, and in euthyroid patients with a history of postpartum thyroiditis, subacute thyroiditis, amiodarone or lithium-induced thyroid disease, or Graves' disease previously treated with thioamides, radioactive iodine, or surgery because they may be particularly sensitive to iodide-induced hypothyroidism.[160–164,166] Patients with nontoxic multinodular goiters may be prone to development of hyperthyroidism.[167] Avoid iodides entirely in patients with toxic nodular goiter or toxic nodules, because thyrotoxicosis may be further aggravated.[167] Iodides are not recommended for use as expectorants because of their potential to induce acneiform eruptions, exacerbate existing lesions, and adversely affect the thyroid. Small-bowel lesions are associated with enteric-coated potassium-containing tablets, which can cause obstruction, hemorrhage, perforation, and possible death. This dosage form is not recommended.

Drug Interactions. Iodide prevents uptake of ^{131}I for several weeks and delays onset of thioamide action if given before the thioamide. Lithium may potentiate the antithyroid action of iodide. Serum iodine may be elevated if potassium-sparing diuretics are taken with potassium iodide.

Parameters to Monitor. Monitor for signs of iodism (*see* Adverse Reactions), hypothyroidism, hyperthyroidism, and parotitis occasionally during long-term use. Monitor thyroid function tests at least q 6–12 months during long-term use in patients with a family history of thyroid disease or goiter. Monitor serum potassium frequently in patients who are taking other drugs that may also affect serum potassium (eg, diuretics).

Notes. Iodide has the most rapid onset of any treatment for hyperthyroidism. In thyroid storm, iodide should theoretically be given 1 hr after the thioamide dose, but should not be withheld if oral thioamides cannot be given.[167] The therapeutic effects of iodide are variable and transient, with "escape" occurring after 10–14 days; do not use iodide alone in the therapy of hyperthyroidism.[168,169] Pharmacologic amounts of iodide can be present in serum from **radiographic contrast agents** and vaginal douches such as **povidone-iodine**.[167,170]

LEVOTHYROXINE SODIUM
Levothroid, Levoxyl, Synthroid, Various

Pharmacology. Levothyroxine is a synthetically prepared hormone identical to the thyroid hormone T_4. Thyroid hormones are responsible for normal growth, development, and energy metabolism.

Administration and Adult Dosage. **PO for replacement in hypothyroidism <6 months in duration** full replacement dosage of 1.6–1.7 μg/kg/day initially, increasing if needed and tolerated in 25–50 μg/day increments at 6- to 8-week intervals to a maintenance dosage that normalizes thyroid-stimulating hormone (TSH).[171–175] **Usual maintenance dosages** 75–100 μg/day for women and 100–150 μg/day for men. Higher mean replacement dosages are required in patients with spontaneous hypothyroidism (1.7–1.8 μg/kg/day) than in those with iatrogenic hypothyroidism after radioiodine therapy for Graves' disease (1.5–1.6 μg/kg/day).[171,174,175] **PO for suppression therapy of nodules** 100–150 μg/day initially, increasing, if necessary and tolerated, in 25–50 μg/day increments at 6- to 8-week intervals to suppress TSH to below normal, detectable limits to prevent further thyroid growth.[171,174,175] Dosages are usually higher than those required for replacement therapy. **PO for suppression therapy of thyroid cancer after thyroidectomy** 2.11 μg/kg/day initially, increasing, if needed and tolerated, in 25–50 μg/day increments at 6- to 8-week intervals to a dosage of 150–250 μg/day to suppress the TSH level to undetectable levels.[171,173–175] **IV for myxedema coma** 300–500 μg or 300 μg/m² to increase serum T_4 levels by 3–5 μg/dL (39–65 nmol/L), then 50–100 μg/day until oral administration is possible; use smaller dosages in cardiovascular disease.[171,173,175–177] **IM** indicated only for replacement therapy if patient cannot take oral medication; parenteral dosage is about 80% of oral dosage because of bioavailability difference.[171,173]

Special Populations. *Pediatric Dosage.* **PO for hypothyroidism** (preterm infants and full-term neonates to 1 yr) 10–15 μg/kg/day to normalize T_4 to greater than 10 μg/dL (129 nmol/L) within 3–4 weeks; (>1 yr) 3–5 μg/kg/day (average 3.5).[171,175,178] Adjust maintenance dosage on the basis of growth, development, and T_4 and TSH values. Replacement by at least 24 months of age corrects short stature by age 5 yr.[179]

Geriatric Dosage. (>50 yr) **PO** start with 25–50 μg/day initially, then increase if tolerated at 6- to 8-week intervals by 12.2–25 μg/day to a maintenance dosage necessary to normalize TSH; (>65 yr) less than 1 μg/kg/day may be required.[171,173,175] Poorly compliant elderly patients (mean age 86 yr) have been maintained on a twice-weekly dosing regimen; however, this regimen may be dangerous in cardiac patients.[180]

Other Conditions. In patients with cardiovascular disease or severe, long-standing (over 6 months) myxedema, **PO** 25–50 μg/day initially, increasing, if tolerated, at 6- to 8-week intervals by 12.5–25 μg/day to a maintenance dosage necessary to normalize TSH.[171,175] In patients with cardiovascular disease, particularly angina, increments should be balanced between exacerbation of angina and maintenance of euthyroidism. In some patients with severe coronary disease, incomplete control of hypothyroidism may be necessary to prevent further exacerbation of angina. During pregnancy, a 20–50% increase in dosage may be required to maintain a normal TSH level.[171–173,175]

Dosage Forms. Tab 25, 50, 75, 88, 100, 112, 125, 137, 150, 175, 200, 300 μg; Inj 200, 500 μg.

Patient Instructions. This medication must be taken regularly to maintain proper hormone levels in the body. Report immediately if chest pain (especially in elderly patients), palpitations, sweating, nervousness, or other signs of overactivity occur.

Missed Doses. Take any missed dose as soon as it is remembered, but if more than 1 dose is missed, do not double dosage.

Pharmacokinetics. *Onset and Duration.* PO onset 3–5 days; peak effect 3–4 weeks; duration after cessation of therapy 7–10 days. IV onset in myxedema coma 6–8 hr, maximum effect in 1 day.[171,176]

Serum Levels. (Physiologic and therapeutic during levothyroxine therapy) free T_4 6–21 ng/L (12–26 pmol/L); total T_4 50–120 μg/L (65–155 nmol/L). Peak free T_4 levels can be 12.7 ± 2.6%, and total T_4 levels 8.1 ± 1.2% higher than trough levels or levels obtained 10 hr after a dose.[181] Many drugs, and pathologic and physiologic states affect binding and hence may affect results of some serum level determinations.[172,182–186]

Fate. Oral bioavailability ranges from 74 ± 11% to 93 ± 25% and is affected by many factors (eg, malabsorption, diet, cholesterol-binding resins, iron, aluminum-containing products).[171,173,175] A dose of 500 μg IV increases serum T_4 levels by 3–5 μg/dL (39–65 nmol/L).[171,176] Only 0.03% is unbound in plasma. V_d is (hypothyroid) 0.17 ± 0.22 L/kg; (euthyroid) 0.16 ± 0.09 L/kg; (hyperthyroid) 0.23 ± 0.44 L/kg. Turnover is (hypothyroid) 9.2 ± 1.7%/day; (euthyroid) 11.2 ± 1.7%/day; (hyperthyroid) 21 ± 4.9%/day. Cl is (hypothyroid) 0.0008 ± 0.0033 L/hr/kg; (euthyroid) 0.00074 ± 0.0017 L/hr/kg; (hyperthyroid) 0.002 ± 0.0007 L/hr/kg.[187] About 80% is deiodinated in the body; 35% is peripherally converted to the more active T_3 and 45% to inactive reverse T_3.[171,175] Another 15–20% is conjugated in the liver to form glucuronides and sulfates, which undergo an enterohepatic recirculation with reabsorption or excretion in the feces.[185,186]

$t_{1/2}$. (Hypothyroid) 7.5 ± 7.1 days; (euthyroid) 6.2 ± 4.7 days; (hyperthyroid) 3.2 ± 1.7 days.[187,188] Protein binding affects half-life (increased binding retards elimination and decreased binding increases elimination).[185]

Adverse Reactions. Most are dose related and can be avoided by increasing the initial dosage slowly to the minimum effective maintenance dosage. Signs of overdosage include headache, palpitations, chest pain, heat intolerance, sweating, leg cramps, weight loss, diarrhea, vomiting, nervousness, and other symptoms of hyperthyroidism. Long-term thyroid administration that results in TSH suppression may predispose to osteoporosis by increasing bone resorption; at greatest risk are postmenopausal women with a past history of hyperthyroidism.[171–173,175,189]

Contraindications. Thyrotoxicosis; uncorrected adrenal insufficiency.

Precautions. Initiate and increase dosage with caution in patients with cardiovascular disease, the elderly, and in long-standing hypothyroidism. In myxedema coma, give a corticosteroid concurrently.[176] The status of other metabolic diseases, including diabetes, adrenal insufficiency, hyperadrenalism, and panhypopituitarism may be affected by changes in thyroid status.

Drug Interactions. Phenytoin, carbamazepine, and other enzyme inducers; iron; aluminum-containing products; sodium polystyrene sulfonate; and cholesterol-binding resins can increase levothyroxine requirements. The action of some drugs (eg, digoxin, warfarin, insulin) may be altered by changing thyroid status.[173,175,182,184–186]

Parameters to Monitor. (Adults) TSH, free T_4 or free T_4 index, and clinical status of the patient q 6–8 weeks initially. Monitor trough levels or obtain levels at least 10 hr after tablet ingestion to avoid transient peak effects.[181] After stabilization, monitor free T_4 or free T_4 index, TSH, and clinical status at 6- to 12-month intervals. (Children) Monitor the parameters above q 4 weeks initially and q 3–4 months after stabilization. In congenital hypothyroidism, monitor T_4 because TSH may remain elevated despite adequate replacement doses.[175,178] (>50 yr) Evaluate the replacement dosage every year and adjust downward as necessary, because dosage requirements decrease with age.[171–175]

Notes. Levothyroxine is the drug of choice for thyroid replacement because of purity, standardization, long half-life, large body pool, and close simulation to normal physiologic hormone levels. Protect from light and moisture. Subpotent levothyroxine tablets are unlikely, because of USP requirements that all tablets be standardized by high-pressure liquid chromatography to be ±10% of the labeled content.[171,175] Bioequivalence between Synthroid, Levothroid, and Levoxyl is likely.[171,173,190,191] Use of adjunctive thyroid hormones for depression and cardiopulmonary bypass is controversial.[175,192] Physiologic dosages of thyroid hormones in euthyroid patients are ineffective for weight reduction, obesity, and premenstrual tension; larger dosages may result in toxicity.[175] (*See* Thyroid Replacement Products Comparison Chart.)

LIOTHYRONINE SODIUM   Cytomel, Triostat, Various

Pharmacology. Liothyronine is a synthetic hormone identical to the thyroid hormone T_3, which is 4 times as potent by weight as T_4. (*See* Levothyroxine.)

Administration and Adult Dosage. **PO for replacement in hypothyroidism <6 months in duration** 25 μg/day initially, increasing, if needed and tolerated, in 12.5–25 μg/day increments at 1- to 2-week intervals to a maintenance dosage of 25–100 μg/day to normalize thyroid-stimulating hormone (TSH). **PO for severe hypothyroidism** 5 μg/day initially, increasing in 5–10 μg/day increments at 1–2-week intervals until 25 μg/day is reached, then increase in 12.5–25 μg/day increments at 1- to 2-week intervals until euthyroid. Dividing daily dosage into 2–3 doses may prevent wide serum level fluctuations.[184,193] **IV for myxedema coma** 25–50 μg initially, then 10–12.5 μg q 4–6 hr to a minimum of 10–15 μg q 12 hr until PO administration is possible; use smaller dosages of 10–20 μg IV initially in cardiovascular disease.[175,177] Limited experience with IV dosages over 100 μg/day. **PO**

for T₃ suppression test 75–100 μg/day in 2–3 divided doses for 7 days, then repeat ¹³¹I thyroid uptake test.

Special Populations. *Pediatric Dosage.* **PO for congenital hypothyroidism** 5 μg/day initially, increasing in 5 μg/day increments at 3- to 4-day intervals until desired effect is obtained. **Usual maintenance dosage** (<1 yr) 20 μg/day; (1–3 yr) 50 μg/day; (>3 yr) 25–100 μg/day. Levothyroxine is the drug of choice in congenital hypothyroidism.[178]

Geriatric Dosage. Not recommended because of greater potential for cardiotoxicity.[175] **PO** if used, start at 5 μg/day and increase in 5 μg/day increments at 2-week intervals, if tolerated, until desired response is obtained. (*See* Levothyroxine.)

Other Conditions. Not recommended in those with cardiovascular disease but, if used, start at PO 5 μg/day and increase in 5 μg/day increments at 2-week intervals, if tolerated, until desired response is obtained. (*Ssee* Levothyroxine.)

Dosage Forms. **Tab** 5, 25, 50 μg; **Inj** 10 μg/mL.

Patient Instructions. This medication must be taken regularly to maintain proper hormone levels in the body. Report immediately if chest pain (especially in elderly patients), palpitations, sweating, nervousness, or other signs of overactivity occur.

Missed Doses. Take any missed dose as soon as it is remembered, but if more than 1 dose is missed, do not double dosage.

Pharmacokinetics. *Onset and Duration.* PO onset 1–3 days; duration after cessation of therapy 3–5 days.

Serum Levels. During T₃ replacement, T₄ is maintained at ≤10 μg/L (13 nmol/L).[175,184,193]

Fate. Oral absorption is usually complete, but may be decreased in CHF.[184] With a typical replacement dose, T₃ has a peak of 4.5–7 μg/L (7–11 nmol/L) 1–2 hr postdose, returning to 0.88–1.6 μg/L (1.4–2.5 nmol/L) before the next dose 24 hr later.[175,184,193] V_d is (hypothyroid) 0.53 ± 0.04 L/kg; (euthyroid) 0.52 ± 0.03 L/kg; (hyperthyroid) 0.94 ± 0.07 L/kg. Turnover is (hypothyroid) 50 ± 5%/day; (euthyroid) 68 ± 11%/day; (hyperthyroid) 110 ± 22%/day. Cl is (hypothyroid) 0.012 ± 0.002 L/hr/kg; (euthyroid) 0.020 ± 0.003 L/hr/kg; (hyperthyroid) 0.043 ± 0.013 L/hr/kg.[187,188] Excreted in urine as deiodinated metabolites and their conjugates.[192]

$t_{1/2}$. (Hypothyroid) 38 ± 6 hr; (euthyroid) 25 ± 3 hr; (hyperthyroid) 17 ± 4.7 hr.[187,188]

Adverse Reactions. (*See* Levothyroxine.) Dose-related adverse effects are more likely and appear more rapidly, because regulation of dosage is more difficult than with levothyroxine. Liothyronine and its mixtures (eg, desiccated thyroid, liotrix) cause "unphysiologic" toxic peaks in serum T₃ levels not found during levothyroxine replacement therapy.[184,193]

Contraindications. (*See* Levothyroxine.)

Precautions. (*See* Levothyroxine.)

Drug Interactions. Normal serum T₃ levels are age related and can be decreased by a wide variety of pharmacologic agents (eg, amiodarone, iodinated contrast dyes, corticosteroids, propylthiouracil) or clinical circumstances (eg, malnutrition, chronic renal, hepatic, pulmonary, or cardiac disease; or acute sepsis) which impair either peripheral or pituitary T_4 to T_3 conversion.[182,184,185] (*See also* Levothyroxine Drug Interactions.)

Parameters to Monitor. Serum TSH level and T_3 level. (*See* Levothyroxine.)

Notes. Liothyronine is not considered the drug of choice for replacement therapy in hypothyroidism because of its greater expense, shorter half-life (necessitating more frequent administration), and greater potential for cardiotoxicity, and the greater difficulty of monitoring.[171–173] Some claim liothyronine to be useful in patients with myxedema coma when impairment of T_4 to T_3 conversion is suspected or in cardiac disease, because adverse effects will dissipate faster.[175–177] **Liothyronine** is the preparation of choice when thyroid supplements must be stopped prior to isotope scanning. After scanning, maintenance therapy with **levothyroxine** is recommended. The use of T_3 for psychiatric disorders and cardiopulmonary bypass is controversial.[175,192] (*See* Thyroid Replacement Products Comparison Chart.)

THYROID REPLACEMENT PRODUCTS COMPARISON CHART

DRUG	DOSAGE FORMS	EQUIVALENT DOSAGE	CONTENTS	RELATIVE ONSET AND DURATION[a]	COMMENTS
Levothyroxine Levothroid Levoxyl Synthroid Various	Tab 25, 50, 75, 88, 100, 112, 125, 137, 150, 175, 200, 300 μg. Inj 200, 500 μg.	60 μg	T_4	Long	Preparation of choice. T_4 content is now standardized using HPLC, and bioequivalence among products is likely.
Liothyronine Cytomel Triostat Various	Tab 5, 25, 50 μg Inj 10 μg/mL.	25 μg	T_3	Short	Expensive; difficult to monitor. Preparation of choice if thyroid supplements are to be stopped for isotope scanning.
Liotrix Thyrolar	Tab ¼, ½, 1, 2, 3.[b]	#1 Tab[c]	T_4 and T_3 in 4:1 ratio	Intermediate	No advantages; more costly and suffers from T_3 content. (See Thyroid, Desiccated.)
Thyroid, Desiccated Various	Tab 15, 30, 60, 90, 120, 180, 240, 300 mg.	60 mg	T_4 and T_3 in variable ratio	Intermediate	Inexpensive; allergy to animal protein rarely occurs; supraphysiologic elevations in T_3 and T_3 toxicosis may occur.

[a]With equivalent dosages.
[b]Numbers represent equivalent dosage of thyroid in grains (ie, 15, 30, 60, 120, 180 mg, respectively).
[c]Thyrolar-1 contains T_4 50 μg and T_3 12.5 μg; other strengths are in the same proportion.
From references 175 and 190.

METHIMAZOLE   Tapasole

Pharmacology. Methimazole is a thioamide antithyroid drug that interferes with the synthesis of thyroid hormones by inhibiting iodide organification. Unlike propylthiouracil (PTU), methimazole does not block peripheral conversion of T_4 to T_3. Titers of thyroid receptor–stimulating antibody (TRab) decline during therapy, suggesting an immunosuppressive effect. Methimazole is 10 times more potent than PTU on a weight basis.

Administration and Adult Dosage. PO for hyperthyroidism 30–40 mg/day as a single dose. If GI intolerance occurs, divide dosage q 8 hr initially until euthyroid (usually 6–8 weeks), then decrease by 33–50% over several weeks to a maintenance dosage of 5–15 mg/day in a single dose. Severe disease might require 2 divided doses. To prevent recurrence of hyperthyroidism, **levothyroxine** 75–100 μg/day may be added after 6 months once the patient is euthyroid; this may improve remission rates, but further study is warranted.[167,169,194–196] **PO for thyroid storm** 40–120 mg/day, divided q 8 hr until euthyroid. Traditional treatment duration for hyperthyroidism is 1–2 yr, although longer or shorter courses (eg, 6 months) might be effective.[167,169,172] Treatment may be continued indefinitely if necessary to control the disease and if no toxicity occurs. **PR** methimazole can be formulated for rectal administration.[197]

Special Populations. *Pediatric Dosage.* **PO** 0.4 mg/kg/day or 15–20 mg/m²/day given in 1–2 divided doses with a maintenance dosage of one-half the initial dosage.[173]

Geriatric Dosage. Same as adult dosage.

Other Conditions. In pregnancy, doses should be as low as possible to maintain maternal T_4 level in approximately the upper normal to mildly thyrotoxic range; initially give a maximum of 30 mg/day orally in single or 3 divided doses for 4–6 weeks, then decrease to 5–15 mg/day in a single dose.[167,169,172,198]

Dosage Forms. Tab 5, 10 mg.

Patient Instructions. Report sore throat, fever, or oral lesions immediately because they may be an early sign of a severe, but rare blood disorder. Also report any skin eruptions, itching, or yellowing of eyes and skin. Be sure to take at prescribed dosage intervals.

Missed Doses. If you miss a dose, take it as soon as possible. If it is time for the next dose, take both doses.

Pharmacokinetics. *Onset and Duration.* **PO** onset about 2–3 weeks, which is consistent with the elimination of existing T_4 stores. Duration intrathyroidally 40 hr.[199]

Serum Levels. <0.2 mg/L (1.8 μmol/L) inhibits iodide organification.[199]

Fate. Well absorbed orally. Considerable interindividual variation in pharmacokinetic parameters. Peak serum levels occur at 2.3 ± 0.8 hr; the peak after 30 mg orally is 0.8 ± 0.2 mg/L (6.8 ± 1.9 μmol/L); after 60 mg orally, 1.5 ± 0.5 mg/L (14 ± 4 μmol/L); after 60 mg rectally, 1.1 ± 0.5 mg/L (10 ± 5 μmol/L).[197,199,200] The drug is actively concentrated in thyroid gland with peak intrathyroidal levels of 0.11–1.1 mg/L (1–10 μmol/L) within 1 hr;[199] there is minimal plasma protein binding; it is distributed into breast milk 10 times greater than PTU.[198] V_d is 1.4 ± 0.6 L/kg; Cl is 0.072 ± 0.018 L/hr/kg. There are no active metabolites; 7–12% is excreted unchanged in urine, 6% excreted as inorganic sulfate, 1.5% as sulfur metabolites, and 50% as unknown metabolites.[199,200]

$t_{\frac{1}{2}}$. α phase 3 ± 1.4 hr; β phase 18.5 ± 13 hr in normal and hyperthyroid patients, increased to 21 hr in cirrhosis.[199] Intrathyroidal half-life is 20 hr.

Adverse Reactions. Maculopapular skin rashes and itching occur frequently and may disappear spontaneously with continued treatment; urticaria requires drug discontinuation.[167,169] Methimazole can be given to patients who develop only a nonurticarial maculopapular rash on PTU. Mild transient leukopenia occurs frequently in untreated Graves' disease, does not predispose to agranulocytosis, and is not an indication to discontinue the drug.[167,169,201,202] Agranulocytosis occurs occasionally, usually in the first 3 months of therapy. Risk increases with dosages over 40 mg/day in patients >40 yr; granulocyte colony-stimulating factors (eg, **filgrastim**) can hasten recovery.[201–204] Rarely, fever, arthralgias, cholestatic or hepatocellular toxicity, vasculitis, lupuslike syndrome, hypoprothrombinemia, aplastic anemia, thrombocytopenia, nephrotic syndrome, loss of taste, and spontaneous appearance of circulating antibodies to insulin or glucagon occur.[167,169,205–208]

Contraindications. Manufacturer states that breastfeeding is a contraindication, but some experts feel that breastfeeding may be performed with dosages of 10 mg/day or less and careful monitoring of infant thyroid function.[209]

Precautions. Although methimazole crosses the placenta at rates 4 times greater than **propylthiouracil** and has been associated with scalp defects (aplasia cutis), recent reports indicate methimazole can be given in pregnant patients intolerant to PTU.[167,198,210] Use with caution during lactation and in patients with severe allergic reactions to other thioamides. A low prevalence of cross-sensitivity occurs between thioamide compounds for nonurticarial skin rashes, so if these occur, another thioamide can be substituted. However, a 50% chance of cross-sensitivity exists for severe reactions (eg, agranulocytosis, hepatitis), so do not substitute another thioamide.[167,202]

Drug Interactions. Iodide given before a thioamide delays the response to the thioamide, especially in thyroid storm. Changes in thyroid status may alter pharmacodynamics and pharmacokinetics of digoxin, warfarin, theophylline, β-blockers, and insulin.

Parameters to Monitor. Monitor clinical status of patient; serum free T_4 or T_4 index, and TSH monthly initially until euthyroid, then q 3–6 months. Obtain occasional liver function tests and CBC with differential (but these are not recommended routinely, because they are not predictive of toxicity, and transient leukopenia and elevations in liver function tests can occur); AST, ALT, total bilirubin, and alkaline phosphatase if patient reports signs of hepatitis; WBC and differential counts if patient reports signs of agranulocytosis such as fever, sore throat, or malaise.

Notes. Methimazole is the drug of choice for treatment of uncomplicated hyperthyroidism, because it is better tolerated and fewer tablets can be given once daily, improving patient compliance.[167,169,172] Remission rates of 20–40% are common after cessation of therapy. Favorable remission rates correlate with longer duration of therapy, higher dosages, mild disease, shrinkage of goiter size with therapy, disappearance of thyroid receptor stimulating antibodies, and initial presentation with T_3 toxicosis.[167,210] Concurrent administration of levothyroxine might also improve remission rates, but further study is required.[167,169,194–196] Most patients eventually require surgery or radioiodine; however, a trial of a thioamide is worthwhile in patients with minimal thyroid enlargement or very mild hyperthyroidism. In thyroid storm, pregnancy, and lactation, PTU is the drug of choice.

PROPYLTHIOURACIL   Various

Pharmacology. Propylthiouracil (PTU) is a thioamide antithyroid drug that blocks the synthesis of thyroid hormones and, at dosages over 450 mg/day, also decreases the peripheral conversion of T_4 to T_3. Titers of thyroid receptor stimulating antibody (TRab) decline during therapy, consistent with an immunosuppressive effect.

Administration and Adult Dosage. PO for hyperthyroidism 100–200 mg (depending on the severity of hyperthyroidism) q 6–8 hr initially until euthyroid (usually 6–8 weeks), then decrease by 33–50% over several weeks to a maintenance dosage of 50–150 mg/day in a single dose. Rarely, initial dosages of 1–1.2 g/day (maximum dosage) in 3–6 doses may be necessary.[167] **PO for thyroid storm** 200–250 mg q 6 hr until euthyroid; maintenance dosage is determined by patient response. Treatment duration for hyperthyroidism is 1–2 yr traditionally, although shorter courses of 6 months may also be effective in mild disease.[167,169,172] Treatment may be continued indefinitely if necessary to control the disease and if no toxicity occurs. To prevent recurrence of hyperthyroidism, **levothyroxine** 75–100 μg/day may be added after 6 months once the patient is euthyroid; this may improve remission rates, but further study is warranted.[167,169,194–196] **PR PTU** can be formulated for rectal administration.[211,212]

Special Populations. *Pediatric Dosage.* Give orally in 3 divided doses. **PO** 150–300 mg/m²/day. Alternatively, (6–10 yr) 5–10 mg/kg/day or 50–150 mg/day initially; (≥10 yr) 150–300 mg/day initially. Maintenance dosage is determined by patient response.

Geriatric Dosage. Same as adult dosage.

Other Conditions. In pregnancy, dosage should be as small as possible to maintain a mildly hyperthyroid maternal state; initially 300 mg/day orally in 3 divided doses for 4–6 weeks, then decrease to 50–150 mg/day in a single dose.[167,172,198]

Dosage Forms. **Tab** 50 mg.

Patient Instructions. Report sore throat, fever, or oral lesions immediately because they may be an early sign of a severe, but rare blood disorder. Also report any skin eruptions, itching, or yellowing of eyes and skin. Be sure to take at prescribed dosage intervals.

Missed Doses. If you miss a dose, take it as soon as possible. If it is time for the next dose, take both doses.

Pharmacokinetics. *Onset and Duration.* PO onset of therapeutic effect 2–3 weeks, consistent with the elimination of existing thyroxine stores.

Serum Levels. Peak PTU levels >4 mg/L (24 μmol/L) produce antithyroid activity; 3 mg/L (18 μmol/L) reduces organification by 50%; 0.8 mg/L (5 μmol/L) reduces peripheral conversion activity by 50%.[200,213]

Fate. Oral bioavailability is 77 ± 13%. Peak levels occur 2 ± 0.3 hr after oral administration, and 4.7 ± 1 hr after rectal administration. Peak serum level after an oral dose of 50 mg is 1 ± 0.2 mg/L (6 ± 1.2 μmol/L); after 200 mg, 4.5 ± 0.7 mg/L (26 ± 4 μmol/L); after 300 mg, 7 ± 0.8 mg/L (42 ± 5 μmol/L); after 400 mg rectally, 3 ± 0.8 mg/L (18 ± 5 μmol/L).[199,211–213] Actively concentrated in the thyroid gland 40% as unknown metabolite, 32% as sulfate, and 20% as unchanged PTU; peak intrathyroidal levels of 0.17 ± 1.7 mg/L (1–10 μmol/L) occur within 1 hr.[167,200] The drug is 80% plasma protein bound; it distributes poorly into breast milk. V_d is 0.29 ± 0.06 L/kg; Cl is 0.23 ± 0.04 L/hr/kg. About 85% is excreted in 24 hr, 61% as glucuronides, 8–9% as inorganic sulfates, 8–10% as unknown sulfur metabolites, and <10% excreted unchanged in urine.[200]

$t_{1/2}$. 1.3 ± 0.6 hr.[167,200,213]

Adverse Reactions. (*See* Methimazole.) However, agranulocytosis is not more prevalent at higher doses as it is with methimazole. Rarely, hepatitis occurs; hepatocellular toxicity is more frequent than cholestatic jaundice.[167,169,214] Transient transaminase elevations can occur in asymptomatic individuals which normalize within 3 months with continued drug administration.[193]

Contraindications. Manufacturer states that breastfeeding is a contraindication, but if necessary, it can be used with infant thyroid monitoring because of low milk levels and lack of effect on infants.[198,209]

Precautions. (*See* Methimazole.) Although it crosses the placenta poorly (one-fourth the rate of methimazole), it can cause fetal hypothyroidism and goiter.[167,169,198] Thyroid dysfunction may diminish as pregnancy progresses, allowing a reduction in dosage and, in some cases, a withdrawal of therapy 2–3 weeks before delivery. Adjunctive thyroid hormone therapy prevents maternal hypothyroidism but, because of minimal placental transfer, has little effect on the fetus.[198] Use with caution prior to surgery or during treatment with anticoagulants because of hypoprothrombinemic effect.

Drug Interactions. (*See* Methimazole.)

Parameters to Monitor. (*See* Methimazole.) Prothrombin time monitoring is advisable, particularly prior to surgery.

Notes. Because propylthiouracil decreases peripheral conversion of T_4 to T_3, it is considered the thioamide of choice in treating thyroid storm; it is also the drug of choice in pregnancy and breastfeeding.[167,198,208] PTU may decrease mortality because of alcoholic liver disease.[215]

■ REFERENCES

1. Kaye TB, Crapo L. The Cushing syndrome: an update on diagnostic tests. *Ann Intern Med* 1990;112:434–44.
2. Axelrod L. Corticosteroid therapy. In, Becker KL, ed. *Principles and practice of endocrinology and metabolism.* Philadelphia: JB Lippincott; 1990:613–23.

3. Schimmer BP, Parker KL. Adrenocorticotropic hormone: adrenocortical steroids and their synthetic analogs; inhibitors of the synthesis and action of adrenal hormones. In, Hardman JG et al., eds. *Goodman and Gilman's the pharmacological basis of therapeutics.* 9th ed. New York: McGraw-Hill; 1996:1459–85.

4. Clayton RN. Diagnosis of adrenal insufficiency. *BMJ* 1989;298:271–2.

5. Cersosimo RJ, Karp DD. Adrenal corticosteroids as antiemetics during cancer chemotherapy. *Pharmacotherapy* 1986;6:118–27.

6. Anon. Ondansetron to prevent vomiting after cancer chemotherapy. *Med Lett Drugs Ther* 1991;33:63–4.

7. The Italian Group for Antiemetic Research. Dexamethasone, granisetron, or both for the prevention of nausea and vomiting during chemotherapy for cancer. *N Engl J Med* 1995;332:1–5.

8. Grunberg SM, Hesketh PJ. Control of chemotherapy-induced emesis. *N Engl J Med* 1993;329:1790–6.

9. Orth DN et al. The adrenal cortex. In, Wilson JD, Foster DW, eds. *Williams textbook of endocrinology.* Philadelphia: WB Saunders; 1992:489–619.

10. Wildenradt SS, Hart LL. Antenatal dexamethasone as prophylaxis of respiratory distress syndrome. *Ann Pharmacother* 1994;28:475–7.

11. Bone RC et al. A controlled clinical trial of high-dose methylprednisolone in the treatment of severe sepsis and shock. *N Engl J Med* 1987;317:653–8.

12. McGowan JE et al. Guidelines for the use of systemic glucocorticoids in the management of selected infections. *J Infect Dis* 1992;165:1–13.

13. Benitz WE, Tatro DS. *The pediatric drug handbook.* 2nd ed. Chicago: Year Book; 1988.

14. Anon. Dexamethasone for bacterial meningitis in children. *Med Lett Drugs Ther* 1989;31:6–7.

15. Prober CG. The role of steroids in the management of children with bacterial meningitis. *Pediatrics* 1995;95:29–31.

16. Baxter JD. Minimizing the side effects of glucocorticoid therapy. *Adv Intern Med* 1990;35:173–94.

17. Tsuei SE et al. Disposition of synthetic glucocorticoids. I. Pharmacokinetics of dexamethasone in healthy adults. *J Pharmacokinet Biopharm* 1979;7:249–64.

18. Gustavson LE, Benet LZ. Pharmacokinetics of natural and synthetic glucocorticoids. In, Anderson DC, Winter JSD, eds. *Butterworth's international medical reviews: clinical endocrinology.* Vol. 4, *Adrenal cortex.* London: Butterworth; 1985:235–81.

19. Baharav E et al. Dexamethasone-induced perineal irritation. *N Engl J Med* 1986;314:515–6. Letter.

20. Health and Public Policy Committee, American College of Physicians. The dexamethasone suppression test for the detection, diagnosis, and management of depression. *Ann Intern Med* 1984;100:307–8.

21. Nierenberg AA, Feinstein AR. How to evaluate a diagnostic marker test: lessons from the rise and fall of dexamethasone suppression test. *JAMA* 1988;259:1699–702.

22. Erstad BL. Severe cardiovascular adverse effects in association with acute, high-dose corticosteroid administration. *DICP* 1989;23:1019–23.

23. Kong AN et al. Pharmacokinetics and pharmacodynamic modeling of direct suppression effects of methylprednisolone on serum cortisol and blood histamine in human subjects. *Clin Pharmacol Ther* 1989;46:616–28.

24. Anon. Drugs for acute spinal cord injury. *Med Lett Drugs Ther* 1993;35:72–3.

25. Truhan AP, Ahmed AR. Corticosteroids: a review with emphasis on complications of prolonged systemic therapy. *Ann Allergy* 1989;62:375–90.

26. Breitenfield RV et al. Stability of renal transplant function with alternate-day corticosteroid therapy. *JAMA* 1980;244:151–6.

27. Bystryn J-C. Adjuvant therapy of pemphigus. *Arch Dermatol* 1984;120:941–51.

28. Siegel SC. Corticosteroid agents: overview of corticosteroid therapy. *J Allergy Clin Immunol* 1985;76:312–20.

29. Iafrate RP et al. Current concepts in clinical therapeutics: asthma. *Clin Pharm* 1986;5:206–27.

30. Haskell RJ et al. A double-blind, randomized clinical trial of methylprednisolone in status asthmaticus. *Arch Intern Med* 1983;143:1324–7.

31. Kelly HW, Murphy S. Corticosteroids for acute, severe asthma. *DICP* 1991;25:72–9.

32. The National Institutes of Health-University of California Expert Panel for Corticosteroids as Adjunctive Therapy for Pneumocystis Pneumonia. Consensus statement of the use of corticosteroids as adjunctive therapy for Pneumocystis pneumonia in the acquired immunodeficiency syndrome. *N Engl J Med* 1990;323:1500–4.

33. Groff GD et al. Systemic steroid therapy for acute gout: a clinical trial and review of the literature. *Semin Arthritis Rheum* 1990;19:329–36.

34. Hill MR et al. Monitoring glucocorticoid therapy: a pharmacokinetic approach. *Clin Pharmacol Ther* 1990;48:390–8.

35. Gambertoglio JG et al. Pharmacokinetics and bioavailability of prednisone and prednisolone in healthy volunteers and patients: a review. *J Pharmacokinet Biopharm* 1980;8:1–52.

36. Lewis GP et al. Prednisone side-effects and serum-protein levels. *Lancet* 1971;2:778–81.

37. Saag KG et al. Low dose long-term corticosteroid therapy in rheumatoid arthritis: an analysis of serious adverse events. *Am J Med* 1994;96:115–23.

38. Klein JF. Adverse psychiatric effects of systemic glucocorticoid therapy. *Am Fam Physician* 1992;46: 1469–74.

39. Anon. Oral corticosteroids. *Med Lett Drugs Ther* 1975;17:99–100.

40. Callahan CM et al. Oral corticosteroid therapy for patients with stable chronic obstructive pulmonary disease: a meta-analysis. *Ann Intern Med* 1991;114:216–23.

41. Weinberger SE. Recent advances in pulmonary medicine. *N Engl J Med* 1993;328:1389–97.

42. Mukwaya G. Immunosuppressive effects and infections associated with corticosteroid therapy. *Pediatr Infect Dis J* 1988;7:499–504.

43. Derendorf H et al. Pharmacokinetics of triamcinolone acetonide after intravenous, oral, and inhaled administration. *J Clin Pharmacol* 1995;35:302–5.

44. United States Pharmacopeial Convention. *USP DI: Drug information for the health care professional.* 18th ed. Rockville, MD: World Color Book Services; 1998.

45. Guzzo CA et al. Dermatological pharmacology. In, Goodman LS et al., eds. *Goodman and Gilman's the pharmacological basis of therapeutics.* 9th ed. New York: McGraw-Hill; 1996:1593–616.

46. Maddin S, Ho VC. Dermatologic therapy. In, Moschella SL, Hurley HJ, eds. *Dermatology.* 3rd ed. Philadelphia: WB Saunders; 1992:2187–215.

47. Stoughton RB, Cornell RC. Corticosteroids. In, Fitzpatrick TB et al., eds. *Dermatology in general medicine.* 4th ed. New York: McGraw-Hill; 1993:2846–50.

48. Hepburn D et al. Topical steroid treatment in infants, children, and adolescents. In, Schachner LA, ed. *Advances in dermatology.* St Louis: Mosby-Year Book; 1994:225–54.

49. Lebovitz HE. α-Glucosidase inhibitors in the treatment of hyperglycemia. In, Lebovitz HE, ed. *Therapy for diabetes mellitus and related disorders.* 2nd ed. Alexandria, VA: American Diabetes Association; 1994.

50. Steele JW et al. Epalrestat: a review of its pharmacology, and therapeutic potential in late-onset complications of diabetes mellitus. *Drugs Aging* 1993;3:532–5.

51. Giugliano D et al. Tolrestat for mild diabetic neuropathy. A 52-week, randomized, placebo-controlled trial. *Ann Intern Med* 1993;118:7–11.

52. Steed DL and the Diabetic Ulcer Study Group. Clinical evaluation of recombinant human platelet-derived growth factor for the treatment of lower extremity diabetic ulcers. *J Vasc Surg* 1995;21:71–81.

53. Santiago JV, ed. *Medical management of insulin-dependent (type I) diabetes.* 2nd ed. Alexandria, VA: American Diabetes Association; 1993.

54. Raskin P, ed. *Medical management of type II diabetes,* 3rd ed. Alexandria, VA: American Diabetes Association; 1994.

55. Koda-Kimble MA. Diabetes mellitus. In, Young LY, Koda-Kimble MA, eds. *Applied therapeutics.* 5th ed. Vancouver, WA: Applied Therapeutics; 1992;72:2–53.

56. The Diabetes Control and Complications Trial Research Group. The effect of intensive treatment of diabetes on the development and progression of long-term complications in insulin-dependent diabetes mellitus. *N Engl J Med* 1993;329:977–86.

57. White JR, Jr., Campbell RK. Pharmacologic therapies in the management of diabetes mellitus. In, Haire-Joshu D, ed. *Management of diabetes mellitus. Perspectives of care across the life span.* St. Louis: Mosby-Year Book; 1994:119–48.

58. Peterson L et al. Insulin adsorbance to polyvinylchloride surfaces with implications for constant-infusion therapy. *Diabetes* 1976;25:72–4.

59. Heinemann L et al. Time-action profile of inhaled insulin. *Diabet Med* 1997;14:63–72.

60. Campbell RK et al. Insulin lispro: its role in the treatment of diabetes mellitus. *Ann Pharmacother* 1996;30:1263–71.

61. Bailey CJ, Turner RC. Metformin. *N Engl J Med* 1996;334:574–9.

62. Somogyi A et al. Reduction of metformin tubular secretion by cimetidine in man. *Br J Clin Pharmacol* 1987;23:545–51.

63. Hermann LS et al. Therapeutic comparison of metformin and sulfonylurea, alone and in various combinations. *Diabetes Care* 1994;17:1100–8.

64. Wolffenbuttel BHR, Graal MB. New treatments for patients with type 2 diabetes mellitus. *Postgrad Med J* 1996;72:657–62.

65. Levien TL, Baker DE. Drug evaluation—repaglinide. Dana Point, CA: The Formulary Monograph Service, April 1998.

66. Gossain VV et al. Management of diabetes in the elderly: a clinical perspective. *J Assoc Acad Minority Physicians* 1996;5:22–31.

67. Davidson MB. Rational use of sulfonylureas. *Postgrad Med* 1992;92:69–85.

68. Gerich JE. Oral hypoglycemic agents. *N Engl J Med* 1989;321:1231–45.

69. White JR Jr et al. Drug interactions and diabetes. The risk of losing glycemic control. *Postgrad Med* 1993;93:131–40.

70. White JR. The pharmacologic management of patients with type II diabetes mellitus in the era of oral agents and insulin analogs. *Diabetes Spectrum* 1996;9:227–34.

71. Spencer CM, Markham A. Troglitazone. *Drugs* 1997;54:89–101.

72. Olgihara T et al. Enhancement of insulin sensitivity by troglitazone lowers blood pressure in diabetic hypertensives. *Am J Hypertens* 1995;8:316–20.

73. Anon. Blood glucose meters and data management. In, *Buyer's guide to diabetes products '98*. Alexandria, VA: American Diabetes Association; 18–27.

74. Hatcher RA et al. *Contraceptive technology*. 16th revised ed. New York: Irvington; 1994.

75. Van Look PFA, von Hertzen H. Emergency contraception. *Br Med Bull* 1993;49:158–70.

76. Weisberg E. Prescribing oral contraceptives. *Drugs* 1995;49:224–31.

77. Bayer SR, DeCherney AH. Clinical manifestations and treatment of dysfunctional uterine bleeding. *JAMA* 1993;269:1823–8.

78. Lu PY, Ory SJ. Endometriosis: current management. *Mayo Clin Proc* 1995;70:453–63.

79. Shenfield GM, Griffin JM. Clinical pharmacokinetics of contraceptive steroids. An update. *Clin Pharmacokinet* 1991;20:15–37.

80. Kuhl H. Pharmacokinetics of oestrogens and progestogens. *Maturitas* 1990;12:171–97.

81. Stanczyk FZ, Roy S. Metabolism of levonorgestrel, norethindrone, and structurally related contraceptive steroids. *Contraception* 1990;42:67–93.

82. Kuhnz W et al. Systemic availability of levonorgestrel after single oral administration of norgestimate-containing combination oral contraceptive to 12 young women. *Contraception* 1994;49:255–63.

83. Fotherby K. Potency and pharmacokinetics of gestagens. *Contraception* 1990;41:533–50.

84. Back DJ et al. Comparative pharmacokinetics of levonorgestrel and ethinyloestradiol following intravenous, oral, and vaginal administration. *Contraception* 1987;36:471–9.

85. Goldzieher JW. Selected aspects of the pharmacokinetics and metabolism of ethinyl estrogens and their clinical implications. *Am J Obstet Gynecol* 1990;163:318–22.

86. Goldzieher JW. Pharmacokinetics and metabolism of ethinyl estrogens. In, Goldzieher JW, Fotherby K, eds. *Pharmacology of the contraceptive steroids*. New York: Raven Press; 1994:140–51.

87. Kuhnz W et al. Pharmacokinetics of levonorgestrel and ethinylestradiol in 14 women during three months of treatment with a tri-step combination oral contraceptive: serum protein binding of levonorgestrel and influence of treatment on free and total testosterone levels in the serum. *Contraception* 1994;50:563–79.

88. Orme ML'E et al. Clinical pharmacokinetics of oral contraceptive steroids. *Clin Pharmacokinet* 1983;8:95–136.

89. Archer DF et al. Pharmacokinetics of a triphasic oral contraceptive containing desogestrel and ethinyl estradiol. *Fertil Steril* 1994;61:645–51.

90. McClamrock HD. Adashi EY. Pharmacokinetics of desogestrel. *Am J Obstet Gynecol* 1993;168:1021–8.

91. Orme M et al. The pharmacokinetics of ethinylestradiol in the presence and absence of gestodene and desogestrel. *Contraception* 1991;43:305–17.

92. Fotherby K. Pharmacokinetics and metabolism of progestins in humans. In, Goldzieher JW, Fotherby K, eds. *Pharmacology of the contraceptive steroids*. New York: Raven Press; 1994:99–126.

93. Kubba A, Guillebaud J. Combined oral contraceptives: acceptability and effective use. *Br Med Bull* 1993;49:140–57.

94. McCann MF, Potter LS. Progestin-only oral contraception: a comprehensive review. *Contraception* 1994;50:S138–48.

95. Speroff L et al. Evaluation of a new generation of oral contraceptives. *Obstet Gynecol* 1993;81:1034–47.

96. Thorogood M, Villard-Mackintosh L. Combined oral contraceptives: risks and benefits. *Br Med Bull* 1993;49:124–39.

97. Upton GV, Corbin A. Contraception for the transitional years of women older than 40 years of age. *Clin Obstet Gynecol* 1992;35:855–64.

98. Schlesselman JJ. Net effect of oral contraceptive use on the risk of cancer in women in the United States. *Obstet Gynecol* 1995;85:793–801.

99. Shenfield GM. Oral contraceptives: are drug interactions of clinical significance. *Drug Safety* 1993;9:21–37.

100. Corson SL. A decade of experience with transdermal estrogen replacement therapy: overview of key pharmacologic and clinical findings. *Int J Fertil* 1993;38:79–91.

101. Kaunitz AM. Long-acting injectable contraception with depot medroxyprogesterone acetate. *Am J Obstet Gynecol* 1994;170:1543–9.

102. Kaunitz AM, Rosenfield A. Injectable contraception with depot medroxyprogesterone acetate. Current status. *Drugs* 1993;45:857–65.
103. Pardthaisong T et al. The long-term growth and development of children exposed to Depo-Provera during pregnancy or lactation. *Contraception* 1992;45:313–24.
104. World Health Organization Task Force for Epidemiological Research on Reproductive Health; Special Programme of Research, Development and Research Training in Human Reproduction. Progestogen-only contraceptives during lactation: I: infant growth. *Contraception* 1994;50:35–53.
105. World Health Organization Task Force for Epidemiological Research on Reproductive Health Special Programme of Research, Development and Research Training in Human Reproduction. Progestogen-only contraceptives during lactation: II: infant development. *Contraception* 1994;50:55–68.
106. Darney PD. Hormonal implants: contraception for a new century. *Am J Obstet Gynecol* 1994;170:1536–43.
107. Skegg DCG et al. Depot medroxyprogesterone acetate and breast cancer. A pooled analysis of the World Health Organization and New Zealand Studies. *JAMA* 1995;273:799–804.
108. Wysowski DK, Green L. Serious adverse events in Norplant users reported to the Food and Drug Administration's Med Watch spontaneous reporting system. *Obstet Gynecol* 1995;85:538–42.
109. Dunson TR et al. Complications and risk factors associated with the removal of Norplant implants. *Obstet Gynecol* 1995;85:543–48.
110. Bagshaw S. The combined oral contraceptive. Risks and adverse effects in perspective. *Drug Safety* 1995;12:91–6.
111. Anon. After the morning after and the morning after that. *Lancet* 1995;345:1381–2. Editorial.
112. Hannaford PC et al. Oral contraception and stroke. Evidence from the Royal College of General Practitioners' Oral Contraception Study. *Stroke* 1994;25:935–42.
113. Lidegaard O. Decline in cerebral thromboembolism among young women after introduction of low-dose oral contraceptives: an incidence study for the period 1980–1993. *Contraception* 1995;52:85–92.
114. Goldzieher JW, Zamah NM. Oral contraceptive side effects: where's the beef? *Contraception* 1995;52:327–35.
115. Anon. Oral contraceptive alert in UK sparks off controversy. *Lancet* 1995;346:1149–50. News.
116. Belchetz PE. Hormonal treatment of postmenopausal women. *N Engl J Med* 1994;330:1062–71.
117. Ettinger B et al. Cyclic hormone replacement therapy using quarterly progestin. *Obstet Gynecol* 1994;83:693–700.
118. The Postmenopausal Estrogen/Progestin Interventions (PEPI) Trial. Effects of estrogen or estrogen/progestin regimens on heart disease risk factors in postmenopausal women. *JAMA* 1995;273:199–208.
119. Lobo RA, Cassidenti DL. Pharmacokinetics of oral 17β-estradiol. *J Reprod Med* 1992;37:77–84.
120. Anderson F. Kinetics and pharmacology of estrogens in pre- and postmenopausal women. *Int J Fertil* 1993; 38(suppl 1):53–64.
121. Handa VL et al. Vaginal administration of low-dose conjugated estrogens: systemic absorption and effects on the endometrium. *Obstet Gynecol* 1994;84:215–8.
122. Pang SC et al. Long-term effects of transdermal estradiol with and without medroxyprogesterone acetate. *Fertil Steril* 1993;59:76–82.
123. Kuhnz W et al. Pharmacokinetics of estradiol free and total estrone, in young women following single intravenous and oral administration of 17 beta-estradiol. *Arzneimittelforschung* 1993;43:966–73.
124. Cobleigh MA et al. Estrogen replacement therapy in breast cancer survivors: a time for change *JAMA* 1994; 272:540–5.
125. Loprinzi CL et al. Megestrol acetate for the prevention of hot flashes. *N Engl J Med* 1994;331:347–52.
126. Campagnoli C et al. Long-term hormone replacement treatment in menopause: new choices, old apprehensions, recent findings. *Maturitas* 1993;18:21–46.
127. Lufkin EG et al. Treatment of postmenopausal osteoporosis with transdermal estrogen. *Ann Intern Med* 1992;117:1–9.
128. Walsh BW et al. Effects of postmenopausal estrogen replacement on the concentrations and metabolism of plasma lipoproteins. *N Engl J Med* 1991;325:1196–204.
129. Lindsay R. Prevention and treatment of osteoporosis. *Lancet* 1993;341:801–5.
130. Liberman UA et al. Effect of oral alendronate on bone mineral density and the incidence of fractures in postmenopausal osteoporosis. The Alendronate Phase III Osteoporosis Treatment Study Group. *N Engl J Med* 1995;333:1437–43.
131. Jeal W et al. Alendronate. A review of its pharmacological properties and therapeutic efficacy in postmenopausal osteoporosis. *Drugs* 1997;53:415–34.
132. Overgaard K et al. Effect of salcatonin given intranasally on bone mass and fracture rates in established osteoporosis: a dose-response study. *BMJ* 1992;305:556–61.
133. Wimalawansa SJ. Combined therapy with estrogen and etidronate has an additive effect on bone mineral density in the hip and vertebrae: four-year randomized study. *Am J Med* 1995;99:36–42.

134. Anon. New drugs for osteoporosis. *Med Lett Drugs Ther* 1996;38:1–3.

135. McCarthy ML, Stoukides CA. Estrogen therapy of uremic bleeding. *Ann Pharmacother* 1994;28:60–2.

136. Zachee P et al. Hematologic aspects of end-stage renal failure. *Ann Hematol* 1994;69:33–40.

137. Bhavnani BR, Cecutti A. Pharmacokinetics of 17β-dihydroequilin sulfate and 17β-dihydroequilin in normal postmenopausal women. *J Clin Endocrinol Metab* 1994;78:197–204.

138. Steinberg KK et al. A meta-analysis of the effect of estrogen replacement therapy on the risk of breast cancer. *JAMA* 1991;265:1985–90. {Erratum JAMA 1991;266:1362}.

139. Anon. Raloxifene for postmenopausal osteoporosis. *Med Lett Drugs Ther* 1998;40:29–30.

140. Ashworth LE. Focus on raloxifene. *Formulary* 1998;33:305–17.

141. Grady D et al. Hormone therapy to prevent disease and prolong life in postmenopausal women. *Ann Intern Med* 1992;117:1016–37.

142. American College of Physicians. Guidelines for counseling postmenopausal women about preventive hormone therapy. *Ann Intern Med* 1992;117:1038–41.

143. Lip GYH et al. Hormone replacement therapy and blood pressure in hypertensive women. *J Humam Hypertens* 1994;8:491–4.

144. Colditz GA et al. The use of estrogens and progestins and the risk of breast cancer in postmenopausal women. *N Engl J Med* 1995;332:1589–93.

145. Stanford JL et al. Combined estrogen and progestin hormone replacement therapy in relation to risk of breast cancer in middle-aged women. *JAMA* 1995;274:137–42.

146. Dupont WD, Page DL. Menopausal estrogen replacement therapy and breast cancer. *Arch Intern Med* 1991;151:67–72.

147. Ettinger B et al. Reduced mortality associated with long-term postmenopausal estrogen therapy. *Obstet Gynecol* 1996;87:6–12.

148. Udoff L et al. Combined continuous hormone replacement therapy: a critical review. *Obstet Gynecol* 1995;86:306–16.

149. Archer DF et al. Bleeding patterns in postmenopausal women taking continuous combined or sequential regimens of conjugated estrogens with medroxyprogesterone acetate. Menopause Study Group. *Obstet Gynecol* 1994;83:686–92.

150. Ravnikar V. Physiology and treatment of hot flushes. *Obstet Gynecol* 1995;75:3S–8.

151. Etienne MC et al. Improved bioavailability of a new oral preparation of medroxyprogesterone acetate. *J Pharm Sci* 1991;80:1130–2.

152. Wright CE et al. Effect of injection volume on the bioavailability of sterile medroxyprogesterone acetate suspension. *Clin Pharm* 1983;2:435–8.

153. Norman TR et al. Comparative bioavailability of orally and vaginally administered progesterone. *Fertil Steril* 1991;56:1034–9.

154. Munk-Jensen N et al. Continuous combined and sequential estradiol and norethindrone acetate treatment of postmenopausal women: effect of plasma lipoproteins in a two-year placebo-controlled trial. *Am J Obstet Gynecol* 1994;171:132–8.

155. Nahoul K et al. Profiles of plasma estrogens, progesterone and their metabolites after oral or vaginal administration of estradiol or progesterone. *Maturitas* 1993;16:185–202.

156. Padwick M et al. Absorption and metabolism of oral progesterone when administered twice daily. *Fertil Steril* 1986;46:402–7.

157. Ottoson UB et al. Serum levels of progesterone and some of its metabolites including deoxycorticosterone after oral and parenteral administration. *Br J Obstet Gynaecol* 1984;91:1111–9.

158. Freeman EW et al. A double-blind trial of oral progesterone, alprazolam, and placebo in treatment of severe premenstrual syndrome. *JAMA* 1995;274:51–7.

159. Freeman E et al. Ineffectiveness of progesterone suppository treatment of premenstrual syndrome. *JAMA* 1990;264:349–53.

160. Sternthal E et al. Suppression of thyroid radioiodine uptake by various doses of stable iodide. *N Engl J Med* 1980;303:1083–8.

161. Braverman LE, Utiger RD. *Werner & Ingbar's the thyroid.* 6th ed. Philadelphia: Lippincott; 1991.

162. Roti E et al. Effects of chronic iodine administration on thyroid status in euthyroid subjects previously treated with antithyroid drugs for Graves' hyperthyroidism. *J Clin Endocrinol Metab* 1993;76:928–32.

163. Roti E et al. Iodine-induced subclinical hypothyroidism in euthyroid subjects with a previous episode of amiodarone-induced thyrotoxicosis. *J Clin Endocrinol Metab* 1992;75:1273–7.

164. Roti E et al. Impaired intrathyroidal iodine organification and iodine-induced hypothyroidism in euthyroid women with a previous episode of postpartum thyroiditis. *J Clin Endocrinol Metab* 1991;73:958–63.

165. Mizukami Y et al. Iodine-induced hypothyroidism: a clinical and histological study of 29 patients. *J Clin Endocrinol Metab* 1993;76:466–71.

166. Delange F. The disorders induced by iodine deficiency. *Thyroid* 1994;4:107–28.

167. Klein I et al. Treatment of hyperthyroid disease. *Ann Intern Med* 1994;121:281–8.

168. Philippou G et al. The effect of iodide on serum thyroid hormone levels in normal persons, in hyperthyroid patients, and in hypothyroid patients on thyroxine replacement. *Clin Endocrinol (Oxf)* 1992;36:573–8.

169. Franklyn JA. The management of hyperthyroidism. *N Engl J Med* 1994;330:1731–8.

170. Mann K et al. Systemic iodine absorption during endoscopic application of radiographic contrast agents for endoscopic retrograde cholangiopancreaticography. *Eur J Endocrinol* 1994;130:498–501.

171. Mandel SJ et al. Levothyroxine therapy in patients with thyroid disease. *Ann Intern Med* 1993;119:492–502.

172. Singer PA et al. Treatment guidelines for patients with hyperthyroidism and hypothyroidism. *JAMA* 1995;273:808–12.

173. Toft AD. Thyroxine therapy. *N Engl J Med* 1994;331:174–81. {Erratum *N Engl J Med* 1994;331:1035}.

174. Burmeister LA et al. Levothyroxine dose requirements for thyrotropin suppression in the treatment of differentiated thyroid cancer. *J Clin Endocrinol Metab* 1992;75:344–50.

175. Roti E et al. The use and misuse of thyroid hormone. *Endocr Rev* 1993;14:401–23.

176. Nicoloff JT, LoPresti JS. Myxedema coma. A form of decompensated hypothyroidism. *Endocrinol Metab Clin North Am* 1993;22:279–90.

177. MacKerrow SD. Myxedema-associated cardiogenic shock treated with intravenous triiodothyronine. *Ann Intern Med* 1992;117:1014–5.

178. Fisher DA. Management of congenital hypothyroidism. *J Clin Endocrinol Metab* 1991;72:523–9.

179. Chiesa A et al. Growth follow-up in 100 children with congenital hypothyroidism before and during treatment. *J Pediatr Endocrinol* 1994;7:211–17.

180. Taylor J et al. Twice-weekly dosing for thyroxine replacement in elderly patients with primary hypothyroidism. *J Intern Med Res* 1994;22:273–7.

181. Ain KA et al. Thyroid hormone levels affected by time of blood sampling in thyroxine-treated patients. *Thyroid* 1993;3:81–5.

182. Davies PH, Franklyn JA. The effects of drugs on test of thyroid function. *Eur J Clin Pharmacol* 1991;40: 439–51.

183. Bishnoi A et al. Effects of commonly prescribed nonsteroidal anti-inflammatory drugs on thyroid hormone measurements. *Am J Med* 1994;96:235–8.

184. Surks MI et al. American Thyroid Association guidelines for use of laboratory tests in thyroid disorders. *JAMA* 1990;263:1529–32.

185. Cavalieri RR, Pitt-Rivers R. The effects of drugs on the distribution and metabolism of thyroid hormones. *Pharmacol Rev* 1981;33:55–80.

186. Curran PG, DeGroot LJ. The effect of hepatic enzyme-inducing drugs on thyroid hormones and the thyroid gland. *Endocr Rev* 1991;12:135–50.

187. Nicoloff JT et al. Simultaneous measurement of thyroxine and triiodothyronine peripheral turnover kinetics in man. *J Clin Invest* 1972;51:473–83.

188. Inada M et al. Estimation of thyroxine and triiodothyronine distribution and of the conversion rate of thyroxine to triiodothyronine in man. *J Clin Invest* 1975;55:1337–48.

189. Faber J, Galloe AM. Changes in bone mass during prolonged subclinical hyperthyroidism due to L-thyroxine treatment: a meta-analysis. *Eur J Endocrinol* 1994;130:350–6.

190. Escalante DA et al. Assessment of interchangeability of two brands of levothyroxine preparation with a third-generation TSH assay. *Am J Med* 1995;98:374–8.

191. Dong BJ et al. Bioequivalence of generic and brand-name levothyroxine products in the treatment of hypothyroidism. *JAMA* 1997;277:1205–13.

192. Pittman CS et al. Urinary metabolites of ^{14}C-labeled thyroxine in man. *J Clin Invest* 1972;51:1759–66.

193. Salter DR et al. Triiodothyronine (T_3) and cardiovascular therapeutics: a review. *J Card Surg* 1992;7:363–74.

194. Hashizume K et al. Administration of thyroxine in treated Graves' disease: effects on the level of antibodies to thyroid-stimulating hormone receptors and on the risk of recurrence of hyperthyroidism. *N Engl J Med* 1991;324:947–53.

195. McIver B et al. Lack of effect of thyroxine in patients with Graves' hyperthyroidism who are treated with an antithyroid drug. *N Engl J Med* 1996;334:220–4.

196. Tamai H et al. Lack of effect of thyroxine administration on elevated thyroid stimulating hormone receptor antibody levels in treated Graves' disease patients. *J Clin Endocrinol Metab* 1995;80:1481–4.

197. Nabil N et al. Methimazole: an alternative route of administration. *J Clin Endocrinol Metab* 1982;54:180–1.

198. Burrow GN. Thyroid function and hyperfunction during gestation. *Endocr Rev* 1993;14:194–202.

199. Cooper DS et al. Methimazole pharmacology in man: studies using a newly developed radioimmunoassay for methimazole. *J Clin Endocrinol Metab* 1984;58:473–9.

200. Kampmann JP, Hansen JM. Clinical pharmacokinetics of antithyroid drugs. *Clin Pharmacokinet* 1981;6: 401–28.

201. Meyer-Gessner H et al. Antithyroid drug-induced agranulocytosis: clinical experience with ten patients treated at one institution and review of the literature. *J Endocrinol Invest* 1994;17:29–36.

202. Tajiri J et al. Antithyroid drug-induced agranulocytosis: the usefulness of routine white blood cell count monitoring. *Arch Intern Med* 1990;150:621–4.

203. Tajiri J et al. Granulocyte colony-stimulating factor treatment of antithyroid drug-induced granulocytopenia. *Arch Intern Med* 1993;153:509–14.

204. Tamai H et al. Treatment of methimazole-induced agranulocytosis using recombinant human granulocyte-colony-stimulating factor (rhG-CSF). *J Clin Endocrinol Metab* 1993;77:1356–60.

205. Dolman KM et al. Vasculitis and antineutrophil cytoplasmic autoantibodies associated with propylthiouracil therapy. *Lancet* 1993;342:651–2.

206. Arab DM et al. Severe cholestatic jaundice in uncomplicated hyperthyroidism treated with methimazole. *J Clin Endocrinol Metab* 1995;80:1083–5.

207. Biswas N et al. Aplastic anemia associated with antithyroid drugs. *Am J Med Sci* 1991;301:190–4.

208. Liaw YF et al. Hepatic injury during propylthiouracil therapy in patients with hyperthyroidism. *Ann Intern Med* 1993;118:424–8.

209. Cooper DS. Antithyroid drugs: to breast-feed or not to breast-feed. *Am J Obstet Gynecol* 1987;157:234–5.

210. Wing DA et al. A comparison of propylthiouracil versus methimazole in the treatment of hyperthyroidism in pregnancy. *Am J Obstet Gynecol* 1994;170:90–5.

211. Walter RM, Bartle WR. Rectal administration of propylthiouracil in the treatment of Graves' disease. *Am J Med* 1990;88:69–70.

212. Bartle WR et al. Rectal absorption of propylthiouracil. *Int J Clin Pharmacol Ther Toxicol* 1988;26:285–7.

213. Cooper DS et al. Acute effects of propylthiouracil (PTU) on a thyroidal iodide organification and peripheral iodothyronine deiodination: correlation with serum PTU levels measured by radioimmunoassay. *J Clin Endocrinol Metab* 1982;54:101–7.

214. Levy M. Propylthiouracil hepatotoxicity. A review and case presentation. *Clin Pediatr (Phila)* 1993;32:25–9.

215. Morgan TR. Treatment of alcoholic hepatitis. *Semin Liver Dis* 1993;13:384–94.

Renal and Electrolytes

Diuretics

Class Instructions: Diuretics. If you are taking more than one dose a day, take the last dose in the afternoon or early evening to avoid having to void urine during the night. Avoid highly salted foods, but rigid salt restriction is not necessary. Avoid excessive water intake. Report any dizziness or lightheadedness (especially upon arising from sitting or lying), muscle cramps, weakness, lethargy, dry mouth, thirst, or low urine output.

Missed Doses. Take this drug at regular intervals. If you miss a dose, take it as soon as you remember. If it is about time for the next dose, take that dose only. Do not double the dose or take extra.

AMILORIDE HYDROCHLORIDE
Midamor, Various

Pharmacology. Amiloride is a potassium-sparing diuretic with a mechanism and site of action resembling triamterene. It has mild antihypertensive activity and a longer duration of action than triamterene.[1-3]

Adult Dosage. PO 10 mg/day in 1–2 doses, to a maximum of 20 mg/day.

Dosage Forms. **Tab** 5 mg and also in Moduretic 5–50 and generic products that contain hydrochlorothiazide 50 mg and amiloride 5 mg.

Pharmacokinetics. Onset is within 2 hr and maximal 6–10 hr after an oral dose; duration is about 24 hr. The drug is about 50% orally absorbed, decreasing to 30% when taken with food. Absorbed drug is excreted unchanged in urine. Half-life is 6–9 hr in normal renal function, increasing up to 144 hr in renal failure.

Adverse Reactions. Adverse reactions are generally similar to triamterene; however, in contrast to triamterene, renal stone formation has not been reported with amiloride.

FUROSEMIDE
Lasix, Various

Pharmacology. Furosemide is actively secreted via the nonspecific organic acid transport system into the lumen of the thick ascending limb of Henle's loop, where it decreases sodium reabsorption by competing for the chloride site on the Na^+-K^+-$2Cl^-$ cotransporter. Medullary hypertonicity is diminished, thereby decreasing the kidney's ability to reabsorb water. Excretion of sodium, chloride, potassium, hydrogen ion, calcium, magnesium, ammonium, bicarbonate, and possibly phosphate is enhanced. IV furosemide increases venous capacitance independent of diuretic effect, producing rapid improvement in pulmonary edema.[2,3]

Administration and Adult Dosage. PO for edema 20–80 mg as a single dose initially; double successive doses q 6–8 hr until response is obtained. The maximum single dose depends on the disease state: 160 mg for hepatic insufficiency; 240 mg for nephrotic syndrome; 80 mg for CHF (with normal kidney function);[4] however, dosages up to 2500 mg/day have been recommended in refractory CHF.[5] After response, effective dosage is given in 1–3 doses daily; usual daily maintenance dosage depends on the single dose to which the patient responded. **PO for chronic renal failure** 80 mg initially, increasing in 80 mg/day increments until response is obtained, to a maximum of 240 mg.[4] (*See* Special Populations.) **PO for hypertension** 40 mg bid. **IV** should be used only when oral administration is not feasible. IV doses can be given over 1–2 min, except the rate should not exceed 4 mg/min when large doses are given. **IM or IV for edema** use one-half the dose of PO furosemide (as outlined above);[4] may double the dose q 2 or more hr until desired response is obtained. This dosage is then given in 1–2 doses daily for maintenance. Dosages up to 4 g/day IV have been used in refractory CHF.[5] **IV for acute pulmonary edema** 40 mg initially, may repeat in 30–60 min with 80 mg, if necessary (assuming relatively normal kidney function). For patients with renal impairment, the initial and subsequent doses must be adjusted based on renal function. For example, if Cl_{cr} is 50 mL/min (about one-half normal), the dose must be doubled; if Cl_{cr} is 25 mL/min, the dose must be quadrupled. **Continuous IV infusion for edema or chronic renal failure** 40 mg loading dose followed by 20–40 mg/hr.

Special Populations. *Pediatric Dosage.* **PO for edema** 2 mg/kg in 1 dose initially, increasing by 1–2 mg/kg in 6–8 hr, if necessary, to a maximum of 6 mg/kg/day. **IM or IV** 1 mg/kg in 1 dose initially, increasing by 1 mg/kg q 2 or more hr until desired response is obtained or to a maximum of 6 mg/kg/day. Maximum single dose depends on renal function. (*See* Notes.)

Geriatric Dosage. Start with a low initial dose and titrate to response.

Other Conditions. For Cl_{cr} <15 mL/min, maximal response is attained with single IV doses of 200 mg (400 mg PO). Hence, there appears to be no need to administer larger single doses to such patients.[4] A diminished response may occur in severe decompensated CHF, caused in part by alterations in oral absorption[6] and decreased renal blood flow (despite relatively normal GFR), resulting in decreased delivery of furosemide to the renal tubule; IV administration circumvents absorption problems. However, decompensated CHF usually affects only the rate, rather than the extent of oral furosemide absorption.[7] Additionally, high-dose therapy may be of benefit in severe, refractory CHF.[6] (*See* Administration and Adult Dosage.) For patients with cirrhosis, dosage is based on renal function.

Dosage Forms. **Soln** 8, 10 mg/mL; **Tab** 20, 40, 80 mg; **Inj** 10 mg/mL.

Patient Instructions. (*See* Class Instructions: Diuretics.)

Pharmacokinetics. *Onset and Duration.* (Venous capacitance) IV onset 5 min, duration >1 hr. (Diuresis) PO onset 30–60 min, peak 1–2 hr, duration <6 hr; IV onset 15 min, peak 30–60 min, duration 1–2 hr; duration may be prolonged in severe renal impairment. (Hypertension) maximum effect on BP may not occur for several days.

Serum Levels. Site of action is within the renal tubules and not the serum; therefore, serum concentrations do not reflect diuretic activity. Serum levels >25 mg/L may be associated with ototoxicity.[8]

Fate. Pharmacokinetics are variable and absorption is erratic; $61 \pm 17\%$ (range 20–100) is bioavailable in normals, 30–100% in renal failure.[8,9] The rate, but not the extent, of absorption may be decreased in patients with edematous bowel caused by decompensated CHF;[7] 96–99% is plasma protein bound, reduced in CHF, renal disease, or cirrhosis.[9] $V_{d\beta}$ is 0.11 L/kg; Cl is 0.12 ± 0.24 L/hr/kg; both V_d and Cl depend on protein binding.[8,9] Two possible inactive metabolites exist: a glucuronide, which is primarily excreted in urine (and to a lesser extent in the feces by passive diffusion into the GI lumen), and saluamine, which may be a true metabolite or an analytical artifact. Renal clearance is primarily by active secretion; 50–80% (IV) and 20–55% (PO) is excreted unchanged in urine. Renal clearance is decreased in renal failure consistent with decreased renal blood flow, a reduction of functioning nephrons, and the presence of competitive inhibitors for secretion.[9]

$t_{\frac{1}{2}}$. 92 ± 7 (range 30–120) min in normals, may be extended in cirrhosis to 81 ± 8 min or CHF to 122 min, and markedly prolonged in end-stage renal disease to 9.7 hr, and in multiorgan failure to 20–24 hr. Mean residence time has been proposed as a more appropriate estimate of duration: 51.4 min (IV); 135–195 min (PO).[8,9]

Adverse Reactions. Dehydration, hypotension, hypochloremic alkalosis, and hypokalemia are frequent. Hyperglycemia and glucose intolerance occur as with thiazides. (*See* Hydrochlorothiazide.) With high-dose therapy (>250 mg/day), hyperuricemia occurs frequently. Tinnitus and hearing loss, occasionally permanent, occur frequently in association with rapid IV injection of large doses in patients with renal impairment.[5,9,10] Rarely, thrombocytopenia, neutropenia, jaundice, pancreatitis, and a variety of skin reactions occur.

Contraindications. Pregnancy; anuria (except for single dose in acute anuria).

Precautions. Use with caution in patients with severe or progressive renal disease; discontinue if renal function worsens. Use with caution in liver disease (may precipitate hepatic encephalopathy), history of diabetes mellitus or gout, and in patients allergic to other sulfonamide derivatives. Use with caution in patients with hypokalemia, hypomagnesemia, or hypocalcemia.

Drug Interactions. Cholestyramine decreases furosemide absorption, and NSAIDs may decrease the diuretic effect of furosemide. Aminoglycoside toxicity may be enhanced in renally impaired patients. IV furosemide may produce flushing, sweating, and blood pressure variations in patients taking chloral hydrate.

Parameters to Monitor. Monitor serum potassium closely, other electrolytes periodically, and serum glucose, uric acid, BUN, and Cr_s occasionally. Observe for clinical signs of fluid or electrolyte depletion such as dry mouth, thirst, weakness, lethargy, muscle pains or cramps, hypotension, oliguria, tachycardia, and GI upset.

Notes. Furosemide is light sensitive; oral solution must be refrigerated and protected from light. In severe proteinuria (>3.5 g/day), urinary albumin binds furosemide and reduces its effectiveness.[7] In general, clinical nonresponders tend to have a decreased fraction of loop diuretics excreted in the urine. For these patients, and for patients with CHF and renal impairment, larger doses may force more drug into the tubule; however, the risk of ototoxicity must be considered. Alternatively, combined use with a **thiazide** or **metolazone** orally may be effective by blocking sodium reabsorption at multiple tubule sites; however, these agents (especially metolazone) have a slow onset of action. If a rapid response is needed, IV **acetazolamide** or **chlorothiazide** can be given followed by the loop diuretic.[3,4,11,12] Combination with theophylline can also enhance diuresis.[12] (*See* Loop Diuretics Comparison Chart.)

			LOOP DIURETICS COMPARISON CHART		
DRUG	DOSAGE FORMS	ADULT DOSAGE[a]	PEDIATRIC DOSAGE[a]	DOSAGE IN RENAL IMPAIRMENT	COMMENTS
Bumetanide Bumex Various	Tab 0.5, 1, 2 mg Inj 0.25 mg/mL.	PO for edema 0.5–2 mg/day, to a maximum of 10 mg/day. IM or IV or 2–3 min 0.5–1 mg, to a maximum of 10 mg/day IV continuous infusion 1 mg, then 1–2 mg/hr.	PO, IM, or IV 0.01–0.02 mg/kg, to a maximum of 0.4 mg/kg or 10 mg total daily dosage.	For Cl_{cr} <15 mL/min, maximal response is attained with single PO or IV doses of 8–10 mg; IV infusion of 12 mg over 12 hr may be more effective and less toxic.	1 mg PO or IV = 40 mg IV furosemide.
Ethacrynic Acid Edecrin	Tab 25, 50 mg Inj 50 mg.	PO minimal dose in the range of 50–200 mg/day initially, to a maximum of 200 mg bid IV 50 mg or 0.5–1 mg/kg, to a maximum of 100 mg.	PO (infants) not established; (children) 25 mg or 1 mg/kg initially, increased in 25 mg increments to desired effect; IV not established; 1 mg/kg has been used.	Not recommended with Cl_{cr} <10 mL/min; for Cl_{cr} of 10–50 mL/min, increase interval to q 8–12 hr.	Nonsulfonamide. Reliable potency data not available; however, 50 mg IV is about equal to furosemide 35 mg IV.
Furosemide Lasix Various	Tab 20, 40, 80 mg Soln 8, 10 mg/mL Inj 10 mg/mL.	(See monograph.)	(See monograph.)	Maximum response occurs with 200 mg IV or an average of 400 mg PO, although quite variable.	IV dose averages 50% of PO dose, with great variability.
Torsemide Demadex	Tab 5, 10, 20, 100 mg Inj 10 mg/mL.	(See monograph.)	(See monograph.)	Maximal response occurs with PO or IV dose of 50–100 mg.	5–10 mg PO or IV = 20 mg IV furosemide.

[a]Higher doses needed for patients with CHF, liver cirrhosis, and nephrotic syndrome.
From references 5–7, 13, 14, and product information.

HYDROCHLOROTHIAZIDE
Esidrix, Hydrodiuril, Oretic, Various

Pharmacology. Thiazides increase sodium and chloride excretion by interfering with their reabsorption in the cortical diluting segment of the nephron; a mild diuresis of slightly concentrated urine results. Potassium, bicarbonate, magnesium, phosphate, and iodide excretion are also increased; calcium excretion is decreased. Decreases in interstitial fluid volume, reductions in intracellular calcium secondary to a fall in smooth muscle sodium concentration, and a change in the affinity of cell surface receptors to vasoconstrictive hormones are thought to be among the mechanisms for the hypotensive effect of the thiazides. Urine output is paradoxically decreased in diabetes insipidus.[2,3]

Administration and Adult Dosage. **PO for edema** 25–200 mg/day in 1–3 doses initially; 25–100 mg/day or intermittently for maintenance, to a maximum of 200 mg/day. **PO for hypertension** 12.5–50 mg/day. Maintenance dosages >50 mg/day provide little additional benefit in controlling essential hypertension and may increase the frequency of dose-related biochemical abnormalities.[15]

Special Populations. *Pediatric Dosage.* **PO** (<6 months) may require up to 3.3 mg/kg/day in 2 divided doses; (>6 months) 2–2.2 mg/kg/day in 2 divided doses.

Geriatric Dosage. Start with a low initial dose and titrate to response.

Other Conditions. At a Cl_{cr} <30 mL/min, usual dosages of thiazides and most related drugs are not very effective as diuretics.[4]

Dosage Forms. **Tab** 25, 50, 100 mg; **Soln** 10, 100 mg/mL.

Patient Instructions. (*See* Class Instructions: Diuretics.) If stomach upset occurs, take drug with meals. Report persistent anorexia, nausea, or vomiting.

Pharmacokinetics. *Onset and Duration.* Onset of diuresis within 2 hr; peak in 4–6 hr; duration 6–12 hr. Onset of hypotensive effect in 3–4 days; duration 1 week or less after discontinuing therapy.

Serum Levels. The site of diuretic action is within the renal tubules and not the serum; therefore, serum concentrations do not reflect diuretic activity.

Fate. Oral bioavailability is 71 ± 15% in healthy individuals, increased when given with an anticholinergic, and decreased by one-half in CHF and after intestinal shunt surgery. There are no differences in absorption among single-entity formulations. The drug is 58 ± 17% plasma protein bound; V_d is 0.83 ± 0.31 L/kg; Cl is 0.29 ± 0.07 L/hr/kg. Over 95% is excreted unchanged in urine by filtration and secretion. In severe renal impairment, renal clearance is prolonged 5-fold, with nonrenal clearance (mechanism as yet unidentified) playing an increased role in elimination.[8,16]

$t_{1/2}$. 2.5 ± 2 hr; prolonged in uncompensated CHF or renal impairment.[8,16,17]

Adverse Reactions. Hypokalemia is frequent; however, its treatment in otherwise healthy hypertensive patients is usually unnecessary. Potassium supplements or potassium-sparing diuretics (*see* Notes) may be indicated in patients with arrhythmias, MI, or severe ischemic heart disease; those with chronic liver disease; elderly eating a poor diet; patients taking digoxin, a corticosteroid, or drugs that interfere with ventricular repolarization such as phenothiazines and heterocyclic antidepressants; and those whose serum potassium falls below 3 mEq/L. Hyperuricemia occurs frequently but is reversible, and treatment is unnecessary unless the patient has renal impairment or a history of gout.[18] Hyperglycemia and alterations in glucose tolerance (usually reversible), loss of diabetic control, or precipitation of diabetes mellitus occur occasionally. Decreased glucose tolerance may increase in prevalence after several years of therapy.[19,20] Thrombocytopenia and pancreatitis occur rarely. Elevation of serum cholesterol and triglycerides occurs; the clinical importance is unknown, but it may increase the risk of coronary heart disease.

Contraindications. Anuria; pregnancy, unless accompanied by severe edema; allergy to sulfonamide derivatives.

Precautions. Use with caution in patients with renal function impairment, liver disease (may precipitate hepatic encephalopathy), history of diabetes mellitus, or gout. Use with caution in patients with diabetes mellitus, because thiazides may increase glucose intolerance.[19,20]

Drug Interactions. Cholestyramine decreases oral absorption of thiazides, and NSAIDs may decrease the diuretic effect of thiazides. Anticholinergics may increase oral bioavailability. Dosage of potent hypotensive agents may have to be reduced if a thiazide is added to the regimen. Concurrent calcium-containing antacids may cause hypercalcemia. Long-term thiazides may reduce lithium excretion.

Parameters to Monitor. Monitor serum potassium weekly to monthly initially; q 3–6 months when stable. Monitor other serum electrolytes periodically. Monitor all electrolytes more closely when other losses occur (eg, vomiting, diarrhea). Observe for clinical signs of fluid or electrolyte depletion such as dry mouth, thirst, weakness, lethargy, muscle pains or cramps, hypotension, oliguria, tachycardia, and GI upset. Monitor blood pressure periodically during antihypertensive therapy and serum glucose in patients with diabetes mellitus.

Notes. For the prevention of hypokalemia during thiazide therapy, a **potassium-sparing diuretic** may be preferred over potassium supplements in alkalotic patients, because these agents decrease hydrogen ion loss, which can correct alkalosis and drive more potassium extracellularly.[21] Potassium-sparing diuretics may also be preferred for patients predisposed to hypomagnesemia and for those with serum potassium <3 mEq/L, because potassium supplements rarely correct hypokalemia of this severity. (*See* Thiazides and Related Diuretics Comparison Chart.) JNC IV guidelines recommend diuretics and β-blockers as initial drugs of choice for patients with hypertension based on demonstrated reductions in morbidity and mortality.

THIAZIDES AND RELATED DIURETICS COMPARISON CHART[a]

DRUG	DOSAGE FORMS	ORAL DIURETIC DOSAGE RANGE (MG/DAY)	EQUIVALENT DIURETIC DOSAGE (MG)	PEAK EFFECT (HR)	DURATION OF DIURESIS (HR)
Bendroflumethiazide Naturetin	Tab 5, 10 mg.	2.5–15	5	4	6–12
Benthiazide Exna Various	Tab 50 mg.	50–150	50	4–6	12–18
Chlorothiazide Diuril Various	Tab 250, 500 mg Susp 50 mg/mL Inj 500 mg.[b]	500–2000	500	2 (PO) 0.5 (IV)	6–12 (PO) 2 (IV)
Chlorthalidone[c] Hygroton Thalitone Various	Tab (Thalitone)[d] 15, 25 mg Tab 25, 50, 100 mg.	15–200	50	2	24–72
Hydrochlorothiazide Various	Cap 12.5 mg Tab 25, 50, 100 mg Soln 10, 100 mg/mL.	25–100	50	4–6	6–12
Hydroflumethiazide Diucardin Saluron Various	Tab 50 mg.	25–100	50	3–4	12–24
Indapamide[c] Lozol Various	Tab 1.25, 2.5 mg.	1.25–5	2.5	2	24–36

(continued)

677

THIAZIDES AND RELATED DIURETICS COMPARISON CHART[a] (continued)

DRUG	DOSAGE FORMS	ORAL DIURETIC DOSAGE RANGE (MG/DAY)	EQUIVALENT DIURETIC DOSAGE (MG)	PEAK EFFECT (HR)	DURATION OF DIURESIS (HR)
Methyclothiazide Aquatensen Enduron Various	Tab 2.5, 5 mg.	2.5–10	5	6	24
Metolazone[c] Mykrox Zaroxolyn	Tab (Mykrox)[d] 0.5 mg Tab 2.5, 5, 10 mg.	5–20 0.5–1 (Mykrox)	5 (Zaroxolyn)	2	12–24
Polythiazide Renese	Tab 1, 2, 4 mg.	1–4	2	6	24–48
Quinethazone[c] Hydromox	Tab 50 mg.	50–200	50	6	18–24
Trichlormethiazide Metahydrin Naqua	Tab 2, 4, mg.	2–4	2	6	24

[a]From USP-DI and product informtion; patients unresponsive to maximal dosage of one agent are unlikely to respond to another agent.
[b]There is no therapeutic advantage in giving the drug parenterally.
[c]Not a thiazide, but similar in structure and mechanism of action.
[d]Thalitone and Mykrox are more bioavailable than other formulations of the respective drugs.

MANNITOL   Osmitrol, Various

Pharmacology. Mannitol and other osmotic diuretics do not act on specific receptors, but rather on tubular fluid composition by distributing into extracellular fluid. Mannitol inhibits sodium and chloride reabsorption in the proximal tubule and ascending loop of Henle. Sodium, potassium, calcium, and phosphate excretion is increased. Renal blood flow is increased, the GFR of superficial nephrons is increased, and that of deep nephrons is decreased.[22] Mannitol increases serum osmolality, expanding intravascular volume and decreasing intraocular and intracranial pressures.[2,22]

Administration and Adult Dosage. *Never administer IM or SC, or add to whole blood for transfusion.* **IV as diagnostic evaluation of acute oliguria** (if blood pressure and CVP are normal and *after* cardiac output is maximized) give test dose of 12.5 g as a 15–20% solution over 3–5 min (often given with **furosemide** 80–120 mg IV), may repeat in1 hr if urine output is less than 30–50 mL/hr. If no response after 2 doses, give no more mannitol and treat for acute tubular necrosis. If response occurs, look for underlying cause of oliguria (eg, hypovolemia). **IV for prevention of acute renal failure** give test dose as above to a total dose of 50 g or more in 1 hr as a loading dose, then maintain urine output at 50 mL/hr with continuous infusion of 5% solution, plus 20 mEq/L sodium chloride and 1 g/L calcium gluconate. **IV for reduction of intracranial or intraocular pressure** 1.5–2 g/kg over 30–60 min as a 15–25% solution. **IV to decrease nephrotoxicity of cisplatin** 12.5 g IV push just prior to cisplatin, then 10 g/hr for 6 hr as a 20% solution. Replace fluids with 0.45% sodium chloride with 20–30 mEq/L potassium chloride at 250 mL/hr for 6 hr. Maintain urine output >100 mL/hr with mannitol infusion.[23] (*See* Notes.)

Special Populations. *Pediatric Dosage.* **IV for oliguria or anuria** give test dose of 20 mg/kg as above; the therapeutic dose is 2 g/kg over 2–6 hr as a 15–20% solution. **IV for reduction of intracranial or intraocular pressure** 2 g/kg over 30–60 min as a 15–25% solution. **IV for intoxications** 2 g/kg as 5–10% solution as needed to maintain a high urinary output. (*See* Notes.)

Geriatric Dosage. Start with a low initial dose and titrate to response.

Dosage Forms. Inj 5, 10, 15, 20, 25%.

Pharmacokinetics. *Onset and Duration.* (Diuresis) onset 1–3 hr, duration depends on half-life. (Decrease in intraocular pressure) onset in 30–60 min, duration 4–6 hr. (Decrease in intracranial pressure) onset within 15 min, peak 60–90 min, duration 3–8 hr after stopping infusion.[24]

Serum Levels. The site of diuretic action is within the renal tubules and not the serum; therefore, serum concentrations do not reflect diuretic activity.

Fate. About 17% is absorbed orally. IV doses of 1 g/kg and 2 g/kg increase serum osmolality by 11 and 32 mOsm/kg, decrease serum sodium by 8.7 and 20.7 mEq/L, and decrease hemoglobin by 2.2 and 2.5 g/dL, respectively.[25] V_c is 0.074 L/kg; $V_{d\beta}$ is 0.23 L/kg; Cl is 0.086 L/hr/kg.[26] Mannitol is virtually completely eliminated unchanged in urine.

$t_{\frac{1}{2}}$. α phase 0.11 ± 0.12 hr; β phase 2.2 ± 1.3 hr.[26]

Adverse Reactions. Most serious and frequent are fluid and electrolyte imbalance, particularly symptoms of fluid overload such as pulmonary edema, hypertension, water intoxication, and CHF. Acute renal failure has been reported occasionally with high doses, especially in patients with renal impairment.[27,28] Dermal necrosis can occur if solution extravasates. Anaphylaxis has been reported rarely.

Contraindications. Patients with well-established anuria caused by severe renal disease or impaired renal function who do not respond to test dose; severe pulmonary congestion, frank pulmonary edema, or severe CHF; severe dehydration; edema not caused by renal, cardiac, or hepatic disease that is associated with abnormal capillary fragility or membrane permeability; active intracranial bleeding, except during craniotomy.

Precautions. Pregnancy. Observe solution for crystals before administering. (*See* Notes.) Water intoxication may occur if fluid input exceeds urine output. Masking of inadequate hydration or hypovolemia may occur by drug-induced sustaining of diuresis. If extravasation occurs, aspirate any accessible extravasated solution, then remove the IV catheter and apply a cold compress to the area.

Drug Interactions. None known.

Parameters to Monitor. Monitor urine output closely and discontinue drug if output is low. Monitor serum electrolytes closely, taking care not to misinterpret low serum sodium as a sign of hypotonicity. (*See* Fate.) If serum sodium is low, measure serum osmolality. Observe for clinical signs of fluid or electrolyte depletion such as dry mouth, thirst, weakness, lethargy, muscle pains or cramps, hypotension, oliguria, tachycardia, and GI upset.

Notes. Mannitol may crystallize out of solution at concentrations above 15%. The crystals may be redissolved by warming containers in hot water and shaking or by autoclaving; cool to body temperature before administration. Administer solutions of 20% or greater through an inline filter. Addition of electrolytes to solutions of 20% or greater concentration may cause precipitation.

SPIRONOLACTONE   Aldactone, Various

Pharmacology. Spironolactone is a steroidal competitive aldosterone antagonist that acts from the interstitial side of the distal and collecting tubular epithelium to block sodium-potassium exchange, producing a delayed and mild diuresis. The diuretic effect is maximal in states of hyperaldosteronism. Sodium, chloride, and calcium excretion is increased; potassium and magnesium excretion is decreased. Spironolactone has mild antihypertensive activity and has a direct positive inotropic action on the heart.[29–31]

Administration and Adult Dosage. **PO for edema** 25–200 mg/day (usually 100 mg) in 2–4 divided doses initially, adjusting dosage after 5 days. If response is inadequate, add a thiazide or loop diuretic to the regimen. **PO for essential hypertension** 50–100 mg/day initially, adjusting dosage after 2 weeks. **PO for ascites** 100 mg/day initially, increasing to 200–400 mg/day in 2–4 divided doses. Restrict sodium to 2 g/day or less and, if necessary, fluid to 1 L/day. To eliminate delay in onset, a loading dose of 2–3 times the daily dosage may be given on the first day of therapy.[32]

Special Populations. *Pediatric Dosage.* PO 3.3 mg/kg/day, readjust dosage after 5 days; dosage may be increased up to triple this value. Restrict duration of therapy to 1 month.

Geriatric Dosage. Start with a low initial dose and titrate to response.

Dosage Forms. **Tab** 25, 50, 100 mg; **Tab** 25 mg with hydrochlorothiazide 25 mg (Aldactazide, various); **Tab** 50 mg with hydrochlorothiazide 50 mg (Aldactazide 50/50).

Patient Instructions. (*See* Class Instructions: Diuretics.) Avoid excessive amounts of high-potassium foods or salt substitutes.

Pharmacokinetics. *Onset and Duration.* Onset gradual, peak 2–3 days with continued administration; onset can be hastened by giving loading dose; duration 2–3 days after cessation of therapy.

Serum Levels. Not established and not used clinically.

Fate. Bioavailability is about 90%;[29] food promotes absorption and possibly decreases first-pass effect.[13] Spironolactone undergoes rapid and extensive metabolism to canrenone (active metabolite), 7α-thiomethylspirolactone (major metabolite), and other sulfur-containing metabolites; together with the parent drug, these metabolites contribute to the overall antimineralocorticoid activity.[14,29] Metabolites are primarily eliminated renally, with minimal biliary excretion. Little or no parent drug is excreted unchanged in urine.[14,33]

$t_{1/2}$. (Spironolactone) 1.4 ± 0.5 hr; (7α-thiomethylspirolactone) 13.8 ± 6.4 hr; (canrenone) 16.5 ± 6.3 hr.[14]

Adverse Reactions. Hyperkalemia may occur, most frequently in patients with renal function impairment (especially those with diabetes mellitus) and those receiving potassium supplements or concomitant ACE inhibitors. Dehydration and hyponatremia occur occasionally, especially when the drug is combined with other diuretics. In patients receiving high dosages, frequent estrogen-like side effects including gynecomastia, decreased libido, and impotence in males occur; menstrual irregularities and breast tenderness occur in females. These effects are reversible after drug discontinuation.[34]

Contraindications. Anuria; acute renal insufficiency; rapidly deteriorating renal function; severe renal failure; serum potassium >5.5 mEq/L or development of hyperkalemia while taking the drug; hypermagnesemia.

Precautions. Pregnancy. Patients with renal impairment, especially those with diabetes mellitus and/or receiving an ACE inhibitor, are at risk for developing hyperkalemia. Use with caution in patients with hepatic disease. Do not use with triamterene or amiloride. Give potassium supplements only to patients with demonstrated hypokalemia who are taking a proximally acting diuretic and a corticosteroid concurrently with spironolactone or only for very short periods in treating cirrhosis and ascites.

Drug Interactions. Use with ACE inhibitors increases risk of hyperkalemia, especially in renal impairment. Spironolactone increases serum concentration of digoxin by reducing renal and possibly nonrenal clearance. Additionally, spironolactone and its metabolites may cross-react with digoxin-binding antibody in some digoxin immunoassays.

Parameters to Monitor. Monitor serum electrolytes, particularly potassium, periodically, especially early in the course of therapy. Monitor BUN and/or Cr_s periodically. In ascites, also obtain daily weight and urinary electrolytes, maintaining weight loss at no greater than 0.5–1 kg/day and urinary Na^+/K^+ ratio at greater than 1. Observe for clinical signs of fluid or electrolyte depletion such as dry mouth, thirst, weakness, lethargy, muscle pains or cramps, hypotension, oliguria, tachycardia, and GI upset.

Notes. Spironolactone is useful in patients with diabetes mellitus (with good renal function) or gout because it causes no impairment of glucose tolerance and minimal hyperuricemia. It is used in the diagnosis of primary aldosteronism and may be used in the management of the condition in patients unable to undergo surgery.

TORSEMIDE   Demadex

Pharmacology. Torsemide is a loop diuretic similar to furosemide. Over the normal dosage range, its diuretic potency by weight is about 2–4 times that of furosemide. Onset of diuresis is similar; however, duration is longer (up to 8–12 hr orally).[35–38]

Adult Dosage. PO for hypertension 5–10 mg/day orally. **Initial PO or IV for edema or chronic renal failure** 20 mg/day; dosage can be doubled until the desired response is obtained, to a usual maximum of 200 mg/day; or, IV by continuous infusion, give 20 mg loading dose, then 10–20 mg/hr. **PO or IV for cirrhosis** 5–10 mg/day initially with a potassium-sparing diuretic, to a usual maximum of 40 mg/day. (*See* Furosemide Notes and Loop Diuretics Comparison Chart.)

Dosage Forms. **Tab** 5, 10, 20, 100 mg; **Inj** 10 mg/mL.

Pharmacokinetics. Oral bioavailability is 79–91% (median 80); V_d is 0.14–0.19 L/kg. In healthy individuals, the elimination half-life of torsemide is dose dependent, ranging from 2.2 to 3.8 hr. Nonrenal Cl remains essentially constant over a dosage range of 5–20 mg, but renal Cl and fraction excreted decrease, suggesting saturable renal clearance. Further studies are needed to clarify whether torsemide undergoes dose-dependent renal elimination. Renal impairment ($Cl_{cr} \leq 60$ mL/min) does not appreciably alter pharmacokinetic parameters; hemodialysis and hemofiltration do not markedly influence serum clearance.

Adverse Reactions. Although the potential for hypokalemia exists, torsemide's kaliuretic potency is less than that of furosemide, suggesting that it may be less potassium wasting during long-term therapy; however, the clinical relevance of this observation is unknown. Precautions and monitoring parameters are the same as for furosemide.

TRIAMTERENE   Dyrenium

Pharmacology. Triamterene acts directly from the distal tubular lumen on active sodium exchange for potassium and hydrogen, producing a mild diuresis that is independent of aldosterone concentration. Sodium, chloride, calcium, and possibly bicarbonate excretion is increased; potassium and possibly magnesium excretion is decreased. Antihypertensive activity is inconsistent and less pronounced than with thiazides or spironolactone.[30,31]

Administration and Adult Dosage. **PO** initially 100 mg bid after meals if used alone; lower dosage if used with another diuretic. Adjust the maintenance dosage to the needs of the patient; it may range from 100 mg/day to 100 mg every other day, to a maximum of 300 mg/day.

Special Populations. *Pediatric Dosage.* **PO** 2–4 mg/kg/day initially, may increase to 6 mg/kg/day in 1–2 doses after meals, to a maximum of 300 mg/day. Decrease dosage if used with another diuretic.

Geriatric Dosage. Start with a low initial dose and titrate to response.

Dosage Forms. **Cap** 50, 100 mg; **Cap** 50 mg with hydrochlorothiazide 25 mg (Dyazide, various); **Tab** 75 mg with hydrochlorothiazide 50 mg (Maxzide, various); 37.5 mg with hydrochlorothiazide 25 mg (Maxzide-25, various).

Patient Instructions. (*See* Class Instructions: Diuretics.) This drug may be taken with food or milk to minimize stomach upset. Report persistent loss of appetite, nausea, or vomiting. Avoid eating excessive amounts of high-potassium foods or salt substitutes.

Pharmacokinetics. *Onset and Duration.* Onset 2–4 hr; full therapeutic effect may not occur for several days; duration 7–9 hr.

Serum Levels. The site of diuretic action is within the renal tubules and not the serum; therefore, serum concentrations do not reflect diuretic activity.

Fate. Variable absorption, depending on formulation,[39,40] bioavailability is $52 \pm 22\%$.[40] When the total urinary excretion of triamterene and its pharmacologically active metabolite is considered, the bioavailability value of triamterene reaches $83.2 \pm 25.9\%$.[40] Triamterene undergoes marked first-pass metabolism with rapid hydroxylation followed by immediate conjugation to the sulfate ester, which is the predominant form in plasma and urine.[40] The sulfate conjugate is nearly equipotent with the parent in causing sodium excretion and sparing of potassium.[41,42] Triamterene is 50–55% plasma protein bound,[30,31] and its sulfate conjugate is 91% protein bound.[40] After oral administration, serum concentrations of both triamterene and its sulfate conjugate undergo a rapid decline over the first 6–8 hr after administration, followed by a slower terminal phase.[41] Both are eliminated renally by filtration and secretion. The fraction of a dose excreted as the parent is $3 \pm 2\%$; that for the sulfate conjugate is $34 \pm 8\%$.[41] The sulfate conjugate may accumulate in renal impairment.[42]

$t_{1/2}$. β phase (healthy adults) 4.3 ± 0.7 hr for triamterene and 3.1 ± 1.2 hr for sulfate;[40] up to 12 hr in cirrhosis.[43] Half-lives may also be prolonged in the elderly.[44]

Adverse Reactions. Nausea, vomiting, diarrhea, and dizziness occur occasionally. Dehydration and hyponatremia with an increase in BUN occur occasionally, especially when the drug is combined with other diuretics. Triamterene renal stones occur occasionally. Hyperkalemia occurs occasionally, especially in diabetics and in patients with renal impairment; metabolic acidosis has been reported. Megaloblastic anemia can occur in alcoholic cirrhosis.

Contraindications. Severe or progressive renal disease or dysfunction (except possibly nephrosis); severe renal failure; severe hepatic disease; serum potassium >5.5 mEq/L or development of hyperkalemia while taking the drug; hypermagnesemia.

Precautions. Pregnancy. Patients with renal impairment, especially those with diabetes mellitus and/or receiving an ACE inhibitor, are at risk for developing hyperkalemia. May cause elevation in serum uric acid in patients predisposed to gout. Do not use with spironolactone or amiloride.

Drug Interactions. Use with ACE inhibitors increases risk of hyperkalemia, especially in renal impairment. Indomethacin (and probably other NSAIDs) may reduce renal function when combined with triamterene.

Parameters to Monitor. Monitor serum electrolytes, particularly potassium, periodically, especially early in the course of therapy. Monitor BUN and/or Cr_s periodically. Observe for clinical signs of fluid or electrolyte depletion such as dry mouth, thirst, weakness, lethargy, muscle pains or cramps, hypotension, oliguria, tachycardia, and GI upset.

DIURETICS OF CHOICE COMPARISON CHART[a]

CONDITION	LOOP DIURETICS	OSMOTIC DIURETICS	THIAZIDES	POTASSIUM-SPARING AGENTS	COMMENTS
Relative potency	>15%	10–15%	5–10%	<5%	Values refer to maximum fraction of filtered sodium excreted following maximally effective dose of drug.
Hypertension	A	—	A	D	Sustained antihypertensive effect of thiazides exhibits a flat dose-response curve and occurs at doses below the threshold for diuresis. Loop diuretics are diuretics of choice with Cl_{cr} <30 mL/min.
Congestive heart failure	A	—	A	D	Begin with thiazide with low dosage; if ineffective, substitute a loop diuretic. Loop diuretics are diuretics of choice with Cl_{cr} <30 mL/min. A loop diuretic plus a thiazide (in a high dose) can evoke a clinically useful diuresis even when Cl_{cr} is <15 mL/min.
Pulmonary edema	A (IV)	—	—	—	Prompt venodilation precedes diuretic effect.
Hepatic ascites	B	—	—	A	Spironolactone is the agent of choice; urine Na:K ratio <1 indicates need for higher dosage (200–1000 mg/day). Rate of diuresis should not exceed 750 mL/day (no peripheral edema), or up to 2 L/day (if edema is present).
Renal failure	A	C	—	—	A loop diuretic plus a thiazide (in a high dose) can evoke a clinically useful diuresis even when Cl_{cr} is <15 mL/min; however, provocative diuretic challenges in oliguric patients can be potentially hazardous, especially if the cause of renal failure is uncertain.

(continued)

DIURETICS OF CHOICE COMPARISON CHART[a] (continued)

CONDITION	LOOP DIURETICS	OSMOTIC DIURETICS	THIAZIDES	POTASSIUM-SPARING AGENTS	COMMENTS
Diabetes insipidus	—	—	A	—	Thiazides are most useful in the nephrogenic form; a long-acting agent is preferred. In pituitary form, oral diuretics may be a useful alternative for patients who prefer oral therapy to the use of intranasal or IV desmopressin.
Hypercalcemia	A	—	—	—	High-dose furosemide (IV 80–100 mg q 1–2 hr) with IV saline for forced diuresis to promote calcium excretion.
Hypercalciuria	—	—	A	—	Thiazides cause marked reduction in urinary calcium excretion; they also appear effective in preventing calcium stone formation irrespective of whether urinary calcium is abnormally elevated.

A = Diuretic of choice; B = diuretic of second choice if patient is unresponsive to first choice; C = useful in some circumstances; D = useful as an adjunct to a more potent diuretic to reduce potassium loss and possibly enhance therapeutic effect.

[a]This table is a guide to the selection of the most appropriate diuretic for the condition listed, but is not an all-inclusive guide to therapy.

From references 30, 31, and 45–47.

Electrolytes

Class Instructions: Oral Electrolytes. Take oral products with (tablets) or diluted in (liquids and powders) 6–8 fl oz of water or juice to avoid GI injury or laxative effect. This medication may be taken with food or after meals if upset stomach occurs.

CALCIUM SALTS
Various

Pharmacology. Calcium plays an important role in neuromuscular activity, pancreatic insulin release, gastric hydrogen secretion, blood coagulation, and platelet aggregation; as a cofactor for some enzyme reactions; and in bone and tooth metabolism.[48]

Administration and Adult Dosage. PO as dietary supplement (elemental calcium) 500–2000 mg bid–qid; RDA 800 mg/day;[49] for mature women, 1 g/day before menopause and 1.5 g/day thereafter has been recommended.[50] **PO to lower serum phosphate in end-stage renal disease (ESRD)** (calcium carbonate) 650 mg with each meal initially, adjust dosage to decrease serum phosphate to less than 6 mg/dL,[51] most patients require more than 1.3 g with each meal; (calcium acetate) 1334 mg with each meal initially, adjust dosage to decrease serum phosphate to <6 mg/dL. (*See* Notes.) **IV for emergency elevation of serum calcium** (calcium gluconate) 15 mg/kg in NS or D5W infused over 8–10 hr (typically raises serum calcium by 2–3 mg/dL),[52] may repeat q 1–3 days depending on response; (calcium gluceptate) 1.1–1.4 g infused at a rate not to exceed 36 mg/min of elemental calcium. **IV for hypocalcemic tetany** 10–20 mL calcium gluconate infused over 10 min, may repeat until tetany is controlled. *Faster IV infusion rates may result in cardiac dysfunction.*[53]

Special Populations. *Pediatric Dosage.* **PO as dietary supplement** (elemental calcium) RDA (<6 months) 400 mg/day; (6 months–1 yr) 600 mg/day; (1–10 yr) 800 mg/day; (11–18 yr) 1200 mg/day.[49] **PO for hypocalcemia** (elemental calcium) (neonates) 50–150 mg/kg/day in 4–6 divided doses, to a maximum of 1 g/day; (children) 20–65 mg/kg/day in 4 divided doses. **IV for emergency elevation of serum calcium** (infants) <1 mEq, may repeat q 1–3 days depending on response; (children) 1–7 mEq, may repeat q 1–3 days depending on response. **IV for hypocalcemic tetany** (infants) 2.4 mEq/day in divided doses; (children) 0.5–0.7 mEq/kg tid–qid, or more until tetany controlled.

Geriatric Dosage. Postmenopausal women may have a requirement of 1.5 g/day.[49] Lower dosage may be required in some patients because of the age-related decrease in renal function; however, requirements may increase with advanced renal insufficiency.

Other Conditions. Adolescence, renal impairment, and pregnancy may increase requirements; base maintenance dosage on serum calcium, serum phosphate, and diet.[49]

Dosage Forms. (*See* Oral Calcium Products Comparison Chart.) **Inj** (chloride) 1 g/10 mL (contains 273 mg or 13.6 mEq Ca); (gluconate) 1 g/10 mL (contains 93 mg or 4.65 mEq Ca); (gluceptate) 1.1 g/5 mL (contains 90 mg or 4.5 mEq Ca).

Patient Instructions. (*See* Class Instructions: Oral Electrolytes.) Do not take within 2 hours of oral tetracycline or fluoroquinolone products. Take calcium tablets with food to maximize absorption. If used as a phosphate binder, calcium must be taken with food. Allow effervescent tablets to degas in a glass of water (about 4 minutes) before taking.

Missed Doses. Take this drug at regular intervals. If you miss a dose, take it as soon as you remember, then return to your normal dosage schedule.

Pharmacokinetics. *Serum Levels.* Normal serum total calcium is 8.4–10.2 mg/dL (2.1–2.6 mmol/L) for an adult with a serum albumin of 4 g/dL. Because a lesser fraction of calcium is protein bound in hypoalbuminemia, the patient's value must be corrected based on serum albumin:

Corrected Serum Ca = Measured Serum Ca + (0.8 × [4 − Serum Albumin]).

Fate. Oral calcium absorption is about 30% and depends on vitamin D and parathyroid hormone. Absorption decreases with age, high intake, achlorhydria, and estrogen loss at menopause;[49] absorption increases when taken with food[50,53] or in divided doses.[54] Bioavailability from various salt forms does not appear to differ substantially in normals;[55] however, differences in disintegration and dissolution among commercial formulations exist.[51,53] About 99% of total body calcium is found in bone; of the 1% in extracellular fluid, 40% is plasma protein bound (mostly to albumin); 9% is complexed to citrate, phosphate, and other anions; and 50% is diffusible and physiologically active. About 135–155 mg/day are secreted into the GI tract, with 85% reabsorbed. Fecal loss of unabsorbed dietary calcium and endogenous excretion is 100–130 mg/day, urine loss is 150 mg/day, and sweat loss is 15 mg/day.[54]

Adverse Reactions. IV calcium solutions, especially calcium chloride, are extremely irritating to the veins.[52] Constipation or flatulence occurs frequently, especially with high dosages; the frequency probably does not differ markedly among salt forms.[50] Calcium overload caused by oral calcium supplements is rare; immobilization, dosages in excess of 3–4 g/day, vitamin D therapy, and renal impairment may contribute to hypercalcemia, hypercalciuria, or nephrolithiasis during oral supplementation. Symptoms of hypercalcemia include nausea, vomiting, constipation, abdominal pain, dry mouth, and polyuria.

Contraindications. Hypercalcemia; sarcoidosis; severe cardiac disease; digitalis glycoside therapy; calcium nephrolithiasis; calcium-phosphate product greater than 70 (to determine calcium-phosphate product, multiply serum phosphate value [in mg/dL] by serum calcium value [in mg/dL]).

Precautions. Avoid extravasation of parenteral calcium products. If extravasation occurs, aspirate any accessible extravasated solution, then remove IV catheter and apply a cold compress to the area.

Drug Interactions. Concomitant thiazide diuretic therapy and sodium depletion or metabolic acidosis may increase tubular reabsorption of calcium. Calcium reduces oral absorption of fluoroquinolones, tetracyclines, and iron salts.

Parameters to Monitor. Serum calcium regularly, with frequency determined by patient's condition; BUN and/or Cr_s, serum phosphate, magnesium, and serum albumin (especially if low) periodically.

Notes. Calcium supplementation can also be achieved by dietary measures: skim milk provides 300 mg calcium/250 mL; cheese 300–400 mg calcium/28 g; and yogurt 43 mg calcium/28 g.[50] Calcium carbonate is inexpensive and a good first-line agent. However, dissolution of calcium from phosphate and carbonate salts is pH dependent. These salts may not be optimal calcium sources for patients with elevated GI pH, such as the elderly or those with achlorhydria. Calcium carbonate as a chewable tablet or nougat or the use of an alternative calcium salt have been recommended.[53] In ESRD, use calcium salts when serum phosphate is <8 mg/dL; when serum phosphate is >8 mg/dL, use aluminum hydroxide. Calcium acetate binds about twice the amount of phosphorus for the same quantity of calcium absorbed; however, the frequency of hypercalcemia does not seem to be diminished. (*See* Oral Calcium Products Comparison Chart.)

ORAL CALCIUM PRODUCTS COMPARISON CHART

PRODUCT	PERCENTAGE CALCIUM	ELEMENTAL CALCIUM CONTENT
Calcium Acetate	25	250 mg Tab = 62.5 mg
Calphron		500 mg Tab = 125 mg
PhosEx		667 mg Tab = 169 mg
PhosLo		1000 mg Tab = 250 mg
Calcium Carbonate	40	5 mL Susp = 500 mg
Calciday-667		650 mg Tab = 260 mg
Cal-Sup		667 mg Tab = 267 mg
Caltrate 600		750 mg Tab = 300 mg
Os-Cal		1250 mg Tab = 500 mg
Titralac		1500 mg Tab = 600 mg
Tums		
Calcium Citrate	21.1	950 mg Tab = 200 mg
Citracal		2376 mg Tab = 500 mg
Calcium Glubionate	6.5	5 mL Syrup = 115 mg
Neo-Calglucon		
Calcium Gluconate	9	500 mg Tab = 45 mg
Various		650 mg Tab = 58.5 mg
		975 mg Tab = 87.8 mg
		1000 mg Tab = 90 mg
Calcium Lactate	13	325 mg Tab = 42.3 mg
Various		650 mg Tab = 84.5 mg
Calcium Phosphate, Tribasic	39	1565 mg Tab = 600 mg
Posture		
Dairy Products	—	Cheese 28 g = 300–400 mg
		Skim Milk 250 mL = 300 mg
		Yogurt 28 g = 43 mg

From references 49–52 and product information.

MAGNESIUM SALTS   Various

Pharmacology. Magnesium is the second most abundant intracellular cation, with an essential role in neuromuscular function and protein and carbohydrate enzymatic systems; it functions as a cofactor for enzymes involved in transfer, storage, and utilization of intracellular energy. Magnesium is also an integral component of bone matrix.[56]

Administration and Adult Dosage. **PO as dietary supplement** (elemental magnesium) 20–130 mg daily–bid.[57] **PO for chronic deficiency** (elemental magnesium) 12–24 mg/kg in divided doses.[58] **IV for prevention of negative balance** (elemental magnesium) 100–200 mg/day in parenteral nutrition solution.[58] **IM for mild deficiency** 1 g $MgSO_4$ q 4–6 hr until serum magnesium is normalized or signs and symptoms abate;[58] **IM for severe hypomagnesemia** 2 g $MgSO_4$ as a 50% solution q 8 hr until serum magnesium is normalized or signs and symptoms abate; because IM injections are painful, continuous IV infusions may be preferred.[59] **IV infusion for severe hypomagnesemia** 48 mEq/day (6 g $MgSO_4$) for 3–7 days by continuous infusion.[59] **IV for life-threatening hypomagnesemia (acute arrhythmias and seizures)** 8–16 mEq (1–2 g $MgSO_4$) over 5–10 min, followed by continuous infusion of 48 mEq magnesium/day.[59] **IV for pre-eclampsia or eclampsia** 4–6 g $MgSO_4$, then 1–2 g/hr by continuous infusion to maintain target serum level. (*See* Notes.)

Special Populations. *Pediatric Dosage.* **IV for hypomagnesemia** 25 mg/kg $MgSO_4$ as a 25% solution over 3–5 min q 6 hr for 3–4 doses. **IM for seizures** 20–40 mg/kg $MgSO_4$ as a 20% solution as needed. **IV for severe seizures** 100–200 mg/kg $MgSO_4$ as a 1–3% solution infused slowly with close monitoring of blood pressure. Administer one-half the dose during the initial 15–20 min and the total dose within 1 hr.

Geriatric Dosage. Lower dosage may be required in some patients because of the age-related decrease in renal function. Magnesium accumulates in advanced renal insufficiency.

Other Conditions. Base maintenance dosage on serum magnesium and diet. Renal impairment decreases requirement. In severe renal failure, reduce dosage by at least 50% of recommended amount and monitor serum magnesium after each dose.[60] Concomitant administration of potassium and calcium may be necessary, because many causes of hypomagnesemia also lead to hypocalcemia and hypokalemia.[58]

Dosage Forms. (*See* Magnesium Products Comparison Chart.)

Patient Instructions. (*See* Oral Electrolytes Class Instructions.)

Missed Doses. Take this drug at regular intervals. If you miss a dose, take it as soon as you remember. Do not double the dose or take extra.

Pharmacokinetics. *Onset and Duration.* Peak levels are achieved immediately after IV, 1 hr after IM. Duration (anticonvulsant) is 30 min with IV, 3–4 hr postonset with IM.

Serum Levels. (Normal) 1.3–2.1 mEq/L (0.65–1.1 mmol/L); (anticonvulsant) 4–7 mEq/L (2–3.5 mmol/L); (pre-eclampsia or eclampsia) 6–8 mEq/L. Intracellular and extracellular concentrations can vary independently; hence, serum magnesium levels may not be indicative of total body stores.

Fate. Oral absorption varies inversely with intake; in general, 24–76% is absorbed,[61] principally in upper small intestine. Total body content is about 24 g,[57] of which 60% is in bone, 39% in tissues, and 1% in extracellular fluid; 30% is plasma protein bound. Elimination is primarily by the kidneys, with only 1–2% in feces. A renal threshold for magnesium excretion exists; therefore, replacement therapy must be continued slowly, usually over 5 days. Raising the serum concentration above normal exceeds the maximum tubular reabsorption capacity with subsequent excretion of excess.

Adverse Reactions. Serum concentration related: (3–5 mEq/L; 1.5–2.5 mmol/L) hypotension; (5–10 mEq/L; 2.5–5 mmol/L) PR interval changes, QRS prolongation, peaked T waves; (10 mEq/L; 5 mmol/L) areflexia; (15 mEq/L; 7.5 mmol/L) respiratory paralysis; (25 mEq/L; 12.5 mmol/L) cardiac arrest.[59] Pain on IM injection occurs very frequently.[60]

Contraindications. Hypermagnesemia; heart block; myocardial damage; severe renal failure.

Precautions. Use with caution in patients with renal impairment (Cl_{cr} <30 mL/min) and those concurrently taking a digitalis glycoside. With bolus $MgSO_4$ administration, 1 g of 10% calcium gluconate IV should be available in case apnea or heart block occurs.[61]

Drug Interactions. IV magnesium may potentiate neuromuscular blocking agents.

Parameters to Monitor. Serum magnesium regularly, frequency determined by condition of patient; BUN and/or Cr_s, serum potassium and calcium periodically. Deep tendon reflexes, respiratory rate, blood pressure, and ECG periodically.

Notes. For mild deficiencies, dietary supplementation may be sufficient to normalize magnesium stores; sources include cereals, nuts, green vegetables, meat, and fish.[61] Magnesium chloride is preferred for oral replacement and supplementation because it may be better absorbed and potentially causes less diarrhea.[62] Patients on long-term diuretic therapy who are prone to hypomagnesemia may benefit from using the minimally effective dose of diuretic and 20–30 mEq/day of magnesium orally or changing to a magnesium-sparing agent (eg, amiloride, spironolactone, triamterene).[63] Drugs known to produce hypomagnesemia include aminoglycoside antibiotics, amphotericin B, diuretics, alcohol, and cisplatin.[59,62] Coadministration of 3 g $MgSO_4$ IV with high-dose **cisplatin** chemotherapy has been recommended.[63] Although controversial, IV magnesium may reduce mortality post-MI.[64,65] Correction of refractory hypocalcemia and hypokalemia with concurrent hypomagnesemia requires magnesium replacement to restore mineral balance.[58] To avoid the precipitation reaction when $MgSO_4$ and calcium chloride are added to parenteral nutrition mixtures, use of calcium glucceptate has been recommended because it reacts more slowly than calcium chloride and a precipitate does not form.[66] (*See* Magnesium Products Comparison Chart.)

MAGNESIUM PRODUCTS COMPARISON CHART

PRODUCT	MAGNESIUM CONTENT[a] (MEQ/G)	DOSAGE FORMS[b]	COMMENTS
Magnesium, Chelated Chelated magnesium	8.3	Tab 500 mg = 100 mg Mg.	Amino acid chelate; sodium free; oral use only.
Magnesium Chloride Slo-Mag Various	9.8 (PO) 20.8 (IV)	SR Tab 535 mg = 64 mg Mg Inj 200 mg/mL = 23.6 mg/mL Mg.	Alternative to parenteral MgSO$_4$.
Magnesium Citrate Various	4.4	Soln 60 mg/mL = 3.2 mg/mL Mg.	Oral use only.
Magnesium Gluconate Almora Magatrate Magonate	4.5–4.8	Tab 500 mg = 27–29 mg Mg Soln 11 mg/mL = 0.5 mg/mL Mg.	Very soluble; well absorbed; produces no diarrhea.
Magnesium Hydroxide Milk of Magnesia	34	Susp 40 mg/mL = 13.6 mg/mL Mg Susp 80 mg/mL = 27 mg/mL Mg Tab 300 mg = 102 mg Mg Tab 600 mg = 205 mg Mg.	Readily available in combination antacid formulations. Start with 5 mL Susp or 1 Tab, increase as tolerated to qid. Requires gastric acid for absorption. Inexpensive.

(continued)

MAGNESIUM PRODUCTS COMPARISON CHART (continued)

PRODUCT	MAGNESIUM CONTENT[a] (MEQ/G)	DOSAGE FORMS[b]	COMMENTS
Magnesium Oxide	60.3	Cap 140 mg = 84 mg Mg. Tab 400 mg = 241 mg Mg.	Poorly soluble; net absorption low, especially in malabsorptive states.
Magnesium Sulfate Epsom salt	8.1	Inj 10% = 9.6 mg/mL Mg. Inj 12.5% = 12 mg/mL Mg. Inj 20% = 23.6 mg/mL Mg. Inj 50% = 48 mg/mL Mg. Pwdr 1 g = 97.2 mg Mg.	Use IV, IM, or PO.

[a] 1 mEq = 12 mg = 0.5 mmol Mg.
[b] Magnesium products exhibit variable oral absorption; increase dosage incrementally until no further rise in serum magnesium occurs or until diarrhea occurs.

PHOSPHATE SALTS   Various

Pharmacology. Phosphate is a structural element of bone and is involved in carbohydrate metabolism, energy transfer, and muscle contraction, and as a buffer in the renal excretion of hydrogen ion.[51] Many of the factors that influence serum calcium concentration also influence serum phosphate directly or indirectly.

Administration and Adult Dosage. **PO** 250–500 mg (8–16 mmol) of phosphorus qid initially, adjusted according to serum phosphate and calcium. **IV replacement (recent and uncomplicated hypophosphatemia)** 0.08 mmol/kg, to a maximum of 0.2 mmol/kg; (prolonged and multiple causes) 0.16 mmol/kg, to a maximum of 0.24 mmol/kg. Infuse doses over 6 hr and additional dosage guided by serum concentrations.[67] **IV for symptomatic hypophosphatemia** 1–3 g (31–94 mmol) of phosphate daily to maintain serum phosphate at 2–3 mg/dL.[68] When serum concentration reaches 2 mg/dL (0.67 mmol/L), and the patient is able to eat a normal diet, change to oral administration and phosphate-rich diet.[69]

Special Populations. *Pediatric Dosage.* **PO** (<4 yr) 250 mg (8 mmol) of phosphorus qid initially; (≥4 yr) same as adult dosage. **IV replacement** (for serum phosphate concentration 0.5–1 mg/dL) 0.05–0.08 mg/kg (0.15–0.25 mmol/kg) per dose over 4–6 hr; (for serum phosphate concentration <0.5 mg/dL) 0.08–0.12 mg/kg (0.25–0.35 mmol/kg) per dose over 6 hr.[55] Repeat doses as needed to achieve desired serum concentration. Actual dosage depends on signs, symptoms, and serum phosphate concentration.

Geriatric Dosage. Lower dosage may be required in some patients because of the age-related decrease in renal function.

Other Conditions. Renal impairment decreases requirement. Choose the appropriate salt form based on patient's sodium and potassium requirements. Requirement is increased during alcohol withdrawal, diabetic ketoacidosis, respiratory alkalosis, aluminum antacid therapy, burns, and anabolism.

Dosage Forms. (*See* Phosphate Products Comparison Chart.)

Patient Instructions. (*See* Class Instructions: Oral Electrolytes.) Do not take capsules whole, but dissolve contents in ¾ glass of water before taking. Powder in packets must be dissolved in one gallon of water before using. Chilling solution may improve palatability. Do not take with calcium-containing products.

Missed Doses. Take this drug at regular intervals. If you miss a dose, take it as soon as you remember. Do not double the dose or take extra.

Pharmacokinetics. *Serum Levels.* (As phosphorus) adults 2.7–4.5 mg/dL (0.9–1.5 mmol/L); children 4.5–5.5 mg/dL (1.5–1.8 mmol/L). Normal serum phosphorus concentrations may vary by as much as 2 mg/dL throughout the day, because of changes in transcellular distribution. Concentrations <1 mg/dL are dangerous and require replacement therapy.

Fate. Normal adult dietary intake is 1–1.5 g/day, of which 60–90% is absorbed, primarily in the jejunum. Most of the absorbed phosphorus is excreted in urine.[67]

Adverse Reactions. Diarrhea and stomach upset occur frequently with oral administration.[67,70] Dose-related hyperphosphatemia, metastatic calcium deposition, dehydration, hypotension, hypomagnesemia, and hyperkalemia or hypernatremia (depending on salt used) can occur.

Contraindications. Hyperphosphatemia; hypocalcemia; hyperkalemia (potassium salt); hypernatremia (sodium salt); severe renal failure.

Precautions. Use cautiously in patients with renal impairment and in those with hypercalcemia. Dilute IV forms before use and administer slowly. Administer the potassium salt peripherally no faster than 10 mEq/hr to avoid vein irritation.[71]

Drug Interactions. None known.

Parameters to Monitor. Serum phosphorus regularly, frequency determined by condition of patient; BUN and/or Cr_s, serum calcium, and magnesium periodically.[72] Monitor serum sodium and/or potassium periodically, depending on salt form used.

Notes. Phosphate salts may precipitate in the presence of calcium salts in IV solutions; add no more than 40 mmol of phosphate and 5 mEq of calcium per liter. Calcium supplementation may be necessary to prevent hypocalcemic tetany during phosphate repletion. IV calcium gluconate or calcium chloride may be given until tetany subsides. Inorganic phosphorus exists in the body as the mono- and dibasic forms, the relative proportions of which are pH dependent. It is therefore preferable to report concentrations as mg/dL or mmol/L, rather than mEq/L.[67] (*See* Phosphate Products Comparison Chart.)

PHOSPHATE PRODUCTS COMPARISON CHART

PRODUCT	DOSAGE FORMS[a]	PHOSPHORUS CONTENT[b]		CATION CONTENT
		mg	mmol	
POTASSIUM SALTS				
K-Phos Original	Tab.	114	3.6	3.7 mEq K$^+$/tablet.
Neutra-Phos K	Pwdr Packet.	250 (per packet)	8	14.3 mEq K$^+$/packet.
Potassium Phosphate	Inj.	94 (per mL)	3	4.4 mEq K$^+$/mL.
SODIUM SALTS				
Fleet's Phospho-Soda	Soln.	128 (per mL)	4.1	111 mg (4.8 mEq) Na$^+$/mL.
Sodium Phosphate	Inj.	94 (per mL)	3	93 mg (4 mEq) Na$^+$/mL.
SODIUM-POTASSIUM SALTS				
K-Phos M.F.	Tab.	125 (per tablet)	4	67 mg (2.9 mEq) Na$^+$ and 1.1 mEq K$^+$/tablet.
K-Phos Neutral	Tab.	250 (per tablet)	8	298 mg (13 mEq) Na$^+$ and 1.1 mEq K$^+$/tablet.
K-Phos No. 2	Tab.	250 (per tablet)	8	134 mg (5.8 mEq) Na$^+$ and 2.3 mEq K$^+$/tablet.
Neutra-Phos Plain	Pwdr Packet.	250 (per packet)	8	164 mg (7.1 mEq) Na$^+$ and 7.1 mEq K$^+$/packet.
Skim Milk	Liquid.	1000 (per quart)	32	552 mg (24 mEq) Na$^+$ and 40 mEq K$^+$/quart.

[a]Contents of capsules, tablets, and powders must be diluted in water before administration.
[b]31.25 mg = 1 mmol.
From references 67–69 and product information.

POTASSIUM SALTS   Various

Pharmacology. Potassium is the major cation of the intracellular space, where its major role is regulating muscle and nerve excitability. Other roles include control of intracellular volume (similar to sodium's control of extracellular volume), protein synthesis, enzymatic reaction, and carbohydrate metabolism.[73] The chloride salt is preferred for most uses, because concomitant chloride loss and metabolic alkalosis frequently accompany hypokalemia. Nonchloride salts are preferred in acidosis (eg, secondary to amphotericin B or carbonic anhydrase inhibitor therapy and in chronic diarrhea with bicarbonate loss).[74,75]

Administration and Adult Dosage. Variable, must be adjusted to needs of patient. **PO for prophylaxis with diuretic therapy** 40 mEq/day of potassium chloride prevents hypokalemia in most patients on long-term diuretic therapy.[74] For nonedematous, ambulatory patients with uncomplicated hypertension, generally no supplementation is needed; however, if serum potassium falls below 3 mEq/L, 50–60 mEq/day is recommended. For edematous patients (eg, CHF, cirrhosis with ascites) give 40–80 mEq/day (mild deficit) or 100–120 mEq/day (severe deficit), with careful monitoring of serum potassium.[76] **IV administration in peripheral vein** (serum potassium greater than 2.5 mEq/L) may be infused at 10–20 mEq/hr;[75] reserve rates faster than 20 mEq/hr for emergency situations; may repeat q 2–3 hr as needed; do not exceed a maximum concentration of 40 mEq/L; **IV administration in central vein** (serum potassium <2.5 mEq/L) up to 60 mEq/hr may be administered;[75] do not exceed a maximum concentration of 80 mEq/L. Infusion into a central vein requires use of a volume control device. Potassium concentration should not exceed 60 mEq/L unless the infusion site is via a large vein distal to the heart (eg, femoral vein) or more than one IV line is available; however, more concentrated solutions (200 mEq/L) infused at a slow rate (20 mEq/hr) have been used with relative safety.[77] (*See* Special Populations, Other Conditions.)

Special Populations. *Pediatric Dosage.* PO 1–2 mEq/kg/day during diuretic therapy.

Geriatric Dosage. Lower dosage may be required in some patients because of the age-related decrease in renal function.

Other Conditions. Base maintenance dosage on serum potassium; renal impairment decreases requirement. For patients with renal impairment or any form of heart block, decrease infusion rate by one-half and do not exceed 5–10 mEq/hr.[75]

Dosage Forms. PO. (*See* Potassium Products Comparison Chart.) **Inj** (potassium chloride) 2 mEq/mL; (potassium acetate) 2, 4 mEq/mL; (potassium phosphate) 4.4 mEq/mL of potassium and 3 mmol/mL of phosphate. (*See* Potassium Products Comparison Chart.)

Patient Instructions. (*See* Class Instructions: Oral Electrolytes.) Do not chew or crush tablets. The expanded wax matrix of sustained-release forms may be found in the stool, but this does not imply a lack of absorption.

Missed Doses. Take this drug at regular intervals. If you miss a dose, take it as soon as you remember, then return to your normal dosage schedule. Do not double the dose or take extra.

Pharmacokinetics. *Onset and Duration.* Peak elevation of serum potassium concentrations following SR preparations is slightly delayed (2 hr) compared to the liquid form (1 hr). Effect on serum potassium is generally limited to the first 3 hr after administration.[78]

Serum Levels. May vary depending on laboratory. Normal serum levels are (newborn) 5–7.5 mEq/L; (adult and child) 3.5–5 mEq/L. Total body stores are about 50 mEq/kg or 3500 mEq. As a general rule, a decrease of 1 mEq/L in serum potassium reflects a 10–20% total body deficit; however, there is considerable variation;[76] signs of hypokalemia appear below 2.5 mEq/L; concentrations >7 mEq/L or <2.5 mEq/mL are dangerous. Clinical signs of hypokalemia or hyperkalemia are not reliable indicators of serum concentrations. Alkalosis decreases concentrations, and acidosis increases concentrations. Any hypokalemia-induced change in ECG must be treated as a medical emergency with IV potassium. Likewise, hyperkalemia-induced changes in ECG must also be treated as a medical emergency.

Fate. When initially administered, the rates of absorption and excretion are more rapid with the liquid than the SR forms; however, bioavailability is the same (78–90%) during long-term administration.[78,79] About 10 mEq/day are eliminated in feces; 60–90 mEq/day in urine, and 7.5 mEq/L in sweat.

Adverse Reactions. Bad taste, nausea, vomiting, diarrhea, and abdominal discomfort occur frequently with oral liquids. Do not use enteric-coated tablets, because they may cause small-bowel and occasionally gastric ulceration.[76] Local tissue necrosis may occur if IV solution extravasates. Hyperkalemia may occur occasionally. Patients with diabetic nephropathy are at an increased risk for hyperkalemia.[80]

Contraindications. Severe renal impairment; untreated Addison's disease; adynamia episodica hereditaria; acute dehydration; heat cramps; hyperkalemia; concurrent ACE inhibitor or potassium-sparing diuretic in patients with renal impairment. Additionally, all solid dosage forms (including SR products) are contraindicated in patients in whom delay or arrest of the tablet through the GI tract may occur.

Precautions. Use with caution (if at all) in patients receiving potassium-sparing diuretics or ACE inhibitors, and in patients with digitalis-induced atrioventricular conduction disturbances or renal failure. Avoid extravasation of parenteral potassium products. If extravasation occurs, aspirate any accessible extravasated solution, then remove IV catheter and apply a cold compress to the area.

Drug Interactions. Use with an ACE inhibitor or potassium-sparing diuretic can result in hyperkalemia.

Parameters to Monitor. Serum potassium weekly to monthly initially, q 3–6 months when stable; BUN and/or Cr_s periodically. For supplementation in patients on long-term diuretic therapy, obtain a pretreatment serum potassium and magnesium, reassess after 2–3 weeks, and then monthly to determine pattern of potassium loss. Once steady state or normokalemia is achieved, assess quarterly or as condition requires.[76]

Notes. Place patient on a cardiac monitor before starting IV potassium.[75] A potassium-sparing diuretic may be preferable to potassium supplementation when large supplements are needed, aldosterone concentrations are elevated, enhanced diuretic response is desired, or magnesium loss is of concern. If large doses of potassium fail to correct hypokalemia, suspect hypomagnesemia, because potassium balance is strongly dependent on magnesium homeostasis.[74,81] If a hypokalemic patient is also hypomagnesemic, as occurs with **amphotericin B** therapy, the patient may not respond to potassium replacement therapy unless magnesium balance is restored. (*See* Potassium Products Comparison Chart.)

POTASSIUM PRODUCTS COMPARISON CHART

PRODUCT	DOSAGE FORMS	COMMENTS
Potassium Acetate Various	Inj 2, 4 mEq/mL.	Useful in metabolic acidosis; avoid in metabolic alkalosis.
Potassium Acetate/ Bicarbonate/ Citrate Trikates Tri-K	Soln 3 mEq/mL.[a]	Preferred form in patients with delayed GI transit time or metabolic acidosis; avoid nonchloride salts in metabolic alkalosis.
Potassium Chloride Kaochlor-Eff Klorvess K-Lyte/Cl Adolph's Morton No Salt NuSalt	Inj 2 mEq/mL Soln 20, 30, 40, 45 mEq/15 mL[a] Pwdr Packet 15, 20, 25 mEq[b] Pwdr Packet 15, 20, 25 mEq[b] SR Cap/Tab 6.7, 8, 10, 20 mEq[c] Salt Substitutes 50– 70 mEq/tsp.[d]	Ideal for hypochloremic metabolic alkalosis.
Potassium Bicarbonate/ Citrate K-Lyte	Pwdr Packet 25, 50 mEq.[b]	Preferred form in patients with delayed GI transit time or metabolic acidosis; avoid nonchloride salts in metabolic alkalosis.
Potassium Gluconate Kaon	Soln 1.33 mEq/mL.[a]	Preferred form in patients with metabolic acidosis; avoid nonchloride salts in metabolic alkalosis.

[a]Liquids have rapid absorption, low frequency of GI ulceration, and unpleasant taste.
[b]Must be dissolved in water before use.
[c]Bioequivalent to liquid forms; avoid in patients with delayed GI transit time.
[d]Salt substitutes may also have large amounts of sodium.
From references 74–76 and product information.

ORAL REHYDRATION SOLUTIONS   Various

Pharmacology. Oral rehydration solutions supply sodium, chloride, potassium, and water to prevent or replace mild to moderate fluid loss (5–10% dehydration) in diarrhea or postoperative states, or when food and liquid intake are temporarily discontinued. A carbohydrate (usually glucose) is present to aid in sodium transport and subsequent water absorption.[82,83]

Administration and Adult Dosage. PO 1900–2850 mL (2–3 quarts)/day. Give only enough solution to supply the calculated water loss plus daily requirement.

Special Populations. *Pediatric Dosage.* Depends primarily on estimated fluid and electrolyte loss.[84] **PO** (infants) 150 mL/kg/day (one-half in the first 8 hr if possible, the remainder over the ensuing 16 hr) offered in frequent, small amounts (not to exceed 100 mL in a 20-min period).[85] Once the solution is well tolerated, it may be given less frequently (q 3–4 hr). For infants who finish the prescribed amount of solution in less than 24 hr, offer plain tap water to avoid hypernatremia.[86] **PO** (5–10 yr) 950–1900 mL (1–2 quarts)/day; (≥11 yr) same as adult dosage.

Geriatric Dosage. Lower dosage may be required in some patients because of the age-related decrease in renal function.

Other Conditions. Adjust intake based on fluid status and serum electrolytes. When electrolyte-containing foods are restarted, adjust solution intake accordingly.

Dosage Forms. (*See* Oral Rehydration Solutions Comparison Chart.)

Patient Instructions. These products are not for fluid replacement in prolonged or severe diarrhea. Reconstitute powdered products in tap water; do not mix with milk or fruit juices. If additional fluids are desired, drink water or other nonelectrolyte-containing fluids to quench thirst.

Adverse Reactions. Hypernatremia, hyperkalemia, and acid-base disturbances may occur occasionally, especially in renal insufficiency or if errors occur in reconstituting bulk powders.

Contraindications. Intractable vomiting; adynamic ileus; intestinal obstruction; perforated bowel; shock; renal dysfunction (anuria, oliguria); monosaccharide malabsorption.[83]

Precautions. Use parenteral replacement to correct electrolyte imbalances caused by severe fluid loss (10–15% of body weight), inability to take oral fluids, severe gastric distention, or severe vomiting. Errors in reconstituting or diluting commercial powders may lead to severe consequences.

Drug Interactions. None known.

Parameters to Monitor. Serum sodium, potassium, chloride, and bicarbonate regularly, with frequency determined by condition of patient; BUN and/or Cr_s and urine-specific gravity periodically; input and output, weight, and signs and symptoms of dehydration daily.

Notes. To prevent dehydration early in the course of diarrhea or to maintain hydration following parenteral replacement in adults and children, 90 mEq/L of sodium is acceptable. For infants, however, who have a higher insensible water loss, dilute solutions containing 50–60 mEq/L of sodium are suggested.[86] Alternatively, solutions of higher sodium concentration may be used in a ratio of 2:1 with additional free water.[82] Vomiting does not preclude use of oral replacement solutions; spooning small quantities into the mouth of the child who is experiencing some vomiting usually results in the administration of sufficient fluid to correct dehydration.[83]

ORAL REHYDRATION SOLUTIONS COMPARISON CHART

SOLUTION	DOSAGE FORMS	ELECTROLYTES (mEq/L)[a]					CARBOHYDRATE
		Na^+	K^+	Cl^-	Base	Other	
Infalyte	Soln 1000 mL.	50	25	45	34 Citrate	—	Rice syrup solids 3%.
Pedialyte	Soln 237, 946 mL.	45	20	35	30 Citrate	—	Dextrose 2.5%.
Rehydralyte	Soln 237 mL.	75	20	65	30 Citrate	—	Dextrose 2.5%.
Resol	Soln 960 mL.	50	20	50	34 Citrate	4 Ca^{++} 4 Mg^{++} 5 $HPO_4^=$	Glucose 2%.
WHO Oral Rehydration Salts[c]	Powder.[b]	90	20	80	30 Bicarbonate	—	Glucose 2%.

[a]Optimal solution (mEq/L): Na^+ 75–100, K^+ 20–30, Cl^- 65–100, base 20–30, carbohydrate 1.5–2%.

[b]Reconstitute powder in tap water; do not mix with milk or fruit juices.

[c]WHO = World Health Organization Oral Rehydration Salts; available from Jianas Brothers Packaging, 2533 SW Boulevard, Kansas City, MO; tel (816) 421–2880.

From references 84–86 and product information.

SODIUM POLYSTYRENE SULFONATE   Kayexalate, Various

Pharmacology. A cation exchange resin that exchanges potassium for sodium. Each gram of resin binds up to 1 mEq of potassium and liberates 1–2 mEq of sodium.[87] Sorbitol is present in some products to induce diarrhea and to reduce the potential for fecal impaction. (*See* Notes.)

Administration and Adult Dosage. **PO** 15–20 g, may repeat as often as q 2 hr,[75] although doses up to 40 g have been recommended;[88] total dosage and duration of therapy depend on patient response. If suspension does not contain sorbitol, give powder with, or suspended in, a sorbitol solution (eg, 15 mL of 70% sorbitol). **PR as enema** 50 g retained for 30 min, if possible, may repeat as often as q 45 min.[75] Follow enema by an irrigation of up to 2 L of nonsodium-containing fluid to remove resin from bowel.

Special Populations. *Pediatric Dosage.* For small children and infants, calculate dosage on the basis of 1 g of resin binding 1 mEq of potassium.

Geriatric Dosage. Lower dosage may be required in some patients because of the age-related decrease in renal function.

Other Conditions. In severe situations, such as ongoing tissue damage or rapidly rising serum potassium in renal failure, a dosage of 80–100 g for every mEq/L of potassium above 5 mEq/L has been recommended.[88] However, under such circumstance, other forms of therapy may be considered.

Dosage Forms. **Pwdr** 454 g; **Susp** (containing sorbitol) 15 g/60 mL.

Pharmacokinetics. *Onset and Duration.* PO onset is 2–12 hr; PR onset is somewhat longer.

Fate. Not absorbed from GI tract; binds potassium and liberates sodium as it passes through intestine.

Adverse Reactions. Anorexia, nausea, and vomiting occur frequently with large doses; gastric irritation, constipation, and fecal impaction (especially in the elderly) occur occasionally. These effects may be avoided by using the enema. However, intestinal necrosis because of the enema has been reported. Use of **sorbitol** in the enema and failure to follow it with a cleansing enema may predispose uremic patients to potentially fatal intestinal necrosis.[87]

Precautions. Use with caution in patients who cannot tolerate any additional sodium load (eg, severe CHF, severe hypertension, marked edema). In addition to potassium, other cations (such as magnesium and calcium) may bind to the resin, causing electrolyte imbalances. If rapid potassium lowering is required, give **insulin** with or without glucose.

Drug Interactions. None known.

Parameters to Monitor. Serum potassium at least daily and more frequently if indicated; serum magnesium and calcium periodically; ECG and patient signs and symptoms may be useful in evaluating status.

Notes. On average, 50 g of resin will lower serum potassium by 0.5–1 mEq/L.[89] Rectal administration is less effective than oral use. Heating may alter the exchange properties of the resin. Sodium polystyrene sulfonate–induced constipation may be treated with 70% **sorbitol** in oral doses (ie, 10–20 mL/2 hr) sufficient to produce 1 or 2 watery stools/day.

Antigout Agents

ALLOPURINOL
Zyloprim, Various

Pharmacology. Allopurinol, a structural analogue of the purine base hypoxanthine, competitively inhibits xanthine oxidase. This reduces both serum and urinary uric acid levels by blocking the conversion of hypoxanthine and xanthine to uric acid and by decreasing urine synthesis.[90–92]

Administration and Adult Dosage. **PO for control of gout** 100 mg/day initially, increasing in 100 mg/day increments at weekly intervals until a serum uric acid level of 6 mg/dL or less is attained. **PO for maintenance of mild gout** 200–300 mg/day in single or divided doses; **PO for maintenance of moderately severe tophaceous gout** 400–600 mg/day, to a maximum of 800 mg/day for resistant cases. Give dosages that exceed 300 mg/day in divided doses. Give prophylactic colchicine 0.5–1.2 mg/day and/or an NSAID starting before allopurinol and continuing for 1 to several months after initiation of therapy because of an initial increased risk of gouty attacks.[90–93] A fluid intake sufficient to yield a daily urinary output of at least 2 L and the maintenance of a neutral or slightly alkaline urine are desirable. In transferring from a uricosuric agent to allopurinol, reduce the uricosuric dosage over a period of several weeks while gradually increasing the dosage of allopurinol. **PO or IV for secondary hyperuricemia associated with vigorous treatment of malignancies** 600–800 mg/day for 2–3 days is advisable with a high fluid intake, then reduce to 300 mg/day. Start at least 2–3 days (preferably 5 days) before initiation of cancer therapy. Discontinue when the potential for uric acid overproduction is no longer present.[94] IV should be used only in those who do not tolerate PO allopurinol. **PO for recurrent calcium oxalate stones in hyperuricosuria** 200–300 mg/day adjusted based on control of hyperuricosuria.

Special Populations. *Pediatric Dosage.* **PO for secondary hyperuricemia associated with malignancies** (<6 yr) 150 mg/day; (6–10 yr) 300 mg/day; alternatively, 2.5 mg/kg q 6 hr, to a maximum of 600 mg/day. Start at least 2–3 days (preferably 5 days) before cancer therapy.[94] Evaluate response 48 hr after cancer therapy is started and adjust dosage as needed.

Geriatric Dosage. Lower dosage may be required in some patients because of the age-related decrease in renal function.

Other Conditions. In renal impairment, reduce initial dosage as follows: with Cl_{cr} of 80 mL/min, give 250 mg/day; with Cl_{cr} of 60 mL/min, give 200 mg/day; with Cl_{cr} of 40 mL/min, give 150 mg/day; with Cl_{cr} of 20 mL/min, give 100 mg/day; with Cl_{cr} of 10 mL/min, give 100 mg q 2 days; with Cl_{cr} <10 mL/min, give 100 mg q 3 days.[95] Base subsequent dosage adjustment on serum uric acid levels.

Dosage Forms. **Tab** 100, 300 mg; **Inj** 500 mg.

Patient Instructions. This drug may be taken with food, milk, or an antacid to minimize stomach upset. Adults should drink at least 10–12 full glasses (8 fl oz each) of fluid each day. Avoid large amounts of alcohol (may increase uric acid in blood) or vitamin C (may increase the possibility of kidney stones by making the urine more acidic). Report any skin rash, painful urination, blood in urine, eye irritation, swelling of lips or mouth, itching, chills, fever, sore throat, nausea, or vomiting while taking this drug. Allopurinol may cause drowsiness; use caution while driving or performing other tasks requiring alertness, coordination, or physical dexterity.

Missed Doses. Take this drug at regular intervals. If you miss a dose, take it as soon as you remember. Do not double the dose or take extra.

Pharmacokinetics. *Onset and Duration.* A measurable decrease in uric acid occurs in 2–3 days; normal serum uric acid is achieved in 1–3 weeks.

Fate. Well absorbed orally (67–81%), but rectal absorption is poor (0–6% of oral bioavailability). Rapidly oxidized to oxypurinol, an active, but less potent, inhibitor of xanthine oxidase. Protein binding of allopurinol or oxypurinol is negligible.[96] Allopurinol V_d is 1.5 ± 0.7 L/kg, Cl is 0.77 ± 0.22 L/hr/kg; oxypurinol V_d is about 1.6 L/kg.[96,97] Oxypurinol and allopurinol are excreted unchanged in urine in a ratio of about 10:1.[96]

$t_{1/2}$. (Allopurinol) 1.4 ± 0.4 hr; (oxypurinol) 19.7 ± 7.3 hr with normal renal function, 5–10 days in renal failure.[96]

Adverse Reactions. A mild maculopapular skin rash occurs in about 2% of patients, but the percentage increases to about 20% with concurrent ampicillin. These rashes may not recur if allopurinol is stopped and restarted at a lower dosage, and oral desensitization to minor rashes from allopurinol in patients has been effective.[92,98] Exfoliative, urticarial, purpuric, and erythema multiforme lesions are also reported occasionally. These more severe reactions require drug discontinuation because severe hypersensitivity reactions such as vasculitis, toxic epidermal necrolysis, Stevens-Johnson syndrome, renal impairment, and hepatic damage can result. An occasional hypersensitivity syndrome (frequently marked by fever, rash, hepatitis, renal failure, and eosinophilia) has a mortality rate reportedly as high as 27%. It may begin 1 day–2 yr (average 6 weeks) after start of therapy and appears related to pre-existing renal dysfunction, elevated oxypurinol serum levels, or concurrent thiazide or other diuretic therapy.[95,99,100] Occasionally, nausea, vomiting, abdominal pain, and drowsiness occur. Rarely, alopecia, cataract formation, hepatotoxicity, bone marrow depression, leukopenia, leukocytosis, or renal xanthine stones occur.

Contraindications. Children (except for hyperuricemia secondary to malignancy). Do not restart the drug in patients who have developed a severe reaction. (*See* Adverse Reactions.)

Precautions. Pregnancy; lactation. Use with caution and in reduced dosage in renal impairment. Adjust dosage conservatively in patients with impaired renal function who are on a diuretic concomitantly.[95,100]

Drug Interactions. Diuretics may contribute to allopurinol toxicity, although a cause-and-effect relationship has not been established. Allopurinol markedly increases the toxicity of oral azathioprine and mercaptopurine. Allopurinol may increase the risk of hypersensitivity reactions to ampicillin and captopril, bone marrow suppression caused by cyclophosphamide, neurotoxicity of vidarabine, and nephrotoxicity of cyclosporine. Allopurinol may also increase the effect of oral anticoagulants. Concurrent use of salicylate for its antirheumatic effect does not compromise the action of allopurinol.

Parameters to Monitor. Monitor serum uric acid levels; pretreatment 24-hr urinary uric acid excretion.[90–92] Periodically determine liver function (particularly in patients with pre-existing liver disease). Monitor renal function tests and CBC, especially during the first few months of therapy. Renal function is particularly important in patients on concurrent diuretic therapy.[95,100]

Notes. Allopurinol is the drug of choice for patients with impaired renal function who respond poorly to uricosuric agents; however, these patients should be monitored closely because of an increased frequency of adverse reactions.[90–93,95] Current data do not support the routine treatment of asymptomatic hyperuricemia in patients other than those receiving vigorous treatment of malignancies and in marked overexcreters.[90–92] Allopurinol has been used investigationally to reduce tissue damage during coronary artery bypass surgery, for organ transplantation storage solutions, and in the treatment of leishmaniasis.[101]

Because of limited studies showing very poor or no absorption of extemporaneously compounded allopurinol suppositories, this dosage form is not recommended.[96] Although preliminary reports indicated that extemporaneously prepared allopurinol mouthwash may be effective in protecting against fluorouracil-induced mucositis, one well-controlled clinical trial found it ineffective for this indication, and it is not recommended.[102]

COLCHICINE   Various

Pharmacology. Colchicine is an anti-inflammatory agent relatively specific for gout, with activity probably because of the impairment of leukocyte chemotaxis, mobility, adhesion, and phagocytosis, and a reduction of the lactic acid production resulting from a decrease in urate crystal deposition.[92]

Administration and Adult Dosage. **PO for acute gout** 1–1.2 mg initially, then 0.5–1.2 mg q 1–2 hr until pain is relieved or GI toxicity occurs (ie, nausea, vomiting, stomach pain, or diarrhea), to a maximum total dosage of 4–8 mg. Pain and swelling typically abate within 12 hr and usually are gone in 24–48 hr. An interval of 3 days is advised if a second course is required. **PO for prophylaxis in chronic gout** 0.5–1.8 mg/day or every other day depending on severity; divided doses are preferred with higher dosages. **PO for surgical prophylaxis in patients with gout** 0.5–0.6 mg tid, 3 days before and after surgery. **Slow IV for acute gout** (if patient cannot take oral preparation) 1–2 mg initially, diluted (if desired) in nonbacteriostatic NS, over 2–5 min, then 0.5 mg q 6–24 hr prn, to a maximum of 4 mg in 24 hr, or a maximum 4 mg for a single course of treatment.[103,104] Some clinicians recommend a single IV dose of 3 mg over 5 min; others recommend an initial dose of 1 mg or less, then 0.5 mg 1–2 times daily prn. If pain recurs, give IV 1–2 mg/day for several days; however, no more colchicine should be given by any route for at least 7 days after a full course (4 mg) of IV therapy.[103,104] IV colchicine is very irritating and extravasation must be avoided to prevent tissue and nerve damage; change to oral therapy as soon as possible. **Do not administer by SC or IM routes.** (*See* Notes.)

Special Populations. *Geriatric Dosage.* Reduce the maximum IV colchicine dosage to 2 mg with at least 3 weeks between courses, and lower the dosage further if previously maintained on oral colchicine.[103,104]

Other Conditions. Reduce the total IV and PO dosage of colchicine in renal impairment in proportion to the remaining renal function.[103–105] The dosage of prophylactic colchicine should not exceed 0.5 mg/day with a Cl_{cr} of $\leq$50 mL/min, because of an increased risk of peripheral neuritis and myopathy.[106] Not recommended in patients who require hemodialysis.[106]

Dosage Forms. **Tab** 500, 600 µg; **Inj** 500 µg/mL.

Patient Instructions. You should always have a supply of this drug at hand, and you should take it promptly at the earliest symptoms of a gouty attack. Relief of gout pain or occurrence of nausea, vomiting, stomach pain, or diarrhea indicate that the full therapeutic dosage has been attained and no more drug should be taken. After treatment of an attack, do not take any more colchicine for at least 3 days. Immediately report black tarry stools or bright red blood in the stools, which may indicate gastrointestinal bleeding. Report any tiredness, weakness, numbness, or tingling. Also immediately report sore throat, fever, or oral lesions, which may be an early sign of a severe, but rare, blood disorder.

Missed Doses. If you are taking this drug at regular intervals, such as daily, and you miss a dose, take it as soon as you remember. If it is about time for the next dose, take that dose only. Do not double the dose or take extra.

Pharmacokinetics. *Fate.* Rapidly but variably absorbed after oral administration (healthy young adults, 44 ± 17%; elderly, 45 ± 19%), with partial hepatic deacetylation. Plasma protein binding is approximately 50%; extensive leukocyte uptake occurs with levels found for up to 9 days. Distribution following IV administration is triphasic; V_d of the terminal phase for healthy young adults is 6.7 ± 1.4 L/kg, and for the elderly is 6.3 ± 2.3 L/kg. Cl for healthy young adults is 0.15 ± 0.02 L/hr/kg, and for the elderly 0.12 ± 0.01 L/hr/kg. Urinary (about 10% unchanged), biliary, and fecal elimination occur.[105,107,108]

$t_{1/2}$. (Healthy young adults) second phase 1.2 ± 0.2 hr; terminal phase 30 ± 6 hr; (elderly) second phase 1.2 ± 0.1 hr; terminal phase 34 ± 8 hr.[107]

Adverse Reactions. Nausea, vomiting, stomach pain, and diarrhea are frequent and may occur several hours after oral or IV drug administration; discontinue drug at first signs. Prolonged administration may occasionally cause bone marrow depression with agranulocytosis or thrombocytopenia, aplastic anemia, and purpura. Peripheral neuritis and myopathy with a characteristically elevated creatine kinase occur occasionally. This reaction usually resolves in 3–4 weeks after drug withdrawal and is associated with standard (unadjusted) dosage in renal insufficiency.[103–106,109] Alopecia, reversible malabsorption of vitamin B_{12}, and reversible azoospermia occur. Tissue and nerve damage may occur with IV extravasation. Overdosage can cause hemorrhagic gastroenteritis, vascular damage leading to shock, nephrotoxicity, and paralysis. As little as 7 mg has proved fatal, but much larger dosages have been survived.[104,105,110]

Contraindications. Serious GI, renal, hepatic, or cardiac disorders; combined hepatic, and renal dysfunction;[103–106] blood dyscrasias.

Precautions. Use with great caution in elderly or debilitated patients, especially those with early manifestations of hepatic, renal, GI, or heart disease. Reduce dosage if weakness, anorexia, nausea, vomiting, stomach pain, or diarrhea occurs.[105]

Drug Interactions. None known.

Notes. Colchicine is most effective when used early in the attack before most WBC chemotaxis takes place.[90,91,111] It may be an effective anti-inflammatory agent in the therapy of the arthritis of pseudogout.[109] For acute gout, an **NSAID** or a **corticosteroid** may be preferred, but daily colchicine is often given for prophylaxis against recurrent gouty attacks before and during the first 1 to several months of allopurinol or uricosuric treatment.[90,91,111] Continuous prophylactic colchicine therapy can be effective in suppressing the acute attacks and renal dysfunction of familial Mediterranean fever.[105,109] Colchicine therapy may also be effective for primary biliary cirrhosis and certain inflammatory dermatoses.[105,109]

PROBENECID Benemid, Various

Pharmacology. Probenecid is an organic acid that inhibits renal tubular reabsorption of urate, thereby increasing the urinary excretion of uric acid and lowering serum urate. Probenecid also interferes with renal tubular secretion of many drugs, causing an increase or prolongation in their serum levels. (*See* Notes.)

Administration and Adult Dosage. **PO for chronic gout** 250 mg bid for 1 week, then 500 mg bid (not to be started during an acute attack). **Colchicine** 0.5–1.2 mg/day started before and continued for 1 to several months after initiation of uricosuric treatment diminishes exacerbation of uricosuric-induced gouty attacks.[90–92] To prevent hematuria, renal colic, costovertebral pain, and urate stone formation, liberal fluid intake and alkalinization of the urine with 3–7.5 g/day sodium bicarbonate or 7.5 g/day potassium citrate is recommended, at least until serum uric acid levels normalize and tophaceous deposits disappear. If an acute gouty attack is precipitated during therapy, increase the dosage of colchicine or add a corticosteroid or an NSAID to control the attack.[90–92] (*See* Precautions.) Decrease daily dosage by 500 mg q 6 months if no acute attacks occur, adjusted to maintain normal serum uric acid levels. **PO to prolong penicillin or cephalosporin action** 2 g/day in 4 divided doses. **PO with procaine penicillin G for neurosyphilis** 2 g/day in 4 divided doses for 10–14 days.[112]

Special Populations. *Pediatric Dosage.* (<2 yr) contraindicated. **PO to prolong penicillin or cephalosporin action** (<50 kg) 25 mg/kg initially, then maintain at 40 mg/kg/day or 1.2 g/m^2/day in 4 divided doses; (>50 kg) same as adult dosage. **PO with amoxicillin for gonorrhea** (<45 kg) 25 mg/kg, to a maximum of 1 g.[112]

Geriatric Dosage. Same as adult dosage.

Other Conditions. For chronic gout in renal impairment (although probably ineffective when Cl_{cr} is ≤30 mL/min), increase initial dosage of 500 mg bid in

500 mg/day increments monthly to the dosage that maintains normal serum uric acid levels, to a maximum of 2 g/day in divided doses.

Dosage Forms. **Tab** 500 mg; **Tab** 500 mg with colchicine 0.5 mg (ColBenemid, various).

Patient Instructions. This drug may be taken with food, milk, or an antacid to minimize stomach upset. Drink a large amount (10–12 full glasses) of fluids each day and avoid the use of aspirin- or salicylate-containing products unless directed otherwise.

Missed Doses. If you are taking this drug at regular intervals, such as daily, and you miss a dose, take it as soon as you remember. If it is about time for the next dose, take that dose only. Do not double the dose or take extra.

Pharmacokinetics. *Fate.* Rapidly and completely absorbed from the GI tract; 74–99% plasma protein bound (decreasing with increasing dose), mostly to albumin.[113] V_d is 0.17 ± 0.03 L/kg.[8] Probenecid is extensively metabolized or conjugated, exhibiting Michaelis-Menten elimination; about 40% is excreted in urine as the monoacylglucuronide, less than 5% as unchanged drug, and the remainder as hydroxylated metabolites, which may have uricosuric activity.[114,115]

$t_{1/2}$. Dose dependent (increases with increasing dose): 4.5 ± 0.6 hr with 0.5 g; 12 hr with 2 g.[8,116]

Adverse Reactions. Headache, nausea, vomiting, urinary frequency, rash, and dizziness occur frequently. Exacerbation of gout and uric acid stones may occur. Nephrotic syndrome, hepatic necrosis, aplastic anemia, hemolytic anemia (possibly related to G-6-PD deficiency), and severe allergic reactions occur rarely.

Contraindications. Children <2 yr; known blood dyscrasias or uric acid kidney stones; initiation during an acute gouty attack.

Precautions. Hypersensitivity reactions require drug discontinuation. Use with caution in patients with a history of peptic ulcer or G-6-PD deficiency. (*See* Notes.)

Drug Interactions. Salicylates and pyrazinamide antagonize the uricosuric action of probenecid. Probenecid may increase the serum concentration of many drugs, including acyclovir, benzodiazepines, some β-lactams, clofibrate, dapsone, methotrexate, NSAIDs, penicillamine, sulfonylureas, thiopental, and zidovudine. NSAID clearance may be decreased by competitively inhibiting either formation or renal excretion of acylglucuronide metabolites.[117]

Parameters to Monitor. Serum uric acid weekly until stable when treating hyperuricemia; pretreatment 24-hr urinary uric acid excretion. If alkali is administered, periodically determine acid-base balance.

Notes. Current data do not support the treatment of patients with asymptomatic hyperuricemia caused by *undersecretion* of uric acid.[90,92,118] Most useful in symptomatic patients with reduced urinary excretion of urate: under 800 mg/day on an unrestricted diet; or under 600 mg/day on a purine-restricted diet.[90] Ineffective in prolonging the half-life of β-lactams that do not undergo renal tubular secretion (eg, ceftazidime, ceftriaxone, moxalactam).[119]

SULFINPYRAZONE   Anturane, Various

Pharmacology. Sulfinpyrazone is an analogue of phenylbutazone that lacks anti-inflammatory and analgesic properties. It is a uricosuric agent with a mechanism and site of action resembling those of probenecid. It also has antiplatelet and antithrombotic activity.[90–92,120–125]

Adult Dosage. PO as a uricosuric 200–400 mg/day orally in 2 divided doses with meals or milk, increasing over 1 week to a maximum of 800 mg/day with adequate fluid intake and alkalization of the urine. Reduce to the lowest dosage needed to control serum uric acid (as low as 200 mg/day). In elderly, azotemic cardiovascular patients, initiate therapy with 200 mg/day, and either increase in 200 mg/day increments q four days or keep constant for another 4 days depending upon Cr_s and serum uric acid, to a maximum maintenance dosage of 800 mg/day.

Dosage Forms. Tab 100 mg; **Cap** 200 mg.

Pharmacokinetics. Oral absorption is rapid and complete, with peak serum levels occurring in 1–2 hr. V_d is 0.73 ± 0.23 L/kg; Cl of the parent compound is 0.14 ± 0.044 L/hr/kg. Hepatic metabolism yields four metabolites. The parent compound is mainly responsible for uricosuric activity; the sulfide metabolite produces the antiplatelet effect. Half-lives are 10 ± 1.3 hr (sulfinpyrazone) and 14.3 ± 4.5 hr (sulfide metabolite).

Adverse Reactions. Adverse effects are similar to probenecid with occasional acute renal insufficiency, possibly caused by precipitation of uric acid in renal tubules or decrease in prostaglandin synthesis. **Colchicine** 0.5–1.2 mg/day started before and continued for 1 to several months after initiation of uricosuric treatment diminishes exacerbation of uricosuric-induced gouty attacks. Treat acute exacerbations of gout by increasing the colchicine dosage or by adding an NSAID or corticosteroid. Sulfinpyrazone is contraindicated in patients with peptic ulcers, symptoms of GI inflammation or ulceration, and blood dyscrasias. Avoid sulfinpyrazone in renal insufficiency because it may not be effective.

■ REFERENCES

1. Macfie HL et al. Amiloride. *Drug Intell Clin Pharm* 1981;15:94–8.
2. Rose BD. Diuretics. *Kidney Int* 1991;39:336–52.
3. Ellison DH. Duiretic drugs and the treatment of edema: from clinic to bench and back again. *Am J Kidney Dis* 1994;23:623–43.
4. Brater DC. Resistance to diuretics: mechanisms and clinical implications. *Adv Nephrol Necker Hosp* 1993;22:349–69.
5. Gerlag PG, van-Meijel JJ. High-dose furosemide in the treatment of refractory congestive heart failure. *Arch Intern Med* 1988;148:286–91.
6. Vasko MR et al. Furosemide absorption altered in decompensated congestive heart failure. *Ann Intern Med* 1985;102:314–8.
7. van Meyel JJ et al. Absorption of high dose furosemide (frusemide) in congestive heart failure. *Clin Pharmacokinet* 1992;22:308–18.
8. Benet LZ et al. Design and optimization of dosage regimens; pharmacokinetic data. In, Hardman JG et al., eds. *Goodman and Gilman's the pharmacological basis of therapeutics.* 9th ed. New York: McGraw-Hill; 1996:1707–92.
9. Ponto LL, Schoenwald RD. Furosemide (frusemide): a pharmacokinetic/pharmacodynamic review (part I). *Clin Pharmacokinet* 1990;18:381–408.

10. Ponto LL, Schoenwald RD. Furosemide (frusemide): a pharmacokinetic/pharmacodynamic review (part II). *Clin Pharmacokinet* 1990;18:460–71.

11. Brater DC. Resistance to loop diuretics: why it happens and what to do about it. *Drugs* 1985;30:427–43.

12. Sica DA, Gehr TWB. Diuretic combinations in refractory oedema states. Pharmacokinetic-pharmacodynamic relationships. *Clin Pharmacokinet* 1996;30:229–49.

13. Overdiek JW, Merkus FW. Spironolactone metabolism and gynaecomastia. *Lancet* 1986;1:1103. Letter.

14. Gardiner P et al. Spironolactone metabolism: steady-state serum levels of the sulfur-containing metabolites. *J Clin Pharmacol* 1989;29:342–7.

15. Myers MG. Hydrochlorothiazide with or without amiloride for hypertension in the elderly: a dose-titration study. *Arch Intern Med* 1987;147:1026–30.

16. Beermann B, Groschinsky g rind M. Clinical pharmacokinetics of diuretics. *Clin Pharmacokinet* 1980;5:221–45.

17. Welling PG. Pharmacokinetics of the thiazide diuretics. *Biopharm Drug Dispos* 1986;7:501–35.

18. Langford HG et al. Is thiazide-produced uric acid elevation harmful? Analysis of data from the Hypertension Detection and Follow-up Program. *Arch Intern Med* 1987;147:645–9.

19. O'Bryne S, Feely J. Effects of drugs on glucose tolerance in non-insulin-dependent diabetes (part II). *Drugs* 1990;40:203–19.

20. O'Bryne S, Feely J. Effects of drugs on glucose tolerance in non-insulin-dependent diabetes (part I). *Drugs* 1990;40:6–18.

21. Womack PL, Hart LL. Potassium supplements vs. potassium-sparing diuretics. *DICP* 1990;24:710–1.

22. Lang F. Osmotic diuresis. *Renal Physiol* 1987;10:160–73.

23. Hoffman DM, Grossano D. Use of mannitol diuresis to reduce cis-platinum nephrotoxicity. *Drug Intell Clin Pharm* 1978;12:489–90. Letter.

24. Nissenson AR. Mannitol. *West J Med* 1979;131:277–84.

25. Manninen PH et al. The effect of high-dose mannitol on serum and urine electrolytes and osmolality in neurosurgical patients. *Can J Anaesth* 1987;34:442–6.

26. Anderson P et al. Use of mannitol during neurosurgery: interpatient variability in the plasma and CSF levels. *Eur J Clin Pharmacol* 1988;35:643–9.

27. Dorman HR et al. Mannitol-induced acute renal failure. *Medicine (Baltimore)* 1990;69:153–9.

28. Horgan KJ et al. Acute renal failure due to mannitol intoxication. *Am J Nephrol* 1989;9:106–9.

29. Skluth HA, Gums JG. Spironolactone: a re-examination. *DICP* 1990;24:52–9.

30. Lant A. Diuretics: clinical pharmacology and therapeutic use (part II). *Drugs* 1985;29:162–88.

31. Lant A. Diuretics: clinical pharmacology and therapeutic use (part I). *Drugs* 1985;29:57–87.

32. Sadee W et al. Multiple dose kinetics of spironolactone and canrenoate-potassium in cardiac and hepatic failure. *Eur J Clin Pharmacol* 1974;7:195–200.

33. Overdiek HW, Merkus FW. Influence of food on the bioavailability of spironolactone. *Clin Pharmacol Ther* 1986;40:531–6.

34. Jeunemaitre X et al. Efficacy and tolerance of spironolactone in essential hypertension. *Am J Cardiol* 1987;60:820–5.

35. Friedel HA, Buckley MM. Torasemide: a review of its pharmacological properties and therapeutic potential. *Drugs* 1991;41:81–103.

36. Brater DC et al. Clinical pharmacology of torsemide, a new loop diuretic. *Clin Pharmacol Ther* 1987;42:187–92.

37. Gehr TW et al. The pharmacokinetics of intravenous and oral torsemide in patients with chronic renal insufficiency. *Clin Pharmacol Ther* 1994;56:31–8.

38. Loute G et al. The influence of haemodialysis and haemofiltration on the clearance of torsemide in renal failure. *Eur J Clin Pharmacol* 1986;31(suppl):53–5.

39. Sharoky M et al. Comparative efficacy and bioequivalence of a brand-name and a generic triamterene-hydrochlorothiazide combination product. *Clin Pharm* 1989;8(7):496–500.

40. Gilfrich H et al. Pharmacokinetics of triamterene after i.v. administration to man: determination of bioavailability. *Eur J Clin Pharmacol* 1983;25:237–41.

41. Muirhead MR et al. Effect of cimetidine on renal and hepatic drug elimination: studies with triamterene. *Clin Pharmacol Ther* 1986;40:400–7.

42. Knauf H et al. Delayed elimination of triamterene and its active metabolite in chronic renal failure. *Eur J Clin Pharmacol* 1983;24:453–6.

43. Mutschler E et al. Pharmacokinetics of triamterene. *Clin Exp Hypertens [A]* 1983;5:249–69.

44. Sica DA, Gehr TW. Triamterene and the kidney. *Nephron* 1989;51:454–61.

45. Alaniz C. Management of cirrhotic ascites. *Clin Pharm* 1989;8:645–54.

46. Burns Schaiff R et al. Medical treatment of hypercalcemia. *Clin Pharm* 1989;8:108–21.

47. Sica DA, Gehr TWB. Diuretic combinations in refractory oedema states. Pharmacokinetic-pharmacodynamic relationships. *Clin Pharmacokinet* 1996;30:229–49.
48. Zaloga GP, Chernow B. Divalent ions: calcium, magnesium, and phosphorus. In, Chernow B, ed. *The pharmacologic approach to the critically ill patient.* 3rd ed. Baltimore: Williams & Wilkins; 1994:777–804.
49. Food and Nutrition Board, NRC. *Recommended dietary allowances.* 10th ed. Washington, DC: National Academy Press; 1989.
50. Anon. Calcium supplements. *Med Lett Drugs Ther* 1989;31:101–3.
51. Delmez JA, Slatopolsky E. Hyperphosphatemia: its consequences and treatment in patients with chronic renal disease. *Am J Kidney Dis* 1992;19:303–17.
52. Tohme JF, Bilezikian JP. Hypocalcemic emergencies. *Endocrinol Metab Clin North Am* 1993;22:363–75.
53. Carr CJ, Shangraw RF. Nutritional and pharmaceutical aspects of calcium supplementation. *Am Pharm* 1987;2:49–50, 54–7.
54. Blanchard J, Aeschlimann JM. Calcium absorption in man: some dosing recommendations. *J Pharmacokinet Biopharm* 1989;17:631–44.
55. Sheikh MS et al. Gastrointestinal absorption of calcium from milk and calcium salts. *N Engl J Med* 1987;317: 532–6.
56. Altura BM. Basic biochemistry and physiology of magnesium: a brief review. *Magnes Trace Elem* 1991;10: 167–71.
57. Gums JG. Clinical significance of magnesium: a review. *Drug Intell Clin Pharm* 1987;21:240–6.
58. Al-Ghandi SMG et al. Magnesium deficiency: pathophysiologic and clinical overview. *Am J Kidney Dis* 1994;5:737–52.
59. Rude RK. Magnesium metabolism and deficiency. *Endocrinol Metab Clin North Am* 1993;22:377–95.
60. Montgomery P. Treatment of magnesium deficiency. *Clin Pharm* 1987;6:834–5.
61. Reinhart RA. Magnesium metabolism: a review with special reference to the relationship between intracellular content and serum levels. *Arch Intern Med* 1988;148:2415–20.
62. Kobrin SM, Goldfarb S. Magnesium deficiency. *Semin Nephrol* 1990;10:525–35.
63. Berkelhammer C, Bear RA. A clinical approach to common electrolyte problems: hypomagnesemia. *Can Med Assoc J* 1985;132:360–8.
64. Yusuf S et al. Intravenous magnesium in acute myocardial infarction: an effective, safe, simple, and inexpensive intervention. *Circulation* 1993;87:2043–6. Editorial.
65. Teo KK, Yusuf S. Role of magnesium in reducing mortality in acute myocardial infarction: a review of the evidence. *Drugs* 1993;46:347–59.
66. Chernow B et al. Hypomagnesemia: implications for the critical care specialist. *Crit Care Med* 1982;10: 193–6.
67. Lloyd CW, Johnson CE. Management of hypophosphatemia. *Clin Pharm* 1988;7:123–8.
68. Rubin MF, Narins RG. Hypophosphatemia: pathophysiological and practical aspect of its therapy. *Semin Nephrol* 1990;10:536–45.
69. Hodgson SF, Hurley DL. Acquired hypophosphatemia. *Endocrinol Metab Clin North Am* 1993;22:397–409.
70. Peppers MP et al. Endocrine crises: hypophosphatemia and hyperphosphatemia. *Crit Care Clin* 1991;7:201–14.
71. Baker WL. Hypophosphatemia. *Am J Nurs* 1985;85:998–1003.
72. Kingston M, Al-Siba'i MB. Treatment of severe hypophosphatemia. *Crit Care Med* 1985;13:16–8.
73. Martin ML et al. Potassium. *Emerg Med Clin North Am* 1986;4:131–44.
74. Krishna GG. Hypokalemic states: current clinical issues. *Semin Nephrol* 1990;10:515–24.
75. Zull DN. Disorders of potassium metabolism. *Emerg Med Clin North Am* 1989;7:771–94.
76. Stanaszek WF, Romankiewicz JA. Current approaches to management of potassium deficiency. *Drug Intell Clin Pharm* 1985;19:176–84.
77. Kruse JA, Carlson RW. Rapid correction of hypokalemia using concentrated intravenous potassium chloride infusions. *Arch Intern Med* 1990;150:613–7.
78. Toner JM, Ramsay LE. Pharmacokinetics of potassium chloride in wax-based and syrup formulations. *Br J Clin Pharmacol* 1985;19:489–94.
79. Skoutakis VA et al. The comparative bioavailability of liquid, wax-matrix, and microencapsulated preparations of potassium chloride. *J Clin Pharmacol* 1985;25:619–21.
80. Breyer JA. Diabetic nephropathy in insulin-dependent patients. *Am J Kidney Dis* 1992;20:533–47.
81. Freedman BI, Burkart JM. Endocrine crises: hypokalemia. *Crit Care Clin* 1991;7:143–53.
82. Finch MH, Younoszai KM. Oral rehydration therapy. *South Med J* 1987;80:609–13.
83. Balistreri WF. Oral rehydration in acute infantile diarrhea. *Am J Med* 1990;88(6A):30S–3S.
84. Grisanti KA, Jaffe DM. Dehydration syndromes: oral rehydration and fluid replacement. *Emerg Med Clin North Am* 1991;9:565–88.
85. Swedberg J, Steiner JF. Oral rehydration therapy in diarrhea: not just for Third World children. *Postgrad Med* 1983;74:335–41.
86. Anon. Oral rehydration solutions. *Med Lett Drugs Ther* 1983;25:19–20.

87. Lillemoe KD et al. Intestinal necrosis due to sodium polystyrene (Kayexalate) in sorbitol enemas: clinical and experimental support for the hypothesis. *Surgery* 1987;101:267–72.

88. Elms JJ. Potassium imbalance: causes and prevention. *Postgrad Med* 1982;72:165–71.

89. Alvo M, Warnock DG. Hyperkalemia. *West J Med* 1984;141:666–71.

90. Star VL, Hochberg MC. Prevention and management of gout. *Drugs* 1993;45:212–22.

91. Conaghan PG, Day RO. Risks and benefits of drugs used in the management and prevention of gout. *Drug Safety* 1994;11:252–8.

92. Emmerson BT. The management of gout. *N Engl J Med* 1996;334:445–51.

93. Campbell SM. Gout: how presentation, diagnosis, and treatment differ in the elderly. *Geriatrics* 1988;43(11):71–7.

94. Conger JD. Acute uric acid nephropathy. *Med Clin North Am* 1990;74:859–71.

95. Hande KR et al. Severe allopurinol toxicity: description and guidelines for prevention in patients with renal insufficiency. *Am J Med* 1984;76:47–56.

96. Murrell GAC, Rapeport WG. Clinical pharmacokinetics of allopurinol. *Clin Pharmacokinet* 1986;11:343–53.

97. Walter-Sack I et al. Disposition and uric acid lowering effect of oxipurinol: comparison of different oxipurinol formulations and allopurinol in healthy individuals. *Eur J Clin Pharmacol* 1995;49:215–20.

98. Fam AG et al. Desensitization to allopurinol in patients with gout and cutaneous reactions. *Am J Med* 1992;93:299–302.

99. Roujeau JC, Stern RS. Severe adverse cutaneous reactions to drugs. *N Engl J Med* 1994;331:1272–85.

100. Arellano F, Sacristán JA. Allopurinol hypersensitivity syndrome: a review. *Ann Pharmacother* 1993;27:337–43.

101. Day RO et al. New uses for allopurinol. *Drugs* 1994;48:339–44.

102. Loprinzi CL et al. A controlled evaluation of an allopurinol mouthwash as prophylaxis against 5-fluorouracil-induced stomatitis. *Cancer* 1990;65:1879–82.

103. Wallace SL, Singer JZ. Review: systemic toxicity associated with the intravenous administration of colchicine—guidelines for use. *J Rheumatol* 1988;15:495–9.

104. Roberts WN et al. Colchicine in acute gout: reassessment of risks and benefits. *JAMA* 1987;257:1920–2.

105. Levy M et al. Colchicine: a state-of-the-art review. *Pharmacotherapy* 1991;11:196–211.

106. Wallace SL et al. Renal function predicts colchicine toxicity: guidelines for the prophylactic use of colchicine in gout. *J Rheumatol* 1991;18:264–9.

107. Rochdi M et al. Pharmacokinetics and absolute bioavailability of colchicine after IV and oral administration in healthy human volunteers and elderly subjects. *Eur J Clin Pharmacol* 1994;46:351–4.

108. Jusko WJ, Gretch M. Plasma and tissue protein binding of drugs in pharmacokinetics. *Drug Metab Rev* 1976;5:43–140.

109. Famaey JP. Colchicine in therapy. State of the art and new perspectives for an old drug. *Clin Exp Rheumatol* 1988;6:305–17.

110. Hood RL. Colchicine poisoning. *J Emerg Med* 1994;12:171–7.

111. Wallace SL, Singer JZ. Therapy in gout. *Rheum Dis Clin North Am* 1988;14:441–57.

112. Anon. Drugs for sexually transmitted diseases. *Med Lett Drugs Ther* 1994;36:1–6.

113. Emanuelsson BM et al. Non-linear elimination and protein binding of probenecid. *Eur J Clin Pharmacol* 1987;32:395–401.

114. Israili ZH et al. Metabolites of probenecid. Chemical, physical, and pharmacological studies. *J Med Chem* 1972;15:709–13.

115. Perel JM et al. Identification and renal excretion of probenecid metabolites in man. *Life Sci* 1970;9:1337–43.

116. Dayton PG et al. The physiological disposition of probenecid, including renal clearance, in man, studied by an improved method for its estimation in biological material. *J Pharmacol Exp Ther* 1963;140:278–86.

117. Smith PC et al. Effect of probenecid on the formation and elimination of acyl glucuronides: studies with zomepirac. *Clin Pharmacol Ther* 1985;38:121–7.

118. Campbell SM. Gout: how presentation, diagnosis, and treatment differ in the elderly. *Geriatrics* 1988;43(11):71–7.

119. Brown GR. Cephalosporin-probenecid drug interactions. *Clin Pharmacokinet* 1993;24:289–300.

120. Hood WB. More on sulfinpyrazone after myocardial infarction. *N Engl J Med* 1982;306:988–9.

121. Palummeri E et al. Sulphinpyrazone in cardiovascular elderly azotemic patients: a proposal of a guided incremental dose schedule. *J Int Med Res* 1984;12:271–6.

122. Mahoney C et al. Kinetics and metabolism of sulfinpyrazone. *Clin Pharmacol Ther* 1983;33:491–7.

123. Schlicht F et al. Pharmacokinetics of sulfinpyrazone and its major metabolites after a single dose and during chronic treatment. *Eur J Clin Pharmacol* 1985;28:97–103.

124. Orlandini G, Brognoli M. Acute renal failure and treatment with sulfinpyrazone. *Clin Nephrol* 1983;20:161–2.

125. Rosenkranz B et al. Effects of sulfinpyrazone on renal function and prostaglandin formation in man. *Nephron* 1985;39:237–43.

℞ Respiratory Drugs

Antiasthmatics

Class Instructions: Antiasthmatic Inhalers. Attach the mouthpiece to the spacer device (which slows the rate of inhalation and thereby increases penetration into airways). To use the inhaler, tilt head up and place mouthpiece of spacer device into mouth, making sure the teeth and tongue are not in the way. While inhaling slowly and deeply, release one dose of aerosolized medication, inhale, remove inhaler from mouth, and hold breath for 5–10 seconds. Wait at least 1 minute between puffs. Do not exceed prescribed dosage. Report if symptoms do not completely clear or the inhaler is required more than prescribed. Clean mouthpiece weekly with hot water and soap. Store away from heat and direct sunlight. Bronchodilators may cause nervousness, tremors (especially with terbutaline or albuterol), or rapid heart rate. Report if these effects continue after dosage reduction; if chest pain, dizziness, or headache occur; or if asthmatic symptoms are not relieved.

Missed Doses. Take missed doses as soon as possible. However, if it is almost time for your next dose, skip the missed dose and go back to your regular schedule. Do not double doses.

ALBUTEROL SULFATE
Epaq, Proventil, Ventolin, Volmax, Various

Pharmacology. Albuterol is a selective β₂-adrenergic agonist that produces bronchodilation, vasodilation, uterine relaxation, skeletal muscle stimulation, peripheral vasodilation, and tachycardia.[1]

Administration and Adult Dosage. Inhal for asthma (metered-dose inhaler) 90–180 μg (1–2 puffs), with 1–5 min between inhalations, q 4–6 hr prn and just before exercise; (inhalation solution) 2.5 mg by nebulization tid–qid; (inhalation capsule) 1–2 inhalation capsule q 4–6 hr or 1 capsule 15 min prior to exercise. **Inhal for severe bronchospasm** nebulized by compressed air or oxygen 2.5–5 mg (0.5–1 mL of 0.5% in 2–3 mL NS) q 4–6 hr prn (q 1–2 hr under medical supervision). **PO for asthma** 2–4 mg q 6–8 hr, increase as tolerated to a maximum of 32 mg/day; **SR Tab** 4–8 mg q 12 hr, to a maximum of 32 mg/day.

Special Populations. *Pediatric Dosage.* **Inhal for asthma** (metered-dose inhaler) (<12 yr) 90–180 μg (1–2 puffs) q 4–6 hr using spacer; (≥12 yr) same as adult dosage; (inhalation solution) (<12 yr) 0.05–0.15 mg/kg q 4–6 hr prn, or (<20 kg) 0.25 mL of 0.5% solution; (>20 kg) 0.5 mL of 0.5% solution to a maximum of 1 mL diluted in 2–3 mL NS q 4–6 hr prn (q 1–2 hr for severe bronchospasm under medical supervision); (≥12 yr) same as adult dosage. **PO for asthma** (2–6 yr) 100–200 μg/kg/dose q 8 hr, to a maximum of 4 mg q 8 hr; (6–12 yr) 2 mg q 6–8 hr, to a maximum of 24 mg/day; (>12 yr) same as adult dosage. **SR Tab** (<12 yr) dosage not established; (>12 yr) same as adult dosage.

Geriatric Dosage. **Inhal for asthma** same as adult dosage. **PO** 2 mg tid–qid initially, increasing prn to a maximum of 8 mg tid–qid.

Dosage Forms. **Inhal** (metered-dose) 90 μg/puff (200 puffs/inhaler); **Inhal** (metered-dose) HFA (Epaq, Proventil HFA) 90 μg/puff (200 puffs/inhaler). *This product does not contain chlorofluorocarbons as a propellant;* **Inhal Soln** 0.5% (5 mg/mL), (unit dose solution, 3 mL) 0.083%; **Inhal Cap** (Rotacap) 200 μg for use with powder inhaler; **Tab** 2, 4 mg; **Syrup** 0.4 mg/mL; **SR Tab** 4, 8 mg. **Inhal** 90 μg plus ipratropium bromide 18 μg/puff (Combivent).

Patient Instructions. (*See* Class Instructions: Antiasthmatic Inhalers.)

Pharmacokinetics. *Onset and Duration.* (Inhal) onset within 15 min, peak 60–90 min or less; (PO) onset 30–60 min, peak 2–3 hr. Duration 4–6 hr, depending on the dose, dosage form, and clinical condition. (*See* Sympathomimetic Bronchodilators Comparison Chart.)

Fate. Peak serum level after 0.15 mg/kg by inhalation is 5.6 μg/L (23 nmol/L). Oral bioavailability is 50% because of hepatic first-pass metabolism; peak after 4 mg tablet is 10 μg/L (42 nmol/L); 50% is excreted in urine as an inactive sulfate conjugate. The drug does not appear to be metabolized in the lung.[2]

$t_{1/2}$. (IV) 2–3 hr; apparent half-life is 5–6 hr after oral and up to 7 hr after inhalation because of prolonged absorption.[2]

Adverse Reactions. Dose-related reflex tachycardia from peripheral vasodilation and from direct stimulation of cardiac β_2-receptors. Tremor, palpitations, and nausea are other dose-related effects that are markedly reduced with aerosol administration. All β_2-agonists lower serum potassium concentrations.

Precautions. Pregnancy; cardiac disorders including coronary insufficiency and hypertension; diabetes. Excessive or prolonged use may lead to tolerance.

Drug Interactions. Concurrent β-blockers may antagonize effects.

Parameters to Monitor. Inhalation technique, asthma symptoms, frequency of use, pulmonary function, and heart rate.

Notes. A relationship between regular (ie, not prn) use of inhaled β_2-agonists and death from asthma has been a concern.[3,4] Regardless of whether β_2-agonists are directly responsible or are simply a marker for more severe asthma, heavy use (over 1 canister/month or 12 puffs/day) of these agents should alert clinicians that it is necessary to re-evaluate the patient's condition. Epaq and Proventil HFA inhalers use a non-CFC propellant; drug delivery is similar, but not identical, to Ventolin and Proventil. **Levalbuterol** (Xopenex) is the active L-isomer of albuterol. It is available as a solution for inhalation.

CROMOLYN SODIUM   Gastrocrom, Intal, Nasalcrom, Opticrom, Various

Pharmacology. Cromolyn stabilizes the membrane of mast cells and other inflammatory cells (eg, eosinophils), inhibiting release and production of soluble mediators (eg, histamine, leukotrienes) that produce inflammation and bronchospasm. The mechanism appears to be the inhibition of calcium ion influx through the cell membrane. Cromolyn inhibits both the early and late responses to specific allergen and exercise challenges. It also prevents the increase in nonspecific bronchial hyperreactivity that occurs during a specific allergen season in atopic asthmatics.[5,6]

Administration and Adult Dosage. Inhal for asthma 20 mg qid at regular intervals in nebulizer (1 ampule inhalant solution) or 0.8–1.6 mg qid via a pressurized metered-dose inhaler. Initiate therapy in conjunction with an aerosolized β_2-agonist. (*See* Notes.) **Inhal for prevention of exercise-induced bronchospasm** single dose (as above) just prior to exercise. **Intranasal for prophylaxis of allergic rhinitis** 5.2 mg/nostril 3–6 times/day at regular intervals. **Ophth for allergic ocular disorders** 1–2 drops (1.6–3.2 mg) in each eye 4–6 times/day at regular intervals. For chronic conditions the drug must be used continuously to be effective. **PO for mastocytosis** 200 mg qid, 30 min before meals and hs.

Special Populations. *Pediatric Dosage.* **Inhal** (<2 yr) dosage not established; (≥2 yr) same as adult dosage. **Intranasal or Ophth** same as adult dosage. **PO for mastocytosis** (term infants–2 yr) 20 mg/kg/day in 4 divided doses, to a maximum of 30 mg/kg/day; (2–12 yr) 100 mg qid, 30 min before meals and hs, increasing if necessary to a maximum of 40 mg/kg/day.

Geriatric Dosage. Same as adult dosage.

Other Conditions. The therapeutic effect is dose dependent, and patients with more severe disease may require more frequent administration initially. After a patient becomes symptom free, the frequency of administration may be reduced to bid–tid.

Dosage Forms. **Inhal Soln** 10 mg/mL; **Inhal** 800 µg/puff (112, 200 doses/inhaler); **Nasal Inhal** 5.2 mg/spray (100 doses/inhaler); **Ophth Drp** 40 mg/mL (250 drops/container); **PO Cap** 100 mg.

Patient Instructions. (Asthma) this medication must be used regularly and continuously to be effective. Do not stop therapy abruptly, except on medical advice. Carefully follow directions for inhaler use included with the device. Actuate metered-dose device during a *slow* deep inhalation, then hold breath for 5–10 seconds. Do not discontinue the use of the nebulizer solution during acute asthmatic attacks. You may mix the nebulizer solution with any bronchodilator inhalant solution. (Mastocytosis) dissolve oral capsules in one-half glass (4 fl oz) of hot water, then add an equal amount of cold water and drink the entire amount. Do not mix with fruit juice, milk, or foods.

Missed Doses. Take this drug at regular intervals. If you miss a dose, take it as soon as you remember. If it is about time for the next dose, take that dose only. Do not double the dose or take extra.

Pharmacokinetics. *Onset and Duration.* (Asthma) onset within 1 min for prevention of allergen-induced mast cell degranulation; duration dose dependent, 2–5 hr.[6] It may require 4–6 weeks to achieve maximal response, although most asthmatics have a response within 2 weeks.[7]

Fate. Oral bioavailability is 0.5–1%. Amount absorbed after inhalation is dependent on the delivery system; about 10% of the dosage for a Spinhaler and less than

2% with the nebulizer solution.[6] Peak serum levels occur 15–20 min after inhalation. V_d is 0.2 ± 0.04 L/kg; Cl is 0.35 ± 0.1 L/hr/kg. Rapidly excreted unchanged in equal portions in the bile and urine.[5,6]

$t_{\frac{1}{2}}$. 22.5 ± 1.6 min.[6]

Adverse Reactions. Mild burning or stinging may occur with ophthalmic solution. Occasionally, headache and diarrhea occur with oral capsules.

Precautions. Use with caution in patients with lactose sensitivity (capsules only). Watch for worsening of asthma in patients discontinuing the drug. Children <5 yr should receive cromolyn as the nebulizer solution. The ophthalmic solution contains 0.01% benzalkonium chloride; therefore, do not wear soft contact lenses during therapy.

Drug Interactions. None known.

Parameters to Monitor. Monitor relief of asthmatic symptoms and the proper dosage and inhalation technique. Patient noncompliance or inappropriate inhalation technique often contribute to treatment failure. The measurement of peak expiratory flow rate with a peak flow meter is useful in severe chronic asthma. Periodic standard pulmonary function tests are indicated q 1–6 months in less severe asthma.

Notes. Comparative studies have shown cromolyn and **theophylline** to be equally effective for the prophylaxis of chronic asthma, although cromolyn produces fewer side effects.[5–7] The inhalant solution is stable with all β_2-agonist and anticholinergic solutions for nebulization.[6] The nasal spray is most effective if started 1 week prior to the allergen season; however, patients receive benefit even if treatment is begun after symptoms occur.[7] Oral cromolyn has been used in the management of GI conditions such as food allergy and irritable bowel syndrome.[8]

IPRATROPIUM BROMIDE
Atrovent, Various

Pharmacology. Ipratropium is a competitive antagonist of acetylcholine at peripheral muscarinic receptors, but not centrally because of its quaternary structure.[9] It is used primarily as a bronchodilator in COPD, emphysema, and bronchitis.

Administration and Adult Dosage. **Inhal for bronchospasm of COPD (including chronic bronchitis)** 36–72 μg (2–4 puffs) qid by metered-dose inhaler, to a maximum of 288 μg (16 puffs)/day.[9,10] **Inhal for acute, severe asthma** 500 μg tid–qid by nebulizer. Combivent or extemporaneous ipratropium/albuterol mixtures have the same dosage as above. **Nasal spray for rhinorrhea of perennial rhinitis** 2 sprays (84 μg)/nostril of 0.03% solution bid–tid; **Nasal spray for rhinorrhea of the common cold** 2 sprays (84 μg)/nostril tid–qid for up to 4 days.

Special Populations. *Pediatric Dosage.* (<12 yr) safety and efficacy not established. **Inhal** (<2 yr) 125 μg/dose by nebulizer;[11] (>2 yr) 18–36 μg (1–2 puffs) q 6–8 hr by metered-dose inhaler or 250 μg q 6–8 hr by nebulizer has been used.[10,12] **Nasal spray for rhinorrhea of perennial rhinitis** (<6 yr) safety and efficacy not established; (6–11 yr) 1 spray (42 μg)/nostril of 0.03% solution bid–tid; (≥12 yr) same as adult dosage.

Geriatric Dosage. Same as adult dosage.

Dosage Forms. **Inhal** 18 μg/puff (200 doses/inhaler); **Inhal Soln** 200 μg/mL (500 μg/vial). **Nasal Spray** 0.03, 0.06%. **Inhal** 18 μg plus 90 μg albuterol/puff (Combivent).

Patient Instructions. (*See* Class Instructions: Antiasthmatic Inhalers.) Temporary blurring of vision may occur if the drug is sprayed into eyes.

Pharmacokinetics. *Onset and Duration.* Onset 3 min; peak 1–2 hr;[10] duration 4–6 hr, depending on intensity of response.[13]

Fate. Only 32% or less is orally absorbed and less than 1% of inhaled dose is absorbed.[10] Metabolized to eight metabolites, which are excreted in the urine and bile. $t_{1/2}$. 1.5–4 hr.[10]

Adverse Reactions. Dryness of the mouth. Because of quaternary nature of the molecule, typical systemic anticholinergic side effects are absent.[10,13] With the nasal spray, epistaxis, nasal dryness, dry mouth, or throat and nasal congestion occur in 1–10% of patients. During long-term use, headache, nausea, and upper respiratory tract infections also occur frequently.

Contraindications. (Aerosol inhaler) hypersensitivity to soy lecithin, soybeans, or related products.

Precautions. Use with caution in narrow-angle glaucoma, prostatic hypertrophy, or bladder neck obstruction.

Drug Interactions. None known.

Parameters to Monitor. Inhalation technique, asthma symptoms, frequency of use, pulmonary function, and anticholinergic symptoms.

Notes. Anticholinergics appear to be as potent bronchodilators as β₂-adrenergic drugs in bronchitis and emphysema, but less potent in asthma.[9,10] Anticholinergics produce an additive bronchodilation with β₂-adrenergic agents in severe asthma.[10,12] Ipratropium and albuterol nebulizer solutions can be mixed if the mixture is used within 1 hr.

MONTELUKAST SODIUM   Singulair

Pharmacology. Montelukast sodium is a selective and orally active leukotriene-receptor antagonist that inhibits the cysteinyl leukotriene $CysLT_1$ receptor.[14,15]

Administration and Adult Dosage. **PO for mild persistent asthma** 10 mg/day in the evening.

Special Populations. *Pediatric Dosage.* **PO for mild persistent asthma** (<6 yr) safety and efficacy not established; (6–14 yr) 5 mg chewable tablet every evening; (≥15 yr) same as adult dosage.

Geriatric Dosage. Same as adult dosage.

Dosage Forms. **Chew Tab** 5 mg; **Tab** 10 mg.

Patient Instructions. This drug is used for long-term control and prevention of mild persistent asthma symptoms. Take this medication daily, even when you are having no symptoms, as well as during periods of worsening asthma. This medication is not for the treatment of acute asthma attacks management of exercise-induced bronchospasm. You should have appropriate short-acting β_2-agonist medication available to treat acute symptoms. Seek medical attention if short-acting inhaled bronchodilators are needed more often than usual, or if the maximum number of inhalations of short-acting bronchodilator treatment prescribed for a 24-hour period is needed.

Missed Doses. Take a missed dose as soon as possible. If it is almost time to take the next dose, skip the missed dose and go back to your regular dosage schedule. Do not double doses.

Pharmacokinetics. *Onset and Duration.* Duration is ≥ 24 hr.[14,15]

Fate. Montelukast is rapidly absorbed after oral administration. Mean oral bioavailability for the film-coated tablet is 64%; for the chewable tablet it is 73% in the fasted state and 63% with a standard morning meal. Peak concentrations occur 3–4 hr following administration of a 10 mg film-coated tablet and 2–2.5 hr after the 5 mg chewable tablet, to fasted adults. Montelukast is >99% protein bound; V_{dss} is 8–11 L; Cl is 2.7 L/hr. CYP3A4 and 2C9 are involved in the metabolism of montelukast. Montelukast and its metabolites are excreted almost exclusively via the bile.

$t_{\frac{1}{2}}$. 2.7–5.5 hr in healthy young adults.

Adverse Reactions. Generally well tolerated. Adverse events which occur with a frequency of ≥ 2% and more frequently in patients on montelukast than placebo were diarrhea, laryngitis, pharyngitis, nausea, otitis, sinusitis, and viral infection.

Contraindications. Patients with known aspirin sensitivity should continue to avoid aspirin or other NSAIDs while taking montelukast. Inform phenylketonurics that the chewable tablets contain phenylalanine (a component of aspartame) 0.824 mg/tablet.

Precautions. (*See* Patient Instructions.) Reduction in systemic corticosteroid dosage in patients on another leukotriene antagonist, zafirlukast, has been followed rarely by eosinophilia, vasculitic rash, worsening pulmonary symptoms, cardiac complications, and/or neuropathy, sometimes presenting as Churg-Strauss syndrome. A causal relationship with leukotriene-receptor antagonists is not established.

Parameters to Monitor. Clinical symptoms of asthma. Appropriate monitoring recommended when systemic corticosteroid reduction is considered.

Notes. Zafirlukast (Accolate) is similar to montelukast, but has the disadvantages of twice-daily administration, the need to take on an empty stomach, and several drug–drug interactions: the anticoagulant effect of warfarin is increased by zafirlukast; erythromycin and theophylline decrease zafirlukast serum concentrations, whereas aspirin increases zafirlukast serum concentrations. Interactions with other drugs are not well studied. (*See* Precautions.) The dosage of zafirlukast in patients ≥ 12 yr is 20 mg bid on an empty stomach; it is available as 20 mg tablets.

NEDOCROMIL SODIUM   Tilade

Pharmacology. Nedocromil sodium is the disodium salt of a pyranoquinolone dicarboxylic acid that is chemically dissimilar, but pharmacologically similar, to cromolyn sodium. Like cromolyn, nedocromil inhibits the activation of and mediator release from inflammatory cells important in asthma and allergy. Nedocromil appears to have more potent in vitro activity against allergic response than cromolyn.[16,17]

Administration and Adult Dosage. Inhal for asthma 2 metered-dose actuations qid. In patients under good control with qid administration (ie, patients requiring inhaled or oral β-agonists not more than twice a week), a lower dosage can be tried. First reduce to a tid regimen, then, after several weeks of continued good control, attempt to reduce to a bid regimen.

Pediatric Dosage. (>12 yr) same as adult dosage.

Dosage Forms. Inhal 16.2 g, containing 112 2 mg doses (1.75 mg reaches the patient).

Pharmacokinetics. Oral bioavailability is only 2–3%. Following inhalation, bioavailability is 5%, with peak serum concentrations occurring in 20–40 min; concentrations fall monoexponentially, with a half-life of 1.5–2.3 hr, reflecting absorption from lungs.

Adverse Reactions. Bronchospasm, headache, distinctive taste, nausea, and vomiting occur frequently. In a limited number of trials, nedocromil was effective for long-term prophylaxis of asthma. Like cromolyn, it can decrease bronchial hyperreactivity but is only partially effective in steroid-dependent asthmatics. Nedocromil sodium is intended for regular maintenance treatment and should not be used in acute asthma attacks.

SALMETEROL XINAFOATE   Serevent

Pharmacology. Salmeterol is a β₂-agonist structurally and pharmacologically similar to albuterol. Salmeterol is intended for regular treatment of reversible airway obstruction and not for immediate symptomatic relief. The place of salmeterol in asthma therapy is being debated, in part because patients in need of regular β₂-agonist therapy should be regarded as candidates for an inhaled corticosteroid to treat underlying inflammation.[18] (*See* Sympathomimetic Bronchodilators Comparison Chart.)

Administration and Adult Dosage. Inhal for asthma prophylaxis or COPD 42 μg (2 puffs) q 12 hr by metered-dose inhaler or 1 dry powder blister inhaled q 12 hr. **Inhal to prevent exercise-induced bronchospasm** 2 puffs 30–60 min before exercise.

Pediatric Dosage. Inhal (<12 yr) safety and efficacy not established; (≥12 yr) same as adult dosage.

Dosage Forms. Inhal 21 μg/metered-dose puff, in 6.5 g (60 actuations) and 13 g (120 actuations) canisters; **Dry Pwdr Inhal** 50 mg/blister.

Patient Instructions. Shake metered-dose cannister well before using. For asthma, use this medication regularly every 12 hours. If asthma symptoms occur between doses, use a short-acting inhaler to treat symptoms. If you regularly need more than 4 inhalations of the short-acting inhaler, see your health care provider.

Pharmacokinetics. Onset of effective bronchodilation is achieved in 20–30 min; peak effect occurs within 3–4 hr. Bronchodilation lasts for at least 12 hr following inhalation of a single dose of 50 μg. After inhalation, salmeterol is extensively metabolized by hydroxylation, with the majority of a dose being eliminated within 72 hr. About 23% of administered radioactivity was recovered in the urine and 57% in the feces over a period of 168 hr.

Adverse Reactions. (*See* Albuterol.)

Notes. **Formoterol** (Foradil–Novartis) is a long-acting β_2-adrenergic agonist that is similar to salmeterol in duration, but may have a more rapid onset. Investigationally, inhaled doses of 12–24 μg once daily have been used.

SYMPATHOMIMETIC BRONCHODILATORS COMPARISON CHART

DRUG	DOSAGE FORMS	DOSAGE Adult	DOSAGE Pediatric[a]	RECEPTOR SELECTIVITY[b] β_1	RECEPTOR SELECTIVITY[b] β_2	RELATIVE β_2 POTENCY[c]	DURATION OF ACTION BY INHALATION (HR)[d]
Albuterol Proventil Ventolin Volmax Various	Inhal (soln) 0.5%; (unit dose) 0.083%, (metered-dose) 0.09 mg/puff; (Rotacaps) 200 µg/cap SR Tab 4, 8 mg Syrup 0.4 mg/mL Tab 2, 4 mg.	Inhal (soln) 2.5–5 mg in 2–3 mL NS q 4–6 hr prm by nebulizer; may use q 1–2 hr prm status asthmaticus under medical supervision; (metered-dose) 1–2 puffs q 4–6 hr prm and prior to exercise; 1 Rotacap is equivalent to 2 metered-dose puffs PO 2–4 mg q 6–8 hr, to a maximum of 32 mg/day SR Tab 4–8 mg q 12 hr, to a maximum of 32 mg/day.	Inhal (soln) 0.05–0.15 mg/kg in 2–3 mL NS q 4–6 hr prm by nebulizer, may use q 1–2 hr prm or 0.5 mg/kg/hr continuously nebulized for status asthmaticus under medical supervision; (metered-dose) 1–2 puffs q 4–6 hr prm and prior to exercise PO 0.1–0.2 mg/kg q 6–8 hr, to a maximum of 24 mg/day.	+	++++	5	4–6
Bitolterol[e] Tornalate Produral	Inhal (metered-dose) 0.37 mg/puff; (soln) 0.2%.	Inhal (metered-dose) 1–3 puffs q 4–6 hr prm.	Inhal (metered-dose) 1–2 puffs q 4–6 hr prm.	+	++++	2.5	4–8

(continued)

722

SYMPATHOMIMETIC BRONCHODILATORS COMPARISON CHART (continued)

DRUG	DOSAGE FORMS	DOSAGE Adult	DOSAGE Pediatric[a]	RECEPTOR SELECTIVITY[b] β_1	β_2	RELATIVE β_2 POTENCY[c]	DURATION OF ACTION BY INHALATION (HR)[d]
Epinephrine Adrenalin Various	Inhal (soln) 1, 1.25, 2.25% (racemic) Inj 0.01, 0.1, 1 mg/mL.	SC 0.2–0.5 mg q 20 min–4 hr prn. Inhal not recommended	SC 0.01 mL/kg of 1:1000 q 15–20 min for 2 doses, then q 4 hr prn. Inhal not recommended for asthma.	+++	+++	5	0.5–2
Epinephrine Aq Suspension Sus-Phrine	Inj 500 mg/mL.	SC 0.5–1.5 mg q 6–10 hr.	SC 0.005 mL/kg q 6–10 hr.	+++	+++	5	0.5–2 (SC)
Isoetharine Various	Inhal (soln)1%.	Inhal (soln) 2.5–10 mg diluted 1:3 in NS q 2–4 hr prn.	Inhal (soln) 0.1–0.2 mg/kg q 2–4 hr prn.	++	+++	1.7	0.5–2
Isoproterenol Isuprel Various	Inhal (soln) 0.25, 0.5, 1%; (metered-dose) 80, 131 μg/puff Inj 0.2 mg/mL SL Tab 10, 15 mg.	Not recommended because of short duration and lack of selectivity.	Not recommended because of short duration and lack of selectivit.	++++	++++	10	0.5–2

(continued)

723

SYMPATHOMIMETIC BRONCHODILATORS COMPARISON CHART (continued)

DRUG	DOSAGE FORMS	DOSAGE Adult	DOSAGE Pediatric[a]	RECEPTOR SELECTIVITY[b] β_1	RECEPTOR SELECTIVITY[b] β_2	RELATIVE β_2 POTENCY[c]	DURATION OF ACTION BY INHALATION (HR)[d]
Metapro-terenol Alupent Metaprel Various	Inhal (soln) 0.4% (unit dose 10 mg), 0.6% (unit dose 15 mg), 5%; (metered-dose) 0.65 mg/puff Syrup 2 mg/mL Tab 10, 20 mg.	Inhal (soln) 5–15 mg q 2–4 hr prn (q 1–2 hr under medical supervision); (metered-dose) 1–3 puffs q 4–6 hr prn and prior to exercise PO 20 mg 3–4 times/day.	Inhal (soln) 0.25–0.5 mg/kg up to 15 mg q 2–4 hr prn; (metered-dose) 1–2 puffs prn and prior to exercise PO 0.5 mg/kg q 4–6 hr, increase by 0.25 mg/kg as tolerated.	++	++	1	3–4
Pirbuterol Maxair	Inhal (metered-dose) 0.2 mg/puff.	Inhal 1–2 puffs q 4–6 hr and prior to exercise.	Inhal 1–2 puffs q 4–6 hr prn and prior to exercise.	+	++++	2.5	4–8
Salmeterol Serevent	Inhal (metered-dose) 21 μg/puff Inhal (dry pwdr) 50 mg/blister.	Inhal (metered-dose) 2 puffs q 12 hr[f] Inhal (dry pwdr) 1 blister q 12 hr.	(<12 yr) not established; (≥12 yr) same as adult dosage.	+	++++	20	12

(continued)

SYMPATHOMIMETIC BRONCHODILATORS COMPARISON CHART (continued)

DRUG	DOSAGE FORMS	DOSAGE Adult	DOSAGE Pediatric[a]	RECEPTOR SELECTIVITY[b] β_1	RECEPTOR SELECTIVITY[b] β_2	RELATIVE β_2 POTENCY[c]	DURATION OF ACTION BY INHALATION (HR)[d]
Terbutaline Brethaire Brethine Bricanyl	Inhal (metered-dose) 0.2 mg/puff Inj 1 mg/mL Tab 2.5, 5 mg.	Inhal 1–3 puffs q 4–6 hr prn; 5–7 mg undiluted by nebulizer q 4–6 hr prn[g] SC 0.25–0.5 mg q 2–6 hr prn PO 5 mg q 6–8 hr.	Inhal 1–2 puffs q 4–6 hr prn; 0.1–0.3 mg/kg q 4–6 hr prn (q 1–2 hr under medical supervision)[g] SC 0.01 mg/kg up to 0.25 mg q 2–6 hr prn PO 0.075 mg/kg q 6–8 hr.	+	++++	2.5	4–8

(continued)

SYMPATHOMIMETIC BRONCHODILATORS COMPARISON CHART (continued)

+ = Minimal effect; +++ = pronounced effect

[a] Isoproterenol and isoetharine are the only metered-dose aerosols labeled for use in children <12 yr.

[b] β_2-selectivity does not equate to bronchoselectivity; β_2-stimulation produces reflex tachycardia from vasodilation as well as stimulation of cardiac β_2-receptors.

[c] Molar potency relative to metaproterenol; large numbers indicate more potent compounds.

[d] Onset and duration data apply to aerosol therapy only. Duration of bronchodilation only applies to otherwise stable asthmatics and is not applicable to acute severe asthma or protection from severe provocation (eg, allergen, exercise, ozone). Duration may be shorter during acute exacerbation or with long-term therapy because of downregulation of β-receptors (tolerance). Oral tablets (especially SR tablets) and syrups are slower in onset, but may be slightly longer acting than aerosols.

[e] Bitolterol is a prodrug converted in the body to **colterol**, the active drug, which is more potent than isoproterenol; the relative potency value because of incomplete conversion.

[f] For prophylaxis only; acute attacks must be treated with a short-acting agent.

[g] Use injectable solution; not a labeled indication.

THEOPHYLLINE
Theo-Dur, Slo-bid, Various

Pharmacology. Theophylline directly relaxes smooth muscle of bronchial airways and pulmonary blood vessels to act as a bronchodilator and pulmonary vasodilator. It is also a diuretic, coronary vasodilator, cardiac stimulant, and cerebral stimulant; it improves diaphragmatic contractility; and it lessens diaphragmatic fatigue. The exact cellular mechanism of smooth muscle relaxation is unknown, but intracellular calcium sequestration, inhibition of specific phosphodiesterase isozymes, adenosine-receptor antagonism, and stimulation of endogenous catecholamine release have all been postulated to play a role.[19] **Aminophylline** is the ethylenediamine salt of theophylline.

Administration and Adult Dosage. **PO (theophylline) or IV (aminophylline) for acute asthma symptoms in the emergency department or in the hospital** no longer recommended because it appears to provide no additional benefit over optimal inhaled β_2-agonist therapy and may increase adverse effects; addition of IV theophylline to other therapies in hospitalized adults remains controversial.[20] The following dosages have been used: 5 mg/kg (6 mg/kg aminophylline), if patient has taken no theophylline in previous 24 hr. In emergencies, 2.5 mg/kg (3 mg/kg aminophylline) may be given if an immediate serum level cannot be obtained. Each 1 mg/kg (1.25 mg/kg aminophylline) results in about a 2 mg/L increase in serum theophylline. Infuse IV aminophylline no faster than 25 mg/min. **Maintenance dosage.** (*See* Theophylline Dosage Adjustment Chart.) **PO for chronic asthma (theophylline)** (*See* Theophylline Dosage Adjustment Chart.) Adjust dosage to achieve serum concentration of 5–15 mg/L.[21,22] **IM, PR Supp** not recommended.

Special Populations. All dosage recommendations are based on the average theophylline clearance for a given population group. There is a wide interpatient variability (often greater than 2-fold) within all patient groups. Therefore, it is essential that serum concentrations be monitored in all patients. If no doses have been missed or extra doses taken during the previous 48 hr, and if peak serum concentrations have been obtained (1–2 hr after liquid or plain uncoated tablet and 4–6 hr after most SR products), adjust dosage using Theophylline Dosage Adjustment Chart.

Pediatric Dosage. **PO or IV for acute symptoms** not recommended for children hospitalized for severe asthma. **PO for chronic asthma** (theophylline) (<1 yr) 0.2 × (age in weeks) + 5 = dosage in mg/kg/day;[20] **IM, PR Supp** not recommended.

Geriatric Dosage. Not established; however, the elderly as a group have slower hepatic clearance. Therefore, use lower initial doses and monitor closely for response and adverse reactions.

Other Conditions. Many factors can alter theophylline dosage requirements. (*See* Precautions and Factors Affecting Serum Theophylline Concentrations Chart.) Use IBW for dosage calculations in obese patients.

THEOPHYLLINE DOSAGE ADJUSTMENT CHART[a]

EVENT	DOSAGE	ACTION
Initial dosage	10 mg/kg/day to a maximum of 300 mg/day.	If initial dosage is tolerated, increase dosage no longer than 3 days to the first increment.
First increment	13 mg/kg/day to a maximum of 450 mg/day.	If the first incremental increase is tolerated, increase dosage no sooner than 3 days to the second increment.
Second increment	16 mg/kg/day to a maximum of 600 mg/day.	If the second incremental increase is tolerated, measure an estimate of the peak serum concentration after at least 3 days.

SERUM THEOPHYLLINE CONCENTRATION		
<10 mg/L	—	Increase dosage by about 25%.
10–15.9 mg/L	—	Maintain dosage if tolerated.
16–19.9 mg/L	—	Consider a 10% dosage reduction.
20–25 mg/L	—	Hold next dose, then resume first incremental dosage.
>25 mg/L	—	Hold next 2 doses, then resume initial dosage.

[a]For children >1 yr and adults with no risk factors for decreased clearance. These recommendations acknowledge interpatient variability in dosage requirements and are based on the principle of not exceeding two-thirds of mean dosage requirements initially and not reaching or exceeding mean dosage requirements without measurement of the serum theophylline concentration. The initial low dosage and spaced increases provide time for the tolerance to caffeine-like effects to occur.
From references 22 and 23.

Dosage Forms. (*See* Theophylline Products Comparison Chart.)

Patient Instructions. Do not chew or crush sustained-release tablets or capsules. Take at equally spaced intervals around the clock. Report any nausea, vomiting, gastrointestinal pain, headache, or restlessness. Contents of sustained-release bead-filled capsules may be mixed with a vehicle (applesauce or jam) and swallowed without chewing for patients who have difficulty swallowing capsules. Take Theo-24 and Uniphyl products at least 1 hour before meals to avoid too rapid absorption of the drug.

Missed Doses. Take missed dose as soon as possible. However, if it is almost time to take the next dose, skip the missed dose and go back to the regular dosage schedule. Do not double doses. Do not have your theophylline levels measured until you have missed no doses for 3 days.

Pharmacokinetics. *Onset and Duration.* IV onset within 15 min with loading dose.

Serum Levels. Well correlated with clinical effects: therapeutic is 10–15 mg/L (56–83 µmol/L); however, improvement in respiratory function can be observed with serum concentrations of 5 mg/L (28 μmol/L).[21,24] A serum concentration of 5–10 mg/L is often adequate for treatment of neonatal apnea. Toxicity increases over 20 mg/L. (*See* Adverse Reactions.)

Fate. Plain uncoated tablets and solution are well absorbed orally; enteric-coated tablets and some SR dosage forms may be unreliably absorbed. Food may affect the rate and extent of absorption of some SR formulations, but has minimal effects on rapid-release forms. Food may either increase the rate of absorption (Theo-24, Uniphyl), producing dose dumping, or impair absorption (Theo-Dur Sprinkle).[25] Rectal suppository absorption is slow and erratic and suppositories (including aminophylline) are not recommended under any circumstances. Rectal solutions may result in serum concentrations comparable to oral solution. About 60% is plasma protein bound (less in neonates); V_d is 0.5 ± 0.1 L/kg (greater in neonates). There may be marked intrapatient variability in clearance over time.[22] Cl is also affected by many factors. (*See* Precautions.) Smoking increases theophylline metabolism; this effect may last for 3 months–2 yr after cessation of smoking. Clearance progressively increases in infants during the first year of life. Dose-dependent pharmacokinetics in therapeutic range occur often in children and rarely in adults.[22] In the elderly, clearance declines with age to about 35 mL/hr/kg.[26] Extensively metabolized in the liver to several inactive metabolites; 10% excreted unchanged in the urine.

$t_{1/2}$. 8 ± 2 hr in adult nonsmokers, 4.4 ± 1 hr in adult smokers (1–2 packs per day); 3.7 ± 1.1 hr in children 1–9 yr. Newborn infants, older patients with COPD or cor pulmonale, and patients with CHF or liver disease may have a half-life >24 hr.

Adverse Reactions. Local GI irritation may occur. Reactions occur more frequently at serum concentrations >20 mg/L and include anorexia, nausea, vomiting, epigastric pain, diarrhea, restlessness, irritability, insomnia, and headache. Serious arrhythmias and convulsions (frequently leading to death or permanent brain damage) usually occur at levels >35 mg/L, but have occurred at lower concentrations and may *not* be preceded by less serious toxicity; cardiovascular reactions include sinus tachycardia and life-threatening ventricular arrhythmias with PVCs. Rapid IV administration may be associated with hypotension, syncope, cardiac arrest (particularly if administered directly into central line), and death.[27] IM administration is painful and offers no advantage.

Contraindications. Active peptic ulcer disease; untreated seizure disorder. (Aminophylline) hypersensitivity to ethylenediamine.

Precautions. Use with caution in severe cardiac disease, hypoxemia, hepatic disease, acute myocardial injury, cor pulmonale, CHF, fever, viral illness, underlying seizure disorder, migraine, hepatic cirrhosis, and neonates. Do not give with other xanthine preparations. The alcohol in some oral liquid preparations may cause side effects in infants.

Drug Interactions. Numerous drugs and conditions can alter theophylline clearance and serum levels. Factors that can decrease serum levels include carbamazepine, charcoal-broiled beef, high-protein/low-carbohydrate diet, isoproterenol (IV), phenytoin, rifampin, and smoking. Factors that can increase serum levels include allopurinol (>600 mg/day), cimetidine, ciprofloxacin, cor pulmonale, macrolides (eg, erythromycin, troleandomycin), oral contraceptives, and propranolol. (*See* Factors Affecting Serum Theophylline Concentrations Chart.)

Parameters to Monitor. (Inpatients) obtain serum theophylline concentrations before starting therapy (if patient previously taking theophylline) and 1, 6, and 24 hr after start of infusion; monitor daily during continuous infusion. (Outpatients) monitor serum concentrations q 6 months, 3–5 days after any dosage change, and whenever there are symptoms of toxicity.[21,22]

Notes. The oral theophylline preparations of choice for long-term use, to achieve both sustained therapeutic concentrations and improved compliance, are completely and slowly absorbed SR formulations that are minimally affected by food and pH.[25] (*See* Theophylline Products Comparison Chart.) Combination products containing **ephedrine** increase CNS toxicity and have no therapeutic advantage over adequate serum concentrations of theophylline alone. **Dyphylline** is chemically related to, but not a salt of, theophylline; the amount of dyphylline equivalent to theophylline is unknown. Because its potency is less than theophylline and it has a short half-life (2 hr), its dosage is greater than theophylline and it must be given more frequently.

FACTORS AFFECTING SERUM THEOPHYLLINE CONCENTRATIONS CHART[a]

FACTOR	DECREASES IN THEOPHYLLINE CONCENTRATIONS	INCREASES IN THEOPHYLLINE CONCENTRATIONS	ACTION
Age	↑ metabolism (1–9 yr)	↓ metabolism (<6 months, elderly)	Adjust dosage according to serum concentration.
Diet	↑ metabolism (high protein)	↓ metabolism (high carbohydrate)	Inform patient that major changes in diet are not recommended while taking theophylline.
Food	↓ or delays absorption of some SR preparations	↑ rate of absorption (fatty food)	Select theophylline product that is not affected by food.
Hypoxia, cor pulmonale, decompensated CHF, cirrhosis	—	↓ metabolism	Decrease dosage according to serum concentration.
Cimetidine	—	↓ metabolism	Use alternative H₂ blocker (eg, famotidine, nizatadine, ranitidine).
Macrolides: troleandomycin, erythromycin, clarithromycin	—	↓ metabolism	Use alternative antibiotic or decrease theophylline dosage.
Phenobarbital, phenytoin, carbamazepine	↑ metabolism	—	Increase dosage according to serum concentration.

(continued)

FACTORS AFFECTING SERUM THEOPHYLLINE CONCENTRATIONS CHART[a] (continued)

FACTOR	DECREASES IN THEOPHYLLINE CONCENTRATIONS	INCREASES IN THEOPHYLLINE CONCENTRATIONS	ACTION
Quinolones: ciprofloxacin, pefloxacin	—	↓ metabolism	Use alternative antibiotic or adjust theophylline dosage. Circumvent with ofloxacin if quinolone therapy is required.
Rifampin	↑ metabolism	—	Increase dosage according to serum concentration.
Smoking	↑ metabolism	—	Advise patient to stop smoking; increase dosage according to serum concentration.
Ticlopidine	—	↓ metabolism	Decrease dosage according to serum concentration.
Viral illness, systemic febrile (eg. influenza)	—	↓ metabolism	Decrease theophylline dosage according to serum concentration. Decrease dosage by 50% if serum concentration is not available.

[a]This chart is not all inclusive; for other factors, *see* Cytochrome P450 Interactions and product information. *From reference 20.*

THEOPHYLLINE PRODUCTS COMPARISON CHART[a]

PRODUCT	ANHYDROUS THEOPHYLLINE CONTENT	MEASURABLE DOSE INCREMENT[b] (MG)	COMMENTS
RAPIDLY ABSORBED			
Plain Uncoated Tablets			
Various	Tab 100 mg scored.	50	Serum level fluctuations are 459%/117%.[c]
	Tab 125 mg scored.	62.5	
	Tab 200 mg scored.	100	
	Tab 250 mg scored.	125	
	Tab 300 mg scored.	150	
Oral Liquids (Alcohol-Free)			
Aerolate	10 mg/mL.	5	Sugar free.
Slo-Phyllin 80 Syrup	5.3 mg/mL.	5	Sugar free.
Intravenous Solution			
Aminophylline[d]	20 mg/mL.	5	Use rubber-stoppered vials to avoid glass particles from the breaking of ampules.
Theophylline	0.4, 0.8, 1.6, 2, 3.2, 4 mg/mL.	—	Available in large volume solutions only.

(continued)

THEOPHYLLINE PRODUCTS COMPARISON CHART[a] (continued)

PRODUCT	ANHYDROUS THEOPHYLLINE CONTENT	MEASURABLE DOSE INCREMENT[b] (MG)	COMMENTS
SLOW-RELEASE PRODUCTS[e]			
Slo-bid Gyrocaps	Cap 50 mg. Cap 75 mg. Cap 100 mg. Cap 125 mg. Cap 200 mg. Cap 300 mg.	25	Excellent bioavailability in young infants; beads can be sprinkled on small amount of food; serum level fluctuations are 43%/18%.[c]
Theo-Dur	Tab 100 mg scored. Tab 200 mg scored. Tab 300 mg scored. Tab 450 mg scored.	25 100 150 225	Serum level fluctuations are 38%/16% for 200, 300, and 450 mg, and 87%/34% for 100 mg tablets;[c] some rapid metabolizers may require 8-hr dosage intervals to avoid breakthrough of symptoms.
Uni-Dur	Tab 400 mg scored. Tab 600 mg scored.	200 300	The extent of absorption of Uni-Dur does not appear to be affected by food; however, large serum level fluctuations (78% in adults) may render this agent unreliable for once-daily administration.[28,29]

[a] Only products with documented bioavailability that are minimally affected by food and with dosage forms that permit incremental changes in dose are listed.

[b] Accuracy of measurement decreases below 0.5 mL with suspensions and syrups, because of viscosity; smaller amounts cannot be accurately measured; measure all liquid dosage forms with a syringe.

[c] Predicted child/adult fluctuation between peak and trough (%) for 12-hr dosage interval; average child $t_{1/2}$ = 3.7 hr, average child $t_{1/2}$ = 8.2 hr.[25]

[d] The ethylenediamine portion of aminophylline may cause urticaria or exfoliative dermatitis rarely.

[e] Only Slo-bid Gyrocaps and Theo-Dur tablets have sufficiently slow and complete absorption to allow bid dosage intervals with minimal serum concentration fluctuations in most patients. Many products advertised for bid dosage do not maintain serum concentrations within the therapeutic range in many patients, especially children.[25] Some once-daily dosage products (eg, Uniphyl) are affected by food and may be unreliable.[21,22]

ZILEUTON   Zyflo

Pharmacology. Zileuton is an inhibitor of leukotriene synthesis. It has anti-inflammatory activity and inhibits the antigen-induced contraction of the trachea and bronchospasm that occurs in asthma.

Adult Dosage. **PO for asthma prophylaxis** 600 mg qid; dosage reduction may be necessary in hepatic dysfunction.

Pediatric Dosage. **PO** (<12 yr) safety and efficacy not established; (≥12 yr) same as adult dosage.

Dosage Forms. **Tab** 600 mg.

Pharmacokinetics. Zileuton is orally absorbed; food has no important effect on absorption. It is 93% plasma protein bound; V_d is about 1.2 L/kg. It is metabolized by CYP1A2, 2C9, and 3A4 and has a half-life of 2.5 hr.

Adverse Reactions. It is generally well tolerated, with headache reported in about 10% of patients in clinical trials. GI effects such as nausea and dyspepsia occur occasionally. Hepatic enzyme abnormalities have been reported. It is contraindicated in patients with active hepatic disease. Low WBC counts occur at a rate greater than placebo-treated patients.

Drug Interactions. Zileuton markedly increases the effects of propranolol, theophylline, and warfarin.

Antihistamines

Class Instructions: Antihistamines. This drug (with the exceptions of astemizole, fexofenadine, and loratadine) may cause drowsiness, dry mouth, or occasional dizziness. Until the extent of drowsiness is known, use caution when driving, operating machinery, or performing other tasks requiring mental alertness or motor coordination. Avoid excessive concurrent use of alcohol and other CNS depressants that cause drowsiness. This drug effectively suppresses seasonal allergic rhinitis only when taken continuously.

Missed Doses. Missed doses should be taken as soon as possible. However, if it is almost time for the next dose, skip the missed dose and go back to the regular dosing schedule. Do not double doses.

CETIRIZINE   Zyrtec

Pharmacology. Cetirizine is a low-sedating, long-acting H_1-receptor antagonist that is a metabolite of hydroxyzine. Cetirizine competitively inhibits the interaction of histamine with H_1 receptors, thereby preventing the allergic response.

Administration and Adult Dosage. **PO for allergic rhinitis or urticaria** 5–10 mg/day depending on symptom severity.

Special Populations. *Pediatric Dosage.* **PO for allergic rhinitis or urticaria** (2–6 yr) 5 mg/day; (>6 yr) same as adult dosage.

Geriatric Dosage. **PO** Same as adult dosage. Reducing dosage in geriatric patients may be necessary because of a 50% increase in cetirizine's half-life and a 40% decrease in clearance.

Other Conditions. In patients with Cl_{cr} of 11–31 mL/min, those on hemodialysis, and in hepatically impaired patients, give 5 mg/day.

Dosage Forms. **Tab** 5, 10 mg; **Syrup** 1 mg/mL.

Patient Instructions. (*See* Class Instructions: Antihistamines.)

Pharmacokinetics. *Onset and Duration.* Onset is within 1 hr; duration is ≥24 hr.

Fate. Cetirizine is rapidly absorbed after oral administration. Peak serum levels are reached within 1 hr. Food does not affect the amount absorbed, but may decrease the absorption rate. Protein binding averages 93%. Cl in normal adults is 0.04–0.05 L/kg/hr. Cetirizine is oxidized to a small extent to inactive metabolites. After a 10 mg dose, 70% of the drug is excreted unchanged in the urine within 72 hr and 10% is excreted in feces. Cetirizine is not appreciably dialyzable.[30–34]

$t_{1/2}$. (Adults) 7–10 hr; (children) 6–7 hr; (elderly/renal insufficiency) 18–21 hr.[30–34]

Adverse Reactions. The most frequent side effects are sedation, headache, dry mouth, fatigue and nausea. Cetirizine 10 mg/day produces more sedation than loratadine 10 mg/day or placebo. Cetirizine has not been implicated in cardiac adverse events. Higher-than-recommended doses of cetirizine (up to 60 mg daily) did not prolong the QT interval in 25 healthy volunteers.

Contraindications. Hypersensitivity to hydroxyzine or cetirizine.

Precautions. Sedative effects may be dose dependent.

Drug Interactions. Exercise caution when cetirizine is combined with anticholinergic agents, alcohol, or other CNS depressants. Since most of cetirizine is eliminated renally, cytochrome P450 interactions are not likely. Clinically important drug interactions have not been found with cetirizine and azithromycin, pseudoephedrine, ketoconazole, or erythromycin. Clearance of cetirizine was reduced slightly by a 400 mg dose of theophylline, but this reduction was not clinically important; however, larger doses may have a greater effect. Therefore, it seems appropriate to monitor patients for increased sedation or other CNS-related side effects when administering theophylline concomitantly with cetirizine.

Parameters to Monitor. (Allergic rhinitis) observe for sneezing, rhinorrhea, itchy nose, and conjunctivitis. Monitor for side effects such as sedation.

Notes. Cetirizine and **loratadine** have the advantages of noncardiotoxicity, once-daily dosing, and commercial availability of liquid dosage forms. (*See* Antihistamines Comparison Chart.)

CHLORPHENIRAMINE MALEATE   Chlor-Trimeton, Various

Pharmacology. Chlorpheniramine is a competitive antagonist of histamine at the H_1-histamine receptor. It also has anticholinergic and transient sedative effects when used intermittently.

Administration and Adult Dosage. **PO for seasonal allergic rhinitis** (effectiveness is maximized if given continuously, starting just prior to the pollen season) 4 mg hs initially, increasing gradually over 10 days as tolerated to 24 mg/day in 1–2 divided doses until the end of the season. **PO for acute allergic reactions** 12 mg in 1–2 divided doses. **SC, IM, or IV for uncomplicated allergic reactions** 5–20 mg. **IV as adjunctive treatment in anaphylaxis** 10–20 mg. **SC, IM, or IV for allergic reactions to blood or plasma** 10–20 mg, to a maximum of 40 mg/day. **SR** (*See* Notes.)

Special Populations. *Pediatric Dosage.* **PO for seasonal allergic rhinitis** (2–6 yr) 1 mg q 4–6 hr up to 4 mg/day; (6–12 yr) 2 mg hs initially, increasing gradually over 10 days as tolerated to 12 mg/day in 1–2 divided doses until the end of the season.[35] **SR** not recommended. (*See* Notes.)

Geriatric Dosage. **PO** (≥60 yr) 4 mg daily–bid. Duration of action may be 36 hr or more, even when serum concentrations are low.[36]

Dosage Forms. **Cap** 12 mg; **Chew Tab** 2 mg; **Tab** 4, 8, 12 mg; **Syrup** 0.4 mg/mL; **SR Cap** 8, 12 mg (*see* Notes); **SR Tab** 8, 12 mg (*see* Notes); **Inj** 10 mg/mL (IM, IV, SC); 100 mg/mL (IM, SC only); **Tab** 4 mg with pseudoephedrine HCl 60 mg (Sudafed Plus, Isoclor, various); 4 mg with phenylpropanolamine HCl 25 mg (Allergy Relief Medicine, various); **Syrup** 0.4 mg/mL with phenylpropanolamine HCl 2.5 mg/mL (Triaminic, various).

Patient Instructions. (*See* Class Instructions: Antihistamines.)

Pharmacokinetics. *Onset and Duration.* Onset is in 0.5–1 hr; duration of suppression of wheal and flare response (IgE mediated) to skin tests with allergenic extract is 2 days.[37] Fast metabolizers have an earlier, greater, and more prolonged antihistaminic response than slow metabolizers because of rapid conversion to active metabolite.[38]

Serum Levels. Serum chlorpheniramine levels do not correlate with histamine antagonist activity because of an unidentified active metabolite.[38] (Children) 2.3–12 μg/L (6–31 nmol/L) suppress allergic rhinitis symptoms; (children) 4–10 μg/L (11–26 nmol/L) suppress histamine-induced wheal and flare.[35]

Fate. Oral bioavailability is about 34%; 72% is plasma protein bound.[36] V_d is (adults) 3.2 ± 0.3 L/kg; (children) 7 ± 2.8 L/kg; Cl is (adults) 0.1 ± 0.006 L/hr/kg; (children) 0.43 ± 0.19 L/hr/kg.[35,39] Rapidly and extensively metabolized by CYP2D6 to mono- and didesmethylchlorpheniramine and unidentified metabolites, one or more of which are active. Metabolites and a small amount of parent drug are excreted in urine.[38,40]

$t_{1/2}$. (Adults) 20 ± 5 hr; (children) 13 ± 6 hr; (chronic renal failure) 280–330 hr.[35,39,40]

Adverse Reactions. Frequent drowsiness, dry mouth, dizziness, and irritability occur with intermittent therapy; however, most patients develop tolerance to these side effects during continuous therapy, particularly if dosage is increased slowly.

Contraindications. Lactation; premature and newborn infants.

Precautions. Use chlorpheniramine with caution in patients ≥60 yr. It may cause paradoxical CNS stimulation in children. OTC labeling states to avoid in patients with narrow-angle glaucoma, symptomatic prostatic hypertrophy, asthma, emphysema, chronic pulmonary disease, shortness of breath, or breathing difficulties except under physician supervision; however, many studies have shown some bronchodilator effect of H_1-receptor antagonists.[37]

Drug Interactions. MAOIs prolong and intensify the anticholinergic effects of antihistamines.[41] Alcohol or sedative-hypnotics may increase CNS depressant effects.

Parameters to Monitor. In seasonal allergic rhinitis, observe for sneezing, rhinorrhea, itchy nose, and conjunctivitis.

Notes. Not effective for nasal stuffiness. SR formulations offer no advantage over syrup or plain, uncoated tablets, because the drug has an inherently long duration of action. (*See* Antihistamines Comparison Chart.)

DIPHENHYDRAMINE HYDROCHLORIDE   Benadryl, Various

Pharmacology. (*See* Chlorpheniramine.)

Administration and Adult Dosage. **PO as an antihistamine or for parkinsonism** 25–50 mg tid–qid. **PO for motion sickness** 50 mg 30 min before exposure, then ac and hs. **PO as a nighttime sleep aid** 25–50 mg hs. **PO as an antitussive** 25 mg q 4–6 hr. **Deep IM or IV as an antihistamine, or for allergic reactions to blood or plasma, motion sickness, adjunctive treatment of anaphylaxis, or parkinsonism** 10–50 mg/dose, 100 mg if required, to a maximum of 400 mg/day.

Special Populations. *Pediatric Dosage.* **PO as an antihistamine** 5 mg/kg/day, or (≤9 kg) 6.25–12.5 mg tid–qid; (>9 kg) 12.5–25 mg tid–qid, to a maximum of 300 mg/day. **PO as an antitussive** (2–6 yr) 6.25 mg q 4 hr, to a maximum of 25 mg/day; (6–12 yr) 12.5 mg q 4 hr, to a maximum of 75 mg/day. **Deep IM or IV** 5 mg/kg/day in 4 divided doses, to a maximum of 300 mg/day.

Geriatric Dosage. **PO as an antihistamine** 25 mg bid–tid initially, then increase as needed.[42] (*See* Notes.)

Other Conditions. In renal impairment, increase dosage interval as follows: Cl_{cr} of 10–50 mL/min, increase to 6–12 hr; Cl_{cr} <10 mL/min, increase to 12–18 hr.[42]

Dosage Forms. **Cap** 25, 50 mg; **Chew Tab** 12.5 mg; **Elxr** 2.5 mg/mL; **Syrup** 2.5 mg/mL; **Tab** 25, 50 mg; **Inj** 50 mg/mL.

Patient Instructions. (*See* Class Instructions: Antihistamines.)

Pharmacokinetics. *Onset and Duration.* Onset is 15 min after single oral dose; duration of suppression of wheal and flare is up to 2 days.[37,43] Duration of effect does not appear to be related to serum levels.

Serum Levels. (Antihistaminic effect) >25 μg/L (0.09 μmol/L); (sedation) 30–50 μg/L (0.1–0.17 μmol/L); (mental impairment) >60 μg/L (0.2 μmol/L).[39,43]

Fate. As a result of first-pass metabolism, oral bioavailability is variable, 61 ± 25%.[39,44] A single 50 mg oral dose in adults usually produces serum concentrations between 25 and 50 μg/L.[43] About 85% is plasma protein bound, lower in Asians and in cirrhosis.[45,46] V_d is 17.4 ± 4.8 L/kg in adults, larger in Asians and in those with cirrhosis. Cl is 1.4 ± 0.6 L/hr/kg in adults, higher in Asians, and

0.7 ± 0.2 L/hr/kg in the elderly.[39,42,44,45] Metabolized to N-dealkylated and acidic metabolites.[44,47] Less than 4% is excreted unchanged in urine.[48]

t½. (Adults) 9.2 ± 2.5 hr; (elderly >65 yr) 13.5 ± 4.2 hr; (children 8–12 yr) 5.4 ± 1.8 hr;[39,44] (cirrhosis) 15 hr.[46]

Adverse Reactions. (*See* Chlorpheniramine.)

Contraindications. (*See* Chlorpheniramine.)

Precautions. (*See* Chlorpheniramine.)

Drug Interactions. (*See* Chlorpheniramine.)

Parameters to Monitor. (*See* Chlorpheniramine.)

Notes. Because of its low degree of efficacy for pruritus, weak suppression of IgE-mediated skin tests, and high sedative potential, diphenhydramine is not the antihistamine of choice for most conditions. In the elderly, diphenhydramine is discouraged as a nighttime sleep aid because of its high anticholinergic potential. **Dimenhydrinate** (Dramamine), used for motion sickness, is the 8-chlorotheophyllinate salt of diphenhydramine; 100 mg dimenhydrinate is about equal to 50 mg diphenhydramine.

FEXOFENADINE   Allegra

Pharmacology. Fexofenadine is a histamine H_1-receptor antagonist that is a metabolite of terfenadine. It causes little sedation and has little anticholinergic activity. (*See* Antihistamines Comparison Chart.)

Adult Dosage. PO for allergic rhinitis 60 mg bid. In renal impairment, reduce dosage to 60 mg/day.

Pediatric Dosage. PO (<12 yr) safety and efficacy not established; (≥12 yr) same as adult dosage.

Dosage Forms. Cap 60 mg; **Cap** 60 mg with pseudoephedrine 120 mg (Allegra D).

Pharmacokinetics. *Onset and Duration.* Onset is rapid; peak serum levels occur at 2.6 hr. Food decreases oral absorption. It is 60–70% plasma protein bound and excreted unchanged in urine and feces. Half-life is about 14 hr in normal renal function and increases to about 19 hr in severe renal impairment.

Adverse Reactions. Drowsiness or fatigue occur in <2% of patients; GI effects occur in about 1.5% and headache in >1%. Pharyngitis and menstrual disturbances have also been reported.

HYDROXYZINE HYDROCHLORIDE   Atarax, Vistaril, Various
HYDROXYZINE PAMOATE   Vistaril, Various

Pharmacology. Hydroxyzine is a competitive antagonist of histamine at the H_1-histamine receptor. It also has antiemetic and sedative effects, thought to be a result of CNS subcortical suppression. Claims of long-term antianxiety properties have not been substantiated by well-designed studies.

Administration and Adult Dosage. **PO for pruritus** 25 mg tid–qid. **PO for seasonal allergic rhinitis** (effectiveness is maximized if given continuously just prior to the pollen season) 25 mg initially q hs until no sedation in morning, then increase dosage q 2–3 days, to a maximum of 150 mg/day in 1–2 divided doses and maintain until end of season. Reduce dosage by one-third or more if sedation persists. Dosage may be increased, if tolerated, for symptoms during peak of pollen season.[49] **IM for sedation before and after general anesthesia** 50–100 mg. **IM for nausea and vomiting, and pre- and postoperative adjunctive medication** 25–100 mg. Preferred IM injection site is upper outer quadrant of gluteus maximus or midlateral thigh. **Not for SC or intra-arterial use.**

Special Populations. *Pediatric Dosage.* **PO for pruritus** (<6 yr) 50 mg/day in 2–3 divided doses; (≥6 yr) 50–100 mg/day in divided doses. **PO for seasonal allergic rhinitis** 10 mg initially q hs until no sedation in morning, then increase dosage q 2–3 days, to a maximum of 75 mg/day in 1–2 divided doses and maintain until end of season. Reduce dosage by one-third or more if sedation persists. Dosage may be increased, if tolerated, for symptoms during peak of pollen season.[49] **IM for pre- and postoperative sedation** 0.7 mg/kg. **IM for nausea and vomiting and pre- and postoperative adjunctive medication** 1.1 mg/kg. Preferred site in children is midlateral muscles of thigh.

Geriatric Dosage. **PO for pruritus** 10 mg tid–qid, increasing to 25 mg tid–qid if necessary.[51]

Dosage Forms. **Cap** (as pamoate equivalent of HCl salt) 25, 50, 100 mg; **Susp** (as pamoate equivalent of HCl salt) 5 mg/mL; **Syrup** (as HCl) 2 mg/mL; **Tab** (as HCl) 10, 25, 50, 100 mg; **Inj** (as HCl) 25, 50 mg/mL (IM only).

Patient Instructions. (*See* Class Instructions: Antihistamines.)

Pharmacokinetics. *Onset and Duration.* Onset 15–30 min after oral administration. Duration of suppression of wheal and flare response to allergenic extract skin test is 4 days.[37,50]

Serum Levels. (Pruritus) 6–42 μg/L (14–102 nmol/L) suppress pruritus in children.[52]

Fate. Peak serum level of 73 ± 11 μg/L occurs 2 ± 0.4 hr after a 0.7 mg/kg dose in healthy adults, 117 ± 61 μg/L at 2.3 ± 0.7 hr in primary biliary cirrhosis (mean dose 44 mg).[53,54] V_d is (healthy adults) 16 ± 3 L/kg,[53] (elderly) 23 ± 6 L/kg, (children) 19 ± 9 L/kg,[52] and (primary biliary cirrhosis) 23 ± 13 L/kg.[54] Cl is (healthy young and elderly adults) 0.6 ± 0.2 L/hr/kg,[51,53] (children) 1.9 L/hr/kg,[52] (primary biliary cirrhosis) 0.5 ± 0.4 L/hr/kg.[54]

$t_{½}$. (Healthy adults) 20 ± 4 hr;[53] (elderly) 29 ± 10 hr;[51] (children) 7 hr, increasing with age;[53] (primary biliary cirrhosis) 37 ± 13 hr.[54]

Adverse Reactions. Transient drowsiness and dry mouth occur frequently when the drug is taken intermittently. Most patients develop tolerance to these effects when the drug is taken continuously, particularly if the dosage is slowly increased over 7–10 days. IM injection may be painful and has caused sterile abscess. Hemolysis has been associated with IV administration and tissue necrosis with SC or intra-arterial administration.

Contraindications. Early pregnancy; SC or intra-arterial use of injectable solution.

Precautions. Use with caution in the elderly.

Drug Interactions. MAO inhibitors prolong and intensify the anticholinergic effects of antihistamines. Alcohol or sedative-hypnotics may increase CNS depressant effects.

Parameters to Monitor. In seasonal allergic rhinitis, observe for sneezing, rhinorrhea, itchy nose, and conjunctivitis.

Notes. Hydroxyzine suppresses wheal and flare response to the greatest degree and for the longest duration of all antihistamines,[37] including the newer nonsedating antihistamines.[50]

LORATADINE   Claritin

Pharmacology. Loratadine is a long-acting piperadine antihistamine that is structurally similar to azatadine, with little or no action at α-adrenergic or cholinergic receptors.[55] (*See* Antihistamines Comparison Chart.)

Adult Dosage. PO for allergic rhinitis or urticaria 10 mg/day on an empty stomach. In patients with hepatic impairment, begin with 10 mg every other day. The dosage of Claritin-D is 1 tablet bid on an empty stomach; Claritin-D 24-hr is given once daily.

Pediatric Dosage. PO (<2 yr) safety and efficacy not established; (2–6 yr) 5 mg/day; (>6 yr) same as adult dosage.

Dosage Forms. Tab 10 mg (conventional and rapidly dissolving); **Syrup** 1 mg/mL; **Tab** 5 mg with pseudoephedrine 120 mg (Claritin-D); **Tab** 10 mg with pseudoephedrine 240 mg (Claritin-D 24-hr).

Pharmacokinetics. The drug is rapidly absorbed; bioavailability and peak serum levels are increased by about 50% in the elderly (66–78 yr) or when taken with food. It is 97% bound to plasma proteins and extensively metabolized to an active metabolite, descarboethoxyloratadine. Approximately 80% of a dose is excreted equally in urine and feces as metabolites after 10 days. The half-life in healthy adults is 8.4 hr (range 3–20) for loratadine and 28 hr (range 8.8–92) for descarboethoxyloratadine.[55,56]

Adverse Reactions. Headache and mild, dose-related drowsiness or fatigue occur occasionally.

ANTIHISTAMINES COMPARISON CHART

DRUG	DOSAGE FORMS	ADULT DOSAGE	PEDIATRIC DOSAGE	HALF-LIFE (HR)	SIDE EFFECTS Sedation[a]	SIDE EFFECTS Anticholinergic
Acrivastine	Tab 8 mg with pseudoephedrine 60 mg (Semprex-D).	PO 1 tab q 4–6 hr, to a maximum of 4/day.	PO (>12 yr) same as adult dosage.	1.5–3	+	±
Astemizole Hismanal	Tab 10 mg.	PO 10 mg/day during allergy season—not for "prn" use.	PO (<6 yr) 0.2 mg/kg/day; (6–12 yr) 5 mg/day.	48+ (metabolites: 4–8 weeks)	±	±
Azatadine Maleate Optimine	Tab 1 mg.	PO 1–2 mg bid.	(<12 yr) safety and efficacy not established.	12	++	++
Azelastine HCl Astelin	Nasal spray 125 µg/spray.	2 sprays/nostril bid.	(≥12 yr) same as adult dosage.	22 (metabolite: 54)	++	++
Brompheniramine Maleate Dimetane Various	Cap 4 mg Inj 10 mg/mL.	PO 4 mg q 4–6 hr, to a maximum of 24 mg/day SC, IM, or slow IV 5–20 mg q 12 hr, to a maximum of 40 mg/day.	PO (<12 yr) 0.5 mg/kg/day in 3–4 doses SC, IM, or slow IV 0.5 mg/kg/day in 3–4 divided doses.	25	+	++

(continued)

742

ANTIHISTAMINES COMPARISON CHART (continued)

DRUG	DOSAGE FORMS	ADULT DOSAGE	PEDIATRIC DOSAGE	HALF-LIFE (HR)	SIDE EFFECTS Sedation[a]	SIDE EFFECTS Anticholinergic
Carbinoxamine Maleate	Drp 2 mg with pseudoephedrine 25 mg/mL Syrup 0.8 mg with pseudoephedrine 12 mg/mL Tab 4 mg with pseudoephedrine 60 mg (Carbodec, Rondec).	PO 1 tab qid.	PO 0.2–0.4 mg/kg/day; (1–3 yr) 2 mg tid–qid; (3–6 yr) 2–4 mg tid–qid; (>6 yr) 4–6 mg tid–qid (dosage refers to carbinoxamine component).	10–20	++	+++
Cetirizine HCl Zyrtec	Tab 5, 10 mg Syrup 1 mg/mL.	PO 5–10 mg/day.	PO (2–6 yr) 5 mg/day; (6–11 yr) 5–10 mg/day.	7–10	+	±
Chlorpheniramine Maleate Chlor-Trimeton Various	Cap 12 mg Syrup 0.4 mg/mL Chew Tab 2 mg Tab 4 mg SR Tab 8, 12 mg Inj 10, 100 mg/mL.	PO (acute allergic reactions) 12 mg/day in 1–2 divided doses; PO (seasonal allergic rhinitis) 24 mg/day in 1–2 divided doses; IV (acute allergic reactions) 5–40 mg.	PO (seasonal allergic rhinitis) (2–6 yr) 1 mg tid up to 4 mg/day, SR not recommended; (6–12 yr) 2 mg tid up to 12 mg/day; SR not recommended.	15–25	+	++

(continued)

743

ANTIHISTAMINES COMPARISON CHART (continued)

DRUG	DOSAGE FORMS	ADULT DOSAGE	PEDIATRIC DOSAGE	HALF-LIFE (HR)	SIDE EFFECTS	
					Sedation[a]	Anticholinergic
Clemastine Fumarate Tavist Various	Syrup 0.13 mg (equivalent to 0.1 mg clemastine/mL Tab 1.34, 2.68 mg (equivalent to 1 and 2 mg clemastine, respectively).	PO 1.34 mg bid–2.68 mg tid, to a maximum of 8.04 mg/day.	PO (6–12 yr) 0.67–1.34 mg bid, to a maximum of 4.02 mg/day.	21	++	+++
Cyproheptadine HCl Periactin Various	Tab 4 mg Syrup 0.4 mg/mL.	PO 4–20 mg/day, usually 4 mg tid–qid, to a maximum of 0.5 mg/kg/day.	PO (2–6 yr) 2 mg bid–tid, to a maximum of 12 mg/day; (7–14 yr) 4 mg bid–tid, to a maximum of 16 mg/day.	—	+	++
Dexchlorphenir-amine Maleate Polaramine Various	Syrup 0.4 mg/mL. Tab 2 mg SR Tab 4, 6 mg.	PO 2 mg q 4–6 hr, to a maximum of 12 mg/day or SR 4–6 mg hs or q 8–10 hr during the day.	PO (2–5 yr) 0.5 mg q 4–6 hr, to a maximum of 3 mg/day, SR not recommended; (6–12 yr) 1 mg q 4–6 hr or SR 4 mg hs.	15–25	+	++

(continued)

ANTIHISTAMINES COMPARISON CHART (continued)

DRUG	DOSAGE FORMS	ADULT DOSAGE	PEDIATRIC DOSAGE	HALF-LIFE (HR)	Sedation[a]	Anticholinergic
Diphenhydramine HCl Benadryl Various	Cap 25, 50 mg Chew Tab 12.5 mg Elxr 2.5 mg/mL Syrup 1.25, 2.5 mg/mL Tab 25, 50 mg Inj 50 mg/mL.	PO (antihistamine) 25–50 mg tid–qid PO (motion sickness) 50 mg 30 min before exposure, ac and hs PO (antitussive) 25 mg q 4–6 hr PO (nighttime sleep aid) 25–50 mg hs IM, IV 10–50 mg, to a maximum of 400 mg/day.	PO (>9 kg) 5 mg/kg/day, usually 12.5–25 mg tid–qid, to a maximum of 300 mg/day PO (antitussive) (6–12 yr) 12.5 mg q 4 hr, to a maximum of 75 mg/day IM, IV 5 mg/kg, to a maximum of 300 mg/day.	9	+++	+++
Ebastine Kestine (Investigational— RPR)	—	PO 10–20 mg/day.	—	15 (metabolite)	±	±
Fexofenadine HCl Allegra	Cap 60 mg.	PO 60 mg bid.	PO (>12 yr) same as adult dosage.	14	±	±

(continued)

ANTIHISTAMINES COMPARISON CHART (continued)

DRUG	DOSAGE FORMS	ADULT DOSAGE	PEDIATRIC DOSAGE	HALF-LIFE (HR)	SIDE EFFECTS Sedation[a]	SIDE EFFECTS Anticholinergic
Hydroxyzine HCl/ Pamoate Atarax Vistaril Various	Cap (as pamoate equivalent of HCl salt) 25, 50, 100 mg Susp (as pamoate equivalent of HCl salt) 5 mg/mL Syrup (as HCl) 2 mg/mL Tab (as HCl) 10, 25, 50, 100 mg Inj (as HCl) 25, 50 mg/mL.	PO (pruritus) 25 mg tid-qid; (seasonal allergic rhinitis) titrate up to 150 mg/ day in 1–2 divided doses IM 25–100 mg.	PO (pruritus) (<6 yr) 50 mg/day in 2–3 divided doses; (≥6 yr) 50–100 mg/day in divided doses; (seasonal allergic rhinitis) 25–75 mg/day in 1–2 divided doses IM (perioperative sedation) 0.7 mg/kg/dose; (nausea, vomiting, perioperative adjunctive medication) 1 mg/kg.	16–24	++	++
Levocabastine HCl Livostin	Ophth Susp 0.05% Nasal Spray (Investigational)	Ophth 1 drop qid.	(>12 yr) same as adult dosage.	35–40	+	+
Loratadine Claritin	Tab 10 mg Syrup 1 mg/mL.	PO 10 mg/day.	PO (2–6 yr) 5 mg/day; (>6 yr) 10 mg/day.	8 (metabolite: 28)	±	±
Phenindamine Tartrate Nolahist	Tab 25 mg.	PO 25 mg q 4–6 hr, to a maximum of 150 mg/day.	PO (6–11 yr) 12.5 mg q 4–6 hr, to a maximum of 75 mg/day.	—	+	++

(continued)

				HALF-LIFE	SIDE EFFECTS	
					Sedation[a]	Anticholinergic
DRUG	DOSAGE FORMS	ADULT DOSAGE	PEDIATRIC DOSAGE	(HR)		
Promethazine HCl Phenergan Various	Syrup 1.25, 5 mg/mL Tab 12.5, 25, 50 mg Inj 25, 50 mg/mL Supp 12.5, 25, 50 mg.	PO (allergy) 25 mg hs or 12.5 mg ac and hs; (nausea and vomiting) 25 mg initial dose, then 12.5–25 mg q 4–6 hr prn; (adjunctive preoperative use) 25–50 mg/dose IM, IV (IV maximum concentration 25 mg/mL, maximum rate 25 mg/min) or PR (allergy) 25 mg, may repeat in 2 hr; (nausea and vomiting) 12.5–25 mg q 4 hr prn; (ad- junctive pre- and postoperative use) 25–50 mg/dose.	PO (allergy) 6.25–12.5 mg qid; (motion sickness or sedation) 12.5–25 mg/bid; IM, IV, or PR (PR not recommended <2 yr); (allergy) 0.5 mg/kg/day in 4 divided doses; (adjunctive preoperative use) 1 mg/kg/dose, maximum dosage not to exceed one-half of adult dosage.	12	++++	++++

(continued)

ANTIHISTAMINES COMPARISON CHART (continued)

DRUG	DOSAGE FORMS	ADULT DOSAGE	PEDIATRIC DOSAGE	HALF-LIFE (HR)	SIDE EFFECTS	
					Sedation[a]	Anticholinergic
Tripelennamine HCl PBZ Various	Tab 25, 50 mg. SR Tab 100 mg.	PO 25–50 mg q 4–6 hr, to a maximum of 600 mg/day.	PO 5 mg/kg/day in 4–6 divided doses, to a maximum of 300 mg/day; SR not recommended.	2–4	++	±
Triprolidine HCl	Syrup 0.25 mg with pseudoephedrine 6 mg/mL Tab 2.5 mg with pseudoephedrine 60 mg (Actifed).	PO 2.5 mg q 4–6 hr, to a maximum of 10 mg/day.	PO (4 months–2 yr) 0.3 mg tid–qid; (2–5 yr) 0.625 mg tid–qid; (6–12 yr) 1.25 mg q 4–6 hr, to a maximum of 4 doses/day.	3	++	++

++++ = Very high; +++ = high; ++ = moderate; + = low; ± = low to none; — = not known

[a]Tolerance usually develops during long-term therapy.
From references 55, 56–60, and product information.

Corticosteroids

BECLOMETHASONE DIPROPIONATE   Beconase, Beclovent, Vancenase, Vanceril

Pharmacology. Potent topical glucocorticoid with little systemic activity because of low systemic bioavailability.

Administration and Adult Dosage. Inhal for asthma 84 µg tid–qid, or 168 µg bid, to a maximum of 840 µg/day. (*See* Notes.) **Intranasal for nasal congestion** 42–84 µg/nostril bid–qid (168–336 µg/day total dosage) for several days, then decrease dosage (if symptoms do not recur) to minimum amount necessary to control stuffiness.

Special Populations. *Pediatric Dosage.* Titrate dosage to the lowest effective dosage. **Inhal for asthma** (6–12 yr) 42–84 µg (1–2 puffs) tid–qid or 168 µg bid, to a maximum of 420 µg/day; (>12 yr) same as adult dosage. **Intranasal for nasal congestion** (<6 yr) not recommended; (6–12 yr) 42 µg/nostril bid or tid.[61]

Geriatric Dosage. Same as adult dosage.

Other Conditions. During a severe asthma attack, patients require supplementary treatment with systemic steroids.

Dosage Forms. Inhal (Beclovent, Vanceril) 42, 84 µg/inhalation (200 doses/inhaler); **Nasal Inhal** (Beconase, Vancenase) 42, 84 µg/spray (200 doses/inhaler); (Beconase AQ, Vancenase AQ); **Aq Susp** 42, 84 µg/spray (200 doses/bottle).

Patient Instructions. Metered-dose oral inhaler. Shake thoroughly; hold mouthpiece approximately two finger-spaces outside mouth with teeth and tongue out of the way. Tilt head back, actuate inhaler during slow deep breath, and hold breath for 5–10 seconds. Allow at least 1 minute between inhalations. Use any inhaled sympathomimetic bronchodilator (if prescribed) a few minutes prior to this drug to prevent bronchospasm and to enhance penetration of the corticosteroid into the bronchial tree. The use of "spacers" with corticosteroid inhalers decreases the frequency of local side effects, hoarseness, and oropharyngeal candidiasis. Rinsing your mouth and gargling with water or mouthwash following administration may also be beneficial. This medication is for preventive therapy and should not be used to treat acute asthma attacks. **Nasal Inhaler.** Blow your nose before use. Shake container well. Remove protective cap and hold inhaler between thumb and forefinger. Tilt head back slightly and insert the end of the inhaler into one nostril. While holding the other nostril closed with one finger, press down once to release 1 dose, and at the same time, inhale gently. Hold breath for a few seconds, then breathe out slowly through your mouth. Repeat the process in the other nostril. Avoid blowing your nose for the next 15 minutes.

Missed Doses. Take missed dose as soon as possible. If it is almost time for the next dose, skip the missed dose and go back to regular dosage schedule. Do not double doses.

Pharmacokinetics. *Onset and Duration.* Effect is usually evident within a few days, but it may take 2–4 weeks for maximum improvement.[62]

Fate. Only 10% or less of an inhaled dose is deposited in the lung; 80% is deposited in the mouth and swallowed. Oral absorption is slow and incomplete (61–90%), and the drug undergoes extensive first-pass metabolism, resulting in oral bioavailability of less than 5%.[63] Well absorbed from the lung and extensively metabolized, with 65% excreted in the bile and less than 10% of unchanged drug and metabolites excreted in urine.[63]

t½. 15 hr.

Adverse Reactions. After oral use, localized growth of *Candida* in the mouth occurs frequently, but clinically apparent infections occur only occasionally. Hoarseness and dry mouth occur occasionally; minimal to no suppression of the pituitary-adrenal axis occurs at the recommended dosage; however, dose-dependent suppression occurs at higher dosages.[62,64–67] After intranasal use, irritation and burning of the nasal mucosa and sneezing occur occasionally; intranasal and pharyngeal *Candida* infections, nasal ulceration, and epistaxis occur rarely. Cases of growth suppression unrelated to suppression of the pituitary-adrenal axis have been reported following use of intranasally or orally inhaled corticosteroids in children. With oral inhalation, the mean reduction in growth velocity is 1 cm/yr (range 0.3 to 1.8 cm/yr). The long-term implications for ultimate adult height are unknown.

Contraindications. Status asthmaticus or other acute episodes of asthma in which intensive measures are required; beclomethasone-exacerbated symptoms.

Precautions. During stress or severe asthmatic attacks, patients withdrawn from systemic corticosteroid should contact their physician immediately. Use the lowest effective dosage possible in children. The potential growth effects of inhaled corticosteroids in children should be weighed against the clinical benefits of the corticosteroids and the availability of nonsteroid alternatives.

Drug Interactions. None known.

Parameters to Monitor. For treatment of asthma, frequency of daytime asthmatic symptoms and nocturnal use of prn sympathomimetic inhaler. For nasal congestion, relief of symptoms. Routinely monitor the growth of children receiving inhaled corticosteroids (eg, via stadiometry).

Notes. Patients needing long-term use of an orally inhaled corticosteroid should be continued on therapeutic doses of a bronchodilator. Prior to use, a patient should be as free of symptoms as possible, which can be achieved with a 1-week course of oral **prednisone.** The nasal inhalation provides effective, prompt relief of nasal congestion when maximally tolerated dosage of oral sympathomimetics is inadequate. (*See also* Inhaled Corticosteroids Comparison Chart.)

INHALED CORTICOSTEROIDS COMPARISON CHART

| DRUG | DOSAGE FORMS[b] | DAILY DOSAGE[a] | | | RECEPTOR BINDING HALF-LIFE | TOPICAL POTENCY[c] | ORAL BIOAVAILABILITY[d] |
		Low (Step 2)	Medium (Step 3)	High (Step 4)			
Beclomethasone Dipropionate Beclovent Vanceril	MDI: 42, 84 µg/puff.	Adult: 168–504 µg Child: 84–336 µg	504–840 µg 336–672 µg	>840 µg >672 µg	7.5 hr	600	20%
Budesonide Pulmicort	DPI: 200 µg/inhalation.	Adult: 200–400 µg Child: 100–200 µg	400–600 µg 200–400 µg	>600 µg >400 µg	5.1 hr	980	11%
Flunisolide Aerobid Aerobid-M	MDI: 250 µg/puff.	Adult: 500–1000 µg Child: 500–750 µg	1000–2000 µg 750–1250 µg	>2000 µg >1250 µg	3.5 hr	330	21%
Fluticasone Propionate Flovent	MDI: 44, 110, 220 µg/puff. DPI: 50, 100, 250 µg/dose.	Adult: 88–264 µg Child: 88–176 µg	264–660 µg 176–440 µg	>660 µg >440 µg	10.5 hr	1200	1%

(continued)

INHALED CORTICOSTEROIDS COMPARISON CHART (continued)

| DRUG | DOSAGE FORMS[b] | DAILY DOSAGE[a] | | | RECEPTOR BINDING HALF-LIFE | TOPICAL POTENCY[c] | ORAL BIOAVAILABILITY[d] |
		Low (Step 2)	Medium (Step 3)	High (Step 4)			
Triamcinolone Acetonide Azmacort	MDI: 100 µg/puff.	Adult: 400–1000 µg Child: 400–800 µg	1000–2000 µg 800–1200 µg	>2000 µg >1200 µg	3.9 hr	330	11%

DPI = dry powder inhaler; MDI = metered-dose inhaler.

[a] Dosage ranges correspond to recommended treatment intensities for steps 2–4 of the NIH guidelines for diagnosis and management of asthma: step 1 = mild intermittent; step 2 = mild persistent; step 3 = moderate persistent; step 4 = severe persistent.[20] The most important determinant of appropriate dosage is the clinician's judgement of the patient's response to therapy; the clinician must monitor the patient's response on several clinical parameters and adjust the dosage accordingly. The stepwise approach to therapy emphasizes that once control of symptoms is achieved, the dosage of medication should be carefully titrated to the minimum dosage required to maintain control, thereby reducing the potential for adverse effects.

[b] MDI dosages are expressed as the actuator dose (the amount of drug leaving the actuator and delivered to the patient), which is the labeling required in the United States. This is different from the dosage expressed as the valve dose (the amount of drug leaving the valve, not all of which is available to the patient), which is used in many European countries and in some of the scientific literature. DPI doses are expressed as the amount of drug in the inhaler following activation.

[c] Potency determined from skin blanching; dexamethasone is the reference drug and has a value of 1 in this assay.

[d] Oral bioavailability of the swallowed portion of the dose received by the patient. About 80% of the dose from an MDI without a spacer is swallowed. Nearly all of the drug delivered to the lungs is bioavailable. From 10–30% of an MDI dose is delivered to the lungs, depending on the product and device. Both the relative potency and the total bioavailability (inhaled + swallowed) determine the systemic activity of the product.

From references 20 and 68–70.

DRUG	DOSAGE FORMS	ADULT DOSAGE	PEDIATRIC DOSAGE
Beclomethasone Dipropionate Beconase Vancenase	Aerosol, Metered-Dose 42, 84 μg/spray Spray, Aqueous 42, 84 μg/spray.	1–2 sprays into each nostril bid–qid.	1 spray into each nostril bid–tid.
Budesonide Rhinocort	Aerosol, Metered-Dose 32 μg/spray.	2 sprays into each nostril bid or 4 sprays into each nostril q AM, to a maximum of 800 μg/day.	2 sprays into each nostril bid or 4 sprays into each nostril q AM, to a maximum of 400 μg/day.
Dexamethasone Sodium Phosphate Turbinaire	Aerosol, Metered-Dose 84 μg/spray.	2 sprays into each nostril bid–tid, to a maximum of 12 sprays/day.	1–2 sprays into each nostril bid, to a max-imum of 8 sprays/day.
Flunisolide Nasalide Nasarel	Spray, Aqueous 25 μg/spray.	2 sprays into each nostril bid, to a max-imum of 8 sprays/day into each nostril.	1 spray into each nostril tid–qid.
Fluticasone Propionate Flonase	Spray, Aqueous 50 μg/spray.	2 sprays into each nostril daily or 1 spray into each nostril bid; main-tenance 1 spray into each nostril daily, to a maximum of 200 μg/day.	(≥4 yr) 1 spray in each nostril daily (100 μg/day); for nonresponders, 2 sprays in each nostril daily or 1 spray in each nostril bid, decrease to 100 μg/day once a response is achieved.
Mometasone Furoate Nasonex	Spray, Aqueous 50 μg/spray.	2 sprays into each nostril once daily.	(<12 yr) not established.
Triamcinolone Acetonide Nasacort Nasarel	Spray, Aqueous 55 μg/spray.	2 sprays into each nostril daily; adjust to a maximum of 4 sprays/day in 1–4 divided doses; maintenance as low as 1 spray/day.	Same as adult dosage.

[a]Unless otherwise stated, pediatric dosage is for patients 6–12 yr; dosages for patients <6 yr have generally not been established.
From references 68–70.

Cough and Cold

DEXTROMETHORPHAN HYDROBROMIDE   Various

Pharmacology. Dextromethorphan is the nonanalgesic, nonaddictive D-isomer of the codeine analogue of levorphanol. With usual antitussive doses, the cough threshold is elevated centrally with little effect on the respiratory, cardiovascular, or GI systems.

Administration and Adult Dosage. PO as cough suppressant 10–30 mg q 4–8 hr, to a maximum of 120 mg/day; **SR** 60 mg q 12 hr.

Special Populations. *Pediatric Dosage.* PO as cough suppressant (<2 yr) not recommended; (2–6 yr) 2.5–7.5 mg q 4–8 hr, to a maximum of 30 mg/day (as syrup); (6–12 yr) 5–10 mg q 4 hr or 15 mg q 6–8 hr, to a maximum of 60 mg/day; (>12 yr) same as adult dosage. SR (2–5 yr) 15 mg q 12 hr; (6–12 yr) 30 mg q 12 hr. (*See* Notes.)

Geriatric Dosage. Same as adult dosage.

Dosage Forms. Cap 30 mg; **Lozenge** 2.5, 5, 7.5 mg; **Syrup** 0.7, 1, 1.5, 2, 3 mg/mL; **SR Susp** 6 mg/mL; (available in many combination products in variable concentrations).

Patient Instructions. Do not use this drug to suppress productive cough, or chronic cough that occurs with smoking, asthma, or emphysema. Report if your cough persists.

Pharmacokinetics. *Onset and Duration.* PO onset 1–2 hr; duration up to 6–8 hr with non-SR, 12 hr for SR suspension.[71]

Fate. Extensively metabolized, including appreciable first-pass effect, mainly to the active metabolite dextrorphan. Genetically determined polymorphic metabolism primarily by CYP2D6 with extensive (93%) and poor (7%) metabolizers.[72]

$t_{\frac{1}{2}}$. (Extensive metabolizers) <4 to about 9 hr; (poor metabolizers) 17–138 hr.[73]

Adverse Reactions. Occasional mild drowsiness and GI upset. Intoxication, bizarre behavior, CNS depression, and respiratory depression can occur with extremely high dosages. Naloxone may be effective in reversing these effects.[74–77] Reports of dextromethorphan abuse have increased, especially among teenagers.[78]

Contraindications. MAO inhibitor therapy.[79]

Precautions. Generally, do not use in patients with chronic cough or cough associated with excessive secretions.

Drug Interactions. Concurrent MAO inhibitors may cause hypotension, hyperpyrexia, nausea, and coma. Drugs that inhibit CYP2D6 may inhibit dextromethorphan metabolism, but serious effects are not reported.

Parameters to Monitor. Observe for relief of cough and CNS side effects.

Notes. Approximately equipotent with **codeine** in antitussive effectiveness in adults.[71,74] One trial of dextromethorphan and codeine for night cough in children found neither superior to placebo, and their efficacies have been questioned for this use.[80] (*See also* Codeine Salts.)

GUAIFENESIN

Pharmacology. Guaifenesin is proposed to have an expectorant action through an increased output of respiratory tract fluid, enhancing the flow of less viscid secretions, promoting ciliary action, and facilitating the removal of inspissated mucus. Evidence of the effectiveness of guaifenesin is largely subjective and not well established clinically.[74,81–85]

Administration and Adult Dosage. PO as an expectorant 100–400 mg q 4 hr; **SR** 600–1200 mg q 12 hr, to a maximum of 2.4 g/day.[84]

Special Populations. *Pediatric Dosage.* PO as an expectorant (2–6 yr) 50–100 mg q 4 hr, to a maximum of 600 mg/day; (6–12 yr) 100–200 mg q 4 hr, to a maximum of 1200 mg/day; (≥12 yr) same as adult dosage. **SR** (2–6 yr) 300 mg q 12 hr; (6–12 yr) 600 mg q 12 hr.

Geriatric Dosage. Same as adult dosage.

Dosage Forms. **Cap** 200 mg; **Syrup** 20, 40 mg/mL; **Tab** 100, 200 mg; **SR Cap** 300 mg; **SR Tab** 600 mg; **SR Tab** 400 mg with phenylpropanolamine 75 mg (Entex LA, various); 600 mg with pseudoephedrine 120 mg (Entex PSE).

Patient Instructions. Take this drug with a large quantity of fluid to ensure proper drug action. Report if your cough persists for more than 1 week, recurs, or is accompanied by a high fever, rash, or persistent headache.

Adverse Reactions. Occasional nausea and vomiting, especially with excessive dosage; dizziness; headache.

Precautions. Generally, do not use in patients with chronic cough or cough associated with excessive secretions.

Drug Interactions. None known.

Notes. May interfere with certain laboratory determinations of 5-hydroxyindoleacetic acid (5-HIAA) and vanilmandelic acid (VMA), but does not cause a positive stool guaiac reaction in normal subjects.[85]

PSEUDOEPHEDRINE HYDROCHLORIDE

Pharmacology. Pseudoephedrine is an indirect-acting agent that stimulates α-, β_1-, and β_2-adrenergic receptors via release of endogenous adrenergic amines. It is used primarily for decongestion of nasal mucosa.

Administration and Adult Dosage. PO as a decongestant 60 mg q 4–6 hr, to a maximum of 240 mg/day. **PO SR Cap/Tab** 120 mg q 12 hr; (Efidac/24) 240 mg once daily.

Special Populations. *Pediatric Dosage.* PO (3–12 months) 3 drops/kg q 4–6 hr, to a maximum of 4 doses/day; (1–2 yr) 7 drops (0.2 mL)/kg q 4–6 hr, to a maximum of 4 doses/day; (2–5 yr) 15 mg (as syrup) q 4–6 hr prn, to a maximum of 60 mg/day; (6–12 yr) 30 mg q 4–6 hr prn, to a maximum of 120 mg/day; (>12 yr) same as adult dosage. Do not give SR Cap/Tab 120 or 240 mg to patients <12 yr.

Geriatric Dosage. Demonstrate safe use of short-acting formulation before using an SR product.

Dosage Forms. **Cap** 60 mg; **SR Cap** 120 mg; **Drp** 9.4 mg/mL; **Syrup** 3, 6 mg/mL; **Tab** 30, 60 mg; **SR Tab** (12-hr) 120, 240 mg; (as sulfate) 120 mg (60 mg as immediate release, 60 mg as delayed release); (Efidac/24) 240 mg. **Tab** 60 mg with triprolidine HCl 2.5 mg (Actifed, various); **SR Cap** 120 mg with chlorpheniramine maleate 8 mg (Deconamine SR, Isoclor Timesules, various).

Patient Instructions. Avoid taking the last dose of the day near bedtime if you have difficulty sleeping. Do not crush or chew SR preparations.

Pharmacokinetics. *Onset and Duration.* Onset within 30 min on an empty stomach, within 1 hr for SR forms; duration 3 hr or longer, 8–12 hr for most SR forms, 24 hr for Efidac/24.[86,87]

Fate. Solution and immediate-release tablets are rapidly and completely absorbed orally. SR dosage forms attain peak serum levels in (12-hr product) 4–6 hr or (24-hr product) 12 hr. Food appears to delay absorption of non-SR forms, but not the SR forms.[88,89] V_d is 2.7 ± 0.2 L/kg; Cl averages 0.44 L/hr/kg. Partially metabolized to inactive metabolite(s), and 6% metabolized to active metabolite, norpseudoephedrine; 45–90% excreted unchanged in urine depending on urinary pH and flow.[89,90]

$t_{\frac{1}{2}}$. Urinary flow and pH dependent; 13 ± 3 hr at pH 8; 6.9 ± 1.2 hr at pH 5.5–6; 4.7 ± 1.4 hr at pH 5.[90,91]

Adverse Reactions. Frequent mild transient nervousness, insomnia, irritability, or headache. Usually negligible pressor effect in normotensive patients.[92,93]

Contraindications. Severe hypertension; coronary artery disease; MAO inhibitor therapy.

Precautions. Use with caution in patients with renal failure,[94] hypertension, diabetes mellitus, ischemic heart disease, increased intraocular pressure, prostatic hypertrophy, urinary retention, or thyroid disease. Elderly patients may be particularly sensitive to CNS effects. If use is necessary in infants with phenylketonuria, reduce dosage to avoid possible increased agitation.[95]

Drug Interactions. Concurrent MAO inhibitors or furazolidone may increase pressor response. Urinary alkalinizers may decrease pseudoephedrine clearance.

Parameters to Monitor. Nasal stuffiness, CNS stimulation, blood pressure in hypertensive patients.

Notes. Combination with an antihistamine may provide additive benefit in seasonal allergic rhinitis, because antihistamines do not relieve nasal stuffiness.[96,97] Neither these combinations nor decongestants alone are of consistent long-term benefit for reduction of middle ear effusion in children with otitis media and are not recommended for this use.[98,99]

■ REFERENCES

1. Tashkin DP, Jenne JW. Beta adrenergic agonists. In, Weiss EB et al., eds. *Bronchial asthma: mechanisms and therapeutics.* 3rd ed. Boston: Little, Brown; 1993:700–48.

2. Hochhaus G, Möllmann H. Pharmacokinetic/pharmacodynamic characteristics of the β_2-agonists terbutaline, salbutamol and fenoterol. *Int J Clin Pharmacol Ther Toxicol* 1992;30:342–62.

3. Spitzer OW et al. The use of β-agonists and the risk of death and near death from asthma. *N Engl J Med* 1992;326:501–6.

4. Mullen M et al. The association between β-agonist use and death from asthma. A meta-analytic integration of case-control studies. *JAMA* 1993;270:1842–5.

5. Shapiro GG, Konig P. Cromolyn sodium: a review. *Pharmacotherapy* 1985;5:156–70.

6. Murphy S, Kelly HW. Cromolyn sodium: a review of its mechanisms and clinical use in asthma. *Drug Intell Clin Pharm* 1987;21:22–35.

7. Berman BA. Cromolyn: past, present, and future. *Pediatr Clin North Am* 1983;30:915–30.

8. Edwards AM. Oral sodium cromoglycate: its use in the management of food allergy. *Clin Exp Allergy* 1995;25 (suppl 1):31–3.

9. Trujillo MH, Bellorin-Font E. Drugs commonly administered by intravenous infusion in intensive care units: a practical guide. *Crit Care Med* 1990;18:232–8.

10. Gross NJ, Skorodin MS. Anticholinergic agents. In, Jenne JW, Murphy S, eds. *Drug therapy for asthma: research and clinical practice.* New York: Marcel Dekker; 1987:615–68.

11. Milner AD. Ipratropium bromide in airways obstruction in childhood. *Postgrad Med J* 1987;63(suppl 1):53–6.

12. Shuk S et al. Efficacy of frequent nebulized ipratropium bromide added to frequent high-dose albuterol therapy in severe childhood asthma. *J Pediatr* 1995;126:639–45.

13. Gross NJ. Ipratropium bromide. *N Engl J Med* 1988;319:486–94.

14. Chung KF. Leukotriene receptor antagonists and biosynthesis inhibitors: potential breakthrough in asthma therapy. *Eur Respir J* 1995;8:1203–13.

15. Larsen JS et al. Antileukotriene therapy for asthma. *Am J Health-Syst Pharm* 1996;53:2821–30.

16. Wasserman SI. A review of some recent clinical studies with nedocromil sodium. *J Allergy Clin Immunol* 1993;92:210–5.

17. Brogden RN, Sorkin EM. Nedocromil sodium. An updated review of its pharmacological properties and therapeutic efficacy in asthma. *Drugs* 1993;45:693–715.

18. Brogden RN, Faulds D. Salmeterol xinafoate. A review of its pharmacological properties and therapeutic potential in reversible obstructive airway disease. *Drugs* 1991;42:895–912.

19. Jenne JW. Physiology and pharmacodynamics of the xanthines. In, Jenne JW, Murphy S, eds. *Drug therapy for asthma: research and clinical practice.* New York: Marcel Dekker; 1987:297–334.

20. Expert Panel Report 2: Guidelines for the diagnosis and management of asthma. Bethesda, MD: National Heart, Lung, and Blood Institute, National Asthma Education and Prevention Program; U.S. Department of Health and Human Services Publication No. 97–4051:1997.

21. Weinberger MM et al. Theophylline in asthma. *N Engl J Med* 1996;334:1380–8.

22. Weinberger MM, Hendeles L. Theophylline. In, Middleton E et al., eds. *Allergy: principles and practice.* St. Louis: Mosby; 1993:816–55.

23. Asmus MJ et al. Pharmacokinetics and drug disposition: apparent decrease in population clearance of theophylline: implications for dosage. *Clin Pharmacol Ther* 1997;62:483–9.

24. Self TH et al. Reassessing the therapeutic range for theophylline on laboratory report forms: the importance of 5–15 μg/ml. *Pharmacotherapy* 1993;13:590–4.

25. Hendeles L, Weinberger M. Selection of a slow-release theophylline product. *J Allergy Clin Immunol* 1986;78: 743–51.

26. Morris JF. Geriatric considerations. In, Weiss EB et al., eds. *Bronchial asthma: mechanisms and therapeutics.* 3rd ed. Boston: Little, Brown; 1993:1017–22.

27. Kelly HW. Theophylline toxicity. In, Jenne JW, Murphy S, eds. *Drug therapy for asthma: research and clinical practice.* New York: Marcel Dekker; 1987:925–51.

28. González MA et al. Pharmacokinetic comparison of a once-daily and twice-daily theophylline delivery system. *Clin Ther* 1994;16:686–92.

29. González MA, Straughn AB. Effect of meals and dosage-form modification on theophylline bioavailability from a 24-hour sustained-release delivery system. *Clin Ther* 1994;16:804–14.

30. Campoli-Richards DM et al. Cetirizine. A review of its pharmacological properties and clinical potential in allergic rhinitis, pollen-induced asthma, and chronic urticaria. *Drugs* 1990;40:762–81.

31. Mansmann HC et al. Efficacy and safety of cetirizine in perennial allergic rhinitis. *Ann Allergy* 1992;68:348–53.

32. Spencer CM et al. Cetirizine. A reappraisal of its pharmacological properties and therapeutic use in selected allergic disorders. *Drugs* 1993;46:1055–80.

33. Barnes CL et al. Cetirizine: a new, nonsedating antihistamine. *Ann Pharmacother* 1993;27:464–70.

34. Sheffer AL et al. Cetirizine: antiallergic therapy beyond traditional H_1 antihistamines. *J Allergy Clin Immunol* 1990;86:1040–6.

35. Simons FER et al. Pharmacokinetics and efficacy of chlorpheniramine in children. *J Allergy Clin Immunol* 1982;69:376–81.

36. Huang SM et al. Pharmacokinetics of chlorpheniramine after intravenous and oral administration in normal adults. *Eur J Clin Pharmacol* 1982;22:359–65.

37. Cook TJ et al. Degree and duration of skin test suppression and side effects with antihistamines. *J Allergy Clin Immunol* 1973;51:71–7.

38. Usdin Yasuda S et al. Chlorpheniramine plasma concentration and histamine H_1-receptor occupancy. *Clin Pharmacol Ther* 1995;58:210–20.

39. Benet LZ et al. Design and optimization of dosage regimens; pharmacokinetic data. In, Hardman JG et al., eds. *Goodman and Gilman's the pharmacological basis of therapeutics*. 9th ed. New York: McGraw-Hill; 1996:1707–92.

40. Paton DM, Webster DR. Clinical pharmacokinetics of H_1-receptor antagonists (the antihistamines). *Clin Pharmacokinet* 1985;10:477–97.

41. Simons FER. H_1-receptor antagonists: clinical pharmacology and therapeutics. *J Allergy Clin Immunol* 1989;84: 845–61.

42. Simons KJ et al. Diphenhydramine: pharmacokinetics and pharmacodynamics in elderly adults, young adults, and children. *J Clin Pharmacol* 1990;30:665–71.

43. Carruthers SG et al. Correlation between plasma diphenhydramine level and sedative and antihistamine effects. *Clin Pharmacol Ther* 1978;23:375–82.

44. Blyden GT et al. Pharmacokinetics of diphenhydramine and a demethylated metabolite following intravenous and oral administration. *J Clin Pharmacol* 1986;26:529–33.

45. Spector R et al. Diphenhydramine in Orientals and Caucasians. *Clin Pharmacol Ther* 1980;28:229–34.

46. Meredith CG et al. Diphenhydramine disposition in chronic liver disease. *Clin Pharmacol Ther* 1984;35:474–9.

47. Glazko AJ et al. Metabolic disposition of diphenhydramine. *Clin Pharmacol Ther* 1974;16:1066–76.

48. Albert KS et al. Pharmacokinetics of diphenhydramine in man. *J Pharmacokinet Biopharm* 1975;3:159–70.

49. Schaaf L et al. Suppression of seasonal allergic rhinitis symptoms with daily hydroxyzine. *J Allergy Clin Immunol* 1979;63:129–33.

50. Gendreau-Reid L et al. Comparison of the suppressive effect of astemizole, terfenadine, and hydroxyzine on histamine-induced wheals and flares in humans. *J Allergy Clin Immunol* 1986;77:335–40.

51. Simons KJ et al. Pharmacokinetic and pharmacodynamic studies of the H_1-receptor antagonist hydroxyzine in the elderly. *Clin Pharmacol Ther* 1989;45:9–14.

52. Simons FER et al. Pharmacokinetics and antipruritic effects of hydroxyzine in children with atopic dermatitis. *J Pediatr* 1984;104:123–7.

53. Simons FE et al. The pharmacokinetics and antihistaminic of the H_1 receptor antagonist hydroxyzine. *J Allergy Clin Immunol* 1984;73(1 pt. 1):69–75.

54. Simons FER et al. The pharmacokinetics and pharmacodynamics of hydroxyzine in patients with primary biliary cirrhosis. *J Clin Pharmacol* 1989;29:809–15.

55. Simons FER, Simons KJ. Antihistamines. In, Middleton E et al., eds. *Allergy. Principles and practice*. St. Louis: Mosby; 1993:856–79.

56. Gonzalez MA, Estes KS. Pharmacokinetic overview of oral second-generation H_1 antihistamines. *Int J Clin Pharmacol Ther* 1998;36:292–300.

57. Corey JP. Advances in the pharmacotherapy of allergic rhinitis: second-generation H_1-receptor antagonists. *Otolaryngol Head Neck Surg* 1993;109:584–92.

58. Krause HF. Antihistamines and decongestants. *Otolaryngol Head Neck Surg* 1992;107:835–40.

59. Korenblat PE, Wedner HJ. *Allergy. Theory and practice*. 2nd ed. Philadelphia: WB Saunders; 1992:300–3.

60. Desager J-P, Horsmans Y. Pharmacokinetic-pharmacodynamic relationships of H_1-antihistamines. *Clin Pharmacokinet* 1995;28:419–32.

61. Kobayaski RH et al. Beclomethasone dipropionate aqueous nasal spray for seasonal allergic rhinitis in children. *Ann Allergy* 1989;62:205–8.

62. Fauci AS et al. Glucocorticoid therapy: mechanisms of action and clinical considerations. *Ann Intern Med* 1976;84:304–15.

63. Azarnoff DL ed. *Steroid therapy*. Philadelphia: WB Saunders, 1975.

64. Barnes PJ. Inhaled glucocorticoids for asthma. *N Engl J Med* 1995;332:868–75.

65. Barnes PJ, Pederson S. Efficacy and safety of inhaled corticosteroid in asthma. *Am Rev Respir Dis* 1993;149: S1–26.

66. Szefler SJ. A comparison of aerosol glucocorticoids in the treatment of chronic bronchial asthma. *Pediatr Asthma Allergy Immunol* 1991;5:227–35.

67. Kamada AK. Therapeutic controversies in the treatment of asthma. *Ann Pharmacother* 1994;28:904–14.

68. Toogood JH et al. Aerosol corticosteroid. In, Weiss EB et al., eds. *Bronchial asthma: mechanisms and therapeutics*. 3rd ed. Boston: Little, Brown; 1993:818–41.

69. McCubbin MM et al. A bioassay for topical and systemic effect of three inhaled steroids. *Clin Pharmacol Ther* 1995;57:455–60.
70. Holliday SM et al. Inhaled fluticasone propionate. A review of its pharmacodynamic and pharmacokinetic properties, and therapeutic use in asthma. *Drugs* 1994;47:318–31.
71. Matthys H et al. Dextromethorphan and codeine: objective assessment of antitussive activity in patients with chronic cough. *J Int Med Res* 1983;11:92–100.
72. Jacqz-Aigrain E et al. CYP2D6- and CYP3A-dependent metabolism of dextromethorphan in humans. *Pharmacokenetics* 1993;3:197–204.
73. Woodworth JR et al. The polymorphic metabolism of dextromethorphan. *J Clin Pharmacol* 1987;27:139–43.
74. Bryant BG, Lombardi TP. Cold, cough, and allergy products. In, Covington TR, ed. *Handbook of nonprescription drugs.* 10th ed. Washington, DC: American Pharmaceutical Association; 1993:89–115.
75. Committee on Drugs. Use of codeine- and dextromethorphan-containing cough syrups in pediatrics. *Pediatrics* 1978;62:118–22.
76. Shaul WL et al. Dextromethorphan toxicity: reversal by naloxone. *Pediatrics* 1977;59:117–9.
77. Katona B, Wason S. Dextromethorphan danger. *N Engl J Med* 1986;314:993. Letter.
78. Bem JL, Peck R. Dextromethorphan. An overview of safety issues. *Drug Safety* 1992;190–9.
79. Nierenberg DW, Semprebon M. The central nervous system serotonin syndrome. *Clin Pharmacol Ther* 1993; 53:84–8.
80. Taylor JA et al. Efficacy of cough suppressants in children. *J Pediatr* 1993;122:799–802.
81. Hirsch SR et al. The expectorant effect of glyceryl guaiacolate in patients with chronic bronchitis. *Chest* 1973; 63:9–14.
82. Heilborn H et al. Effect of bromhexine and guaiphenesine on clinical state, ventilatory capacity and sputum viscosity in chronic asthma. *Scand J Respir Dis* 1976;57:88–96.
83. Anon. Guaiphenesin and iodide. *Drug Ther Bull* 1985;23:62–4.
84. Anon. Cold, cough, allergy, bronchodilator, and antiasthmatic drug products for over-the-counter human use; expectorant drug products for over-the-counter human use; final monograph. *Fed Regist* 1989;54:8494–509.
85. Ziment I. Drugs modifying the sol-layer and the hydration of mucus. In, Braga PC, Allegra L, eds. *Drugs in bronchial mucology.* New York: Raven Press; 1989:293–322.
86. Roth RP et al. Nasal decongestant activity of pseudoephedrine. *Ann Otol Rhinol Laryngol* 1977;86:235–42.
87. Hamilton LH et al. A study of sustained action pseudoephedrine in allergic rhinitis. *Ann Allergy* 1982;48:87–92.
88. Hwang SS et al. In vitro and in vivo evaluation of a once-daily controlled-release pseudoephedrine product. *J Clin Pharmacol* 1995;35:259–67.
89. Kanfer I et al. Pharmacokinetics of oral decongestants. *Pharmacotherapy* 1993;13(6 pt 2):116S–28S.
90. Brater DC et al. Renal excretion of pseudoephedrine. *Clin Pharmacol Ther* 1980;28:690–4.
91. Kuntzman RG et al. The influence of urinary pH on the plasma half-life of pseudoephedrine in man and dog and a sensitive assay for its determination in human plasma. *Clin Pharmacol Ther* 1971;12:62–7.
92. Chua SS, Benrimoj SI. Non-prescription sympathomimetic agents and hypertension. *Med Toxicol* 1988;3: 387–417.
93. Beck RA et al. Cardiovascular effects of pseudoephedrine in medically controlled hypertensive patients. *Arch Intern Med* 1992;152:1242–5.
94. Sica DA, Comstock TJ. Case report: pseudoephedrine accumulation in renal failure. *Am J Med Sci* 1989;298: 261–3.
95. Spielberg SP, Schulman JD. A possible reaction to pseudoephedrine in a patient with phenylketonuria. *J Pediatr* 1977;90:1026.
96. Hendeles L. Selecting a decongestant. *Pharmacotherapy* 1993;13(6 pt 2):129S–34.
97. Bryant BG, Lombardi TP. Cold, cough, and allergy products. In, Covington TR, ed. *Handbook of nonprescription drugs.* 10th ed. Washington, DC: American Pharmaceutical Association; 1993:89–115.
98. Thoene DE, Johnson CE. Pharmacotherapy of otitis media. *Pharmacotherapy* 1991;11:212–21.
99. Bahal N, Nahata MC. Recent advances in the treatment of otitis media. *J Clin Pharm Ther* 1992;17:201–15.

CLINICAL INFORMATION

- DRUG-INDUCED DISEASES
- DRUG INTERACTIONS AND INTERFERENCES
- DRUG USE IN SPECIAL POPULATIONS
- IMMUNIZATION
- MEDICAL EMERGENCIES
- NUTRITION SUPPORT

Drug-Induced Diseases

William G. Troutman

BLOOD DYSCRASIAS, HEPATOTOXICITY, NEPHROTOXICITY, OCULOTOXICITY, OTOTOXICITY, PANCREATITIS, SEXUAL DYSFUNCTION, SKIN DISORDERS

The tables in the following sections provide information on specific drug-induced diseases. The tables identify drugs of major importance that are thought to be most frequently implicated in causing the disorder in question and thus do not include all drugs reported to cause the drug-induced disease.

When several members of a drug class are known to be similarly capable of producing a disorder, the class name (eg, phenothiazines, sulfonamides) is used, although individual agents may also be listed in boldface type for ease of location. Each entry briefly describes the clinical nature of the drug's toxicity and, when possible, gives its prevalence. Occasionally, the available literature reports that a drug is a possible cause of a disorder, but fails to adequately characterize the frequency and severity of the adverse reaction. In these cases, the phrase "scattered reports only" appears in the discussion section of the table. References are provided after each table for literature discussions and case reports of each particular drug-induced disorder.

Prior to using a table, it is important to read the introductory statement to become familiar with any general information, inclusion criteria, and abbreviations which pertain to that table.

DRUG-INDUCED BLOOD DYSCRASIAS

This table does not include all drugs capable of causing the specified dyscrasias and excludes cancer chemotherapeutic agents, which are known for producing dose-related bone marrow suppression. Five major types of blood dyscrasias have been selected for inclusion in this table: the following abbreviations are used to indicate the specific blood dyscrasia:

AA – Aplastic Anemia
AGN – Agranulocytosis, Granulocytopenia, or Neutropenia
HA – Hemolytic Anemia
MA – Macrocytic Anemia
Th – Thrombocytopenia

(continued)

DRUG AND DYSCRASIA	NATURE OF DYSCRASIA

Acetaminophen

Th — Scattered reports only; observed in 6 of 174 overdose patients in one report; may be an immune reaction.[1,2]

Alcohol

HA — Most commonly encountered in chronic alcoholism.[3]

MA — Results from malnutrition and decreased folate absorption and/or utilization. Responds rapidly to folic acid administration.[3]

Th — Transient in many drinkers; persistent thrombocytopenia may accompany advanced alcoholic liver disease.[3]

Amphotericin B

AGN — Scattered reports only.[3,4]

Th — Scattered reports only.[3–5]

Amrinone

Th — 18.6% prevalence in one study of oral therapy (oral form not marketed in the United States); the prevalence during parenteral therapy has been estimated at 2.4%, although 8 of 16 children receiving parenteral amrinone developed thrombocytopenia in one report. Thrombocytopenia may be caused by nonimmune peripheral platelet destruction.[6–8]

Antidepressants, Heterocyclic

AGN — Idiosyncratic reaction, probably resulting from a direct toxic effect rather than allergy. Most commonly occurs between the second and eighth weeks of therapy.[3,9,10]

Ascorbic Acid

HA — In G-6-PD deficiency with large doses.[3]

Aspirin

HA — Almost always encountered in patients with G-6-PD deficiency, usually in conjunction with infection or other complicating factors.[3,11]

Th — May occur in addition to the drug's effects on platelet adhesiveness. Some evidence for an immune reaction.[1,3,12]

Azathioprine

AGN — WBC counts $<2.5 \times 10^9$/L occur in about 3% of rheumatoid arthritis patients treated with azathioprine; an additional 15% develop some lesser degree of leukopenia.[13]

Captopril

AGN — Prevalence estimated at 1/5000 patients. The prevalence increases greatly in patients with reduced renal function or collagen-vascular diseases and reaches 7% in patients with both renal impairment and a collagen-vascular disease. Most common during the first 3 weeks of therapy.[14]

(continued)

DRUG AND DYSCRASIA	NATURE OF DYSCRASIA

Carbamazepine

AA   27 cases reported from 1964–1988; onset may be delayed until weeks or months after the initiation of therapy.[3,15]

AGN   Transient leukopenia occurs in about 10% of patients, usually during the first month of therapy. Recovery usually occurs within a week of drug withdrawal. Persistent leukopenia occurs in 2%.[15,16]

Th   Prevalence estimated at 2%.[15,17]

Cephalosporins

AGN   Rare; possibly the result of an immune reaction, but occurs most often with high dosages.[3,18]

HA   Positive direct Coombs' test occurs frequently and may persist for up to 2 months after discontinuation of therapy. Hemolysis is rare.[3,18]

Th   Rare; possibly the result of an immune reaction. Usually occurs late in the course of therapy.[3,18]

Chloramphenicol

AA   Prevalence estimated at 1/12,000 to 1/50,000 patients. Most cases develop with oral administration and after discontinuation of therapy, suggesting the development of a toxic metabolite. An association between the ophthalmic use of chloramphenicol and the development of aplastic anemia is weak, if it exists at all. Blacks may be more susceptible than whites. Aplastic anemia should not be confused with the dose-related anemia seen with chloramphenicol. (Note: one case report suggests that a patient's dose-related anemia may have progressed to aplastic anemia, but most sources separate the two dyscrasias.)[3,19–23]

AGN   Rare when compared with the prevalence of aplastic anemia.[3,19]

HA   In G-6-PD deficiency.[3]

Chloroquine

AGN   Scattered reports only; may be dose related.[3]

HA   Only a few cases have been reported; some association with G-6-PD deficiency is suspected.[3]

Cimetidine

AA   Scattered reports only; however, at least two fatalities reported (one fatality was also receiving chloramphenicol).[24]

AGN   Usually occurs in patients with systemic disease or other drug therapy which may have contributed to the dyscrasia.[24]

Clozapine

AGN   Frequency of granulocytopenia is calculated to be 0.4–0.8% among closely monitored patients. Mild to moderate neutropenia occurs in 3–20%. Most cases occur in the first 4 months. Recovery usually occurs 2–3 weeks after drug withdrawal. Weekly WBC counts are mandated.[25–27]

Cocaine

Th   Reported with both IV and inhalational use.[28]

(continued)

DRUG AND DYSCRASIA	NATURE OF DYSCRASIA

Contraceptives, Oral

MA — Results from impaired absorption and/or utilization of folate; of consequence only if the patient's folate status is markedly impaired.[3]

Dapsone

AGN — Many cases have occurred during combination therapy, so it is difficult to determine if dapsone alone is the causative agent.[3,29]

HA — In G-6-PD deficiency; may also have other mechanism(s). May be dose related; uncommon at 100 mg/day, but frequent at 200–300 mg/day.[3]

Digitoxin

Th — Scattered reports only; evidence of an immune mechanism.[1,30]

Digoxin

Th — Scattered reports only; evidence of an immune mechanism.[1,31]

Dimercaprol

HA — In G-6-PD deficiency.[3]

Dipyridamole

Th — Relative risk of thrombocytopenia calculated to be 14 times higher than in untreated individuals, but needs confirmation.[32]

Diuretics, Thiazide

HA — Exact mechanism is unclear; may be an immune reaction.[3,33]

Th — Mild thrombocytopenia occurs frequently, but severe cases are rare. May be caused by an immune reaction.[1,3,34]

Eflornithine

AA — Deaths caused by aplastic anemia have been reported.[35]

AGN — Leukopenia is reported in 18–37% of patients.[35]

MA — Megaloblastic anemia is frequently reported.[35]

Th — Thrombocytopenia is frequently reported.[35]

Felbamate

AA — More than 30 cases were reported shortly after the introduction of felbamate, resulting in the manufacturer and FDA urging withdrawal of patients from therapy. When a strict definition of aplastic anemia is applied and when confounding factors are accounted for, the risk of aplastic anemia from felbamate may not be markedly different from the risk posed by carbamazepine. Most cases developed 2–6 months after initiation of therapy. Monitoring has not been effective for the early identification of cases.[36,37]

Fluconazole

Th — Scattered reports only.[38]

Flucytosine

AGN — Dose related; usually requires plasma level of 125 mg/L or greater.[39]

Th — Dose related; usually requires plasma level of 125 mg/L or greater.[39]

(continued)

DRUG AND DYSCRASIA	NATURE OF DYSCRASIA

Foscarnet

AGN — Neutropenia occurs in 14% of patients treated for cytomegalovirus retinitis.[40]

Furosemide

Th — Uncommon, mild and asymptomatic.[3]

Ganciclovir

AGN — Granulocytopenia occurs in about 40% of patients; it is usually reversible upon drug discontinuation, but irreversible neutropenia and deaths have occurred.[40,41]

Th — Thrombocytopenia occurs in about 20% of patients.[41]

Gold Salts

AA — Not dose dependent; while this reaction is not common, numerous fatalities have been reported.[13,42]

AGN — Often brief and self-limiting; usually responds to withdrawal of therapy.[43,44]

Th — Not dose or duration dependent; prevalence estimated at 1–3%; onset usually during the loading phase (first 1000 mg), but may be delayed until after the drug has been discontinued. Mechanism is unclear, but it often appears to be immunologically mediated. Up to 85% of patients with gold-induced thrombocytopenia are HLA-DR3 compared with 30% of all rheumatoid arthritis patients.[1,3,13,45,46]

Heparin

Th — Many patients demonstrate a mild to moderate transient decrease in platelets after 5–8 days of heparin therapy. Up to 3% experience immune-mediated, persistent thrombocytopenia, which is associated with increased thrombin generation and development of life-threatening thrombosis. Intermittent, continuous infusion and "minidose" regimens have all been implicated; this is uncommon with SC administration. Prompt cessation of heparin minimizes serious complications; platelet count usually returns to normal within 48 hr. Low-molecular-weight heparins (eg, **dalteparin, enoxaparin**) are much less likely than unfractionated heparin to stimulate the formation of immune complexes leading to thrombocytopenia. Low-molecular-weight heparins offer very little protection from thrombocytopenia in patients who have already formed heparin-associated antibodies. The antithrombin activity of **danaparoid,** its much lower risk of cross-reactivity, and positive clinical experience have led some authors to recommend its use in patients with heparin-induced thrombocytopenia.[47–50]

Immune Globulin

AGN — Transient neutropenia frequently accompanies IV use.[51]

HA — Acute Coombs' positive hemolysis has been reported in patients receiving high-dose therapy.[51]

(continued)

DRUG AND DYSCRASIA	NATURE OF DYSCRASIA

Indomethacin

AA Although rare, indomethacin has been associated with a risk 12.7 times higher than in untreated individuals, especially when used regularly and for a long duration.[52]

AGN Although rare, risk may be 8.9 times higher than in untreated individuals.[52]

Interferon Alfa

Th Scattered reports only.[53]

Isoniazid

AGN Scattered reports only; some evidence of an immune reaction.[3,54]

Th Scattered reports only; some evidence of an immune reaction.[1,3,54]

Lamotrigine

AGN Scattered reports only; too early to establish a pattern of risk.[55]

Levamisole

AGN May be the result of an autoimmune reaction with a prevalence of 4% or more in some series. Presence of the HLA-B27 phenotype in sero-positive rheumatoid arthritis may be an important predisposing factor.[9,52,56]

Th Scattered reports only.[1,57]

Levodopa

HA Autoimmune reaction; positive direct and indirect Coombs' tests are frequent, but hemolysis is rare. **Carbidopa-levodopa** combinations have also produced hemolysis.[3]

Mefenamic Acid

HA Thought to be autoimmune.[3,11]

Methimazole

AA Scattered reports only; however, some increased risk is present. Most cases occur during the first 3 months of therapy.[58,59]

AGN Prevalence estimated at 0.31%. Encountered overwhelmingly in women and appears to increase with age. Most cases occur in the first 3 months of therapy, and monitoring during this time may detect agranulocytosis before it becomes clinically apparent.[3,58,60,61]

Methyldopa

HA Autoimmune reaction; positive direct Coombs' test occurs in 5–25% of patients, depending on dosage; hemolysis occurs in less than 1%, and its onset is gradual after 4 months or more of therapy. Recovery is rapid after discontinuation of the drug.[3,11,62]

Th Rare; may be caused by an immune reaction.[1,3,63]

Methylene Blue

HA In G-6-PD deficiency.[3]

Nalidixic Acid

HA In G-6-PD deficiency; may also have other mechanisms.[3]

Th Scattered reports only; possibly associated with renal impairment in one series.[64]

(continued)

DRUG AND DYSCRASIA	NATURE OF DYSCRASIA

Nitrofurantoin

HA   In G-6-PD deficiency; also encountered with enolase deficiency (mechanism unknown).[3]

Penicillamine

AA   Rare; develops after several months of therapy; due to direct marrow toxicity.[65,66]

AGN   Rare; most cases occur during the first month of therapy.[3,66]

HA   Scattered reports only; may be caused by G-6-PD deficiency or fluctuations in copper levels during therapy of Wilson's disease.[66,67]

Th   Prevalence estimated at 10%; some decrease in platelet counts occurs in 75% of penicillamine-treated patients. May be the result of an immune reaction; most commonly occurs during the first 6 months of therapy.[3,66,68]

Penicillins

AA   Prevalence very low when extent of use is considered.[3]

AGN   Uncommon with most penicillins, but frequent with **methicillin;** in one report, neutropenia developed in 23 of 68 methicillin-treated patients; resolution occurred within 3–7 days after drug withdrawal.[3,9,69]

HA   Positive direct Coombs' test occurs with large IV doses; hemolysis rare.[3,11]

Phenazopyridine

HA   Prevalence and mechanism unknown; renal insufficiency and overdose may be contributing factors. Often accompanied by methemoglobinemia.[3,70]

Phenobarbital

MA   Over 100 cases reported; usually responds to folic acid.[3]

Phenothiazines

AGN   Most common during the first 2 months of therapy and in older patients (>85% are >40 yr). Rapid onset and general lack of dose dependence suggest an idiosyncratic mechanism. Prevalence estimated as high as 1/1200.[3,9,71,72]

Phenytoin

AA   Fewer than 25 reported cases, but the association with phenytoin is strong.[3]

AGN   Scattered reports only; onset after days to years of therapy.[3,9]

MA   Caused by impaired absorption and/or utilization of folate and responds to folic acid therapy (although folate replacement may lower phenytoin levels). Mild macrocytosis is very common (25% or more); onset is unpredictable, but usually appears after 6 months or more of therapy.[3]

Th   Scattered reports only; may be the result of an immune reaction.[1,3,73]

Primaquine

HA   In G-6-PD deficiency.[3]

(*continued*)

DRUG AND DYSCRASIA	NATURE OF DYSCRASIA

Primidone

MA Similar to phenobarbital, but prevalence may be lower; onset is unpredictable and may be delayed for several years during therapy. Some cases have responded to folic acid.[3]

Procainamide

AGN Prevalence usually estimated at less than 1%, but with a 25% fatal outcome. Occurs with both conventional and sustained-release products; usually occurs within the first 90 days of use. No relationship with daily or total dosage.[3,9,74–76]

Propylthiouracil

AA Scattered reports only; however, some increased risk is present. Most cases occur within the first 3 months of therapy.[58,59]

AGN Prevalence estimated at 0.55%. Occurs overwhelmingly in women and appears to increase with age. Most cases occur in the first 3 months of therapy, and monitoring during this time may detect agranulocytosis before it becomes clinically apparent. Some evidence for an immune reaction.[3,9,58–61,77]

Quinacrine

AA About one-half of reported cases were preceded by a rash or lichenoid eruption; prevalence estimated at 3/100,000.[3,78]

HA In G-6-PD deficiency; usually requires concurrent infection or other complicating factors.[3]

Quinidine

AGN Scattered reports only; an immune mechanism has been described.[9,79]

HA In G-6-PD deficiency (but not in blacks). A rapid onset immune mechanism has also been described.[3,9,11,80]

Th Caused by quinidine-specific antibodies; little or no cross-reactivity with quinine. Accounts for a large portion of drug-induced thrombocytopenia.[1,3,32,73,81]

Quinine

AGN Scattered reports only.[3]

HA In G-6-PD deficiency (but not in blacks). An immune mechanism is also suspected because quinine-dependent antibodies to RBCs have been demonstrated in cases of quinine-induced hemolytic-uremic syndrome.[3,82]

Th Caused by quinine-specific antibodies; little or no cross-reactivity with quinidine. Fatalities have been reported. It has occurred in people drinking quinine-containing tonic water.[1,3,32,83–85]

Rifabutin

AGN In a study of the pharmacokinetic interactions between rifabutin and azithromycin or clarithromycin, rifabutin, alone or in combination with either of the other two drugs, produced neutropenia in most of the patients. Neutropenia was not seen when either of the other drugs was used without rifabutin.[86]

(continued)

DRUG AND DYSCRASIA	NATURE OF DYSCRASIA

Rifampin

HA Rare, but many patients develop a positive Coombs' test; onset in hours in some sensitized patients.[3,54,87]

Th Peripheral destruction of platelets appears to result from an immune reaction; difficult to separate rifampin contribution from that of other drugs, because it is usually used in combination therapy.[1,3,54]

Sulfasalazine

AGN Leukopenia reported in 5.6% of patients receiving the drug for rheumatoid arthritis and agranulocytosis/neutropenia in 4 of 1000 patients; prevalence of agranulocytosis/neutropenia among inflammatory bowel disease patients is considerably lower (0.3 of 1000 patients). Onset is usually during the first 3 months of therapy; recovery takes 2 weeks after drug discontinuation.[13,88,89]

HA In G-6-PD deficiency, but also occurs in nondeficient patients. Hemolysis may be more common in slow acetylators.[3,89–91]

MA One series of 130 arthritis patients reported macrocytosis in 21% and macrocytic anemia in 3%.[92]

Sulfonamides

AA Historically, an important cause of aplastic anemia, but most cases were reported following use of older sulfonamides; rarely occurs with products currently in use.[3]

AGN Occurs mostly with older products; rarely occurs with products currently in use. Most current cases are in combined use with trimethoprim; also reported with **silver sulfadiazine**. Onset is usually rapid.[3,11,93,94]

HA In G-6-PD deficiency; but also occurs in nondeficient patients.[3,95]

Th Scattered reports only; probably an immune reaction. (*See also* Trimethoprim.)[1,32,73]

Ticlopidine

AGN Neutropenia developed in 13 of 1518 patients in one study; onset was most common in the first 3 months of therapy. Neutropenia resolved within 3 weeks of drug discontinuation.[96]

Tocainide

AGN Prevalence estimated at 0.07–0.18% of patients.[97,98]

Triamterene

MA Few cases reported, but it is a potent inhibitor of dihydrofolate reductase; greatest risk in those with folate deficiency prior to therapy (eg, alcoholics).[3]

Trimethoprim

AGN Rare; occurs when used alone and in combination with sulfonamides, with the latter numerically more common.[3,94,99]

MA Most cases occur after 1–2 weeks of therapy; this drug may have small antifolate action in humans, which becomes important only in those with folate deficiency prior to therapy (eg, alcoholics).[3]

Th Thrombocytopenia is common, but severe cases are rare. Most commonly occurs in combination therapy with sulfonamides. Relative risk calculated at 124 times that of untreated individuals.[1,3,32]

(*continued*)

DRUG AND DYSCRASIA	NATURE OF DYSCRASIA

Vaccines

Th   A study of 9 million doses of measles, rubella, and mumps vaccines administered to children determined that the prevalence of thrombocytopenia was 0.17 cases/100,000 doses for measles vaccine and 0.23, 0.87, and 0.95 cases/100,000 doses for rubella, measles-rubella, and mumps-measles-rubella vaccines, respectively. These rates are similar to the rates of thrombocytopenia following the natural courses of the disease in unvaccinated children. Most of the cases had platelet counts >0.01×10^{12}/L.[100]

Valproic Acid

MA   Macrocytosis occurs in 11 of 60 patients in one report.[101]

Th   Thrombocytopenia occurred in 12 of 60 patients in one report. Both immune and dose-dependent mechanisms have been suggested.[1,101]

Vancomycin

AGN   Scattered reports only; however, prevalence may be as high as 2%; mechanism unknown.[2,102,103]

Vesnarinone

AGN   Reversible neutropenia occurs in about 3%, mostly in the first 16–24 weeks of treatment. Absolute granulocyte count <1×10^9/L occur in 0.85% with counts <0.1×10^9/L in 0.25%.[104,105]

Vitamin K

HA   In G-6-PD deficiency; usually requires concurrent infection or other complicating factors. Hemolysis from high doses can contribute to jaundice in neonates; rarely toxic in older children and adults.[3]

Zidovudine

AGN   Most patients experience at least a 25% reduction in neutrophil count; absolute neutrophil counts of <0.5×10^9/L occur in 16% of patients. Usual onset is during the first 3 months of therapy.[106,107]

MA   Macrocytosis develops in most patients, usually beginning during the first few weeks of therapy. Zidovudine is now the leading cause of drug-induced macrocytosis.[106–108]

■ REFERENCES

1. Hackett T et al. Drug-induced platelet destruction. *Semin Thromb Hemost* 1982;8:116–37.
2. Fischereder M, Jaffe JP. Thrombocytopenia following acute acetaminophen overdose. *Am J Hematol* 1994;45:258–9.
3. Swanson M, Cook R. *Drugs chemicals and blood dyscrasias.* Hamilton, IL: Drug Intelligence Publications; 1977.
4. Wilson R, Feldman S. Toxicity of amphotericin B in children with cancer. *Am J Dis Child* 1979;133:731–4.
5. Chan CSP et al. Amphotericin-B-induced thrombocytopenia. *Ann Intern Med* 1982;96:332–3.
6. Ansell J et al. Amrinone-induced thrombocytopenia. *Arch Intern Med* 1984;144:949–52.
7. Treadway G. Clinical safety of intravenous amrinone—a review. *Am J Cardiol* 1985;56:39B–40B.
8. Ross MP et al. Amrinone-associated thrombocytopenia: pharmacokinetic analysis. *Clin Pharmacol Ther* 1993;53:661–7.
9. Heimpel H. Drug-induced agranulocytosis. *Med Toxicol Adverse Drug Exp* 1988;3:449–62.
10. Levin GM, DeVane CL. A review of cyclic antidepressant-induced blood dyscrasias. *Ann Pharmacother* 1992;26:378–83.

11. Sanford-Driscoll M, Knodel LC. Induction of hemolytic anemia by nonsteroidal anti-inflammatory drugs. *Drug Intell Clin Pharm* 1986;20:925–34.

12. Garg SK, Sarker CR. Aspirin-induced thrombocytopenia on an immune basis. *Am J Med Sci* 1974;267: 129–32.

13. George CS, Lichtin AE. Hematologic complications of rheumatic disease therapies. *Rheum Dis Clin North Am* 1997;23:425–37.

14. Cooper RA. Captopril-associated neutropenia. Who is at risk? *Arch Intern Med* 1983;143:659–60. Editorial.

15. Sobotka JL et al. A review of carbamazepine's hematologic reactions and monitoring recommendations. *DICP* 1990;24:1214–9.

16. Tohen M et al. Blood dyscrasias with carbamazepine and valproate: a pharmacoepidemiological study of 2,228 patients at risk. *Am J Psychiatry* 1995;152:413–8.

17. Bradley JM et al. Carbamazepine-induced thrombocytopenia in a young child. *Clin Pharm* 1985;4:221–3.

18. Thompson JW, Jacobs RF. Adverse effects of newer cephalosporins. An update. *Drug Saf* 1993;9:132–42.

19. Chaplin S. Bone marrow depression due to mianserin, phenylbutazone, oxyphenbutazone, and chloramphenicol—part I. *Adverse Drug React Acute Poisoning Rev* 1986;2:97–136.

20. Chaplin S. Bone marrow depression due to mianserin, phenylbutazone, oxyphenbutazone, and chloramphenicol—part II. *Adverse Drug React Acute Poisoning Rev* 1986;3:181–96.

21. Rayner SA, Buckley RJ. Ocular chloramphenicol and aplastic anemia. Is there a link? *Drug Saf* 1996; 14:273–6.

22. Fraunfelder FT et al. Blood dyscrasias and topical ophthalmic chloramphenicol. *Am J Ophthalmol* 1993; 115:812–3. Letter.

23. Flegg P et al. Chloramphenicol. Are concerns about aplastic anemia justified? *Drug Saf* 1992;7:167–9.

24. Aymard J-P et al. Haematological adverse effects of histamine H₂-receptor antagonists. *Med Toxicol Adverse Drug Exp* 1988;3:430–48.

25. Alvir JMJ et al. Clozapine-induced agranulocytosis. Incidence and risk factors in the United States. *N Engl J Med* 1993;329:162–7.

26. Atkin K et al. Neutropenia and agranulocytosis in patients receiving clozapine in the UK and Ireland. *Br J Psychiatr* 1996;169:483–8.

27. Honigfeld G. Effects of the Clozapine National Registry System on incidence of deaths related to agranulocytosis. *Psychiatr Serv* 1996;47:52–6.

28. Leissinger CA. Severe thrombocytopenia associated with cocaine use. *Ann Intern Med* 1990;112:708–10.

29. Cockburn EM et al. Dapsone-induced agranulocytosis: spontaneous reporting data. *Br J Dermatol* 1993;128: 702–3. Letter.

30. Young RC et al. Thrombocytopenia due to digitoxin. Demonstration of antibody and mechanisms of action. *Am J Med* 1966;41:605–14.

31. Pirovino M et al. Digoxin-associated thrombocytopaenia. *Eur J Clin Pharmacol* 1981;19:205–7.

32. Kaufman DW et al. Acute thrombocytopenic purpura in relation to the use of drugs. *Blood* 1993;82:2714–8.

33. Beck ML et al. Fatal intravascular immune hemolysis induced by hydrochlorothiazide. *Am J Clin Pathol* 1984;81:791–4.

34. Okafor KC et al. Hydrochlorothiazide-induced thrombocytopenic purpura. *Drug Intell Clin Pharm* 1986;20: 60–1.

35. Sahai J, Berry AJ. Eflornithine for the treatment of *Pneumocystis carinii* pneumonia in patients with the acquired immunodeficiency syndrome: a preliminary review. *Pharmacotherapy* 1989;9:29–33.

36. Pennell PB et al. Aplastic anemia in a patient receiving felbamate for complex partial seizures. *Neurology* 1995;45:456–60.

37. Kaufman DW et al. Aplastic anemia among users of felbamate. *Pharmacoepidemiol Drug Saf* 1996;5(suppl): S106. Abstract.

38. Mercurio MG et al. Thrombocytopenia caused by fluconazole therapy. *J Am Acad Dermatol* 1995;32:525–6.

39. Kauffman CA, Frame PT. Bone marrow toxicity associated with 5-fluorocytosine therapy. *Antimicrob Agents Chemother* 1977;11:244–7.

40. Morbidity and toxic effects associated with ganciclovir or foscarnet therapy in a randomized cytomegalovirus retinitis trial. Studies of Ocular Complications of AIDS Research Group, in collaboration with the AIDS Clinical Trials Group. *Intern Med* 1995;155:65–74.

41. Cytovene product information. Palo Alto, CA: Syntex Laboratories; 1994.

42. Gibson J et al. Aplastic anemia in association with gold therapy for rheumatoid arthritis. *Aust N Z J Med* 1983;13:130–4.

43. Gibbons RB. Complications of chryotherapy. A review of recent studies. *Arch Intern Med* 1979;139:343–6.

44. Gottlieb NL et al. The course of severe gold-associated granulocytopenia. *Clin Res* 1982;30:659A. Abstract.

45. Coblyn JS et al. Gold-induced thrombocytopenia. A clinical and immunogenetic study of twenty-three patients. *Ann Intern Med* 1981;95:178–81.

46. Adachi JD et al. Gold induced thrombocytopenia: platelet associated IgG and HLA typing in three patients. *J Rheumatol* 1984;11:355–7.

47. Warkentin TE et al. Heparin-induced thrombocytopenia in patients treated with low-molecular-weight heparin or unfractionated heparin. *N Engl J Med* 1995;332:1330–5.

48. Warkentin TE. Heparin-induced thrombocytopenia. *Drug Saf* 1997;17:325–41.

49. Schmitt BP, Adelman B. Heparin-associated thrombocytopenia: a critical review and pooled analysis. *Am J Med Sci* 1993;305:208–15.

50. Phillips DE et al. Heparin-induced thrombotic thrombocytopenia. *Ann Pharmacother* 1994;28:43–6.

51. Misbah SA, Chapel HM. Adverse effects of intravenous immunoglobulin. *Drug Saf* 1993;9:254–62.

52. Risks of agranulocytosis and aplastic anemia. A first report of their relation to drug use with special reference to analgesics. The International Agranulocytosis and Aplastic Anemia Study. *JAMA* 1986;256:1749–57.

53. Murakami CS et al. Idiopathic thrombocytopenic purpura during interferon-α_{2B} treatment for chronic hepatitis. *Am J Gastroenterol* 1994;89:2244–5.

54. Holdiness MR. A review of blood dyscrasias induced by the antituberculosis drugs. *Tubercle* 1987;68:301–9.

55. Nicholson RJ et al. Leucopenia associated with lamotrigine. *BMJ* 1995;310:504.

56. Mielants H, Veys EM. A study of the hematological side effects of levamisole in rheumatoid arthritis with recommendations. *J Rheumatol* 1978;5(suppl 4):77–83.

57. El-Ghobarey AF, Capell HA. Levamisole-induced thrombocytopenia. *Br Med J* 1977;2:555–6.

58. Risk of agranulocytosis and aplastic anemia in relation to use of antithyroid drugs. International Agranulocytosis and Aplastic Anaemia Study. *BMJ* 1988;297:262–5.

59. Biswas N et al. Case report: aplastic anemia associated with antithyroid drugs. *Am J Med Sci* 1991;301:190–4.

60. Tajiri J et al. Antithyroid drug-induced agranulocytosis. The usefulness of routine white blood cell count monitoring. *Arch Intern Med* 1990;150:621–4.

61. Meyer-Gebner M et al. Antithyroid drug-induced agranulocytosis: clinical experience with ten patients treated at one institution and review of the literature. *J Endocrinol Invest* 1994;17:29–36.

62. Kelton JG. Impaired reticuloendothelial function in patients treated with methyldopa. *N Engl J Med* 1985; 313:596–600.

63. Manohitharajah SM et al. Methyldopa and associated thrombocytopenia. *Br Med J* 1971;1:494.

64. Meyboom RHB. Thrombocytopenia induced by nalidixic acid. *Br Med J* 1984;289:962.

65. Kay AGL. Myelotoxicity of D-penicillamine. *Ann Rheum Dis* 1979;38:232–6.

66. Camp AV. Hematologic toxicity from penicillamine in rheumatoid arthritis. *J Rheumatol* 1981;8(suppl 7): 164–5.

67. Lyle WH. D-penicillamine and haemolytic anaemia. *Lancet* 1976;1:428. Letter.

68. Thomas D et al. A study of D-penicillamine induced thrombocytopenia in rheumatoid arthritis with Cr^{51}-labelled autologous platelets. *Aust N Z J Med* 1981;11:722. Abstract.

69. Mallouh AA. Methicillin-induced neutropenia. *Pediatr Infect Dis J* 1985;4:262–4.

70. Jeffery WH et al. Acquired methemoglobinemia and hemolytic anemia after usual doses of phenazopyridine. *Drug Intell Clin Pharm* 1982;16:157–9.

71. Hollister LE. Allergic reactions to tranquilizing drugs. *Ann Intern Med* 1958;49:17–29.

72. Pisciotta AV et al. Agranulocytosis following administration of phenothiazine derivatives. *Am J Med* 1958; 25:210–23.

73. Cimo PL et al. Detection of drug-dependent antibodies by the ^{51}Cr platelet lysis test: documentation of immune thrombocytopenia induced by diphenylhydantoin diazepam, and sulfisoxazole. *Am J Hematol* 1977; 2:65–72.

74. Meyers DG et al. Severe neutropenia associated with procainamide: comparison of sustained release and conventional preparations. *Am Heart J* 1985;109:1393–5.

75. Thompson JF et al. Procainamide agranulocytosis: a case report and review of the literature. *Curr Ther Res* 1988;44:872–81.

76. Danielly J et al. Procainamide-associated blood dyscrasias. *Am J Cardiol* 1994;74:1179–80.

77. Fibbe WE et al. Agranulocytosis induced by propylthiouracil: evidence of a drug dependent antibody reacting with granulocytes, monocytes and haematopoietic progenitor cells. *Br J Haematol* 1986;64:363–73.

78. Custer RP. Aplastic anemia in soldiers treated with atabrine (quinacrine). *Am J Med Sci* 1946;212:211–24.

79. Ascensao JL et al. Quinidine-induced neutropenia: report of a case with drug-dependent inhibition of granulocyte colony generation. *Acta Haematol* 1984;72:349–54.

80. Geltner D et al. Quinidine hypersensitivity and liver involvement. A survey of 32 patients. *Gastroenterology* 1976;70:650–2.

81. Reid DM, Shulman NR. Drug purpura due to surreptitious quinidine intake. *Ann Intern Med* 1988;108:206–8.

82. Webb RF et al. Acute intravascular haemolysis due to quinine. *N Z Med J* 1980;91:14–6.

83. McDonald SP et al. Quinine-induced hemolytic uremic syndrome. *Clin Nephrol* 1977;47:397–400.

84. Murray JA et al. Bitter lemon purpura. *Br Med J* 1979;2:1551–2.

85. Freiman JP. Fatal quinine-induced thrombocytopenia. *Ann Intern Med* 1990;112:308–9. Letter.

86. Apseloff G et al. Severe neutropenia caused by recommended prophylactic doses of rifabutin. *Lancet* 1996;348:685. Letter.

87. Tahan SR et al. Acute hemolysis and renal failure with rifampicin-dependent antibodies after discontinuous administration. *Transfusion* 1985;25:124–7.

88. Marabani M et al. Leucopenia during sulfasalazine treatment for rheumatoid arthritis. *Ann Rheum Dis* 1989; 48:505–7.

89. Jick H et al. The risk of sulfasalazine- and mesalazine-associated blood disorders. *Pharmacotherapy* 1995;15: 176–81.

90. Cohen SM et al. Ulcerative colitis and erythrocyte G6PD deficiency. Salicylazosulfapyridine-provoked hemolysis. *JAMA* 1968;205:528–30.

91. Das KM et al. Adverse reactions during salicylazosulfapyridine therapy and the relation with drug metabolism and acetylator phenotype. *N Engl J Med* 1973;289:491–5.

92. Hopkinson ND et al. Haematological side-effects of sulphasalazine in inflammatory arthritis. *Br J Rheumatol* 1989;28:414–7.

93. Jarrett F et al. Acute leukopenia during topical burn therapy with silver sulfadiazine. *Am J Surg* 1978;135: 818–9.

94. Anti-infective drug use in relation to the risk of agranulocytosis and aplastic anemia. The International Agranulocytosis and Aplastic Anemia Study. *Arch Intern Med* 1989;149:1036–40.

95. Zinkham WH. Unstable hemoglobins and the selective hemolytic action of sulfonamides. The International Agranulocytosis and Aplastic Anemia Study. *Arch Intern Med* 1977;137:1365–6. Editorial.

96. Hass WK et al. A randomized trial comparing ticlopidine hydrochloride with aspirin for the prevention of stroke in high-risk patients. *N Engl J Med* 1989;321:501–7.

97. Volosin K et al. Tocainide associated agranulocytosis. *Am Heart J* 1985;109:1392–3.

98. Roden DM, Woosley RL. Tocainide. *N Engl J Med* 1986;315:41–5.

99. Hawkins T et al. Severe trimethoprim induced neutropenia and thrombocytopenia. *N Z Med J* 1993;106: 251–2.

100. Jonville-Béra AP et al. Thrombocytopenic purpura after measles, mumps and rubella vaccination: a retrospective survey by the French Regional Pharmacovigilance Centres and Pasteur-Mérieux Sérums et Vaccins. *Pediatr Infect Dis J* 1996;15:44–8.

101. May RB, Sunder TR. Hematologic manifestations of long-term valproate therapy. *Epilepsia* 1993;34: 1098–101.

102. Mackett RL, Guay DRP. Vancomycin-induced neutropenia. *Can Med Assoc J* 1985;132:39–40.

103. Sacho H, Moore PJ. Vancomycin-induced neutropenia. *S Afr Med J* 1989;76:701. Letter.

104. Bertolet BD et al. Neutropenia occurring during treatment with vesnarinone (OPC-8212). *Am J Cardiol* 1994; 74:968–70.

105. Furusawa S et al. Vesnarinone-induced granulocytopenia: incidence in Japan and recommendations for safety. *J Clin Pharmacol* 1996;36:477–81.

106. Richman DD et al. The toxicity of azidothymidine (AZT) in the treatment of patients with AIDS and AIDS-related complex. A double-blind, placebo-controlled trial. *N Engl J Med* 1987;317:192–7.

107. Rachlis A, Fanning MM. Zidovudine toxicity. Clinical features and management. *Drug Saf* 1993;8:312–20.

108. Snower DP, Weil SC. Changing etiology of macrocytosis. Zidovudine as a frequent causative factor. *Am J Clin Pathol* 1993;99:57–60.

DRUG-INDUCED HEPATOTOXICITY

This table includes only those drugs with well-established records of hepatotoxicity. Absence of a drug should not be interpreted to mean that a drug is incapable of producing liver damage, because virtually all drugs have been reported to produce elevations of serum liver enzymes. Combining drugs that have hepatotoxic potential commonly results in greater than additive liver damage. In general, drug-induced hepatotoxicity is most prevalent in older patients, women, and those with pre-existing hepatic impairment.

ACE Inhibitors

Hepatic injury occurs occasionally with angiotensin converting enzyme (ACE) inhibitors. **Captopril** and **enalapril** are implicated in most reported cases, but other ACE inhibitors likely have similar hepatotoxic potential. Most cases show cholestatic injury, but mixed and hepatocellular damage are also reported.[1-3]

Acetaminophen

Centrilobular hepatic necrosis may follow acute overdose with ≥140 mg/kg in children, or ≥6 g in adults. These doses saturate the normal metabolic pathways, producing large quantities of a hepatotoxic metabolite. Children appear to have a lower risk than adults of developing acetaminophen-induced hepatitis. Laboratory evidence of hepatotoxicity peaks 3–4 days after the acute exposure. Therapy with **acetylcysteine** to bind the metabolite is indicated when the 4-hr postingestion serum acetaminophen level is over 150 mg/L. Even without acetylcysteine, fatalities are uncommon following acetaminophen overdose. Nonfatal cases usually recover fully in a few weeks. Chronic **alcohol** ingestion increases acetaminophen toxicity as does recent fasting. Acute alcohol ingestion is thought by some to have a protective action. Less destructive, but still detectable, hepatitis is reported in patients taking large acetaminophen doses for therapeutic purposes.[1,3-5]

Alcohol

Fatty infiltration of the liver occurs in 70–100% of alcoholics. Fatty liver is generally without clinical manifestation, but 30% of alcoholics progress to develop alcoholic hepatitis and about 10% develop cirrhosis. Malnutrition may potentiate alcoholic liver disease, and alcohol may enhance the hepatotoxicity of other drugs.[2]

Aldesleukin

Increases in serum bilirubin, alkaline phosphatase, and transaminases occur frequently. These primarily cholestatic changes are rapidly reversible after drug discontinuation.[6]

Allopurinol

Hepatitis and hepatic necrosis may accompany other symptoms (especially rash, fever, eosinophilia, and vasculitis) of allopurinol hypersensitivity. Damage is usually focal, but widespread damage is also reported. This reaction is rare, but serious when it occurs. Renal impairment may be a predisposing factor for allopurinol-induced hepatitis. Cholestasis has also been attributed to allopurinol.[1,2,7,8]

Aminoglutethimide

Laboratory evidence of hepatic dysfunction is common, but clinical evidence is rare.[1,7,9]

Aminosalicylic Acid

Up to 5% of patients develop a generalized hypersensitivity reaction. About 25% of these patients have evidence of mixed cholestatic and hepatocellular injury as part of their hypersensitivity reaction. Fatalities have been reported.[1,2,10]

(continued)

Amiodarone

Mild increases in transaminases and LDH levels occur in up to one-half of patients, while phospholipidosis occurs in virtually all; normal values often return despite continued therapy. Symptoms of liver injury (eg, jaundice, nausea and vomiting, hepatomegaly, or weight loss) occur in 1–4% of patients. Onset is typically after 2–4 months of therapy, but may be delayed for 1 yr or more. Recovery after drug discontinuation may take from several months to 1 yr or more. The dose-related hepatotoxicity of amiodarone is reminiscent of alcoholic hepatitis. Cirrhosis and fatalities have also been reported.[1,2,11–13]

Amoxicillin and Clavulanic Acid

Based on an extensive review of medical records, the frequency of acute hepatic injury with amoxicillin and clavulanic acid is 1.7 cases/10,000 prescriptions (compared with 0.3 for amoxicillin alone). In most cases, the hepatic injury is cholestatic. The risk of hepatic injury is increased by repeated prescriptions for amoxicillin and clavulanic acid and by advancing age.[2,14]

Androgens

(*See* Steroids, C–17–α-Alkyl.)

Antidepressants, Heterocyclic

The prevalence of hepatic injury is estimated at about 1%, with most of the cases presenting as cholestasis. This idiosyncratic reaction resembles the cholestasis associated with phenothiazines.[1,2,7]

Asparaginase

Slowly reversible steatosis occurs in 50–90% of patients, apparently as a result of the drug's influence on protein synthesis. Daily administration may be more hepatotoxic than weekly administration.[1,2,15–17]

Azathioprine

This drug is less hepatotoxic than its metabolite mercaptopurine. Azathioprine's hepatotoxicity is predominantly cholestatic rather than hepatocellular. Vascular lesions, including venous occlusion and peliosis hepatis, have been reported, but their prevalence is unknown. Nodular regenerative hyperplasia has followed use in kidney and liver transplantation.[2,8,15,18]

Busulfan

Use of this drug in bone marrow transplant patients is associated with apparently dose-related veno-occlusive disease of the liver. Although the exact contribution of the drug is difficult to discern, this syndrome occurs in 20% of adults and in 5% of children treated with total doses of 16 mg/kg or more.[2,15,19,20]

Carbamazepine

Hepatic necrosis, granulomas, and cholestasis have all occurred, with some cases showing signs of hypersensitivity. Onset is most often in the first 4 weeks of therapy. Fatalities have been reported.[1,2,21]

Carmustine

Changes in liver function tests are found in 20–30% of patients, from a few days to several weeks after drug administration. These changes are usually mild and resolve quickly with drug discontinuation.[15]

Cephalosporins

Transient minor increases in AST, ALT, and alkaline phosphatase occur frequently. **Ceftriaxone** use is associated with development of "gallbladder sludge" in up to 25% of patients.[22]

(*continued*)

Chenodiol

Dose-related elevations in hepatic enzymes and a 0.4–3% prevalence of "clinically significant" hepatic injury occur.[1,23]

Chlorpropamide

Most reported hepatotoxic reactions are cholestatic, and are probably caused by an immune mechanism. Prevalence is estimated at 0.5–1.5%, with the onset usually within the first 2 months of therapy.[1,7]

Chlorzoxazone

Idiosyncratic hepatocellular damage occurs rarely, but fatalities have been reported. Discontinue the drug if elevated transaminases or bilirubin are detected.[24]

Cisplatin

Transient, dose-related elevations of hepatic enzymes occur frequently.[1,16]

Clozapine

Transient elevations of hepatic enzymes occur frequently during the first 3 months of clozapine use. While several cases of fulminant hepatitis have been reported, the risk of serious clozapine-induced hepatotoxicity remains small and some authors recommend against routine testing.[25,26]

Cocaine

Hepatic necrosis has been reported in cases of cocaine abuse, including at least one fatality. The prevalence of this reaction is not known.[2,11,27]

Contraceptives, Oral

Data from two large, long-term cohort studies (about 33,000 users) did not detect any association between oral contraceptive use and serious liver disease. One of the studies detected an increase in the frequency of mild liver disease among users of older, high-estrogen (>50 µg) products. Older combination oral contraceptives were associated with an increase in the annual incidence of hepatic adenomas (3.4/100,000 vs. 1.3/100,000 in nonusers), especially after 5 or more years of use. The frequency of gallbladder disease was also increased by older oral contraceptives.[1,2,7,28,29]

Cyclosporine

Elevated serum levels of alkaline phosphatase and conjugated hyperbilirubin occur in 50–60% of patients. These changes are usually mild and pose little threat.[1,30,31]

Dantrolene

At least 1.8% of patients develop laboratory evidence of hepatic dysfunction, with symptomatic hepatitis in about 0.6%; the fatality rate among jaundiced patients is about 25%. Predisposing factors seem to include dosage (>300 mg/day), sex (women more than men), age (>30 yr), and duration of therapy (≥2 months).[1,32,33]

Dapsone

Hepatitis may occur as part of the "dapsone syndrome," which is a generalized hypersensitivity reaction including rash, fever, and lymphadenopathy. The true prevalence is unknown, but has been estimated to be as high as 5%. The onset is usually during the first 2 months of therapy. Although most dapsone-associated liver injury is hepatocellular, some cases of cholestasis have occurred.[1,2,7,34–36]

(*continued*)

Disulfiram

This drug is occasionally associated with hepatitis, which may be caused by hypersensitivity. Most cases develop during the first few weeks of treatment. Deaths have been reported.[2,37,38]

Erythromycin

Erythromycin was thought to be a frequent cause of jaundice, but recent studies indicate that jaundice occurs only occasionally. Cholestasis apparently results from hypersensitivity (60% have eosinophilia and 50% have fever), which appears after 10–14 days of initial therapy or after 1–2 days in patients with a previous history of erythromycin exposure. Despite extensive use of the drug in children, most cases are reported in adults. Rapid reversal of symptoms follows drug discontinuation, but laboratory changes may persist for up to 6 months. Although most cases involve the estolate salt, hepatotoxicity has occurred with the ethylsuccinate, stearate, and propionate salts, and with erythromycin base.[1,2,7,39–41]

Ethionamide

Hepatitis may occur in 3–5% of patients, and serum enzyme elevations in 30% or more. Onset of hepatitis is usually after several months of therapy.[1,2,42]

Etretinate

Elevated hepatic enzymes occur in up to one-third of patients, but further evidence of hepatocellular damage is rare. Onset occurs most often 3–6 months after the start of therapy. Liver function tests should be monitored every 2–4 weeks for the first 4–6 months of therapy.[1,2,43]

Felbamate

Although the prevalence of hepatocellular destruction is unclear, it is of sufficient concern to limit the use of felbamate to carefully selected patients. At least six cases of fatal felbamate-induced hepatic necrosis have been reported.[44]

Ferrous Salts

Hepatic necrosis may appear within 1–3 days of an acute overdose. The fatality rate is high if the patient is not treated promptly.

Floxuridine

Hepatic arterial infusion of floxuridine results in 9% sclerosing cholangitis at 9 months and 26% after 1 yr. Elevations of liver enzyme levels are common, but are not predictive of greater hepatotoxicity.[2,16,45]

Flutamide

Through 1994, there were as least 20 reported deaths reasonably attributed to flutamide-induced hepatotoxicity. The deaths, typically the result of massive hepatic necrosis, occurred between 5 days and 9 months (mean 3 months) after the initiation of flutamide therapy. At the same time, the hospitalization rate for noninfectious liver disease in flutamide-treated patients was 10 times the expected rate. Flutamide use should be accompanied by regular liver function testing.[2,46]

Gold Salts

Cholestasis occurs occasionally with normal doses of parenteral gold salts; hypersensitivity is the suspected mechanism. Onset is commonly within the first few weeks of therapy, and recovery usually occurs within 3 months after drug discontinuation. Lipogranulomas are frequently found in liver biopsies of parenteral gold-treated patients. These may persist long after drug withdrawal, but do not seem to impair liver function. Hepatic necrosis may result from overdose.[1,7,47,48]

(continued)

Halothane

As many as 30% of patients may have increased serum transaminases or other evidence of mild hepatic impairment. Despite extensive publicity, the actual frequency of severe halothane hepatitis is low, ranging from 1/3500 to 1/35,000, with reported fatality rates of 17–96%. Susceptibility is greatest in adults, women, obese patients, and especially in patients with prior exposure to halothane. The mechanism of halothane hepatitis is poorly understood, but hypersensitivity is the most likely explanation. Fever precedes jaundice in most patients. The onset of jaundice is usually 5–8.5 days after exposure, but can occur between 1 and 26 days; shorter latent periods are associated with prior halothane exposure. **Methoxyflurane** and **enflurane** produce similar hepatotoxic reactions, although less frequently.[1,3,49,50]

Histamine H₂-Receptor Antagonists

Cimetidine and **ranitidine** have been associated with increased liver enzymes. The risk of acute liver injury with cimetidine is about 1/5000, with most cases occurring during the first 2 months of use.[51]

Isoniazid

Elevated serum transaminase levels occur frequently, are presumed to be associated with subclinical hepatitis, resolve rapidly after drug discontinuation, and may resolve despite continued isoniazid therapy. A syndrome resembling viral hepatitis occurs in 1–2% of patients, with the onset usually during the first 20 weeks of therapy. The fatality rate from isoniazid hepatitis has fallen steadily over the past 2 decades, probably in response to more aggressive monitoring, and is now estimated to be 1.7/100,000 patients starting isoniazid and 2.9/100,000 patients completing a course of therapy. Most fatalities occur in women. Despite the widespread assumption that patients under 35 yr are unlikely to develop isoniazid-induced fatal hepatotoxicity, reported deaths indicate otherwise. **Alcohol** consumption increases the risk of hepatotoxicity, while the contribution of concomitant administration of **rifampin** is poorly defined. The role of acetylator phenotype remains unclear, but a case-control study found that patients admitted to the hospital for suspected isoniazid-induced hepatotoxicity were significantly more likely to be slow acetylators than isoniazid-treated patients who completed their courses of therapy without hepatotoxicity.[1,2,11,52,53]

Ketoconazole

Elevated hepatic enzyme levels occur in about 20% of ketoconazole-treated patients with overt hepatitis in 3%. The typical onset for overt hepatitis is 30–60 days after initiation of ketoconazole therapy. There have been a few deaths attributed to ketoconazole hepatotoxicity.[1,2,7,54]

Mercaptopurine

Jaundice associated with cholestasis, hepatic necrosis, and mixed reactions occurs in 6–40% of patients, with the highest prevalence associated with doses of 2 mg/kg/day or more. Onset is usually during the first 2 months of therapy.[1,2,15,55]

Methotrexate

Hepatic injury (macrovesicular steatosis, necrosis, and bridging fibrosis) occurs frequently, depends on dose and duration of therapy, and may progress to cirrhosis if the drug is not stopped. Intermittent high doses pose less risk than daily low doses. Cirrhosis is reported in up to 24% of patients receiving long-term daily doses; other contributing factors include alcoholism and pre-existing liver or kidney disease. Hepatic fibrosis is not reflected by standard liver function tests and is best detected by biopsy. Biopsy has been recommended at intervals of up to 36 months, after every 1.5 g of

(continued)

methotrexate, if 6 of 12 monthly transaminase levels are elevated, or if the serum albumin level drops below normal. Isolated elevations of transaminase levels do not preclude continued methotrexate therapy.[1–3,15,56–58]

Methyldopa

Mild changes in liver function tests occur in up to 35% of patients taking methyldopa, but the prevalence of clinical hepatitis is probably less than 1%. Most cases occur during the first 3 months of therapy. Hepatitis is more common in women, and most patients have rapid recovery after drug discontinuation. The fatality rate is less than 10% among patients who develop hepatitis. There is evidence to support a hypersensitivity mechanism in some patients.[1,59]

Minocycline

The long-term use of minocycline for acne and arthritis has resulted in a growing number of cases of minocycline-induced hepatitis. The presence of fever, rash, and eosinophilia strongly implies a hypersensitivity mechanism. Onset of clinical symptoms ranges from 4 weeks to 2 years after the initiation of minocycline therapy.[60,61]

Niacin

Elevations of hepatic enzyme and bilirubin levels occur in 30–50% of patients taking sustained-release niacin in therapeutic doses. Symptomatic hepatic dysfunction occurs frequently and limits the use of the sustained-release product. Immediate-release niacin is also hepatotoxic, but to a lesser extent than sustained-release.[1,2,62]

Nitrofurantoin

Hepatic damage occurs occasionally, usually during the first month of therapy. Cholestasis is the most common presentation; hepatic necrosis is also reported. Hypersensitivity is the suspected mechanism, and the onset is frequently associated with fever, rash, and eosinophilia. Several late-developing cases of chronic active hepatitis have been reported; almost all are in women and after >6 months of therapy.[1,2,63]

Nonsteroidal Anti-inflammatory Drugs

The incidence of clinically apparent hepatic injury from nonsalicylate NSAIDs is estimated to be about 1/10,000 patient–years. The incidence for **sulindac** may be 5–10 times higher than for the other nonsalicylate NSAIDs; despite previous reports to the contrary, current data analysis does not support a higher incidence of hepatotoxicity with **diclofenac**.[2,4,64]

Octreotide

The majority of patients receiving long-term octreotide therapy develop cholelithiasis and/or gallbladder sludge; some require cholecystectomy. The prevalence and speed of onset of symptoms may be dosage related.[65]

Papaverine

Numerous reports of hepatocellular injury and elevated liver enzymes in 27–43% of patients indicate a marked hepatotoxic potential.[1,2,66]

Pemoline

Pemoline occasionally causes elevated liver enzymes. The prescribing information for pemoline includes a boxed warning describing 13 cases of acute hepatic failure reported to the FDA between 1975 and 1996; 11 cases resulted in death or required liver transplantation. The earliest onset of hepatic abnormalities in these cases occurred 6 months after the start of pemoline therapy. The few published reports of possible pemoline-induced fulminant hepatic failure do not hold up well under close scrutiny.[67]

(*continued*)

Penicillamine
Cholestasis occurs occasionally.[1,2,8,68]

Penicillins
Cloxacillin and **flucloxacillin** are rarely associated with cholestatic hepatitis. The effect is reversible, but it may persist for months after drug discontinuation.[1–3,69–71]

Phenothiazines
Most reports of liver damage involve **chlorpromazine.** The prevalence of hepatic enzyme elevation with this drug has been estimated to be as high as 42%, although 10% is probably more realistic. Similarly, cholestatic jaundice has been projected to occur in up to 5% of patients receiving chlorpromazine, but the actual prevalence is closer to 1%. The onset of cholestasis is generally in the first month of therapy and usually follows a prodrome of GI or influenza-like symptoms. About 70% of affected patients show signs of hypersensitivity, most frequently fever and eosinophilia, while only 5% have rash. Cholestasis usually follows a benign course, and most patients recover 1–2 months after drug discontinuation. A syndrome resembling primary biliary cirrhosis may occasionally occur. Despite the dominance of chlorpromazine in the reported cases, other phenothiazines are capable of producing similar hepatic damage.[1–3,72]

Phenytoin
Hepatocellular necrosis has been occasionally associated with phenytoin therapy. It is usually accompanied by other signs of hypersensitivity (eg, eosinophilia, fever, rash, lymphadenopathy). Onset usually occurs during the first 6 weeks of therapy. Reported fatality rates have been as high as 30%.[1,2,11,73,74]

Plicamycin
Laboratory evidence of dose-related hepatotoxicity occurs in virtually all patients. A common lesion is perivenous necrosis.[1–3,75]

Progestins
(*See* Steroids, C–17–α–Alkyl.)

Propoxyphene
A small number of cases of propoxyphene-induced cholestasis have been reported; these are thought to be the result of hypersensitivity.[1,2,7,76]

Propylthiouracil
Increases in ALT levels occur in up to 30% of patients. Onset is usually within the first 2 months of therapy, and ALT levels commonly return to normal with dosage reduction. Clinical hepatitis occurs rarely.[1,2,77]

Pyrazinamide
Pyrazinamide-induced hepatitis depends on dose and duration of therapy. Daily administration appears to present a greater risk than weekly administration.[1,78,79]

Riluzole
Elevated hepatic enzymes occur frequently, and the prevalence appears to be dosage related.[80]

Quinidine
Hepatic damage is rare and is usually accompanied by other signs of hypersensitivity, especially fever. Most reactions occur in the first month of therapy. The pathology is usually a mixture of hepatocellular necrosis and cholestasis; granulomas have also been reported.[1,81]

(*continued*)

Salicylates

Up to 50% of patients taking antiarthritic dosages have laboratory evidence of liver damage. The risk of liver damage is greatest in patients with connective tissue disorders such as SLE or juvenile rheumatoid arthritis. Clinically apparent salicylate-induced hepatitis is uncommon, usually mild, and readily reversible. Hepatotoxicity most often occurs at serum salicylate levels >250 mg/L, and only 7% of cases have serum salicylate levels <150 mg/L. Salicylates may cause microvesicular steatosis following intentional overdose.[1,2]

Steroids, C–17–α-Alkyl

Canalicular cholestasis occurs with a minimal amount of hepatic inflammation. The prevalence appears to be dose related; although laboratory changes are common (occurring in almost all patients taking anabolic steroids), jaundice is not. Jaundice may or may not be preceded by other clinical signs and usually follows 1–6 months of therapy. Peliosis hepatis has also been associated with these compounds, especially the anabolic steroids. Examples include **methyltestosterone, norethandrolone, methandrostenolone, fluoxymesterone, oxandrolone, oxymetholone,** and **stanozolol.** C–17–α-ethinyl steroids such as **ethinyl estradiol, mestranol, norethindrone,** and **norethynodrel** may produce similar reactions. An association between C–17–α-alkyl steroids and an increase in the prevalence of hepatocellular carcinoma is unclear.[1,2,7,82]

Sulfasalazine

A small number of cases of sulfasalazine-associated hepatic damage, including fatalities, have been reported in both children and adults. Hepatic necrosis is apparently part of a generalized hypersensitivity reaction that includes rash, fever, and lymphadenopathy. Onset is usually within the first 4 weeks of therapy.[1,2,83]

Sulfonamides, Antibacterial

The sulfonamides currently in use appear to have a lower prevalence of hepatitis than their predecessors, with most reported cases appearing before 1947. Most cases of hepatotoxicity develop during the first 2 weeks of therapy and many are accompanied by other signs of hypersensitivity.[1,2,41,84] (*See also* Trimethoprim-Sulfamethoxazole.)

Tacrine

In a study of 2446 patients receiving tacrine, 25% had serum ALT levels at least 3 times greater than the upper limit of normal (ULN), 6% had levels at least 10 times greater than the ULN, and 2% had levels at least 25 times greater than the ULN. Most increases were detected in the first week of therapy. Most patients' ALT levels returned to no more than twice the ULN within 1 month after drug discontinuation, and no patients developed jaundice. Only 33% developed ALT levels more than 3 times the ULN on rechallenge.[85]

Tetracycline

Microvesicular steatosis may occur in patients receiving large doses of tetracycline IV, usually in excess of 1.5 g/day. Contributing factors include pregnancy, malnutrition, and impaired renal function, but hepatotoxicity has been reported in patients with none of these. Onset is most often during the first 10 days of therapy. Most cases of overt liver disease have resulted in death. Oral therapy may also produce signs of hepatotoxicity, although far less frequently.[1,2,41]

(*continued*)

Tizanidine
Increases in liver enzymes described by the authors as "clinically significant" occurred in 5–7% of patients treated with tizanidine. These increases resolved after drug discontinuation.[86]

Tolcapone
ALT levels increase to >3 times the upper limit of normal in about 8% of tolcapone-treated patients. These elevations usually develop 6–12 weeks after the start of tolcapone use and may resolve despite continued therapy.[87]

Trimethoprim-Sulfamethoxazole
"Clinically important" liver disease occurs in at least 5.2/100,000 patients (3.8/100,000 with trimethoprim alone). The available evidence supports hypersensitivity as the mechanism and cholestasis as the predominant form of injury. Fulminant hepatic failure has been reported.[2,41,88]

Troglitazone
Mild, asymptomatic hepatocellular injury occurs frequently with troglitazone; usually after 3–7 months of use. Severe liver injury occurs occasionally.[89]

Troleandomycin
From 30 to 50% of patients receiving the drug show some laboratory evidence of abnormal liver function, and up to 4% develop jaundice.[1,2]

Valproic Acid
Hepatic enzyme elevations occur in 6–44% of patients, with clinically apparent liver disease in 0.05–1%. Fatal hepatotoxicity occurs most often in children ≤2 yr old on polydrug therapy (1/600); 3–10 yr olds on monotherapy (1/16,000) or polytherapy (1/8300). The diffuse hepatocellular injury, microvesicular steatosis, and hepatic necrosis do not appear to be dose related and most commonly occur in the first 2–3 months of therapy. Serial liver function tests in asymptomatic patients do not predict patients at risk, but are commonly recommended because immediate discontinuation may reverse the condition.[1,2,74,90,91]

Vitamin A
Hepatomegaly, portal hypertension, and mild increases in liver enzyme levels are common features of chronic vitamin A toxicity. Central vein sclerosis and perisinusoidal fibrosis, which may progress to cirrhosis, have been reported in cases of chronic intoxication. These effects are associated with doses over 50,000 IU/day (sometimes with doses as low as 25,000 IU/day). Hepatotoxicity is also possible with acute doses over 600,000 IU.[1,2,92]

■ REFERENCES

1. Stricker BHCh. *Drug-induced hepatic injury.* 2nd ed. Amsterdam: Elsevier; 1992.
2. Zimmerman HJ. Hepatotoxicity. *Dis Mon* 1993;39:675–787.
3. Hagley MT et al. Hepatotoxicity associated with angiotensin-converting enzyme inhibitors. *Ann Pharmacother* 1993;27:228–31.
4. Whitcomb DC, Block GD. Association of acetaminophen hepatotoxicity with fasting and ethanol use. *JAMA* 1994;272:1845–50.
5. Heubi JE et al. Therapeutic misadventures with acetaminophen: hepatotoxicity after multiple doses in children. *J Pediatr* 1998;132:22–7.
6. Fisher B et al. Interleukin-2 induces profound reversible cholestasis: a detailed analysis in treated cancer patients. *J Clin Oncol* 1989;7:1852–62.
7. Zimmerman HJ, Lewis JH. Drug-induced cholestasis. *Med Toxicol* 1987;2:112–60.
8. Arellano F, Sacristán JA. Allopurinol hypersensitivity syndrome: a review. *Ann Pharmacother* 1993;27:337–43.

9. Nagel GA et al. Phase II study of aminoglutethimide and medroxyprogesterone acetate in the treatment of patients with advanced breast cancer. *Cancer Res* 1982;42(suppl):3442S–4S.

10. Simpson DG, Walker JH. Hypersensitivity to para-aminosalicylic acid. *Am J Med* 1960;29:297–306.

11. Lee WM. Drug-induced hepatotoxicity. *N Engl J Med* 1995;333:1118–27.

12. Guigui B et al. Amiodarone-induced hepatic phospholipidosis: a morphological alteration independent of pseudoalcoholic liver disease. *Hepatology* 1988;8:1063–8.

13. Richer M, Robert S. Fatal hepatotoxicity following oral administration of amiodarone. *Ann Pharmacother* 1995; 29:582–6.

14. Garcia Rodriguez LA et al. Risk of acute liver injury associated with combination of amoxicillin and clavulanic acid. *Arch Intern Med* 1996;156:1327–32.

15. Perry MC. Chemotherapeutic agents and hepatotoxicity. *Semin Oncol* 1992;19:551–65.

16. Pratt CB et al. Comparison of daily versus weekly L-asparaginase for the treatment of childhood acute leukemia. *J Pediatr* 1970;77:474–83.

17. Pratt CB, Johnson WW. Duration and severity of fatty metamorphosis of the liver following L-asparaginase therapy. *Cancer* 1971;28:361–4.

18. Gane E et al. Nodular regenerative hyperplasia of the liver graft after liver transplantation. *Hepatology* 1994; 20:88–94.

19. Grochow LB et al. Pharmacokinetics of busulfan: correlation with veno-occlusive disease in patients undergoing bone marrow transplantation. *Cancer Chemother Pharmacol* 1989;25:55–61.

20. Vassal G et al. Busulfan and veno-occlusive disease of the liver. *Ann Intern Med* 1990;112:881. Letter.

21. Horowitz S et al. Hepatotoxic reactions associated with carbamazepine therapy. *Epilepsia* 1988;29:149–54.

22. Thompson JW, Jacobs RF. Adverse effects of newer cephalosporins. An update. *Drug Saf* 1993;9:132–42.

23. Schoenfield LJ et al. Chenodiol (chenodeoxycholic acid) for dissolution of gallstones: The National Cooperative Gallstone Study. A controlled trial of efficacy and safety. *Ann Intern Med* 1981;95:257–82.

24. Labeling change. *FDA Med Bull* 1996;26(1):3.

25. MacFarlane B et al. Fatal fulminant liver failure due to clozapine: a case report and review of clozapine-induced hepatotoxicity. *Gastroenterology* 1997;112:1707–9.

26. Hummer M et al. Hepatotoxicity of clozapine. *J Clin Psychopharmacol* 1997;17:314–7.

27. Wanless IR et al. Histopathology of cocaine hepatotoxicity. Report of four patients. *Gastroenterology* 1990;98:497–501.

28. Lindberg MC. Hepatobiliary complications of oral contraceptives. *J Gen Intern Med* 1992;7:199–209.

29. Hannaford PC et al. Combined oral contraceptives and liver disease. *Contraception* 1997;55:145–51.

30. Atkinson K et al. Cyclosporine-associated hepatotoxicity after allogeneic marrow transplantation in man: differentiation from other causes of posttransplant liver disease. *Transplant Proc* 1983;15(suppl 1):2761–7.

31. Kassianides C et al. Liver injury from cyclosporine A. *Dig Dis Sci* 1990;35:693–7.

32. Utili R et al. Dantrolene-associated hepatic injury. Incidence and character. *Gastroenterology* 1977;72:610–6.

33. Ward A et al. Dantrolene. A review of its pharmacodynamic and pharmacokinetic properties and therapeutic use in malignant hyperthermia, the neuroleptic malignant syndrome and an update of its use in muscle spasticity. *Drugs* 1986;32:130–68.

34. Tomecki KJ, Catalano CJ. Dapsone hypersensitivity. The sulfone syndrome revisited. *Arch Dermatol* 1981;117: 38–9.

35. Kromann NP et al. The dapsone syndrome. *Arch Dermatol* 1982;118:531–2.

36. Mohle-Boetani J et al. The sulfone syndrome in a patient receiving dapsone prophylaxis for *Pneumocystis carinii* pneumonia. *West J Med* 1992;156:303–6.

37. Wright C et al. Disulfiram-induced fulminating hepatitis: guidelines for liver-panel monitoring. *J Clin Psychiatry* 1988;49:430–4.

38. Mason NA. Disulfiram-induced hepatitis: case report and review of the literature. *DICP* 1989;23:872–5.

39. Inman WHW, Rawson NSB. Erythromycin estolate and jaundice. *Br Med J* 1983;286:1954–5.

40. Derby LE et al. Erythromycin-associated cholestatic hepatitis. *Med J Aust* 1993;158:600–2.

41. Carson JL et al. Acute liver disease associated with erythromycins, sulfonamides, and tetracyclines. *Ann Intern Med* 1993;119:576–83.

42. Conn HO et al. Ethionamide-induced hepatitis. A review with a report of an additional case. *Am Rev Resp Dis* 1964;90:542–52.

43. Sanchez MR et al. Retinoid hepatitis. *J Am Acad Dermatol* 1993;28:853–8.

44. O'Neil MG et al. Felbamate associated fatal acute hepatic necrosis. *Neurology* 1996;46:1457–9.

45. Rougier P et al. Hepatic arterial infusion of floxuridine in patients with liver metastases from colorectal carcinoma: long-term results of a prospective randomized trial. *J Clin Oncol* 1992;10:1112–8.

46. Wysowski DK, Fourcroy JL. Flutamide hepatotoxicity. *J Urol* 1996;155:209–12.

47. Howrie DL, Gartner JC. Gold-induced hepatotoxicity: case report and review of the literature. *J Rheumatol* 1982;9:727–9.

48. Landas SK et al. Lipogranulomas and gold in the liver in rheumatoid arthritis. *Am J Surg Pathol* 1992;16:171–4.

49. Neuberger JM. Halothane and hepatitis. Incidence, predisposing factors and exposure guidelines. *Drug Saf* 1990;5:28–38.

50. Elliott RH, Strunin L. Hepatotoxicity of volatile anaesthetics. *Br J Anaesth* 1993;70:339–48.

51. Garcia Rodriguez LA et al. The risk of acute liver injury associated with cimetidine and other acid-suppressing anti-ulcer drugs. *Br J Clin Pharmacol* 1997;43:183–8.

52. Millard PS et al. Isoniazid-related fatal hepatitis. *West J Med* 1996;164:486–91.

53. Pande JN et al. Risk factors for hepatotoxicity from antituberculosis drugs: a case-control study. *Thorax* 1996; 51:132–6.

54. Chien R-N et al. Hepatic injury during ketoconazole therapy in patients with onychomycosis: a controlled cohort study. *Hepatology* 1997;25:103–7.

55. Einhorn M, Davidsohn I. Hepatotoxicity of mercaptopurine. *JAMA* 1964;188:802–6.

56. Lewis JH, Schiff E. Methotrexate-induced chronic liver injury: guidelines for detection and prevention. *Am J Gastroenterol* 1988;88:1337–45.

57. Kremer JM et al. Methotrexate for rheumatoid arthritis. Suggested guidelines for monitoring liver toxicity. *Arthritis Rheum* 1994;37:316–28.

58. Farrow AC et al. Serum aminotransferase elevation during and following treatment of childhood acute lymphoblastic leukemia. *J Clin Oncol* 1997;15:1560–6.

59. Rodman JS et al. Methyldopa hepatitis. A report of six cases and review of the literature. *Am J Med* 1976; 60:941–8.

60. Malcolm A et al. Minocycline-induced liver injury. *Am J Gastroenterol* 1996;91:1641–3.

61. Gough A et al. Minocycline induced autoimmune hepatitis and systemic lupus erythematosis-like syndrome. *BMJ* 1996;312:169–72.

62. McKenney JM et al. A comparison of the efficacy and toxic effects of sustained- vs immediate-release niacin in hypercholesterolemic patients. *JAMA* 1994;271:672–7.

63. Stricker BH et al. Hepatic injury associated with the use of nitrofurans: a clinicopathological study of 52 reported cases. *Hepatology* 1988;8:599–606.

64. Walker AM. Quantitative studies of the risk of serious hepatic injury in persons using nonsteroidal anti-inflammatory drugs. *Arthritis Rheum* 1997;40:201–8.

65. Trendle MC et al. Incidence and morbidity of cholestasis in patients receiving chronic octreotide for metastatic carcinoid and malignant islet cell tumors. *Cancer* 1997;79:830–4.

66. Pathy MS, Reynolds AJ. Papaverine and hepatotoxicity. *Postgrad Med J* 1980;56:488–90.

67. Shevell M, Schreiber R. Pemoline-associated hepatic failure: a critical analysis of the literature. *Pediatr Neurol* 1997;16:14–6.

68. Seibold JR et al. Cholestasis associated with D-penicillamine therapy: case report and review of the literature. *Arthritis Rheum* 1981;24:554–6.

69. Olsson R et al. Liver damage from flucloxacillin, cloxacillin, and dicloxacillin. *J Hepatol* 1992;15:154–61.

70. Derby LE et al. Cholestatic hepatitis associated with flucloxacillin. *Med J Aust* 1993;158:596–600.

71. Presti ME et al. Nafcillin-associated hepatotoxicity. Report of a case and review of the literature. *Dig Dis Sci* 1996;41:180–4.

72. Regal RE et al. Phenothiazine-induced cholestatic jaundice. *Clin Pharm* 1987;6:787–94.

73. Smythe MA, Umstead GS. Phenytoin hepatotoxicity: a review of the literature. *DICP* 1989;23:13–8.

74. Wyllie E, Wyllie R. Routine laboratory monitoring for serious adverse effects of antiepileptic medications: the controversy. *Epilepsia* 1991;32(suppl 5):S74–9.

75. Green L, Donehower RC. Hepatic toxicity of low doses of mithramycin in hypercalcemia. *Cancer Treat Rep* 1984;68:1379–81.

76. Bassendine MF et al. Dextropropoxyphene induced hepatotoxicity mimicking biliary tract disease. *Gut* 1986;27:444–9.

77. Liaw Y-F et al. Hepatic injury during propylthiouracil therapy in patients with hyperthyroidism. A cohort study. *Ann Intern Med* 1993;118:424–8.

78. Hong Kong Chest Service/British Medical Research Council. Controlled trial of four thrice-weekly regimens and a daily regimen all given for 6 months for pulmonary tuberculosis. *Lancet* 1981;1:171–4.

79. Cohen CD et al. Hepatic complications of antituberculosis therapy revisited. *S Afr Med J* 1983;63:960–3.

80. Miller RG et al. Clinical trials of riluzole in patients with ALS. ALS/Riluzole Study Group-II. *Neurology* 1996; 47(suppl 2):S86–92.

81. Geltner D et al. Quinidine hypersensitivity and liver involvement. A survey of 32 patients. *Gastroenterology* 1976;70:650–2.

82. Haupt HA, Rovere GD. Anabolic steroids: a review of the literature. *Am J Sports Med* 1984;12:469–84.
83. Boyer DL et al. Sulfasalazine-induced hepatotoxicity in children with inflammatory bowel disease. *J Pediatr Gastroenterol Nutr* 1989;8:528–32.
84. Dujovne CA et al. Sulfonamide hepatic injury. Review of the literature and report of a case due to sulfamethoxazole. *N Engl J Med* 1967;277:785–8.
85. Watkins PB et al. Hepatotoxic effects of tacrine administration in patients with Alzheimer's disease. *JAMA* 1994;271:992–8.
86. Wagstaff AJ, Bryson HM. Tizanidine. A review of its pharmacology, clinical efficacy and tolerability in the management of spasticity associated with cerebral and spinal disorders. *Drugs* 1997;53:435–52.
87. Waters CH et al. Tolcapone in stable Parkinson's disease: efficacy and safety of long-term treatment. The Tolcapone Stable Study Group. *Neurology* 1997;49:665–71.
88. Jick H, Derby LE. A large population-based follow-up study of trimethoprim-sulfamethoxazole, trimethoprim, and cephalexin for uncommon serious drug toxicity. *Pharmacotherapy* 1995;15:428–32.
89. Watkins PB, Whitcomb RW. Hepatic dysfunction association with troglitazone. *N Engl J Med* 1998;338:916–7.
90. Siemes H et al. Valproate (VPA) metabolites in various clinical conditions of probable VPA-associated hepatotoxicity. *Epilepsia* 1993;34:332–46.
91. Bryant AE, Dreifuss FE. Valproic acid hepatic fatalities. III. U.S. experience since 1986. *Neurology* 1996;46:465–9.
92. Kowalski TE et al. Vitamin A hepatotoxicity: a cautionary note regarding 25,000 IU supplements. *Am J Med* 1994;97:523–8.

DRUG-INDUCED NEPHROTOXICITY

This table includes agents that are associated with drug-induced nephrotoxicity, but excludes drugs that produce nephrotoxicity as a result of damage to tissues other than the kidney (eg, liver or skeletal muscle). The following abbreviations are used in the table:

Cl$_{er}$ – Creatinine Clearance
Cr$_s$ – Serum Creatinine
GFR   – Glomerular Filtration Rate
mOsm   – Milliosmoles

Acetaminophen

Tubular necrosis has been reported, usually in association with hepatotoxicity from acute overdose. Whether nephrotoxicity is a direct effect of acetaminophen or the result of the liver damage is the subject of controversy. There is a possible association between prolonged acetaminophen use (1–5 kg cumulative dosage) and the development of chronic renal failure. There is insufficient evidence to associate acetaminophen use alone with analgesic nephropathy. (*See* Analgesics.)[1–7]

ACE Inhibitors

Angiotensin-converting enzyme (ACE) inhibitors are frequently associated with the development of proteinuria and renal insufficiency. The prevalence of proteinuria in **captopril**-treated patients is estimated at 1%. The risks of renal insufficiency are greater with long-acting ACE inhibitors such as **enalapril** or **lisinopril** than with captopril. Immune complex glomerulopathy is a major contributor to ACE inhibitor nephrotoxicity. Hyponatremia, diuretic therapy (as well as other causes of hypovolemia), pre-existing renal impairment, CHF, and diabetes mellitus contribute to an increased risk of nephrotoxicity. Recovery of renal function usually follows ACE inhibitor discontinuation.[1,2,8–12]

Acetazolamide

Glaucoma therapy with acetazolamide is associated with a 10-fold increase in the risk of renal stone formation. Both calcium phosphate and calcium oxalate stones have been identified.[13,14]

(*continued*)

Acyclovir

Acyclovir is concentrated in the urine and its precipitation in the collecting tubules with subsequent obstructive nephropathy may accompany high-dose (500 mg/m^2) IV use; oral therapy is apparently free from this problem. Adequate hydration should minimize the risk. Normal renal function usually returns within 6 weeks after drug withdrawal.[2,8,15]

Aldesleukin

Almost all patients receiving aldesleukin develop acute renal impairment marked by decreased Cl$_{cr}$, oliguria or anuria, and fluid retention. Most patients recover within 1 week after drug discontinuation, but some require 1 month or more.[16]

Allopurinol

Glomerulonephritis, interstitial nephritis, and interstitial fibrosis occur rarely in allopurinol-treated patients. Most cases are associated with generalized hypersensitivity reactions to allopurinol (allopurinol hypersensitivity syndrome).[17,18]

Aminoglycosides

Proximal tubular necrosis occurs in up to 30% of patients treated with aminoglycosides for more than 7 days. Because of slow clearance of these drugs from renal tissue, they may still be present in high concentrations in the kidney after serum levels are undetectable, but there does not appear to be a good correlation between renal tissue concentrations of individual aminoglycosides and their nephrotoxic potential. Aminoglycoside-induced acute renal failure is usually nonoliguric, which may delay its recognition. It is often first detected as an asymptomatic increase in Cr$_s$. Detectable changes in GFR usually occur at least 5 days after initiation of therapy and may progress after drug discontinuation. Aminoglycoside-induced renal damage is related to total dosage and duration of treatment. Administration of single daily doses does not markedly affect the frequency of nephrotoxicity. Recovery of some to all lost renal function may occur over several weeks after drug discontinuation. Monitoring of aminoglycoside plasma levels and serial renal function tests may be of value in recognizing nephrotoxicity. **Neomycin** has the greatest and **streptomycin** the least nephrotoxic potential of the aminoglycosides. All other currently marketed aminoglycosides have intermediate nephrotoxic potentials. Concomitant therapy with other nephrotoxic drugs should be avoided.[1,2,8,9,19–22]

Amphotericin B

Some degree of nephrotoxicity occurs in almost all patients treated with amphotericin B. The drug causes a reduction in renal plasma flow as well as glomerular and tubular damage. Most patients experience a rapid decline in GFR, which often stabilizes at 20–60% of normal, and may not return to normal until several months after drug discontinuation. Distal tubular damage may lead to loss of concentrating ability, renal tubular acidosis, and electrolyte disturbances (most commonly hypokalemia, but also hyponatremia and hypomagnesemia). These effects appear to be dosage related, and many patients respond favorably to temporary drug discontinuation or a reduction in dosage. Some authors suggest that the total dosage of amphotericin B should be kept below 3–5 g to minimize permanent nephrotoxicity. Sodium loading (eg, 1 L normal saline IV daily) reduces the frequency and severity of amphotericin B–induced nephrotoxicity. Newer dosage forms (eg, liposomal amphotericin B) may also offer some protection.[1,2,8,9,23–25]

(*continued*)

Analgesics

Analgesic nephropathy is a syndrome of papillary necrosis and progressive renal medullary impairment that occurs in persons with long-term consumption of large quantities of oral analgesic products, especially combination products. Most reported patients are 30–70 yr old, and women greatly outnumber men. The syndrome is characterized by proteinuria, reduced renal concentrating ability, and the presence of RBCs and WBCs in the urine. Analgesic nephropathy has been historically attributed to **phenacetin,** but the removal of phenacetin from nonprescription analgesic products has not been consistently associated with a decline in analgesic nephropathy mortality. **Acetaminophen** or **salicylates** taken alone do not seem to cause analgesic nephropathy. Historically, this syndrome has been responsible for a large percentage of chronic renal failure deaths, with a considerable variation in prevalence among nations (high in Australia and Germany, low in the United States), apparently reflecting analgesic abuse patterns. Mild cases are reversible, but severe cases may continue to deteriorate after the discontinuation of analgesics. The prevalence of urinary tract cancer appears higher than normal among chronic analgesic abusers.[1,2,5–8]

Azacitidine

Proximal and distal tubular dysfunction, polyuria, glucosuria, and decreases in serum bicarbonate occur occasionally during azacitidine therapy.[26]

Carboplatin

Although apparently less nephrotoxic than cisplatin, carboplatin therapy is frequently associated with reductions in GFR and increased electrolyte losses (especially calcium and magnesium). Patients with pre-existing renal impairment and those who receive inadequate hydration during drug administration are at greatest risk.[27]

Cephalosporins

The cephalosporin (and cephamycin) antibiotics are capable of producing rare interstitial nephritis similar to the penicillins. Increases in BUN and Cr_s occur occasionally. The nephrotoxicity of the newer cephalosporins is minimal compared to older drugs such as **cephalothin.**[28–30]

Cidofovir

Proteinuria occurs frequently during cidofovir therapy. **Probenecid** decreases the prevalence and magnitude of proteinuria and must be given with cidofovir.[31]

Cisplatin

Dosage-related proximal tubular impairment is the major limiting factor in cisplatin therapy, and may occur in 50–75% of patients. Cl_{cr} is typically reduced to 60–80% of baseline with repeated courses of therapy. The greatest damage occurs in the first month of therapy, and it appears to be more likely when the drug is administered repetitively at close time intervals. Forced hydration and mannitol diuresis may reduce renal toxicity, at least for the first cycle of therapy. Magnesium and calcium loss are common manifestations of cisplatin-induced nephrotoxicity. Cisplatin-induced renal effects may be detected as long as 6 months after the end of therapy.[1,18,27,32]

Contrast Media, Iodinated

Increased Cr_s occurs frequently in patients receiving iodine-containing contrast media. In unselected patients, the prevalence of Cr_s >0.5 mg/dL or greater than 50% above pretreatment is 2–7%. A variety of renal lesions are described including medullary necrosis and proximal tubular vacuolation and necrosis as well as the deposition of urate and oxalate crystals. The most common pattern is acute oliguric renal failure

(*continued*)

developing within 24 hr after the administration of the contrast agent and lasting 2–5 days; nonoliguric renal failure has also been reported. Most patients recover fully, but permanent renal impairment has been reported. Cr_s usually peaks 3–5 days after exposure and returns to baseline in 10–14 days. Patients with pre-existing renal impairment are at much greater risk and constitute 60% of patients experiencing nephrotoxicity. Vigorous hydration before, during, and after drug administration reduces the risk of nephrotoxicity, but mannitol or furosemide diuresis does not. High-osmolality ionic contrast media may be more nephrotoxic than low-osmolality ionic contrast media. Newer, nonionic contrast agents may be less nephrotoxic than ionic agents.[1,2,9,33–36]

Cyclosporine

Dose-related nephrotoxicity occurs in 30–50% of cyclosporine-treated patients and frequently limits the usefulness of the drug. Reduction in dosage usually reduces the renal toxicity. The drug produces a decrease in GFR, impaired tubular function, interstitial nephritis, hypertension, fluid retention, and hyperkalemia. Cyclosporine causes vasoconstriction in preglomerular arterioles, which may lead to chronic arteriopathy and tubular atrophy if the dosage is not reduced. Cyclosporine nephrotoxicity is usually reversible during the first 6 months of therapy, but the risk of permanent renal impairment increases with time. Calcium-channel blockers appear to reduce the prevalence of cyclosporine-induced nephrotoxicity in renal transplant patients.[1,2,8,19,37,38]

Demeclocycline

This drug is capable of producing nephrogenic diabetes insipidus, which is usually, but not always, dosage related. For this reason, it has been used in the management of the syndrome of inappropriate antidiuretic hormone secretion.[19,39] (*See also* Tetracyclines.)

Diuretics, Thiazide

Occasional cases of interstitial nephritis have been reported, which may be the result of hypersensitivity reactions.[2]

Fluoroquinolones

Acute interstitial nephritis is associated with fluoroquinolone antibiotics, most commonly **ciprofloxacin.** A hypersensitivity mechanism is suspected, but remains to be confirmed.[40,41]

Foscarnet

Acute tubular necrosis occurs frequently with foscarnet. Cr_s increased during 35 of 56 courses of therapy in one retrospective study. Hydration with normal saline appears to markedly decrease the severity and frequency of nephrotoxicity.[42]

Furosemide

Use of high-dose furosemide (5–10 mg/kg/day) in adults with refractory CHF is associated with a 40% decrease in Cl_{cr}. Nephrocalcinosis and nephrolithiasis occur in up to 64% of low-birthweight infants treated with furosemide. These effects usually resolve following drug discontinuation.[43,44]

Gallium Nitrate

Nephrotoxicity is the most frequent adverse effect of gallium, and elevations in BUN and Cr_s may occur after only 1 dose. At least one death has been associated with gallium-induced nephrotoxicity.[45,46]

(*continued*)

Gold Salts

A lesion resembling membranous glomerulonephritis with proteinuria may occur in 3–10% of patients receiving parenteral gold therapy. Microhematuria and nephrotic syndrome are less frequent. One-half of the cases of proteinuria develop in the first 6 months of therapy. Occasionally, acute tubular necrosis and interstitial nephritis are reported. Although recovery may take up to 18 months, permanent renal impairment after drug withdrawal is uncommon. There is evidence for both immune and direct toxic mechanisms for gold nephrotoxicity. Oral **auranofin** appears to be less nephrotoxic than parenteral gold products.[1,2,8,9,47,48]

Ifosamide

Reversible, subclinical nephrotoxicity occurs in almost all ifosamide-treated patients, with clinically important nephrotoxicity in many. Renal damage may correlate with total dosage, and cumulative doses >100 g/m^2 should be avoided, especially in children. Fanconi syndrome-like symptoms including renal loss of glucose, electrolytes, and small proteins occur in 4%.[27,49,50]

Immune Globulin

Intravenous administration of immune globulin can produce reversible acute renal failure after the first or repeated exposures. The origin of the acute renal failure is not the immune globulin, but rather the large amount of sucrose used in some immune globulin products to reduce the formation of immunoglobulin aggregates. The damage is probably due to the delivery of a high-osmotic solute load to the kidneys. Maltose- and dextrose-stabilized products may have the same capacity, but there are no case reports in the published literature.[51]

Indinavir

Crystalluria occurs in 20% of indinavir-treated patients; many develop nephrolithiasis, back pain, or flank pain. The crystals contain indinavir and good hydration (>1.5 L fluid/day) reduces their formation.[52]

Lithium

Lithium frequently produces nephrogenic diabetes insipidus, which is at least in part dosage related. This typically mild effect is usually reversible upon drug withdrawal. It appears that long-term therapy (10–15 yr) is associated with an increased prevalence of reduced Cl_{cr} and renal concentrating ability beyond what would be explained by aging alone. Interstitial nephritis and nephrotic syndrome have also been reported.[1,2,8,9,19,53–56]

Mannitol

High doses (>200 g/day or >400 g/2 days) are associated with the development of acute oliguric renal failure. Although low doses act as renal vasodilators, high doses produce renal vasoconstriction. Keeping the osmolal gap to no more than 55 mOsm/kg should minimize the risk. Acute renal failure may require 7–10 days for recovery; dialysis shortens the recovery period to 1–2 days.[57,58]

Methotrexate

This drug is directly toxic to the kidney in large doses, producing acute tubular necrosis. Methotrexate is primarily eliminated through the kidney, and its nephrotoxicity compounds itself by causing the serum level of the drug to rise. About 20% of deaths associated with methotrexate therapy are caused by acute renal failure. The drug and its metabolites may precipitate in the distal tubule. Close monitoring of methotrexate serum levels and adjustment of dosage may help to minimize the risk of nephrotoxicity, as do vigorous hydration and alkalinization during drug administration.[2,59,60]

(*continued*)

Methoxyflurane

Nephrogenic diabetes insipidus, proximal tubular damage, and interstitial nephritis are reported. The nephrotoxicity of methoxyflurane appears to be dose related and may be caused by increased circulating fluoride ion concentrations. Fluoride causes distal tubular dysfunction by inhibiting sodium and chloride transport in the ascending loop of Henle, and reducing the response to antidiuretic hormone. Urinary oxalate crystallization has also been reported following methoxyflurane anesthesia.[19,61,62]

Mitomycin

Tubular necrosis occurs most frequently with daily therapy, but is also reported with the intermittent therapy now recommended. Nephrotoxicity appears to be related to the total dosage administered, with the risk of renal impairment rising when the total dosage exceeds 30 mg/m^2. Onset may be delayed for many months.[63,64]

Nitrosoureas

The nitrosoureas can produce insidious nephrotoxicity in patients on long-term therapy. **Lomustine** seems to have the greatest nephrotoxic potential. Some cases of permanent renal function impairment have been reported.[65]

Nonsteroidal Anti-inflammatory Drugs

NSAIDs can reduce Cl_{cr} and produce renal insufficiency as a result of renal circulatory changes caused by inhibition of prostaglandin synthesis. These effects tend to be relatively minor and usually reversible. The prevalence is usually low (0.5–1% of patients), but some patients are at increased risk; predisposing factors include advanced age, pre-existing renal impairment, and states of renal hypoperfusion (eg, sodium depletion, hypotension, diuretic use, hepatic cirrhosis, and CHF). Reversible acute interstitial nephritis and necrosis occur occasionally. It is not possible at this time to accurately categorize the prevalence associated with each NSAID. **Fenoprofen** is the NSAID most commonly associated with interstitial nephritis and nephrotic syndrome.[1,2,6–9,19,66–68]

Omeprazole

Interstitial nephritis occurs rarely during omeprazole therapy. At least 13 cases have been published, 10 with positive biopsies; 5 cases were rechallenged with recurrence of interstitial nephritis in all. Onset is usually after 2 weeks to 6 months of omeprazole therapy.[69]

Penicillamine

Slight to moderate proteinuria occurs in 7–30% of patients on long-term (>6 months) therapy with penicillamine for rheumatoid arthritis. Most cases develop in the first year. Proteinuria is usually benign and slowly reversible over 6–12 months, but nephrotic syndrome is occasionally encountered. The lesions appear to be perimembranous glomerulonephritis resulting from the deposition of antigen-antibody complexes on the renal basement membrane.[1,2,9,19,70]

Penicillins

Interstitial nephritis has been reported with most penicillins. **Methicillin** is by far the most frequently implicated penicillin (frequency 10–16%); the reason for its dominance in unknown. Penicillin-induced interstitial nephritis is an immune reaction that most commonly occurs during a long course of therapy. The reaction is usually accompanied by other signs of hypersensitivity such as fever, rash, and eosinophilia; hematuria may also occur. The reduction of renal function may not be oliguric, so urine volume is not a reliable parameter to monitor. Recovery usually occurs within weeks to months after drug discontinuation.[1,2,19,71]

(continued)

Pentamidine

Prospective trials of IV pentamidine for the treatment of *Pneumocystis carinii* pneumonia show nephrotoxicity in 4–66% of patients. Onset is usually 8–12 days after the start of pentamidine use.[72]

Plicamycin

High doses (50 µg/kg/day) produced renal impairment in 40% of patients, including some who died of acute renal failure. Nephrotoxicity is far less likely at the 25–30-µg/kg/day (or lower) dosage used most often.[73]

Polymyxins

Adverse reactions involving the kidney occur in about 20% of patients receiving **colistimethate** parenterally. Tubular necrosis is the most frequently described lesion, but interstitial nephritis is also reported. High dosage, long duration of therapy, and renal impairment are predisposing factors. Polymyxin-induced renal damage is usually reversible, but some patients continue to deteriorate after drug withdrawal.[74]

Rifampin

There are at least 49 published cases of rifampin-induced acute renal failure. Acute tubular necrosis is the most common lesion. This appears to be a hypersensitivity reaction and most often occurs with intermittent or interrupted dosage regimens, but has also accompanied continuous therapy.[75]

Streptozocin

Nephrotoxicity is the most common dosage-limiting side effect. The prevalence increases with prolonged administration until virtually all patients demonstrate renal impairment. Dosages below 1.5 g/m^2/week are less toxic. The damage is both glomerular and tubular. The drug should be discontinued as soon as renal damage is detected.[27,73]

Sulfonamides, Antibacterial

Early sulfonamides were poorly soluble, and urinary crystallization was a common problem. Crystalluria occurs in 8–29% of **sulfadiazine**-treated patients; symptomatic renal impairment resulting largely from nephrolithiasis occurs in 2–8%. Today crystallization occurs in fewer than 0.3% of patients receiving the more soluble sulfonamides and adequate hydration. Interstitial nephritis, glomerulonephritis, and tubular necrosis are reported rarely. These reactions are probably allergic in origin.[2,8,76,77]

Tacrolimus

Acute nephrotoxicity occurs with a prevalence similar to that of cyclosporine. Progressive nephrotoxicity is reported with long-term (>1 yr) therapy.[37,78]

Tetracyclines

Fanconi syndrome, characterized by tubular damage with proteinuria, glycosuria, aminoaciduria, and electrolyte disturbances, was associated with the use of outdated tetracycline products. Because of changes in the manufacturing process, this syndrome is now unlikely to occur. The antianabolic effects of tetracyclines can contribute to azotemia in patients with pre-existing renal impairment.[79] (*See also* Demeclocycline.)

Topiramate

Nephrolithiasis occurs in 1.5% of topiramate-treated patients.[80]

(*continued*)

Triamterene

Triamterene therapy is associated with an increase in urinary sediment, and the drug may be incorporated into existing renal calculi. One report suggests that 1 in 1500 users of the drug will develop triamterene-associated calculi during the course of 1 yr. As a precaution, the drug should probably not be used in patients with a history of renal calculi. Triamterene may also be associated with the development of interstitial nephritis.[81,82]

Vancomycin

Nephrotoxicity from vancomycin was commonly reported early in its history. Currently, the prevalence of vancomycin-induced renal impairment (usually mild) is 5–17%. It is usually reversible after discontinuation of the drug. Concomitant administration of **aminoglycosides** results in at least additive nephrotoxicity.[2,83–86]

■ REFERENCES

1. Koren G. The nephrotoxic potential of drugs and chemicals. Pharmacological basis and clinical relevance. *Med Toxicol Adverse Drug Exp* 1989;4:59–72.
2. Wang AYM, Lai KN. Drug-induced renal diseases. *Adverse Drug React Bull* 1994;Oct(168):635–8.
3. Blantz RC. Acetaminophen: acute and chronic effects on renal function. *Am J Kidney Dis* 1996;28(suppl 1): S3–6.
4. Barrett BJ. Acetaminophen and adverse chronic renal outcomes: an appraisal of the epidemiological evidence. *Am J Kidney Dis* 1996;28(suppl 1):S14–9.
5. De Broe ME, Elseviers MM. Analgesic nephropathy. *N Engl J Med* 1998;338:446–52.
6. Perneger TV et al. Risk of kidney failure associated with the use of acetaminophen, aspirin, and nonsteroidal anti-inflammatory drugs. *N Engl J Med* 1994;331:1675–9.
7. Whelton A. Renal effects of over-the-counter analgesics. *J Clin Pharmacol* 1995;35:454–63.
8. Choudhury D, Ahmed Z. Drug-induced nephrotoxicity. *Med Clin North Am* 1997;81:705–17.
9. Hoitsma AJ et al. Drug-induced nephrotoxicity. Aetiology, clinical features and management. *Drug Saf* 1991; 61:131–47.
10. Packer M. Identification of risk factors predisposing to the development of functional renal insufficiency during treatment with converting-enzyme inhibitors in chronic heart failure. *Cardiology* 1989;76(suppl 2):50–5.
11. Mandal AK et al. Diuretics potentiate angiotensin converting enzyme inhibitor-induced acute renal failure. *Clin Nephrol* 1994;42:170–4.
12. Textor SC. Renal failure related to angiotensin-converting enzyme inhibitors. *Semin Nephrol* 1997;17:67–76.
13. Kass MA et al. Acetazolamide and urolithiasis. *Ophthalmology* 1981;88:261–5.
14. Tawil R et al. Acetazolamide-induced nephrolithiasis: implications for treatment of neuromuscular disorders. *Neurology* 1993;43:1105–6.
15. Sawyer MH et al. Acyclovir-induced renal failure. Clinical course and histology. *Am J Med* 1988;84:1067–71.
16. Vial T, Descotes J. Clinical toxicity of interleukin-2. *Drug Saf* 1992;7:417–33.
17. Elasy T et al. Allopurinol hypersensitivity syndrome revisited. *West J Med* 1995;162:360–1.
18. Arellano F, Sacristán JA. Allopurinol hypersensitivity syndrome: a review. *Ann Pharmacother* 1993;27:337–43.
19. Werner M, Costa MJ. Nephrotoxicity of xenobiotics. *Clin Chim Acta* 1995;237:107–54.
20. Barclay ML, Begg EJ. Aminoglycoside toxicity and relation to dose regimen. *Adverse Drug React Toxicol Rev* 1994;13:207–34.
21. Ali MZ, Goetz MB. A meta-analysis of the relative efficacy and toxicity of single daily dosing versus multiple daily dosing of aminoglycosides. *Clin Infect Dis* 1997;24:796–809.
22. Swan SK. Aminoglycoside nephrotoxicity. *Semin Nephrol* 1997;17:27–33.
23. Sabra R, Branch RA. Amphotericin B nephrotoxicity. *Drug Saf* 1990;5:94–108.
24. Anderson CM. Sodium chloride treatment of amphotericin B nephrotoxicity—standard of care? *West J Med* 1995;162:313–7.
25. Sorkine P et al. Administration of amphotericin B in lipid emulsion decreases nephrotoxicity: results of a prospective, randomized, controlled study in critically ill patients. *Crit Care Med* 1996;24:1311–5.
26. Kintzel PE, Dorr RT. Anticancer drug renal toxicity and elimination: dosing guidelines for altered renal function. *Cancer Treat Rev* 1995;21:33–64.

27. Cornelison TL, Reed E. Nephrotoxicity and hydration management for cisplatin, carboplatin, and ormaplatin. *Gynecol Oncol* 1993;50:147–58.
28. Quin JD. The nephrotoxicity of cephalosporins. *Adverse Drug React Acute Poisoning Rev* 1989;8:63–72.
29. Zhanel GG. Cephalosporin-induced nephrotoxicity: does it exist? *DICP* 1990;24:262–5.
30. Thompson JW, Jacobs RF. Adverse effects of newer cephalosporins. An update. *Drug Saf* 1993;9:132–42.
31. Polis MA et al. Anticytomegaloviral activity and safety of cidofovir in patients with human immunodeficiency virus infection and cytomegalovirus viuria. *Antimicrob Agents Chemother* 1995;39:882–6.
32. Anand AJ, Bashey B. Newer insights into cisplatin nephrotoxicity. *Ann Pharmacother* 1993;27;1519–25.
33. Spinler SA, Goldfarb S. Nephrotoxicity of contrast media following cardiac angiography: pathogenesis, clinical course, and preventive measures, including the role of low-osmolality contrast media. *Ann Pharmacother* 1992; 26:56–64.
34. Porter GA. Contrast medium-associated nephrotoxicity. Recognition and management. *Invest Radiol* 1993;28 (suppl 4):S11–8.
35. Rudnick MR et al. Contrast media-associated nephrotoxicity. *Semin Nephrol* 1997;17:15–26.
36. Katzberg RW. Urography into the 21st century: new contrast media, renal handling, imaging characteristics, and nephrotoxicity. *Radiology* 1997;204:297–312.
37. Andoh TF et al. Nephrotoxicity of immunosuppressive drugs: experimental and clinical observations. *Semin Nephrol* 1997;17:34–45.
38. Rossi SJ et al. Prevention and management of the adverse effects associated with immunosuppressive therapy. *Drug Saf* 1993;9:104–31.
39. Forrest JN et al. Superiority of demeclocycline over lithium in the treatment of chronic syndrome of inappropriate secretion of antidiuretic hormone. *N Engl J Med* 1978;298:173–7.
40. Hadimeri H et al. Allergic nephropathy associated with norfloxacin and ciprofloxacin therapy. Report of two cases and review of the literature. *Scand J Urol Nephrol* 1997;31:481–5.
41. Reece RJ, Nicholls AJ. Ciprofloxacin-induced acute interstitial nephritis. *Nephrol Dial Transplant* 1996;11:393. Letter.
42. Deray G et al. Foscarnet nephrotoxicity: mechanism, incidence and prevention. *Am J Nephrol* 1989;9:316–21.
43. Alon US et al. Nephrocalcinosis and nephrolithiasis in infants with congestive heart failure treated with furosemide. *J Pediatr* 1994;125:149–51.
44. Cotter G et al. Increased toxicity of high-dose furosemide versus low-dose dopamine in the treatment of refractory congestive heart failure. *Clin Pharmacol Ther* 1997;62:187–93.
45. Samson MK et al. Phase I-II clinical trial of gallium nitrate (NSC–15200). *Cancer Clin Trials* 1980;3:131–6.
46. Warrell RP et al. Treatment of patients with advanced malignant lymphoma using gallium nitrate administered as a seven-day continuous infusion. *Cancer* 1983;51:1982–7.
47. Hall CL. Gold nephropathy. *Nephron* 1988;50:265–72.
48. Newton P et al. Proteinuria with gold therapy: when should gold be permanently stopped? *Br J Rheumatol* 1983;22:11–7.
49. Skinner R et al. Risk factors for ifosamide nephrotoxicity in children. *Lancet* 1996;348:578–80.
50. Ho PTC et al. A prospective evaluation of ifosamide-related nephrotoxicity in children and young adults. *Cancer* 1995;76:2557–64.
51. Ahsan N et al. Acute renal failure following immunoglobulin therapy. *Am J Nephrol* 1996;16:532–6.
52. Kopp JB. Crystalluria and urinary tract abnormalities associated with indinavir. *Ann Intern Med* 1997;127: 119–25.
53. Jorkasky DK et al. Lithium-induced renal disease: a prospective study. *Clin Nephrol* 1988;30:293–302.
54. Schou M. Effects of long-term lithium treatment on kidney function: an overview. *J Psychiatr Res* 1988;22:287–96.
55. Bendz H et al. Kidney damage in long-term lithium patients: a cross-sectional study of patients with 15 years or more on lithium. *Nephrol Dial Transplant* 1994;9:1250–4.
56. Walker RG. Lithium nephrotoxicity. *Kidney Int* 1993;44(suppl 42):S93–8.
57. Dorman HR et al. Mannitol-induced acute renal failure. *Medicine* 1990;69:153–9.
58. Gadallah MF et al. Case report: mannitol nephrotoxicity syndrome: role of hemodialysis and postulate of mechanisms. *Am J Med Sci* 1995;309:219–22.
59. Condit PT et al. Renal toxicity of methotrexate. *Cancer* 1969;23:126–31.
60. Stoller RG et al. Use of plasma pharmacokinetics to predict and prevent methotrexate toxicity. *N Engl J Med* 1997;297:630–4.
61. Cousins MJ, Mazze RI. Methoxyflurane nephrotoxicity. A study of dose response in man. *JAMA* 1973;225: 1611–6.
62. Desmond JW. Methoxyflurane nephrotoxicity. *Can Anaesth Soc J* 1974;21:294–307.

63. Valavaara R, Nordman E. Renal complications of mitomycin C therapy with special reference to the total dose. *Cancer* 1985;55:47–50.
64. Verwey J et al. Mitomycin C-induced renal toxicity, a dose-dependent side effect? *Eur J Cancer Clin Oncol* 1987;23:195–9.
65. Weiss RB et al. Nephrotoxicity of semustine. *Cancer Treat Rep* 1983;67:1105–12.
66. Stillman MT, Schlesinger PA. Nonsteroidal anti-inflammtory drug nephrotoxicity. Should we be concerned? *Arch Intern Med* 1990;150:268–70.
67. Porile JL et al. Acute interstitial nephritis with glomerulopathy due to nonsteroidal anti-inflammatory agents: a review of its clinical spectrum and effects of steroid therapy. *J Clin Pharmacol* 1990;30:468–75.
68. Bennett WM et al. The renal effects of nonsteroidal anti-inflammatory drugs: summary and recommendations. *Am J Kidney Dis* 1996;28(suppl 1):S56–62.
69. Yip D et al. Omeprazole-induced interstitial nephritis. *J Clin Gastroenterol* 1997;25:450–2.
70. Hall CL et al. Natural course of penicillamine nephropathy: a long term study of 33 patients. *Br Med J* 1988; 296:1083–6.
71. Appel GB. A decade of penicillin related acute interstitial nephritis—more questions than answers. *Clin Nephrol* 1980;13:151–4.
72. O'Brien JG et al. A 5-year retrospective review of adverse drug reactions and their risk factors in human immunodeficiency virus-infected patients who are receiving intravenous pentamidine therapy for *Pneumocystis carinii* pneumonia. *Clin Infect Dis* 1997;24:854–9.
73. Ries F. Nephrotoxicity of chemotherapy. *Eur J Cancer Clin Oncol* 1988;24:951–3.
74. Koch-Weser J et al. Adverse effects of sodium colistimethate. Manifestations and specific reaction rates during 317 courses of therapy. *Ann Intern Med* 1970;72:857–68.
75. De Vriese AS et al. Rifampicin-associated acute renal failure: pathophysiologic, immunologic, and clinical features. *Am J Kidney Dis* 1998;31:108–15.
76. Appel GB, Neu HC. The nephrotoxicity of antimicrobial agents (third of three parts). *N Engl J Med* 1977; 296:784–7.
77. Becker K et al. Sulfadiazine-associated nephrotoxicity in patients with the acquired immunodeficiency syndrome. *Medicine* 1996;75:185–94.
78. Porayko MK et al. Nephrotoxicity of FK 506 and cyclosporine when used as primary immunosuppression in liver transplant recipients. *Transplant Proc* 1993;25:665–8.
79. Appel GB, Neu HC. The nephrotoxicity of antimicrobial agents (second of three parts). *N Engl J Med* 1977; 296:722–8.
80. Shorvon SD. Safety of topiramate: adverse events and relationships to dosing. *Epilepsia* 1996;37(suppl 2): S18–22.
81. Ettinger B et al. Triamterene nephrolithiasis. *JAMA* 1980;244:2443–5.
82. Sica DA, Gehr TWB. Triamterene and the kidney. *Nephron* 1989;51:454–61.
83. Bailie GR, Neal D. Vancomycin ototoxicity and nephrotoxicity. A review. *Med Toxicol Adverse Drug Exp* 1988;3:376–86.
84. Eng RHK et al. Effect of intravenous vancomycin on renal function. *Chemotherapy* 1989;35:320–5.
85. Rybak MJ et al. Nephrotoxicity of vancomycin, alone and with an aminoglycoside. *J Antimicrob Chemother* 1990;25:679–87.
86. Duffull SB, Begg EJ. Vancomycin toxicity. What is the evidence for dose dependency? *Adverse Drug React Toxicol Rev* 1994;13:103–14.

DRUG-INDUCED OCULOTOXICITY

Occasionally, nonspecific blurred vision occurs with almost all drugs. The agents in this table are associated with a specific pattern of drug-induced oculotoxicity when administered *systemically.*

Allopurinol

Despite the discovery of allopurinol in cataractous lenses taken from patients on long-term (>2 yr) therapy, there is no clinical evidence for an increased risk of cataracts in allopurinol-treated patients.[1–3]

Amantadine

At least 9 cases of diffuse, white, subendothelial corneal opacities have been reported. These opacities usually resolved within a few weeks after amantadine discontinuation.[4]

Amiodarone

Most patients treated with amiodarone develop bilateral corneal microdeposits (75% after 1 yr of therapy). Visual symptoms occur in 6–14%. Halo vision at night is most commonly reported, but patients may also complain of photophobia and blurred vision. The deposits are apparently dose related and reversible, disappearing 3–7 months after drug discontinuation. Minute lens opacities occurred in 7 of 14 amiodarone-treated patients in one study.[5–7]

Anticholinergic Agents

Blurring of vision can result from paralysis of accommodation (cycloplegia). These drugs also dilate the pupil (mydriasis), which may produce photophobia and precipitate narrow-angle glaucoma. With systemic administration, large doses are usually required to produce mydriasis, which is most commonly associated with potent anticholinergics such as **atropine, scopolamine,** or **benztropine.** Patients being treated for narrow-angle glaucoma can usually tolerate systemic anticholinergic therapy, but should nevertheless avoid these drugs unless absolutely necessary. Patients with open-angle glaucoma, particularly if treated, can receive anticholinergic medications without much risk. Patients receiving nebulized **ipratropium** by face mask are at risk for developing increased intraocular pressure and precipitation of narrow-angle glaucoma, probably from the drug escaping from beneath ill-fitting masks and directly affecting the eyes. All of the ocular effects of anticholinergics are dose related and reversible.[5,8–10]

Anticonvulsants

Diplopia and nystagmus occur frequently. Blurred vision may be caused by mydriasis (**phenytoin**) or cycloplegia (**carbamazepine**). All of these effects are dose related.[11]

Antidepressants, Heterocyclic

These drugs have anticholinergic properties and are capable of precipitating narrow-angle glaucoma and cycloplegia at usual doses. (*See* Anticholinergic Agents.) There is a 10–30% prevalence of blurred vision resulting from cycloplegia, but it is rarely troublesome and is reversible upon drug discontinuation. Blurred vision usually resolves despite continued antidepressant use as the eye becomes tolerant to the drug's effects. SSRIs do not seem to produce any important ocular effects.[5,12,13]

Antihistamine Drugs (H₁-Blockers)

With the exception of **astemizole, loratadine,** and **fexofenadine,** these drugs have some anticholinergic properties and are capable of precipitating narrow-angle glaucoma and cycloplegia. (*See* Anticholinergic Agents.) These effects are minor and are

(*continued*)

reversible upon drug discontinuation. Antihistamines (most notably **diphenhy-dramine**) may reduce night vision.[5,9,14]

β-Adrenergic Blocking Agents

A reduction in tear production occurs, which can produce a hot, dry, gritty sensation in the eyes. This is rapidly reversible upon drug discontinuation.

Bromocriptine

Myopia is a frequent complication of long-term bromocriptine therapy and often goes unappreciated until the patient complains of blurred vision. The cause is not fully determined, but it may be due to lens swelling. Myopia is reversible within 1–2 weeks after drug discontinuation.[5,15,16]

Busulfan

Long-term therapy (usually ≥1 yr) with busulfan is associated with the development of posterior subcapsular cataracts in about 10% of patients.[3,17–19]

Chloramphenicol

Optic neuritis, papilledema, and visual field defects are occasionally reported. These effects can occur after weeks or years of therapy, but are most common after several months of chloramphenicol use. Most cases are reported in children with cystic fibrosis, but the association with this disorder is unclear and may only reflect the types of patients who received long-term chloramphenicol therapy. Both permanent visual impairment and recovery are reported after drug discontinuation. There is anecdotal reports that large doses of vitamins B_6 and B_{12} may have a beneficial impact on these adverse effects.[5,19–22]

Chloroquine

The oculotoxicity of chloroquine limits its usefulness; two general types of ocular change occur: corneal deposits and retinopathy. About 50% of patients demonstrate corneal deposits, less than one-half of whom have visual impairment resulting from these deposits. Opacities present as punctate or whirling patterns. They may appear after as little as 2 months and usually do not interfere with vision. They are usually reversible in 6–8 weeks after drug discontinuation. Early changes in the retina (deposition of pigment in the macula) are usually asymptomatic and reversible. More advanced damage includes hyperpigmentation of the macula surrounded by a depigmented ring and hyperpigmented retina ("bull's-eye" retinopathy). Patients complain of reading difficulty, blurred vision, visual field defects, and photophobia; some may also report defective color vision and light flashes. The prevalence ranges from 3–45% in various reports. The drug should be discontinued if these symptoms develop. Patients receiving long-term therapy with chloroquine ≤3 mg/kg/day should have ophthalmologic examinations at least every 6 months initially and then annually if their vision remains stable. Those receiving >3 mg/kg/day should be examined every 6 months.[27] Daily dosage seems to be more important than the total dosage or duration of therapy for the development of retinopathy; limiting the daily dosage to 4 mg/kg up to a maximum of 250 mg in adults minimizes the risk. The prognosis of chloroquine-induced retinopathy is uncertain. Weekly use of chloroquine for malarial prophylaxis does not seem to cause retinopathy.[15,23–27]

(*continued*)

Cidofovir

Anterior uveitis occurs in about one-third of AIDS patients receiving the drug intravenously for treatment of cytomegalovirus retinitis. The onset is usually after 4–5 days of treatment. Uveitis usually responds to topical cycloplegics and corticosteroids, and does not require discontinuation of cidofovir.[28]

Cisplatin

Blurred vision and altered color perception are frequently associated with high-dose cisplatin. Blurred vision gradually improves after drug discontinuation, while altered color vision may persist. Pigmentary retinopathy is also reported.[3,18,19]

Clomiphene

Visual disturbances, most commonly blurred vision, occur frequently with clomiphene. These disturbances usually disappear after the drug is withdrawn, but one report of three patients describes prolonged afterimages, shimmering of the peripheral visual field, and photophobia.[29]

Contraceptives, Oral

A variety of retinal vascular disorders have been attributed to oral contraceptives, but the association remains unproved. It is purported that some oral contraceptive users cannot tolerate contact lenses, possibly because of ocular edema or dryness; however, a prospective study failed to show any differences in lens tolerance between oral contraceptive users and nonusers.[30,31]

Corticosteroids

These drugs can produce a variety of ocular disorders with long-term therapy, most notably glaucoma and cataracts. Corticosteroid-induced increases in intraocular pressure occur in approximately 30% of long-term users and appear to be dose related. Glaucoma may persist for several months after drug discontinuation. Corticosteroid-induced cataracts (usually posterior subcapsular) are found in 10–40% of patients on long-term, systemic therapy and are correlated with total dosage and duration of therapy. Outcome is variable, ranging from improvement despite continued therapy to rare loss of sight. Most patients have no vision impairment. Although they most commonly occur with large oral doses, increased intraocular pressure and cataracts are reported in patients receiving corticosteroids by the topical ophthalmic, inhalation, and intranasal routes. Children develop cataracts more frequently than adults; Hispanics may be affected more often than blacks or non-Hispanic whites.[2,3,5,18,19,32–34]

Cyclophosphamide

Keratoconjunctivitis occurs in up to 50%. One report showed a 17% prevalence of transient reversible blurred vision during high-dose cyclophosphamide therapy. Recovery took from 1 hr to 14 days.[3,18,19,35]

Cyclosporine

Retinopathy occurs frequently with cyclosporine and severe visual disturbances, including cortical blindness, occur occasionally. Oculotoxicity appears to be dose related and resolves after drug discontinuation.[19,36]

Cytarabine

Keratoconjunctivitis, corneal damage, ocular pain, and photophobia are frequent, dose-related side effects of cytarabine. These symptoms usually resolve 1–2 weeks after drug discontinuation. Pretreatment with corticosteroid eye drops may be beneficial, but should be used with caution in patients with corneal damage.[3,18,19,37,38]

(*continued*)

Deferoxamine

Oculotoxicity, including blurred vision, impaired color vision, night blindness, and retinal deposits, occurs in 4–11% of patients receiving deferoxamine for chronic iron overload. These effects appear to be dose related and may be because of the chelation of trace minerals.[39–42]

Digitalis Glycosides

The most unique ocular effect is the frosted or snowy appearance of objects or colored halos around them. These effects are most noticeable in bright light. Color vision may be affected such that objects appear yellow (green or other colors are reported, but far less frequently). With **digoxin,** color changes usually occur when the plasma level exceeds 1.5 µg/L. Digitalis glycosides are also reported to produce photophobia, blurred vision, central scotomas, and flickering or light flashes before the eyes. Reversible ocular side effects occur in up to 25% of patients with digitalis intoxication.[5,43,44]

Disopyramide

The anticholinergic effects of disopyramide frequently produce blurred vision.[45]

Disulfiram

A few cases of retrobulbar neuritis have occurred, manifested by a dramatic decline in visual acuity and impairment of color vision. In most patients, vision returns to normal after drug discontinuation.[5,46]

Doxorubicin

This drug stimulates excessive lacrimation shortly after administration in about 25% of patients. Conjunctivitis has also been reported.[18,19,47]

Ethambutol

Retrobulbar neuritis is the primary ocular complication. Symptoms include blurred vision, scotoma, and reduction of the visual field. Color vision defects also occur, usually presenting as a reduction in green perception. Retrobulbar neuritis is dose related, occurring most frequently with dosages of 25 mg/kg/day or more. Its onset is usually after 3–6 months of therapy and it is slowly reversible after drug discontinuation. Dosages up to 15 mg/kg/day appear relatively free of ocular side effects.[5]

Fenoldopam

Treatment of hypertensive emergencies with fenoldopam results in dose-dependent, mild increases in intraocular pressure during the infusion. Increases in intraocular pressure occur in patients with and without ocular hypertension. The importance of these findings is yet to be established.[48,49]

Fluorouracil

Adverse ocular effects occur in 25–50% of patients receiving fluorouracil systemically. Blurred vision, ocular irritation and pain, conjunctivitis, keratitis, and excessive lacrimation occur frequently. These effects resolve in 1–2 weeks after drug discontinuation. Some patients may develop eversion of the eyelid margin (cicatricial ectropion) or potentially irreversible fibrosis of the tear duct (dacryostenosis) with prolonged therapy.[3,5,18,19,50,51]

Gold Salts

Parenteral gold can produce microscopic crystalline deposits in the cornea, most commonly in the superficial layers. These deposits are dose related and rarely occur until the total dosage of parenteral gold exceeds 1 g. The deposits slowly resolve after drug discontinuation, do not appear to affect vision, and are not a reason to stop gold therapy. **Auranofin** does not seem to produce these ocular effects.[5,52,53]

(*continued*)

Hydroxychloroquine

This drug can produce the same spectrum of ocular toxicity as **chloroquine.** (*See* Chloroquine.) Corneal deposits occur only with high daily doses. Limiting the daily dosage to 6.5 mg/kg up to a maximum of 400 mg in adults minimizes the risk of retinopathy.[5,24,25,27,54,55]

Interferon Alfa

Although the prevalence cannot be accurately determined, retinal vascular complications have been reported. Onset is usually after 2–3 months of treatment. These effects appear to be reversible after drug discontinuation.[56]

Isoniazid

Optic neuritis occurs occasionally, most commonly in malnourished or alcoholic patients, and often manifests itself as impaired red-green perception. It responds to **pyridoxine** therapy.[5]

Methotrexate

Adverse ocular effects associated with systemic methotrexate occur in up to 25% and include conjunctivitis, increased or decreased lacrimation, photophobia, and eye pain. Onset is during the first week of therapy, and resolution usually occurs in 1–2 weeks after drug discontinuation.[13,18,19]

Minocycline

Dark blue discoloration of the sclera has been reported. While the prevalence cannot be accurately estimated, the growing use of minocycline as an antiarthritic drug should increase the number of cases. It is not known if the discoloration is reversible.[57]

Muromonab-CD3

Conjunctivitis and photophobia occur frequently.[58]

Oprelvekin

Transient blurred vision and conjunctival injection occur frequently during oprelvekin therapy. Papilledema occurs in 1.5%.

Oxygen

Retrolental fibroplasia is an important complication of oxygen therapy in neonates, particularly premature or other low-birthweight neonates. The risk of retrolental fibroplasia in these patients increases whenever the concentration of inspired oxygen exceeds normal.[59-61]

Paclitaxel

Scintillating scotomas or photopsia occur frequently during paclitaxel infusions. The onset of these short-lived effects is usually during the last hour of the infusion. They do not always recur during subsequent infusions.[19,62,63]

Pamidronate

Reversible anterior uveitis and conjunctivitis are occasional complications of pamidronate therapy. Onset is usually 24–48 hr after IV infusion.[28,64]

Pentostatin

Conjunctivitis and keratitis frequently occur during pentostatin therapy. Although conjunctivitis is usually mild, keratitis can be severe.[3]

(*continued*)

Phenothiazines

Lesions of the lens, cornea, and retina are the most important features of pheno-thiazine-induced oculotoxicity. White to yellow-brown deposits in the lens most frequently occur with long-term, high-total-dose (over 600 g) **chlorpromazine** therapy. Epithelial keratopathy, possibly resulting from a photosensitivity reaction, can occur after only a few months of high-dose therapy. It is characterized by a diffuse opacification of the corneal epithelium. The consistent use of sunglasses may reduce the risk of keratopathy. Lens and corneal deposits usually do not interfere with vision, and all of these effects may be slowly reversible. **Thioridazine** is most noted for producing pigmentary retinopathy. As with most phenothiazine-induced ocular effects, pigmentary retinopathy is dose related. Patients may complain of blurred vision, decreased night vision, brown discoloration of vision, and central scotoma. Vision may improve if the drug is withdrawn soon enough; however, some cases continue to deteriorate despite drug discontinuation. Other phenothiazines may cause pigmentary retinopathy, but the supporting data are limited to case reports. Phenothiazines (especially thioridazine) have anticholinergic effects and may precipitate narrow-angle glaucoma. Corneal edema is a rare, but dangerous, complication of phenothiazine use requiring immediate discontinuation of therapy.[12,65,66]

Psoralens

The combination of psoralens and long-wave ultraviolet light (PUVA therapy) radiation is associated with the development of conjunctivitis, photophobia, and other signs of ocular irritation. The use of UVA protective lenses during therapy greatly reduces the prevalence. An experimentally demonstrated connection between PUVA therapy and cataracts has not been confirmed clinically.[5,67,68]

Quinine

Loss of visual acuity and reduction of the visual field to the point of blindness can occur with quinine therapy or (especially) overdose. Other reported ocular effects include impaired color vision and night blindness. These effects are usually reversible, but permanent constriction of the visual field and blindness are reported. The ocular effects of quinine may be the result of changes in the retinal vasculature.[5,69,70]

Retinoids

Blepharoconjunctivitis occurs in >50% of patients receiving **isotretinoin.** This painful condition appears to be dose related, and its onset is usually during the first 2 months of therapy. Dry eyes may occur with or without blepharoconjunctivitis. Corneal opacities, which clear in 6–7 weeks after drug discontinuation, are also reported. Similar effects are reported with **etretinate.** Other effects associated with retinoid therapy include papilledema and night blindness. Resolution usually occurs within a week after retinoid discontinuation.[5,19,71–74]

Rifabutin

Uveitis occurs frequently during rifabutin treatment and prophylaxis of *Mycobacterium avium* complex infection in AIDS patients. Its onset is variable (2 weeks to 7 months after starting treatment). Uveitis may be unilateral or bilateral, and responds to topical corticosteroid therapy.[28,75,76]

Rifampin

Exudative conjunctivitis, ocular pain, and orange staining of tears (and consequent staining of soft contact lenses) are occasionally reported with rifampin. These effects are rapidly reversible when the drug is withdrawn.[77–79]

(continued)

Sympathomimetic Agents

These drugs are capable of dilating the pupil and precipitating narrow-angle glaucoma. Sympathomimetics with marked α-adrenergic activity (eg, **ephedrine, phenylpropanolamine, tetrahydrozoline**) should be avoided. The risk of this reaction is slight unless large doses are taken orally or the drugs are applied topically.[9]

Tamoxifen

Fine, refractile retinal opacities and retinopathy occur frequently; corneal opacities are also reported. The prevalence of retinopathy has been 1.5–11.8% in prospective studies. While these lesions may occur with any dosage, they occur most often with daily dosages >180 mg or cumulative dosages >100 g. They may result in reduced visual acuity and are slowly reversible after drug discontinuation.[3,5,18,19,80]

Vinca Alkaloids

Various ocular disorders occur frequently. Most (ptosis, blurred vision, night blindness) are thought to be the result of cranial nerve impairment. Ptosis occurs in up to 50% of vincristine-treated patients. Time to onset ranges widely (2–44 weeks) as does resolution after drug discontinuation (2–24 weeks). **Vincristine** may be more oculotoxic than **vinblastine**.[3,5,18,19,81]

■ REFERENCES

1. Lerman S et al. Further studies on allopurinol therapy and human cataractogenesis. *Am J Ophthalmol* 1984;97:205–9.
2. Clair WK et al. Allopurinol use and the risk of cataract formation. *Br J Ophthalmol* 1989;73:173–6.
3. Burns LJ. Ocular toxicities of chemotherapy. *Semin Oncol* 1992;19:492–500.
4. Fraunfelder FT, Meyer SM. Amantadine and corneal deposits. *Am J Ophthalmol* 1990;110:96–7. Letter.
5. Davidson SI, Rennie IG. Ocular toxicity from systemic drug therapy. An overview of clinically important adverse reactions. *Med Toxicol* 1986;1:217–24.
6. Flach AJ et al. Amiodarone-induced lens opacities. *Arch Ophthalmol* 1983;101:1554–6.
7. Naccarelli GV et al. Adverse effects of amiodarone. Pathogenesis, incidence and management. *Med Toxicol Adverse Drug Esp* 1989;4:246–53.
8. Hiatt RL et al. Systemically administered anticholinergic drugs and intraocular pressure. *Arch Ophthalmol* 1970;84:735–40.
9. Durkee DP, Bryant BG. Drug therapy reviews: drug therapy of glaucoma. *Am J Hosp Pharm* 1978;35:682–90.
10. Singh J et al. Nebulized bronchodilator therapy causes acute angle closure glaucoma in predisposed individuals. *Respir Med* 1993;87:559–61. Letter.
11. Goldman MJ, Schultz-Ross RA. Adverse ocular effects of anticonvulsants. *Psychosomatics* 1993;34:154–8.
12. Oshika T. Ocular adverse effects of neuropsychiatric agents. Incidence and management. *Drug Saf* 1995;12:256–63.
13. Ritch R et al. Oral imipramine and acute angle closure glaucoma. *Arch Ophthalmol* 1994;112:67–8.
14. Luria SM et al. Effects of aspirin and dimenhydrinate (Dramamine) on visual processes. *Br J Clin Pharmacol* 1979;7:585–93.
15. Calne DB et al. Long-term treatment of parkinsonism with bromocriptine. *Lancet* 1978;1:735–8.
16. Manor RS et al. Myopia during bromocriptine treatment. *Lancet* 1981;1:102. Letter.
17. Podos SM, Canellos GP. Lens changes in chronic granulocytic leukemia. Possible relationship to chemotherapy. *Am J Ophthalmol* 1969;68:500–4.
18. Imperia PS et al. Ocular complications of systemic cancer chemotherapy. *Surv Ophthalmol* 1989;34:209–30.
19. Al-Tweigeri T et al. Ocular toxicity and cancer chemotherapy. A review. *Cancer* 1996;78:1359–73.
20. Cocke JG et al. Optic neuritis with prolonged use of chloramphenicol. Case report and relationship to fundus changes in cystic fibrosis. *J Pediatr* 1966;68:27–31.
21. Huang NN et al. Visual disturbances in cystic fibrosis following chloramphenicol administration. *J Pediatr* 1966;68:32–44.

22. Cocke JG. Chloramphenicol optic neuritis. Apparent protective effects of very high daily doses of pyridoxine and cyanocobalamin. *Am J Dis Child* 1967;114:424–6.

23. Harley RD et al. Optic neuritis and optic atrophy following chloramphenicol in cystic fibrosis patients. *Trans Am Acad Ophthalmol Otolaryngol* 1970;74:1011–31.

24. Easterbrook M. Ocular effects and safety of antimalarial agents. *Am J Med* 1988;85(suppl 4A):23–9.

25. Kerdel F et al. Antimalarial agents and the eye. *Dermatol Clin* 1992;10:513–9.

26. Lange WR et al. No evidence for chloroquine-associated retinopathy among missionaries on long-term malaria chemoprophylaxis. *Am J Trop Med Hyg* 1994;51:389–92.

27. Easterbrook MA, Bernstein H. Ophthalmological monitoring of patients taking antimalarials: preferred practice patterns. *J Rheumatol* 1997;24:1390–2.

28. Fraunfelder FW, Rosenbaum JT. Drug-induced uveitis. Incidence, prevention and treatment. *Drug Saf* 1997;17:197–207.

29. Purvin VA. Visual disturbance secondary to clomiphene citrate. *Arch Ophthalmol* 1995;113:482–4.

30. De Vries Reilingh A et al. Contact lens tolerance and oral contraceptives. *Ann Ophthalmol* 1978;10:947–52.

31. Petursson GJ et al. Oral contraceptives. *Ophthalmology* 1981;88:368–71.

32. Renfro L, Snow JS. Ocular effects of topical and systemic steroids. *Dermatol Clin* 1992;10:505–12.

33. Toogood JH et al. Association of ocular cataracts with inhaled and oral steroid therapy during long-term treatment of asthma. *J Allergy Clin Immunol* 1993;91:571–9.

34. Opatowsky I et al. Intraocular pressure elevation associated with inhalation and nasal corticosteroids. *Ophthalmology* 1995;102:177–9.

35. Kende G et al. Blurring of vision. A previously undescribed complication of cyclophosphamide therapy. *Cancer* 1979;44:69–71.

36. Memon M et al. Reversible cyclosporine-induced cortical blindness in allogenic bone marrow transplant recipients. *Bone Marrow Transplant* 1995;15:283–6.

37. Lass JH et al. Topical corticosteroid therapy for corneal toxicity from systemically administered cytarabine. *Am J Ophthalmol* 1982;94:617–21.

38. Herzig RH et al. High-dose cytosine arabinoside therapy for refractory leukemia. *Blood* 1983;62:361–9.

39. Olivieri NF et al. Visual and auditory neurotoxicity in patients receiving subcutaneous deferoxamine infusions. *N Engl J Med* 1986;314:869–73.

40. De Virgiliis S et al. Depletion of trace elements and acute ocular toxicity induced by desferrioxamine in patients with thalassemia. *Arch Dis Child* 1988;63:250–5.

41. Cases A et al. Acute visual and auditory neurotoxicity in patients with end-stage renal disease receiving desferrioxamine. *Clin Nephrol* 1988;29:176–8.

42. Cases A et al. Ocular and auditory toxicity in hemodialyzed patients receiving desferrioxamine. *Nephron* 1990;56:19–23.

43. Robertson DM et al. Ocular manifestations of digitalis toxicity. Discussion and report of three cases of central scotomas. *Arch Ophthalmol* 1966;76:640–5.

44. Aronson JK, Ford AR. The use of colour vision measurement in the diagnosis of digoxin toxicity. *Q J Med* 1980;49:273–82.

45. Bauman JL. Long-term therapy with disopyramide phosphate: side effects and effectiveness. *Am Heart J* 1986;111:654–60.

46. Norton AL, Walsh FB. Disulfiram-induced optic neuritis. *Trans Am Acad Ophthalmol Otolaryngol* 1972;76:1263–5.

47. Curran CF, Luce JK. Ocular adverse reactions associated with Adriamycin (doxorubicin). *Am J Ophthalmol* 1989;108:709–11.

48. Everitt DE et al. Effect of intravenous fenoldopam on intraocular pressure in ocular hypertension. *J Clin Pharmacol* 1997;37:312–20.

49. Elliott WJ et al. Intraocular pressure increases with fenoldopam, but not nitroprusside, in hypertensive humans. *Clin Pharmacol Ther* 1991;49:285–93.

50. Straus DJ et al. Cicatricial ectropion secondary to 5-fluorouracil therapy. *Med Pediatr Oncol* 1977;3:15–9.

51. Haidak DJ et al. Tear-duct fibrosis (dacryostenosis) due to 5-fluorouracil. *Ann Intern Med* 1978;88:657.

52. Bron AJ et al. Epithelial deposition of gold in the cornea in patients receiving systemic therapy. *Am J Ophthalmol* 1979;88:354–60.

53. Kincaid MC et al. Ocular chrysiasis. *Arch Ophthalmol* 1982;100:1791–4.

54. Easterbrook M. The ocular safety of hydroxychloroquine. *Semin Arthritis Rheum* 1993;23(suppl 1):62–7.

55. Bernstein HN. Ocular safety of hydroxychloroquine sulfate (Plaquenil). *South Med J* 1992;85:274–9.

56. Guyer DR et al. Interferon-associated retinopathy. *Arch Ophthalmol* 1993;111:350–6.

57. Fraunfelder FW, Randall JA. Minocycline-induced scleral pigmentation. *Ophthalmology* 1997;104:936–8.

58. Dukar O, Barr CC. Visual loss complicating OKT3 monoclonal antibody therapy. *Am J Ophthalmol* 1993;115:781–5.

59. Committee on Fetus and Newborn, American Academy of Pediatrics. History of oxygen therapy and retrolental fibroplasia. *Pediatrics* 1976;57(suppl):591–642.

60. Betts EK et al. Retrolental fibroplasia and oxygen administration during general anesthesia. *Anesthesiology* 1977;47:518–20.

61. Naiman J et al. Retrolental fibroplasia in hypoxic newborn. *Am J Ophthalmol* 1979;88:55–8.

62. Capri G et al. Optic nerve disturbances: a new form of paclitaxel neurotoxicity. *J Natl Cancer Inst* 1994;86:1099–101.

63. Seidman AD, Barrett S. Photopsia during 3-hour paclitaxel administration at doses ≥250 mg/m². *J Clin Oncol* 1994;12:1741–2. Letter.

64. Macarol V, Fraunfelder FT. Pamidronate disodium and possible ocular adverse drug reactions. *Am J Ophthalmol* 1994;118:220–4.

65. Bond WS, Yee GC. Ocular and cutaneous effects of chronic phenothiazine therapy. *Am J Hosp Pharm* 1980;37:74–8.

66. Ngen CC, Singh P. Long-term phenothiazine administration and the eye in 100 Malaysians. *Br J Psychiatry* 1988;152:278–80.

67. Farber EM et al. Current status of oral PUVA therapy for psoriasis. Eye protection revisions. *J Am Acad Dermatol* 1982;6:851–5.

68. Stern RS. Ocular lens findings in patients treated with PUVA. Photochemotherapy follow-up-study. *J Invest Dermatol* 1994;103:534–8.

69. Gangitano JL, Keltner JL. Abnormalities of the pupil and visual-evoked potential in quinine amblyopia. *Am J Ophthalmol* 1980;89:425–30.

70. Dyson EH et al. Death and blindness due to overdose of quinine. *Br Med J* 1985;291:31–3.

71. Fraunfelder FT et al. Adverse ocular reactions possibly associated with isotretinoin. *Am J Ophthalmol* 1985;100:534–7.

72. Lebowitz MA, Berson DS. Ocular effects of oral retinoids. *J Am Acad Dermatol* 1988;19:209–11.

73. Gold JA et al. Ocular side effects of the retinoids. *Intern J Dermatol* 1989;28:218–25.

74. Gross EG, Helfgott MA. Retinoids and the eye. *Dermatol Clin* 1992;10:521–31.

75. Saran BR et al. Hypopyon uveitis in patients with acquired immunodeficiency syndrome treated for systemic *Mycobacterium avium* complex infection with rifabutin. *Arch Ophthalmol* 1994;112:1159–65.

76. Karbassi M, Nikou S. Acute uveitis in patients with acquired immunodeficiency syndrome receiving prophylactic rifabutin. *Arch Ophthalmol* 1995;113:699–701.

77. Cayley FE, Majumdar SK. Ocular toxicity due to rifampicin. *Br Med J* 1976;1:199–200.

78. Lyons RW. Orange contact lenses from rifampin. *N Engl J Med* 1979;300:372–3. Letter.

79. Harris J, Jenkins P. Discoloration of soft contact lenses by rifampicin. *Lancet* 1985;2:1133. Letter.

80. Nayfield SG, Gorin MB. Tamoxifen-associated eye disease: a review. *J Clin Oncol* 1996;14:1018–26.

81. Albert DM et al. Ocular complications of vincristine therapy. *Arch Ophthalmol* 1967;78:709–13.

DRUG-INDUCED OTOTOXICITY

Drug-induced ototoxicity can affect hearing (auditory or cochlear function), balance (vestibular function), or both, depending on the drug. Drugs of almost every class have been reported to produce tinnitus, as have placebos. The agents in this table are associated with a measurable change in hearing or vestibular defect when administered *systemically*.

Aminoglycosides

Aminoglycoside antibiotics can cause both cochlear and vestibular toxicity. Cochlear toxicity presents as progressive hearing loss starting with the highest tones and advancing to lower tones. Thus, considerable damage may occur before the patient is cognizant of it. Vestibular damage presents as dizziness, vertigo, or ataxia. Both forms of ototoxicity are usually bilateral and potentially reversible, but permanent damage is common and may progress after aminoglycoside discontinuation. Estimates of the prevalence of aminoglycoside-induced ototoxicity vary widely depending on the criteria applied. Clinically detectable ototoxicity probably occurs in as many as 5% of patients, with a much higher percentage demonstrating audiometrically detectable dam-

(continued)

age. Most aminoglycoside-induced ototoxicity is associated with parenteral therapy, but it has followed topical, oral, and irrigation use of these drugs, especially **neomycin.** A patient should receive dosages by these routes that are no greater than the dosages given by injection. Possible predisposing factors for ototoxicity include decreased renal function, long duration of therapy, large total dosage, plasma levels exceeding the therapeutic range, previous aminoglycoside use, concurrent use of other ototoxic drugs, dehydration, and old age. There is some evidence of an inherited susceptibility to aminoglycoside-induced ototoxicity. Hearing impairment is less common in neonates and children. Two meta-analyses found no difference in the effects on hearing of single daily dosing and multiple daily dosing of aminoglycosides. The comparative effects on vestibular function have not been adequately investigated. Serial audiometry may be useful in early detection of ototoxicity. Each aminoglycoside has a slightly different spectrum of ototoxicity; the table below serves as a general guide to their relative ototoxic potential.[1–9]

RELATIVE OTOTOXIC POTENTIAL

DRUG	COCHLEAR	VESTIBULAR
Amikacin	++	+
Gentamicin	++	++
Kanamycin	+++	+
Neomycin	+++	+
Netilmicin	+	+
Streptomycin	++	+++
Tobramycin	++	++

Antidepressants, Heterocyclic

The prevalence of **tricyclic antidepressant**–associated tinnitus is estimated to be 1%. Tinnitus may subside despite continued therapy.[2,4,10]

Azithromycin

In elderly patients or patients with AIDS treated with 600 mg/day for *Mycobacterium avium* complex or toxoplasmosis, hearing loss occurs in 15–25%. Hearing loss occurs at all frequencies, but lower frequencies, including the speech range, are most often affected. Drug withdrawal or reduction of the dose to 300 mg/day resolves the hearing loss. Tinnitus and vestibular disturbances also occur frequently.[11,12]

Carboplatin

Although carboplatin is generally considered to be far less ototoxic than **cisplatin,** it can contribute to hearing loss when used in consolidation-phase treatment following cisplatin-containing induction.[4,13,14]

Chloroquine

Nerve deafness is a rare but consistent feature of chloroquine therapy. Its onset is usually delayed and is usually thought of as irreversible and accompanying long-term therapy. A partially reversible case and a case resulting from only 1 g of chloroquine have been reported.[2–4,15]

Cisplatin

Tinnitus occurs frequently and usually subsides within 1 week of drug discontinuation. It cannot be relied on to predict further ototoxicity. Hearing loss occurs fre-

(*continued*)

quently in patients receiving cisplatin and may be dose limiting. Audiometric abnormalities can be detected in most patients and may appear within a few days after the drug is started. High frequencies are lost first, and hearing loss occurs early or not at all. If therapy continues despite early hearing loss, the majority of patients experience hearing loss in the speech frequencies. Effects are cumulative, dose related, and probably irreversible. Prolonged, low-dose therapy may produce less ototoxicity than short-term, high-dose treatment. Ototoxicity occurs more frequently in children and the elderly, and those with pre-existing hearing loss appear to be at increased risk.[1-4,14,16-20]

Deferoxamine

Dosage-related hearing impairment occurs during long-term deferoxamine therapy. The prevalence is difficult to estimate, but it occurs frequently. High-frequency hearing is affected first, and both reversible and irreversible hearing loss have been reported.[4,21-23]

Diuretics, Loop

Rapid-onset hearing loss is a frequent feature of high-dose, rapid IV administration of **furosemide.** The onset may be more gradual with **ethacrynic acid.** Renal failure is usually listed as a predisposing factor, but only renal failure patients are likely to receive large IV doses. Coadministration with **aminoglycoside antibiotics** is often said to result in increased ototoxicity, but one study failed to confirm this. The hearing loss is usually transient, but permanent loss has been reported, more often with ethacrynic acid than with furosemide. Hearing loss and vestibular toxicity after oral therapy have been reported. **Bumetanide** or **torsemide** produce less ototoxicity than ethacrynic acid or furosemide.[1-4,24,25]

Eflornithine

High- and low-frequency hearing impairment is reported frequently and dizziness occurs occasionally.[18]

Erythromycin

Hearing loss has occasionally followed high-dose (>4 g/day) parenteral or oral therapy, and does not seem to be caused by any particular salt form. Impaired hepatic or renal function and advanced age may increase the risk. The loss occurs at speech frequencies and is usually reversible, but irreversible hearing loss has been reported. Recovery usually begins within 24 hr of drug discontinuation.[1,3,4,26,27]

Interferons

Tinnitus and hearing loss occur frequently during parenteral interferon therapy. These effects usually resolve 1–2 weeks after drug discontinuation. Interferon beta is more ototoxic than interferon alfa.[4,28]

Minocycline

Reversible vestibular toxicity, manifested primarily by dizziness, loss of balance, and lightheadedness, is a frequent occurrence. This adverse effect was noted in an average of 76% of patients in 6 studies and required 12–52% of affected patients to either discontinue the drug or to stop working. Other studies have found lower, but still large, percentages of patients with vestibular toxicity. Women are more susceptible than men. Onset is often during the first 2 days of therapy, and recovery begins soon after minocycline discontinuation.[1,4,29-31]

(*continued*)

Nonsteroidal Anti-inflammatory Drugs

Although not as common as with salicylates, NSAIDs have been associated with hearing impairment and deafness, including some cases of permanent damage. Tinnitus and vestibular dysfunction have also been reported.[1–4, 32]

Quinine

Tinnitus and high-frequency hearing impairment occur frequently. Although these effects are usually reversible, permanent hearing impairment has occurred with long-term therapy. Vestibular effects have also been described.[1,4,32]

Salicylates

Tinnitus, high-frequency hearing loss, and occasional vertigo are common features of salicylate intoxication. Hearing loss appears to be related to the unbound plasma salicylate level, explaining the marked interpatient variability in the total salicylate serum level at which it is first detected. Most patients demonstrating ototoxicity from salicylates are receiving long-term, high-dose therapy, such as for rheumatoid arthritis. Salicylate ototoxicity, even if severe, is almost always reversible in 48–72 hr, but permanent hearing loss has been reported.[1–4,32,33]

Vancomycin

Transient and permanent hearing loss, tinnitus, and dizziness have occurred. Hearing impairment is rare with plasma levels <30 mg/L (<21 μmol/L). In many of the reported cases, the patient had also been exposed to other ototoxic drugs, especially **aminoglycoside antibiotics.** The prevalence of purely vancomycin-induced ototoxicity is unknown, but it is probably low.[1,4,34,35]

Zidovudine

Audiometry determined that hearing loss occurred in 29% of 99 patients receiving antiretroviral drugs, with most cases associated with zidovudine. The prevalence of hearing loss was marked for patients >35 years.[36]

■ REFERENCES

1. Huang MY, Schacht J. Drug-induced ototoxicity. Pathogenesis and prevention. *Med Toxicol Adverse Drug Exp* 1989;4:452–67.
2. Griffin JP. Drug-induced ototoxicity. *Br J Audiol* 1988;22:195–210.
3. Norris CH. Drugs affecting the inner ear. A review of their clinical efficacy, mechanisms of action, toxicity, and place in therapy. *Drugs* 1988;36:754–72.
4. Seligmann H et al. Drug-induced tinnitus and other hearing disorders. *Drug Saf* 1996;14:198–212.
5. Brummett RE, Fox KE. Aminoglycoside-induced hearing loss in humans. *Antimicrob Agents Chemother* 1989;33:797–800.
6. Garrison MW et al. Aminoglycosides: another perspective. *DICP* 1990;24:267–72.
7. Matz GJ. Aminoglycoside cochlear ototoxicity. *Otolaryngol Clin North Am* 1993;26:705–12.
8. Bailey TC et al. A meta-analysis of extended-interval dosing versus multiple daily dosing of aminoglycosides. *Clin Infect Dis* 1997;24:786–95.
9. Ali MZ et al. A meta-analysis of the relative efficacy and toxicity of single daily dosing versus multiple daily dosing of aminoglycosides. *Clin Infect Dis* 1997;24:798–809.
10. Tandon R et al. Imipramine and tinnitus. *J Clin Psychiatry* 1987;48:109–11.
11. Tseng AL et al. Azithromycin-related ototoxicity in patients infected with human immunodeficiency virus. *Clin Infect Dis* 1997;24:76–7.
12. Brown BA et al. Relationship of adverse events to serum drug levels in patients receiving high-dose azithromycin for mycobacterial lung disease. *Clin Infect Dis* 1997;24:958–64.
13. Freilich RJ et al. Hearing loss in children with brain tumors treated with cisplatin and carboplatin-based high-dose chemotherapy with autologous bone marrow rescue. *Med Pediatr Oncol* 1996;26:95–100.
14. van der Hulst RJAM et al. High frequency audiometry in prospective clinical research of ototoxicity due to platinum derivatives. *Ann Otol Rhinol Laryngol* 1988;97:133–7.
15. Mukherjee DK. Chloroquine ototoxicity—a reversible phenomenon? *J Laryngol Otol* 1979;93:809–15.

16. Skinner R et al. Ototoxicity of cisplatinum in children and adolescents. *Br J Cancer* 1990;61:927–31.

17. Blakley BW, Myers SF. Patterns of hearing loss resulting from *cis*-platinum therapy. *Otolaryngol Head Neck Surg* 1993;109:385–91.

18. Schweitzer VG. Ototoxicity of chemotherapeutic agents. *Otolaryngol Clin North Am* 1993;26:759–89.

19. Kennedy ICS et al. Carboplatin is ototoxic. *Cancer Chemother Pharmacol* 1990;26:232–4.

20. Ilveskoski I et al. Ototoxicity in children with malignant brain tumors treated with the "8 in 1" chemotherapy protocol. *Med Pediatr Oncol* 1996;27:26–31.

21. Olivieri NF et al. Visual and auditory neurotoxicity in patients receiving subcutaneous deferoxamine infusions. *N Eng J Med* 1986;314:869–73.

22. Gallant T et al. Serial studies of auditory neurotoxicity in patients receiving deferoxamine therapy. *Am J Med* 1987;83:1085–90.

23. Cases A et al. Ocular and auditory toxicity in hemodialyzed patients receiving desferrioxamine. *Nephron* 1990;56:19–23.

24. Rybak LP. Ototoxicity of loop diuretics. *Otolaryngol Clin North Am* 1993;26:829–44.

25. Smith CR, Lietman PS. Effect of furosemide on aminoglycoside-induced nephrotoxicity and auditory toxicity in humans. *Antimicrob Agents Chemother* 1983;23:133–7.

26. Brummett RE. Ototoxic liability of erythromycin and analogues. *Otolaryngol Clin North Am* 1993;26:811–9.

27. Sacristán JA et al. Erythromycin-induced hypoacusis: 11 new cases and literature review. *Ann Pharmacother* 1993;27:950–5.

28. Kanda Y et al. Sudden hearing loss associated with interferon. *Lancet* 1994;343:1134–5.

29. Schofield CBS, Masterton G. Vestibular reactions to minocycline. *MMWR* 1976;25:31.

30. Gump DW et al. Side effects of minocycline: different dosage regimens. *Antimicrob Agents Chemother* 1977;12:642–6.

31. Greco TP et al. Minocycline toxicity: experience with an altered dosage regimen. *Curr Ther Res* 1979;25:193–201.

32. Jung TTK et al. Ototoxicity of salicylate, nonsteroidal anti-inflammatory drugs, and quinine. *Otolaryngol Clin North Am* 1993;26:791–810.

33. Brien J. Ototoxicity associated with salicylates. A brief review. *Drug Saf* 1993;9:143–8.

34. Brummett RE. Ototoxicity of vancomycin and analogues. *Otolaryngol Clin North Am* 1993;26:821–8.

35. Duffull SB, Begg EJ. Vancomycin toxicity. What is the evidence for dose dependency? *Adverse Drug React Toxicol Rev* 1994;13:103–14.

36. Marra CM et al. Hearing loss and antiretroviral therapy in patients infected with HIV-1. *Arch Neurol* 1997;54:407–10.

DRUG-INDUCED PANCREATITIS

Pancreatitis may be either acute or chronic, with most drug-induced cases being acute. The diagnosis of acute drug-induced pancreatitis requires both laboratory (elevated serum amylase and lipase levels) and clinical (abdominal pain) evidence. The strongest associations are made when readmnistration of the drug results in a recurrence of pancreatitis (ie, a positive rechallenge). Pancreatitis has occurred during therapy with many drugs; the drugs included in this table are those that present sufficient evidence to establish themselves as probable causes of pancreatitis.

ACE Inhibitors

There are numerous cases of ACE inhibitor–induced pancreatitis in the literature and in the files of manufacturers. **Captopril, enalapril,** and **lisonipril** have all been implicated. It is not possible to estimate a prevalence. A few of the cases have been confirmed by rechallenge.[1,3–5]

Alcohol

Alcohol is the greatest cause of drug-induced pancreatitis, easily exceeding the number of cases caused by all other drugs. Acute pancreatitis occurs in about 5% of alco-

(*continued*)

holics and usually develops after several years of alcohol abuse. It probably represents an acute flare of chronic pancreatitis.[6]

Asparaginase

The estimated prevalence of asparaginase-induced acute pancreatitis ranges from 1–26%, with fatalities in 1.8–4.6% of cases. Many patients who develop pancreatitis during asparaginase therapy are in poor condition and are also receiving other chemotherapeutic agents. Asparaginase inhibits amylase and lipase production, complicating the diagnosis and evaluation of asparaginase-induced pancreatitis.[1,2,7–9]

Azathioprine

There are many published cases of azathioprine-induced pancreatitis including at least 11 with positive rechallenge. Most cases occur in transplant recipients who are receiving other drugs implicated in causing pancreatitis.[1,2]

Calcium Salts

Pancreatitis is associated with hypercalcemia from pathologic causes, and it is likely that hypercalcemia resulting from the administration of exogenous calcium can also produce pancreatitis. There are at least 6 published cases of pancreatitis from parenteral nutrition–induced hypercalcemia.[1,10]

Contrast Media

Up to 11% of patients receiving contrast media through endoscopic retrograde cholangiopancreatography develop pancreatitis. Use of lower-osmolarity agents reduces the prevalence of pancreatitis.[2,11]

Corticosteroids

Although corticosteroids are commonly implicated as causes of pancreatitis, most of the reported cases involve disease states which predispose to pancreatitis. The weak evidence against corticosteroids is further complicated by data supporting the use of corticosteroids in the treatment of acute pancreatitis.[1,2,12]

Cyclosporine

Cyclosporine-induced pancreatitis was identified in 5 of 143 heart and heart-lung transplant recipients in one study. In another, 4 of 105 cyclosporine-treated renal transplant recipients developed panceatitis, compared with only 2 of 180 **azathioprine**-treated patients. All cases occurred within 4 months of the start of cyclosporine therapy.[1,2,13,14]

Didanosine

Estimates of the prevalence of pancreatitis in didanosine-treated patients range from 3–26%. A published report of didanosine treatment of 51 adult males with AIDS (10–12 mg/kg/day) found clinical pancreatitis in 12 (24%) and asymptomatic elevations of amylase and lipase levels in 10 others. Two patients died from fulminant pancreatitis. Pancreatitis may be dose related because in one study pancreatitis developed in 7 of 60 HIV-positive children receiving doses ≥ 360 mg/m^2/day, but not in any of the 35 patients receiving ≤ 270 mg/m^2/day.[1,2,15,16]

Diuretics, Thiazide

Although there are at least 25 published case reports of thiazide-associated pancreatitis, the quality of the evidence is poor. Some of the cases are complicated by hypercalcemia, a known risk factor for pancreatitis.[1,2]

Estrogens

Estrogen therapy increases the risk of pancreatitis in patients with pre-existing hyperlipidemia, especially hypertriglyceridemia. Hypertriglyceridemia is a known cause of pancreatitis and estrogen therapy raises serum triglyceride levels. In one report, 4 of 7

(continued)

women with serum triglycerides above 1500 mg/dL (17 mmol/L) while receiving postmenopausal estrogen replacement therapy (ERT) developed pancreatitis. Cases have also been reported in younger patients taking **oral contraceptives.** ERT is relatively contraindicated when serum triglycerides are >350 mg/dL (4 mmol/L) and absolutely contraindicated at >750 mg/dL (8.5 mmol/L).[1,2,17,18]

Furosemide

There are a small number of published cases of furosemide-associated pancreatitis. The dosage range for these cases is 40–160 mg/day and most cases occurred during the first few weeks of treatment. The evidence for furosemide-associated pancreatitis is weakened by the small number of positive rechallenges.[1,2,19]

Mercaptopurine

Inflammatory bowel disease is associated with pancreatitis. In one study of 400 patients with inflammatory bowel disease, 13 (4.25%) developed pancreatitis while receiving mercaptopurine (50–100 mg/day). Seven of the 13 were rechallenged and all developed recurrent pancreatitis, establishing a strong cause-and-effect relationship. Pancreatitis developed during the first month of initial treatment in all patients, and within 24 hours for 4 of the 7 rechallenges.[1,2,20]

Mesalamine Derivatives

Inflammatory bowel disease is associated with pancreatitis, but **mesalamine, sulfasalazine,** and **olsalazine** have been implicated in cases of acute pancreatitis confirmed by rechallenge. Positive rechallenge can occur after rectal administration.[1,2,21,22]

Metronidazole

Pancreatitis occurs occasionally with metronidazole. One study of 6485 HMO patients found a rate of pancreatitis requiring hospitalization of 3.9–4.6/10,000 in patients receiving metronidazole. The study was not able to capture nonhospitalized cases.[1,2,23]

Nonsteroidal Anti-inflammatory Drugs

There are isolated case reports of pancreatitis associated with most NSAIDs, but **sulindac** is clearly the most commonly reported. Many cases have positive rechallenges. The onset of symptoms is from 2 weeks to 9 months after initiation of therapy.[1,2]

Octreotide

When placebo or 100-µg doses of octreotide were administered before and immediately after endoscopic retrograde cholangiopancreatography in 84 patients, the frequency of pancreatitis within the first 24 hr after the procedure was 11% in the placebo group and 35% in the octreotide group. Despite the higher frequency of pancreatitis, the octreotide patients were NPO for fewer days.[1,2,24]

Pentamidine

Both injected and aerosolized pentamidine have been implicated in causing pancreatitis; a few fatalities have been reported. Most of the patients had AIDS, which may have contributed to their pancreatitis.[2]

Valproic Acid

Five of 72 valproate-treated, mentally retarded patients in one series developed pancreatitis. There are at least 50 other published cases, including some fatalities. The prevalence of asymptomatic elevations of serum amylase may be as high as 20%. There is no obvious connection with dosage or duration of therapy although one-half

(*continued*)

of the cases occur in the first 3 months of therapy and two-thirds occur during the first year. When detected, pancreatitis is rapidly reversible following drug withdrawal.[1,2,25–27]

Vinca Alkaloids

Pancreatitis with vinca alkaloid (ie, **vincristine**) therapy occurs primarily in patients receiving multiple-drug therapy, making the establishment of a cause-and-effect association difficult. Animal data show that vinca alkaloids can severely disrupt pancreatic architecture.[1]

■ REFERENCES

1. Wilmink T, Frick TW. Drug-induced pancreatitis. *Drug Saf* 1996;14:406–23.
2. Underwood TW, Frye CB. Drug-induced pancreatitis. *Clin Pharm* 1993;12:440–8.
3. Maringhini A et al. Enalapril-associated acute pancreatitis: recurrence after rechallenge. *Am J Gastroenterol* 1997;92:166–7.
4. Jeandidier N et al. Captopril-induced acute pancreatitis. *Diabetes Care* 1995;18:410–1.
5. Dabaghi S. ACE inhibitors and pancreatitis. *Ann Intern Med* 1991;115:330–1. Letter.
6. Steinberg W, Tenner S. Acute pancreatitis. *N Engl J Med* 1994;330:1198–210.
7. Haskell CM et al. L-Asparaginase. Therapeutic and toxic effects in patients with neoplastic disease. *N Engl J Med* 1969;281:1028–34.
8. Nguyen DL et al. Serial sonograms to detect pancreatitis in children receiving L-asparaginase. *South Med J* 1987;80:1133–6.
9. Sadoff J et al. Surgical pancreatic complications induced by L-asparaginase. *J Pediatr Surg* 1997;32:860–3.
10. Izsak EM et al. Pancreatitis in association with hypercalcemia in patients receiving total parenteral nutrition. *Gastroenterology* 1980;79:555–8.
11. Banerjee AK et al. Trial of low versus high osmolar contrast media in endoscopic retrograde cholangiopancreatography. *Br J Clin Pract* 1990;44:445–7.
12. Steinberg WM, Lewis JH. Steroid-induced pancreatitis: does it really exist? *Gastroenterology* 1981;81:799–808.
13. Steed DL et al. General surgical complications in heart and heart-lung transplantation. *Surgery* 1985;98:739–45.
14. Yoshimura N et al. Effect of cyclosporine on the endocrine and exocrine pancreas in kidney transplant recipients. *Am J Kidney Dis* 1988;12:11–7.
15. Maxson CJ et al. Acute pancreatitis as a common complication of 2', 3'-dideoxyinosine therapy in the acquired immunodeficiency syndrome. *Am J Gastroenterol* 1992;87:708–13.
16. Butler KM et al. Pancreatitis in human immunodeficiency virus-infected children receiving dideoxyinosine. *Pediatrics* 1993;91:747–51.
17. Parker WA. Estrogen-induced pancreatitis. *Clin Pharm* 1983;2:75–9.
18. Glueck CJ et al. Severe hypertriglyceridemia and pancreatitis when estrogen replacement therapy is given to hypertriglyceridemic women. *J Lab Clin Med* 1994;123:59–64.
19. Banerjee AK et al. Drug-induced pancreatitis. A critical review. *Med Toxicol Adv Drug Exp* 1989;4:186–98.
20. Haber CJ et al. Nature and course of pancreatitis caused by 6-mercaptopurine in the treatment of inflammatory bowel disease. *Gastroenterology* 1986;91:982–6.
21. Poldermans D, van Blankenstein M. Pancreatitis induced by disodium azodisalicylate. *Am J Gastroenterol* 1988; 83:578–80.
22. Isaacs KL, Murphy D. Pancreatitis after rectal administration of 5-aminosalicylic acid. *J Clin Gastroenterol* 1990;12:198–9.
23. Friedman GD, Selby JV. How often does metronidazole induce pancreatitis? *Gastroenterology* 1990;98:1702–3.
24. Sternlieb JM et al. A multicenter, randomized, controlled trial to evaluate the effect of prophylactic octreotide on ERCP-induced pancreatitis. *Am J Gastroenterol* 1992;87:1561–6.
25. Binek J et al. Valproic-acid-induced pancreatitis. Case report and review of the literature. *J Clin Gastroenterol* 1991;13:690–3.
26. Asconapé JJ et al. Valproate-associated pancreatitis. *Epilepsia* 1993;34:177–83.
27. Buzan RD et al. Valproate-associated pancreatitis and cholecystitis in six mentally retarded adults. *J Clin Psychiatry* 1995;56:529–32.

DRUG-INDUCED SEXUAL DYSFUNCTION

The large subjective component of human sexual response makes the evaluation of drug-induced sexual dysfunction difficult. Variations in study design have produced widely divergent reported rates of sexual dysfunction in the "normal" or control populations. Common drug-induced sexual dysfunctions include decreased libido or sexual drive, impotence (failure to achieve or maintain an erection in men), priapism (persistent and often painful erection), delayed ejaculation or failure of ejaculation, retrograde ejaculation (into the urinary bladder), and, in women, failure to achieve orgasm and decreased vaginal lubrication. Gynecomastia (enlargement of the male breast) has also been included in this table. Although it is not life threatening, drug-induced sexual dysfunction has a negative impact on quality of life and is an important contributor to noncompliance with prescribed drug regimens.

Alcohol
Low doses result in behavioral disinhibition. With higher doses, sexual response is impaired, frequently resulting in failure of erection in men and reduced vaginal vasodilation and delayed orgasm in women. In chronic alcoholics, sexual dysfunction frequently persists long after alcohol withdrawal and is permanent in some. The long-term effects are probably both neurologic and endocrine in origin; alcohol reduces testosterone levels and increases luteinizing hormone levels. Long-term effects are independent of liver disease.[1-8]

Alprostadil
Intracavernous injection of alprostadil produces penile pain in 20–30% of patients and priapism in 2%. Fibrotic nodules or scarring occur frequently. Intraurethral administration does not appear to cause priapism or fibrosis, but 36% experience penile pain.[9-11]

Aminocaproic Acid
This drug may inhibit ejaculation without affecting libido and has produced "dry" ejaculation. Effects are rapidly reversible upon drug discontinuation.[1,2,12,13]

Amphetamines
Low doses may increase libido and produce a delay in male orgasm. High doses have been associated with failure to achieve an erection in men and loss of orgasm in both sexes.[2,14-16]

Anabolic Steroids
Impotence and gynecomastia occur frequently in men and may be the result of reduction in the circulating levels of natural testosterone.[1,3,17]

Anticonvulsants
Both female and male libido may be reduced. Self-reported sexual dysfunction has been described in a widely varying percentage of patients. Social and psychological aspects of epilepsy probably play an important role in these findings. Some effects may be caused by a reduction in the level of free testosterone, resulting from hepatic enzyme induction and higher concentrations of sex hormone–binding globulins.[1,4,18-20]

Antidepressants, Heterocyclic
Impotence, delayed ejaculation, and painful ejaculation have been reported in men. Women and men have reported delayed orgasm and anorgasmia. **Clomipramine** is the worst offender. Both increased and, more commonly, decreased libido have been reported in men and women. The frequency of these effects varies considerably among published reports, perhaps reflecting the influence of the underlying depressive illness.[1-4,16,21-24] (See also Selective Serotonin Reuptake Inhibitors, and Trazodone.)

(continued)

β-Adrenergic Blocking Agents

These drugs are associated with a variety of sexual problems, most commonly impotence. In a study of 46 men taking **propranolol,** 7 experienced "complete" impotence, 13 noted reduced potency, and 2 complained of reduced libido. In a larger trial, the frequencies of impotence during propranolol therapy were 13.8% and 13.2% after 12 weeks and 2 years, respectively. However, these figures did not differ significantly from placebo. Most of the published reports implicate propranolol; other more cardioselective β-blockers are less frequently associated with complaints of adverse sexual effects. There have been at least 25 reported patients who complained of sexual dysfunction (18 impotence, 9 decreased libido) while receiving topical ophthalmic treatment with **timolol.** Some of these patients were rechallenged with positive results.[1,4,12,25–31]

Calcium-Channel Blockers

Although these drugs are generally thought to be free of adverse effects on sexual function, they are associated with gynecomastia. **Verapamil** is the most commonly implicated calcium-channel blocker, but **nifedipine** and **diltiazem** can also produce gynecomastia. Other calcium-channel blockers seem to be less likely to cause gynecomastia.[1,32]

Carbonic Anhydrase Inhibitors

Many patients receiving carbonic anhydrase inhibitors (eg, **acetazolamide, methazolamide**) develop a syndrome of malaise, fatigue, weight loss, and depression that often includes loss of libido. These patients appear to be more acidotic than those without the syndrome and some respond to therapy with sodium bicarbonate. Decreased libido has occurred in both men and women and usually requires 2 weeks of carbonic anhydrase inhibitor therapy to develop.[1,2]

Cimetidine

In a group of 22 men treated with high dosages of cimetidine for hypersecretory states, 11 developed gynecomastia and 9 experienced impotence. These effects appear to be dose related and readily reversible, and are not an important problem at dosages used for peptic ulcers. Cimetidine has some antiandrogenic effects, possibly the result of hyperprolactinemia, which are thought to be responsible for sexual dysfunction. Displacement of androgens from breast androgen receptors may contribute to the development of gynecomastia. **Ranitidine** does not appear to be associated with as high a prevalence of sexual dysfunction, and **famotidine** is not antiandrogenic.[1–4,12,17,32,33]

Clofibrate

In large multicenter trials, impotence has been reported more frequently than with placebo.[1–4,12,34,35]

Clonidine

Although some reports have indicated no sexual problems, others have indicated problems in up to 24% of patients. Impotence is the most frequently noted effect, but delayed or retrograde ejaculation in men and failure of arousal and orgasm in women have also been described.[1–4,12,28,36,37]

Cocaine

Although cocaine is often perceived as a sexual stimulant, its use is associated with difficulty in establishing an erection and delayed ejaculation.[2,16,38,39]

Cyproterone

Gynecomastia results from the antiandrogen effects of cyproterone.[17]

(*continued*)

Danazol

Most women treated with danazol for endometriosis experience reversible decreased libido.

Digoxin

Digitalis glycosides have some estrogen-like activity, and digoxin has been associated with decreased libido, impotence, and gynecomastia in men. In one study, digoxin use was associated with a 60% decrease in testosterone and a similar increase in estrogen in men.[1-4,12,41]

Diuretics, Thiazide

Thiazide diuretics and **chlorthalidone** are thought to produce adverse sexual effects, but the prevalence remains difficult to quantify. In one large study, the prevalence of impotence was reported to be significantly higher with **bendroflumethiazide** than with placebo (23% after 2 years compared with 10% for placebo), and in another, **hydrochlorothiazide** was reported to produce more impotence and loss of libido than **propranolol**. In a well-designed study, 14% of men taking **chlorothiazide** complained of impotence as did 14% of placebo-treated men. In two studies, chlorthalidone therapy resulted in more impotence than placebo.[1-4,12,27-29,36,42,43]

Estrogens

Impotence and gynecomastia occur frequently in men taking estrogens for prostate cancer. Estrogens have been used to reduce libido and sexual activity of male sex offenders.[1-4,44]

Finasteride

Gynecomastia occurs in 0.4% of finasteride-treated men. Onset is usually delayed until after 5-6 months of treatment.[45]

Flutamide

Gynecomastia may result from the antiandrogen effects of flutamide.[17]

Gonadotropin-Releasing Hormone Analogues

Most men and women treated with **goserelin** experience reversible decreased libido. It is likely that **leuprolide**-treated patients react similarly.[40]

Growth Hormone

(*See* Somatropin.)

Guanethidine

Up to 54% of men have reported impotence and up to 71% have reported ejaculatory impairment. Guanethidine does not affect parasympathetic function and would not be expected to produce impotence, leading some to suggest that the impotence is secondary to the inhibition of ejaculation. Retrograde ejaculation occurs as a result of the failure of the internal urethral sphincter to close; this action is sympathetically mediated. Although it is not well characterized, decreased libido in women taking guanethidine has been reported. Guanethidine effects are reversible upon drug discontinuation and may be alleviated by a reduction in dosage.[1-4,12,36]

HMG-CoA Reductase Inhibitors

At least 47 cases of **simvastatin**-associated impotence have been reported, including some with positive rechallenge. There are scattered reports of impotence with **lovastatin** and **pravastatin**.[46,47]

(*continued*)

Ketoconazole

Gynecomastia has been reported, apparently the result of the inhibition of testosterone synthesis.[1,17,32]

Marijuana

Both positive and negative effects on sexual function are possible. Low doses may have a disinhibiting effect, while large doses have been associated with decreased libido and impotence. Long-term use may also result in gynecomastia.[2,32,48]

Methyldopa

Impotence and ejaculatory failure in men, and reduced libido in both sexes have been described. The frequency of sexual dysfunction varies from quite low in some reports to greater than 50% in response to direct questioning. These effects are dose related and reversible. They may be the result of drug-induced sympathetic inhibition and mild CNS depression. Gynecomastia in men and painful breast enlargement in women have occurred.[1-4,12,29,36]

Metoclopramide

Gynecomastia and galactorrhea have been reported in adults and children receiving metoclopramide. These effects are probably due to metoclopramide-induced hyperprolactinemia.[49]

Monoamine Oxidase Inhibitors

Reported adverse sexual effects of MAOIs are highly variable. Impotence, spontaneous erections, and ejaculatory delay, as well as orgasmic failure in both men and women, have been described. The true prevalence of these effects cannot be determined from available data, but MAOIs may be associated with more sexual dysfunction than heterocyclic antidepressants.[1,2,4,16]

Narcotics

Long-term narcotic use (especially abuse) is frequently associated with decreased libido and orgasmic failure in both sexes, and impotence in men. These effects are dose related, with the highest frequency of impotence reported in narcotic addicts (80–90% in some series), and are reversible upon drug discontinuation.[2,50-52]

Nitrates and Nitrites

These vasodilators have been used (primarily by inhalation) to enhance the perception of orgasm. When they are used too soon before orgasm, however, the vasodilation rapidly produces loss of erection. This effect has been used therapeutically to reduce spontaneous erections in men undergoing urologic procedures.[2,53,54]

Omeprazole

Although the prevalence is unclear, impotence and gynecomastia in men and breast enlargement in women have been described.[1,55]

Papaverine

Intracavernous injection of papaverine resulted in priapism (defined as an erection lasting longer than 3 hr) in 17% of 400 patients. Those with psychogenic or neurogenic impotence were more likely to experience priapism than those with vasculogenic impotence.[9,56]

Phenothiazines

These drugs have been implicated in producing a wide variety of adverse sexual effects including impotence and priapism, absent and spontaneous ejaculation, painful ejaculation, retrograde ejaculation, menstrual irregularities, and decreased libido.

(continued)

These effects result from the complex actions of the drugs on the patient's hormonal balance and central sympathetic and parasympathetic pathways. With the exception of priapism, these effects are usually benign and respond to drug discontinuation. **Thioridazine** is the most commonly implicated drug. The possible contribution of the underlying disease state cannot be overlooked.[1–4,16,25,57]

Phenoxybenzamine

This α-adrenergic blocker is associated with dosage-related failure of ejaculation, but not interference with orgasm. This effect was present in all 19 patients in one study and reversed 24–48 hr after drug discontinuation.[1–3,58]

Progestins

Impotence has been reported in 25–70% of men receiving progestins for prostatic hypertrophy. Progestins have been used to reduce libido and sexual activity of male sex offenders.[2,44,59]

Reserpine

Impotence (33%) and failure of ejaculation (14%) in men and reduced libido in both sexes occur frequently.[1,2,4,12,36]

Sedative-Hypnotics

In a manner similar to alcohol, low doses may produce some disinhibition, whereas large doses may reduce sexual performance.[1–4]

Selective Serotonin Reuptake Inhibitors

Anorgasmia and delay of orgasm are frequent adverse effects of SSRIs, affecting the majority of patients in some studies. Although **fluoxetine** and **sertraline** are the most frequently mentioned, all of the SSRIs have been implicated. Some patients have benefited from dosage reduction. **Bupropion, mirtazapine,** and **nefazodone** have limited, if any, adverse effects on sexual function and should be considered in patients with SSRI-induced dysfunction.[1,3,24,60,61]

Somatropin

Benign gynecomastia may occur in prepubertal and adult males receiving somatropin. Onset may not occur until after months or years of treatment.[62]

Spironolactone

Gynecomastia in men and painful breast enlargement or menstrual irregularities in women are frequent with large dosages. Less frequently reported effects are impotence, inhibition of vaginal lubrication, and loss of libido. The structural similarity of the drug to estrogens and progestins is thought to be a key factor in the genesis of adverse sexual effects. Spironolactone may inhibit the formation of testosterone and its breast receptor binding. It may also increase the metabolic clearance of testosterone and its rate of peripheral conversion to estradiol. These effects appear to be dosage related.[1,2,4,12,17,32,36]

Trazodone

Numerous cases of priapism have been reported, usually during the first month of therapy.[1,4,12,57,63]

■ REFERENCES

1. Forman R et al. *Drug-induced infertility and sexual dysfunction.* Cambridge: Cambridge University; 1996.
2. Buffum J. Pharmacosexology: the effects of drugs on sexual function. A review. *J Psychoact Drugs* 1982;14:5–44.

3. Brock GB, Lue TF. Drug-induced male sexual dysfunction. An update. *Drug Saf* 1993;8:414–26.

4. McWaine DE, Procci WR. Drug-induced sexual dysfunction. *Med Toxicol Adverse Drug Exp* 1988;3:289–306.

5. Lemere F, Smith JW. Alcohol-induced sexual impotence. *Am J Psychiatry* 1973;130:212–3.

6. Wilson GT, Lawson DM. Effects of alcohol on sexual arousal in women. *J Abnorm Psychol* 1976;85:489–97.

7. Gordon GG et al. Effect of alcohol (ethanol) administration on sex-hormone metabolism in normal men. *N Engl J Med* 1976;295:793–7.

8. Dudek FA, Turner DS. Alcoholism and sexual functioning. *J Psychoact Drugs* 1982;14:47–54.

9. Fallon B. Intracavernous injection therapy for male erectile dysfunction. *Urol Clin North Am* 1995;22:833–45.

10. Chen RN et al. Penile scarring with intracavernous injection therapy using prostaglandin E1: a risk factor analysis. *J Urol* 1996;155:138–40.

11. Padma-Nathan H et al. Treatment of men with erectile dysfunction with transurethral alprostadil. *N Engl J Med* 1997;336:1–7.

12. Buffum J. Pharmacosexology update: prescription drugs and sexual function. *J Psychoact Drugs* 1986;18: 97–106.

13. Evans BE, Aledort LM. Inhibition of ejaculation due to epsilon aminocaproic acid. *N Engl J Med* 1978;298: 166–7. Letter.

14. Greaves G. Sexual disturbances among chronic amphetamine users. *J Nerv Ment Dis* 1972;155:363–5.

15. Smith DE et al. *Amphetamine abuse and sexual dysfunction: clinical and research considerations.* In, Smith DE et al, eds. Amphetamine use, misuse, and abuse: proceedings of the National Amphetamine Conference, 1978. Boston: GK Hall; 1979:228–48.

16. Segraves RT. Effects of psychotropic drugs on human erection and ejaculation. *Arch Gen Psychiatry* 1989; 46:275–84.

17. Braunstein GD. Gynecomastia. *N Engl J Med* 1993;328:490–5.

18. Toone BK et al. Sex hormone changes in male epileptics. *Clin Endocrinol* 1980;12:391–5.

19. Dana-Haeri J et al. Reduction of free testosterone by antiepileptic drugs. *Br Med J* 1982;284:85–6.

20. Morrell MJ. Sexual dysfunction in epilepsy. *Epilepsia* 1991;32(suppl 6):S38–45.

21. Harrison WM et al. Effects of antidepressant medication on sexual function: a controlled study. *J Clin Psychopharmacol* 1986;6:144–9.

22. Shen WW, Sata LS. Inhibited female orgasm resulting from psychotropic drugs. A five-year, updated, clinical review. *J Reprod Med* 1990;35:11–4.

23. Balon R et al. Sexual dysfunction during antidepressant treatment. *J Clin Psychiatry* 1993;54:209–12.

24. Segraves RT. Antidepressant-induced sexual dysfunction. *J Clin Psychiatry* 1998;59(suppl 4):48–54.

25. Pollack MH et al. Genitourinary and sexual adverse effects of psychotropic medication. *Int J Psychiatry Med* 1992;22:305–27.

26. Fraunfelder FT, Meyer SM. Sexual dysfunction secondary to topical ophthalmic timolol. *JAMA* 1985;253: 3092–3. Letter.

27. Medical Research Council Working Party on Mild to Moderate Hypertension. Adverse reactions to bendrofluazide and propranolol for the treatment of mild hypertension. *Lancet* 1981;2:539–42.

28. Veterans Administration Cooperative Study Group on Antihypertensive Agents. Comparison of propranolol and hydrochlorothiazide for the initial treatment of hypertension. II. Results of long-term therapy. *JAMA* 1982;248:2004–11.

29. Bansal S. Sexual dysfunction in hypertensive men. A critical review of the literature. *Hypertension* 1988; 12:1–10.

30. Prisant LM et al. Sexual dysfunction with antihypertensive drugs. *Arch Intern Med* 1994;154:730–6.

31. Grimm RH Jr et al. Long-term effects on sexual function of five antihypertensive drugs and nutritional hygienic treatment in hypertensive men and women. Treatment of Mild Hypertension Study (TOMHS). *Hypertension* 1997;29:8–14.

32. Thompson DF, Carter JR. Drug-induced gynecomastia. *Pharmacotherapy* 1993;13:37–45.

33. Jensen RT et al. Cimetidine-induced impotence and breast changes in patients with gastric hypersecretory states. *N Engl J Med* 1983;308:883–7.

34. The Coronary Drug Project Research Group. Clofibrate and niacin in coronary heart disease. *JAMA* 1975;231:360–81.

35. Oliver MF et al. A co-operative trial in the primary prevention of ischaemic heart disease using clofibrate. Report from the Committee of Principal Investigators. *Br Heart J* 1978;40:1069–118.

36. Duncan L, Bateman DN. Sexual function in women. Do antihypertensive drugs have an impact? *Drug Saf* 1993;8:225–34.

37. Meston CM. Inhibition of subjective and physiological sexual arousal in women by clonidine. *Psychosom Med* 1997;59:399–407.

38. Siegel RK. Cocaine and sexual dysfunction: the curse of mama coca. *J Psychoact Drugs* 1982;14:71–4.

39. Wesson DR. Cocaine use by masseuses. *J Psychoact Drugs* 1982;14:75–6.

40. Shaw RW. An open randomized comparative study of the effect of goserelin depot and danazol in the treatment of endometriosis. Zoladex Endometriosis Study Team. *Fertil Steril* 1992;58:265–72.

41. Neri A et al. Subjective assessment of sexual dysfunction of patients on long-term administration of digoxin. *Arch Sex Behav* 1980;9:343–7.

42. Wassertheil-Smoller S et al. Effect of antihypertensives on sexual function and quality of life: the TAIM study. *Ann Intern Med* 1991;114:613–20.

43. Chang SW et al. The impact of diuretic therapy on reported sexual function. *Arch Intern Med* 1991;151:2402–8.

44. Bancroft J et al. The control of deviant sexual behavior by drugs: I. Behavioural changes following oestrogens and anti-androgens. *Br J Psychiatry* 1974;125:310–5.

45. Wilton L et al. The safety of finasteride used in benign prostatic hypertrophy: a non-interventional observational cohort study in 14,772 patients. *Br J Urol* 1996;78:379–84.

46. Boyd IW. HMG-CoA reductase inhibitor-induced impotence. *Ann Pharmacother* 1996;30:1199. Letter.

47. Jackson G. Simvastatin and impotence. *BMJ* 1997;315:31.

48. Halikas J et al. Effects of regular marijuana use on sexual performance. *J Psychoact Drugs* 1982;14:59–70.

49. Madani S, Tolia V. Gynecomastia with metoclopramide use in pediatric patients. *J Clin Gastroenterol* 1997;24: 79–81.

50. Cushman P. Sexual behavior in heroin addiction and methadone maintenance. Correlation with plasma luteinizing hormone. *N Y State J Med* 1972;72:1261–5.

51. Langrod J et al. Methadone treatment and physical complaints: a clinical analysis. *Int J Addict* 1981;16:947–52.

52. Rosenbaum M. When drugs come into the picture, love flies out the window: women addicts' love relationships. *Int J Addict* 1981;16:1197–206.

53. Sigell LT et al. Popping and snorting volatile nitrites: a current fad for getting high. *Am J Psychiatry* 1978; 135:1216–8.

54. Welti RS, Brodsky JB. Treatment of intraoperative penile tumescence. *J Urol* 1980;124:925–6.

55. Lindquist M, Edwards IR. Endocrine adverse effects of omeprazole. *BMJ* 1992;305:451–2.

56. Lomas GM, Jarow JP. Risk factors for papaverine-induced priapism. *J Urol* 1992;147:1280–1.

57. Thompson JW et al. Psychotropic medication and priapism: a comprehensive review. *J Clin Psychiatry* 1990; 51:430–3.

58. Kedia KR, Persky L. Effect of phenoxybenzamine (dibenzyline) on sexual function in man. *Urology* 1981;18: 620–2.

59. Meiraz D et al. Treatment of benign prostatic hyperplasia with hydroxyprogesterone-caproate: placebo-controlled study. *Urology* 1977;9:144–8.

60. Piazza LA et al. Sexual functioning in chronically depressed patients treated with SSRI antidepressants: a pilot study. *Am J Psychiatry* 1997;154:1757–9.

61. Modell JG et al. Comparative sexual side effects of bupropion, fluoxetine, paroxetine, and sertraline. *Clin Pharmacol Ther* 1997;61:476–87.

62. Malozowski S, Stadel BV. Prepubertal gynecomastia during growth hormone therapy. *J Pediatrics* 1995;126: 659–61.

63. Warner MD et al. Trazodone and priapism. *J Clin Psychiatry* 1987;48:244–5.

DRUG-INDUCED SKIN DISORDERS

Most drugs occasionally have been associated with rashes or other dermatologic reactions. The difficulty of determining a correct diagnosis of a skin disorder and the complexity of establishing a causal relationship with drug therapy make estimating the frequency of occurrence of these reactions virtually impossible. Only skin disorders resulting from *systemic* administration of drugs are represented in this table. Drugs believed to be among the most common causes of a particular drug-induced skin disorder are designated by "XX" in the table. Stevens–Johnson syndrome and toxic epidermal necrolysis have been combined into a single column because of their similarity in histopathology and because they are usually caused by the same drugs. The following abbreviations are used to indicate specific skin disorders:

(*continued*)

AE – Acneiforms Eruptions
AL – Alopecia
ED – Exfoliative Dermatitis
FE – Fixed Eruptions
LE – Lupus Erythematosus-Like Reactions
Ph – Photosensitivity and Phototoxicity Reactions
SJ/TN – Stevens–Johnson Syndrome/Toxic Epidermal Necrolysis

DRUG	AE	AL	ED	FE	LE	PH	SJ/TN	REFERENCES
Acetaminophen		X		X			X	1–3
Allopurinol				X			XX	1–6
Amantadine		X				X		1
Aminosalicylic Acid			X					5
Amiodarone		X				X		1,4,7
Amphetamines		X						2
Androgens	XX	X						1,2,4,5
Antidepressants, Heterocyclic	X					X		1,4,7
Auranofin		X						1
Azathioprine		X						1
Barbiturates	X			X			XX	1–6,8
Bleomycin		XX						1,2
Bromocriptine		X						1,2,4
Captopril		X	X					1
Carbamazepine			X	X			X	1–3,5,8
Carboplatin		X						1
Chloral Hydrate	X			X				1,2
Chlordiazepoxide				X				1
Chloroquine				X		X	X	2,4,7
Cimetidine							X	2,4
Clofibrate		X						2,5
Colchicine		XX					X	1–3,5
Contraceptives, Oral	X	X		X	X	X		1,2,4,5,7
Corticosteroids	XX							1,2,4,5
Cyclophosphamide		XX					X	1,2
Cyclosporine	X	X						1
Cytarabine		XX						1
Dacarbazine						X		1,2,7
Dactinomycin	XX						X	1,2,5
Danazol	XX							1,2
Dapsone				X		X	X	1,2,7
Daunorubicin		X						1,2

(*continued*)

DRUG	AE	AL	ED	FE	LE	PH	SJ/TN	REFERENCES
Disulfiram	X							1
Diuretics, Thiazide						XX		1,2,4,5,7
Doxorubicin		XX						1
Ethionamide	X							1
Etoposide		XX						1
Etretinate		XX				X		1,2,4,7
Fluoroquinolones						XX	X	1,7,8
Fluorouracil		XX				X		1,2,4,7
Gold Salts		X	XX	X		X	X	1,2,5,7
Griseofulvin				X		X		2,4,7
Heparin		X						1,2
Hydralazine					XX			1,2,5,9
Ifosfamide		XX						1
Interferon Alfa (2a, 2b)		XX						1,2
Isoniazid	X	X	X	X	X	X	X	1,2,4,5,9
Isotretinoin		XX				X		1,2,4,7
Ketoconazole		X						1
Lamotrigine							XX	10
Levodopa		X						2,5
Lithium	XX	X	X					1,2,4,5
Meprobamate				X				1
Methotrexate		XX				X	X	1,2,4,7
Methyldopa					X			1,5,9
Methysergide		X						1
Metronidazole				X				1,2
Minocycline					X	X		7,11
Mitomycin		X						1
Nalidixic Acid						X		2,7
Nitrofurantoin		X		X			X	2,4
NSAIDs		X		X		X	X	1–4,7
Paclitaxel		XX						1
Penicillamine		X		X	X			1,2,4,9
Penicillins			XX	X			X	1–6,8
Phenolphthalein				X			X	1,2,4,5
Phenothiazines			X	X	X	XX		1,2,4,5,7,9
Phenytoin	X		X	X	X		X	1,2,4,5,8,9
Plicamycin							X	2,4
Procainamide					XX			1,5,9
Propranolol		X		X				4,5

(continued)

DRUG	AE	AL	ED	FE	LE	PH	SJ/TN	REFERENCES
Propylthiouracil		X			X			1,2,5
Psoralens	X				X	XX		1,2
Quinacrine		X						2,5
Quinidine	X		X	X	X	X		2,5,7,9
Quinine	X			X		X		1,2
Rifampin	X						X	1,8
Salicylates			X				X	1–4
Streptomycin			XX	X			X	1,2,4
Sulfonamides			XX	X	X	XX	XX	1–9
Sulfonylureas						X	X	1,2,4–7
Tamoxifen		X						1
Tetracyclines			X			XX		1,2,4–7
Tretinoin						X		1,7
Trimethadione	X	X			X			1,2,5
Valproic Acid		X						1,2,5,6
Vinblastine		XX				X		1,2,4,7
Vincristine		XX						1
Vitamin A		X						1,2,4,5
Warfarin		X						1,2,4,5

■ REFERENCES

1. Zürcher K, Krebs A. *Cutaneous drug reactions,* 2nd ed. Basel: S Karger; 1992.
2. Bork K. *Cutaneous side effects of drugs.* Philadelphia: WB Saunders; 1988.
3. Roujeau J-C et al. Toxic epidermal necrolysis (Lyell syndrome). Incidence and drug etiology in France, 1981–1985. *Arch Dermatol* 1990;126:37–42.
4. Blacker KL et al. Cutaneous reactions to drugs. In Fitzpatrick TB et al, eds. *Dermatology in general medicine,* 4th ed. New York: McGraw-Hill; 1993:1783–806.
5. Millikan LE. Drug eruptions (dermatitis medicamentosa). In Moschella SL, Hurley HJ, eds. *Dermatology,* 3rd ed. Philadelphia: WB Saunders; 1992:535–73.
6. Chan H-L et al. The incidence of erythema multiforme, Stevens–Johnson syndrome, and toxic epidermal necrolysis. A population-based study with particular reference to reactions caused by drugs among outpatients. *Arch Dermatol* 1990;126:43–7.
7. Drugs that cause photosensitivity. *Med Lett Drugs Ther* 1995;37:35–6.
8. Roujeau JC, Stern RS. Severe adverse cutaneous reactions to drugs. *N Engl J Med* 1994;331:1272–85.
9. Price EJ, Venables PJW. Drug-induced lupus. *Drug Saf* 1995;12:283–90.
10. Mackay FJ et al. Safety of long-term lamotrigine in epilepsy. *Epilepsia* 1997;38:881–6.
11. Shapiro LE et al. Comparative safety of tetracycline, minocycline, and doxycycline. *Arch Dermatol* 1997;133:1224–30.

Drug Interactions and Interferences

Cytochrome P450 Enzyme Interactions

Philip D. Hansten

Cytochrome P450 enzymes are found throughout the body and play an important role in the metabolism of many drugs, catalyzing α-hydroxylation, N-demethylation, ring oxidation, and more.[1,2] Most substrates are metabolized by a specific enzyme, whereas each cytochrome P450 enzyme is generally capable of metabolizing many different compounds.[2,3] Induction or inhibition of these enzymes can drastically affect the outcome of drug therapy.

Cytochrome P450 enzymes are identified by the prefix "CYP" followed by an Arabic number identifying the family, although Roman numerals are still sometimes used. The three important enzyme families in humans are CYP1, CYP2, and CYP3. Subfamilies are given letters (eg, CYP2B, CYP2C). This is followed by a number identifying the specific enzyme.

Although most concentrated in the liver, cytochrome P450 enzymes exist in all tissues of the human body.[2,3] Intestinal mucosal cytochrome P450 enzymes appear to be primarily from the CYP3A family, probably CYP3A4 in humans.[3] These enzymes affect the bioavailability of some drugs.

■ INDUCTION AND INHIBITION

When the amount of enzyme present in the body is increased by a drug or chemical, the enzyme is said to be "induced." Although most inducers are P450 substrates, this is not always the case. Induction can increase the rate of clearance of a drug, decreasing its efficacy. It can also increase the rate of formation of an active or toxic metabolite, resulting in exaggeration of therapeutic effect or increased toxicity.

Theoretically, all substrates metabolized by the same enzyme can compete for the same binding site, causing competitive inhibition. However, the clinical relevance depends on the concentration, relative affinities, and other elimination pathways of each substrate. Like inducers, not all inhibitors are enzyme substrates. Some drugs or their metabolites can form an inactive complex with a cytochrome P450 enzyme or its heme group. Inhibition may lead to increased toxic effects by causing drug accumulation, or it can lower toxic or therapeutic effects by decreasing the amount of toxic or active metabolite(s).

■ DRUG INTERACTIONS

Knowing which drugs are metabolized by each cytochrome P450 enzyme and the drugs that influence those enzymes can help in predicting drug-drug interactions. However, there are additional points to consider when predicting drug interactions.

The effect of inhibition on drug elimination depends on whether a substrate has alternate elimination pathways. Inhibition of an enzyme may not be clinically important if there are alternative metabolic pathways.

Therapeutic range is also important. If a drug has a wide therapeutic range, factors such as induction or inhibition can become clinically unimportant. The opposite is true for drugs with a narrow therapeutic range, such as tricyclic antidepressants and antiarrhythmics.[4,5]

Last, consider metabolites. Not only does inhibition and induction of cytochrome P450 enzymes influence the formation of active metabolites, the formation of active metabolites may enhance inhibition or induction. Fluoxetine, an inhibitor of CYP2D6, has an active metabolite norfluoxetine, which also inhibits CYP2D6.[6,7]

The following table is meant to serve as an aid in the prediction of drug-drug interactions. However, it is also important to consider many other parameters: whether the patient is a poor or extensive metabolizer, the affinity of the drug for the binding site, the concentration of drug in the liver, the presence of alternate elimination pathways, and the therapeutic range. Because research on P450 metabolism is currently being published at a rapid rate, the table is not complete. The absence of a drug from the table does not necessarily imply that it is not metabolized by one of the P450 enzymes. When using the table, consider the following principles:

- Inhibition of drug metabolism tends to be substrate independent. That is, a potent inhibitor of CYP2D6 is likely to inhibit the metabolism of any drug metabolized by CYP2D6.
- The magnitude of cytochrome P450 enzyme inhibition is usually dose related over the dosage range of the inhibitor. For example, fluconazole 100 mg/day is usually a modest inhibitor of CYP3A4, but at 400 mg/day it can substantially inhibit the isozyme.
- Some cytochrome P450 inhibitors affect more than one enzyme. For example, ritonavir inhibits both CYP2D6 and CYP3A4.
- Drug enantiomers may be metabolized by different cytochrome P450 isozymes. For example, (R)-warfarin is metabolized by CYP1A2 and CYP3A4, while the more potent (S)-warfarin is metabolized primarily by CYP2C9. Thus, CYP1A2 or CYP3A4 inhibitors tend to produce only small increases in the hypoprothrombinemic response to warfarin, while potent CYP2C9 inhibitors produce large increases in warfarin effect.

COMMON DRUGS THAT INTERACT WITH P450 ENZYMES

	SUBFAMILY SUBSTRATES	INDUCERS	INHIBITORS
1A2	acetaminophen, amitriptyline, antipyrine, caffeine, clomipramine, clozapine, imipramine, olanzapine, propranolol, tacrine, theophylline, (R)-warfarin, zileuton	charcoal-broiled food, omeprazole, smoking	ciprofloxacin, enoxacin, fluvoxamine, macrolides,[a] mexiletine, tacrine, zileuton
2B6	cyclophosphamide, ifosfamide	phenobarbital, phenytoin	
2C8	benzphetamine, diazepam, diclofenac, (R)-mephenytoin, paclitaxel, tolbutamide		
2C9/10	diclofenac, dronabinol, flubiprofen, hexobarbital, ibuprofen, (R)-mephenytoin, naproxen, phenytoin, piroxicam, tolbutamide, (S)-warfarin	barbiturates, carbamazepine, phenytoin, primidone, rifampin	amiodarone, disulfiram, fluconazole, fluoxetine, fluvastatin, metronidazole, ritonavir, sulfa-phenazole, zafirlukast
2C18	cimetidine, (S)-mephenytoin, propranolol, retinoic acid	omeprazole, piroxicam	
2C19	amitriptyline, clomipramine, diazepam, hexo-barbital, imipramine, mephenytoin, mepho-barbital, omeprazole, propranolol		fluoxetine, fluvoxamine, omeprazole, ritonavir
2D6	chlorpheniramine, codeine, debrisoquine, dextromethorphan, flecainide, fluoxetine, haloperidol, loratadine, metoprolol, mexiletine, paroxetine, perphenazine, propafenone, propranolol, risperidone, thioridazine, timolol, tramadol, trazodone, tricyclic antidepressants, venlafaxine		amiodarone, chloroquine, cimetidine, haloperidol, perphenazine, propoxyphene, quinidine, ritonavir, SSRIs,[b] thioridazine

(*continued*)

COMMON DRUGS THAT INTERACT WITH P450 ENZYMES (continued)

SUBFAMILY SUBSTRATES	INDUCERS	INHIBITORS
2E1	acetaminophen, alcohol, chlorzoxazone, dapsone, halothane, isoflurane, methoxy-flurane, sevoflurane	alcohol (chronic), isoniazid	disulfiram
3A3/4	alfentanil, alprazolam, amlodipine, amiodarone, amitriptyline, androgens, astemizole, atorvastatin, benzphetamine, bromocriptine, carbamazepine, cisapride, clomipramine, clonazepam, cocaine, corticosteroids, cyclosporine, dapsone, dexamethasone, diazepam, diltiazem, disopyramide, ergotamine, erythromycin, ethinyl estradiol, ethosuximide, etoposide, felodipine, fentanyl, fexofenadine, finasteride, ifosfamide, imipramine, indinavir, isradipine, itraconazole, ketoconazole, lidocaine, loratadine, lovastatin, miconazole (IV), midazolam, nefazodone, nicardipine, nifedipine, nimodipine, nisoldipine, nitrendipine, omeprazole, paclitaxel, pimozide, progesterone, propafenone, quinidine, quinine, rifabutin, ritonavir, saquinavir, sertraline, tacrolimus, tamoxifen, teniposide, terfenadine, testosterone, theophylline, triazolam, troleandomycin, verapamil, vinca alkaloids, (R)-warfarin, zolpidem	aminoglutethimide, barbiturates, carbamazepine, glucocorticoids, griseofulvin, phenytoin, primidone, rifabutin, rifampin, sulfinpyrazone, troglitazone	cyclophosphamide, cyclosporine, delavirdine, diltiazem, fluvoxamine, grapefruit juice, ifosfamide, indinavir, itraconazole, ketoconazole, macrolides,[a] metronidazole, miconazole (IV), nefazodone, nicardipine, nifedipine, quinidine, ritonavir, verapamil, zafirlukast

[a]CYP3A4 enzyme inhibition by macrolide antibiotics varies by drug: troleandomycin > erythromycin > clarithromycin > azithromycin = dirithromycin = 0.
[b]CYP2D6 enzyme inhibition by SSRI varies by drug: paroxetine = fluoxetine >> sertraline > fluvoxamine.
Compiled from references 3, 8–27.

■ REFERENCES

1. Almira M. Drug biotransformation. In, Katzung BG, ed. *Basic and clinical pharmacology*. Norwalk, CT: Appleton & Lange; 1992:49–59.

2. Watkins PB. Role of cytochromes P450 in drug metabolism and hepatotoxicity. *Semin Liver Dis* 1990;10:235–50.

3. Watkins PB. Drug metabolism by cytochromes P450 in the liver and small bowel. *Gastroenterol Clin North Am* 1992;21:511–26.

4. DeVane CL. Pharmacogenetics and drug metabolism of newer antidepressant agents. *J Clin Psychiatry* 1994;55(suppl):38-4-5.

5. Lennard M. Genetically determined adverse drug reactions involving metabolism. *Drug Saf* 1993;9:60–77.

6. Crewe HK et al. The effect of selective serotonin reuptake inhibitors on cytochrome P4502D6 (CYP2D6) activity in human liver microsomes. *Br J Clin Pharmacol* 1992;34:262–5.

7. Otton SV et al. Inhibition by fluoxetine of cytochrome P4502D6 activity. *Clin Pharmacol Ther* 1993;53:401–9.

8. Spinler SA et al. Possible inhibition of hepatic metabolism of quinidine by erythromycin. *Clin Pharmacol Ther* 1995;57:89–94.

9. Ereshefsky L et al. Antidepressant drug interactions and the cytochrome P450 system, the role of cytochrome P4502D6. *Clin Pharmacokinet* 1995;29(suppl):10–9.

10. von Moltke LL et al. Metabolism of drugs by cytochrome P450 3A isoforms. *Clin Pharmacokinet* 1995;29 (suppl):33–44.

11. Flockhart DA. Drug interactions and the cytochrome P450 system. *Clin Pharmacokinet* 1995;29(suppl):45–52.

12. Slaughter RL, Edwards DJ. Recent advances: the cytochrome P450 enzymes. *Ann Pharmacother* 1995;29: 619–24.

13. Pollock BG. Recent developments in drug metabolism of relevance to psychiatrists. *Harvard Rev Psychiatr* 1994;2:204–13.

14. Gonzalez FJ. Human cytochromes P450: problems and prospects. *Trends Pharmacol Sci* 1992;13:346–52.

15. Tatro DS, ed. *Drug interactions facts*. St. Louis: Facts and Comparisons; 1995.

16. Riesenman C. Antidepressant drug interactions and the cytochrome P450 system: a critical appraisal. *Pharmacotherapy* 1995;6(pt 2):84S–99S.

17. Kivisto KT et al. The role of human cytochrome P450 enzymes in the metabolism of anticancer agents: implications for drug interactions. *Br J Clin Pharmacol* 1995;40:523–30.

18. Schein JR. Cigarette smoking and clinically significant drug interactions. *Ann Pharmacother* 1995;29:1139–48.

19. Mitra AK et al. Metabolism of dapsone to its hydroxylamine by CYP2E1 in vitro and in vivo. *Clin Pharmacol Ther* 1995;58:556–66.

20. Transon C et al. In vivo inhibition profile of cytochrome P450TB (CYP2C9) by (+/−)-fluvastatin. *Clin Pharmacol Ther* 1995;58:412–7.

21. Periti P et al. Pharmacokinetic drug interactions of macrolides. *Clin Pharmacokinet* 1992;23:106–31.

22. Crewe HK et al. The effect of selective serotonin re-uptake inhibitors on cytochrome P4502D6 (CYP2D6) activity in human liver microsomes. *Br J Clin Pharmacol* 1992;34:262–5.

23. Manufacturer's Product Information.

24. Ketter TA et al. The emerging role of cytochrome P4503A in psychopharmacology. *J Clin Psychopharmacol* 1995;15:387–98.

25. Bertz RJ, Granneman GR. Use of in vitro and in vivo data to estimate the likelihood of metabolic pharmacokinetic interactions. *Clin Pharmacokinet* 1997;32:210–58.

26. Rendic S, Di Carlo FJ. Human cytochrome P450 enzymes: a status report summarizing their reactions, substrates, inducers and inhibitors. *Drug Metab Rev* 1997;29:413–580.

27. Michalets EL. Update: clinically significant cytochrome P-450 drug interactions. *Pharmacotherapy* 1998;18:84–112.

Drug-Induced Discoloration
of Feces and Urine

The drugs and drug classes in the following tables have been associated with the discoloration of feces or urine. Drugs and drug classes are listed generically.

DRUGS THAT MAY DISCOLOR FECES

DRUG/DRUG CLASS	COLOR PRODUCED
Antacids, Aluminum Hydroxide Types	Whitish or speckling
Anthraquinones	Brownish staining of rectal mucosa
Antibiotics, Oral	Greenish gray
Anticoagulants	Pink to red or black*
Bismuth Salts	Greenish black
Charcoal	Black
Clofazimine	Red to brownish black
Ferrous Salts	Black
Heparin	Pink to red or black*
Indocyanine Green	Green
Indomethacin	Green because of biliverdinemia
NSAIDs	Pink to red or black*
Omeprazole	Discoloration
Phenazopyridine	Orange-red
Pyrvinium Pamoate	Red
Rifampin	Red-orange
Risperidone	Discoloration
Salicylates (especially Aspirin)	Pink to red or black*

*These colors may indicate intestinal bleeding.

DRUGS THAT MAY DISCOLOR URINE

DRUG/DRUG CLASS	COLOR PRODUCED
Aminopyrine	Red
Aminosalicylic Acid	Discoloration; red in hypochlorite solution*
Amitriptyline	Blue-green
Anthraquinones	Yellow-brown in acid urine; yellow-pink-red in alkaline urine
Antipyrine	Red-brown
Azuresin	Blue or green
Chloroquine	Rust yellow to brown
Chlorzoxazone	Orange or purplish red
Cimetidine (injection)	Green†
Clofazimine	Red to brownish black

(continued)

DRUGS THAT MAY DISCOLOR URINE (continued)

DRUG/DRUG CLASS	COLOR PRODUCED
Daunorubicin	Red
Deferoxamine	Reddish
Doxorubicin	Red
Ethoxazene	Orange to orange-brown
Ferrous Salts	Black
Flutamide	Amber or yellow-green
Furazolidone	Brown
Idarubicin	Red
Indandiones	Orange-red in alkaline urine
Indomethacin	Green because of biliverdinemia
Iron Sorbitex	Brown-black
Levodopa	Red-brown; dark on standing in hypochlorite solution*
Loratadine	Discoloration
Methocarbamol	Dark to brown, black or green on standing
Methyldopa	Dark on standing in hypochlorite solution*
Methylene Blue	Blue or green
Metronidazole	Dark, brown
Mitoxantrone	Blue-green
Niacin	Dark
Nitrofurantoin	Rust yellow to brown
Pamaquine	Rust yellow to brown
Phenacetin	Dark brown to black on standing
Phenazopyridine	Orange to red
Phenolphthalein	Pink to purplish red in alkaline urine
Phenothiazines	Pink to red or red-brown
Phensuximide	Pink to red or red-brown
Phenytoin	Pink to red or red-brown
Primaquine	Rust yellow to brown
Promethazine (injection)	Green[†]
Propofol (injection)	Green,[†] white
Quinacrine	Deep yellow in acidic urine
Quinine	Brown to black
Resorcinol	Dark green
Riboflavin	Yellow fluorescence
Rifabutin	Discoloration
Rifampin	Red-orange
Sulfasalazine	Orange-yellow in alkaline urine
Sulfonamides, Antibacterial	Rust yellow to brown

(continued)

DRUGS THAT MAY DISCOLOR URINE (continued)

DRUG/DRUG CLASS	COLOR PRODUCED
Sulindac	Discoloration
Tolcapone	Bright yellow
Tolonium	Blue-green
Triamterene	Pale blue fluorescence
Warfarin	Orange

*Hypochlorite solution in toilet bowl from prior use of chlorine bleach.
†Caused by phenol as a preservative in the injectable formulation.

■ REFERENCES

1. *Physicians' desk reference,* 49th ed. Montvale, NJ: Medical Economics Data Production; 1995.
2. Baran RB, Rowles B. Factors affecting coloration of urine and feces. *J Am Pharm Assoc* 1973;NS13:139–42.
3. Bodenham A et al. Propofol infusion and green urine. *Lancet* 1987;2:740. Letter.
4. Bowling P et al. Intravenous medications and green urine. *JAMA* 1981;246:216. Letter.
5. Devereaux MW, Mancall EL. Brown urine, bleach, and L-DOPA. *N Engl J Med* 1974;291:1142. Letter.
6. Michaels RM, ed. Discolored urine. *Physicians' Drug Alert* 1981;2(9):71.
7. Nates J et al. Appearance of white urine during propofol anesthesia. *Anesth Analg* 1995;81:204–13. Letter.
8. Raymond JR, Yarger WE. Abnormal urine color: differential diagnosis. *South Med J* 1988;81:837–41.
9. Wallach J. *Interpretation of diagnostic tests,* 6th ed. Boston: Little, Brown; 1996;867–8, 879.

Drug Use in Special Populations

Drugs and Pregnancy

Andrea J. Anderson

In the United States, fetal malformations occur in 3–6% of pregnancies. These include major and minor malformations from any cause, be it drug, infection, maternal disease state, genetic, or pollutant.[1,2] Drug use during pregnancy may be associated with risk to the developing fetus as well as to the pregnant woman. Drugs are probably responsible for only about 1–5% of fetal malformations; 60–70% of malformations have unknown causes.[2–4]

The genetic makeup of both the fetus and the mother influences the extent to which an agent may affect the developing fetus. For example, the rates of absorption, metabolism, and elimination of an agent by the mother, its rate of placental transfer, or the way it interacts with cells and tissues of the embryo are all genetically determined factors. Thus, human teratogenicity cannot be predicted based only on animal data or extrapolated from one pregnancy to another.

■ PHYSIOLOGIC AND DEVELOPMENTAL FACTORS

Teratogenic substances rarely cause a single defect. Most often, a spectrum of defects occurs that corresponds with the systems undergoing major development at the time of exposure. Major malformations are usually the result of first trimester exposure during critical periods of organogenesis. Exposures during the second and third trimesters may result in alterations or damage in fine structure and function. Intrauterine growth retardation is perhaps the most reliable indicator that a teratogen was present during the second and third trimesters of fetal development. Several organs and systems continue to develop after birth. Therefore, exposure to agents late in pregnancy carries some risk and may result in debilitating alterations in development such as mental retardation. Figure 3–1 depicts the stages of human structural development in relation to teratogenic potential.[5]

■ DRUG FACTORS

Most chemicals in the maternal bloodstream cross the placenta. Movement of compounds across the placenta is generally bidirectional, although the net transfer occurs from mother to fetus in most instances.[6,7] Although active and facilitated

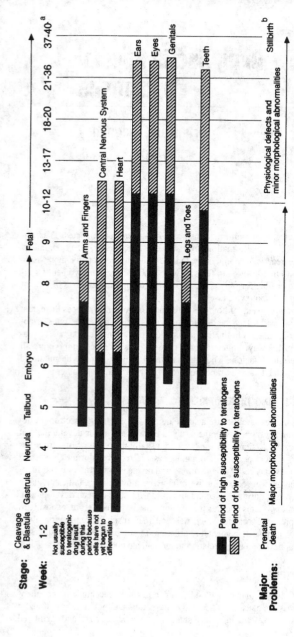

Figure 3–1. Variation in teratogenic susceptibility of organ systems during stages of human intrauterine development. (From Pagliaro LA, Pagliaro AM. *Problems in pediatric drug therapy*. 3rd ed. Hamilton, IL: Drug Intelligence Publications; 1995, reproduced with permission.)

[a] Average time for fertilization to parturition is 38 weeks.

[b] Drugs administered during this period may cause neonatal depression at birth (or other effects directly related to the pharmacological effect of the administered drug).

transport of some substances across the placenta have been demonstrated, the transplacental passage of most agents occurs primarily by simple diffusion.[6,8,9] Only the unbound (free) fraction of a drug is subject to placental transfer; therefore, the greater the degree of protein binding of a drug, the less will be transferred to the fetus.[6,8,9] Early in pregnancy, the placental membrane is relatively thick, and this characteristic tends to reduce permeability.[6] The thickness of the trophoblastic epithelium decreases and surface area increases in the last trimester. The passage of drugs is increased during this stage of pregnancy.[6,10]

The rate-limiting factors in placental transfer of drugs are the same as those that govern membrane diffusion by molecules in general. Thus, the rate of diffusion across the placental barrier is directly proportional to the maternal–fetal concentration gradient and the surface area of the placenta.[6,8,9] Higher concentrations are generally attained in fetal serum and amniotic fluid after bolus than after continuous infusion of drug into the mother, and by multiple-dose rather than single-dose therapy.[6] Certain physicochemical properties of drugs or chemicals favor transport to the fetus, including low molecular weight, lipid solubility, and nonionization at pH 7.4.[7,9,10]

Each drug has a threshold above which fetal defects can occur and below which no effects are discernible. Whether an agent reaches a "threshold concentration" in the fetus depends on maternal factors (eg, rates of absorption and clearance) as well as the chemical nature of the agent.

Administration of drugs near term poses another potential threat to the fetus. Before birth, the fetus relies on maternal systems for drug elimination. After birth, the infant must rely on its own metabolic and excretory capabilities, which have not yet fully developed. Drugs given near term or during birth, especially those with long half-lives, may have an even more prolonged action in the neonate. Drugs that cause maternal addiction are also known to cause fetal addiction. Neonatal withdrawal symptoms may occur when mothers have been addicted to drugs during pregnancy or when they have taken addicting drugs near term, even though the mothers themselves are not addicted.

■ EFFECTS OF PREGNANCY ON THE MOTHER

Maternal physiology changes as pregnancy progresses and may have an effect on drug disposition and clearance. Maternal plasma volume increases by about 20% at midgestation and 50% at term,[9] and then falls toward prepregnancy levels postpartum. The apparent volume of distribution for many drugs increases as the fetal compartment enlarges, causing changes in maternal serum drug concentrations. Drugs with narrow therapeutic ranges require careful monitoring during pregnancy, and possibly dosage increases. As postpartum maternal plasma volume returns to normal, dosages of many drugs require reduction. Changes in plasma protein concentrations during pregnancy may affect the degree of binding and thus the amount of unbound drug.[8,9] Despite an increase in production of serum albumin, the increased intracellular and intravascular volumes cause serum albumin concentrations to decline.[11] A decrease in total plasma protein concentrations of about 10 g/L occurs during pregnancy.[8] Body fat increases by 3–4 kg during pregnancy and may act as a depot for fat-soluble drugs, thereby increasing their apparent volume of distribution (V_d).[9] Renal blood flow and glomerular filtration rate increase by almost 50% during pregnancy because of increased cardiac output. Renally excreted drugs may therefore have increased rates of clearance.[9]

■ INTERPRETATION OF STUDIES

There are few controlled, prospective studies of drug use in pregnancy. Most of the available information comes from case reports or case-control studies. Cause-and-effect relationships between drugs and teratogenicity are difficult to establish retrospectively because of the numerous variables in each report. These include maternal drug dosage, time of ingestion relative to the date of conception, duration of therapy, concomitant exposure to other potential teratogens, and questionable study design or methodology. Because studies cannot disprove that a slight teratogenic risk may occur with in utero exposure to drugs, drugs should be used during pregnancy only when absolutely necessary. The following table provides information concerning the effects of drugs used during pregnancy on the pregnant woman and on pregnancy outcome. For a more thorough discussion of the principles of teratology, the reader should consult reference 1.

The following abbreviation is used in the table:

- IUGR—intrauterine growth retardation, less than the tenth percentile (of an appropriate standard) birthweight for gestational age.[12]

DRUGS AND PREGNANCY

ANALGESIC AND ANTI-INFLAMMATORY DRUGS

ANTIMIGRAINE DRUGS
Ergotamine
Ergotamine can stimulate uterine contraction and potentially cause abortion.[13]

Sumatriptan
Preliminary evidence collected by the manufacturer indicates no increased risk of birth defects in 124 pregnancies with early drug exposure.[13] Sumatriptan does not have the oxytocic effect of the ergot alkaloids.

NONSTEROIDAL ANTI-INFLAMMATORY DRUGS
Acetaminophen
Acetaminophen does not cause congenital malformations and is the analgesic-antipyretic of choice for use near term, because it does not affect platelet function or peripheral prostaglandin synthesis.[14,15] In maternal acetaminophen overdose, most infants are normal at birth,[16–19] but there have been a few cases of neonatal liver toxicity.[16,20] Acetaminophen may prevent fetal distress in laboring women with chorioamnionitis and fever.[21]

Nonsteroidal Anti-inflammatory Drugs
Early case reports implicating **indomethacin** as a cause of prenatal closure of the ductus arteriosus are inconclusive.[22–25] Indomethacin may cause oligohydramnios because of decreased fetal urine output, placing the fetus at risk for pulmonary hypoplasia and umbilical cord compromise.[13,24–27]

(continued)

ANALGESIC AND ANTI-INFLAMMATORY DRUGS

First trimester **aspirin** use does not increase the risk of congenital heart defects relative to that of other structural malformations.[28] Repeated third trimester administration of aspirin 325 mg may result in prolonged constriction of the ductus arteriosus and pulmonary hypertension.[29] Maternal ingestion of aspirin 325 mg during the third trimester may interfere with uterine contractility and prolong gestation and labor.[29] Maternal and neonatal platelet function may be affected, resulting in increased maternal blood loss at delivery and abnormal platelet function tests and clinical bleeding in newborns, including intracranial hemorrhage.[13,30] Second or third trimester use of low-dose (20–100 mg/day) aspirin in mothers at risk of developing pregnancy-related hypertension decreases the frequency of this disorder and its complications.[31,32] A follow-up 18 months after delivery of infants exposed in utero to aspirin 50 mg/day showed no increase in malformations and normal physical and neurologic development.[33]

Systematic evaluations of other commonly used NSAIDs have not been conducted in humans, but no substantive reports of NSAID teratogenicity exist.[13,22,30] However, caution is warranted because of their similarity to indomethacin and aspirin. **Ibuprofen** may cause mild oligohydramnios and mild constriction of the fetal ductus arteriosus.[13] Similar effects are likely with **naproxen**.[13] Persistent pulmonary hypertension occurred in a neonate whose mother had ingested 5 g **naproxen** 8 hr before delivery.[22] **Ketorolac** should be avoided during pregnancy.[13]

OPIOIDS

Narcotics

Narcotic analgesics do not cause fetal malformations, but narcotic abuse during pregnancy or use near term may lead to fetal addiction and neonatal withdrawal. Meconium may be present in the amniotic fluid, caused most likely by increased bowel activity during periods of fetal withdrawal and/or hypoxia, putting the fetus at risk for meconium aspiration.[34] (*See* Heroin.) Withdrawal symptoms, including irritability, increased muscle tone, sleep disturbances, vague autonomic nervous system symptoms, tremulousness, high-pitched crying, frantic and uncoordinated sucking, and seizures may occur in neonates born to narcotic-addicted women and nonaddicted women using narcotics near term. Neonatal respiratory depression may occur when narcotic analgesics are given during labor and is dependent on the drug, dose, dosing interval, and route of administration (IV > IM).[35] Epidural **alfentanil** does not provide good analgesia and can cause neonatal hypotonus.[36] **Meperidine** crosses the placenta rapidly and can cause a sinusoidal fetal heart rate pattern. It is eliminated by the fetus at a rate much slower than the mother's; its metabolite, normeperidine, is long acting.[37] Meperidine given during delivery can interfere with the early establishment of breastfeeding because of infant sedation.[38,39] Meperidine by patient-controlled analgesia (PCA) for postcesarean pain causes a much greater decrease in neonatal alertness and sucking than an equivalent dosage of PCA **morphine.** Infants born to narcotic-dependent women maintained on **methadone** during pregnancy may have smaller birth weights, lengths, and head circumferences than nonexposed infants, but they are usually not growth retarded.[13] Divided doses of methadone better stabilize the fetal activity pattern (which may indicate fetal withdrawal) before and after drug administration than do single daily doses.[40] Prolonged thrombocytosis has occurred in infants born to women taking methadone alone or with other addictive drugs.[35] Maternal **propoxyphene** use may cause neonatal withdrawal symptoms.[35]

(*continued*)

ANALGESIC AND ANTI-INFLAMMATORY DRUGS

Narcotic Partial Agonists

Buprenorphine used by a pregnant woman daily near term resulted in a mild narcoticlike withdrawal syndrome in her newborn.[41] **Butorphanol**[42] and **nalbuphine**[43] during labor can cause a sinusoidal fetal heart rate pattern. Nalbuphine offers no advantage over pure narcotics and may cause more abnormal Apgar scores (<7) at 1 min.[13,40] Nalbuphine with **pentazocine** use throughout pregnancy has caused infant withdrawal symptoms similar to those reported in offspring of heroin and methadone addicts.[13,35] Small-for-gestational-age infants, prematurity, and fetal distress have also been observed.[44] **Tramadol** withdrawal has been reported in a neonate exposed in utero throughout pregnancy.[45]

OTHER ANTI-INFLAMMATORY DRUGS

Gold Salts

Although teratogenic in animals, reports have described normal children born to women using gold salts during pregnancy. A few cases of musculoskeletal problems and one case of IUGR occurred among 128 infants exposed to injectable gold during pregnancy.[22,46] Six women given **auranofin** during pregnancy delivered normal infants.[46]

Penicillamine

Data on the teratogenicity of penicillamine are contradictory. Most pregnant women taking penicillamine deliver normal healthy babies, even at the high dosages used in treating Wilson's disease.[22,46] However, there have been cases of fetal connective tissue disease, contracted joints, poor wound healing, and cutis laxa.[22,46] Penicillamine is best avoided during pregnancy.[46]

ANTIMICROBIAL DRUGS

AMINOGLYCOSIDES

Streptomycin may cause congenital hearing loss, ranging from minor high-frequency loss to total deafness, when given to pregnant women for the treatment of tuberculosis. Prevalence is low, especially with careful dosage calculation and limited duration of therapy.[6,35,47,48] Other aminoglycosides may pose a similar risk.[6,35,49]

ANTIMYCOBACTERIAL DRUGS

Antituberculars

Ethambutol does not appear to cause malformations, but several anomalies involving the CNS occurred in 655 reported exposures.[6,35,47,48] Of the reported **isoniazid** exposures during pregnancy, only 1% demonstrated any malformations. No pattern of malformation was revealed, but several abnormalities involved the CNS.[6,35,47,48] Exposures were confounded by concomitant ethambutol therapy. Isoniazid is the safest and most effective antitubercular during pregnancy,[6] although there may be an increased risk of hepatotoxicity in pregnant women. **Rifampin** safety during pregnancy is less well established; however, it has not been associated with an increased risk of fetal malformations. In most reports, rifampin was taken with either isoniazid or ethambutol. Neonatal hypoprothrombinemia has been reported and raises some concern about the use of rifampin, especially near term.[6,35,47,48] If rifampin is given during pregnancy, maternal oral prophylaxis with vitamin K 20 mg/day for 2 weeks prior to delivery is recommended.[6,35,47] Infants should receive 0.5–1 mg of vitamin K IM or SC immediately after delivery and again 6–8 hr later.[35]

(continued)

ANTIMICROBIAL DRUGS

Sulfones

Dapsone does not appear to increase the risk of fetal abnormalities.[50] A woman on dapsone throughout her first pregnancy delivered a male infant who developed hyperbilirubinemia necessitating phototherapy. In a subsequent pregnancy, dapsone was discontinued 1 month prior to delivery and the infant did not develop hyperbilirubinemia. Because dapsone is similar to sulfonamides, it may displace bilirubin from albumin binding sites.[6,47,51] (*See* Sulfonamides.)

Thalidomide

Thalidomide causes bilateral limb reduction defects, facial hemangioma, esophageal or duodenal atresia, and anomalies of the kidneys, heart, and external ears. The time of greatest risk is between gestational days 22 and 32. If exposure occurs between days 27 and 30, the arms are most often affected; with exposure between days 30 and 33, the legs and arms are affected.[2]

ANTIPARASITIC DRUGS

Antimalarials

Chloroquine or **hydroxychloroquine** malaria prophylaxis does not cause adverse fetal effects; however, larger anti-inflammatory doses have resulted in spontaneous abortion and fetal retinal and vestibular damage.[6,46,47,52] These drugs are best avoided in anti-inflammatory dosages during pregnancy. There are no reports of **primaquine** teratogenicity, but it may induce hemolysis in neonates by the same mechanism as in adults.[35] **Pyrimethamine** is a microbial folate antagonist and should be used cautiously because the mammalian folate antagonist methotrexate is teratogenic; folic acid supplementation may be warranted during treatment.[6,35,46,47,53] **Quinine** has been used as a folk medicine abortifacient, despite its poor efficacy. Maternal deaths have been reported. Fetal anomalies include blindness, optic nerve hypoplasia, deafness, and hearing impairment.[6,35,46,47]

ANTIVIRAL DRUGS

Acyclovir

Maternal acyclovir during the second and third trimesters does not cause fetal toxicity.[47,54–61] Acyclovir may mediate a delay in maternal humoral antibody response that could result in delayed transfer of IgG to the fetus, thereby increasing the risk of neonatal HSV infection and treatment is recommended for HIV-infected pregnant women.[56]

Zidovudine

Use of zidovudine in pregnant women does not cause an increased rate of birth defects.[62–64] Concentrations of zidovudine are 2.5–7 times higher in amniotic fluid than in cord blood; concentrations in cord blood are higher (113–140%) than those in maternal blood.[65,66] Transmission of HIV from mother to fetus is substantially reduced with zidovudine treatment, and treatment is recommended for HIV-infected pregnant women.[63]

β-LACTAMS

Cephalosporins and **penicillins** are thought to be without teratogenic risk.[6,8,47,49,67] Treatment of early syphilis with penicillin (or other drugs) during pregnancy may produce the Jarisch–Herxheimer reaction, resulting in uterine cramping, decreased fetal movement, and, in some cases, fetal death.[68]

(*continued*)

ANTIMICROBIAL DRUGS

MACROLIDES

About 10–15% of women treated with **erythromycin estolate** in the second trimester develop abnormally elevated AST concentrations which normalize when therapy is discontinued.[35] There is no evidence that erythromycin is harmful to the fetus.[6,35,47,67]

QUINOLONES

Nalidixic acid use during pregnancy can cause increased intracranial pressure, papilledema, and bulging fontanelles in the newborn. Avoid first trimester use.[6,47,49] **Fluoroquinolones** (eg, **ciprofloxacin, norfloxacin, ofloxacin**) cause arthropathy in immature animals and, therefore, are not recommended for use in pregnancy.[47]

SULFONAMIDES

There are occasional reports of abnormalities, but no malformation pattern has emerged. Evidence associating sulfonamide use near term with neonatal kernicterus is lacking, despite sulfonamide displacement of bilirubin from albumin binding sites.[6,47,49,67,69–71] There is a theoretical risk for hemolysis in the fetus or neonate because of their relative deficiencies of G-6-PD and glutathione.[6,47]

TETRACYCLINES

Tetracyclines can cause hypoplasia and permanent staining of the teeth when taken after the 12th week of pregnancy. The risk of discoloration increases with dose, duration of therapy, and advancing pregnancy; one-third to one-half of third trimester exposures may be affected. Tetracyclines are also incorporated into calcifying bone, and inhibition of bone growth may occur. As bone is resorbed, the tetracycline is released.[6,47,49,67] Pregnant women with pyelonephritis or underlying renal disease, or following an overdose, are at risk for developing acute fatty necrosis of the liver and azotemia.[6,47,49,67]

MISCELLANEOUS ANTIMICROBIALS

Chloramphenicol

Although reports of fetal abnormality or toxicity from maternal chloramphenicol are lacking, there is a theoretical risk of blood dyscrasias. Particular caution should be exercised near term because the "gray baby" syndrome is a result of toxic accumulation of chloramphenicol in neonates caused by their slow elimination of the drug.[6,47,49]

Metronidazole

Twenty years' experience and several studies demonstrate no association of metronidazole with congenital malformations, abortions, or stillbirths.[72–75] However, a few cases of facial clefting have been reported.[76]

Nitrofurantoin

No fetal abnormalities or neonatal hemolytic anemia have been observed with nitrofurantoin use during pregnancy.[6,49,77–79] A theoretical risk for the development of hemolysis in neonates exists if the drug is taken by the mother near term because of infants' relative G-6-PD and glutathione deficiencies.[79]

Trimethoprim

Because it is a folate antagonist, caution is advised in pregnancy.[6,54] (*See* Methotrexate and Pyrimethamine.) However, data suggest a lack of teratogenicity.[6,49,67,70,71,80–82] Neither single-dose trimethoprim 600 mg nor the usual 5-day course (300 mg/day) for asymptomatic bacteriuria caused any detrimental effects on pregnancy outcome when given between the 16th and 30th weeks of gestation.[82]

(*continued*)

ANTIMICROBIAL DRUGS

Vancomycin

There is a theoretical risk for auditory and renal toxicity in the fetus.[6,47] However, in one small prospective trial, IV vancomycin during the second or third trimesters produced no cases of fetal renal toxicity or hearing impairment.[83]

ANTINEOPLASTICS AND IMMUNOSUPPRESSANTS

ANTINEOPLASTICS

Antineoplastic agents have both teratogenic and mutagenic potential, and reports of infertility and congenital defects exist. Nevertheless, several studies indicate that fertility is preserved, with normal pregnancy outcome, among both women and men treated for cancer prior to conception. Although aggressive treatment of malignancy is necessary on occasion, avoidance or minimum use of these drugs, especially during the first trimester, is recommended. However, normal pregnancy outcome has occurred, particularly if exposure is early in gestation (first 2 weeks after conception).[84] Chemotherapy generally produces a decrease in birthweight, but not IUGR.[85] Use of antineoplastics near delivery may cause neonatal bone marrow suppression,[86] because the drug may not have been eliminated prior to delivery. Chemotherapy should be avoided within 3 weeks of delivery if possible.[84]

ALKYLATING AGENTS

Busulfan

Use during pregnancy has been associated with IUGR and multiple malformations, although no specific pattern is evident.

Chlorambucil

Treatment in the first and second trimesters may cause spontaneous abortion, or cleft palate, renal aplasia, and skeletal abnormalities.[84]

Cyclophosphamide

Use in the first trimester has resulted in fetal malformations, particularly of the toes; syndactyly; cleft palate; facial anomalies; IUGR; and possible developmental delay. The overall risk of malformation is estimated to be 16–22%. No malformations have been reported with second or third trimester use, but pancytopenia occurred in neonates exposed late in pregnancy. A report of malignancies in a child that occurred 10 and 14 yr after exposure in utero raises the question whether intrauterine exposure to cyclophosphamide can cause iatrogenic or secondary cancers.[87] Cyclophosphamide should be avoided in pregnancy.

Procarbazine

Use in pregnancy is limited, but several fetal abnormalities have occurred, all with first trimester exposure.[35]

ANTIMETABOLITES

Fluorouracil

Use may cause malformations consistent with inhibition of cell division and cell growth.[35] Inadvertent first trimester topical administration of 5% fluorouracil to the lower genital tract did not result in abnormal-appearing infants in 10 pregnancies.[88,89]

(continued)

ANTINEOPLASTICS AND IMMUNOSUPPRESSANTS

Methotrexate

Use in the first trimester causes spontaneous abortion and congenital abnormalities, including cranial anomalies, left palate, syndactyly, growth retardation, and developmental abnormalities.[2] One study of 10 pregnancies in eight women taking methotrexate 7.5–10 mg/week during the first trimester for arthritis resulted in three spontaneous abortions, two elective abortions, and the birth of five full-term normal infants who had no medical illnesses or learning disabilities. Normal pregnancy outcome has occurred after use in the second and third trimesters.[2,90] It is recommended that methotrexate be discontinued for at least one menstrual cycle before conception and that the mother be taking folic acid.

Thioguanine

Use in both the first and second trimesters has been associated with abnormalities.[35,91]

DNA INTERCALATING DRUGS

Daunorubicin and **doxorubicin** have been given without fetal malformation, although some spontaneous abortions have occurred.[84]

MITOTIC INHIBITORS

Vinblastine and **vincristine** have reportedly been given in 21 pregnancies (13 in the first trimester) with no resultant congenital malformations.[84]

IMMUNOSUPPRESSANTS

Azathioprine

Normal pregnancy outcome has occurred with azathioprine taken for renal transplantation, SLE, or acute or chronic leukemias.[92] However, IUGR, neonatal lymphopenia, hypogammaglobulinemia, thymic hypoplasia, fetal bone marrow suppression, leukopenia, and thrombocytopenia have occurred.[93] Azathioprine for inflammatory bowel disease with or without a corticosteroid plus sulfasalazine resulted in no congenital anomalies or developmental problems.[93] Older studies showed some abnormal chromosomal aberrations; however, there is no evidence of permanent genomal or gonadal damage.

Cyclosporine

Use of cyclosporine throughout pregnancy following renal or hepatic transplant does not appear to cause malformations, although experience is limited.[46] IUGR occurred in 11 of 20 infants, and 6 had severe IUGR (below the third percentile). However, normal-size-for-gestational-age infants are often delivered. No neonatal distress or increased mortality has been reported.[94,95]

Tacrolimus

Use in pregnancy following liver transplant resulted in preterm deliveries of 27 infants of 21 mothers.[96] However, prenatal and postnatal growth were appropriate for age. One infant was born with unilateral polycystic kidney disease.

CARDIOVASCULAR DRUGS

ANTIARRHYTHMIC DRUGS

Amiodarone

Neonatal hypothyroidism with and without goiter, as well as hyperthyroidism, has occurred with amiodarone use.[97] A child with transient congenital hypothyroidism showed some delay in motor development and impaired speech performance at age 5.[97]

(continued)

CARDIOVASCULAR DRUGS

Digoxin

Digoxin is not a teratogen. It may be given to pregnant women to treat fetal CHF and supraventricular tachycardia. Maternal digitalis toxicity has caused fetal toxicity and miscarriage in one case and neonatal ECG changes with subsequent infant death in another. As pregnancy progresses, renal clearance of digoxin increases and bioavailability may also increase. Therefore, maternal serum concentrations may decrease or increase and should be monitored.[98,99]

Disopyramide

Use during pregnancy has not been well studied, but in one report, uterine contractions were precipitated by disopyramide which subsided when the drug was discontinued.[98]

Procainamide

Use during pregnancy is probably safe. However, because of the potential for SLE, caution is advised.[98]

Quinidine

Use during pregnancy is not teratogenic.[35,98] Neonatal thrombocytopenia has occurred after maternal use of quinidine.[35]

ANTIHYPERTENSIVE DRUGS

ACE Inhibitors

Several cases of IUGR and prolonged neonatal anuria and hypotension with resultant renal failure have occurred following maternal **captopril** or **enalapril** use.[100–103] Oligohydramnios or anhydramnios was present in seven of nine cases (not recorded in the other two cases) and led to pulmonary hypoplasia and death in some. Respiratory problems occurred in several neonates. Some infants had altered or absent skull formation with dysmorphic facial features, microcephaly, and occipital encephalocele. One infant exposed during the second and third trimesters had prolonged anuria and hypotension requiring dialysis, and one infant exposed throughout pregnancy had hypoglycemia; others have had persistent ductus arteriosus (this may have been caused by low birthweight).[102–104] There may be an increased frequency of fetal loss with ACE inhibitors.[103] The FDA warns against their use in the second and third trimesters.

Diazoxide

When given by rapid IV bolus, diazoxide can cause excessive maternal hypotension and fetal distress. Slow IV infusion or minibolus administration may prevent these effects. Other reported effects include inhibition of labor, neonatal hyperglycemia when exposure preceded delivery, alopecia, hypertrichosis languinosa, and decreased bone age after exposure in the last 19–70 days of gestation. Other investigators report no problems after long-term oral administration of diazoxide.[98,105,106]

Hydralazine

Use in pregnancy may cause reduced uteroplacental blood flow, fetal heart rate changes after acute administration, and neonatal hypothermia and thrombocytopenia.[98,105,106] There is little information concerning first trimester use.

Methyldopa

Methyldopa in pregnancy is more extensively studied than any other antihypertensive. Available data show no teratogenicity. Transient reduction in neonatal blood pressure may occur after maternal methyldopa ingestion. There is a questionable association of IUGR and maternal treatment with methyldopa. One study suggested IUGR was caused by chronic hypertension rather than by methyldopa.[98,105,106]

(*continued*)

CARDIOVASCULAR DRUGS

Reserpine

When given to mothers within 24 hr of delivery, reserpine produces edema of the neonatal nasal mucosa. This effect is especially important because newborns are obligate nose breathers. Lethargy, hypothermia, and bradycardia have also been reported in infants whose mothers received antenatal reserpine.[105,107]

β-ADRENERGIC BLOCKING DRUGS

Atenolol, pindolol, metoprolol, and **propranolol** are generally safe in pregnancy. Maternal hypertension can cause IUGR, decreased placental size, neonatal respiratory depression, and hypoglycemia. IUGR and neonatal hypoglycemia and hypotension have also occurred following β-blockers. Whether these effects are caused by the drugs or by maternal disease has not been established. Neonatal bradycardia may be caused by these agents; it is usually mild, but was severe following an IV **esmolol** infusion in one case.[108] β-blockers may adversely affect fetal adaptation to intrauterine hypoxia, such as that associated with umbilical cord compression.[98,100,105,109–113] Although generally regarded as safe during pregnancy, **labetalol** given IV to control severe hypertension has caused neonatal bradycardia, weak femoral pulses, inadequate breathing, hypotonia, hypotension, and hypoglycemia.[105,106,113,114]

CALCIUM-CHANNEL BLOCKING DRUGS

No malformations have been associated with use of calcium-channel blocking agents during pregnancy.[115–117] Bolus doses of IV **isradipine** during labor effectively reduce maternal blood pressure while causing an increased fetal heart rate.[115] **Nifedipine** does not appear to alter uterine arterial resistance when given at 17–22 weeks,[116] or 26–35 weeks' gestational age.[117]

INOTROPIC DRUGS

The treatment of hypotension during pregnancy with sympathomimetic agents (eg, **dopamine, dobutamine, norepinephrine**) is complicated by the fact that the uterine vasculature is supplied solely with α-adrenergic receptors and is maximally dilated under basal conditions. Pure α-adrenergic agents markedly constrict uterine vessels and decrease blood flow, thereby compromising the fetus. β-Adrenergic agents cause peripheral vasodilation and tend to shunt blood away from the uterus and also may cause fetal compromise. Volume-expanding agents seem to be the most prudent treatment for sudden hypotension in pregnancy.

CENTRAL NERVOUS SYSTEM DRUGS

ANTICONVULSANTS

Many congenital malformations have been reported in children of epileptic mothers, and all anticonvulsants for which data are adequate have been implicated as possible causes of malformations. Epileptic mothers have an increased frequency of fetal malformation compared with nonepileptic mothers, and anticonvulsant drugs appear to increase this frequency.[118] Major malformations seem to be more common following combination therapy than with monotherapy.[118] Fetal deficiency of epoxide hydrolase, a major enzyme in the metabolic pathway of many anticonvulsants (eg, **carbamazepine, phenytoin,** and **valproic acid**) that helps eliminate toxic intermediates, may mediate teratogenic effects. Deficient function of this enzyme may be inherited as an autosomal recessive trait.[119–123] Total concentrations of carbamazepine, phenytoin, phenobarbital, and valproic acid decline as pregnancy progresses, caused mainly by changes in plasma protein binding.[118] However, free or unbound drug concentrations

(*continued*)

CENTRAL NERVOUS SYSTEM DRUGS

fall appreciably only for phenobarbital. Free concentrations of valproic acid increase. Measurement of free anticonvulsant drug concentrations allows for appropriate dosage adjustment.[118] Decreased fetal **folic acid** concentrations have been reported with several anticonvulsants (eg, carbamazepine, phenobarbital, phenytoin, and valproic acid). Folic acid supplementation during pregnancy may decrease the risk of abnormal offspring.[124]

Carbamazepine

Carbamazepine increases the risk for certain abnormalities, including spina bifida.[118,124] The malformations are similar to those ascribed to other anticonvulsants: specific facial features, nail hypoplasia, and smaller head circumference. Data concerning developmental delay or impairment require substantiation.[118] Higher serum concentrations of carbamazepine were found in mothers of abnormal offspring than in mothers of normal offspring.[125] Mothers receiving carbamazepine should receive supplemental folic acid.[124]

Gabapentin

There is little information about gabapentin in pregnancy. Of nine exposed women reported to the manufacturer, four had elective abortions, four had normal infants, and one infant had pyloric stenosis and an inguinal hernia.

Oxazolidinediones

Long-term use of **trimethadione** or **paramethadione** during pregnancy has resulted in children with abnormalities, including mental deficiency, prominent forehead with V-shaped eyebrows, epicanthal folds, microcephaly, low-set ears with anteriorly folded helices, short stature, and hypospadias. The frequency of spontaneous abortion may also be increased.[2,35,118]

Phenobarbital

Abnormalities have been reported with phenobarbital alone and in combination, but causality is not established. Malformations similar to those of phenytoin and alcohol have been reported with phenobarbital and may be related to the folate deficiency that each of these can cause.[118] These effects may be more likely when maternal serum concentrations exceed usual therapeutic concentrations. Barbiturates can cause a decrease in vitamin K–dependent clotting factors, leading to bleeding in the newborn.[35,118] Neonatal withdrawal may occur after phenobarbital use during pregnancy.

Phenytoin

Phenytoin serum concentrations may decrease during pregnancy because of increased plasma clearance. Adjustment of phenytoin dosage to maintain serum free drug concentrations seems to improve seizure control.[126] Phenytoin is a teratogen, causing a cluster of anomalies called the fetal hydantoin syndrome (FHS), the principal features of which are craniofacial anomalies (eg, bowed upper lip, ocular hypertelorism, broad nasal bridge, short nose, epicanthal folds), digital hypoplasia with small or absent nails, and pre- and postnatal growth deficiency.[2,118,127] The risk of developing the full-blown FHS is about 5–10% when phenytoin is taken throughout pregnancy; the risk of a less serious effect is 30%.[128] Serum anticonvulsant concentrations were higher in mothers of malformed infants than in mothers of normal infants in some studies.[129] Maternal phenytoin use may also result in developmental delay and intellectual impairment.[129] Phenytoin can cause a decrease in vitamin K–dependent clotting factors, leading to bleeding in the newborn.[35,118]

(*continued*)

CENTRAL NERVOUS SYSTEM DRUGS

Primidone

The teratogenicity of primidone alone is difficult to assess, because few cases have been reported and primidone is often taken with other anticonvulsants, primarily phenytoin. Although no specific pattern is established, reported malformations include craniofacial alterations, hirsute forehead, cardiac defects, pre- and postnatal growth retardation, digital hypoplasia with small or flat nails, inguinal hernias, and hypospadias.[35,118] Some cases of developmental delay have also been reported. These effects may be more likely when maternal serum concentrations exceed usual therapeutic concentrations. Phenobarbital is one metabolite of primidone. (*See* Phenobarbital.)

Valproic Acid

Neural tube defects (eg, spina bifida) occurred in 1–2% of valproic acid–exposed fetuses compared with 0.4% in fetuses exposed to other anticonvulsants.[118,128] The risk for neural tube defects may be 5- to 10-fold higher with valproic acid compared with the background frequency.[119] The rate of spina bifida appears to be related to valproate serum levels. Serum levels should be kept as low as possible during pregnancy and the mother given supplemental folic acid.[118] External ear anomalies, congenital heart defects, hypospadias, craniofacial anomalies, low birthweight, and small head circumference have been reported.[118,125,128,130–132] Cases of limb reduction defects, radial ray aplasia, talipes equinovarus, developmental delay, neurologic abnormality, and brain atrophy have also been reported.[128,130]

ANTIDEPRESSANTS

Selective Serotonin Reuptake Inhibitors

Prospective follow-up of exposed pregnancies, including first trimester exposure and spontaneous reports to the manufacturer, do not implicate **fluoxetine** as a teratogen.[133] However, a prospective study found increased risks of multiple minor malformations, prematurity, large for gestational age, admission to a special care nursery, and poor neonatal adaptation.[133] Several case reports of neonatal withdrawal following maternal fluoxetine or **sertraline** use during the third trimester have been reported.[133,134] Symptoms include restlessness, irritability, crying, tremors, increased muscle tone, poor feeding, and sleep disturbance.

Tricyclic Antidepressants

Although there are several case reports of varied fetal anomalies after maternal use of tricyclic antidepressants (TCAs) during pregnancy, no consistent pattern of malformation has been observed. Maternal use of TCAs during pregnancy has occasionally produced neonatal symptoms of breathlessness, respiratory distress, hypertonia with tremor, clonus, spasm, cyanosis, tachypnea, irritability, and feeding difficulties. In one case, neonatal urinary retention occurred following maternal **nortriptyline** use.[135]

ANTIPSYCHOTIC DRUGS

There is some evidence that women with psychoses have twice the rate of fetal malformation as the general population.[136] Most data do not implicate **phenothiazines, haloperidol,** or **clozapine** as teratogens.[136] Phenothiazine use near term has resulted in some cases of extrapyramidal effects in the neonate, which have persisted up to 9 months.[136,137] Leukemia, hyperbilirubinemia, and jaundice (primarily in premature neonates), decreased gastric motility, poor sucking, and respiratory depression have also been reported. If drug therapy is necessary during pregnancy, high-potency agents (eg, **haloperidol, fluphenazine**) are preferred over low-potency agents (eg, **chlorpromazine, thioridazine**) because the latter may cause maternal hypotension.[136]

(*continued*)

CENTRAL NERVOUS SYSTEM DRUGS

ANXIOLYTICS, SEDATIVES, AND HYPNOTICS

High dosages of any sedative-hypnotic close to or during delivery may result in neonatal CNS and respiratory depression.

Anesthetics, General

There is a possible association between general anesthesia for surgery performed between gestational weeks 4 and 5 and neural tube defects,[138] and first trimester exposure to general anesthesia is associated with hydrocephalus and eye defects.[139] However, not all patients in these studies received the same preoperative medications or inhalation anesthetics, although **nitrous oxide** was received by over 98% in one study.[140] Definitive conclusions await further study. **Halothane**, teratogenic in rats, has questionable effects on the developing human embryo.[140] Although a two- to four-fold increase in the rate of spontaneous abortion in pregnant women with long-term exposure to inhalation anesthetics (eg, operating room and dental personnel) has been suggested, poor study design makes conclusions suspect.[140,141] CNS and respiratory depression in the neonate may occur following inhalation anesthetic use during labor. When given intermittently during labor, equilibrium between mother and fetus is usually not reached. However, when inhaled continuously, high fetal tissue concentrations may occur causing neonatal depression, especially in the premature or poor-risk infant.[251] During labor, halothane is not recommended due to its low analgesic activity. Nitrous oxide, **methoxyflurane**, and **enflurane** are commonly used.[142] Neonatal EEG recordings have documented that **thiopental** general anesthesia has more neonatal depressant effects than 0.5% **bupivacaine** epidural anesthesia when used for cesarean section.[143]

Barbiturates

Barbiturate addiction during pregnancy can result in neonatal withdrawal. Symptoms include tremors, irritability, restlessness, high-pitched crying, increased tone, hyperphagia, and overreaction to stimuli, which may persist for up to 6 months.[35] (*See* Anticonvulsants, Phenobarbital.)

Benzodiazepines

Recent data do not support an earlier reported association between **diazepam** or **chlordiazepoxide** and oral clefting.[12,35,135,144,145] However, there is a case report describing an acentric craniofacial cleft in a child whose mother took 580 mg diazepam as a single dose about 43 days after her last menstrual period.[146] Infants of mothers using benzodiazepines near term may exhibit withdrawal symptoms (including tremors, irritability, and hypertonicity) and cardiovascular, respiratory, and CNS effects consistent with benzodiazepine pharmacology. Many exhibit the "floppy baby syndrome" characterized by muscular relaxation, poor sucking, disturbances in thermoregulation, and regurgitation.[13,35,142,144,147-149] **Oxazepam, lorazepam,** and **temazepam** are short acting and predominantly metabolized into inactive glucuronides and subsequently excreted via the kidneys; they therefore may be preferred over diazepam, although irritability, feeding difficulties, and muscle tone disorders lasting 2 months were reported in two infants of mothers who used lorazepam 2–3 mg/day throughout pregnancy.[148,150] It seems best to avoid benzodiazepines during the period of organogenesis and near delivery.[13]

Meprobamate

In one study, meprobamate ingestion during the first 42 days of pregnancy resulted in 8 of 66 exposed children having abnormalities, 5 of whom had cardiovascular malformations. Other large-scale investigations have not confirmed these findings.[35] Alternative agents are advised, especially during the first trimester.

(*continued*)

CENTRAL NERVOUS SYSTEM DRUGS

LITHIUM

Lithium use during the first trimester of pregnancy, particularly from the third to eighth weeks, may cause an increased risk of cardiovascular abnormalities, including Ebstein's anomaly.[151–155] Anomalies of the external ear, ureters, CNS, and endocrine system, as well as macrosomia, have also been reported.[153,154] A case of polyhydramnios possibly caused by lithium-induced fetal polyuria has occurred.[156] Of lithium-exposed pregnancies followed by the Lithium Registry, 39% delivered prematurely, 36% had macrosomia (>90th percentile body weight for gestational age), and there was an 8.3% perinatal mortality rate. Symptoms of lithium toxicity, including lethargy, hypotonia, poor sucking reflex, respiratory distress, cyanosis, arrhythmias, and hypothermia, have been reported in newborns of women on long-term lithium therapy. Newborn blood concentrations were 0.6–1 mEq/L. Monitor maternal serum concentrations frequently during pregnancy, because lithium clearance varies as pregnancy progresses.[135,151–153]

GASTROINTESTINAL DRUGS

ACID-PEPTIC THERAPY
Antacids

The safety of antacid use during the first trimester of pregnancy has not been established.[69] Second and third trimester use appears to be without adverse effects.

Histamine H₂-Receptor Antagonists

No reports link **cimetidine** or **ranitidine** to adverse pregnancy outcome.[157] Manufacturer data on cimetidine use in 50 pregnant women reveal no increased risk to the developing fetus, although time of exposure was not noted. The use of H₂-antagonists as preanesthetic agents to prevent aspiration of acidic stomach contents has no reported adverse effects on the course of delivery or on the neonate.[69,158,159]

Sucralfate

There have been no adequate studies of sucralfate in pregnant women. Because little of the drug is absorbed, little risk is expected.[69]

ANTIEMETICS

One study of 120 women with hyperemesis gravidarum treated with **metoclopramide, prochlorperazine,** or placebo found no malformations or neonatal problems.[160] However, a reanalysis of some early data questions the initial negative findings and suggests an increased risk of malformations with first trimester antinauseant phenothiazine use during the fourth to tenth week of gestation.[137]

GASTROINTESTINAL MOTILITY
Cisapride

A prospective study of cisapride use in pregnancy found no increased risks of major or minor malformations, spontaneous abortion, or decreased birthweight in 88 pregnancies.[161]

Metoclopramide

There are no reports of adverse fetal outcome with use of metoclopramide during pregnancy; however, the drug has not been used widely in this setting.[69,160] The use of metoclopramide during labor, anesthesia, or cesarean section to prevent acid aspiration has not resulted in adverse maternal, fetal, or neonatal outcome.[69,160]

(*continued*)

GASTROINTESTINAL DRUGS

MISCELLANEOUS GASTROINTESTINAL DRUGS
Mesalamine Derivatives
Sulfasalazine has been associated with IUGR. However, one large survey found the prevalence of IUGR, prematurity, pregnancy loss, and developmental defects to be lower in women taking sulfasalazine for Crohn's disease than in the general population.[46,69,162,163] (*See also* Antimicrobial Drugs, Sulfonamides.)

HEMATOLOGIC DRUGS

COAGULANTS AND ANTICOAGULANTS
Heparin
Heparin has not been associated with an increased risk for structural or functional defects or with IUGR. Maternal thrombocytopenia and hemorrhage may occur.[164–167]

Warfarin
Warfarin and related anticoagulants may produce the "fetal warfarin syndrome" or "warfarin embryopathy." The critical period of risk appears to be between 6 and 12 weeks of gestation. Features include nasal hypoplasia, neonatal respiratory distress from upper airway obstruction, stippled epiphyses, IUGR, and varying degrees of hypoplasia of the extremities. Eye abnormalities, including blindness, have also been reported. About one-third of exposed cases result in adverse pregnancy outcomes. One-half of these are spontaneous abortions or stillbirths, and the other half exhibit some type of congenital abnormality.[2,128,164–171] A few cases of diaphragmatic malformation have been reported when warfarin was used early in pregnancy.[172] CNS defects occur in about 3% of those exposed and appear to occur independent of the fetal warfarin syndrome. Critical periods of risk for CNS effects appear to be during the second and third trimesters.[171] Warfarin also increases the risk for fetal as well as maternal hemorrhage, especially when used near term.[164,168]

HORMONAL DRUGS

ADRENAL HORMONES
Corticosteroid use during pregnancy may cause an increased risk for maternal gestational diabetes, hypertension, and excessive weight gain.[95] Although teratogenic in animals, corticosteroids have not been demonstrated to be teratogenic in humans. Large prospective investigations, together with cases of pregnant women with inflammatory bowel disease, asthma, or rheumatoid arthritis, do not show an increase in spontaneous abortions or congenital defects in infants exposed prenatally. Some studies show decreased birthweight and increased rates of prematurity, although these effects may have been due to the underlying maternal disease.[95,173] Women who had status asthmaticus during pregnancy were more likely to have infants with low birthweight or IUGR.[173] A placental enzyme (11-β-OH-dehydrogenase) inactivates certain corticosteroids, leading to low fetal concentrations. This inactivation is greater with **hydrocortisone, prednisone,** or **prednisolone** compared to that with **betamethasone** or **beclomethasone.** The fetal liver is relatively ineffective in converting prednisone into the active prednisolone, even at term. Therefore, prednisone or hydrocortisone may be preferred during pregnancy. When appropriate, corticosteroids can be administered by aerosol inhalation or intrasynovial injection to minimize systemic availability.[23,95,173] Neonates born to women taking long-term coticosteroids should be monitored for adrenal insufficiency, although this rarely occurs. Maternal betamethasone

(*continued*)

HORMONAL DRUGS

therapy is used to prevent respiratory distress in infants born between 28 and 34 weeks of gestation with no apparent adverse effects.[174,175] No differences in psychologic or physical development, pulmonary function, ophthalmologic findings, or neurologic function were noted between exposed and nonexposed children between 10 and 12 years of age.[176] However, there was a significantly increased frequency of hospitalizations for infections during early childhood in the exposed group.

ANDROGENS

Androgen (eg, **testosterone, methyltestosterone,** and **danazol**) exposure during the first week of gestation may cause masculinization of the female embryo. Clitoromegaly, with or without fusion of the labia minora, may occur. In some cases, a urogenital sinus opening at the base of the clitoris has been observed. The extent of the defect is correlated with the time of exposure and dosage.[2,177,178] Although danazol dosages under 400 mg/day may carry a lower risk, virilization was observed with 200 mg/day in one case.[178] Because differentiation of external genitalia occurs 8–12 weeks postconception, exposure beyond the 12th week of gestation is expected to produce only clitoral hypertrophy. If danazol is discontinued by the 8th week of gestation, the risk is substantially lower. Internal genitalia are unaffected because they are not androgen responsive. The male fetus does not appear to be adversely affected.

ANTIDIABETIC DRUGS

Maternal diabetes is known to increase the rate of malformations and perinatal mortality.[179,180] Pregnancy in 20 women exposed to an oral hypoglycemic (16 to a sulfonylurea, 3 to a biguanide, 1 unknown) during organogenesis resulted in a higher proportion of major and minor malformations than a similar unexposed control group.[180] A retrospective case review did not find a similar increase in malformations.[181] Malformations reported included auricular, vertebral, cardiac, neural tube, and limb defects.[180–182] Complicating the issue is a study that shows **glyburide** does not cross the human placenta ex vivo in appreciable amounts.[183] Sulfonylureas (eg, **chlorpropamide, glyburide,** and **glipizide**) and biguanides (eg, **metformin**) may cause prolonged hypoglycemia or hyperinsulinism in the newborn.[2,35,128,180,184] Pregnant diabetics should be treated with **insulin.**

FEMALE SEX HORMONES

Clomiphene

Clomiphene-induced ovulation results in an increased frequency of multiple ovulations (primarily twinning), delayed follicular rupture, ectopic pregnancy, and female fetuses. There is also an increase in abnormal karyotypes in oocytes and abortuses. The high proportion of abnormal karyotypes could be related to the increase in spontaneous abortions and low pregnancy rate noted after ovulation induction and in vitro fertilization.[185,186] The rate of birth defects reported after ovulation induction in most studies has been within the expected range.[185,187,188]

Diethylstilbestrol (DES)

Daughters of DES-exposed mothers have an increased frequency of vaginal adenosis; structural defects of the cervix, vagina, uterus, and fallopian tubes; and reproductive complications such as infertility, spontaneous abortion, ectopic pregnancy, premature deliveries, and perinatal deaths.[2,189–192] Two large cohort studies do not confirm the relation of DES to clear cell carcinoma. Early studies showing such an association were retrospective and had serious methodologic flaws.[193] If an association exists,

(continued)

HORMONAL DRUGS

the risk of developing this cancer in exposed females is very low. Data on DES-exposed males suggest an increased risk for infertility, various urogenital abnormalities, and testicular cancer.[194]

Progestins

High doses of progestins (eg, **medroxyprogesterone, norethindrone,** and **norethynodrel**) during pregnancy may cause masculinization of female external genitalia (clitoral hypertrophy or labioscrotal fusion). Hypospadias has occurred in males.[195,196] This most likely occurs during the period of external genitalia development (8–12 weeks postconception).[2,35,197–199] Doses used in oral or implantable contraceptives do not appear to carry these risks.[200]

THYROID AND ANTITHYROID DRUGS

Propylthiouracil and **methimazole** were associated with neonatal goiter in early reports, possibly because of the use of iodine in addition to unnecessarily high dosages of antithyroid medication. However, even conservative management does not completely eliminate the risk of congenital goiter. Transient neonatal hypothyroidism and neonatal thyrotoxicosis may occur. Hypothyroidism may be prevented by discontinuing the drug 4–6 weeks before delivery if the mother has remained euthyroid. Monitor infants for thyrotoxicosis, because it may be masked by the antithyroid agent. Four cases of infants with ulcer-like midline scalp defects have been associated with maternal methimazole. Mothers with moderate to severe hyperthyroidism not receiving treatment have an increased risk of complications including toxemia, small-for-gestational-age babies, and neonatal morbidity.[201–203] Excessive **iodine** use during pregnancy can cause congenital goiter and hypothyroidism. Goiters may be large enough to cause tracheal compression and interfere with delivery. Severe maternal iodine deficiency produces hypothyroidism and cretinism.[201,202]

No adverse effects have been reported after inadvertent exposure to ^{131}I prior to 10 weeks' gestation. After 10 weeks' gestation, the fetal thyroid actively concentrates iodine; any radioactive iodine ingested by the mother will cross the placenta and destroy fetal thyroid tissue.[2,201]

MISCELLANEOUS HORMONAL AGENTS

Oxytocin

Oxytocin given for induction of labor may cause tetanic uterine contractions, causing decreased uterine blood flow and fetal distress. The risk of neonatal hyperbilirubinemia may be increased 1.6-fold following oxytocin-induced labor compared with spontaneous labor, and neonatal jaundice has occurred.[204]

Prostaglandins

Misoprostol has uterotonic effects and should not be used during pregnancy. In 56 pregnant women who requested first trimester abortions, 1 or 2 oral doses of misoprostol 400 μg resulted in spontaneous fetal expulsions.[205] Twenty-five women had uterine bleeding. High doses of misoprostol in early pregnancy, such as those used to induce abortion, cause defects. Anomalies reported include paralysis of cranial nerves VI and VII.[206–208] Misoprostol is used with **methotrexate** for first trimester pregnancy termination. (*See* Methotrexate monograph.) **Dinoprostone,** when administered as vaginal tablets to mildly hypertensive women at term to induce labor, produces significant decreases in the percentage of time occupied by fetal body and breathing movements 3–4 hr later.[209] Fetal outcome is normal. Dinoprostone may shorten labor more than oxytocin.[210,211]

(*continued*)

RENAL AND ELECTROLYTES

DIURETICS

Diuretics should be used with great caution during pregnancy because they can decrease maternal intravascular volume and consequently diminish uteroplacental perfusion, thereby compromising fetal oxygenation. This effect is most rapid and severe with loop diuretics (eg, **bumetanide, furosemide**, and **torsemide**). IV furosemide administration to the pregnant woman has enabled ultrasonic imaging of the fetal bladder because of increased fetal urine output. **Thiazide diuretic** use in pregnancy may produce neonatal hypoglycemia, hyponatremia, hypokalemia, and thrombocytopenia.[98,105,106,212]

ELECTROLYTES

Long-term infusion of **magnesium sulfate** during the second trimester occasionally causes bone abnormalities and dental enamel hypoplasia.[213,214] However, infusions between 24 and 34 weeks' gestation in women with preterm labor generally does not cause adverse neonatal outcomes.[215] Use of magnesium sulfate as a tocolytic agent near term may cause dosage-related neonatal hypotonia, hyporeflexia, respiratory distress, hypocalcemia, and hypermagnesemia.[213,216] Serial serum magnesium levels should be used to guide therapy.

RESPIRATORY DRUGS

ANTIALLERGICS

Cromolyn sodium use during pregnancy is not known to have any teratogenic effects. A prescription event monitoring study of **nedocromil** in the United Kingdom identified 79 exposed pregnancies.[219] Routine follow-up showed no abnormalities among the 33 infants with first trimester exposure.

ANTIASTHMATICS

β-Adrenergic Agonists

Aerosol inhalation of **metaproterenol, albuterol, isoetharine**, or **terbutaline** is probably safe during pregnancy. Less is known about the oral use of these products, but experience suggests no adverse outcome. In one series, **salmeterol** was taken during the first trimester during 64 pregnancies and only during the second and third trimesters in three pregnancies.[220] The 67 pregnancies resulted in 50 live births, 6 spontaneous abortions, 2 ectopic pregnancies, 4 elective terminations, and 5 unknown outcomes. The small number of fetuses exposed to salmeterol during this study precludes any definitive conclusions about its safety. **Albuterol, terbutaline**, and **ritodrine** have been given in large IV or PO doses for their tocolytic effects in the third trimester without permanent harm to the fetus, although hypertension, hypoglycemia, hypokalemia, and hypocalcemia have been reported.[216] **Ephedrine** use during labor may cause altered neonatal sleep patterns.[143]

Theophylline

Maternal theophylline pharmacokinetics may change during the second and third trimesters, with decreased theophylline protein binding, decreased nonrenal clearance, and increased renal clearance.[221] Both V_d and half-life increase during the third trimester.[221] Pregnant women should have theophylline concentrations monitored frequently for dosage adjustments. No adverse fetal effects from long-term theophylline use during pregnancy are known.[222] Theophylline toxicity occurred in three newborns whose mothers received theophylline or **aminophylline** in late pregnancy and during labor. Symptoms included jitteriness, vomiting, tachycardia, and irritability, all of which resolved.[35]

(continued)

RESPIRATORY DRUGS

Inhaled Corticosteroids

This route is preferred during pregnancy to minimize fetal exposure. (*See* Corticosteroids.)

ANTIHISTAMINES

Despite reports implicating both **meclizine** and Bendectin (**doxylamine** and **pyridoxine** with or without **dicyclomine**) as teratogens, large-scale studies and two meta-analyses have shown no association between antihistamines and fetal malformation.[3,35,217,218] A prospective study of **hydroxyzine** and **cetirizine** found no increase in major or minor malformations, or birth-related difficulties.[218] **Dimenhydrinate** may have an oxytocic effect on the term uterus, causing shortened labor. The same concerns as with oxytocin (hyperstimulation and the possibility of uterine rupture) apply.[160]

COUGH AND COLD

Use of **sympathomimetics** (eg, **pseudoephedrine**) for treatment of nasal congestion may cause increased fetal activity and fetal tachycardia. Systemically administered sympathomimetics should be avoided in patients with hypertension or eclampsia, or situations in which there is poor fetal cardiac reserve.[35,223]

MISCELLANEOUS DRUGS

ANESTHETICS, LOCAL

Maternal exposure to local anesthetics during the first 4 months of pregnancy does not cause fetal malformations.[142,143,224] However, local anesthetics have resulted in fetal and neonatal CNS and myocardial depression following maternal use during labor. Fetal bradycardia may occur after paracervical blocks. Epidural administration of **bupivacaine** or **lidocaine** may be the safest method for obstetric analgesia. Epidural lidocaine was shown to decrease neonatal neurobehavioral performance, but the effect was short lived and of minimal clinical consequence.[142] High-concentration (0.75%) bupivacaine is not recommended for use in obstetrics because of the profound neonatal myocardial depression and prolonged difficult resuscitation following accidental intravascular injection.[142,224] Lower concentrations are popular because of the high quality of analgesia with minimal degree of motor block.[142] **Mepivacaine** should not be used in obstetric anesthesia because the neonate is unable to metabolize it.[142,143]

ERGOT ALKALOIDS

The use of **ergonovine** or **methylergonovine** before delivery carries the same risk of uterine stimulation as oxytocin.[13,216] (*See* Hormones and Synthetic Substitutes, Oxytocin.)

PODOPHYLLIN

Podophyllotoxins are antimitotic agents, and their use during pregnancy is contraindicated. Maternal oral use during the 5th through 9th weeks of gestation is associated with congenital malformation. High doses used topically at the 34th week resulted in severe maternal toxicity and a stillborn fetus. There are several cases in which topical podophyllin use during pregnancy produced no adverse outcome.[225–228]

(*continued*)

MISCELLANEOUS DRUGS

RETINOIDS
Etretinate

Etretinate is a known teratogen in humans. Fetal abnormalities include facial dysmorphia; syndactylies; absence of terminal phalanges; neural tube closure defects; malformations of the hip, ankle, and forearm; low-set ears; high palate; decreased cranial volume; and alterations of the cervical vertebrae and skull.[229] Etretinate accumulates in adipose tissue with repeated administration and has been detected in the serum of some patients up to 3 yr after discontinuing therapy. The importance of this, relative to the risk of teratogenicity, is unknown. An effective form of contraception must be used for at least 1 month before etretinate therapy, during therapy, and for an indefinite time following therapy, some say for at least 2 yr.[229–234] Unpublished data from the manufacturer indicate suspected teratogenicity in 8 of 95 fetuses reportedly exposed 1–24 months following drug discontinuation.[231]

Isotretinoin

Use during pregnancy causes defects of the CNS, heart, external ear, and thymus.[128,235–243] Other reported malformations include cleft palate, microphthalmia, micrognathia, facial dysmorphia, and limb reduction defects. Infants may exhibit hearing and visual impairment and mental retardation.[241] One report estimates the relative risk for major birth defects from isotretinoin to be 25.6.[235] Data suggest that the risk is substantial even when exposure to isotretinoin is brief or dosage is low.[242] The risk for spontaneous abortion is also increased.[236,237,242] In an analysis of cases reported to the manufacturer, 28% of exposed fetuses were malformed.[242] Exposures before day 14 of gestation resulted in the same rates of malformation and spontaneous/missed abortion as exposures between days 14 and 83.[242]

Tretinoin

Topical application of tretinoin results in absorption of vitamin A with equivalent activity less than that of a prenatal vitamin. Therefore, teratogenicity of this retinoid, although theoretically possible, is unlikely when used topically as directed.[244,245] Both studies of first trimester use of topical retinoids and a review of cases of malformations typical of retinoids failed to implicate topical retinoids in malformations.[244–246] However, two cases of malformations similar to those of isotretinoin after first trimester tretinoin exposure have occurred.[247,248]

Vitamin A

Retinol or retinyl esters (but not beta carotene) in toxic doses are teratogenic in experimental animals, producing defects in almost all organ systems. Human data on vitamin A teratogenicity consist of only a few anecdotal reports and epidemiologic studies. Epidemiologic studies show that doses of vitamin A contained in prenatal vitamin supplements (ie, $\leq$10,000 IU/day) do not increase the risk of fetal malformation.[249–252] However, because of methodologic flaws and incomplete data, the degree of risk with higher daily dosages of vitamin A is unclear. Further research is warranted. Defects observed when mothers ingested $\geq$25,000 IU/day of vitamin A during pregnancy include craniofacial, CNS, cardiac, urinary, vertebral, and other skeletal malformations.[2,253,254]

VAGINAL SPERMICIDES

Use of vaginal spermicides was associated with major congenital anomalies in two retrospective analyses, but there were many flaws in the studies, casting doubt on the results.[255,256] Subsequent studies, including a meta-analysis of nine studies, fail to implicate these agents as teratogens.[200,257–260]

(*continued*)

MISCELLANEOUS DRUGS

VACCINES

See Immunization, page 960, for information regarding vaccination during pregnancy.

VITAMIN D

Excessive use has been associated with an idiopathic hypercalcemic syndrome including cardiovascular malformation, abnormal bone mineralization, elfin facies, mental retardation, hypercalcemia, and nephrocalcinosis. Definitive conclusions await further investigation.[2,261,262]

DRUGS FOR NONMEDICAL USE

Alcohol

Animal studies show that alcohol and **acetaldehyde** exposure in utero results in morphologic changes in the structure as well as in protein and endocrine content of the CNS.[263–265] As many as 5% of human congenital anomalies may be due to maternal alcohol consumption,[266] and it may be responsible for 10% of all cases of mental retardation. (Alcohol is the most frequent recognizable cause of mental retardation.[266,267]) A 2-fold increase in spontaneous abortion was noted among women who drank one to two drinks daily for the first 2 months of pregnancy; the rate was higher in those who drank more than two drinks daily. Moderate drinking (1–13 fl oz of absolute alcohol per week) results in an increase in some of the features of the fetal alcohol syndrome (FAS), including IUGR.[267,268] Chronic heavy alcohol consumption causes the full-blown FAS in 10–50% of children exposed in utero. Features of FAS include IUGR, microcephaly, postnatal growth deficiency, developmental delay, mental retardation, and craniofacial anomalies. Joint, limb, cardiac, ocular, brain, and urogenital defects, along with eustachian tube dysfunction, also occur. Neonates may have withdrawal symptoms similar to those of adults.[128,263–277] Alcohol-related birth defects may occur at rates higher than that of full-blown FAS, and CNS dysfunction may occur with lower alcohol exposure than that required to produce the FAS.[267] Alcohol consumption during pregnancy should be avoided because the minimum dosage that may produce adverse fetal effects has not been established. One author proposes that the threshold dosage for alcohol teratogenesis may be 1 fl oz of absolute alcohol per day.[267]

Amphetamines

Data on the effect of prenatal amphetamines, both prescribed and abused, are conflicting; however, no consistent pattern of abnormalities has emerged.[35,278] Most studies found no increase in severe congenital malformations, but others report biliary atresia, congenital heart disease, and eye and CNS defects.[35,278] Reports of decreased birthweight and length, head circumference, and IUGR may reflect poor maternal nutrition, but use of other drugs and alcohol may have confounded these findings. Investigations with term neonates exposed antenatally to methamphetamine, with or without cocaine, document an increased prevalence of prematurity, IUGR, altered behavioral patterns (abnormal sleep patterns, poor feeding, tremors, and hypertonia), and the presence of cerebral injury as detected by ultrasonography.[278–280] (*See also* Cocaine.)

Caffeine

Caffeine is not suspected of causing fetal malformations. Data suggest that caffeine use before and during pregnancy may increase the rate of spontaneous abortion.[281,282] A small reduction in birthweight may occur when caffeine consumption during pregnancy exceeds 300 mg/day, although cigarette smoking may contribute. There are

(*continued*)

DRUGS FOR NONMEDICAL USE

conflicting data about whether 400–600 mg/day of caffeine increases the risk of miscarriage, stillbirth, or prematurity.[282–287] One study showed that rates of infant central and obstructive apnea positively correlated with increasing maternal caffeine consumption.[288]

Cocaine

Maternal cocaine use during pregnancy can cause adverse fetal and maternal outcomes. Although most data relate to use near term, preliminary findings suggest some risks from exposure early in pregnancy. Poor health care and nutrition, a high infection rate, and frequent concomitant drug (eg, narcotics, nicotine, or marijuana) and alcohol use complicate risk evaluation. A meta-analysis of 20 papers found no significant differences in adverse fetal effects between cocaine users and polydrug users.[289] Maternal cocaine use results in an increase in the frequency of spontaneous abortion, placental hemorrhage, abruptio placentae, and stillbirths. There is also an increase in frequency of prematurity as well as premature rupture of the membranes. A few cases of precipitate delivery have been reported, as well as two cases of precipitate rupture of ectopic pregnancy. Fetal genitourinary malformations and intrauterine death have been reported when mothers used cocaine.[289–294] Cocaine most likely disrupts morphogenesis by vasoconstriction of uterine and fetal circulation. Interruption of calcium metabolism may also contribute to hydronephrosis.[291,293,295,296] Infants may experience a withdrawal syndrome consisting of jitteriness, tremor, hyperreflexia, hypertonia, irritability, high-pitched crying, frantic sucking, poor feeding, tachypnea, abnormal sleep patterns, vomiting, or loose stools. Neurologic signs of toxicity, including seizures, have also been reported. Exposed infants have an increased frequency of abnormal pneumograms, respiratory distress, or other cardiorespiratory abnormalities. Some authors feel these abnormalities may predispose infants to sudden infant death syndrome (SIDS). Retrospective population-based studies found that the risk of SIDS in cocaine-exposed infants was higher than that of infants whose mothers did not abuse any drugs; however, several confounding independent risks for SIDS were not controlled.[297,298] Several reports of neonatal or fetal cerebral infarction or intracranial hemorrhage exist.[289,290,295,299–327]

Heroin

Poor nutrition and health care, lack of prenatal care, high infection rates, and frequent concomitant nicotine, nonmedical drug, and alcohol use complicate risk assessment. No specific pattern of fetal malformation has been noted. Some studies have associated maternal heroin use with a decrease in birthweight and length, reduced head circumference, small-for-gestational-age infants, low Apgar scores, meconium staining, neonatal respiratory distress, jaundice, and increased neonatal mortality. A narcotic withdrawal syndrome occurs frequently, usually within the first 24–48 hr after birth, although it can be delayed for as long as 6 days. The symptoms, which may persist for as long as 20 days, include irritability; feeding and sleeping problems; hyperactivity; and excessive sneezing, yawning, vomiting, mucous secretion, sweating, and face scratching. Other withdrawal symptoms including increased muscle tone, vague autonomic nervous system symptoms, tremulousness, high-pitched crying, frantic and uncoordinated sucking, and seizures may occur in neonates born to narcotic-addicted women and nonaddicted women who use narcotics near term. The frequency of withdrawal is directly related to the daily dosage and duration of maternal heroin use. The results of studies evaluating development show conflicting results ranging from no effect to problems with behavior and perceptual and organizational abilities.[35,328] One retrospective, population-based study found that the relative risk of SIDS was 15.5 in infants of mothers who abused illicit opiates during all or part of pregnancy.[297]

(*continued*)

DRUGS FOR NONMEDICAL USE

Marijuana

Marijuana smoke contains carbon monoxide and may cause constriction of uterine and placental vessels resulting in fetal hypoxia and decreased nutrient supply.[325,329] Marijuana use during pregnancy has not resulted in any specific pattern of malformation, but exposures were confounded by nicotine and other nonmedical drug and alcohol use.[325,327,329–331]

Phencyclidine

Long-term phencyclidine use during pregnancy, especially near term, may produce neonatal withdrawal symptoms of hypertonicity, occasional darting eye movements, and lethargy, as well as coarse flappy tremors after stimulation. These infants have a marked increase in lability of behavioral states and poor consolability.[332,333] Some children at 9 and 18 months of age exhibited fine motor, adaptive, and language scores in the low-normal range. Motor movements in the lower extremities were also awkward.[325,332]

Tobacco

Cigarette smoke contains numerous toxins, including carbon monoxide and nicotine, which are probably responsible for reported fetal hypoxia because of decreased oxygen exchange and placental vasoconstriction.[334,335] Smoking during pregnancy causes increased rates of IUGR or low birthweight (5% decrease/pack smoked daily), prematurity, spontaneous abortion, neonatal and postnatal deaths, abruptio placentae, premature rupture of membranes, and placenta previa.[2,184,335–339] Women exposed to second-hand smoke may also be at risk for delivering a growth-retarded or preterm infant.[336] If a woman stops smoking by the 20th week of pregnancy, the risk of a low-birthweight infant is similar to that of the general population.[334] Cigarette smoking alters the placental arterial linings as well as accelerating placental senescence, which may explain the placental complications of smoking.[335,338–340] One study involving 17,152 infants (15.7% of the mothers were smokers) found an increased frequency of minor malformations in infants of mothers aged 35 yr or older who smoked.[341] Some data suggest infants of smokers have increased nervous system excitation, hypertonicity, and altered breathing patterns with an increased rate of central apnea.[288,342] These children have also been shown to have altered language, auditory, and lower cognitive functions. Some studies suggest an increased risk of childhood acute lymphocytic and lymphoblastic leukemias and lymphoma in those whose fathers and/or mothers smoked before or during pregnancy.[343,344] Tobacco chewing during pregnancy also results in a greatly increased rate of stillbirth, IUGR, and prematurity.[336]

■ REFERENCES

1. Wilson JG, Fraser RC, eds. *Handbook of teratology.* Vol I. General principles and etiology. New York: Plenum Press; 1977.

2. Beckman DA, Brent RL. Mechanism of known environmental teratogens: drugs and chemicals. *Clin Perinatol* 1986;13:649–87.

3. Brent RL. The complexities of solving the problem of human malformations. *Clin Perinatol* 1986;13:491–503.

4. Friedman JM et al. Potential human teratogenicity of frequently prescribed drugs. *Obstet Gynecol* 1990;75:594–9.

5. Pagliaro LA, Pagliaro AM, eds. *Problems in pediatric drug therapy.* 3rd ed. Hamilton, IL: Drug Intelligence Publications; 1995.

6. Chow AW, Jewesson PJ. Pharmacokinetics and safety of antimicrobial agents during pregnancy. *Rev Infect Dis* 1985;7:287–313.

7. Berlin CM. Effects of drugs on the fetus. *Pediatr Rev* 1991;12:282–7.

8. Landers DV et al. Antibiotic use during pregnancy and the postpartum period. *Clin Obstet Gynecol* 1983;26: 391–406.

9. Murray L, Seger D. Drug therapy during pregnancy and lactation. *Emerg Med Clin North Am* 1994;12:129–49.

10. Pacifici GM, Nottoli R. Placental transfer of drugs administered to the mother. *Clin Pharmacokinet* 1995;28: 235–69.

11. Frey BM, O'Donnell J. Drug therapy in pregnancy and lactation. *J Pharm Pract* 1989;2:2–12.

12. Kramer MS. Intrauterine growth and gestational duration determinants. *Pediatrics* 1987;80:502–11.

13. Rathmell JP et al. Management of nonobstetric pain during pregnancy and lactation. *Anesth Analg* 1997;85:1074–87.

14. Streissguth AP et al. Aspirin and acetaminophen use by pregnant women and subsequent child IQ and attention decrements. *Teratology* 1987;35:211–9.

15. Heymann MA. Non-narcotic analgesics: use in pregnancy and fetal and perinatal effects. *Drugs* 1986;32 (suppl 4):164–76.

16. Ludmir J et al. Maternal acetaminophen overdose at 15 weeks of gestation. *Obstet Gynecol* 1986;67:750–1.

17. McElhatton PR et al. Paracetamol poisoning in pregnancy: an analysis of the outcomes of cases referred to the teratology information service of the national poisons information service. *Human Exp Toxicol* 1990;9:147–53.

18. Rosevear SK, Hope PL. Favourable neonatal outcome following maternal paracetamol overdose and severe fetal distress: case report. *Br J Obstet Gynaecol* 1989;96:491–3.

19. Robertson RG et al. Acetaminophen overdose in the second trimester of pregnancy. *J Fam Pract* 1986; 23:267–8.

20. Kurzel RB. Can acetaminophen excess result in maternal and fetal toxicity? *South Med J* 1990;83:953–5.

21. Kirshon B et al. Effect of acetaminophen on fetal acid–base balance in chorioamnionitis. *J Reprod Med* 1989; 34:955–9.

22. Brooks PM, Needs CJ. The use of antirheumatic medication during pregnancy and in the puerperium. *Rheum Dis Clin North Am* 1989;15:789–806.

23. Kirshon B et al. Influence of short-term indomethacin therapy on fetal urine output. *Obstet Gynecol* 1988; 72:51–3.

24. Morales WJ et al. Efficacy and safety of indomethacin versus ritodrine in the management of preterm labor: a randomized study. *Obstet Gynecol* 1989;74:567–72.

25. Hallak M et al. Indomethacin for preterm labor: fetal toxicity in a dizygotic twin gestation. *Obstet Gynecol* 1991;78:911–3.

26. Wurtzel D. Prenatal administration of indomethacin as a tocolytic agent: effect on neonatal renal function. *Obstet Gynecol* 1990;76:689–92.

27. Hickok DE et al. The association between decreased amniotic fluid volume and treatment with nonsteroidal anti-inflammatory agents for preterm labor. *Am J Obstet Gynecol* 1989;160:1525–31.

28. Werler MM et al. The relation of aspirin use during the first trimester of pregnancy to congenital cardiac defects. *N Engl J Med* 1989;321:1639–42.

29. Rudolph AM. Effects of aspirin and acetaminophen in pregnancy and in the newborn. *Arch Intern Med* 1981; 141:358–63.

30. Barry WS et al. Ibuprofen overdose and exposure in utero: results from a postmarketing voluntary reporting system. *Am J Med* 1984;77(suppl 1a):35–9.

31. Sibai BM et al. Low-dose aspirin in pregnancy. *Obstet Gynecol* 1989;74:551–7.

32. Schiff E et al. The use of aspirin to prevent pregnancy-induced hypertension and lower the ratio of thromboxane A2 to prostacyclin in relatively high risk pregnancies. *N Engl J Med* 1989;321:351–6.

33. Parazzini F et al. Follow-up of children in the Italian Study of Aspirin in Pregnancy. *Lancet* 1994;343:1235. Letter.

34. Edelin KC et al. Methadone maintenance in pregnancy: consequences to care and outcome. *Obstet Gynecol* 1988;71:399–404.

35. Briggs GG et al. *Drugs in pregnancy and lactation.* 3rd ed. Baltimore: Williams & Wilkins; 1990.

36. Curran MJA. Options for labor analgesia: techniques of epidural and spinal analgesia. *Semin Perinatol* 1991; 15:348–57.

37. Savona-Ventura C et al. Pethidine blood concentrations at time of birth. *Int J Gynecol Obstet* 1991;36:103–7.

38. Wittels B et al. Postcesarean analagesia with both epidural morphine and intravenous patient-controlled analgesia: neurobehavioral outcomes among nursing infants. *Anesth Analg* 1997;85:600–6.

39. Nissen E et al. Effects of routinely given pethidine during labour on infants' developing breastfeeding behaviour. *Acta Paediatr* 1997;86:201–8.

40. Wittmann BK, Segal S. Comparison of the effects of single- and split-dose methadone administration on the fetus: ultrasound evaluation. *Int J Addiction* 1991;26:213–8.

41. Marquet P et al. Buprenorphine withdrawal syndrome in a newborn. *Clin Pharmacol Ther* 1997;62:569–71.
42. Hatjis CG, Meis PJ. Sinusoidal fetal heart rate pattern associated with butorphanol administration. *Obstet Gynecol* 1986;67:377–80.
43. Dan U et al. Intravenous pethidine and nalbuphine during labor: a prospective double-blind comparative study. *Gynecol Obstet Invest* 1991;32:39–43.
44. Little BB et al. Effects of T's and blues abuse on pregnancy outcome and infant health status. *Ann J Perinatol* 1990;7:359–62.
45. Meyer FP et al. Tramadol withdrawal in a neonate. *Eur J Clin Pharmacol* 1997;53:159–60.
46. Ramsey-Goldman R, Schilling E. Optimum use of disease-modifying and immunosuppressive antirheumatic agents during pregnancy and lactation. *Clin Immunother* 1996;1:40–58.
47. Anon. Safety of antimicrobial drugs in pregnancy. *Med Lett Drugs Ther* 1987;29:61–3.
48. Holdiness MR. Teratology of the antituberculosis drugs. *Early Hum Dev* 1987;15:61–74.
49. Pedler SJ, Bint AJ. Management of bacteriuria in pregnancy. *Drugs* 1987;33:413–21.
50. Barnhart ER, ed. Dapsone. In, *Physicians' desk reference*. 44th ed. Oradell, NJ: Medical Economics; 1990: 1079–80.
51. Thornton YS, Bowe ET. Neonatal hyperbilirubinemia after treatment of maternal leprosy. *South Med J* 1989; 82:668.
52. Levy M et al. Pregnancy outcome following first trimester exposure to chloroquine. *Am J Perinatol* 1991; 8:174–8.
53. Pajor A. Pancytopenia in a patient given pyrimethamine and sulphamethoxidiazine during pregnancy. *Arch Gynecol Obstet* 1990;247:247:215–7.
54. Landsberger EJ et al. Successful management of varicella pneumonia complicating pregnancy: a report of three cases. *J Reprod Med* 1986;31:311–4.
55. Brown ZA, Baker DA. Acyclovir therapy during pregnancy. *Obstet Gynecol* 1989;73:526–31.
56. Leen CLS et al. Acyclovir and pregnancy. *Br Med J* 1987;294:308. Letter.
57. Hankins GDV et al. Acyclovir treatment of varicella pneumonia in pregnancy. *Crit Care Med* 1987;15:336–7.
58. Boyd K, Walker E. Use of acyclovir to treat chickenpox in pregnancy. *Br Med J* 1988;296:393–4.
59. Eder SE et al. Varicella pneumonia during pregnancy: treatment of two cases with acyclovir. *Am J Perinatol* 1988;5:16–8.
60. Klein NA et al. Herpes simplex virus hepatitis in pregnancy. Two patients successfully treated with acyclovir. *Gastroenterology* 1991;100:239–44.
61. Anons. Pregnancy outcomes following systemic prenatal acyclovir exposure—June 1, 1984–June 30, 1993. *MMWR* 1993;42:806–9.
62. Sperling RS et al. A survey of zidovudine use in pregnant women with human immunodeficiency virus infection. *N Engl J Med* 1992;326:857–61.
63. Anons. Birth outcomes following zidovudine therapy in pregnant women. *MMWR* 1994;43:409, 415–6.
64. Kumar RM et al. Zidovudine use in pregnancy: a report on 104 cases and the occurrence of birth defects. *J Acquir Immune Defic Syndr* 1994;7:1034–9.
65. Chavanet P et al. Perinatal pharmacokinetics of zidovudine. *N Engl J Med* 1989;321:1548–9. Letter.
66. Watts DH et al. Pharmacokinetic disposition of zidovudine during pregnancy. *J Infect Dis* 1991;163:226–32.
67. Chapman ST. Bacterial infections in pregnancy. *Clin Obstet Gynecol* 1986;13:397–417.
68. Klein VR et al. The Jarisch–Herxheimer reaction complicating syphilotherapy in pregnancy. *Obstet Gynecol* 1990;75:375–80.
69. Lewis JH et al. The use of gastrointestinal drugs during pregnancy and lactation. *Am J Gastroenterol* 1985; 80:912–23.
70. Soper DE, Merrill-Nach S. Successful therapy of penicillinase-producing *Neisseria gonorrhoeae* pharyngeal infection during pregnancy. *Obstet Gynecol* 1986;68:290–1.
71. Czeizel A. A case-control analysis of the teratogenic effects of co-trimoxazole. *Reprod Toxicol* 1990;4: 305–13.
72. Amon I. Placental transfer of metronidazole. *J Perinat Med* 1985;13:97–8. Letter.
73. Drinkwater P. Metronidazole. *Aust N Z J Obstet Gynaecol* 1987;27:228–30.
74. Roe FJC. Safety of nitroimidazoles. *Scand J Infect Dis* 1985;46(suppl):72–81.
75. Piper JM et al. Prenatal use of metronidazole and birth defects: no association. *Obstet Gynecol* 1993;82: 348–52.
76. Greenberg F. Possible metronidazole teratogenicity and clefting. *Am J Med Genetics* 1985;22:825. Letter.
77. Hailey FJ et al. Fetal safety of nitrofurantoin macrocrystals therapy during pregnancy: a retrospective analysis. *J Int Med Res* 1983;11:364–9.
78. D'Arcy PF. Nitrofurantoin. *Drug Intell Clin Pharm* 1985;19:540–7.
79. Personal communication, Carol A. Bixler, Norwich Eaton Pharmaceuticals, February 12, 1991.

80. Cruikshank DP, Warenski JC. First-trimester maternal *Listeria monocytogenes* sepsis and chorioamnionitis with normal neonatal outcome. *Obstet Gynecol* 1989;73:469–71.

81. Kelly RT, Bibbins B. Pregnancy and brucellosis. *Tex Med* 1987;83:39–41.

82. Bailey RR et al. Comparison of single dose with a five-day course of trimethoprim for asymptomatic (covert) bacteriuria of pregnancy. *N Z Med J* 1986;99:501–3.

83. Reyes MP et al. Vancomycin during pregnancy: does it cause hearing loss or nephrotoxicity in the infant? *Am J Obstet Gynecol* 1989;161:977–81.

84. Sorosky JI et al. The use of chemotherapeutic agents during pregnancy. *Obstet Gynecol Clin North Am* 1997;24:591–9.

85. Kim DS, Park MI. Maternal and fetal survival following surgery and chemotherapy of endodermal sinus tumor of the ovary during pregnancy: a case report. *Obstet Gynecol* 1989;73:503–7.

86. Raffles A et al. Transplacental effects of maternal cancer chemotherapy. Case report. *Br J Obstet Gynaecol* 1989;96;1099–100.

87. Zemlickis D et al. Teratogenicity and carcinogenicity in a twin exposed in utero to cyclophosphamide. *Teratog Carcinog Mutagen* 1993;13:139–43.

88. Kopelman JN, Miyazawa K. Inadvertent 5-fluorouracil treatment in early pregnancy: a report of three cases. *Reprod Toxicol* 1990;4:233–5.

89. Van Le L et al. Accidental use of low-dose 5-fluorouracil in pregnancy. *J Reprod Med* 1991;36:872–4.

90. Blatt J et al. Pregnancy outcome following cancer chemotherapy. *Am J Med* 1980;69:828–32.

91. Artlich A et al. Teratogenic effects in a case of maternal treatment for acute myelocytic leukaemia—neonatal and infantile course. *Eur J Pediatr* 1994;153:488–91.

92. Korelitz BI. Pregnancy, fertility, and inflammatory bowel disease. *Am J Gastroenterol* 1985;80:365–70.

93. Alstead EM et al. Safety of azathioprine in pregnancy in inflammatory bowel disease. *Gastroenterology* 1990; 99:443–6.

94. Pickrell MD et al. Pregnancy after renal transplantation: severe intrauterine growth retardation during treatment with cyclosporin A. *Br Med J* 1988;296:825.

95. Burrows DA et al. Successful twin pregnancy after renal transplant maintained on cyclosporine A immunosuppression. *Obstet Gynecol* 1988;72:459–61.

96. Jain A et al. Pregnancy after liver transplantation under tacrolimus. *Transplantation* 1997;64:559–65.

97. Plomp TA et al. Use of amiodarone during pregnancy. *Eur J Obstet Gynecol Reprod Biol* 1992;43:201–7.

98. Lees KR, Rubin PC. Treatment of cardiovascular diseases. *Br Med J* 1987;294:358–60.

99. Moriguchi Mitani G et al. The pharmacokinetics of antiarrhythmic agents in pregnancy and lactation. *Clin Pharmacokinet* 1987;12:253–91.

100. Kaler SG et al. Hypertrichosis and congenital anomalies associated with maternal use of minoxidil. *Pediatrics* 1987;79:434–6.

101. Rosa FW et al. Neonatal anuria with maternal angiotensin-converting enzyme inhibition. *Obstet Gynecol* 1989;74:371–4.

102. Mehta N, Modi N. ACE inhibitors in pregnancy. *Lancet* 1989;2:96. Letter.

103. Cunniff C et al. Oligohydramnios sequence and renal tubular malformation associated with maternal enalapril use. *Am J Obstet Gynecol* 1990;162:187–9.

104. Piper JM et al. Pregnancy outcome following exposure to angiotensin-converting enzyme inhibitors. *Obstet Gynecol* 1992;80:429–32.

105. Lubbe WF. Hypertension in pregnancy: pathophysiology and management. *Drugs* 1984;28:170–88.

106. Naden RP, Redman CWG. Antihypertensive drugs in pregnancy. *Clin Perinatol* 1985;12:521–38.

107. Mabie WC et al. Chronic hypertension in pregnancy. *Obstet Gynecol* 1986;67:197–205.

108. Ducey JP, Knape KG. Maternal esmolol administration resulting in fetal distress and cesarean section in a term pregnancy. *Anesthesiology* 1992;77:829–32.

109. Al Kasab SM et al. β-Adrenergic receptor blockage in the management of pregnant women with mitral stenosis. *Am J Obstet Gynecol* 1990;163:37–40.

110. Ellenbogen A et al. Metabolic effects of pindolol on both mother and fetus. *Curr Ther Res* 1988;43:1038–41.

111. Lyons CW, Colmorgen GHC. Medical management of pheochromocytoma in pregnancy. *Obstet Gynecol* 1988;72:450–1.

112. Devoe LD et al. Metastatic pheochromocytoma in pregnancy and fetal biophysical assessment after maternal administration of alpha-adrenergic, beta-adrenergic, and dopamine antagonists. *Obstet Gynecol* 1986;68 (suppl):15S–8.

113. Haraldsson A, Geven W. Severe adverse effects of maternal labetalol in a premature infant. *Acta Paediatr Scand* 1989;78:956–8.

114. Haraldsson A, Geven W. Half-life of maternal labetalol in a premature infant. *Pharm Weekbl Sci* 1989;11: 229–31.

115. Wide-Swensson D et al. Effects of isradipine, a new calcium antagonist, on maternal cardiovascular system and uterine activity in labour. *Br J Obstet Gynaecol* 1990;97:945–9.

116. Thaler I et al. Effect of calcium channel blocker nifedipine on uterine artery flow velocity waveforms. *J Ultrasound Med* 1991;10:301–4.

117. Moretti MM et al. The effect of nifedipine therapy on fetal and placental Doppler waveforms in preeclampsia remote from term. *Am J Obstet Gynecol* 1990;163:1844–8.

118. Yerby MS. Contraception, pregnancy and lactation in women with epilepsy. *Baillieres Clin Neurol* 1996;5:887–908.

119. Kaneko S. Antiepileptic drug therapy and reproductive consequences: functional and morphologic effects. *Reprod Toxicol* 1991;5:179–98.

120. Sharony R, Graham JM. Identification of fetal problems associated with anticonvulsant usage and maternal epilepsy. *Obstet Gynecol Clin North Am* 1991;18:933–51.

121. Finnell RH et al. Clinical and experimental studies linking oxidative metabolism to phenytoin-induced teratogenesis. *Neurology* 1992;42(suppl 5):25–31.

122. Omtzigt JGC et al. The 10,11-epoxide-10,11-diol pathway of carbamazepine in early pregnancy in maternal serum, urine, and amniotic fluid: effect of dose, comedication, and relation to outcome of pregnancy. *Ther Drug Monit* 1993;15:1–10.

123. Van Dyke DC et al. Differences in phenytoin biotransformation and susceptibility to congenital malformations: a review. *DICP* 1991;25:987–92.

124. Eller DP et al. Maternal and fetal implications of anticonvulsive therapy. *Obstet Gynecol Clin North Am* 1997;24:523–34.

125. Lindhout D. Antiepileptic drugs and teratogenesis in two consecutive cohorts: changes in prescription policy paralleled by changes in pattern of malformations. *Neurology* 1992;42(suppl 5):94–110.

126. Dickinson RG et al. The effect of pregnancy in humans on the pharmacokinetics of stable isotope labelled phenytoin. *Br J Clin Pharmacol* 1989;28:17–27.

127. Dravet C et al. Epilepsy, antiepileptic drugs, and malformations in children of women with epilepsy: a French prospective cohort study. *Neurology* 1992;42(suppl 5):75–82.

128. Cohen MM. Syndromology: an updated conceptual overview. VII. Aspects of teratogenesis. *Int J Oral Maxillofac Surg* 1990;19:26–32.

129. Scolnik D et al. Neurodevelopment of children exposed in utero to phenytoin and carbamazepine monotherapy. *JAMA* 1994;271:767–70.

130. Verloes A et al. Proximal phocomelia and radial ray aplasia in fetal valproic syndrome. *Eur J Pediatr* 1990;149:266–7.

131. Hubert A et al. Aplasia cutis congenita of the scalp in an infant exposed to valproic acid in utero. *Acta Paediatr* 1994;83:789–90.

132. Sharony R et al. Preaxial ray reduction defects as part of valproic acid embryofetopathy. *Prenatal Diag* 1993;13:909–18.

133. Baum AL, Misri S. Selective serotonin-reuptake inhibitors in pregnancy and lactation. *Harvard Rev Psychiatry* 1996;4:117–25.

134. Kent LSW, Laidlaw JDD. Suspected congenital sertraline dependence. *Br J Psychiatry* 1995;167:412–3. Letter.

135. Calabrese JR, Gulledge AD. Psychotropics during pregnancy and lactation: a review. *Psychosomatics* 1985;26:413–29.

136. Trixler M, Tényi T. Antipsychotic use in pregnancy. *Drug Saf* 1997;16:403–10.

137. Marken PA et al. Treatment of psychosis in pregnancy. *DICP* 1989;23:598–9.

138. Kallen B, Mazze RI. Neural tube defects and first trimester operations. *Teratology* 1990;41:717–20.

139. Sylvester GC et al. First-trimester anesthesia exposure and the risk of central nervous system defects: a population-based case-control study. *Am J Public Health* 1994;84:1757–60.

140. Baeder C, Albrecht M. Embryotoxic/teratogenic potential of halothane. *Int Arch Occup Environ Health* 1990;62:263–71.

141. Tannenbaum TN, Goldberg RJ. Exposure to anesthetic gases and reproductive outcome. A review of the epidemiologic literature. *J Occup Med* 1985;27:659–68.

142. Kanto J. Obstetric analgesia: clinical pharmacokinetic considerations. *Clin Pharmacokinet* 1986;11:283–98.

143. Janowsky EC. Pharmacologic aspects of local anesthetic use. *Anesthesiol Clin North Am* 1990;8:1–25.

144. Shiono PH, Mills JL. Oral clefts and diazepam use during pregnancy. *N Engl J Med* 1984;311:919–20. Letter.

145. Bergman U et al. Teratogenic effects of benzodiazepine use during pregnancy. *J Pediatr* 1990;116:490–1. Letter.

146. Rivas F et al. Acentric craniofacial cleft in a newborn female prenatally exposed to a high dose of diazepam. *Teratology* 1984;30:179–80.

147. Laegreid L et al. Congenital malformations and maternal consumption of benzodiazepines: a case-control study. *Dev Med Child Neurol* 1990;32:432–41.

860   DRUG USE IN SPECIAL POPULATIONS

148. St Clair SM, Schirmer RG. First-trimester exposure to alprazolam. *Obstet Gynecol* 1992;80:843–6.
149. Laegreid L et al. The effect of benzodiazepines on the fetus and the newborn. *Neuropediatrics* 1992;23:18–23.
150. Sanchis A et al. Adverse effects of maternal lorazepam on neonates. *DICP* 1991;25:1137–8.
151. Zalzstein E et al. A case-control study on the association between first trimester exposure to lithium and Ebstein's anomaly. *Am J Cardiol* 1990;65:817–8.
152. Warkany J. Teratogen update: lithium. *Teratology* 1988;38:593–6.
153. Chapman WS. Lithium use during pregnancy. *J Fla Med Assoc* 1989;76:454–8.
154. Jacobson SJ et al. Prospective multicentre study of pregnancy outcome after lithium exposure during first trimester. *Lancet* 1992;339:530–3.
155. Cohen LS et al. A reevaluation of risk of in utero exposure to lithium. *JAMA* 1994;271:146–50.
156. Ang MS et al. Maternal lithium therapy and polyhydramnios. *Obstet Gynecol* 1990;76:517–9.
157. Koren G, Zemlickis DM. Outcome of pregnancy after first trimester exposure to H$_2$ receptor antagonists. *Am J Perinatol* 1991;8:37–8.
158. Qvist N et al. Cimetidine as pre-anesthetic agent for cesarean section: perinatal effects on the infant, the placental transfer of cimetidine and its elimination in the infants. *J Perinat Med* 1985;13:179–83.
159. Ikenoue T et al. Effects of ranitidine on maternal gastric juice and neonates when administered prior to caesarean section. *Aliment Pharmacol Ther* 1991;5:315–8.
160. Seto A et al. Pregnancy outcome following first trimester exposure to antihistamines: a meta-analysis. *Am J Perinatol* 1997;14:119–24.
161. Bailey B et al. Cisapride use during human pregnancy: a prospective, controlled, multicenter study. *Dig Dis Sci* 1997;42:1848–52.
162. Baiocco PJ, Korelitz BI. The influence of inflammatory bowel disease and its treatment on pregnancy and fetal outcome. *J Clin Gastroenterol* 1984;6:211–6.
163. Meyers S, Sacher DB. Medical management of Crohn's disease. *Hepatogastroenterology* 1990;37:42–55.
164. Hall JG et al. Maternal and fetal sequelae of anticoagulation during pregnancy. *Am J Med* 1980;68:122–40.
165. Ginsberg JS et al. Risks to the fetus of anticoagulant therapy during pregnancy. *Thromb Haemost* 1989;61:197–203.
166. Ginsberg JS, Hirsh J. Use of anticoagulants during pregnancy. *Chest* 1989;95(suppl):156S–60.
167. Nageotte MP et al. Anticoagulation in pregnancy. *Am J Obstet Gynecol* 1981;141:472–3.
168. Iturbe-Alessio I et al. Risks of anticoagulant therapy in pregnant women with artificial heart valves. *N Engl J Med* 1986;315:1390–3.
169. Born D et al. Pregnancy in patients with prosthetic heart valves: the effects of anticoagulation on mother, fetus, and neonate. *Am Heart J* 1992;124:413–7.
170. Gärtner BC et al. Phenprocoumon therapy during pregnancy: case report and comparison of the teratogenic risk of different coumarin derivatives. *Z Geburtshilfe Perinatol* 1993;197:262–5.
171. Pati S, Helmbrecht GD. Congenital schizencephaly associated with in utero warfarin exposure. *Reprod Toxicol* 1994;8:115–20.
172. Normann EK, Stray-Pedersen B. Warfarin-induced fetal diaphragmatic hernia: case report. *Br J Obstet Gynaecol* 1989;96:729–30.
173. Fitzsimons R et al. Outcome of pregnancy in women requiring corticosteroids for severe asthma. *J Allergy Clin Immunol* 1986;78:349–53.
174. Avery ME et al. Update on prenatal steroid for prevention of respiratory distress. *Am J Obstet Gynecol* 1986;155:2–5.
175. Van Marter LJ et al. Maternal glucocorticoid therapy and reduced risk of bronchopulmonary dysplasia. *Pediatrics* 1990;86:331–6.
176. Smolder-de Haas H et al. Physical development and medical history of children who were treated antenatally with corticosteroids to prevent respiratory distress syndrome: a 10- to 12-year follow-up. *Pediatrics* 1990;85:65–70.
177. Saenger P. Abnormal sex differentiation. *J Pediatr* 1984;104:1–17.
178. Brunskill PJ. The effect of fetal exposure to danazol. *Br J Obstet Gynaecol* 1992;99:212–5.
179. Rosenn B et al. Minor congenital malformations in infants of insulin-dependent diabetic women: association with poor glycemic control. *Obstet Gynecol* 1990;70:745–9.
180. Piacquadio K et al. Effects of in-utero exposure to oral hypoglycaemic drugs. *Lancet* 1991;338:866–9.
181. Hellmuth E et al. Congenital malformations in offspring of diabetic women treated with oral hypoglycaemic agents during embryogenesis. *Diabetic Med* 1994;11:471–4.
182. Saili A, Sarna MS. Tolbutamide: teratogenic effects. *Indian Pediatr* 1991;28:936–40.
183. Elliott BD et al. Insignificant transfer of glyburide occurs across the human placenta. *Am J Obstet Gynecol* 1991;165:807–12.
184. Kramer MS et al. Determinants of fetal growth and body proportionality. *Pediatrics* 1990;86:18–26.

185. Fischer K. A rapid evolution mechanism may contribute to changes in sex ratio, multiple birth incidence, frequency of autoimmune disease and frequency of birth defects in Clomid conceptions. *Med Hypotheses* 1990;31:59–65.

186. Wramsby H et al. Chromosome analysis of human oocytes recovered from preovulatory follicles in stimulated cycles. *N Engl J Med* 1987;316:121–4.

187. Shoham Z et al. Early miscarriage and fetal malformations after induction of ovulation (by clomiphene citrate and/or human menotropins), in vitro fertilization, and gamete intrafallopian transfer. *Fertil Steril* 1991;55:1–11.

188. Mills JL et al. Risk of neural tube defects in relation to maternal fertility and fertility drug use. *Lancet* 1990;336:103–4.

189. Melnick S et al. Rates and risks of diethylstilbestrol-related clear-cell adenocarcinoma of the vagina and cervix. An update. *N Engl J Med* 1987;316:514–6.

190. Anons. Infertility among daughters exposed to diethylstilbestrol. *Drug Newsl* 1988;7:59. Abstract.

191. Adams DM et al. Intrapartum uterine rupture. *Obstet Gynecol* 1989;73:471–3.

192. Claman P, Berger MJ. Phenotypic differences in upper genital tract abnormalities and reproductive history in dizygotic twins exposed to diethylstilbestrol. *J Reprod Med* 1990;35:431–3.

193. McFarlane MJ et al. Diethylstilbestrol and clear cell vaginal carcinoma: reappraisal of the epidemiologic evidence. *Am J Med* 1986;81:855–63.

194. Leary FJ et al. Males exposed in utero to diethylstilbestrol. *JAMA* 1984;252:2984–9.

195. Harris EL. Genetic epidemiology of hypospadias. *Epidemiol Rev* 1990;12:29–40.

196. Blickstein I, Katz Z. Possible relationship of bladder exstrophy and epispadias with progestins taken during early pregnancy. *Br J Urol* 1991;68:105–6.

197. Stoll C et al. Genetic and environmental factors in hypospadias. *J Med Genet* 1990;27:559–63.

198. Progestational drug birth defects warning statement. *FDC Rep* 1987;49:T&G1–2.

199. Lammer EJ, Cordero JF. Exogenous sex hormone exposure and the risk for major malformations. *JAMA* 1986;255:3128–32.

200. Simpson JL, Phillips OP. Spermicides, hormonal contraception and congenital malformations. *Adv Contraception* 1990;6:141–67.

201. Mestman JH. Thyroid disease in pregnancy. *Clin Perinatol* 1985;12:651–7.

202. Momotani N et al. Antithyroid drug therapy for Graves' disease during pregnancy. *N Engl J Med* 1986;315:24–8.

203. Martinez-Frias ML et al. Methimazole in animal feed and congenital aplasia cutis. *Lancet* 1992;339:742–3. Letter.

204. Singhi S et al. Iatrogenic neonatal and maternal hyponatremia following oxytocin and aqueous glucose infusion during labour. *Br J Obstet Gynaecol* 1985;92:356–63.

205. Schönhöfer PS. Brazil: misuse of misoprostol as an abortifacient may induce malformations. *Lancet* 1991;337;1534–5.

206. Gonzalez CH et al. Limb deficiency with or without Möbius sequence in seven Brazilian children associated with misoprostol use in the first trimester of pregnancy. *Am J Med Genet* 1993;47:59–64.

207. Pastuszak AL et al. Use of misoprostol during pregnancy and Möbius' syndrome in infants. *N Engl J Med* 1998;338:1881–5.

208. Schuller L et al. Pregnancy outcome after abortion attempt with misoprostol. *Teratology* 1997;55:36. Abstract

209. Sorokin Y et al. Effects of induction of labor with prostaglandin E_2 on fetal breathing and body movements: controlled, randomized, double-blind study. *Obstet Gynecol* 1992;80:788–91.

210. Papageorgiou I et al. Labor characteristics of uncomplicated prolonged pregnancies after induction with intracervical prostaglandin E_2 gel versus intravenous oxytocin. *Gynecol Obstet Invest* 1992;34:92–6.

211. Ray DA, Garite TJ. Prostaglandin E_2 for induction of labor in patients with premature rupture of membranes at term. *Am J Obstet Gynecol* 1992;166:836–43.

212. Sibai BM et al. Effects of diuretics on plasma volume in pregnancies with long-term hypertension. *Am J Obstet Gynecol* 1984;150:831–5.

213. Lamm CI et al. Congenital rickets associated with magnesium sulfate infusion for tocolysis. *J Pediatr* 1988;113:1078–82.

214. Holcomb WL et al. Magnesium tocolysis and neonatal bone abnormalities: a controlled study. *Obstet Gynecol* 1991;78:611–4.

215. Cox SM et al. Randomized investigation of magnesium sulfate for prevention of preterm birth. *Am J Obstet Gynecol* 1990;163:767–72.

216. Doan-Wiggins L. Drug therapy for obstetric emergencies. *Emerg Med Clin North Am* 1994;12:257–3.

217. McKeigue PM et al. Bendectin and birth defects: I. a meta-analysis of the epidemiologic studies. *Teratology* 1994;50:27–37.

218. Einarson A et al. Prospective controlled study of hydroxyzine and cetirizine in pregnancy. *Ann Allergy Asthma Immunol* 1997;78:183–6.

219. Asthma. *PEM News*, no. 7. Drug Safety Research Unit, Southampton, England, August 1990.

220. Mann RD et al. Salmeterol. *PEM Report*, no. 25. Drug Safety Research Unit, Southampton, England, July 1994.

221. Frederiksen MC et al. Theophylline pharmacokinetics in pregnancy. *Clin Pharmacol Ther* 1986;40:321–8.

222. Stenius-Aarniala B et al. Slow-release theophylline in pregnant asthmatics. *Chest* 1995;107:642–7.

223. Wright JW et al. Effect of tocolytic agents on fetal umbilical velocimetry. *Am J Obstet Gynecol* 1990;163: 748–50.

224. Gormley DE. Cutaneous surgery and the pregnant patient. *J Am Acad Dermatol* 1990;23:269–79.

225. Chamberlain MJ et al. Toxic effect of podophyllum application in pregnancy. *Br Med J* 1972;3:391–2.

226. Ridley CM. Toxicity of podophyllum. *Br Med J* 1972;3:698. Letter.

227. Karol MD et al. Podophyllum: suspected teratogenicity from topical application. *Clin Toxicol* 1980;16:283–6.

228. Sundharam JA. Is podophyllin safe for use in pregnancy? *Arch Dermatol* 1989;125:1000–1.

229. Stamatos MN. *The most important step forward in years (etretinate)*. Nutley, NJ: Roche Laboratories; 1986. Promotional letter.

230. Etretinate approved. *FDA Drug Bull* 1986;16:16–7.

231. Vahlquist A, Rollman O. Etretinate and the risk for teratogenicity: drug monitoring in a pregnant woman for 9 months after stopping treatment. *Br J Dermatol* 1990;123:131. Letter.

232. Personal communication, Joseph B. Laudano, Roche Laboratories, January 29, 1987.

233. Anons. Etretinate for psoriasis. *Med Lett Drugs Ther* 1987;29:9–10.

234. Geiger J-M et al. Teratogenic risk with etretinate and acitretin treatment. *Dermatology* 1994;189:109–16.

235. Lammer EJ et al. Retinoic acid embryopathy. *N Engl J Med* 1985;313:837–41.

236. Holmes A, Wolfe S. When a uniquely effective drug is teratogenic: the case of isotretinoin. *N Engl J Med* 1989;321:756. Letter.

237. Faich G, Rosa F. When a uniquely effective drug is teratogenic: the case of isotretinoin. *N Engl J Med* 1989; 321:756–7. Letter.

238. Rappaport EB, Knapp M. Isotretinoin embryopathy—a continuing problem. *J Clin Pharmacol* 1989;29: 463–5.

239. Hansen LA, Pearl GS. Isotretinoin teratogenicity. Case report with neuropathologic findings. *Acta Neuropathol* 1985;65:335–7.

240. McBride WG. Limb reduction deformities in child exposed to isotretinoin in utero on gestation days 26–40 only. *Lancet* 1985;1:1276. Letter.

241. Anons. Birth defects caused by isotretinoin—New Jersey. *MMWR* 1988;37:171–2, 177.

242. Dai WS et al. Epidemiology of isotretinoin exposure during pregnancy. *J Am Acad Dermatol* 1992;26: 599–606.

243. Rizzo R et al. Limb reduction defects in humans associated with prenatal isotretinoin exposure. *Teratology* 1991;44:599–604.

244. deWals P et al. Association between holoprosencephaly and exposure to topical retinoids: results of the EUROCAT survey. *Paediatr Perinat Epidemiol* 1991;5:445–7.

245. Jick SS et al. First trimester topical tretinoin and congenital disorders. *Lancet* 1993;341:1181–2.

246. Shapiro L et al. Safety of first-trimester exposure to topical tretinoin: prospective cohort study. *Lancet* 1997;350:1143–4.

247. Camera G, Pregliasco P. Ear malformation in baby born to mother using tretinoin cream. *Lancet* 1992; 339:687. Letter.

248. Lipson AH et al. Multiple congenital defects associated with maternal use of topical tretinoin. *Lancet* 1993; 341:1352–3. Letter.

249. Martínez-Frías ML, Salvador J. Epidemiological aspects of prenatal exposure to high doses of vitamin A in Spain. *Eur J Epidemiol* 1990;6:118–23.

250. Werler MM et al. Maternal vitamin A supplementation in relation to selected birth defects. *Teratology* 1990; 42:497–503.

251. Rothman KJ et al. Teratogenicity of high vitamin A intake. *N Engl J Med* 1995;333:1369–73.

252. Oakley GP, Erickson JD. Vitamin A and birth defects. Continuing caution is needed. *N Engl J Med* 1995; 333:1414–5. Editorial.

253. Anons. Use of supplements containing high-dose vitamin A–New York State, 1983–1984. *MMWR* 1987; 36:80–2.

254. Committee on Safety of Medicines. Vitamin A and teratogenesis. *Lancet* 1985;1:319–20.

255. Shapiro S et al. Birth defects and vaginal spermicides. *JAMA* 1982;247:2381–4.

256. Jick H et al. Vaginal spermicides and congenital disorders. *JAMA* 1981;245:1329–32.

257. Louik C et al. Maternal exposure to spermicides in relation to certain birth defects. *N Engl J Med* 1987;317:474–8.

258. Warburton D et al. Lack of association between spermicide use and trisomy. *N Engl J Med* 1987;317:478–82.

259. Einarson TR et al. Maternal spermicide use and adverse reproductive outcome: a meta-analysis. *Am J Obstet Gynecol* 1990;162:655–60.

260. Data do not support association between spermicides, birth defects. *FDA Drug Bull* 1986;16:21.

261. Martin NDT et al. Increased plasma 1,25-dihydroxyvitamin D in infants with hypercalcemia and elfin facies. *N Engl J Med* 1985;313:888–9. Letter.

262. Chesney RW et al. Increased plasma 1,25-dihydroxyvitamin D in infants with hypercalcemia and elfin facies. *N Engl J Med* 1985;313:889–90. Letter.

263. Rudeen PK, Creighton JA. Mechanisms of central nervous system alcohol-related birth defects. In, Sun G-Y et al, eds. *Molecular mechanisms of alcohol.* Clifton, NJ: Humana Press; 1989;147–65.

264. Goodwin FK. Acetaldehyde produced and transferred by human placenta. *JAMA* 1988;260:3563.

265. Blakley PM, Scott WJ. Determination of the proximate teratogen of the mouse fetal alcohol syndrome. 1. Teratogenicity of ethanol and acetaldehyde. *Toxicol Applied Pharmacol* 1984;72:355–63.

266. Little BB et al. Alcohol abuse during pregnancy: changes in frequency in a large urban hospital. *Obstet Gynecol* 1989;74:547–50.

267. Clarren SK. Fetal alcohol syndrome: diagnosis, treatment, and mechanisms of teratogenesis. In Transplacental disorders: perinatal detection, treatment, and management (including pediatric AIDS). *Proceedings of the 1988 Albany Birth Defects Symposium XIX.* New York: Alan R. Liss; 1990:37–55.

268. Virji SK. The relationship between alcohol consumption during pregnancy and infant birthweight. An epidemiologic study. *Acta Obstet Gynecol Scand* 1991;70:303–8.

269. Kline J et al. Drinking during pregnancy and spontaneous abortion. *Lancet* 1980;2:176–80.

270. Harlap S, Shiono PH. Alcohol, smoking, and incidence of spontaneous abortions in the first and second trimester. *Lancet* 1980;2:173–6.

271. Streissguth AP et al. Natural history of the fetal alcohol syndrome: a 10–year follow-up of eleven patients. *Lancet* 1985;2:85–91.

272. Halmesmaki E et al. Low somatomedin C and high growth hormone levels in newborns: damages by maternal alcohol abuse. *Obstet Gynecol* 1989;74:366–70.

273. Strömland K. Contribution of ocular examination to the diagnosis of foetal alcohol syndrome in mentally retarded children. *J Mental Defic Res* 1990;34:429–35.

274. Froster UG, Baird PA. Congenital defects of the limbs and alcohol exposure in pregnancy: data from a population based study. *Am J Med Genet* 1992;44:782–5.

275. Ronen GM, Andrews WL. Holoprosencephaly as a possible embryonic alcohol effect. *Am J Med Genet* 1991;40:151–4.

276. Bonnemann C, Meinecke P. Holoprosencephaly as a possible embryonic alcohol effect: another observation. *Am J Med Genet* 1990;37:431–2.

277. Astley SJ et al. Analysis of facial shape in children gestationally exposed to marijuana, alcohol, and/or cocaine. *Pediatrics* 1992;89:67–77.

278. Little BB et al. Methamphetamine abuse during pregnancy: outcome and fetal effects. *Obstet Gynecol* 1988; 72:541–4.

279. Oro AS, Dixon SD. Perinatal cocaine and methamphetamine exposure: maternal and neonatal correlates. *J Pediatr* 1987;111:571–8.

280. Dixon SD, Bejar R. Echoencephalographic findings in neonates associated with maternal cocaine and methamphetamine use: incidence and clinical correlates. *J Pediatr* 1989;115:770–8.

281. Infante-Rivard C et al. Fetal loss associated with caffeine intake before and during pregnancy. *JAMA* 1993; 270:2940–3.

282. Dlugosz L, Bracken MB. Reproductive effects of caffeine: a review and theoretical analysis. *Epidemiol Rev* 1992;14:83–100.

283. Watkinson B, Fried PA. Maternal caffeine use before, during and after pregnancy and effects upon offspring. *Neurobehav Toxicol Teratol* 1985;7:9–17.

284. Cerrato PL. Caffeine: how much is too much? *RN* 1990;53:77–80.

285. Szucs Myers VA, Miwa LJ. Caffeine consumption during pregnancy. *Drug Intell Clin Pharm* 1988;22:614–6.

286. Olsen J et al. Coffee consumption, birthweight, and reproductive failures. *Epidemiology* 1991;2:370–4.

287. Narod SA et al. Coffee during pregnancy: a reproductive hazard? *Am J Obstet Gynecol* 1991;164:1109–14.

288. Toubas PL et al. Effects of maternal smoking and caffeine habits on infantile apnea: a retrospective study. *Pediatrics* 1986;78:159–63.

289. Lutiger B et al. Relationship between gestational cocaine use and pregnancy outcome: a meta-analysis. *Teratology* 1991;44:405–14.

290. Chen C et al. Respiratory instability in neonates with in utero exposure to cocaine. *J Pediatr* 1991;119:111–3.

291. Ho J et al. Renal vascular abnormalities associated with prenatal cocaine exposure. *Clin Pediatr* 1994; 33:155–6.

292. Lezcano L et al. Crossed renal ectopia associated with maternal alkaloid cocaine abuse: a case report. *J Perinatol* 1994;14:230–3.

293. Viscarello RR et al. Limb–body wall complex associated with cocaine abuse: further evidence of cocaine's teratogenicity. *Obstet Gynecol* 1992;80:523–6.

294. Hume RF Jr et al. Ultrasound diagnosis of fetal anomalies associated with in utero cocaine exposure: further support for cocaine-induced vascular disruption teratogenesis. *Fetal Diagn Ther* 1994;9:239–45.

295. Hoyme HE et al. Prenatal cocaine exposure and fetal vascular disruption. *Pediatrics* 1990;85:743–7.

296. Greenfield SP et al. Genitourinary tract malformations and maternal cocaine abuse. *Urology* 1991;37:455–9.

297. Davidson Ward SL et al. Sudden infant death syndrome in infants of substance-abusing mothers. *J Pediatr* 1990;117:876–81.

298. Durand DJ et al. Association between prenatal cocaine exposure and sudden infant death syndrome. *J Pediatr* 1990;117:909–11.

299. Lowenstein DH et al. Acute neurologic and psychiatric complications associated with cocaine abuse. *Am J Med* 1987;83:841–6.

300. Chasnoff IJ et al. Perinatal cerebral infarction and maternal cocaine use. *J Pediatr* 1986;108:456–9.

301. Chasnoff IJ et al. Cocaine use in pregnancy. *N Engl J Med* 1985;313:666–9.

302. Oro AS, Dixon SD. Perinatal cocaine and methamphetamine exposure: maternal and neonatal correlates. *J Pediatr* 1987;111:571–8.

303. Burkett G et al. Perinatal implications of cocaine exposure. *J Reprod Med* 1990;35:35–42.

304. Collins E et al. Perinatal cocaine intoxication. *Med J Aust* 1989;150:331–4.

305. Cherukuri R et al. A cohort study of alkaloidal cocaine ("crack") in pregnancy. *Obstet Gynecol* 1988; 72:147–51.

306. Kaye K et al. Birth outcomes for infants of drug abusing mothers. *NY State J Med* 1989;89:256–61.

307. Bingol N et al. Teratogenicity of cocaine in humans. *J Pediatr* 1987;110:93–6.

308. Keith LG et al. Substance abuse in pregnant women: recent experience at the Perinatal Center for Chemical Dependence of Northwestern Memorial Hospital. *Obstet Gynecol* 1989;73:715–20.

309. Roland EH, Volpe JJ. Effect of maternal cocaine use on the fetus and newborn: review of the literature. *Pediatr Neurosci* 1989;15:88–94.

310. Doering PL. Effects of cocaine on the human fetus: a review of clinical studies. *DICP* 1989;23:639–45.

311. Mastrogiannis DS et al. Perinatal outcome after recent cocaine usage. *Obstet Gynecol* 1990;76:8–11.

312. Cravey RH. Cocaine deaths in infants. *J Anal Toxicol* 1988;12:354–5.

313. Chouteau M et al. The effect of cocaine abuse on birth weight and gestational age. *Obstet Gynecol* 1988;72: 351–4.

314. Little BB et al. Cocaine abuse during pregnancy: maternal and fetal implications. *Obstet Gynecol* 1989;73: 157–60.

315. Mercado A et al. Cocaine, pregnancy, and postpartum intracerebral hemorrhage. *Obstet Gynecol* 1989;73: 467–8.

316. Ney JA et al. The prevalence of substance abuse in patients with suspected preterm labor. *Am J Obstet Gynecol* 1990;162:1562–7.

317. Thatcher SS et al. Cocaine use and acute rupture of ectopic pregnancies. *Obstet Gynecol* 1989;74:478–9.

318. Gonsoulin W et al. Rupture of unscarred uterus in primigravid woman in association with cocaine abuse. *Am J Obstet Gynecol* 1990;163:526–7.

319. Madden JD et al. Maternal cocaine abuse and effect on the newborn. *Pediatrics* 1986;77:209–11.

320. Rosenstein BJ et al. Congenital renal abnormalities in infants with in utero cocaine exposure. *J Urol* 1990; 144:110–2.

321. Chavez GF et al. Maternal cocaine use during early pregnancy as a risk factor for congenital urogenital anomalies. *JAMA* 1989;262:795–8.

322. Ward SLD et al. Abnormal sleeping ventilatory pattern in infants of substance-abusing mothers. *Am J Dis Child* 1986;140:1015–20.

323. Chasnoff IJ et al. Prenatal cocaine exposure is associated with respiratory pattern abnormalities. *Am J Dis Child* 1989;143:583–7.

324. Cregler LL, Mark H. Medical complications of cocaine abuse. *N Engl J Med* 1986;315:1495–500.

325. Braude MC et al. Perinatal effects of drugs of abuse. *Fed Proc* 1987;46:2446–53.

326. Feldman JG et al. A cohort study of the impact of perinatal drug use on prematurity in an inner-city population. *Am J Public Health* 1992;82:726–8.

327. Zuckerman B et al. Effects of maternal marijuana and cocaine use on fetal growth. *N Engl J Med* 1989;320: 762–8.

328. Klenka HM. Babies born in a district general hospital to mothers taking heroin. *Br Med J* 1986;293:745–6.

329. Fried PA. Cigarettes and marijuana: are there measurable long-term neurobehavioral teratogenic effects? *Neurotoxicology* 1989;10:577–84.

330. Hatch EE, Bracken MB. Effect of marijuana use in pregnancy on fetal growth. *Am J Epidemiol* 1986;124:986–93.

331. Tansley BW et al. Visual processing in children exposed prenatally to marijuana and nicotine: a preliminary report. *Can J Public Health* 1986;77(suppl 1):72–8.

332. Chasnoff IJ et al. Phencyclidine: effects on the fetus and neonate. *Dev Pharmacol Ther* 1983;6:404–8.

333. Golden NL et al. Phencyclidine use during pregnancy. *Am J Obstet Gynecol* 1984;148:254–9.

334. Lindblad A et al. Effect of nicotine on human fetal blood flow. *Obstet Gynecol* 1988;72:371–82.

335. Pinette MG et al. Maternal smoking and accelerated placental maturation. *Obstet Gynecol* 1989;73:379–82.

336. Cole H. Studying reproductive risks, smoking. *JAMA* 1986;255:22–3.

337. Shiono PH et al. Smoking and drinking during pregnancy: their effects on preterm birth. *JAMA* 1986;255: 82–4.

338. Brown HL et al. Premature placental calcification in maternal cigarette smokers. *Obstet Gynecol* 1988;71: 914–7.

339. Newnham JP et al. Effects of maternal cigarette smoking on ultrasonic measurements of fetal growth and on Doppler flow velocity waveforms. *Early Hum Dev* 1990;24:23–6.

340. Jauniaux E, Burton GJ. The effect of smoking in pregnancy on early placental morphology. *Obstet Gynecol* 1992;79:645–8.

341. Seidman DS et al. Effect of maternal smoking and age on congenital anomalies. *Obstet Gynecol* 1990;76: 1046–50.

342. Brown RW et al. Effect of maternal smoking during pregnancy on passive respiratory mechanics in early infancy. *Pediatr Pulmonol* 1995;19:23–8.

343. John EM et al. Prenatal exposure to parents' smoking and childhood cancer. *Am J Epidemiol* 1991;133: 123–32.

344. Stjernfeldt M et al. Maternal smoking and irradiation during pregnancy as risk factors for child leukemia. *Cancer Detect Prev* 1992;16:129–35.

Drugs and Breastfeeding

Philip O. Anderson

With the increasing recognition of the benefits of breastfeeding, the clinician must often weigh the benefits versus risks of drug therapy in lactating women. The physicochemical, pharmacokinetic, and clinical factors involved with drug use in nursing women have been described.[1-7] These factors are summarized as follows.

■ PHYSICOCHEMICAL FACTORS

Small water-soluble nonelectrolytes pass into milk by simple diffusion through pores in the mammary epithelial membrane that separates plasma from milk. Equilibration between the two fluids is rapid, and milk levels of drugs approximate plasma levels. For larger molecules, only the lipid-soluble, nonionized forms pass through the membrane by crossing the cell wall and diffusing across the interior of the cell to reach the milk. Because the pH of milk is generally lower than that of plasma, milk can act as an "ion trap" for basic drugs. At equilibrium, these compounds may be concentrated in milk relative to plasma. Conversely, acidic drugs are inhibited from entering milk. The pKa of weak electrolytes is an important determinant of their equilibrium concentration in milk.

Protein binding is also an important determinant because plasma proteins bind drugs much more avidly than do milk proteins. Highly protein-bound drugs do not pass into milk in high concentrations. Lipid solubility favors passage of drugs into milk, because the fat component of milk can concentrate lipid-soluble drugs. However, because milk contains only 3–5% fat, its capacity for concentrating drugs is limited. Active transport of drugs into breastmilk may occur, but it is rare.[8]

■ PHARMACOKINETIC FACTORS

Because the breast is periodically emptied and refilled with newly formed milk, equilibrium between plasma and milk is rarely reached. The rate of drug passage from plasma into milk is therefore important in determining the concentration of a drug in milk. Factors favoring rapid passage into milk are high lipid solubility and low molecular weight.

Passage of drugs between plasma and milk occurs in both directions. When the concentration of nonionized free drug in milk is higher than it is in plasma, net transfer of drug from milk to plasma occurs. Thus, pumping and discarding milk does not appreciably hasten the elimination of most drugs from milk, and it does not have a marked effect on overall clearance of the drug from the mother's body.

■ METHODS OF EXPRESSING THE EXTENT OF PASSAGE

The ratio of concentrations of a drug in milk and plasma (the milk/plasma or M/P ratio) has often been used as a measure of a drug's passage into breastmilk. However, the M/P ratio has shortcomings that make it meaningless as a measure of drug safety during nursing. There is no standard method of calculating the value, and the value is not constant, as often calculated, but varies with the time after the dose and with the number of doses given. It also does not take into account the potential toxicity of the drug.

The percentage of the maternal dosage that is excreted into milk is also used to express the extent of passage. This value alone is not predictive of safety in a nursing infant, but can be used to calculate the actual dosage received by the infant. Usually a weight-adjusted (ie, mg/kg) infant dosage less than 10% of the mother's is considered safe; of 205 drugs reported in the literature, 87% of drugs fell into this category.[9] The likelihood of an adverse effect in the infant increases markedly in those few drugs that have a dosage in milk that approaches the maternal weight-adjusted dosage.[9]

Drug clearance can be a useful factor for identifying drugs that may accumulate in infants and have a pharmacologic effect.[10,11] Drugs with a total body clearance of 0.6 L/hr/kg or greater and that have no active metabolites are unlikely to cause a pharmacologic effect in a nursing infant because they are rapidly eliminated from both the mother and infant, and accumulation does not occur.

Knowledge of the actual dosage received by an infant via milk, either from the literature or by calculation, and comparison of this dosage with the therapeutic infant dosage is the most reliable way to measure drug safety in the nursing infant.

All of the above methods fall short of providing a complete assessment of the safety of a drug during breastfeeding in a specific mother–infant pair. Several other factors must be considered in addition.

■ CLINICAL CONSIDERATIONS

Factors that should be considered when determining the advisability of using a particular drug in a nursing mother include the potential acute toxicity of the drug, dosage and duration of therapy, age of the infant, quantity of milk consumed, experience with the drug in infants, oral absorption of the drug by the infant, potential long-term effects, and possible interference with lactation.[1,7]

A stepwise approach to using medications in breastfeeding women can be followed in order to minimize infant exposure to medications in milk.[1] Starting from the strategies that are least disruptive to nursing and progressing to those that are most disruptive, the prescriber can consider the following steps: Withhold the drug; delay drug therapy temporarily; choose drugs that pass poorly into milk; use alternative routes of administration (eg, topical, inhalation); avoid nursing at times of peak milk levels; administer the drug before the infant's longest sleep period; withhold breastfeeding temporarily; and, infrequently, discontinue breastfeeding.

Another consideration is non–dose-related adverse effects, such as allergic reactions and some hemolytic anemias; however, these are relatively uncommon. GI intolerance caused by antimicrobial agents in breastmilk can occur whether or not the drugs are absorbed by the infant. Antimicrobial agents are among the most commonly used maternal medications during nursing. Although serious side effects are rare, diarrhea occurs in about 12% of infants.[12] Disruption of the infant's GI flora is uncommon, but it can occasionally lead to thrush and rarely to pseudomembranous colitis.[13] Severe diarrhea or blood in the infant's stool during maternal antimicrobial use is an indication to stop nursing and seek medical attention.

Although the above considerations are important, follow-up of mothers who took medications while breastfeeding their infants has shown that serious side effects are uncommon.[12] Nursing seldom must be discontinued completely because of concern of acute toxicity from maternal drug therapy.

The following table contains information on the use of specific drugs during nursing. The risks are assessed and alternatives are presented based on the principles discussed. Information in the table is from reference 1 unless noted otherwise.

DRUGS AND BREASTFEEDING

ANALGESICS AND ANTI-INFLAMMATORY DRUGS

ANTIMIGRANE DRUGS
Ergotamine
When given daily for 6 days postpartum ergotamine did not affect lactation or infant weight in one study; however, the excretion of ergotamine into milk during lactation has not been studied. Avoid its use during lactation, because older ergot preparations have produced toxicity in infants.

Sumatriptan
Minimally excreted in milk, sumatriptan has poor oral absorption by the infant. It poses little risk during breastfeeding.[14]

NONSTEROIDAL ANTI-INFLAMMATORY DRUGS
Acetaminophen
The amount of acetaminophen excreted into milk is small. Acetaminophen is a good analgesic choice during nursing.

Nonsteroidal Anti-inflammatory Drugs
Amounts of most NSAIDs in milk are low because they are weak acids that are extensively plasma protein bound. However, short-acting agents are preferred, particularly in the case of breast-fed neonates. Some agents have active metabolites (eg, **sulindac**) or glucuronide metabolites (eg, **salicylate, fenoprofen,** and **ketoprofen**) that can add to infant intake. Because of the increased likelihood of accumulation, avoid long-acting agents such as **diflunisal, naproxen, piroxicam,** and **sulindac** in mothers of neonates, although amounts of piroxicam in milk are low.[1,7] The more toxic NSAIDs such as **mefenamic acid** and **indomethacin** should also be avoided, although recent studies on indomethacin indicate that it may not be contraindicated.[15,16] **Ketorolac** is contraindicated during nursing. **Diclofenac** was not detected in milk after a single dose of 50 mg IM, or 100 mg/day for 1 week, and the amount of **tolmetin** in one woman's milk was low. **Ibuprofen** and **flurbiprofen** have the best documentation of safety during breastfeeding; the dose of ibuprofen that an infant receives in milk is less than 0.001% of the mother's dosage,[17] and flurbiprofen levels are low to undetectable after dosages up to 50 mg tid.[1]

Salicylates
Salicylate enters milk in a low concentration relative to that in plasma, although its glucuronide metabolite increases the overall infant dosage. Doses over 1 g yield markedly higher salicylate concentrations in milk and may result in high infant plasma concentrations. The risk of Reye syndrome caused by salicylate in milk is unknown. NSAIDs such as ibuprofen are preferred over aspirin for long-term therapy. Although acetaminophen or ibuprofen is preferred, occasional **aspirin** in analgesic doses probably poses a minimal risk to the infant except for the potential antiplatelet effect. Avoidance of breastfeeding for 1–2 hr after a dose should minimize this effect.

(continued)

ANALGESICS AND ANTI-INFLAMMATORY DRUGS

OTHER ANTI-INFLAMMATORY DRUGS (*SEE ALSO* ANTIMALARIALS)
Gold

During maternal administration of **aurothioglucose** and **gold sodium thiomalate,** gold was detected in the blood and urine of some nursing infants. The weight-adjusted infant dosage may be greater than the maternal dosage, but the amount of gold that infants absorb is not clear. Sufficient amounts are absorbed, however, to potentially cause adverse effects. Opinions vary, but gold therapy is a reason to very carefully monitor the breast-fed infant, and may be a reason for withholding breastfeeding.[1,18]

Penicillamine
Penicillamine was used during 3 months of breastfeeding in one woman, but it is not recommended.[18]

OPIOIDS
Neonates are particularly susceptible to narcotics in breastmilk.[7] Postpartum maternal opioids (oral **codeine** or **propoxyphene** with or without prior IM **meperidine**) may be a causative factor in episodes of apnea, bradycardia, and cyanosis during the first week of life. Avoid maternal narcotics when the breast-fed neonate has experienced such an episode.[7] Although single analgesic doses of most narcotics are excreted into milk in small amounts, infant drowsiness caused by repeated administration of postpartum oral narcotics in milk is more prevalent than commonly thought—about 20% in one study.[12] Drowsiness is dose related and can be severe with the maximum dosage. Limiting oral dosage to 1 tablet (eg, **codeine** 30 mg, **hydrocodone** 5 mg, or **oxycodone** 5 mg) q 4 hr is advisable; analgesia can be supplemented with additional acetaminophen or ibuprofen.[7]

Meperidine
Meperidine is particularly likely to interfere with infant nursing behavior when given during labor.[19,20] Furthermore, repeated postpartum meperidine doses, including patient-controlled analgesia, cause diminished alertness and orientation in breast-fed neonates compared with equivalent doses of **morphine.**[1,21] Meperidine is best avoided during labor and nursing, although a single small dose for anesthesia or conscious sedation may not cause problems in older breastfeeding infants.[22]

Morphine
Morphine 10–15 mg in single parenteral doses produces only low concentrations in milk, but repeated doses may result in drug accumulation in infant plasma to near therapeutic concentrations. Morphine glucuronides in milk contribute an additional 50–100% to the infant dose via deconjugation in the infant's gut to the active drug. Epidural administration and patient-controlled analgesia cause fewer infant effects than IV administration and are preferred.[7,21]

Fentanyl and Sufentanil
IV or epidural fentanyl and epidural sufentanil produce low milk levels.[23,24] Additionally, these drugs have poor oral bioavailability, so they are good choices for maternal analgesia during nursing.

Narcotic Partial Agonists
IV narcotic agonist/antagonists given during labor can interfere with establishment of lactation.[18,19,25] Extradural spinal **buprenorphine** infusion begun postpartum caused decreases in milk production and infant weight gain that persisted after discontinuation of the drug.[26] Despite breastfeeding and relatively high infant serum drug levels, mild

(*continued*)

ANALGESICS AND ANTI-INFLAMMATORY DRUGS

buprenorphine withdrawal occurred in the neonate of a mother taking the drug long term for heroin addiction.[27] **Butorphanol** and **nalbuphine** levels in milk are low, and oral bioavailability in the infant should be low.[28,29] Only about 0.1% of the maternal dose of **tramadol** is found in milk according to the manufacturer.[30]

ANTIMICROBIAL DRUGS

AMINOGLYCOSIDES

Systemic effects in infants are unlikely because of the small amounts in milk and poor oral absorption; however, observe infants for disruptions of the GI flora, such as diarrhea and thrush.

ANTIFUNGAL DRUGS

Amphotericin B and **nystatin** are virtually unabsorbed orally, and the latter is frequently used orally for treating thrush in infants; therefore, both are safe for use in nursing mothers, including topical application to the nipples. Likewise, **clotrimazole** has poor oral bioavailability and has also been used orally in infants with thrush, sometimes successfully after nystatin has failed.[31] **Miconazole** has efficacy and safety similar to clotrimazole.[32] These two imidazoles are preferred for topical or vaginal application during nursing. **Fluconazole** amounts in milk are much less than the dosage prescribed for infants and can be used for recalcitrant *Candida* infections,[33,34] given to both the mother and infant simultaneously. **Ketoconazole** levels in milk are low,[35] but it is best avoided in nursing mothers either orally or topically to the nipples because of its oral absorption, occasional hepatotoxicity, and the availability of safer alternatives. Other imidazole antifungals have not been studied. **Gentian violet** is potentially toxic (toxic to mucous membranes, potential tattooing of the skin, and carcinogenic and mutagenic in rodents) and is best avoided topically on the nipples or in the infant's mouth.[36,37]

ANTIMYCOBACTERIAL DRUGS

Clofazimine

Clofazimine is excreted into milk, reportedly coloring it bright pink.[38] Infants receive about 15–30% of the maternal mg/kg dose.[39] Breast-fed infants can develop the typical skin discoloration.[1,38] The skin color returned to normal 5 months after the end of maternal therapy in one infant.

Antituberculars

Antituberculars pass into milk in small quantities. Use caution in nursing mothers because many of these drugs can cause hepatic damage. However, inadequate maternal therapy poses a much greater risk to the infant than the drugs in milk. The mother may take single daily doses of many of these drugs at bedtime and substitute a bottle for a nighttime feeding to minimize infant exposure. **Isoniazid** is excreted into milk in amounts that are less than those given to treat an infant. **Pyrazinamide** concentrations in milk in one woman were low and would give the baby less than a therapeutic dosage. **Rifampin** has not been well studied, but amounts in milk are small. **Cycloserine** is excreted in small amounts, and no adverse reactions have been reported in infants. **Ethambutol** has not been adequately studied.

Sulfones

Newborns and G-6-PD–deficient infants are particularly susceptible to **dapsone** hemolysis. Older infants may tolerate the amounts of sulfones excreted into milk.

(*continued*)

ANTIMICROBIAL DRUGS

ANTIPARASITIC DRUGS
Anthelmintics
Mebendazole was undetectable in milk in one woman and is poorly absorbed orally; therefore, it is unlikely to cause adverse effects in a breast-fed infant. Contrary to an earlier report, it does not inhibit lactation.[40] Only a small amount of **praziquantel** reaches the infant, and the drug appears safe during nursing.

Antimalarials
Undertake breastfeeding cautiously during long-term daily therapy with **chloroquine** or **hydroxychloroquine,** because the importance of the small amounts of drug and metabolites in milk is unclear and accumulation may occur. Weekly prophylactic doses are probably safe, because the amount of drug in milk is less than the infant prophylactic dose.[1,17] Small amounts of **quinine** in milk are unlikely to harm the infant, although allergic reactions may occur. **Pyrimethamine** appears to be safe and may be excreted into milk in quantities sufficient to treat or protect infants <6 months of age against malaria; however, breastfeeding is not a reliable method of drug administration. **Mefloquine** appears in milk in small amounts after a single dose, but has not been studied after repeated weekly administration for malaria prophylaxis.

Lindane
Lindane was excreted into milk at up to 30 times the typical background concentration (from environmental pollution) after maternal topical application of a 0.3% emulsion daily for 3 days. Milk concentrations remained elevated over background concentrations for at least 7 days. Although they have not been studied, alternative drugs (eg, **permethrin,** and **pyrethrins**) are preferred for nursing mothers because of their low order of toxicity.

ANTIVIRAL DRUGS
Acyclovir
Acyclovir has not been well studied, but a breast-fed infant would receive about 1% of the mother's weight-adjusted oral dosage. Some controversy exists, but the low dosage in milk and its poor oral bioavailability mean that it may be well tolerated by the nursing infant, even with large IV doses.[41,42] Topical acyclovir applied to small areas of the mother's body away from the breast should pose no risk to the infant.

Amantadine
Amantadine is a dopamine agonist that decreases serum prolactin, and theoretically decreases lactation. The drug is best avoided during nursing. It is not known if **rimantadine** has the same effect, so use it cautiously during nursing.

β-LACTAMS
Cephalosporins
Cephalosporins appear in trace amounts in milk and can lead to disruption of the GI flora or, rarely, allergic sensitization. Breastfeeding is safe with first- and second-generation agents. The risk may be greater with the third-generation cephalosporins and similar agents (eg, **aztreonam** and **moxalactam**) that are more active against GI flora. Observe infants for diarrhea, thrush, and rashes.

(continued)

ANTIMICROBIAL DRUGS

Penicillins

Penicillins appear in trace amounts in milk that can occasionally lead to allergic sensitization, allergic reactions in previously sensitized infants, or disruption of the GI flora, especially with the broader-spectrum agents. Unless the infant is allergic to penicillin, breastfeeding is generally safe with penicillins. Observe infants for diarrhea, rashes, and thrush.

MACROLIDES

Erythromycin, clarithromycin, and **azithromycin** are excreted into the milk in amounts much smaller than a typical infant dosage and are usually safe.[1,43,44]

QUINOLONES

Ciprofloxacin, ofloxacin, and **pefloxacin** are concentrated in milk; **nalidixic acid** and **fleroxacin** have also been detected.[45,46] Ciprofloxacin appears to have caused pseudomembranous colitis in a breast-fed infant via breastmilk,[13] and nalidixic acid caused hemolytic anemia in a breast-fed neonate. Most fluoroquinolones are best avoided during nursing. **Norfloxacin** was undetectable in milk after a 200-mg dose, and may be acceptable for maternal UTI treatment because of its low milk excretion and poor oral bioavailability.

SULFONAMIDES

Some sulfonamides may cause hemolysis in G-6-PD–deficient infants; theoretically, sulfonamides may increase the risk of kernicterus in neonates. **Sulfamethoxazole,** with or without trimethoprim, and **sulfisoxazole** can be used by mothers of healthy, full-term infants over 2 months of age.

TETRACYCLINES

Tooth staining caused by a tetracycline in breastmilk has not been reported. Milk calcium apparently inhibits absorption of the small amounts of **tetracycline** in milk. Infant absorption and plasma concentrations have not been reported with other tetracyclines, but infants would only receive a few milligrams per day of **demeclocycline, doxycycline,** or **minocycline** with usual maternal dosages. Doxycycline concentrations in milk progressively increased with duration of therapy in one study. Although other drugs are preferred for most infections, tetracyclines can be used for a short time (7–14 days); avoid prolonged or repeat courses during nursing. Minocycline has caused black milk.[47]

MISCELLANEOUS ANTIMICROBIALS

Chloramphenicol

Breastfeeding is contraindicated during maternal chloramphenicol treatment. Milk concentrations are not sufficient to induce "gray baby" syndrome, but theoretically may be enough to cause the rare, idiosyncratic aplastic anemia. Adverse reactions in infants, including refusal of the breast, falling asleep during feeding, and vomiting after feeding, have occurred.

Clindamycin

Clindamycin is excreted variably in small amounts into milk. It is not certain what effects these amounts may have on infants' GI flora (eg, pseudomembranous colitis), but a single case of bloody stools in an infant with normal stool flora was reported during maternal clindamycin use. Clindamycin is best avoided if possible, but a few days of therapy with close monitoring of the infant is acceptable. Vaginal clindamycin presents less infant risk than oral or IV use.

(continued)

ANTIMICROBIAL DRUGS

Metronidazole
Both metronidazole and its hydroxy metabolite are found in the plasma of nursing infants in concentrations that are 10–20% of maternal plasma concentrations. Anecdotal cases of diarrhea and isolation of *Candida* species from breast-fed infants have been reported, but most infants do not have immediate reactions. Because of the carcinogenicity in animals, possible mutagenicity, and the relatively high infant plasma concentrations achieved, metronidazole should probably be avoided in nursing mothers.[1,48] When essential to treat trichomoniasis, metronidazole may be given as a single 2-g dose, and an alternative feeding method used for the next 24 hr. After longer courses for anaerobic infections, nursing can resume 12–24 hr after the final dose. **Furazolidone,** which is poorly absorbed orally, can be used to treat maternal giardiasis if the infant is over 1 month of age.

Methenamine
Both the hippurate and methenamine salts of methenamine pass into milk in small quantities and seem safe to use.

Nitrofurantoin
Nitrofurantoin is excreted into milk in pharmacologically unimportant amounts, but avoid it in infants under 1 month of age and those with G-6-PD deficiency.

Trimethoprim
Trimethoprim is excreted into milk in amounts that are not harmful.

Vancomycin
Because it is excreted into milk in only small amounts[49] and is not orally absorbed, vancomycin is safe during nursing.

ANTINEOPLASTICS AND IMMUNOSUPPRESSANTS

Breastfeeding is generally considered to be contraindicated in women receiving antineoplastics because of the potential for immunosuppression and carcinogenicity.[18]

ALKYLATING AGENTS
Busulfan
Busulfan in a dosage of 4 mg/day for 5 weeks was taken by one woman while breastfeeding, with no apparent adverse effects on her infant's leukocytes or hemoglobin. This case is by no means conclusive, however, and breastfeeding is not recommended.

Cisplatin
Platinum was not detected in the milk of one patient at any time after an IV infusion of 100 mg/m^2 of cisplatin. In another patient, milk platinum was 0.9 mg/L 19.5 hr after her third daily dose of 20 mg/m^2. Because the platinum may be in a reactive form, nursing is not recommended during cisplatin therapy.

Cyclophosphamide
Cyclophosphamide is detectable in milk, and has caused bone marrow depression in infants of women who nursed while receiving the drug. Breastfeeding is contraindicated during cyclophosphamide therapy.

(*continued*)

ANTINEOPLASTICS AND IMMUNOSUPPRESSANTS

ANTIMETABOLITES
Methotrexate
Low amounts of methotrexate were found in milk in one patient; however, this case is not conclusive. Low weekly doses for arthritis probably pose only a slight risk to the infant.

DNA INTERCALATING DRUGS
Doxorubicin
Doxorubicin and its primary active metabolite, **doxorubicinol,** appear in milk, with their highest milk concentrations occurring 24 hr after a dose.

Mitoxantrone
Measurable levels of mitoxantrone occurred in milk for at least 28 days after 6 mg/kg was given daily for 3 days.[50]

MITOTIC INHIBITORS
Etoposide
Etoposide milk levels are undetectable 24 hr after a dose.[50]

MISCELLANEOUS ANTINEOPLASTICS
Hydroxyurea
Only small amounts of hydroxyurea are found in milk, but breastfeeding is not advised.

IMMUNOSUPPRESSANTS
Three infants were reportedly breastfed safely during maternal **azathioprine** use (75–100 mg/day) after renal transplantation. Low concentrations of the azathioprine metabolite, **mercaptopurine,** were found in milk. Breastfeeding can be undertaken with close infant monitoring for infection or other signs of immunosuppression during azathioprine therapy, although there is concern over potential carcinogenicity.[1,18] Maternal **cyclosporine** therapy results in the infant receiving 2% or less of the mother's mg/kg dosage.[51,52] Eight infants have been breastfed safely for 4–12 months during maternal therapy with cyclosporine, prednisone, and azathioprine. Infant serum cyclosporine levels were undetectable (<30 μg/L), renal function was unaffected, and they grew normally.[51] **Tacrolimus** colostrum levels are about 50% of maternal serum levels.[53] The implications of these low levels for the infant are not known.

CARDIOVASCULAR DRUGS

ANTIARRHYTHMIC DRUGS
Some antiarrhythmics reach near-therapeutic concentrations in breast-fed infants. **Amiodarone** is excreted in amounts that may pose a hazard to the infant and it should not be used during nursing.[1,54] Data on **disopyramide** indicate that infants may receive relatively large amounts of the drug and its active metabolite, with plasma concentrations near the therapeutic range. Disopyramide may be used cautiously during lactation when other alternatives are unacceptable. Observe the infant for anticholinergic symptoms, and monitor infant plasma concentrations if there is a concern. The anticholinergic activity of disopyramide may also suppress lactation. (*See* Anticholinergics.) Sparse data from one patient indicate that **tocainide** may be concentrated in milk and it should be used with caution during nursing. Because of its low oral

(*continued*)

CARDIOVASCULAR DRUGS

bioavailability, maternal **bretylium** is unlikely to harm nursing infants; 400 mg q 8 hr was taken orally by one mother while nursing, with no apparent effects on her infant. Infants receive trivial doses of **digoxin** via breastmilk. Amounts of **flecainide** in milk are small and unlikely to affect the infant. **Lidocaine** concentrations in milk during continuous IV infusion and as a local anesthetic are low and poorly absorbed by the infant, so it poses no hazard to the infant.[55,56] Concentrations of **mexiletine** in milk are too low to be detected in the plasma of breast-fed infants. **Procainamide** and its active metabolite, **N-acetylprocainamide,** are concentrated in milk, but absolute amounts are small; procainamide may be used with caution in nursing mothers. **Propafenone** milk levels are very low, but no clinical experience has been reported.[57] **Quinidine** excretion seems inconsequential.

ANTIHYPERTENSIVE DRUGS

Certain antihypertensives are less desirable than others during nursing. Milk concentrations of **clonidine** are much higher than maternal plasma concentrations, and breast-fed infants have plasma concentrations approaching those of the mother.[1,58] Clonidine and **guanfacine** may also decrease prolactin secretion. These drugs must be used with caution during breastfeeding, and should be avoided if possible. Avoid **reserpine** because it causes nasal stuffiness and increased tracheobronchial secretions in the infant. The angiotensin-converting enzyme (ACE) inhibitors, **benazepril, captopril,** and **enalapril,** are found in small amounts and no adverse effects have occurred in breast-fed infants.[1,59] Additionally, milk ACE activity was in the normal range after a dose of enalapril. These ACE inhibitors are good choices during lactation; others have not been studied. Limited data indicate that low-dose, short-term use of **hydralazine** (ie, a few days postpartum) is safe. There is limited information on **minoxidil** in milk, but amounts are small. However, use minoxidil with caution, particularly when therapy involves large dosages and long-term use. Several studies indicate that **methyldopa** is excreted in unimportant amounts.

β-ADRENERGIC BLOCKING DRUGS

The excretion of β-blockers into breastmilk has been extensively studied. The infant's dosage varies greatly among the different compounds, allowing a range of choices. The most water-soluble drugs reach the infant in the greatest amounts because of low plasma protein binding. Additionally, the water-soluble agents have the longest half-lives, are renally eliminated, and are therefore more likely to accumulate in infants. Maternal therapy with **atenolol** and **acebutolol** have resulted in adverse effects (eg, bradycardia, hypotension, tachypnea, and cyanosis) in breast-fed infants. These two drugs, as well as **betaxolol, nadolol, sotalol,** and **timolol,** should be avoided in mothers of newborn infants or when high dosage is required. **Oxprenolol** and **mepindolol** excretion is intermediate and they should be avoided during the early neonatal period. **Propranolol, metoprolol,** and **labetalol** (and its isomer, **dilevalol**) are excreted in low enough quantities to allow nursing even in the neonatal period.

CALCIUM-CHANNEL BLOCKING DRUGS

Case reports indicate that only small amounts of **diltiazem, nifedipine, nimodipine,** and **nitrendipine** are excreted into milk.[1,60] More data are needed to judge the safety of these drugs during nursing. Several case reports indicate that the amounts of **verapamil** and **norverapamil** in milk and infant plasma are low. Verapamil appears to be safe during nursing.

(continued)

CENTRAL NERVOUS SYSTEM DRUGS

ANTICONVULSANTS

Breast-fed infants may achieve plasma anticonvulsant concentrations that produce pharmacologic effects; mild drowsiness, irritability, and feeding difficulties are common in the infants of mothers taking anticonvulsants, especially during the early neonatal period.[1,61] Breastfeeding can mitigate withdrawal symptoms in infants whose mothers took anticonvulsants during pregnancy, and withdrawal symptoms have been observed after abrupt weaning. Plasma concentration monitoring in breast-fed infants may be indicated, particularly in infants who are excessively drowsy, feed poorly, or gain weight inadequately. Long-term effects of exposure are not well studied. Infants of mothers taking anticonvulsants may have more difficulty nursing and may breast-feed for a shorter duration.[62,63]

Carbamazepine

Both carbamazepine and its major active metabolite are excreted into milk and can be detected in nursing infants' plasma; concentrations are usually low, but near the therapeutic range in some infants. Two cases of hepatic dysfunction in breast-fed neonates have been reported.[64,65] Carbamazepine can be used during lactation, but close observation of the infant for jaundice and other signs of possible adverse idiosyncratic effects is advisable. Measurement of infant plasma concentration may be indicated if symptoms occur.

Clonazepam

Plasma concentrations of clonazepam were low in two nursing infants, and no effects were noted.[1] In another infant, breastfeeding increased plasma levels over those present at birth.[66] Observation of the infant for drowsiness and monitoring of the infant's plasma concentration may be indicated.

Ethosuximide

Breast-fed infants may attain ethosuximide plasma concentrations near the therapeutic range, and some infants may show signs of drowsiness or fussiness. Breastfeed with caution, and keep the mother's plasma concentrations as low as possible while remaining in the therapeutic range. Infant plasma drug concentration monitoring is indicated.

Lamotrigine

Serum lamotrigine levels in two infants breastfed during maternal lamotrigine therapy were 25–70% of the maternal serum level. No adverse effects occurred.[67]

Phenobarbital

The effect of phenobarbital is unpredictable: Drowsiness leading to feeding difficulties can occur; breastfeeding can prevent withdrawal symptoms in infants whose mothers took phenobarbital during pregnancy; and withdrawal symptoms have been observed after abrupt weaning. Phenobarbital can be used in low to moderate dosages, but monitor infant behavior, weight gain, and, if there is concern, plasma concentrations. Sometimes breastfeeding may have to be discontinued because of excessive drowsiness and poor weight gain.

Phenytoin

Only small amounts of phenytoin are excreted into milk. Rarely, infants may experience idiosyncratic reactions such as cyanosis and methemoglobinemia, but infants generally tolerate phenytoin in milk well.

(continued)

CENTRAL NERVOUS SYSTEM DRUGS

Primidone

Primidone and its metabolites (**phenylethylmalonamide, phenobarbital,** and **para-hydroxyphenobarbital**) appear in milk in large amounts. Considerations are the same as for phenobarbital. (*See* Phenobarbital.)

Valproic Acid

Milk concentrations of valproate are low, and usually no effects occur in infants. One case of probable infant thrombocytopenic purpura from valproate in milk has been reported.[68] Observe infants for rare idiosyncratic effects such as thrombocytopenia and hepatotoxicity.

Vigabatrin

Limited data from two mothers indicate that a breast-fed infant would receive <4% of the mother's mg/kg dose of vigabatrin.[69]

ANTIDEPRESSANTS

Heterocyclic Antidepressants

Most of these drugs have not been well studied during lactation. Some authors recommend against use of antidepressants because of theoretical (but undemonstrated) long-term effects on infants' neurologic development; others consider **tricyclic antidepressants** (TCAs) to be acceptable. Follow-up for 1–3 yr in a small group of breast-fed infants indicates no adverse effects on growth and development. Sedating TCAs and those with active metabolites (eg, **amitriptyline, doxepin,** and **imipramine**) are less desirable than other TCAs. Respiratory depression was reported in one breast-fed infant whose mother was taking **doxepin** 25 mg tid, but an infant whose mother was taking 150 mg at night had no problems. Maternal dosages of **amitriptyline** up to 150 mg/day, **clomipramine** 150 mg/day, **desipramine** 300 mg/day, **imipramine** 200 mg/day, or **nortriptyline** 125 mg/day have not caused observable effects in the infants studied. In several infants, nortriptyline plasma levels were undetectable with maternal nortriptyline dosages of up to 125 mg/day or amitriptyline 175 mg/day.[1,70,71] One nortriptyline metabolite has been detected in low levels in the serum of breast-fed infants without adverse consequences.[70,72] Nortriptyline (and probably the other secondary amine, desipramine) is the TCA of choice during breastfeeding. Giving the drug as a single dose at bedtime and skipping nighttime feeding(s) may further minimize infant exposure. A dose of 250 mg/day of **amoxapine** or 100–150 mg/day of **maprotiline** produce low drug concentrations in milk, but effects of these drugs on infants have not been well studied.

Selective Serotonin Reuptake Inhibitors

Fluoxetine use during nursing is inadvisable. Although daily dosage of the drug and metabolite in milk are less than 10% of the mother's weight-adjusted dosage,[73] their half-lives are very long. One case of colic (increased crying, decreased sleep, watery stools, and vomiting) and unexplained high serum levels was reported in a breast-fed 6 week old.[74] The infant improved after switching to formula and colic reappeared upon rechallenge. Data from 4 infants indicate that fluoxetine in breastmilk has no effect on neurological development,[75] but a larger retrospective study found that fluoxetine may reduce the growth rate of infants who are exposed via breastmilk from birth.[76] Older infants may be less susceptible to fluoxetine's effects than newborns who eliminate the drug more slowly. **Citalopram** reaches the infant in dosages similar to those of fluoxetine.[77,78] The manufacturer states that drowsiness and weight loss

(*continued*)

CENTRAL NERVOUS SYSTEM DRUGS

in breast-fed infants has occurred; citalopram is not a good choice during breastfeeding. **Paroxetine** and **fluvoxamine** appear in milk in amounts similar to or less than fluoxetine,[75,79] but there is much less experience with them. One infant developed normally up to 21 months of age after 5 months of exposure to fluvoxamine in breastmilk.[79] **Sertraline** concentrations in the serum of breast-fed infants are usually low to undetectable, platelet serotonin is unaffected, and no adverse effects on growth have been seen on follow-up.[80–82] Neonatal sertraline withdrawal symptoms from intrauterine exposure are not improved by breastfeeding, indicating minimal drug passage into milk.[83] Sertraline is the SSRI of choice during breastfeeding.

Monoamine Oxidase Inhibitors

There are no data on the amounts of MAOIs excreted into milk. Because of their potential for toxicity and lactation inhibition, avoid MAOIs during nursing.

Other Antidepressants

Bupropion and its metabolites are concentrated in milk, but were undetectable in one 14-month-old infant whose mother was taking 300 mg/day and nursing twice daily.[84] A single 50-mg dose of **trazodone** produces low drug concentrations in milk, but the effect on infants has not been reported.[84] Infants receive **venlafaxine** doses of up to 9.2% of the mother's mg/kg dosage and the active metabolite is detectable in infant's serum. Although adverse effects were not seen in 3 breast-fed infants, caution should be used with venlafaxine until more experience is gained.[85]

ANTIPSYCHOTIC DRUGS

Data on the use of antipsychotics during lactation are sparse.[84,86] **Phenothiazines** and **thioxanthenes** pass into milk somewhat unpredictably, but usually in small amounts. Drowsiness can occur with the more sedating agents, such as **chlorpromazine.** Other effects, such as extrapyramidal symptoms, may be possible, but have not been reported. Limited follow-up, ranging from 15 months to 6 yr, indicates no long-term effects on infant development in most infants. However, three infants whose mothers were taking large dosages of chlorpromazine (200–600 mg/day) and **haloperidol** (20–40 mg/day) in combination showed a deterioration of mental and psychomotor developmental scores over the first 12–18 months of life.[87] Nine other infants whose mothers were taking lower dosages of a single antipsychotic (including haloperidol up to 20 mg/day) showed normal development. Breastfeeding during **clozapine** use in four infants resulted in sedation in one and agranulocytosis in another which resolved upon discontinuation;[86] nursing is not recommended during clozapine use.[84,88]

ANXIOLYTICS, SEDATIVES, AND HYPNOTICS

Many sedatives and hypnotics pass into breastmilk in measurable and potentially important amounts. Minimize sedative and hypnotic intake during lactation.

Anesthetics, General

Compared with epidural anesthesia, general anesthesia used during cesarean delivery can decrease both the frequency and duration of breastfeeding.[88] Excretion of most inhalation anesthetics in breastmilk has not been well studied. Blood levels of anesthetic gases such as **desflurane, enflurane, halothane, isoflurane, nitrous oxide,** and **sevoflurane** drop rapidly following termination of anesthesia, are predicted to pass poorly into milk, and are probably poorly absorbed by the infant.[89,90] **Etomidate** milk levels drop rapidly after a dose and should pose little risk to the infant.[91] Amounts of **propofol** in milk are small and do not have good oral bioavailability in the infant. Typical IV doses of **methohexital** or **thiopental** for induction of anesthesia produce

(*continued*)

CENTRAL NERVOUS SYSTEM DRUGS

low concentrations in milk that do not cause effects in the infant.[1,22,91] Current opinion suggests that breastfeeding can be resumed as soon as the mother has recovered sufficiently from general anesthesia to nurse.[89,90]

Barbiturates

These drugs may stimulate metabolism of endogenous compounds in the infant when small amounts pass into milk. Short-acting agents are preferable to long-acting agents, because smaller amounts are excreted into milk. Large single doses may have more potential for causing infant drowsiness than multiple small doses. (*See also* Anesthetics and Anticonvulsants.)

Benzodiazepines

Long-acting benzodiazepines and those with active metabolites (eg, **diazepam**) can accumulate and cause adverse effects in infants, especially with repeated doses, and in neonates, because of their immature excretory mechanisms. A single dose of diazepam for short dental, surgical, or diagnostic procedures is not likely to cause sedation in infants past the neonatal period.[22] Milk **alprazolam** levels are low,[92] but infant drowsiness and withdrawal symptoms have been reported with alprazolam use during nursing.[1,12] When oral therapy is essential, the short-acting agents, **oxazepam** or **lorazepam,** are preferred; **temazepam** may also be acceptable.[86,93] **Midazolam** concentrations in milk are low and unlikely to affect the infant after a single dose or short course of therapy.[89,90]

Chloral Hydrate

Chloral hydrate and its active metabolite, **trichloroethanol,** appear in milk in dosages that approximate an infant sedative dosage and are detectable for up to 24 hr after a single dose.

Meprobamate

Concentrations peak in milk at 4 hr, which is 2 hr after peak maternal plasma concentrations.

Zolpidem

Zolpidem milk levels are low for 3 hr after a dose and undetectable thereafter.[94]

LITHIUM

Lithium in milk can adversely affect the infant when its elimination is impaired, as in dehydration or in neonates or premature infants. Neonates may also have transplacentally acquired plasma lithium levels. The long-term effects of lithium on infants are not known; many authors consider lithium therapy a contraindication to breastfeeding, but others do not. Lithium may be used cautiously in mothers who are carefully selected for their ability to monitor their full-term infants. Discontinue breastfeeding immediately if the infant appears restless or looks ill. Measurement of plasma lithium concentrations in the infant can help rule out lithium toxicity.[1,72]

PARKINSONISM DRUGS
Dopamine Agonists

Some ergot alkaloids have dopaminergic activity that can suppress prolactin release and lactation. **Bromocriptine** was used therapeutically for this purpose, but has lost this indication in the United States because of potentially serious maternal toxicity.

(*continued*)

CENTRAL NERVOUS SYSTEM DRUGS

Levodopa

Lithium decreases serum prolactin in nonnursing women with hyperprolactinemia and galactorrhea in a dose-dependent fashion and inhibits lactation in animals at high dosages. It is likely that levodopa interferes with lactation in nursing mothers. Effects in breast-fed infants have not been studied.

GASTROINTESTINAL DRUGS

ACID-PEPTIC THERAPY

Antacids

Although **aluminum, calcium,** and **magnesium** antacids are partially absorbed, they are unlikely to appreciably increase concentrations of these ions in milk and are safe to use.

Histamine H_2 Blockers

Cimetidine is concentrated in milk because of ion trapping and possibly active secretion;[8] **ranitidine** is also concentrated, but to a lesser extent. Cimetidine and ranitidine are best taken as a single dose at bedtime with avoidance of night feedings. **Famotidine** and **nizatidine** are less concentrated in milk and are preferred during nursing.

Proton Pump Inhibitors

Omeprazole and **lansoprazole** have not been adequately studied. In one mother, omeprazole milk levels were low and her newborn infant breastfed without harm.[95]

Sucralfate

Because sucralfate is virtually nonabsorbable, it may be preferable to H_2-receptor antagonists.

GASTROINTESTINAL MOTILITY

Antidiarrheals

Nonabsorbable products such as **kaolin-pectin** are preferred in nursing mothers. The **loperamide** prodrug loperamide oxide results in only small amounts of loperamide in breastmilk. **Diphenoxylate** excretion into milk has not been studied. One or two small doses of loperamide or diphenoxylate daily should pose little risk to the nursing infant. Avoid **bismuth subsalicylate** because the salicylate in the product is absorbable.

Gastrokinetic Agents

Milk **cisapride** concentrations are low, but its effects on maternal prolactin or infants are not known. **Metoclopramide** elevates serum prolactin via central dopaminergic antagonism and results in increased milk production and a more rapid transition from colostrum to mature milk. It may be used therapeutically in mothers who are producing insufficient quantities of milk, such as the mothers of premature or sick infants, or adoptive mothers. However, metoclopramide may induce or worsen depression, so caution is warranted. Although infant dosages of metoclopramide from milk are low, the infant's serum prolactin concentrations may sometimes be elevated. Limiting the duration of metoclopramide therapy to 14 days is essential.

Cathartics and Laxatives

Some **anthraquinone** derivatives, such as **aloe** and **cascara,** and other stimulant cathartics (eg, **phenolphthalein**) should be avoided during nursing because of a laxative effect in breast-fed infants. Laxatives that are nonabsorbable or poorly absorbed,

(*continued*)

GASTROINTESTINAL DRUGS

such as bulk-forming (eg, **psyllium**), osmotic (eg, **magnesium** or **phosphate salts**), or stool-softening (eg, **docusate**) types, are preferred during lactation. **Senna** in moderate dosages is acceptable if other measures fail. **Bisacodyl** is virtually unabsorbed from the GI tract and should be safe.

MISCELLANEOUS GASTROINTESTINAL DRUGS

Mesalamine Derivatives

Small amounts of **sulfasalazine** and **sulfapyridine** have been found in milk and infant's plasma after oral sulfasalazine use. The small amount of sulfapyridine released should cause no bilirubin displacement. **Olsalazine** is not detectable in milk, but its metabolite N-acetyl-5-ASA is found in small amounts.[96] Small amounts of **mesalamine** and larger amounts of its metabolite are found in milk after oral administration.[97] Diarrhea (bloody in one case) has occurred in infants of mothers using mesalamine derivatives. Sulfasalazine, mesalamine, and its derivatives may be used cautiously during nursing with close infant observation.

Ursodiol

Ursodiol was undetectable in the milk of one lactating mother, and her nursing infant developed normally during therapy.[98]

HEMATOLOGIC DRUGS

COAGULANTS AND ANTICOAGULANTS

Indandiones

Anisindione and **phenindione** are contraindicated because infant hemorrhage has occurred.

Heparins

Although minimal documentation exists, it is unlikely that **heparin** or low-molecular-weight heparins (eg, **enoxaparin, dalteparin**) pass into milk or are absorbed orally by the infant; anticoagulant activity was undetectable in one breast-fed infant whose mother received 20–40 mg/day of enoxaparin.[99]

Coumarins

Amounts of **warfarin** in milk are of no clinical consequence with maternal dosage of 12 mg/day or less, because of extensive protein binding,[1,9] higher dosages have not been studied. Other coumarin derivatives (eg, **acenocoumarol, dicumarol,** and **phenprocoumon**) also appear safe.[1,100]

HORMONES AND SYNTHETIC SUBSTITUTES

ADRENAL HORMONES

Corticosteroids

Prednisone and **prednisolone** excretion into milk is minimal even with large oral doses.[101] The infant dosage can be reduced even further by using prednisolone rather than prednisone and avoiding nursing for 3–4 hr after a dose. Three infants have been breastfed during long-term maternal use of **methylprednisolone** 6–8 mg/day with apparent safety. Large IV doses of corticosteroids or use of long-acting agents such as **dexamethasone** have not been studied, and caution is warranted. Depot injections, inhaled corticosteroids (eg, **beclomethasone, fluticasone**), or topical corticosteroids should present little or no risk to the infant because of low maternal plasma concentra-

(continued)

HORMONES AND SYNTHETIC SUBSTITUTES

tions. However, topical application to the nipple has caused effects in the infant because of direct ingestion.[102]

ANTIDIABETIC DRUGS
Insulin
Diabetic mothers using insulin may nurse their infants. However, it has been empirically found that the mother may need to reduce her insulin dosage to about 75% of the prepregnancy dosage.

Sulfonylureas
Tolbutamide is excreted in milk in small amounts that should cause no harm. The manufacturer reports that **chlorpropamide** levels in milk are low, but no published clinical data are available. No information is available on the other oral sulfonylurea agents.

CONTRACEPTIVES
Estrogen-Progestin Combinations
Although present in milk in small amounts, estrogens and progestins are readily metabolized by nursing infants. Rare case reports of breast enlargement in infants and proliferation of the vaginal epithelium in female infants have been attributed to combination oral contraceptives. These effects occur primarily with products containing >50 μg of estrogen. These high-estrogen contraceptives also markedly suppress lactation, especially when administered immediately postpartum. When currently available low-dose estrogen-progestin combination contraceptives are begun 6 or more weeks postpartum, a dramatic immediate effect on milk supply is usually not seen, but long-term negative effects on milk yield lead to early feeding supplementation and discontinuation of breastfeeding, and in one study, decreased infant growth. An 8-year follow-up of breast-fed infants of mothers taking contraceptives containing **ethinyl estradiol** 50 μg found no adverse effects on the infants' development or behavior. Progestin-only contraceptives are preferred during lactation.

Progestin-Only
No immediate effects have been reported with progestin-only contraceptives, such as **levonorgestrel** implants, depot **medroxyprogesterone** acetate, or oral **norethindrone** or **norgestrel.** Progestin-only contraceptives generally have no effect on, or enhance, milk supply and may extend the duration of lactation. Although infant growth may undergo a slight, transient depression after insertion of levonorgestrel implants, large, multicenter studies have found no effect of progestin-only contraceptives on growth and development of infants and children up to puberty.[103,106] Early (ie, immediately postpartum) initiation of these agents is controversial. Because physiologic postpartum progesterone withdrawal is a primary stimulus for lactation, it appears best to wait for at least 3 days postpartum before starting a progestin-only contraceptive.[107] However, one study found no adverse effects on lactation or infant growth when depot medroxyprogesterone was given immediately postpartum.[108] Progestin-only contraceptives started 6 weeks postpartum are the preferred hormonal contraceptives during lactation.[109,110] (See also Progesterone.)

(continued)

HORMONES AND SYNTHETIC SUBSTITUTES

FEMALE SEX HORMONES

Progesterone

Contraceptive use via implants (investigationally) or intrauterine devices transfers little progesterone to the breast-fed infant, and any drug in milk is minimally absorbed by the infant.[1,109,110] Milk progesterone concentrations have not been measured after higher doses used to treat premenstrual syndrome.

THYROID AND ANTITHYROID DRUGS

Iodides

Inorganic iodide is contraindicated during breastfeeding, because of possible thyroid suppression and rash. Topical and vaginal **povidone-iodine** in nursing mothers results in elevated milk iodine concentrations and occasional thyroid suppression in nursing infants. Avoid povidone-iodine preparations while nursing and minimize their use during delivery.

Thioamides

Propylthiouracil in dosages of ≤300 mg/day is the antithyroid drug of choice during lactation. **Methimazole** ≤20 mg/day or **carbimazole** (a methimazole prodrug) ≤15 mg/day may also be used, but these drugs pass into milk in greater quantities and have longer half-lives than propylthiouracil; thus, they are less desirable alternatives.[111] A potential for idiosyncratic reactions (eg, agranulocytosis) and hypothyroidism exists, and measurement of the infant's serum thyroxine and TSH concentrations at 2–4-week intervals is prudent during maternal antithyroid drug use.

Thyroid Hormones

Normal lactation requires thyroid hormones. **Levothyroxine** (T_4) passes into milk poorly, although **liothyronine** (T_3) may pass in more physiologically relevant amounts. Milk concentrations of thyroid hormones have not been measured after exogenous administration, but a physiologic replacement dosage of levothyroxine to a breastfeeding mother is not expected to result in excessive thyroid administration to the infant. Replacement therapy with liothyronine or supraphysiologic maternal levothyroxine dosage may transfer larger amounts of liothyronine to the infant.

Protirelin

Protirelin (thyrotropin-releasing hormone [TRH]) causes an increase in prolactin secretion and may enhance milk yield.[112]

MISCELLANEOUS HORMONAL AGENTS

Ergot Alkaloids

Ergonovine can lower postpartum serum prolactin concentrations, but **methylergonovine** apparently does not. Methylergonovine is not found in milk in important quantities. Short-term, low-dose regimens of these agents immediately postpartum pose no hazard to the infant, but methylergonovine is preferred because it does not inhibit lactation. Courses of these drugs given several days postpartum may expose the infant to greater risk of ergot side effects because of the larger amount of milk consumed at this age.

Calcitriol

Calcitriol requirements in hypoparathyroid women decrease during lactation. Failure to substantially decrease (by up to 2/3) the calcitriol dosage results in maternal hypercalcemia.[113,114]

(*continued*)

HORMONES AND SYNTHETIC SUBSTITUTES

Desmopressin
Desmopressin is excreted in negligible amounts into milk and is poorly absorbed orally by the infant, so it appears safe to use.

Human Growth Hormone
Somatropin can increase insufficient milk production in the mothers of preterm infants.[115]

RENAL AND ELECTROLYTES

DIURETICS
Large dosages of short-acting thiazide-type (eg, **hydrochlorothiazide**), usual dosages of loop diuretics (eg, **furosemide**), or long-acting thiazide-type diuretics (eg, **chlorthalidone** and **bendroflumethiazide**) can suppress lactation and should be avoided. Long-acting agents may also accumulate in infants' plasma. Low dosages of short-acting thiazide-type diuretics should pose no problems to the infant or suppress lactation, although theoretically, thrombocytopenia or allergic reactions to **sulfonamide** diuretics might occur. **Acetazolamide** appears in milk in small amounts that are unlikely to harm the infant. The amounts of **spironolactone** and its metabolites in milk are inconsequential.

ELECTROLYTES
Fluoride
Fluoride supplementation is not recommended during the first 6 months after birth; from 6 months to 3 yr of age, fluoride supplementation of the breast-fed infant is recommended only if the mother's water supply contains less than 0.3 ppm fluoride.[116]

Magnesium Sulfate
When given IV, magnesium sulfate increases milk magnesium concentrations only slightly. Oral absorption of magnesium is poor, so maternal magnesium therapy is not a contraindication to breastfeeding. Difficulty in establishing a milk supply by the mother and difficulty in nursing by the infant are sometimes observed after mothers have received magnesium sulfate infusions for the treatment of pre-eclampsia or eclampsia, although the frequency and cause are not clear.

ANTIGOUT AGENTS
Allopurinol
This drug and its active metabolite, **oxypurinol**, are excreted into milk in nearly therapeutic amounts, and oxypurinol is detectable in the nursing infant's plasma in near-therapeutic levels.[117] Although one infant breastfed without harm during maternal allopurinol therapy, observe infants for side effects, especially hypersensitivity reactions. If possible, give allopurinol to the mother in a single dose after the last nursing of the day.

Colchicine
Several infants have been breastfed safely during long-term, low-dose administration of colchicine for familial Mediterranean fever.[118,119] The amount excreted in milk indicates that toxicity might occur with higher dosages.[119] Colchicine is known to decrease milk production and alter milk composition in animals when infused into the udder. Use it with great caution and in low dosages when breastfeeding.

(continued)

RESPIRATORY DRUGS

ANTIASTHMATICS
Anticholinergics
Excretion of anticholinergics into milk has not been studied. Theoretical hazards of the orally absorbable compounds include anticholinergic effects such as drying of secretions, temperature elevations, and CNS disturbances in the infant. Anticholinergics can inhibit lactation by inhibiting growth hormone and oxytocin secretion.[1,121,122] Observe infants carefully for anticholinergic symptoms and signs of decreased lactation (eg, insatiety, poor weight gain) when anticholinergics are given to the mother. It is unlikely that inhaled **ipratropium** affects the infant or milk production.

Terbutaline
Oral administration results in low milk terbutaline concentrations, causes no symptoms in breast-fed infants, and is not expected to decrease milk supply. Other β_2-receptor agonists (eg, **albuterol**) appear safe to use orally, but inhaler products should transfer less drug to the infant and are preferred.

Theophylline
Maternal theophylline use may occasionally cause irritability and fretful sleep in infants. Newborn infants are most likely to be affected because of their slow elimination and low plasma protein binding of theophylline. There is no need to avoid theophylline products; however, keep maternal plasma concentrations in the lower part of the therapeutic range and measure infant plasma concentrations if side effects occur. The related drug **dyphylline** is excreted into milk in greater amounts and is best avoided.

ANTIHISTAMINES
There are few studies on antihistamine use during lactation. One study found drowsiness or irritability occurred in 12% of breast-fed infants whose mothers took antihistamines.[12] Older sedating (and more anticholinergic) antihistamines are more problematic because they may both affect the infant and suppress lactation. (*See* Anticholinergics.) Nonsedating antihistamines are preferred agents for long-term therapy. However, single bedtime doses of a sedating antihistamine after the last feeding of the day may be adequate for many women and minimize the amount the infant receives. Avoid sedating antihistamines in high dosages, in SR formulations, or in combinations with a sympathomimetic agent.

Cetirizine
Cetirizine has not been studied, but is not a preferred agent because of its sedative and anticholinergic effects.

Cyproheptadine
Cyproheptadine lowers maternal serum prolactin and should be avoided during lactation.

Fexofenadine
Based on terfenadine experience, fexofenadine is likely to be well tolerated.[12,120]

Loratadine
Loratadine is excreted into milk in seemingly unimportant amounts.

Triprolidine
Only small amounts of triprolidine are found in breastmilk.

RESPIRATORY DRUGS

COUGH AND COLD

α-Adrenergic **sympathomimetics** decrease milk flow in animals by central inhibition of secretion and release of oxytocin, and by peripheral vasoconstriction, which limits the access of oxytocin to myoepithelial cells in the mammary glands. **Norepinephrine** may also decrease prolactin release. Although these effects are not well documented in humans, lactation inhibition seems to occur with oral decongestant (eg, **pseudoephedrine**) use; therefore, sympathomimetic nasal sprays (eg, **oxymetazoline**) are recommended over oral decongestant products. Pseudoephedrine may also cause irritability in some infants.[12]

MISCELLANEOUS DRUGS

CHOLINERGIC DRUGS

Six infants of mothers treated with **neostigmine** for myasthenia gravis were reportedly breastfed successfully. Neostigmine was not found in milk, but one infant appeared to have abdominal cramps after each breastfeeding. **Pyridostigmine** has been used safely during breastfeeding in three patients with myasthenia gravis.

Baclofen

Only small amounts of baclofen appear in milk, and it may be used in nursing mothers with caution.

Bupivacaine

Bupivacaine is undetectable in milk when administered to the mother by intrapleural or epidural routes. Epidural analgesia with bupivacaine post-cesarean section improved breastfeeding performance in one study.[26] (*See also* Lidocaine in Antiarrhythmics.)

Pyridoxine

In high doses (200–600 mg/day), pyridoxine has been used therapeutically to suppress lactation, although it is often not effective. With usual dosages found in foods and low-dose vitamin supplements, pyridoxine has no effect on prolactin or lactation.

Radiopharmaceuticals

Exposure of the infant to excessive amounts of radioactivity is usually the primary concern raised by administration of radiopharmaceuticals to nursing mothers, rather than any pharmacologic toxicity of the agent. Discontinue breastfeeding, at least temporarily, after administration of a radiopharmaceutical to a nursing mother. The length of time needed for milk radioactivity to decline (by means of both radioactive decay and maternal excretion) to a safe exposure level depends on several factors: dosage, biological half-life, radionuclide half-life, and "contamination" with other isotopes. The age of the infant, potential for oral absorption of the radionuclide from the infant's GI tract, and threshold level that is considered safe are also important factors. Two reviews deal comprehensively with the topic of radiopharmaceutical use in nursing mothers and provide more detailed information.[123,124]

Retinoids

Acitretin passes into breastmilk in a quantity sufficient to merit avoidance of nursing while taking it. Although there is no information on use during lactation, the manufacturers of oral **isotretinoin** and topical **tretinoin** state that they are not compatible with nursing. Based on the systemic bioavailability of tretinoin applied topically to a small area such as the face, it seems unlikely that harmful amounts reach the infant via breastmilk. Avoid contact of the infant's skin with treated areas of the mother's skin, regardless of whether she is nursing.

(*continued*)

MISCELLANEOUS DRUGS

Vaccines

Breastfeeding is not a contraindication to the use of any vaccine (live or inactivated) in the nursing mother.[125]

DIAGNOSTIC AGENTS

Iodinated Contrast Media

Iopanoic acid contains free iodide that can be detected in milk. (*See* Iodides.) **Diatrizoate, iodamide, iohexol, metrizoate,** and **metrizamide** are detectable in milk after IV administration. Although no adverse effects have been reported in infants, breastfeeding should probably be withheld for a period of time after administration of most iodinated contrast media, the time depending on its rate of elimination. A few hours is probably adequate following an IV pyelogram. Large amounts of iodine are excreted into milk for weeks after lymphangiography with **ethiodized oil,** and nursing should be discontinued after this procedure.

Fluorescein

Fluorescein is detectable in milk after IV or topical administration. After IV administration, it had a milk half-life of 62 hr in one mother. The drug may present a risk to neonates who are undergoing phototherapy. Temporarily withholding nursing after fluorescein use (especially IV) seems appropriate in this situation.

Gadolinium

Gadodiamide and **gadopentetate,** used in magnetic resonance imaging, are detectable in milk, but have poor oral absorption and are rapidly excreted renally. Withholding nursing for 6–12 hr should provide adequate safety.

DRUGS FOR NONMEDICAL USE

Alcohol

Alcohol equilibrates rapidly between blood and milk, resulting in milk concentrations equivalent to simultaneous blood concentrations. Peak maternal plasma alcohol levels occur later in nursing mothers than in nonnursing women[126]; alteration in milk odor parallels milk alcohol levels.[126,127] Potential effects on infants vary, depending on the pattern of use. Drunkenness (deep, unarousable sleep with snoring, deep respiration, no reaction to pain, inability to suck, excessive perspiration, and a feeble pulse) was reported after maternal binge drinking. Pseudo-Cushing syndrome was reported in the infant of a chronic alcoholic mother. One prospective study suggests that as little as one drink daily can cause slight impairment of the infant's motor development; the impairment increases in a dose-dependent fashion.[1] Infants suck more, but consume less milk after maternal alcohol ingestion.[127] Alcohol also affects lactation; it inhibits the milk ejection reflex in a dose-dependent fashion, with single doses over 2 g/kg completely blocking suckling-induced oxytocin release. Animal studies show that alcohol consumption results in a reduced suckling-induced prolactin release and reduced milk yield. An unknown substance in beer increases maternal serum prolactin; this effect also occurs with nonalcoholic beer.[1,128] Use alcohol in moderation during lactation and withhold nursing temporarily after alcohol consumption, with the duration dependent on the amount consumed—at least 2 hr per drink is suggested.[129]

(*continued*)

DRUGS FOR NONMEDICAL USE

Amphetamine

In a mother taking amphetamine 20 mg/day therapeutically, amphetamine concentrations in milk were less than those in plasma and no adverse effects on the infant were noted. However, there is likely to be substantial intersubject variation in excretion, and concentrations in milk have not been measured during high-dose abuse of amphetamines. Anecdotally, infants breastfed by amphetamine abusers seem to experience drug-induced behavioral abnormalities, such as agitation and crying. Amphetamine also inhibits prolactin release and, in high dosages, may interfere with lactation.

Caffeine

Anecdotal reports of infant jitteriness and difficulty sleeping have been reported with very high maternal intake of caffeine, but infant serum caffeine concentrations were not measured. Systematic studies have indicated that caffeine and its metabolites are excreted into milk in relatively small amounts with usual maternal intake and infants are usually not affected, even with rather high maternal intake.[1,130,131] Effects are more likely in premature and newborn infants, because of their greatly diminished ability to metabolize caffeine.

Cocaine

Although not well studied in humans, the chemical nature of cocaine, and results from animal studies, indicate that it probably appears in milk in amounts that affect the infant.[1,132] In addition, plasma cholinesterase, which is needed to metabolize the drug, is low in newborns. Cocaine and its toxic metabolite can be detected in milk and can cause adverse effects (vomiting, diarrhea, irritability, and dilated pupils) in breast-fed infants.[1,132] Cocaine was detectable in milk for 24–36 hr after use. Convulsions occurred in an infant whose mother used topical cocaine to treat sore nipples. Breast-feeding is not recommended when the mother is a chronic cocaine user, and even occasional use of cocaine is discouraged during breastfeeding. Withhold breastfeeding for at least 24 hr after occasional cocaine use.

Heroin

Abuse can result in high enough concentrations in milk to cause addiction or alleviate withdrawal symptoms in infants; however, breastfeeding is not a reliable method of preventing withdrawal. Most authorities consider breastfeeding safe during **methadone** maintenance in doses up to 80 mg/day.[1,133]

Marijuana

Marijuana excretion into milk is not well studied, but **dronabinol** (tetrahydrocannabinol) may reach high concentrations in milk and may be detected in the infant, particularly with heavy maternal use. Short-term effects in infants have not been reported, but a decrement in motor development at 1 yr in the infants of marijuana-smoking mothers was reported in one study. Marijuana lowers serum prolactin slightly in nonlactating women and oxytocin release in rodents. One survey indicated that women who smoke marijuana breastfeed for a shorter duration than nonusers and that the effect appears to be dose related.[134] Avoid breastfeeding in heavy marijuana users and during therapeutic dronabinol use. Withhold breastfeeding for several hours after occasional marijuana use and use caution to avoid exposing the infant to marijuana smoke.

Phencyclidine

Phencyclidine is concentrated in milk and remains detectable in milk for weeks after heavy use. Avoid breastfeeding after phencyclidine use; a sufficient duration of abstinence has not been defined.

(*continued*)

DRUGS FOR NONMEDICAL USE

Tobacco

Nicotine and its metabolite, **cotinine,** are excreted into breastmilk in amounts proportional to the number of cigarettes smoked by the mother.[1,135] The milk of smokers contains higher concentrations of cadmium than the milk of nonsmokers; other toxins in smoke have not been measured. Smokers also produce lower milk volumes, have lower milkfat content, use formula supplements more often, and wean their infants from breastfeeding earlier than nonsmokers, in part because nicotine lowers maternal basal prolactin concentrations.[136,137] Infants of smoking mothers have an increased frequency of infantile colic, large postnursing decreases in respiratory rate and oxygen saturation, and more respiratory infections.[135] However, among infants of smokers, those who are not breastfed have almost double the risk of respiratory illness of breast-fed infants.[138] In nonsmokers, breastfeeding reduces the risk of sudden infant death syndrome compared to bottle feeding, but smoking negates this advantage.[139] Advise nursing mothers to (1) stop or decrease smoking to the greatest degree possible, (2) not breastfeed right after smoking, and (3) not smoke in the same room with the infant.[140] The use of nicotine chewing gum, topical patches, or nasal spray has not been studied during lactation. Although they are not recommended by the manufacturer during nursing, these products are likely to be less hazardous to the nursing infant than maternal smoking.

■ REFERENCES

1. Anderson PO. Drug use during breast feeding. *Clin Pharm* 1991;10:594–624.
2. Rasmussen F. The mechanisms of drug secretion into milk. In, Galli C et al, eds. *Dietary lipids and postnatal development.* New York: Raven Press; 1973;231:45.
3. Richter O, Reinhardt D. The transference of drugs from breast-feeding mothers to their infants: a pharmacokinetic model. *Biol Res Preg* 1980;1:112–7.
4. Wilson JT et al. Pharmacokinetic pitfalls in the estimation of the breast milk/plasma ratio for drugs. *Ann Rev Pharmacol Toxicol* 1985;25:667–89.
5. Fleishaker JC et al. Factors affecting the milk-to-plasma drug concentration ratio in lactating women: physical interactions with protein and fat. *J Pharm Sci* 1987;76:189–93.
6. Atkinson HC, Begg EJ. Prediction of drug distribution into human milk from physicochemical characteristics. *Clin Pharmacokinet* 1990;18:151–67.
7. Anderson PO. Medication use while breast feeding a neonate. *Neonatal Pharmacol Q* 1993;2:3–14.
8. Oo CY et al. Active transport of cimetidine into human milk. *Clin Pharmacol Ther* 1995;58:548–55.
9. Bennett PN, Notarianni LJ. Risk from drugs in breast milk: an analysis by relative dose. *Br J Clin Pharmacol* 1996;42:673P–4P. Abstract.
10. Ito S, Koren G. A novel index for expressing exposure of the infant to drugs in breast milk. *Br J Clin Pharmacol* 1994;38:99–102.
11. Bailey B, Ito S. Breast-feeding and maternal drug use. *Pediatr Clin North Am* 1997;44:41–54.
12. Ito S et al. Prospective follow-up of adverse reactions in breast-fed infants exposed to maternal medication. *Am J Obstet Gynecol* 1993;168:1393–9.
13. Harmon T et al. Perforated pseudomembranous colitis in the breast-fed infant. *J Pediatr Surg* 1992;27:744–46.
14. Wojnar-Horton RE et al. Distribution and excretion of sumatriptan in human milk. *Br J Clin Pharmacol* 1996;41:217–21.
15. Lebedevs TH et al. Excretion of indomethacin in breast milk. *Br J Clin Pharmacol* 1991;32:751–4.
16. Beaulac-Baillargeon L, Allard G. Distribution of indomethacin in human milk and estimation of its milk to plasma ratio in vitro. *Br J Clin Pharmacol* 1993;36:413–6.
17. Walter K, Dilger C. Ibuprofen in human milk. *Br J Clin Pharmacol* 1997;44:211–2. Letter.
18. Ramsey-Goldman R, Schilling E. Optimum use of disease-modifying and immunosuppressive antirheumatic agents during pregnancy and lactation. *Clin Immunother* 1996;5:40–58.

19. Rajan L. The impact of obstetric procedures and analgesia/anesthesia during labour and delivery on breast feeding. *Midwifery* 1994;10:87–103.

20. Nissen E et al. Effects of routinely given pethidine during labour on infants' developing breastfeeding behaviour. *Acta Paediatr* 1997;86:201–8.

21. Wittels B et al. Postcesarean analgesia with both epidural morphine and intravenous patient-controlled analgesia: neurobehavioral outcomes among nursing neonates. *Anesth Analg* 1997;85:600–6.

22. Borgatta L et al. Clinical significance of methohexital, meperidine, and diazepam in breastmilk. *J Clin Pharmacol* 1997;37:186–92.

23. Madej TH, Strunin L. Comparison of epidural fentanyl with sufentanil. *Anaesthesia* 1987;42:1156–61.

24. Steer PL et al. Concentration of fentanyl in colostrum after an analgesic dose. *Can J Anaesth* 1992;39:231–5.

25. Crowell MK et al. Relationship between obstetric analgesia and time of effective breast feeding. *J Nurse Midwifery* 1994;39:150–5.

26. Hirose M et al. The effect of postoperative analgesia with continuous epidural bupivacaine after cesarean section on the amount of breast feeding and infant weight gain. *Anesth Analg* 1996;82:1166–9.

27. Marquet P et al. Buprenorphine withdrawal syndrome in a newborn. *Clin Pharmacol Ther* 1997;62:569–71.

28. Pittman KA et al. Human perinatal distribution of butorphanol. *Am J Obstet Gynecol* 1980;138:797–800.

29. Wischnik A et al. Elimination von nalbuphin in die muttermilch. *Arzneimittelforschung* 1988;38:1496–8.

30. Lee CR et al. Tramadol. *Drugs* 1993;46:313–40.

31. Johnstone HA, Marcinak JF. Candidiasis in the breastfeeding mother and infant. *J Obstet Gynecol Neonatal Nurs* 1990;19:171–3.

32. Amir LH, Pakula S. Nipple pain, mastalgia and candidiasis in the lactating breast. *Aust NZ J Obstet Gynecol* 1991;31:378–80.

33. Schilling CG et al. Excretion of fluconazole in human breast milk. *Pharmacotherapy* 1993;13:387. Abstract.

34. Force RW. Fluconazole concentrations in breast milk. *Pediatr Infect Dis J* 1995;14:235–6.

35. Moretti ME et al. Disposition of maternal ketoconazole in breast milk. *Am J Obstet Gynecol* 1995;173:1625–6.

36. Utter AR. Gentian violet treatment for thrush: can its use cause breastfeeding problems? *J Human Lact* 1990;6:178–80.

37. USP-DI, 16th ed. Vol. I. *Drug information for the health care professional*. Rockville, MD: U.S. Pharmacopoeial Convention; 1996:1539–60.

38. Waters MFR. G 30 320 or B 663–Lampren (Geigy). *Lepr Rev* 1969;40:21–47.

39. Venkatesan K et al. Excretion of clofazimine in human milk in leprosy patients. *Lepr Rev* 1997;68:242–6.

40. Kurzel RB et al. Mebendazole and postpartum lactation. *NZ J Med* 1994;107:439. Letter.

41. Taddio A et al. Acyclovir excretion in human breast milk. *Ann Pharmacother* 1994;28:585–7.

42. Bork K, Benes P. Concentration and kinetic studies of intravenous acyclovir in serum and breast milk of a patient with eczema herpeticum. *J Am Acad Dermatol* 1995;32:1053–5.

43. Sedlmayr T et al. Clarithromycin, ein neues makrolid-antibiotikum. *Geburtshilfe Frauenheilkd* 1993;53:488–91.

44. Kelsey JJ et al. Presence of azithromycin breast milk concentrations: a case report. *Am J Obstet Gynecol* 1994;170:1375–6.

45. Dan M et al. Penetration of fleroxacin into breast milk and pharmacokinetics in lactating women. *Antimicrob Agents Chemother* 1993;37:293–6.

46. Gardner DK et al. Simultaneous concentrations of ciprofloxacin in breast milk and in serum in mother and breast-fed infant. *Clin Pharm* 1992;11:352–4.

47. Hunt MJ. Black breast milk due to minocycline therapy. *Br J Dermatol* 1996;134:943–4.

48. Dobias L et al. Genotoxicity and carcinogenicity of metronidazole. *Mutation Res* 1994;317:177–94.

49. Reyes MP et al. Vancomycin during pregnancy: does it cause hearing loss or nephrotoxicity in the infant? *Am J Obstet Gynecol* 1989;161:977–81.

50. Azuno Y et al. Mitoxantrone and etoposide in breast milk. *Am J Hematol* 1995;48:131–2.

51. Nyberg G. et al. Breast-feeding during treatment with cyclosporine. *Transplantation* 1998;65:253–5.

52. Thiru Y et al. Successful breast feeding while mother was taking cyclosporin. *BMJ* 1997;315:463.

53. Jain A et al. Pregnancy after liver transplantation under tacrolimus. *Transplantation* 1997;64:559–65.

54. Plomp TA et al. Use of amiodarone during pregnancy. *Eur J Obstet Gynecol Reprod Biol* 1992;43:201–7.

55. Zeisler JA et al. Lidocaine excretion in breast milk. *Drug Intell Clin Pharm* 1981;57:691–3.

56. Lebedevs TH et al. Excretion of lignocaine and its metabolite monoethylglycinexylidide in breast milk following its use in a dental procedure. *J Clin Periodontol* 1993;20:606–8.

57. Libardoni M et al. Transfer of propafenone and 5-OH-propafenone to foetal plasma and maternal milk. *Br J Clin Pharmacol* 1991;32:527–8. Letter.

58. Bunjes R et al. Clonidine and breast feeding. *Clin Pharm* 1993;12:178–9. Letter.

59. Kaiser G et al. Benazepril and benazeprilat in human plasma and breast milk. *Eur J Clin Pharmacol* 1989;36(suppl):A303. Abstract.

60. Carcas AJ et al. Nimodipine transfer into human breast milk and cerebrospinal fluid. *Ann Pharmacother* 1996;30:148–50.

61. Yerby MS. Contraception, pregnancy and lactation in women with epilepsy. *Baillieres Clin Neurol* 1996;5:887–908.

62. Ito S et al. Initiation and duration of breast-feeding in women receiving antiepileptics. *Am J Obstet Gynecol* 1995;172:881–6.

63. Hartmann AM et al. Stillen, gewichtszunanme und verhalten bei neugeborenen epileptischer frauen. *Monatsschr Kinderheilkd* 1994;142:505–12.

64. Frey B et al. Transient cholestatic hepatitis in a neonate associated with carbamazepine exposure during pregnancy and breast-feeding. *Eur J Pediatr* 1990;150:136–8.

65. Merlob P et al. Transient hepatic dysfunction in an infant of an epileptic mother treated with carbamazepine during pregnancy and breastfeeding. *Ann Pharmacother* 1992;26:1563–5.

66. Bossi L et al. Pharmacokinetics and clinical effects of antiepileptic drugs in newborns of chronically treated epileptic mothers. In, Janz D et al, eds. *Epilepsy, pregnancy and the child*. New York: Raven Press; 1982:373–81.

67. Tomsen T et al. Lamotrigine in pregnancy and lactation. A case report. *Epilepsia* 1997;38:1039–41.

68. Stahl MMS et al. Thrombocytopenic purpura and anemia in a breast-fed infant whose mother was treated with valproic acid. *J Pediatr* 1997;130:1001–3.

69. Tran A et al. Vigabatrin: placental transfer in vivo and excretion into breast milk of the enantiomers. *Br J Clin Pharmacol* 1998;45:409–11.

70. Wisner KL et al. Nortriptyline and its hydroxymetabolites in breastfeeding mothers and newborns. *Psychopharmacol Bull* 1997;33:249–51.

71. Yoshida K et al. Investigation of pharmacokinetics and of possible adverse effects in infants exposed to tricyclic antidepressants in breast-milk. *J Affect Disord* 1997;43:225–37.

72. Mammen O et al. Antidepressants and breast-feeding. *Am J Psychiatr* 1997;154:1174–5. Letter.

73. Taddio A et al. Excretion of fluoxetine and its metabolite, norfluoxetine, in human breast milk. *J Clin Pharmacol* 1996;36:42–7.

74. Baum AL, Misri S. Selective serotonin-reuptake inhibitors in pregnancy and lactation. *Harvard Rev Psychiatr* 1996;4:117–25.

75. Yoshida K et al. Fluoxetine in breast milk and developmental outcome of breast-fed infants. *Br J Psychiatr* 1998;172:175–9.

76. Chambers CD et al. Weight gain in infants breastfed by mothers who take fluoxetine. Presented at the 38th annual Teratology Society meeting, San Diego, June 1998.

77. Jensen PN et al. Citalopram and desmethylcitalopram concentrations in breast milk and serum of mother and infant. *Ther Drug Monit* 1997;19:236–9.

78. Spigset O et al. Excretion of citalopram in breast milk. *Br J Clin Pharmacol* 1997;44:295–8.

79. Yoshida K et al. Fluvoxamine in breast-milk and infant development. *Br J Clin Pharmacol* 1997;44:210–1. Letter.

80. Wisner KL et al. Serum sertraline and *N*-desmethylsertraline levels in breast-feeding mother-infant pairs. *Am J Psychiatr* 1998;155:690–2.

81. Mammen OK et al. Sertraline and norsertraline levels in three breastfed infants. *J Clin Psychiatr* 1997;58:100–3.

82. Kristensen JH et al. Distribution and excretion of sertraline and *N*-desmethylsertraline in human milk. *Br J Clin Pharmacol* 1998;45:453–7.

83. Kent LSW, Laidlaw JDD. Suspected congenital sertraline dependence. *Br J Psychiatr* 1995;167:412–3. Letter.

84. Spigset O, Hägg S. Excretion of psychotropic drugs into human milk. *CNS Drugs* 1998;9:111–34.

85. Ilett KF et al. Distribution and excretion of venlafaxine and *O*-desmethylvenlafaxine in human milk. *Br J Clin Pharmacol* 1998;45:459–62.

86. Pons G et al. Excretion of psychoactive drugs into breast milk. *Clin Pharmacokinet* 1994;27:270–89.

87. Yoshida K et al. Neuroleptic drugs in breast-milk: a study of pharmacokinetics and of possible adverse effects in breast-fed infants. *Psychol Med* 1998;28:81–91.

88. Dev VJ, Krupp P. Adverse event profile and safety of clozapine. *Rev Contemp Pharmacother* 1995;6:197–208.

89. Lee JJ, Rubin AP. Breast feeding and anaesthesia. *Anaesthesia* 1993;48:616:25.

90. Spigset O. Anaesthetic agents and excretion in breast milk. *Acta Anaesthesiol Scand* 1994;38:94–103.

91. Esener Z et al. Thiopentone and etomidate concentrations in maternal and umbilical plasma, and in colostrum. *Br J Anaesthesia* 1992;69:586–8.

92. Oo Cy et al. Pharmacokinetics in lactating women; prediction of alprazolam transfer into milk. *Br J Clin Pharmacol* 1995;40:231–6.

93. Lebedevs TH et al. Excretion of temazepam in breast milk. *Br J Clin Pharmacol* 1992;33:204–6. Letter.

94. Pons G et al. Zolpidem excretion in breast milk. *Eur J Clin Pharmacol* 1989;37:245–8.

95. Marshall JK et al. Omeprazole for refractory gastroesophageal reflux disease during pregnancy and lactation. *Can J Gastroenterol* 1998;12:225–7.

96. Miller LG et al. Disposition of olsalazine and metabolites in breast milk. *J Clin Pharmacol* 1993;33:703–6.

97. Klotz U, Harings-Kaim A. Negligible amounts of 5-aminosalicylic acid in breast milk. *Lancet* 1993;342:618–9. Letter.

98. Rudi J et al. Therapie mit ursodeoxycholsäure bei primär biliärer zirrhose während der schwangerschaft. *Z Gastroenterol* 1996;34:188–91.

99. Guillonneau M et al. L'allaitement est possible en cas de traitement maternel par l'enoxaparine. *Arch Pediatr* 1996;4:513–4.

100. von Kries R et al. Transfer von phenprocoumon in die muttermilch. *Monatsschr Kinderheilkd* 1993;141:505–7.

101. Greenberger PA et al. Pharmacokinetics of prednisolone transfer to breastmilk. *Clin Pharmacol Ther* 1993;53:324–8.

102. DeStefano P et al. Factitious hypertension with mineralocorticoid excess in an infant. *Helv Paediatr Acta* 1983;38:185–9.

103. Pardthaisong T et al. The long-term growth and development of children exposed to Depo-Provera during pregnancy or lactation. *Contraception* 1992;45:313–24.

104. Dunson TR et al. A multicenter clinical trial of a progestin-only oral contraceptive in lactating women. *Contraception* 1993;47:23–35.

105. Progestogen-only contraceptives during lactation: I. Infant growth. World Health Organization Task Force for Epidemiological Research on Reproductive Health; Special Programme of Research, Development and Research Training in Human Reproduction. *Contraception* 1994;50:35–53.

106. Progestogen-only contraceptives during lactation: II. Infant development. World Health Organization Task Force for Epidemiological Research on Reproductive Health; Special Programme of Research, Development and Research Training in Human Reproduction. *Contraception* 1994;50:55–68.

107. Kennedy KI et al. Premature introduction of progestin-only contraceptive methods during lactation. *Contraception* 1997;55:347–50.

108. Hannon PR et al. The influence of medroxyprogesterone on the duration of breast-feeding in mothers in an urban community. *Arch Pediatr Adolesc Med* 1997;151:490–6.

109. Chi I-C et al. The progestin-only oral contraceptive–its place in postpartum contraception. *Adv Contraception* 1992;8:93–103.

110. Diáz S, Croxatto HB. Contraception in lactating women. *Curr Opin Obstet Gynecol* 1993;5:815–22.

111. Aziz F. Effect of methimazole treatment of maternal thyrotoxicosis on thyroid function in breast-feeding infants. *J Pediatr* 1996;128:855–8.

112. Hanew K et al. Simultaneous administration of TRH and sulpiride caused additive but not synergistic PRL responses in normal subjects. *Endocrinol Jpn* 1992;39:465–8.

113. Caplan RH, Wickus GG. Reduced calcitriol requirements for treating hypoparathyroidism during lactation. A case report. *J Reprod Med* 1993;38:914–8.

114. Cathébras P et al. Hypercalcémie induite par la lactation chez deux patientes hypoparathyroïdiennes traitées. *Rev Med Intern* 1996;17:675–6.

115. Gunn AJ et al. Growth hormone increases breast milk volumes in mothers of preterm infants. *Pediatrics* 1996;98:279–82.

116. American Academy of Pediatrics Work Group on Breastfeeding. Breastfeeding and the use of human milk. *Pediatrics* 1997;100:1035–9.

117. Kamilli I, Gresser U. Allopurinol and oxypurinol in human breast milk. *Clin Invest* 1993;71:161–4.

118. Ben-Chetrit E et al. Colchicine in breast milk of patients with familial Mediterranean fever. *Arth Rheum* 1996;39:1213–7.

119. Guillonneau M et al. Colchicine is excreted at high concentrations in human breast milk. *Eur J Obstet Gynecol* 1995;61:177–8.

120. Lucas BD Jr et al. Terfenadine breast milk excretion and pharmacokinetic in lactating women. *Pharmacotherapy* 1992;12:506. Abstract.

121. Aaron DK et al. Reducing milk production in ewes at weaning using restricted feeding and methscopolamine bromide. *J Anim Sci* 1997;75:1434–42.

122. Daniel JA et al. Methscopolamine bromide blocks hypothalamic-stimulated release of growth hormone in ewes. *J Anim Sci* 1997;75:1359–62.

123. Romney BM et al. Radionuclide administration to nursing mothers; mathematically derived guidelines. *Radiology* 1986;160:549–54.

124. Mountford PJ, Coakley AJ. A review of the secretion of radioactivity in human breast milk: data, quantitative analysis and recommendations. *Nucl Med Commun* 1989;10:15–27.

125. Gizurarson S. Optimal delivery of vaccines. Clinical pharmacokinetic considerations. *Clin Pharmacokinet* 1996;30:1–15.

126. da-Silva VA et al. Ethanol pharmacokinetics in lactating women. *Braz J Med Biol Res* 1993;26:1097–103.

127. Mennella JA, Beauchamp GK. The transfer of alcohol in human milk. Effects on flavor and the infant's behavior. *N Engl J Med* 1991;325:981–5.

128. Menella JA, Beauchamp GK. Beer, breastfeeding, and folklore. *Dev Psychobiol* 1993;16:459–66.

129. Anderson PO. Alcohol and breast feeding. *J Human Lact* 1995;11:321–3.

130. Blanchard J et al. Methylxanthine levels in breast milk of lactating women in different ethnic and socioeconomic classes. *Biopharm Drug Dispos* 1992;13:187–96.

131. Oo CY et al. Pharmacokinetics of caffeine and its demethylated metabolites in lactation: predictions of milk to serum concentration ratios. *Pharm Res* 1995;12:313–6.

132. Dickson PH et al. The routine analysis of breast milk for drugs of abuse in a clinical toxicology laboratory. *J Forensic Sci* 1994;39:207–14.

133. Wojnar-Horton RC et al. Methadone distribution and excretion into breast milk of clients in a methadone maintenance programme. *Br J Clin Pharmacol* 1997;44:543–7.

134. Howard CR, Lawrence RA. Breast-feeding and drug exposure. *Obstet Gynecol Clin North Am* 1998;25: 195–217.

135. Stephans MBF, Wilkerson N. Physiologic effects of maternal smoking on breast-feeding infants. *J Acad Nurse Pract* 1993;5:105–13.

136. Mansbach IK et al. Onset and duration of breast feeding among Israeli mothers: relationships with smoking and types of delivery. *Soc Sci Med* 1991;33:1391–7.

137. Hopkinson LM et al. Milk production by mothers of premature infants: influence of cigarette smoking. *Pediatrics* 1992;90:934–8.

138. Jin C, Rossignol AM. Effects of passive smoking on respiratory illness from birth to eighteen months, in Shanghai, People's Republic of China. *J Pediatr* 1993;123:553–8.

139. Klonoff-Cohen HS et al. The effect of passive smoking and tobacco exposure through breast milk on sudden infant death syndrome. *JAMA* 1995;273:795–8.

140. Hakansson A, Cars H. Maternal cigarette smoking; breast-feeding, and respiratory tract infections in infancy; a matched-pairs study. *Scand J Prim Health Care* 1991;9:115–9.

Pediatric Drug Therapy

William E. Murray

Pediatric drug therapy presents a challenge to the practitioner in many respects. The pediatric population is comprised of a range of patient weights and organ maturity. There is often a lack of pediatric-specific data in the literature from which to derive appropriate dosage regimens. At times, medications must be used for which data are extrapolated on the basis of limited pharmacokinetic knowledge about the pediatric population. It must be remembered that children should not be treated as "little adults" when designing dosage regimens. Dosage administration nomograms derived from adult data should not be used in the pediatric population. Pharmacodynamic responses for the majority of medications used in children are even less well known. Children often react much differently from adults to certain medications. Examples are the use of stimulants such as methylphenidate to control hyperactivity common with attention deficit disorders, and paradoxical hyperactivity, which may be observed in children taking phenobarbital. With therapeutically monitored medications, the standard adult therapeutic range is typically used, because age-specific, concentration-effect information is scarce. Because of protein binding differences, infants may respond to lower total drug concentrations than adults for certain medications (eg, phenytoin, theophylline).

One of the problems facing the clinician and caregiver of small children is the administration of medications. Dosage forms are usually designed with the adult population in mind, and the dosage cannot easily be individualized in small patients. This is especially true for most sustained-release products. Most young children cannot swallow tablets and capsules; thus, liquid preparations are generally preferred in this age group. For many drugs, liquid forms are not commercially available and must be extemporaneously compounded. Stability of these preparations is often unknown or of limited duration. Even when appropriate dosage forms suitable for young children are available, palatability, resistance to taking medications, and compliance issues may hinder optimal therapy.

■ PHARMACOKINETICS

ABSORPTION

At birth, gastric pH is neutral but falls to values of 1–3 in the first day of life. Subsequently, gastric pH returns toward neutrality, because gastric acid secretion is low in the first several weeks to months. Adult values are usually achieved after the age of 2 yr.[1,2] Medications that require gastric acidity for absorption may have poor bioavailability in this age group, rendering them ineffective or requiring much higher doses than normal in order for therapeutic serum concentrations to be reached. Examples of medications in this group include phenytoin, ketoconazole, and itraconazole.[1,3] Alternative agents may have to be used if adequate serum levels cannot be documented when these drugs are administered orally. Certain medications that are acid labile may actually have increased bioavailability in infants. These include antibiotics such as penicillin G and ampicillin.[4]

Gastric emptying time can be delayed in infants, especially premature infants.[1,3,5] Peak drug concentrations may occur much later in infancy than in older children and adults. Other factors that may influence overall bioavailability of a particular medication in infants include the relatively high frequencies of gastroesophageal reflux, which may cause the dose to be spit up or vomited, and acute gastroenteritis (diarrhea), which may considerably shorten intestinal transit time. The oral route must be used with caution in these instances, especially in critically ill patients.

Other routes of administration can also pose difficulties in the pediatric population. Overall muscle mass is decreased, and intramuscular administration may not be practical and is certainly not appreciated by most children. Most adults still remember their first injections in the doctor's office when they were children. Also, the dose of drug to be administered may require multiple injections.

Rectal administration may be used in situations where the oral route is not practical or available; however, absorption may be incomplete and/or erratic. Topical administration of medications can lead to undesired systemic absorption, especially in infants in whom the skin thickness is less and the total skin surface area is proportionally greater than in adults.[1,2,4]

DISTRIBUTION

Rapid changes in body composition can dramatically alter the V_d for many medications during the first several months of life. Newborns have a higher percentage of total body water and extracellular fluid than older children and adults.[1,3,6] Hydrophilic drugs such as the aminoglycosides have a much larger V_d in newborns; this gradually decreases over the first year of life to approach adult values.

Total body fat in newborns (especially premature infants) is much lower than in older children and adults.[6] Medications that are lipophilic may have a lower weight-adjusted V_d in the very young.

Protein binding is an important determinant of the V_d for drugs that are bound by albumin and other plasma proteins. In the neonatal period, the binding affinity of albumin is decreased compared with older children and adults (because of the persistence of fetal albumin).[1-3] Highly protein-bound drugs such as phenytoin have a higher free fraction in neonates, and there may be an increased pharmacodynamic response at lower concentrations of total drug. The V_d of these drugs is inversely related to the degree of protein binding.

Additionally, the clinician must be aware of the potential for highly protein-bound substances to displace bilirubin from binding sites on albumin, particularly in the newborn.[1-3,7] The blood-brain barrier in newborns is more permeable than in older patients, and free bilirubin can readily cross into the CNS and cause kernicterus.

Tissue-binding for many medications is unknown, but can vary dramatically from that in adults. One example is digoxin, which binds to erythrocytes in pediatric patients to a much greater extent than in adult patients.[2,4] Digoxin has a much larger V_d in pediatric patients, and recommended loading dose regimens in this age group are much larger on a mg/kg basis than in adult patients. Generally, drug distribution volumes are larger in neonates and gradually approach adult values (in L/kg) by the first year of life.

METABOLISM

Metabolic processes show dramatic changes in the first weeks to months of life. At birth, most hepatic enzymes are immature and drug metabolizing capacity is greatly reduced. Phase I reactions (ie, oxidation) are largely controlled by the mixed-function oxidase system, of which the cytochrome P450 enzymes are the major determinant. These enzymes are largely undeveloped in newborns, especially premature infants, but maturation may take place quickly in the first weeks to months of life. Phase II reactions (ie, conjugation) include glucuronidation, sulfation, and acetylation. These reactions are also immature at birth, and drug toxicity has resulted (eg, with chloramphenicol) because of the absence of knowledge about reduced dosage requirements in newborns.[1-3,6]

The liver size relative to body weight in newborns is much larger than in adults.[1] Rapid weight gain, with subsequent increases in liver size and metabolic capacity, may require many dosage adjustments to prevent newborns from growing out of their dosages for many medications. When full metabolic capacity is reached in the pediatric patient, the hepatic clearance may greatly exceed that observed in adult patients on a weight-adjusted basis. Pediatric dosages of many medications on a mg/kg basis are often much greater than in adults. Figure 3–2 illustrates the change in clearance with age for theophylline.[6] Most medications have similar curves, but may be shifted to the left or have different relative peaks compared with adult values. A decrease in hepatic clearance relative to body weight typically begins after a child weighs approximately 30 kg.[8] Thereafter, the increase in total body weight in proportion to liver size becomes greater. Thus in adolescence, drug dosages typically begin to approach adult values. Drug toxicity can be observed in the adolescent patient if drug dosages on a mg/kg basis (designed for younger patients) are used.

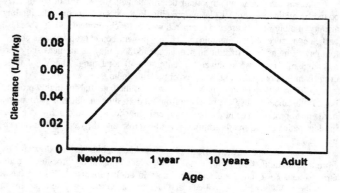

Figure 3–2. Maturation of Theophylline Metabolism.

RENAL ELIMINATION

The kidneys are the major route of drug elimination for many drugs. The kidneys are functionally immature at birth with regard to both glomerular filtration and tubular secretion. Glomerular filtration at birth adjusted for body surface area is only 30–40% of values in older infants and healthy young adults.[1–3] Premature infants often have even lower values during the first few weeks of life. Dosages of many medications (eg, aminoglycosides, vancomycin) that are eliminated largely by glomerular filtration must be decreased on the basis of the relative immaturity of the kidneys at birth. Maturation of glomerular filtration occurs over the first several weeks to months of life. The dosages of most medications are similar to those in older children by 4–6 months of age. Although the frequency of renal disease in children is much lower than in the adult population, factors that may alter renal function, such as shock, nonsteroidal anti-inflammatory drugs, or hypoxia, must by considered when evaluating dosage regimens. Serum creatinine, the usual marker for renal function, is usually lower in young children compared with adults. This is because of children's lower muscle mass. Thus, a serum creatinine that indicates normal renal function in an adult may indicate renal impairment in a young child.

Tubular secretion is also diminished in the newborn. Drugs that have a component of tubular secretion (eg, penicillin) are typically administered at reduced dosages in the newborn. Maturation of tubular secretion occurs somewhat more slowly than glomerular filtration, but approaches adult values by 8–12 months of age.[1–3]

EVALUATING DRUG DATA IN CHILDREN

With the numerous maturational changes observed in children from birth through adolescence, results of pediatric drug studies must be used with caution in children whose age differs from that in the study. Dosages extrapolated only on a weight basis have the potential to underdose or overdose other age groups, depending on the population studied. Body surface area may correlate better with total body water and extracellular water than body weight, and may be useful in certain instances in calculating dosage regimens. With the exception of cancer chemotherapeutic agents, information on drug dosage is more widely available in mg/kg than by body surface area.[5] Medications with narrow therapeutic ranges should have serum concentrations measured to aid in individualizing drug therapy, especially in critically ill children or those with known decreased renal or hepatic function.

Pharmacodynamic changes are poorly studied in the pediatric population, and responses to specific drug concentrations may be much different than in the adult population. Diseases of childhood often differ from those in adults. Medications that may be tolerated by adult patients may be inappropriate for the pediatric population (eg, aspirin for fever).

Caution must be used in the interpretation of drug levels, because there may be much greater fluctuation in serum concentrations because of shorter drug half-lives in children than in adults. Additionally, the total volume of blood needed for drug level monitoring in small children may limit serum level monitoring.

Detailed information on specific drugs can be found in the Pediatric Dosage sections of the individual drug monographs.

■ REFERENCES

1. Stewart CF, Hampton EM. Effect of maturation on drug disposition in pediatric patients. *Clin Pharm* 1987;6:548–64.
2. Besunder JB et al. Principles of drug biodisposition in the neonate. A critical evaluation of the pharmacokinetic-pharmacodynamic interface (part I). *Clin Pharmacokinet* 1988;14:189–216.
3. Milsap RL et al. Special pharmacokinetic considerations in children. In, Evans WE et al, eds. *Applied pharmacokinetics. Principles of therapeutic drug monitoring,* 3rd ed. Vancouver, WA: Applied Therapeutics; 1992: 10-1–32.
4. Morselli PL et al. Clinical pharmacokinetics in newborns and infants. Age-related differences and therapeutic implications. In, Gibaldi M, Prescott LF, eds. *Handbook of clinical pharmacokinetics,* Section II. Balgowlah, NSW, Australia: ADIS Health Science Press; 1983:98–141.
5. Maxwell GM. Paediatric drug dosing. Bodyweight versus surface area. *Drugs* 1989;37:113–5.
6. McLeod HL, Evans WE. Pediatric pharmacokinetics and therapeutic drug monitoring. *Pediatr Rev* 1992;13:413–21.
7. Morselli PL. Clinical pharmacokinetics in neonates. In, Gibaldi M, Prescott LF, eds. *Handbook of clinical pharmacokinetics,* Section II. Balgowlah, NSW, Australia: ADIS Health Science Press; 1983:79–97.
8. Rane A, Wilson JT. Clinical pharmacokinetics in infants and children. In, Gibaldi M, Prescott LF, eds. *Handbook of clinical pharmacokinetics,* Section II. Balgowlah, NSW, Australia: ADIS Health Science Press; 1983:142–68.

Geriatric Drug Therapy

Dianne E. Tobias

Geriatric drug therapy is an important area of therapeutics and research, because of the growing elderly population, their disproportionately high use of medications, and their increased risk of drug misadventures. Although they represent approximately 12% of the U.S. population, the elderly consume more than 30% of all medications.[1] Trends include increasing numbers of the extreme elderly (over age 80) and elderly with functional disabilities. It is estimated that the number of elderly who are dependent in their activities of daily living will triple from 1985 to 2060. Ethical considerations, such as a patient's right to exercise decisions regarding treatment, are particularly relevant to the elderly population.[2,3] As the number of elderly increases and health care resources diminish, cost–benefit considerations will become increasingly important.[4]

The elderly are the most physiologically heterogeneous category of the adult population. The rate of normal aging varies considerably, and comparing data from persons of chronologically similar age can be misleading; health status is probably as important as age. Optimization of drug therapy in the elderly requires an understanding of how aging and concomitant pathology affect the pharmacokinetics and pharmacodynamics of drugs, the need to assess elderly patients individually, and elderly patients' expectations of therapy.[5]

Compliance issues leading to misuse and medication errors can be important in the elderly.[6] The cost of medications, physical difficulty in opening medication containers, swallowing large tablets, reading the prescription label, and the presence of depression or cognitive impairment can contribute to compliance problems.[7–9]

Adverse drug reactions are more common in the elderly,[10–13] although the correlation with age alone is debatable.[1,14] Increased medication use, especially medications with greater potential for toxicity, and chronic pathology with intermittent acute exacerbations are thought to contribute to the higher frequency and severity of adverse drug reactions. Most reactions in the elderly are dose related rather than idiosyncratic as a result of changes in pharmacokinetics and/or pharmacodynamics. Given the wide physiologic variability in the elderly population, the contribution of pharmacokinetic and pharmacodynamic changes can vary considerably. Additionally, the elderly are more sensitive to specific adverse reactions. For example, they have an increased sensitivity to anticholinergic side effects, especially central effects such as disorientation and memory impairment. These effects can be additive because many drugs commonly taken by the elderly are centrally active.[15–17] Varying degrees of cognitive impairment or even delirium can be induced by drugs in several classes including benzodiazepines, centrally acting antihypertensive agents, and antidepressants.[15,18] The onset can be insidious and mistakenly attributed solely to the aging process.

■ PHARMACOKINETICS

ABSORPTION

With aging there is some decrease in gastric secretions, acidity, gastric emptying, peristalsis, absorptive surface area, and splanchnic blood flow,[9,19] although the effect on gastric pH may not be as pronounced as once believed.[20,21] Taken together, the changes predict an altered extent or rate of absorption of orally administered drugs, yet most formal studies show no difference in oral bioavailability. Some factors might counterbalance each other (eg, acidity and gastric emptying; decreased absorptive surface and longer transit time). Some drugs (eg, digoxin) have shown a clinically unimportant slowed rate of absorption with equivalent quantities absorbed. Drugs with high extraction ratios may have increased bioavailability in the elderly compared with young patients, because of a decreased first-pass effect secondary to reduced hepatic blood flow. Decreased first-pass metabolism in the elderly has been shown for labetalol, propranolol, lidocaine, and verapamil.[22] It is known that the elderly have drier skin with lower lipid content, which is expected to be less permeable to hydrophilic compounds. Although neither conclusively nor well studied, percutaneous drug absorption appears to decrease with age.[23]

DISTRIBUTION

Body weight generally decreases, but more important, body composition changes with age. Total body water and lean body mass decrease, while body fat increases in proportion to total body weight. The percentage of body weight contributed by fat changes from 18% and 33% in young men and women, respectively, to 36% and 45% in their elderly counterparts.[24] These factors can alter the apparent volume of distribution (V_d) of drugs in the elderly, although other aspects of drug disposition (binding, metabolism, elimination) can be additive or negate the effect. The V_d changes are most marked for highly lipophilic and hydrophilic drugs, and elderly patients are particularly susceptible to overdosage from drugs that should be dosed on ideal body weight or lean body weight.[25] Theoretically, highly lipid-soluble drugs (eg, long-acting benzodiazepines, lidocaine) may have an increased V_d and a prolonged effect if drug clearance remains constant. Conversely, water-soluble drugs (eg, gentamicin) may have a decreased V_d, and at least transiently increased serum levels, leading to possible toxicity if initial doses are not conservative.[9] Although cardiac output does not appear to decrease with age,[26] some chronic diseases affecting the elderly do contribute to a decrease in cardiac output and regional blood flow. There is some evidence that blood is preferentially shunted away from the liver and kidneys to the brain, heart, and muscles.[15,27] These changes could explain the slowed elimination of some drugs and the heightened sensitivity to others.

PROTEIN BINDING

The proportion of albumin among total plasma proteins decreases with frailty, catabolic disease states, and immobility seen in many elderly,[28] but it is no longer believed that serum albumin decreases with age alone.[23] Serum albumin determinations should be performed to aid monitoring and dosage adjustment of drugs that are highly protein bound in the chronically immobile or ill elderly. A decrease in serum albumin can increase the percentage of free drug available for pharmacologic effect and elimination. Changes in albumin binding are more important with highly bound (greater than 90%) acidic drugs such as salicylates, phenytoin, and warfarin.[9] Conversely, basic drugs, including lidocaine, propranolol, and meperidine, have affinity for α_1-acid-glycoprotein, which may increase with age, especially when associated with conditions such as inflammatory diseases and malignancies.[9] Protein binding theoretically may be increased and result in less free drug available, although the clinical relevance of this is unclear.[23] With both types of binding, the net effect on clearance varies, depending on metabolism and elimination. Although not always available, free drug concentration measurements are often desirable in the elderly. There is also some evidence that the elderly may have a greater potential for protein displacement drug interactions.[29,30]

METABOLISM

Liver size and hepatic blood flow decrease with age and especially with disease. Studies show hepatic blood flow decreases by 35%, and liver volume by 44% and 28% in elderly women and men, respectively, when compared to younger counterparts.[13] Such a decrease in hepatic blood flow can limit the first-pass effect of drugs with high extraction ratios and markedly reduce their systemic clearance. Studies on phase I drug metabolism (ie, oxidation) do not consistently show a correlation with age,[23] although most show that the elderly, especially men, have prolonged elimination. Differences may be explained by environmental factors such as smoking habits and genetics. Phase II metabolism (ie, conjugation) does not appear to be influenced as much by age, although there has been less study in this area.[9,13,23] The effect of aging on drug acetylation is inconsistent and the importance unclear.[9,23] There does not appear to be any age difference in the degree of inhibition or induction of cytochrome P450 isozymes.[13,31] Monitoring and management of interactions with drugs such as cimetidine should be handled in the same manner as in younger patients. The changes described in liver size and metabolic function help to explain why certain drugs may have prolonged elimination; however, the variability of data cautions against generalizing about the effect of age alone. The initial dosage of metabolized drugs should be conservative and subsequent dosage adjustments based on careful monitoring of therapeutic and toxic parameters.

RENAL ELIMINATION

The effect of aging on the renal elimination of drugs is probably the most completely understood and important aspect affecting geriatric drug therapy. Glomerular filtration, tubular secretion, and renal blood flow all decrease with age. Creatinine clearance (Cl_{cr}) decreases approximately 1% per year after age 40;[32] the effect is variable, and volume depletion, congestive heart failure, and renal disease can further decrease organ function. Because creatinine production also decreases with age, serum creatinine may be normal despite a substantial decrease in renal function. It is therefore recommended that Cl_{cr} be measured or estimated using a method that incorporates age and weight.[33,34] The dosage of renally excreted drugs with low therapeutic indices should be conservative initially, with subsequent dosage titrated by close clinical and serum drug level monitoring, if applicable.

■ PHARMACODYNAMICS

Heightened drug effects that cannot be explained by altered pharmacokinetic variables alone have been hypothesized to be caused by changes in compensatory homeostasis, drug receptor sensitivity, or complications of chronic diseases that occur in the elderly. There is a gradual decrease in homeostatic reserve with aging. Postural control and orthostatic circulatory response are examples of compensatory mechanisms that are slowed in aging. Adequate postural blood pressure control relies on several factors, including central coordination, muscle tone, and proprioception, all of which can be blunted in the elderly.[15] As a result, side effects that are minimal or absent in a young patient with normal compensatory response can be marked in the elderly. The administration of long-acting anxiolytics, hypnotics, or antipsychotics can further alter these mechanisms and lead to an increased risk of falls in the elderly.[9,35] Similarly, symptomatic postural hypotension can result from the administration of a variety of antihypertensive agents (especially calcium-channel blockers and ACE inhibitors) and other drugs (eg, antipsychotics, antidepressants) that affect vasomotor tone. Physiologic mechanisms such as vasoconstriction and tachycardia cannot fully compensate for postural hypotension in the elderly.[15] Temperature regulation and intestinal motility are other homeostatic mechanisms that change with aging and can explain heightened effects of certain drugs.

The number and characteristics of drug receptors can change with aging and produce altered, often heightened, drug response. Research has shown age-related decreases in several autonomic receptors. There is some evidence of increased sensitivity to oral anticoagulants and digoxin, apart from the alterations in pharmacokinetics, which might contribute to the higher frequency of adverse reactions to these two agents in the elderly.[15]

Preliminary data indicate a possible increase in brain sensitivity to certain drugs with aging. It is unknown whether this effect is caused by changes in blood-brain permeability or tissue receptor sensitivity.[9] More research into drug pharmacodynamics in the elderly is needed, especially the interrelationship with pharmacokinetic alterations. The presence and impact of multiple concurrent pathologies and their treatments cannot be overemphasized in their contribution to the various drug effects seen in the elderly.

■ OTHER FACTORS

Cigarette smoking can cause clinically important induction of the metabolism of some drugs to a similar degree in both the elderly and the young.[23,36] This, and the fact that many published studies do not indicate smoking history, could explain some interpatient variability of pharmacokinetic data.

Nutritional intake is sometimes diminished in the elderly and can lead to nutritional and vitamin deficiencies. Nutritional status of the elderly can impact the outcome of drug therapy, and, conversely, drug therapy can affect nutritional status.[19,36,37]

■ EVALUATING DRUG DATA FOR THE ELDERLY

Because of age-related changes that may impact the outcome of drug therapy as outlined in this chapter, the results of drug studies using young subjects cannot always be extrapolated accurately to the elderly. Studies on diseases and drugs in the elderly do not always include sufficient numbers of elderly, especially extremely aged subjects, to draw appropriate conclusions.[38] Studies that include the elderly do not always separate results by decade of age and health status, two criteria that are helpful in assessing applicability of data in this heterogeneous population. Many studies also do not mention data on nutrition, alcohol, and smoking, which might explain some variability of results.[19] Although single-dose studies in healthy volunteers can be useful, long-term studies in afflicted elderly patients often yield data more applicable to therapeutics. Drugs are often not studied over a wide dosage range, so a minimal effective dosage in the elderly cannot be determined.[39]

When reviewing studies that include the elderly, one should consider the following potential problems: numbers of subjects must be sufficient to allow for high attrition rates and the typically wide variation in this population; study lengths must be sufficient for a chronic disease; concomitant diseases and medications must be acknowledged and their impact assessed; and "normal" values can be different from those of a younger population.[40–42]

■ CONCLUSION

The effects of aging as related to drug therapy illustrate the challenges in caring for the elderly. Clinical practice guidelines that have been developed for conditions commonly afflicting the elderly, such as those published by the Agency for Health Care Policy and Research, can be a helpful guide.[43] Conservative dosage, especially initially, with close clinical monitoring for dose-dependent effects is critical and should be emphasized by all health care practitioners caring for the elderly. For detailed information on specific drugs in the elderly, refer to the Geriatric Dosage section of the individual drug monographs.

■ REFERENCES

1. Gerety MB et al. Adverse events related to drugs and drug withdrawal in nursing home residents. *J Am Geriatr Soc* 1993;41:1326–32.
2. Faden R, German PS. Quality of life. Considerations in geriatrics. *Clin Geriatr Med* 1994;10:541–55.
3. Goldstein MK. Ethical considerations in pharmacotherapy of the aged. *Drugs Aging* 1991;1:91–7.
4. Livesley B. Cost-benefit considerations in the treatment of elderly people. *Drugs Aging* 1991;1:249–53.
5. Tobias DE. Ensuring and documenting the quality of drug therapy in the elderly. *Generations* 1994;18:40–2.
6. Burns JMA et al. Elderly patients and their medication: a post-discharge follow-up study. *Age Aging* 1992;21: 178–81.

7. Honig PK, Cantilena LR. Polypharmacy. Pharmacokinetic perspectives. *Clin Pharmacokinet* 1994;26:85–90.
8. Botelho RJ, Dudrak R. Home assessment of adherence to long-term medication in the elderly. *J Fam Pract* 1992;35:61–5.
9. Tregaskis BF, Stevenson IH. Pharmacokinetics in old age. *Br Med Bull* 1990;46:9–21.
10. Denham MJ. Adverse drug reactions. *Br Med Bull* 1990;46:53–62.
11. Beard K. Adverse reactions as a cause of hospital admission in the aged. *Drugs Aging* 1992;2:356–67.
12. Owens NJ et al. Distinguishing between the fit and frail elderly, and optimising pharmacotherapy. *Drugs Aging* 1994;4:47–55.
13. Woodhouse KW, James OFW. Hepatic drug metabolism and ageing. *Br Med Bull* 1990;46:22–35.
14. Walker J, Wynne H. Review: the frequency and severity of adverse drug reactions in elderly people. *Age Ageing* 1994;23:255–9.
15. Hämmerlein A et al. Pharmacokinetic and pharmacodynamic changes in the elderly. Clinical implications. *Clin Pharmacokinet* 1998;35:49–64.
16. Feinberg M. The problems of anticholinergic adverse effects in older patients. *Drugs Aging* 1993;3:335–48.
17. Nolan L, O'Malley K. Adverse effects of antidepressants in the elderly. *Drugs Aging* 1992;2:450–8.
18. Bowen JD, Larson EB. Drug-induced cognitive impairment. Defining the problem and finding solutions. *Drugs Aging* 1993;3:349–57.
19. Iber FL et al. Age-related changes in the gastrointestinal system. Effects on drug therapy. *Drugs Aging* 1994;5:34–48.
20. Gainsborough N et al. The association of age with gastric emptying. *Age Aging* 1993;22:37–40.
21. Russell TL et al. Upper gastrointestinal pH in seventy-nine healthy, elderly, North American men and women. *Pharm Res* 1993;10:187–96.
22. Durnas C et al. Hepatic drug metabolism and aging. *Clin Pharmacokinet* 1990;19:359–89.
23. Roskos KV, Maibach HI. Percutaneous absorption and age. Implications for therapy. *Drugs Aging* 1992;2:432–49.
24. Novak LP. Aging, total body potassium, fat-free mass, and cell mass in males and females between ages 18 and 85 years. *J Gerontol* 1972;27:438–43.
25. Morgan DJ, Bray KM. Lean body mass as a predictor of drug dosage. Implications for drug therapy. *Clin Pharmacokinet* 1994;26:292–307.
26. Rodeheffer RJ et al. Exercise cardiac output is maintained with advancing age in healthy human subjects: cardiac dilatation and increased stroke volume compensate for a diminished heart rate. *Circulation* 1984; 69:208–13.
27. Schumacher GE. Using pharmacokinetics in drug therapy. VII: pharmacokinetic factors influencing drug therapy in the aged. *Am J Hosp Pharm* 1980;37:559–62.
28. Woo J et al. Effect of age and disease on two drug binding proteins: albumin and α-1-acid glycoprotein. *Clin Biochem* 1994;27:289–92.
29. Wallace S et al. Factors affecting drug binding in plasma of elderly patients. *Br J Clin Pharmacol* 1976;3:327–30.
30. Ritschel WA. Drug disposition in the elderly: gerontokinetics. *Methods Find Exp Clin Pharmacol* 1992;14:555–72.
31. Vestal RE et al. Aging and the response to inhibition and induction of theophylline metabolism. *Exp Gerontol* 1993;28:421–33.
32. Lindeman RD. Changes in renal function with aging. Implications for treatment. *Drugs Aging* 1992;2:423–31.
33. Siersbaek-Nielsen K et al. Rapid evaluation of creatinine clearance. *Lancet* 1971;1:1133–4.
34. Cockcroft DW, Gault MH. Prediction of creatinine clearance from serum creatinine. *Nephron* 1976;16:31–41.
35. Campbell AJ. Drug treatment as a cause of falls in old age. A review of the offending agents. *Drugs Aging* 1991;1:289–302.
36. O'Mahony MS, Woodhouse KW. Age, environmental factors and drug metabolism. *Pharmacol Ther* 1994;61:279–87.
37. Roe DA. Medications and nutrition in the elderly. *Prim Care* 1994;21:135–47.
38. Gurwitz JH et al. The exclusion of the elderly and women from clinical trials in acute myocardial infarction. *JAMA* 1992;268:1417–22.
39. Kitler ME. Clinical trials and clinical practice in the elderly. A focus on hypertension. *Drugs Aging* 1992;2:86–94.
40. Zimmer AW et al. Conducting clinical research in geriatric populations. *Ann Intern Med* 1985;103:276–83.
41. Butler RN. The importance of basic research in gerontology. *Age Aging* 1993;22:S53–4.
42. Fraser CG. Age-related changes in laboratory test results. Clinical implications. *Drugs Aging* 1993;3:246–57.
43. Agency for Health Care Policy and Research. Guidelines for pressure ulcer prevention: improving practice and a stimulus for research. *J Gerontol* 1993;48:M3–5.

Genetic and Ethnic Considerations in Pharmacotherapy

Ernest J. Dole

There are well-documented differences in the metabolism of some medications in different populations.[1–6] This field of study is called pharmacogenetics, and includes approximately 100 diverse, monogenically transmitted conditions. Included in this group are polymorphisms of cytochrome P450 enzymes, N-acetyltransferase, G-6-PD, and thiopurine methyltransferase.[2] Although less well studied, there also appears to be some differences in the pharmacodynamic response of some populations to some drugs.

Pharmacogenomics is a term used for the application of pharmacogenetics prospectively to individual patients or groups of patients. Genetic testing of patients before treatment would identify patients who are likely either to be responders or to have adverse outcomes with a particular therapy. Drug therapy would then be given only to those who will respond favorably. This is a new and rapidly evolving area and will not be covered specifically in this chapter.

■ METABOLIC DIFFERENCES

CYTOCHROME P450 ENZYMES

The human cytochrome P450 enzyme CYP2C19 catalyzes the oxidation of numerous medications including mephenytoin, imipramine, and benzodiazepines. This enzyme is under monogenic control. The poor metabolizer (PM) phenotype for mephenytoin and related medications is inherited as an autosomal recessive trait.[1] The phenotype for PM of mephenytoin is present in 2–5% of non-Hispanic whites (NHWs) and 18–23% of Japanese. Additionally, 5–17% of those of Chinese descent fall into this category, whereas there are no PMs among Panamanian Indians.[2,3,5,6] Patients with the PM phenotype may require decreased dosages of the medications that are metabolized by CYP2C19.[2,7] (*See* Cytochrome P450 Enzyme Interactions.)

The human cytochrome P450 enzyme CYP2D6 also catalyzes the oxidation of numerous medications, including debrisoquin and many psychotropic agents.[1–3,5] The enzyme is also under monogenic control, and its phenotypic expression is polymorphic in most populations. CYP2D6 exhibits bimodal distribution with people classified as either PMs or as fast metabolizers (FMs). The FM phenotype for debrisoquin and related drugs occurs in about 93% of NHWs.[2,3,5] The proportion of CYP2D6 FM is higher, approximately 98%, in African-American populations than in NHWs or Hispanics. PMs may exhibit markedly higher serum concentrations of tricyclic antidepressants, SSRIs, and antipsychotics when given in comparable doses.[1,2,6,7] (*See* Cytochrome P450 Enzyme Interactions.)

N-ACETYLTRANSFERASE

N-acetyltransferase (NAT) is a hepatic enzyme responsible for the acetylation of a number of medications, including clonazepam, hydralazine, isoniazid, and phenelzine.[1,2] PM status is an autosomal recessive trait. Ethnic variation in PM status is important because (1) slow acetylators are at a higher risk for developing drug-induced SLE such as that seen with isoniazid and hydralazine; (2) slow acetylators may be more likely to have a good response than fast acetylators to phenelzine, hydralazine, and isoniazid at similar doses; and (3) slow acetylators are thought by some to be at increased risk of developing isoniazid hepatitis.[1,2,6]

Of NHWs, 52–58% are slow acetylators, compared with 7–12% of Japanese.[2] The most exhaustive study of differences in NAT activity found African-Americans to have greater NAT activity than NHWs.[8]

ACETALDEHYDE DEHYDROGENASE

There are variations in the ethnic distribution of acetaldehyde dehydrogenase (ALDH). NHWs show no ALDH deficiency while American Indians show marked dissimilarity. ALDH deficiency may result in a disulfiram-like reaction when alcohol is consumed. This disulfiram-like reaction has been documented in American Indian populations.[3,6]

GLUCOSE-6-PHOSPHATE DEHYDROGENASE

G-6-PD exists as at least 80 variant forms. The enzyme maintains the integrity of RBCs, especially in the presence of oxidant medications (eg, sulfonamides, nitrofurans, and primaquine). Persons of Middle Eastern descent, Romanians, Sardinians, southern Chinese, and Thais all have a prevalence of G-6-PD deficiency of greater than 1%.[2] The prevalence of G-6-PD in African-American males is 13%. A striking example of the effects of G-6-PD deficiency occurred during World War II. American soldiers fighting in the Pacific theater were routinely administered primaquine for the prevention of malaria. Subsequently, many soldiers of African-American descent suffered from hemolysis.[6] Patients at risk for G-6-PD deficiency should be given oxidant medications with caution. (*See* Drug-Induced Blood Dyscrasias.)

THIOPURINE METHYLTRANSFERASE

Thiopurine methyltransferase (TPMT) is integral to the metabolism of at least three medications: mercaptopurine, azathioprine, and thioguanine.[1,2,4] The prevalence of TPMT with maximum activity is approximately 90% for African-Americans and NHWs, with the remainder having intermediate activity.[2,9] Patients with intermediate activity of TPMT accumulate about 50% more thioguanine metabolites than do patients with maximum TPMT activity.[9] Patients with TPMT deficiency may need to have their mercaptopurine dosage reduced to 6-10% of normal to avoid toxicity.[4,9]

α_1-ACID GLYCOPROTEIN

In addition to enzymes, drug-binding proteins may vary by ethnicity. Ethnic differences in plasma protein binding of medications appear to be common.[3,5] α_1-acid glycoprotein (AGP) is found in blood and avidly binds basic compounds. Medications that bind to this protein include carbamazepine, imipramine, fluphenazine, thiothixene, and triazolam. AGP variation is genetically controlled, resulting in the increased binding of, and decreased free fraction of, amitriptyline, methadone, and nortriptyline to a slow-variant (S-variant) of AGP.[3] The decreased free fraction of these medications may result in a change in the clinical response to the medications.

Interethnic variation has been demonstrated in the absolute level of AGP as well as the two variants slow (S) and fast (F). African-Americans and NHWs demonstrate a range of 34–67% of the S-variant, while American Indians have a slightly narrower observed prevalence of the S-variant, 43–45%. These differences may influence the response to tricyclic antidepressants, antipsychotics, and benzodiazepines.[3] NHWs have higher binding to AGP than do other ethnic groups, apparently the result of higher plasma AGP concentrations.[5]

■ PHARMACODYNAMIC DIFFERENCES

HYPERTENSION

African-Americans have increased blood pressures, a higher prevalence of hypertension, and higher risk of cardiovascular disease than do NHWs. Evidence exists that African-Americans may, at equivalent blood pressures, suffer greater harm than NHWs and that their response to therapy may be less.[1,10–12] It has been proposed that the prevalence of hypertension in African-Americans may be caused by a genetic sensitivity to the blood-pressure effects of salt.[1] The Veterans Administration Cooperative Study Group on Antihypertensive Agents demonstrated that fewer African-American than NHW patients reached their goal blood pressure while receiving β-adrenergic blockers. These findings, coupled with the understanding that hypertension in African-Americans is typified by low plasma renin levels, persuaded many clinicians to avoid β-blockers in African-American patients.[13] African-Americans clear propranolol more quickly than NHWs.[1,6] African-American patients respond better to calcium-channel blockers (CCBs) than to β-blockers.[1] The 1997 Joint National Committee on Prevention, Detection, Evaluation, and Treatment of High Blood Pressure recommendations state that diuretics and CCBs may be better choices than angiotensin converting enzyme inhibitors (ACEIs) or β-blockers for antihypertensive therapy in African-Americans.[11–14] However, in African-American patients with diabetes mellitus, ACEIs, angiotensin II–receptor antagonists, or CCBs may be the agents of choice for the treatment of hypertension.[15] However, β-blocker therapy should not be withheld from African-American patients when there is a clear indication for such therapy such as in migraine, hyperthyroidism, arrhythmia control, and after myocardial infarction.[16] Additionally, many of the ethnic differences in response to β-blockers disappear with the addition of a diuretic.[12–16]

STROKE

Stroke is a major cause of mortality among African-Americans, possibly because of the high prevalence of cigarette use and hypertension.[1] African-Americans had greater than twice the risk of subarachnoid hemorrhages of NHWs and 1.4 times the risk of intracerebral hemorrhage in one study.[17] In patients under 75 years of age, the risk of intracerebral hemorrhage among African-Americans was 2.3 times that of NHWs. Thirty-day mortality following subarachnoid hemorrhage was similar in both groups. The potential life lost because of intracerebral bleeding was 1.9 years/1000 African-Americans under 65 years old, compared with 0.5 year/1000 NHWs of the same age.

PSYCHOTROPIC MEDICATIONS

A retrospective chart review evaluated 41 Hispanic females and 21 NHW females with appropriately diagnosed depression.[18] All patients were receiving tricyclic antidepressants. Hispanic females received half the dosage of medication, yet reported similar treatment outcomes when compared to NHWs. However, despite the lower dosages, Hispanic patients reported adverse drug events much more frequently, 78% for the Hispanic group versus 33% for the NHW group. Additionally, over three times as many Hispanic patients discontinued their medication because of adverse drug events than did NHW patients. The authors postulated that the typical adverse drug event profile of tricyclic antidepressants often mimicked the somatic symptoms of the depression. Therefore, the Hispanic patients may have decreased their medication dosage or discontinued the medication because they perceived the adverse effects of the drugs as a worsening of their conditions.

One study evaluated the pharmacotherapeutic regimens and mental health diagnoses of Hispanic, NHW, and African-American patients.[19] Approximately 1800 charts were retrospectively reviewed from patients in five public community mental health clinics. African-American patients in this population were more often diagnosed with schizophrenia (67%) than were the NHW patients (49%) or the Hispanic patients (42%). However, Hispanic patients were more likely to be diagnosed with other mental illness. With regard to prescribed medications, Hispanics were prescribed medication less often than the other two groups. Seventy-seven percent of Hispanics were taking medications, compared with greater than 88% of NHW and 94% of African-American patients. However, when medications were prescribed, there were no differences in the number of medications or the dosages of prescribed neuroleptics.

■ MEDICATION COMPLIANCE

Noncompliance with medication regimens is a major barrier to the treatment of illness, especially chronic disease states. Barriers to communication have been cited as a primary reason of medication noncompliance.

Hispanics and Asian populations have been documented to expect rapid relief from symptoms. Additionally, these patients have been documented to have increased concerns about detrimental adverse drug events from "powerful" Western medicines.[19] These beliefs may interfere with the acceptance and use of medications with a delayed onset of action such as antidepressants. Patients who are not from the primary culture may not be familiar with the practice of taking long-term medication for the treatment of chronic illness, or are not willing to tolerate adverse reactions as the price for poorly understood benefits of treatment.[20,21]

FACTOR	DRUGS[a,b]	CLINICAL EFFECTS	FREQUENCY	TRANSMISSION
CYP2C19	a	Increased toxicity with PM[c]	PM: 2–5% NHWs, 5% Hispanics, 5–17% Chinese, 18% African-Americans, 18–30% Japanese	Autosomal recessive
CYP2D6	a	Increased toxicity with PM	PM: <1% Asian descent, 2% African-Americans, 5% American Indians, 5–8% NHWs	Autosomal recessive
N-acetyltransferase (NAT)	Amrinone, caffeine, clonazepam, dapsone, hydralazine, isoniazid, phenelzine, procainamide, sulfasalazine	Increased toxicity with PM	PM: 52–58% NHWs, 56% Spanish, 45% African-American, 22% Chinese, 20% American Indians, 7–12% Japanese, 5–59% Alaskan Natives	Autosomal recessive
Acetaldehyde dehydrogenase (ALDH) deficiency	Ethanol	Increased ethanol toxicity	44% Japanese, 43–45% American Indians, 25–45% Chinese	—
G-6-PD deficiency	b	Hemolytic anemia	13% African-American males, ≥1% African-American females, ≥1% of persons of Middle Eastern descent, Romanians, Sardinians, southern Chinese, Thais	X-linked incomplete codominant

(continued)

909

GENETIC AND ETHNIC FACTORS AFFECTING DRUG THERAPY (continued)

FACTOR	DRUGS[a,b]	CLINICAL EFFECTS	FREQUENCY	TRANSMISSION
Thiopurine methyl-transferase	Azathioprine, mercaptopurine, thioguanine	Increased toxicity of mercaptopurine, azathioprine, and thioguanine	PM: 10% African-Americans	
α_1-acid glycoprotein S-Var[d]	Amitriptyline, methadone, nortriptyline, propranolol	Increased protein binding and lower plasma free fractions of basic medications	34–67% African-Americans and NHWs, 43–45% American Indians	

[a]For lists of drugs metabolized by CYP2C19 and CYP2D6 *see* Cytochrome P450 Enzyme Interactions, page 823.
[b]For drugs *see* Drug-Induced Blood Dyscrasias, page 763.
[c]PM = poor metabolizer.
[d]S-Var = slow variant status.
From references 1–3, 5, 6, and 9.

■ REFERENCES

1. Gibaldi M. Ethic differences in the assessment and treatment of disease. *Pharmacotherapy* 1993;13:170–6.
2. West WL et al. Interpatient variability: genetic predisposition and other genetic factors. *J Clin Pharmacol* 1997;37:635–48.
3. Mendoza R et al. Ethnic psychopharmacology: the Hispanic and Native American perspective. *Psychopharmacol Bull* 1991;27:449–61.
4. Vesell ES. Therapeutic lessons from pharmacogenetics. *Ann Intern Med* 1997;126:653–5. Commentary.
5. Johnson JA. Influence of race or ethnicity on pharmacokinetics of drugs. *J Pharm Sci* 1997;86:1328–33.
6. Lin KM et al. Psychopharmacology, ethnicity and culture. *Transcultural Psychiatr Res Rev* 1995;32:3–40.
7. DeVane LC. Pharmacogenetics and drug metabolism of newer antidepressant agents. *J Clin Psychiatry* 1994;55(12 suppl):38–45.
8. Relling MV et al. Racial and gender differences in N-acetyltransferase, xanthine oxidase, and CYP1A2 activities. *Clin Pharmacol Ther* 1992;52:643–58.
9. Yates CR et al. Molecular diagnosis of thiopurine S-methyltransferase deficiency: genetic basis for azathioprine and mercaptopurine intolerance. *Ann Intern Med* 1997;126:608–14.
10. Jandt FE. *Intercultural communication: an introduction.* Thousand Oaks, CA: Sage Publications; 1995.
11. Moser M. Black-white differences in response to antihypertensive medication. *J Natl Med Assoc* 1985; 87(suppl):612–3.
12. The Sixth Report of the Joint National Committee on Prevention, Detection, Evaluation, and Treatment of High Blood Pressure. *Arch Intern Med* 1997;157:2413–44.
13. Veterans Administration Cooperative Study Group on Antihypertensive Agents. Comparison of propanolol and hydrochlorothiazide for the initial treatment of hypertension I. Results of short-term titration with emphasis of racial differences in responses. *JAMA* 1982;248:1996–2003.
14. Materson BJ. Lessons on the interaction of race and antihypertensive drug therapy from the VA Cooperative Study Group. *Am J Hypertens* 1995;8(12 part 2):91S–93S.
15. Powers DR, Wallin JD. End-stage renal disease in specific ethnic and racial groups. Risk factors and benefits of antihypertensive therapy. *Arch Int Med* 1998;158:793–800.
16. Prisant LM. Use of β-adrenergic receptor blockers in blacks. *J Clin Pharmacol* 1996;36:967–73.
17. Otten MW et al. The effect of known risk factors on the excess mortality of black adults in the United States. *JAMA* 1990;263:845–50.
18. Marcos LR et al. Pharmacotherapy of Hispanic depressed patients: clinical observations. *Am J Psychother* 1982;36:505–12.
19. Adams GL et al. Diagnosis and pharmacotherapy issues in the care of Hispanics in the public sector. *Am J Psychiatry* 1984;141:970–4.
20. Levy RA, Hawks JW. Multicultural medicine and pharmacy management II. Compliance with medications. *Drug Benefit Trends* 1995(July):13–4, 24.
21. Patcher LE. Culture and clinical care. Folk illness beliefs and behaviors and their implications for health care delivery. *JAMA* 1994;271:690–4.

Renal Disease

John G. Gambertoglio
Brian P. Kearney

■ DOSAGE MODIFICATION IN RENAL IMPAIRMENT

The number of individuals with impaired kidney function is increasing steadily. In the United States, over 100,000 patients with end-stage renal disease are undergoing either hemodialysis or continuous ambulatory peritoneal dialysis, and over 1000 patients each year undergo kidney transplantation. Therapeutic advances in immunosuppressive drugs and dialysis techniques have made increased survival and a reasonable quality of life possible for patients with kidney diseases.

Invariably, these patients have multiple medical problems that either contributed to the development of their renal dysfunction or are sequelae of having chronic renal disease. Hypertension, diabetes, infection, bone disease, neurologic dysfunction, GI disturbances, and bleeding abnormalities are but a few of the frequently encountered medical conditions in renal failure patients. These patients are prescribed a number of medications; in one survey of dialysis patients, it was determined that they received an average of over eight drugs per patient.[1] Thus, renal patients are at increased risk for adverse reactions to drugs because of the number of drugs received, concurrent medical problems, and the impaired drug excretory pathway.[2,3] Complications resulting from drug administration can be minimized by the rational use of drugs and knowledge of their pharmacokinetic and pharmacodynamic characteristics in renal failure patients.

Since the advent of specific and sensitive methods for measuring drug concentrations in biological fluids, a voluminous literature has evolved concerning drug disposition in renal disease and the effects of dialysis.[4-6] This section provides a conceptual discussion of how renal disease alters drug disposition. It also describes an approach for determining the appropriate dosage adjustment necessary in the presence of renal disease to achieve the optimal therapeutic effect with minimal toxicity. The section, Dialysis of Drugs, discusses the concepts of drug removal by dialysis and provides specific data on the amount removed by dialysis and dosage modification for a number of drugs during dialysis.

FOUR BASIC QUESTIONS

A practical approach to drug therapy in patients with renal insufficiency is to answer the following questions:

1. What is the patient's renal function status?
2. What alterations exist in the pharmacokinetics or pharmacodynamics of the specific drug in renal failure?
3. What approaches to dosage modification are useful for a specific drug?
4. What is the dialysis removal of the drug and is dosage supplementation necessary?

DETERMINING RENAL FUNCTION

The usual tests to measure a patient's renal function include blood urea nitrogen (BUN), serum creatinine (Cr_s), and creatinine clearance (Cl_{cr}).[7]

The BUN is useful as a correlate of uremic symptoms and helps the clinician determine the adequacy of treatment modalities such as dialysis. However, the level of BUN can change because of many factors in addition to changes in renal function. Urea is both filtered and reabsorbed by the nephron, and its renal excretion is a function of urine flow. For example, excessive diuretic use, dehydration, or bleeding can all increase the BUN without there being a decline in renal function.[7]

For adults, creatinine production and elimination are constant at approximately 20 mg/kg/day under steady-state conditions.[8] Creatinine is filtered by the glomerulus with little renal tubular secretion; however, secretion becomes important at low levels of renal function. Decreases in renal function are reflected by increases in Cr_s and corresponding decreases in Cl_{cr}. Nonrenal factors that can affect the BUN do not alter Cr_s, so Cr_s and Cl_{cr} serve as better markers of changing renal function. The relationship between Cr_s and Cl_{cr} is a hyperbolic one, as is shown in Figure 3–3. Initial small increases in Cr_s represent larger decreases in renal func-

Figure 3–3. The Relationship Between Steady-State Values for Serum Creatinine, Blood Urea Nitrogen, and Glomerular Filtration Rate (GFR). It is assumed that creatinine clearance is equal to GFR and that creatinine production is constant, even under conditions of severe impairment of glomerular function.
From Kassirer JP. Clinical evaluation of kidney function-glomerular function. N Engl J Med 1971;285:385–9. *Reproduced with permission.*

tion (flatter part of the curve) than do similar increases in Cr_s at higher levels of Cr_s. Furthermore, for every doubling in Cr_s there is a halving in Cl_{cr} (ie, as Cr_s changes from 1 to 2 mg/dL, the Cl_{cr} declines from 120 to 60 mL/min; 2–4 mg/dL represents a decrease in Cl_{cr} from 60 to 30 mL/min). This approach can be used as a rough clinical guide in monitoring the progress of a patient's renal function and determining drug dosage adjustments.

Although Cr_s is easy to determine, requiring collection of only a single blood sample, measurement of Cl_{cr} is more difficult. The standard method consists of a continuous 24-hr urine collection for urine creatinine with a single blood sample for Cr_s at approximately the middle of the urine collection period. The most difficult problem from a practical standpoint is obtaining a complete urine collection. Almost invariably, urine collection is incomplete and consequently the Cl_{cr} is underestimated. However, the accuracy of the Cl_{cr} and urine collection can be estimated by determining the creatinine index. This is simply done by calculating the amount of creatinine (in mg/day) excreted in the urine over the 24-hr collection period. This total amount should be compared to the expected amount of creatinine to be excreted, which is approximately 20–25 mg/kg/day ideal body weight in males and 15–20 mg/kg/day in females. For example, in a 70-kg man, the expected creatinine production and excretion in the urine is approximately 1.4 g/day. If the patient's total creatinine excretion is less than this value, the possibility exists of an inadequate urine collection and correspondingly underestimated Cl_{cr}. The use of the creatinine index applies only under steady-state conditions, that is, when creatinine production and excretion are equivalent. Therefore, even if a patient's creatinine clearance were only 25% of normal (approximately 30 mL/min) at steady state, the production and excretion of creatinine are the same. At this level of renal function, the patient's Cr_s would be approximately 4 mg/dL and the excretion of creatinine would still be 1.4 g/day, matching creatinine production.

Another approach for estimating a patient's renal function is to use equations based on the patient's age and physical data. Many of these equations exist, however, the one that is most frequently used for adults is by Cockcroft and Gault, which requires knowing the patient's age, weight, and Cr_s.[9] Equations are given for men, women, and children in Appendix 2, Anthropometrics. These equations assume steady-state serum creatinine values and are not considered valid under conditions of fluctuating renal function. Also, in patients undergoing hemodialysis, the Cr_s can vary widely during and between dialyses, thereby limiting the usefulness of these equations.

■ PHARMACOKINETIC/PHARMACODYNAMIC ALTERATIONS OF DRUGS IN RENAL FAILURE

The presence of decreased renal function may affect the disposition of drugs by altering the processes of absorption, distribution, protein binding, metabolism, or excretion. Furthermore, the pharmacologic effect of a drug may be different in patients with renal impairment, because of biochemical or pathophysiologic changes associated with renal disease.

The bioavailability of drugs may be altered in renal failure because of associated GI disturbances such as nausea, vomiting, and diarrhea. Furthermore, patients with decreased renal function have an increased gastric pH because of increased salivary urea levels caused by their increased BUN. Drugs best absorbed in an acidic medium, such as ferrous sulfate, may have diminished absorption. In addition, these patients routinely take aluminum or calcium antacids (for calcium-phosphorus abnormalities), which may also alter drug bioavailability. Finally, certain drugs, such as propoxyphene and possibly some β-blockers, may have an altered first-pass effect in renal failure that can lead to increased bioavailability compared with control subjects.[10–13]

The plasma protein binding of drugs in renal failure may be altered. This may be caused by hypoalbuminemia; accumulation of acidic byproducts of uremia, resulting in competitive displacement of drugs from binding sites; or changes in the structure of albumin, resulting in a decreased number of effective binding sites.[10,12–14] Most weak organic acid drugs, such as cefazolin, phenytoin, salicylate, valproic acid, and warfarin, exhibit decreased plasma protein binding in uremia. Weak organic basic drugs have either decreased or unchanged binding in uremia. For example, the binding of carbamazepine, dapsone, diazepam, and morphine is decreased, whereas the binding of propranolol, quinidine, verapamil, and trimethoprim is unchanged. Some of these drugs, such as propranolol and lidocaine, are primarily bound to α_1-acid glycoprotein from which little displacement occurs in renal disease or hypoalbuminemia. The effects of altered protein binding of drugs may lead to an increased pharmacologic effect, an increased V_d, and either increased or unchanged total body clearance depending on whether it is a high or low extraction ratio drug.

The V_d of drugs may be increased, decreased, or unchanged in renal failure patients.[11,14] Examples of drugs with an increased V_d include cefazolin, furosemide, naproxen, and phenytoin. Digoxin exhibits a decreased V_d in renal impairment. Gentamicin, minoxidil, and procainamide are examples of drugs whose V_d does not change markedly in uremia.

Phenytoin is an example of a drug with altered protein binding in uremia that results in important differences in dosage.[15] The percentage of unbound phenytoin in plasma is normally 10%, but is 20–35% in renal failure patients. This results in an increase in the V_d from 0.65 L/kg in those with normal kidney function to 1–1.8 L/kg in renal failure patients. Furthermore, the apparent half-life decreases from 11–16 hr to 6–10 hr and the apparent plasma clearance increases from 28–41 mL/hr/kg to 64–225 mL/hr/kg in controls and renal failure patients, respectively. These pharmacokinetic changes in phenytoin result in a change in its therapeutic concentration range. In patients with normal kidney function, the usual therapeutic plasma concentration range for phenytoin is 10–20 mg/L, while in those with end-stage renal disease, it is approximately 4–8 mg/L. Both of these ranges of total drug yield the same concentration of unbound drug, which is approximately 1–2 mg/L.

Drugs are eliminated from the body by two primary pathways: renal excretion and nonrenal elimination (predominantly through hepatic metabolism).[4] The degree to which renal failure impairs drug elimination depends largely on the percentage of drug excreted unchanged by the kidney. For example, the aminoglycoside antibiotics are greater than 95% excreted unchanged by the kidney; cephalosporins range from 70–100%; penicillins from 85–100%; vancomycin from 95–100%; acyclovir from 75–80%; lithium from 95–100%; and ranitidine 80%. For many of these drugs, linear correlations have been established between the half-life of the drug and serum creatinine or between plasma clearance of the drug and Cl_{cr}. These specific correlations are then used as guides to determine drug dosage in renal failure. For example, the linear correlation between gentamicin serum half-life and Cr_s demonstrates that the half-life of gentamicin can change from 2 hr in normals to as much as 60 hr in renal failure patients. This correlation has led to a simple dosage guide, which indicates that the half-life of gentamicin can be estimated by multiplying the Cr_s by 3 or 4. This can then be used to determine the dosage of gentamicin in patients with varying degrees of renal insufficiency.

Drug metabolism typically involves enzymatic conversion of drugs to more water-soluble compounds. These metabolites are formed through processes of oxidation, reduction, synthesis (eg, conjugation), or hydrolysis and are, to a large extent, excreted by the kidney.[4,14] Most metabolites are inactive or have minimal pharmacologic activity. However, some metabolites that are active may accumulate in renal impairment and lead to toxicity. Examples of drugs metabolized to active or toxic compounds that are excreted by the kidney include allopurinol to oxypurinol, which is an active inhibitor of xanthine oxidase; cefotaxime to desacetylcefotaxime, which is microbiologically active; meperidine to normeperidine, which may cause seizure activity in renal failure; and procainamide to N-acetylprocainamide, which has antiarrhythmic properties. These metabolites may accumulate to toxic levels in renal failure patients unless appropriate dosage reductions are made.

The presence of renal failure may also lead to alterations in drug metabolism because of the abnormalities associated with the uremic state. For example, both the antiviral agent acyclovir and the antihypertensive agent captopril demonstrate a 50% decrease in nonrenal clearance in patients with end-stage renal disease.[16,17] As a consequence, the elimination half-life for both these drugs is unexpectedly increased sixfold in the presence of renal failure. This shows that predictions of the disposition of drugs in renal failure based on general principles and nomograms are subject to unexpected error. The pharmacokinetics of several newer drugs and changes caused by renal failure have been reviewed.[18,19]

The pharmacodynamics of a drug may be altered in uremia, causing its pharmacologic effects to be different from those expected in patients with normal renal function. One well-defined example is that of nifedipine, where marked differences in E_{max} (maximal effect change in diastolic blood pressure) were observed with averages of 12% and 29% in control and severe renal failure patients, respectively.[20,21] Thus, at the same plasma concentration of unbound nifedipine, a greater effect on blood pressure lowering occurs in patients with renal insufficiency. The response of these patients to nifedipine may be different than anticipated, requiring dosage modification because of drug effect changes rather than pharmacokinetic changes.

■ DOSAGE APPROACHES THAT ARE USEFUL AND PRACTICAL FOR SPECIFIC DRUGS

The general approaches for dosage adjustments of drugs in renal insufficiency are to (1) decrease the dose and maintain the usual dosage interval, (2) lengthen the dosage interval and maintain the usual dose, or (3) use a combination of modifying both the dose and interval. The primary goal of these approaches is to provide similar average steady-state plasma concentrations or AUCs for a drug in renal failure compared with normal kidney function. The choice of approach depends on the type of drug and the desirability, from a therapeutic or toxic standpoint, of having small or large fluctuations in peak and trough plasma drug concentrations. Other considerations are that the dosage regimen adjustment should be practical and the reduced dose or prolonged dosage interval should be relatively easy to implement.

When presented with a patient with impaired renal function for whom drug dosage regimen decisions must be made, the most practical and efficient approach is to first consult published tables or guidelines on specific drugs.[4,12,18,19] This may be accomplished by referring to tables by Bennett and colleagues,[5] which provides a quick reference source for drug dosage in renal failure. Additional sources are the appendices of *Handbook of Drug Therapy in Liver and Kidney Disease*[4] and "Use of Drugs in Renal Failure" in *Diseases of the Kidney,*[12] which describe specific pharmacokinetic alterations of drugs in kidney disease, recommended dosage, and the effects of dialysis. The reader is also advised to refer to specific drug monographs in this book, which briefly describe the effect of renal failure on drug disposition and dosage recommendations. These sources allow the user to determine whether dosage adjustments are necessary and whether there are any important toxicities or precautions in using a particular drug in the renal failure patient. These sources, however, serve only as general guidelines.

For drugs requiring dosage adjustment in renal insufficiency, the reader should consult the original publications, which provide specific data on individual drugs. Consulting the original publications will provide details regarding the relationship of renal function and drug elimination, and may provide a dosage nomogram or specific dosage recommendations and precautions for the use of a drug with varying degrees of renal insufficiency.

A final approach for dosage of drugs in renal impairment is to use general dosage equations provided by Rowland and Tozer.[22] This approach is recommended when specific guidelines for the use of a drug in renal failure have not been established. Basic pharmacokinetic information about the drug is needed—primarily the fraction of available dose that is normally excreted unchanged in the urine, f_e (normal), and the fraction of normal renal function (RF) in a given patient. The RF is the ratio of the diseased patient's Cl_{cr} to that of a normal value: RF = Cl_{cr} (failure)/Cl_{cr}(normal). The patient's Cl_{cr} may be determined from Cr_s values at steady state using the method of Cockcroft and Gault.[9]

Next, the following equation, which takes into consideration the renal unbound clearance and the extrarenal unbound clearance of the drug, is used:

$$R_d = \frac{RF \times f_e \text{ (normal)} + [1 - f_e \text{ (normal)}] \times [(140 - age) \times \text{weight in kg}^{0.7}]}{1660}$$

where R_d is the ratio of the unbound drug clearance in the patient to that normally observed, or Cl_u (failure)/Cl_u (normal), and age and weight are that of the patient. Once the value of R_d is obtained, the dosage regimen adjustment can be made using the following equation:

$$(D_M / \tau)(\text{failure}) = R_d \times (D_M / \tau)(\text{normal})$$

where D_M/τ is the maintenance dosage rate in the renal failure patient (failure) and under normal circumstances (normal). An example will clarify the use of this approach. An 80-kg, 45-year-old man with a serum creatinine of 5.4 mg/dL requires treatment with ceftazidime for a pseudomonal infection. This drug is 70% excreted unchanged in the urine, and the usual dosage is 1 g q 8 hr IV. Using the equation of Cockcroft and Gault, his Cl_{cr} is calculated as

$$Cl_{cr} = \frac{(140 - 45) \times 80}{(5.4 \times 72)} = 20 \text{ mL} / \min$$

Therefore

$$RF = \frac{20 \text{ mL} / \min}{120 \text{ mL} / \min} = 0.17$$

so

$$R_d = \frac{0.17 \times 0.7 + (1 - 0.7) \times ([140 - 45] \times 80^{0.7})}{1660}$$

$$R_d = 0.12 + 0.3 \times 1.2 = 0.49$$

and

$$(D_M / \tau)(\text{failure}) = 0.49 \times (D_M / \tau)(\text{normal})$$

which means that in this patient, the maintenance dosage of ceftazidime should be halved. Thus, the maintenance regimen could be 0.5 g q 8 hr or 1 g q 16 hr for this patient. The dosage could also be modified for practical reasons to 1.5 g q 24 hr.

This general equation approach provides a reasonable initial method for adjusting the dosage in patients with renal insufficiency until more specific guidelines can be consulted. This method is based on several assumptions: (1) bioavailability is unchanged in renal failure; (2) metabolites are not therapeutically active or toxic; (3) decreased renal function does not alter metabolism of the drug; (4) metabolism or renal excretion does not exhibit concentration-dependent pharmacokinetics; (5) renal function is constant with time; and (6) the renal clearance of the drug is directly proportional to the renal clearance of the compound used to measure renal function. The method above provides the best mathematical estimate of dosage in renal impairment. A simpler, but less complete, nomogram method has also been published (Fig. 3–4). All of the above limitations also apply to the nomogram.

For the drugs having a much longer half-life than usual in renal failure, the time to reach steady state is much longer than in a patient with normal renal function. Consequently, it is common to initiate therapy for many drugs with a loading dose in order to shorten the time to reach therapeutic plasma concentrations. The amount of the loading dose will obviously depend on the particular drug being used and the desired therapeutic objectives.

Figure 3–4. Estimation of Dosage Regimens in Patients with Renal Function Impairment. For Conditions for Use of Nomogram, How to Use Nomogram, and Modification of Dosage Regimen, see below.
From Rowland M, Tozer TN. Clinical pharmacokinetics: concepts and application. *Philadelphia: Lea & Febiger; 1980, reproduced with permission. To be used to determine how to change a normal dosage regimen. The normal dosage regimen depends on age, weight, and condition being treated.*

Finally, it should be stated that any dosage modification in renal failure may require plasma concentration determination of the drug, if available, and necessitates close clinical observation for assessment of toxicity and achievement of maximum therapeutic effect.

CONDITIONS FOR USE OF NOMOGRAM (FIG. 3–4)

This nomogram should be used only if the following conditions are met:

1. Metabolites are inactive and nontoxic.
2. Individual variation in metabolism or response are not significant.
3. Altered protein binding, metabolism, or distribution do not occur.
4. Cardiac output, hepatic function, and all other physiologic factors that might affect absorption or distribution are normal.
5. Renal function is reasonably constant.
6. Pharmacokinetics of the drug are linear.
7. The renal clearance of the drug is proportional to Cl_{cr}.

HOW TO USE NOMOGRAM

With a ruler, connect the fraction of drug normally excreted unchanged and the patient's kidney function, expressed as a fraction or normal value in a person of the same age. Read off from the center line the clearance of unbound drug (Cl_u) and the half-life relative to their normal values in a patient of the same age.

MODIFICATION OF DOSAGE REGIMEN

I. Initial dose—no change (*see* text).
II. Adjustment in rate of administration for maintenance of drug in body.
   A. Change in dosage interval, τ, only:

$$\tau(\text{failure}) = \frac{t_{1/2}\ (\text{failure})}{t_{1/2}\ (\text{normal})} \times \tau(\text{normal})$$

   B. Change in maintenance dose, D, only:

$$D(\text{failure}) = \frac{Cl_u\ (\text{failure})}{Cl_u\ (\text{normal})} \times D(\text{normal})$$

   C. Change in rate of administration D/τ:

$$\frac{D}{\tau}(\text{failure}) = \frac{Cl_u(\text{failure})}{Cl_u(\text{normal})} \times \frac{D}{\tau}(\text{normal})$$

■ REFERENCES

1. Anderson RJ et al. Prescribing medication in long-term dialysis units. *Arch Intern Med* 1982;142:1305–8.
2. Smith JW et al. Studies on the epidemiology of adverse drug reactions: V. Clinical factors affecting susceptibility. *Ann Intern Med* 1966;65:629–40.
3. Jick H. Adverse drug effects in relation to renal function. *Am J Med* 1977;62:514–7.

4. Schrier RW, Gambertoglio JG, eds. *Handbook of drug therapy in liver and kidney disease.* Boston: Little, Brown; 1991.

5. Bennett WM. Guide to drug dosage in renal failure. In Holford NHG, ed. *Drug data handbook,* 3rd ed. Auckland, NZ: ADIS International; 1998:49–119.

6. Benet LZ et al. Design and optimization of dosage regimens: pharmacokinetic data. In, Hardman JG, et al. eds. *Goodman and Gilman's the pharmacological basis of therapeutics.* 9th ed. New York: McGraw-Hill; 1996: 1707–9.

7. LaFayette RA et al. Laboratory evaluation of renal function. In, Schrier RW, Gottschalk CW, eds. *Diseases of the kidney.* Boston: Little, Brown; 1997:307–54.

8. Wesson LE. Electrolyte excretion in relation to diurnal cycles of renal function. *Medicine* 1964;43:547–92.

9. Cockcroft DW, Gault MH. Prediction of creatinine clearance from serum creatinine. *Nephron* 1976;16:31–41.

10. Matzke GR, Millikin SP. Influence of renal disease and dialysis on pharmacokinetics. In, Evans WE et al, eds. *Applied pharmacokinetics.* 2nd ed. Vancouver, WA: Applied Therapeutics; 1991.

11. Gambertoglio JG. Effects of renal disease: altered pharmacokinetics. In, Benet LZ et al, eds. *Pharmacokinetic basis for drug treatment.* New York: Raven Press; 1984:149–71.

12. Gambertoglio JG et al. Use of drugs in patients with renal failure. In, Schrier RW, Gottschalk CW, eds. *Diseases of the kidney,* Boston: Little, Brown; 1993:3211–68.

13. Talbert RL. Drug dosing in renal insufficiency. *J Clin Pharmacol* 1994;34:99–110.

14. Aweeka F. Drug dosing in renal failure. In, Young LY, Koda-Kimble MA, eds. *Applied therapeutics: the clinical use of drugs.* 5th ed. Vancouver, WA: Applied Therapeutics; 1992.

15. Flaherty JF et al. Neuropsychiatric drugs. In, Schrier RW, Gambertoglio JG, eds. *Handbook of drug therapy in liver and kidney disease.* Boston: Little, Brown; 1991.

16. Laskin OL et al. Acyclovir kinetics in end-stage renal disease. *Clin Pharmacol Ther* 1982;31:594–600.

17. Duchin KL et al. Elimination kinetics of captopril in patients with renal failure. *Kidney Intern* 1984;25:942–7.

18. Fillastre JP, Singlas E. Pharmacokinetics of newer drugs in patients with renal impairment (part I). *Clin Pharmacokinet* 1991;20:293–310.

19. Singlas E, Fillastre JP. Pharmacokinetics of newer drugs in patients with renal impairment (part II). *Clin Pharmacokinet* 1991;20:389–410.

20. Kleinbloesem CH et al. Nifedipine: relationship between pharmacokinetics and pharmacodynamics. *Clin Pharmacokinet* 1987;12:12–29.

21. Kleinbloesem CH. Nifedipine: influence of renal function on pharmacokinetic/hemodynamic relationship. *Clin Pharmacol Ther* 1985;37:563–74.

22. Rowland M, Tozer TN. Disease. In, *Clinical pharmacokinetics, concepts and applications.* 2nd ed. Philadelphia: Lea & Febiger; 1989:238–54.

■ DIALYSIS OF DRUGS

DIALYSIS REMOVAL OF DRUGS AND DOSAGE SUPPLEMENTATION

As noted in the previous section, this is the fourth area involved in formulating a practical approach to drug therapy in patients with renal insufficiency. Dialysis is an important therapy in the treatment of patients with end-stage renal disease. These patients are primarily managed with hemodialysis, but the use of continuous ambulatory peritoneal dialysis is now common. Although the purpose of dialysis is to remove unwanted toxic waste products from the body, it also has the effect of removing drugs used therapeutically. Thus, it is important to know to what extent a drug is removed by dialysis, because this may affect the patient's therapy. Supplemental doses or a revised dosage regimen may be required under these circumstances.

Dialysis procedures, including hemoperfusion, have also been used in the drug overdose situation as a means of eliminating drugs from the body. It is therefore important to consider how effective these procedures are and whether they offer any substantial advantage over conventional means of treating overdoses.

The objectives of this section are to review various factors involved in assessing the removal of drugs by dialysis and to illustrate how the use of pharmacokinetic information can be useful for determining the dialyzability of a drug. Additionally, the accompanying table lists the effect of hemodialysis and peritoneal dialysis on the removal of specific drugs.

METHODOLOGIC PROBLEMS

Several problems are encountered in attempting to assess the literature on removal of drugs by dialysis. First, for some drugs, only anecdotal reports are available. This is primarily true in the overdose setting, in which the effect of dialysis on drug removal is determined primarily by clinical response. For example, a comatose patient awakens during or shortly after dialysis and it is assumed that dialysis removed the drug, accounting for the improved clinical status. Second, the amount of drug ingested and/or the amount of drug recovered in the dialysate are often unknown. Third, the type of dialysis system employed is frequently not specified—this is important when comparing the system being used with published data. With advances in newer dialysis technology such as high-flux hemodialysis, earlier data evaluating conventional methods are not applicable. Fourth, there is often a lack of patient data, such as weight, hematocrit, and renal and liver function. The method used to calculate drug clearance is often unspecified. For example, was clearance determined from the amount of drug recovered in the dialysate or from differences in arterial and venous plasma concentrations across the dialyzer? The proper method for clearance calculations in hemodialysis has been described.[1]

A common error is misinterpretation of plasma drug concentrations obtained before and after dialysis. A declining plasma level during dialysis is often believed to be the result of the dialysis procedure. However, a declining level could be caused by drug elimination by metabolism or renal excretion, and the contribution of dialysis to this decline may be very small. The situation in which drug concentrations are relatively unchanged during dialysis usually means that little or no drug is being removed by dialysis. However, it is also possible that the drug continues to be absorbed from the GI tract as dialysis is being carried out, as in the delayed and prolonged absorption observed in drug overdose cases.[2] Another problem is that of interpreting drug removal rate by dialysis. If 200 mg of a drug were removed in the first hour of dialysis, one might assume that 5 hr of dialysis would remove five times as much (ie, 1000 mg). This is incorrect, because drug removal by dialysis occurs by a first-order process; as the amount of drug in the body declines, so does its removal rate. Thus, the total amount removed is less than that calculated from the initial estimates.

For many drugs, there is a lack of correlation between plasma drug concentrations and clinical response. Some drugs have been found to have active or toxic metabolites that correlate well with the toxic effects of the drug.[2] In attempting to collect information on dialysis removal of drugs, attention must be given to metabolites as well. A final point relative to the overdose situation is that the pharmacokinetic disposition of a drug may be altered.[2] In making predictions of drug dialyzability, pharmacokinetic data are usually derived from healthy subjects receiving therapeutic dosages. However, during an overdose, there may be changes in drug metabolism, V_d, or protein binding. For example, large amounts of drug in the body may saturate plasma protein binding, which could in turn alter drug distribution and metabolism.

PHARMACOKINETIC FACTORS

Certain properties of a drug can be used to make some predictions about drug dialyzability.[3–12] Drugs with small molecular weights, usually less than 500, cross conventional cuprophane dialysis membranes readily. Large-molecular-weight drugs, such as vancomycin (MW 1486) and amphotericin B (MW 924) cross these membranes poorly and are not effectively removed by conventional hemodialysis. The use of high-flux dialysis systems with polysulfone membranes, however, allows for removal of large-molecular-weight compounds such as vancomycin.

Drugs with high water solubility are more easily removed to the aqueous dialysate than more lipid-soluble compounds. In addition, the latter usually have a larger V_d than more water-soluble drugs. A large V_d such as that of digoxin (approximately 500 L) impairs the ability of dialysis to remove a drug from the body. Because the majority of drug is contained in tissue compartments rather than in the blood, it is not accessible for removal. A large V_d limits the use of hemoperfusion as well.[13] Hemoperfusion may rapidly clear the blood compartment of a drug (evidenced by a dramatic decrease in plasma levels); however, once hemoperfusion has ended, plasma drug concentrations can increase as a result of re-equilibration of drug from tissue stores.

Plasma protein binding of a drug also determines how effectively it can be dialyzed.[12] Drugs with a high degree of protein binding, such as propranolol (90–94%) and warfarin (99%), are poorly removed by dialysis because the drug-protein complex is too large to cross most dialysis membranes. This is not a limitation of hemoperfusion, because the drug is removed from plasma proteins as the complex passes through the high surface area adsorbent material.[9]

The clearance of a drug by dialysis can be compared to the clearance of the drug by the body. Clearance terms are additive:

$$Cl_{TD} = Cl_T + Cl_D,$$

where

Cl_{TD} = total body clearance of drug during dialysis
Cl_T = total body clearance of drug
Cl_D = dialysis clearance of drug.

Thus, if dialysis clearance adds substantially to body clearance, forming a much larger total clearance, then the drug will be eliminated that much faster. For example, if the dialysis clearance of a drug is 50 mL/min and the body clearance is 50 mL/min, then the drug would be eliminated from the body twice as fast during the dialysis period. In order to relate clearance to drug half-life ($t_{1/2}$), the following equations are useful:

$$t_{1/2} = \frac{0.693 \times V_d}{Cl_T} \text{ (off dialysis)}$$

$$t_{1/2} = \frac{0.693 \times V_d}{Cl_T + Cl_D} \quad \text{(on dialysis)}$$

Thus, the more the dialysis clearance adds to the body's clearance, the shorter the drug half-life will be on dialysis (assuming V_d remains constant). A further extension of this gives the following equation:

$$\text{Fraction lost during a dialysis period} = 1 - e^{-(Cl_T + Cl_D)(\tau/V_d)}$$

where τ is the duration of the dialysis period.

This allows calculation of the fraction of drug in the body that is lost during a dialysis period by all routes of elimination (ie, dialysis, metabolism, and renal excretion). Thus, it is necessary to acquire from literature sources (keeping in mind the limitations discussed previously) values for V_d, Cl_T, and Cl_D. If renal or liver function is diminished, this must be taken into consideration. In addition, changes in V_d in certain disease states (eg, the decreased V_d of digoxin in renal failure) must also be taken into account.

Clearance data are not always available in the literature. Many authors report only the half-lives of the drugs, on and off dialysis. The following equation may be used to estimate the fraction of drug removed by dialysis alone using half-life data;[13]

$$f = \frac{t_{1/2(\text{off})} - t_{1/2(\text{on})} \times (1 - e^{([0.693/t_{1/2(\text{on})}] \times \tau)})}{t_{1/2(\text{off})}}$$

where

f = fraction of drug removed by dialysis
$t_{1/2(\text{on})}$ = half-life on dialysis
$t_{1/2(\text{off})}$ = half-life off dialysis
τ = duration of dialysis.

The assumptions made when using this equation are that

1. All drug elimination (including dialysis removal) occurs by first-order processes.
2. Dialysis is initiated after the completion of the absorption and distribution phases.

The primary limitation of this equation is that inaccurate values of half-lives result in incorrect estimates of drug removal by dialysis. It is important to note the duration of dialysis in relation to the estimate of $t_{1/2(\text{on})}$. For example, if the $t_{1/2(\text{on})}$ is reported as 24 hr, but the dialysis duration is only 4 hr, the half-life value is probably not accurate. On the other hand, if the $t_{1/2(\text{on})}$ is reported as 1 hr during a 4-hr dialysis period, the half-life value might be more reliable.

Two examples illustrate the use of pharmacokinetic data to calculate drug clearance during dialysis. Phenobarbital has a V_d of approximately 50 L, a total body clearance of 0.3 L/hr, and a hemodialysis clearance of 4.2 L/hr. The half-life off dialysis is 115 hr and would decrease to 8 hr with dialysis. Approximately 50% of the drug would be removed from the body during 8 hr of dialysis. As another example, digoxin has a V_d of about 300 L and Cl_T of 2.4 L/hr in an anephric patient. The hemodialysis clearance of digoxin is 1.2 L/hr. Therefore, the half-life of digoxin in this patient off dialysis is 86 hr, while on dialysis it declines to 58 hr. Although this appears to be a substantial decrease in half-life, it means that the patient would have to be dialyzed 58 hr continuously in order to remove one-half the digoxin in the body. The fraction of drug lost during a routine hemodialysis period of 4 hr would be only 5%. Thus, a supplemental dose of digoxin following hemodialysis is not warranted.

HIGH-FLUX HEMODIALYSIS

High-flux dialyzers, which use more permeable polysulfone membranes, allow for greater removal of middle-molecular-weight compounds. For example, data are available comparing the dialysis clearance of vancomycin (MW 1486) using a conventional cuprophane membrane and the new polysulfone membranes. Conventional methods resulted in a dialysis clearance of 0.58 L/hr whereas high-flux dialysis produced a mean vancomycin dialysis clearance ranging from 2.7 to 5.1 L/hr. With conventional methods, only 7% of a dose of vancomycin was removed, compared to 26–50% using the polysulfone dialyzers. This enhanced removal of vancomycin by high-flux dialysis could be used as an effective means of drug removal in the overdose setting and suggests the need for vancomycin dosage supplementation posthemodialysis in the renal failure patient. Other antibiotics studied, such as ceftazidime and gentamicin, have also demonstrated increased removal using high-flux polysulfone dialyzers. (*See* Dialysis of Drugs table.)

USE OF THE TABLE

The table that follows provides data on specific drugs. For each drug, a qualitative statement of the range of drug removal by dialysis was derived using pharmacokinetic parameters taken from the literature. Drug removal is intentionally described in a qualitative fashion for a number of reasons. First, much of this information changes quite rapidly (eg, as new dialysis techniques are developed). Second, a given value for the amount of drug removed or the dialysis clearance determined in one study may differ from that found in another study, because of differences in dialysate or blood flow during dialysis, or the duration of the dialysis. The usual duration of dialysis has changed since earlier studies. Most conventional hemodialysis runs are 4 hr, whereas high-flux dialysis procedures last 2–2.5 hr. Also, data vary on the amount of drug removed by peritoneal dialysis, because estimates of removal were determined from the literature in which both constant dialysis for long periods of time (such as in an overdose situation) and intermittent dialysis for shorter periods each day were used. Finally, the table contains comments for clarification of certain points and selected references are provided for more specific information.

Dialysis information is *not* currently available for the following drugs: alprazolam, amlodipine, betaxolol, bumetanide, carteolol, chlorpheniramine, cisplatin, clarithromycin, clofazimine, clorazepate, clozapine, codeine, cytarabine, dapsone, diltiazem, dopamine, ethacrynic acid, felbamate, fluorouracil, glipizide, griseo-fulvin, guanethidine, hydralazine, hydrochlorothiazide, indomethacin, lamivudine, levodopa, lovastatin, melphalan, metolazone, milrinone, misoprostol, morphine, muromonab-CD3, nevirapine, nitrofurantoin, ondansetron, paromomycin, penicil-lamine, pentazocine, piroxicam, pravastatin, prazepam, primaquine, probenecid, ramipril, simvastatin, spironolactone, stavudine, sulfisoxazole, sulindac, tamoxi-fen, triamterene, and zalcitabine.

The following abbreviations and drug removal ranges are used in the table beginning on page 927:

- D — Dialyzed, 50–100%
- HD — Hemodialysis
- MD — Moderately Dialyzed, 20–50%
- ND — Not Dialyzed, 0–5%
- PD — Peritoneal Dialysis
- SD — Slightly Dialyzed, 5–20%

DIALYSIS OF DRUGS

DRUG	HEMODIALYSIS	PERITONEAL DIALYSIS	COMMENTS AND REFERENCES
Acebutolol	SD–MD		[Ref. 15,16]
Acetaminophen	SD–MD	ND	HD has not been shown to prevent hepatic or renal toxicity. Concentration-dependent kinetics. [Ref. 14]
Acetazolamide	MD		Data from single case study. [Ref. 14]
Acetohexamide		ND	Active metabolite also not dialyzed. [Ref. 14]
Acyclovir	D	SD	Give one-half usual dose post-HD. [Ref. 14,17–19]
Alcohol	D		[Ref. 14]
Allopurinol Oxypurinol (active metabolite)	MD		Oxypurinol dialyzed as well as creatinine. [Ref. 14]
Amantadine	ND–SD	SD	[Ref. 14]
Amikacin	D	SD–MD	Give 50–75% of the loading dose postdialysis; use plasma levels as a guide. [Ref. 14,20]
Amiloride			No data; this drug is not recommended for patients on dialysis.
Amiodarone	ND	ND	[Ref. 14,21]
Amitriptyline			No data; limited removal because of high protein binding and large V_d. [Ref. 22–26]
Amoxicillin	MD	SD	Give 1 g dose post-HD. [Ref. 14]
Amphotericin B	ND		[Ref. 14]
Ampicillin	MD	ND–SD	Give 1 g dose post-HD. [Ref. 14,20]
Antidepressants, Heterocyclic	ND	ND	Multiple metabolites. [Ref. 12]
Aspirin	D	MD	Concentration-dependent kinetics. [Ref. 14]
Astemizole	ND		Limited data for HD. [Ref. 27]
Atenolol	MD	ND	[Ref. 14,28–30]
Atovaquone			No data; limited HD removal due to high protein binding.
Azathioprine Mercaptopurine (active metabolite)	SD–MD		Data for azathioprine and metabolites using a nonspecific assay. [Ref. 14]

(continued)

DIALYSIS OF DRUGS (continued)

DRUG	HEMODIALYSIS	PERITONEAL DIALYSIS	COMMENTS AND REFERENCES
Azithromycin			No data; limited removal because of large V_d.
Aztreonam	MD	SD	Give one-half usual dose post-HD. [Ref. 14]
Bacampicillin	MD	ND–SD	(See Ampicillin.)
Baclofen			No data; toxicity has been reported in patients on dialysis.
Bleomycin			No data; probably poorly dialyzed because of large MW.
Bretylium	MD		[Ref. 14]
Captopril	MD	SD	[Ref. 14,31]
Carbamazepine	SD		Active epoxide metabolite. [Ref. 14]
Carisoprodol			No data; mulitple metabolites, one of which is meprobamate.
Cefaclor	MD		Give usual dose post-HD. [Ref. 14,32]
Cefadroxil	D		[Ref. 33]
Cefamandole	MD		Give one-half usual dose post-HD. [Ref. 14]
Cefazolin	MD	SD	Give a 0.5–1 g dose post-HD. [Ref. 14,34]
Cefixime	ND	ND	[Ref. 35]
Cefmetazole	D		[Ref. 36]
Cefonicid	ND–SD	ND–SD	No supplemental dose post-dialysis. [Ref. 14]
Cefoperazone	SD	ND	[Ref. 14,37]
Cefotaxime	MD	SD	Give one-half usual dose post-HD. [Ref. 14,38–41]
Desacetylcefotaxime (active metabolite)	MD	SD	
Cefoxitin	MD	SD	Give one-half usual dose post-HD. [Ref. 14,42]
Cefpodoxime	MD	ND–SD	[Ref. 43,44]
Cefprozil	MD		[Ref. 45]
Ceftazidime	D	SD	Give one-half usual dose post-HD. [Ref. 14,46–48]
Ceftizoxime	SD	ND	[Ref. 49–51]
Ceftriaxone	MD	ND	Give usual dose post-HD. [Ref. 20,52–56]

(continued)

DIALYSIS OF DRUGS (continued)

DRUG	HEMODIALYSIS	PERITONEAL DIALYSIS	COMMENTS AND REFERENCES
Cefuroxime	MD	SD	[Ref. 57–59]
Cephalexin	MD	SD	Give usual dose post-HD. [Ref. 14,60]
Cephalothin	MD	SD	Give one-half usual dose post-HD; slightly active desacetyl metabolite. [Ref. 14,61,62]
Cephapirin	MD		Give one-half usual dose post-HD; slightly active desacetyl metabolite. [Ref. 14]
Cephradine	MD	SD	[Ref. 14]
Chloral Hydrate	MD–D		[Ref. 14]
Trichloroethanol (*active metabolite*)	MD–D		[Ref. 14]
Chloramphenicol	SD	ND	No supplemental dose required; increased dialysis removal in hepatic failure. [Ref. 14]
Chlordiazepoxide	ND–SD		Active metabolites. [Ref. 14]
Chloroquine	ND	ND	[Ref. 14,63]
Chlorpromazine			No data; because of high protein binding and large V_d, little removal expected.
Chlorpropamide		ND	Active metabolite; single case of PD did not decrease plasma levels. [Ref. 14,64]
Cimetidine	SD	ND–SD	Supplemental postdialysis dose unnecessary; schedule doses around dialysis. [Ref. 14]
Ciprofloxacin	SD	ND–SD	Therapeutic levels achieved in the peritoneal fluid following oral doses. [Ref. 14,65]
Clindamycin	ND	ND	[Ref. 14,66]
Clonidine	ND		[Ref. 14,30]
Cloxacillin	ND		[Ref. 14]
Colchicine	ND		Insufficient data. [Ref. 67]
Cyclophosphamide	MD		[Ref. 14]
Cyclosporine	ND		Because of large MW and large V_d, little removal expected. [Ref. 14]
Desipramine			No data; because of high protein binding and large V_d, little removal expected.
Diazepam	ND		Active metabolites. [Ref. 68, 69]

(continued)

DIALYSIS OF DRUGS (continued)

DRUG	HEMODIALYSIS	PERITONEAL DIALYSIS	COMMENTS AND REFERENCES
Dicloxacillin	ND		[Ref. 14]
Didanosine	MD	ND	[Ref. 70,71]
Digitoxin	ND	ND	[Ref. 14]
Digoxin	ND	ND	Post-HD rebound in plasma levels. [Ref. 14]
Diltiazem		ND	[Ref. 72]
Dipyridamole			No data; because of extensive protein binding, little removal by HD expected.
Disopyramide	ND		Concentration-dependent kinetics. [Ref. 14]
Doxepin	ND		[Ref. 73]
Doxycycline	ND	ND–SD	[Ref. 14]
Enalapril	SD–MD		[Ref. 14,74–76]
Enoxacin	ND		[Ref. 77–78]
Epoetin Alfa		ND	Limited removal expected by HD because of large MW. [Ref. 79–81]
Erythromycin	SD	ND	[Ref. 14,82]
Esmolol	ND	ND	[Ref. 83]
Ethambutol	SD		No supplemental dose after HD. [Ref. 14]
Ethchlorvynol	ND–SD	ND	Concentration-dependent kinetics. [Ref. 14]
Ethosuximide	MD–D		Administer dose after dialysis. [Ref. 14]
Ethylene Glycol	D		Toxic metabolites formed. [Ref. 14]
Etodolac	ND		Limited data. [Ref. 84]
Famotidine	SD	ND	[Ref. 14,85–87]
Felodipine	SD		[Ref. 88]
Fenoprofen			Probably not removed by HD because of high protein binding.
Filgrastim	ND		Limited removal because of large MW. [Ref. 89]
Flecainide	ND	ND	[Ref. 14,90]
Fluconazole	MD	SD	Administer daily dose post-HD. [Ref. 14,91–93]
Flucytosine	D	MD	Give 20 mg/kg post-HD. [Ref. 14]
Flurazepam			No data; probably not dialyzed.

(continued)

DIALYSIS OF DRUGS (continued)

DRUG	HEMODIALYSIS	PERITONEAL DIALYSIS	COMMENTS AND REFERENCES
Flurbiprofen	ND		High protein binding likely to limit HD removal. [Ref. 94]
Foscarnet	MD	MD	[Ref. 95–99]
Furosemide	ND		[Ref. 14]
Ganciclovir	D		Administer dose post-HD. [Ref. 14,100]
Gemfibrozil	ND		Data limited to one patient on HD. [Ref. 101]
Gentamicin	D	SD–MD	(*See* Amikacin.) Increased clearance with high-flux dialysis (unpublished). Clinically important plasma levels achieved following intra-peritoneal doses. [Ref. 14,102–104]
Glutethimide	ND–SD	ND	Active metabolite formed. [Ref. 14]
Glyburide	ND		[Ref. 105]
Haloperidol			No data; probably minimal removal because of large V_d.
Heparin			No data; probably poorly dialyzed because of large MW.
Ibuprofen	ND		Two metabolites (believed inactive) well dialyzed [Ref. 14,106]
Imipenem/ Cilastatin	MD–D MD	SD SD	Give one-half usual dose post-HD. [Ref. 14]
Indinavir			No data; large MW, 60% protein bound.
Insulin			No data; probably poorly dialyzed because of large MW.
Isoniazid	D	MD	Give usual dose post-HD. [Ref. 14]
Isopropyl Alcohol	D		Major toxic metabolite is acetone. [Ref. 14]
Isradipine	ND		Little removal by PD expected because of high plasma clearance and V_d. [Ref. 107]
Itraconazole	ND	ND	[Ref. 108]
Kanamycin	D	SD–MD	(*See* Amikacin.) [Ref. 14]
Ketoconazole	ND	ND	[Ref. 14,109]
Labetalol	ND	ND	[Ref. 14]

(*continued*)

DIALYSIS OF DRUGS (continued)

DRUG	HEMODIALYSIS	PERITONEAL DIALYSIS	COMMENTS AND REFERENCES
Lidocaine	ND		Active metabolites. [Ref. 14]
Lisinopril	MD		[Ref. 70,110]
Lithium	MD–D	MD	Rebound rise in plasma levels postdialysis; case reports suggest 300–600 mg lithium carbonate after each HD. [Ref. 14,111–113]
Lomefloxacin	ND		[Ref. 114,115]
Lorazepam	SD		[Ref. 116]
Meperidine			No data; active metabolite accumulates in renal failure.
Meprobamate	SD–MD	ND–SD	Limited information; mostly case reports. [Ref. 14]
Mercaptopurine			(*See* Azathioprine.)
Methadone	ND	ND	[Ref. 14]
Methanol	D		[Ref. 14]
Methaqualone	SD	SD	Insufficient data. [Ref. 14]
Methicillin	ND		[Ref. 14]
Methotrexate *(conventional)* *(high-flux)*	ND–SD D	ND	Removal depends on type of dialysis. [Ref. 14,117]
Methyldopa	SD–MD	SD	Parent drug and metabolite data. [Ref. 14]
Methylprednisolone	SD		[Ref. 14]
Metoprolol	ND		Data indicate HD removal of metabolites. [Ref. 14,30]
Metronidazole	MD	SD	Adjust dosage to administer post-HD; active hydroxy metabolite removed by HD to same extent. [Ref. 14,118–121]
Mezlocillin	MD	SD	Give dose post-HD. [Ref. 14,20,122,123]
Miconazole	ND		[Ref. 14]
Midazolam			No data; because of high protein binding, little removal by HD expected.
Minocycline	ND	ND	Insufficient data. [Ref. 14]
Minoxidil	MD		[Ref. 124]
Nadolol	MD		[Ref. 14]
Nafcillin	ND		[Ref. 14]

(*continued*)

DIALYSIS OF DRUGS (continued)

DRUG	HEMODIALYSIS	PERITONEAL DIALYSIS	COMMENTS AND REFERENCES
Naproxen	ND		[Ref. 14]
Nelfinavir			No data; little removal expected due to large MW and high protein binding (>90%).
Neomycin	D		(*See* Amikacin.) [Ref. 14]
Netilmicin	D		(*See* Amikacin.) [Ref. 14,125]
Nifedipine	ND	ND	[Ref. 126–128]
Nitroprusside			HD useful in overdose. [Ref. 14]
Cyanide	ND		
Thiocyanate	MD		
(toxic metabolites)			
Norfloxacin	ND		Insufficient data. [Ref. 14]
Nortriptyline			No data; because of high protein binding and large V_d, little removal expected. [Ref. 129]
Ofloxacin	MD	ND	[Ref. 130–133]
Omeprazole	SD–MD		HD data limited to one patient. [Ref. 134]
Oxacillin	ND	ND	[Ref. 14,135]
Oxazepam	ND		(*See* Diazepam.) [Ref. 14]
Penicillin G	MD		Give 500,000 units post-HD. [Ref. 14]
Pentamidine			No data; probably not dialyzed because of very large V_d.
Pentobarbital	SD	ND–SD	[Ref. 14]
Pentoxifylline	MD		Limited data from one patient on HD. [Ref. 136]
Phenobarbital	MD–D	SD–MD	Administer dose after dialysis. [Ref. 14,137]
Phenothiazines	ND		Numerous metabolites; toxicity and dialyzability unknown. [Ref. 14]
Phenytoin	ND	ND	Concentration-dependent kinetics. [Ref. 14]
Piperacillin	MD	ND	[Ref. 14,138–140]
Prazosin			Insufficient data; probably not dialyzed. [Ref. 14]
Prednisone			
Prednisolone *(active metabolite)*	SD		[Ref. 14]

(continued)

DIALYSIS OF DRUGS (continued)

DRUG	HEMODIALYSIS	PERITONEAL DIALYSIS	COMMENTS AND REFERENCES
Primidone	MD		Partly metabolized to pheno-barbital. [Ref. 14]
Procainamide	MD	ND	Post-HD dose may be necessary to maintain therapeutic levels. [Ref. 14]
N-Acetylprocain-amide (*active metabolite*)	MD	ND	Has class III antiarrhythmic activity.
Propoxyphene	ND	ND	Active metabolite poorly dialyzed. [Ref. 14]
Propranolol	ND		[Ref. 14]
Pseudoephedrine		SD	Limited data. [Ref. 141]
Pyrazinamide	D		[Ref. 142]
Quinapril	ND	ND	[Ref. 143,144]
Quinidine	ND–SD	ND	[Ref. 14]
Ranitidine	SD	ND	[Ref. 14,145]
Reserpine			Insufficient data; probably not dialyzed. [Ref. 14]
Rifabutin	ND		No data; little removal by dialysis is expected because of large V_d.
Rifampin			Not dialyzed because of large MW and V_d.
Rimantadine	ND		[Ref. 146]
Ritonavir			No data; little removal expected due to large MW and high protein binding (>90%).
Saquinavir			No data; little removal expected due to large MW and high protein binding (>90%).
Sargramostim			No data; little removal is expected by HD because of large MW.
Secobarbital	SD	ND–SD	[Ref. 14]
Sotalol	MD		[Ref. 147–149]
Streptomycin	MD–D		(*See* Amikacin.) [Ref. 14]
Sulfadiazine	MD		Limited data. [Ref. 150,151]
Sulfamethoxazole	MD	ND	Give in 2 divided doses, 1 pre- and 1 post-dialyis. [Ref. 14,152–154]

(*continued*)

DIALYSIS OF DRUGS (continued)

DRUG	HEMODIALYSIS	PERITONEAL DIALYSIS	COMMENTS AND REFERENCES
Sulindac	ND		[Ref. 155]
Tacrolimus	ND		Limited data available for HD. High degree of protein binding and large MW limit HD removal. [Ref. 156]
Temazepam	ND	ND	[Ref. 157]
Tetracycline	SD	SD	[Ref. 14]
Theophylline	D	SD–MD	Nonlinear disposition; supplemental doses needed post-HD. [Ref. 14,158–163]
Thiabendazole	ND		Slight removal of metabolites by HD. [Ref. 164–166]
Ticarcillin	MD	ND–SD	Give a 0.75–1.5 g dose post-HD. [Ref. 14]
Timolol	ND		[Ref. 167]
Tobramycin	D	MD	(*See* Amikacin.) [Ref. 14,104]
Tocainide	SD–MD	ND	[Ref. 14,168]
Tolazamide	ND		Inactive and less active metabolites. [Ref. 14]
Tolmetin			No data; high protein binding limits removal by HD.
Torsemide	ND		Data from the manufacturer.
Triazolam	ND	ND	[Ref. 169]
Trimethoprim	SD–MD	ND	Give daily dose after dialysis. [Ref. 14,152–154]
Valproic Acid	SD	ND	[Ref. 14]
Vancomycin			
(*conventional*)	ND–SD		Removal depends on type of dialysis. [Ref. 14,170–186]
(*high-flux*)	MD		
Verapamil	ND		[Ref. 14,187–189]
Vinblastine			No data; probably poorly dialyzed because of large V_d.
Vincristine			No data; probably poorly dialyzed because of large V_d.
Warfarin			Probably poorly dialyzed because of high protein binding.
Zidovudine	ND	ND	[Ref. 14,190]

■ REFERENCES

1. Lee CS et al. Clearance calculations in hemodialysis: application to blood, plasma, and dialysate measurements for ethambutol. *J Pharmacokinet Biopharm* 1980;8:69–82.

2. Rosenberg J et al. Pharmacokinetics of drug overdose *Clin Pharmacokinet* 1981;6:161–92.

3. Takki S et al. Pharmacokinetic evaluation of hemodialysis in acute drug overdose. *J Pharmacokinet Biopharm* 1978;6:427–42.

4. Gibson TP, Nelson HA. Drug kinetics and artificial kidneys. *Clin Pharmacokinet* 1977;2:403–26.

5. Tilstone WJ et al. The use of pharmacokinetic principles in determining the effectiveness of removal of toxins from blood. *Clin Pharmacokinet* 1979;4:23–37.

6. Gwilt PR. General equation for assessing drug removal by extracorporeal devices. *J Pharm Sci* 1981;70: 345–50.

7. Lee CS. The assessment of fractional drug removal by extracorporeal dialysis. *Biopharm Drug Disp* 1982;3: 165–73. Abstract.

8. Gibson TP et al. Artificial kidneys and clearance calculations. *Clin Pharmacol Ther* 1976;20:720–3.

9. Reetze-Bonorden P et al. Drug dosage in patients during continuous renal replacement therapy. Pharmacokinetic and therapeutic considerations. *Clin Pharmacokinet* 1993;24:362–79.

10. Paton T et al. Drug therapy in patients undergoing peritoneal dialysis. Clinical pharmacokinetic considerations. *Clin Pharmacokinet* 1985;10:404–25.

11. Keller E. Peritoneal kinetics of different drugs. *Clin Nephrol* 1988;30:(suppl 1):S24–8.

12. Gwilt PR, Perrier D. Plasma protein binding and distribution characteristics of drugs as indices of their hemodialyzability. *Clin Pharmacol Ther* 1978;24:154–61.

13. Pond S et al. Pharmacokinetics of haemoperfusion for drug overdose. *Clin Pharmacokinet* 1979;4:329–54.

14. Aweeka FT, Gambertoglio JG. Drug overdose and pharmacologic considerations in dialysis. In, Cogan MG, Schoenfeld P, eds. *Introduction to dialysis.* 2nd ed. New York: Churchill Livingstone; 1991.

15. Roux A et al. Pharmacokinetics of acebutolol after intravenous bolus administration. *Br J Clin Pharmacol* 1980;9:215–7.

16. Roux A et al. Pharmacokinetics of acebutolol in patients with all grades of renal failure. *Eur J Clin Pharmacol* 1980;17:339–48.

17. Almond MK et al. Avoiding acyclovir neurotoxicity in patients with chronic renal failure undergoing haemodialysis. *Nephron* 1995;69:428–32.

18. Leikin JB et al. Hemodialysis removal of acyclovir. *Vet Hum Toxicol* 1995;37:233–4.

19. Stathoulopoulou F et al. Clinical pharmacokinetics of oral acyclovir in patients on continuous ambulatory peritoneal dialysis. *Nephron* 1996;74:337–41.

20. Keane WF et al. Peritoneal dialysis-related peritonitis treatment recommendations. 1993 update. *Perit Dial Int* 1993;13:14–28.

21. Ujhelyi MR et al. Disposition of intravenous amiodarone in subjects with normal and impaired renal function. *J Clin Pharmacol* 1996;36:122–30.

22. Oreopoulos DG, Lal S. Recovery from massive amitriptyline overdosage. *Lancet* 1968;2:221. Letter.

23. Halle MA, Collipp PJ. Amitriptyline hydrochloride poisoning. Unsuccessful treatment by peritoneal dialysis. *N Y State J Med* 1969;69:1434–6.

24. Sunshine P, Yaffe SJ. Amitriptyline poisoning: clinical and pathological findings in a fatal case. *Am J Dis Child* 1963;106:501–6.

25. Comstock TJ et al. Severe amitriptyline intoxication and the use of charcoal hemoperfusion. *Clin Pharm* 1983;2:85–8.

26. Bailey RR et al. Haemodialysis and forced diuresis for tricyclic antidepressant poisoning. *Br Med J* 1974; 4:230–1. Letter.

27. Zazgornik J et al. Plasma concentrations of astemizole in patients with terminal renal insufficiency, before, during, and after hemodialysis. *Int J Clin Pharmacol Ther Toxicol* 1986;24:246–8.

28. Salahudeen AK et al. Atenolol pharmacokinetics in patients on continuous ambulatory peritoneal dialysis. *Br J Clin Pharmacol* 1984;18:457–60.

29. Campese VM et al. Pharmacokinetics of atenolol in patients with chronic hemodialysis or peritoneal dialysis. *J Clin Pharmacol* 1985;25:393–5.

30. Niedermayer W et al. Pharmacokinetics of antihypertensive drugs (atenolol, metoprolol, propranolol and clonidine) and their metabolites during intermittent hemodialysis in humans. *Proc Eur Dial Transplant Assoc* 1978;15:607–9.

31. Drummer OH et al. The pharmacokinetics of captopril and captopril disulfide conjugates in uraemic patients on maintenance dialysis: comparison with patients with normal renal function. *Eur J Clin Pharmacol* 1987; 32:267–71.

32. Spyker DA et al. Pharmacokinetics of cefaclor in renal failure: effects of multiple doses and hemodialysis. *Antimicrob Agents Chemother* 1982;21:278–81.

33. Leroy A et al. Pharmacokinetics of cefadroxil in patients with impaired renal function. *J Antimicrob Chemother* 1982;10(suppl B):39–46.

34. Paton TW et al. The disposition of cefazolin and tobramycin following intraperitoneal administration in patients on CAPD. *Perit Dial Bull* 1983;3:73–6.

35. Guay DR et al. Pharmacokinetics of cefixime (CL284,635; FK 027) in healthy subjects and patients with renal insufficiency. *Antimicrob Agents Chemother* 1986;30:485–90.

36. Halstenson CE et al. Disposition of cefmetazole in healthy volunteers and patients with impaired renal function. *Antimicrob Agents Chemother* 1990;34:519–23.

37. Hodler JE et al. Pharmacokinetics of cefoperazone in patients undergoing chronic ambulatory peritoneal dialysis: clinical and pathophysiological implications. *Eur J Clin Pharmacol* 1984;26:609–12.

38. Heim KL et al. Disposition of cefotaxime and desacetyl cefotaxime during continuous ambulatory peritoneal dialysis. *Antimicrob Agents Chemother* 1986;30:15–9.

39. Petersen J et al. Pharmacokinetics of intraperitoneal cefotaxime treatment of peritonitis in patients on continuous ambulatory dialysis. *Nephron* 1985;40:79–82.

40. Overgaard S et al. Cefotaxime disposition pharmacokinetics during peritoneal dialysis. *Pharmacol Toxicol* 1987;60:321–4.

41. Hasegawa H et al. Pharmacokinetics of cefotaxime in patients undergoing haemodialysis and continuous ambulatory peritoneal dialysis. *J Antimicrob Chemother* 1984;14(suppl B):135–42.

42. Vlasses PH et al. Disposition of intravenous and intraperitoneal cefoxitin during chronic intermittent peritoneal dialysis. *Am J Kidney Dis* 1983;3:67–70.

43. Hoffler D et al. Cefpodoxime proxetil in patients with endstage renal failure on hemodialysis. *Infection* 1990; 18:157–62.

44. Johnson CA et al. Pharmacokinetics and ex vivo susceptibility of cefpodoxime proxetil in patients receiving continuous ambulatory peritoneal dialysis. *Antimicrob Agents Chemother* 1993;37:2650–5.

45. Shyu WC et al. Pharmacokinetics of cefprozil in healthy subjects and patients with renal impairment. *J Clin Pharmacol* 1991;31:362–71.

46. Ohkawa M et al. Pharmacokinetics of ceftazidime in patients with renal insufficiency and in those undergoing hemodialysis. *Chemotherapy* 1985;31:410–6.

47. Comstock TJ et al. Ceftazidime pharmacokinetics during continuous ambulatory peritoneal dialysis (CAPD) and intermittent peritoneal dialysis (IPD). *Drug Intell Clin Pharm* 1983;17:453.

48. Demotes-Mainard F et al. Pharmacokinetics of intravenous and intraperitoneal ceftazidime in chronic ambulatory peritoneal dialysis. *J Clin Pharmacol* 1993;33:475–9.

49. Gross ML et al. Ceftizoxime elimination kinetics in continuous ambulatory peritoneal dialysis. *Clin Pharmacol Ther* 1983;34:673–4.

50. Johnson CA et al. Pharmacokinetics of intravenous ceftizoxime in patients on continuous ambulatory peritoneal dialysis. *Clin Nephrol* 1985;23:120–4.

51. Cutler RE et al. Pharmacokinetics of ceftizoxime. *J Antimicrob Chemother* 1982;10(suppl C):91–7.

52. Albin H et al. Pharmacokinetics of intravenous and intraperitoneal ceftriaxone in chronic ambulatory peritoneal dialysis. *Eur J Clin Pharmacol* 1986;31:479–83.

53. Koup JR et al. Ceftriaxone pharmacokinetics during peritoneal dialysis. *Eur J Clin Pharmacol* 1986;30:303–7.

54. Losno Garcia R et al. Single-dose pharmacokinetics of ceftriaxone in patients with end-stage renal disease and hemodialysis. *Chemotherapy* 1988;34:261–6.

55. Ti T-Y et al. Kinetic disposition of intravenous ceftriaxone in normal subjects and patients with renal failure on hemodialysis or peritoneal dialysis. *Antimicrob Agents Chemother* 1984;25:83–7.

56. Cohen D et al. Pharmacokinetics of ceftriaxone in patients with renal failure and in those undergoing hemodialysis. *Antimicrob Agents Chemother* 1983;24:529–32.

57. Weiss LG et al. Pharmacokinetics of intravenous cefuroxime during intermittent and continuous arteriovenous hemofiltration. *Clin Nephrol* 1988;30:282–6.

58. Chan MK et al. Cefuroxime pharmacokinetics in continuous and intermittent peritoneal dialysis. *Nephron* 1985;41:161–5.

59. Local FK et al. Pharmacokinetics of intravenous and intraperitoneal cefuroxime in patients undergoing peritoneal dialysis. *Clin Nephrol* 1981;16:40–3.

60. Bunke CM et al. Pharmacokinetics of common antibiotics used in continuous ambulatory peritoneal dialysis. *Am J Kidney Dis* 1983;3:114–7.

61. Imada A et al. Comparative study of the pharmacokinetics of various beta-lactams after intravenous and intraperitoneal administration in patients undergoing continuous ambulatory peritoneal dialysis. *Drugs* 1988;35(suppl 2):82–7.

62. Aziz NS et al. Pharmacokinetics of cephalothin and its metabolite in uremic patients undergoing hemodialysis using an HPLC assay. *Perubatan UKM* (Medical Journal, National Univ. of Malaysia) 1980;2:82–9.

63. Akintonwa A et al. Hemodialysis clearance of chloroquine in uremic patients. *Ther Drug Monit* 1986;8:285–7.

64. Ludwig SM et al. Chlorpropamide overdose in renal failure: management with charcoal hemoperfusion. *Am J Kidney Dis* 1987;10:457–60.

65. Drusano GL et al. Pharmacokinetics of intravenously administered ciprofloxacin in patients with various degrees of renal function. *Antimicrob Agents Chemother* 1987;37:860–4.

66. Schwartz MT et al. Clindamycin phosphate kinetics in subjects undergoing CAPD. *Clin Nephrol* 1986;26:303–6.

67. Ellwood MG, Robb GH. Self-poisoning with colchicine. *Postgrad Med J* 1971;47:129–38.

68. Cutler RE, Blair AD. Pharmacokinetics of diazepam in normal and uremic humans. *Clin Pharmacol Ther* 1979;25:219–20. Abstract.

69. Ochs HR et al. Diazepam kinetics in patients with renal insufficiency or hyperthyroidism. *Br J Clin Pharmacol* 1981;12:829–32.

70. Knupp CA et al. Disposition of didanosine in HIV-seropositive patients with normal renal function or chronic renal failure: influence of hemodialysis and continuous ambulatory peritoneal dialysis. *Clin Pharmacol Ther* 1996;60:535–42.

71. Singlas E et al. Didanosine pharmacokinetics in patients with normal and impaired renal function: influence of hemodialysis. *Antimicrob Agents Chemother* 1992;36:1519–24.

72. Grech-Belanger O et al. Pharmacokinetics of diltiazem in patients undergoing continuous ambulatory peritoneal dialysis. *J Clin Pharmacol* 1988;28:477–80.

73. Faulkner RD et al. Hemodialysis of doxepin and desmethyldoxepin in uremic patients. *Artif Organs* 1984; 8:151–5.

74. Kelly J et al. Chronic dose pharmacokinetics of enalapril in renal impairment. *Proc Br Paedod Soc* 1985; Apr:264.

75. Sica DA et al. Comparison of the steady-state pharmacokinetics of fosinopril, lisinopril and enalapril in patients with chronic renal insufficiency. *Clin Pharmacokinet* 1991;20:420–7.

76. Kelly JG et al. Pharmacokinetics of lisinopril, enalapril and enalaprilat in renal failure: effects of haemodialysis. *Br J Clin Pharmacol* 1988;26:781–6.

77. van der Auwera P et al. Pharmacokinetics of enoxacin and its oxometabolite following intravenous administration to patients with different degrees of renal impairment. *Antimicrob Agents Chemother* 1990;34:1491–7.

78. Nix DE et al. The effect of renal impairment and haemodialysis on single dose pharmacokinetics or oral enoxacin. *J Antimicrob Chemother* 1988;21(suppl B):87–95.

79. Stockenhuber F et al. Pharmacokinetics and dose response after intravenous and subcutaneous administration of recombinant erythropoietin in patients on regular haemodialysis treatment or continuous ambulatory peritoneal dialysis. *Nephron* 1991;59:399–402.

80. Macdougal IC et al. Pharmacokinetics of recombinant human erythropoietin in patients on continuous ambulatory peritoneal dialysis. *Lancet* 1989;1:425–7.

81. Keen ML. Epoetin alfa—focus on dialyzability. Case study of the anemic patient. *Anna Journal* 1995;22:610–3.

82. Kroboth PD et al. Hearing loss and erythromycin pharmacokinetics in a patient receiving hemodialysis. *Arch Intern Med* 1983;143:1263–5.

83. Covinsky JO. Esmolol: a novel cardioselective, titratable, intravenous beta-blocker with ultrashort half-life. *Drug Intell Clin Pharm* 1987;21:316–21.

84. Brater DC. Evaluation of etodolac in subjects with renal impairment. *Eur J Rheumatol Inflamm* 1990;10:44–5.

85. Halstenson CE et al. Disposition of famotidine in renal insufficiency. *J Clin Pharmacol* 1987;27:782–7.

86. Gladziwa U et al. Pharmacokinetics and dynamics of famotidine in patients with renal failure. *Br J Clin Pharmacol* 1988;26:315–21.

87. Hachisu T et al. Optimal therapeutic regimen of famotidine based on plasma concentrations in patients with chronic renal failure. *Clin Ther* 1988;10:656–63.

88. Buur T et al. Pharmacokinetics of felodipine in chronic hemodialysis patients. *J Clin Pharmacol* 1991;31: 709–13.

89. Shishido K et al. The effects and pharmacokinetics of rhG-CSF on the treatment of neutropenia in patients with renal failure. *Nippon Jinzo Gakkai Shi* 1991;33:973–81.

90. Bailie GR, Waldek S. Pharmacokinetics of flecainide in a patient undergoing continuous ambulatory peritoneal dialysis. *J Clin Pharm Ther* 1988;13:121–4.

91. Toon S et al. An assessment of the effects of impaired renal function and haemodialysis on the pharmacokinetics of fluconazole. *Br J Clin Pharmacol* 1990;29:221–6.

92. Debruyne D et al. Pharmacokinetics of fluconazole in patients undergoing continuous ambulatory peritoneal dialysis. *Clin Pharmacokinet* 1990;18:491–9.

93. Berl T et al. Pharmacokinetics of fluconazole in renal failure. *J Am Soc Nephrol* 1995;6:242–7.

94. Cefali EA et al. Pharmacokinetic comparison of flurbiprofen in end-stage renal disease subjects and subjects with normal renal function. *J Clin Pharmacol* 1991;31:808–14.

95. MacGragor RR et al. Successful foscarnet therapy for cytomegalovirus retinitis in an AIDS patient undergoing hemodialysis: rationale for empiric dosing and plasma level monitoring. *J Infect Dis* 1991;164:785–7.

96. Aweeka FT et al. Pharmacokinetics (PK) of foscarnet in patients (PTS) with varying degrees of renal function *Int Conf AIDS* 1993:485. Abstract PO-B26–2097.

97. Alexander AC et al. Disposition of foscarnet during peritoneal dialysis. *Ann Pharmacother* 1996;30:1106–9.

98. Aweeka FT et al. Foscarnet pharmacokinetics: dosing in patients maintained on continuous ambulatory peritoneal dialysis. *J AIDS*. In press.

99. Aweeka FT et al. Pharmacokinetics of foscarnet in patients with varying degrees of renal function and hemodialysis. *Clin Pharmacol Ther*. In press.

100. Swan SK et al. Pharmacokinetics of ganciclovir in a patient undergoing hemodialysis. *Am J Kidney Dis* 1991; 17:69–72.

101. Knauf H et al. Gemfibrozil absorption and elimination in kidney and liver disease. *Klin Wochenschr* 1990;68:692–8.

102. Indraprasit S et al. Gentamicin removal during intermittent peritoneal dialysis. *Nephron* 1986;44:18–21.

103. Lockwood WR, Bower JD. Tobramycin and gentamicin concentrations in the serum of normal and anephric patients. *Antimicrob Agents Chemother* 1973;3:125–9.

104. Matzke GR et al. Hemodialysis elimination rates and clearance of gentamicin and tobramycin. *Antimicrob Agents Chemother* 1984;25:128–30.

105. Pearson JG et al. Pharmacokinetic disposition of ^{14}C-glyburide in patients with varying renal function. *Clin Pharmacol Ther* 1986;39:318–24.

106. Senekjian HO et al. Absorption and disposition of ibuprofen in hemodialyzed uremic patients. *Eur J Rheumatol Inflamm* 1983;6:155–62.

107. Schonholzer K, Marone C. Pharmacokinetics and dialysability of isradipine in chronic haemodialysis patients *Eur J Clin Pharmacol* 1991;42:231–3.

108. Boelaert J et al. Itraconazole pharmacokinetics in patients with renal dysfunction. *Antimicrob Agents Chemother* 1988;32:1595–7.

109. Daneshmend TK, Warnock DW. Clinical pharmacokinetics of ketoconazole. *Clin Pharmacokinet* 1988;14:13–34.

110. Gautam PC et al. Pharmacokinetics of lisinopril (MK521) in healthy young and elderly subjects and in elderly patients with cardiac failure. *J Pharm Pharmacol* 1987;39:929–31.

111. Jaeger A et al. Toxicokinetics of lithium intoxication treated by hemodialysis. *Clin Toxicol* 1985–1986;23: 501–17.

112. Jaeger A et al. When should dialysis be performed in lithium poisoning? A kinetic study in 14 cases of lithium poisoning. *J Toxicol Clin Toxicol* 1993;31:429–47.

113. Leblanc M et al. Lithium poisoning treated by high-performance continuous arteriovenous and venovenous hemodiafiltration. *Am J Kidney Dis* 1996;27:365–72.

114. Blum RA et al. Pharmacokinetics of lomefloxacin in renally compromised patients. *Antimicrob Agents Chemother* 1990;34:2364–8.

115. Leroy A et al. Lomefloxacin pharmacokinetics in subjects with normal and impaired renal function. *Antimicrob Agents Chemother* 1990;34:17–20.

116. Morrison G et al. Effect of renal impairment and hemodialysis on lorazepam kinetics. *Clin Pharmacol Ther* 1984;35:646–52.

117. Wall SM. Effective clearance of methotrexate using high-flux hemodialysis membranes. *Am J Kidney Dis* 1996;28:846–54.

118. Roux AF et al. Metronidazole kinetics in patients with acute renal failure on dialysis: a cumulative study. *Clin Pharmacol Ther* 1984;36:363–8.

119. Kreeft JH et al. Metronidazole kinetics in dialysis patients. *Surgery* 1983;93(1 pt 2):149–53.

120. Lau AH et al. Hemodialysis clearance of metronidazole and its metabolites. *Antimicrob Agents Chemother* 1986;29:235–8.

121. Cassey JG et al. Pharmacokinetics of metronidazole in patients undergoing peritoneal dialysis. *Antimicrob Agents Chemother* 1983;24:950–1.

122. Thorsteinsson SB et al. Pharmacokinetics of mezlocillin during hemodialysis. *Scand J Infect Dis* 1981;29 (suppl):59–63.

123. Brogard JM et al. Pharmacokinetics of mezlocillin in patients with kidney impairment: special reference to hemodialysis and dosage adjustments in relation to renal function. *Chemotherapy* 1982;28:318–26.

124. Lowenthal DT, Affrime MB. Pharmacology and pharmacokinetics of minoxidil. *J Cardiovasc Pharmacol* 1980;2(suppl 2):S93–106.

125. Were AJ et al. Netilmicin and vancomycin in the treatment of peritonitis in CAPD patients. *Clin Nephrol* 1992;37:209–13.

126. Spital A et al. Nifedipine in continuous ambulatory peritoneal dialysis. *Arch Intern Med* 1983;143:2025. Letter.

127. Martre H et al. Haemodialysis does not affect the pharmacokinetics of nifedipine. *Br J Clin Pharmacol* 1985;20:155–8.

128. Kleinbloesem CH et al. Influence of haemodialysis on the pharmacokinetics and haemodynamic effects of nifedipine during continuous intravenous infusion. *Clin Pharmacokinet* 1986;11:316–22.

129. Dawling S et al. Nortriptyline metabolism in chronic renal failure: metabolite elimination. *Clin Pharmacol Ther* 1982;32:322–9.

130. Kampf D et al. Multiple dose kinetics of ofloxacin and ofloxacin metabolites in haemodialysis patients. *Eur J Clin Pharmacol* 1992;42:95–9.

131. Dorfler A et al. Pharmacokinetics of ofloxacin in patients on haemodialysis treatment. *Drugs* 1987;34 (suppl 1):62–70.

132. Chan MK et al. Ofloxacin pharmacokinetics in patients on continuous ambulatory peritoneal dialysis. *Clin Nephrol* 1987;28:277–80.

133. Bandai H et al. Pharmacokinetics of ofloxacin in severe chronic renal failure. *Clin Ther* 1989;11:210–8.

134. Roggo A et al. The effect of hemodialysis on omeprazole plasma concentrations in the anuric patient: a case report. *Int J Clin Pharmacol Ther Toxicol* 1990;28:115–7.

135. Bulger RJ et al. Effect of uremia on methicillin and oxacillin blood levels. *JAMA* 1964;187:319–22.

136. Silver MR, Kroboth PD. Pentoxifylline in end-stage renal disease. *Drug Intell Clin Pharm* 1987;21:976–8.

137. Porto I et al. Removal of phenobarbital during continuous cycling peritoneal dialysis in a child. *Pharmacotherapy* 1997;17:832–5.

138. Giron JA et al. Pharmacokinetics of piperacillin in patients with moderate renal failure and in patients undergoing hemodialysis. *Antimicrob Agents Chemother* 1981;19:279–83.

139. Heim KL. The effect of hemodialysis on piperacillin pharmacokinetics. *Drug Intell Clin Pharm* 1985;19:455.

140. Johnson CA et al. Single-dose pharmacokinetics of piperacillin and tazobactam in patients with renal disease. *Clin Pharmacol Ther* 1992;51:32–41.

141. Sica DA, Comstock TJ. Pseudoephedrine accumulation in renal failure. *Am J Med Sci* 1989;298:261–3.

142. Stamatakis G et al. Pyrazinamide and pyrazinoic acid pharmacokinetics in patients with chronic renal failure. *Clin Nephrol* 1988;30:230–4.

143. Swartz RD et al. Pharmacokinetics of quinapril and its active metabolite quinaprilat during continuous ambulatory peritoneal dialysis. *J Clin Pharmacol* 1990;30:1136–41.

144. Blum RA et al. Pharmacokinetics of quinapril and its active metabolite, quinaprilat, in patients on chronic hemodialysis. *J Clin Pharmacol* 1990;30:938–42.

145. Comstock TJ et al. Ranitidine bioavailability and disposition kinetics in patients undergoing chronic hemodialysis. *Nephron* 1989;52:15–9.

146. Capparelli EV et al. Rimantadine pharmacokinetics in healthy subjects and patients with end-stage renal failure. *Clin Pharmacol Ther* 1988;43:536–41.

147. Blair AD et al. Sotalol kinetics in renal insufficiency. *Clin Pharmacol Ther* 1981;29:457–63.

148. Tjandramaga TB et al. The effect of end-stage renal failure and haemodialysis on the elimination kinetics of sotalol. *Br J Clin Pharmacol* 1976;3:259–65.

149. Singh SN et al. Sotalol-induced torsades de pointes successfully treated with hemodialysis after failure of conventional therapy. *Am Heart J* 1991;121(2 pt 1):601–2.

150. Canfield CJ et al. Acute renal failure in *Plasmodium falciparum* malaria. Treatment of peritoneal dialysis. *Arch Intern Med* 1968;122:199–203.

151. Adam W, Dawborn J. Urinary excretion and plasma levels of sulphonamides in patients with renal impairment. *Australas Ann Med* 1970;19:240–4.

152. Nissenson AR et al. Pharmacokinetics of intravenous trimethoprim-sulfamethoxazole during hemodialysis. *Am J Nephrol* 1987;7:270–4.

153. Svirbley JE et al. Co-trimoxazole (sulfamethoxazole plus trimethoprim) peritoneal barrier transfer pharmacokinetics. *Clin Pharmacokinet* 1989;16:317–25.

154. Halstenson CE et al. Trimethoprim-sulfamethoxazole pharmacokinetics during continuous ambulatory peritoneal dialysis. *Clin Nephrol* 1984;22:239–43.

155. Ravis WR et al. Pharmacokinetics and dialyzability of sulindac and metabolites in patients with end-stage renal failure. *J Clin Pharmacol* 1993;33:527–34.

156. Venkataramanan R et al. Pharmacokinetics of FK 506: preclinical and clinical studies. *Transplant Proc* 1990;22:52–6.

157. Kroboth PD et al. Effects of end-stage renal disease and aluminum hydroxide of temazepam kinetics. *Clin Pharmacol Ther* 1985;37:453–9.

158. Anderson JR et al. Effects of hemodialysis on theophylline kinetics. *J Clin Pharmacol* 1983;23:428–32.
159. Lee CS et al. Comparative pharmacokinetics of theophylline in peritoneal dialysis and hemodialysis. *J Clin Pharmacol* 1983;23:274–80.
160. Slaughter RL et al. Hemodialysis clearance of theophylline. *Ther Drug Monit* 1982;4:191–3.
161. Blouin RA et al. Theophylline hemodialysis clearance. *Ther Drug Monit* 1980;2:221–3.
162. Colanna F. Peritoneal dialysis in a 6-weeks old preterm infant with severe theophylline intoxication. *Minerva Pediatr* 1996;48:383–5.
163. Higgins RM et al. Severe theophylline poisoning: charcoal haemoperfusion or haemodialysis? *Postgrad Med J* 1995;71:224–6.
164. Bauer LA et al. The pharmacokinetics of thiabendazole and its metabolites in an anephric patient undergoing hemodialysis and hemoperfusion. *J Clin Pharmacol* 1982;22:276–80.
165. Schumaker JD et al. Thiabendazole treatment of severe strongyloidiasis in a hemodialyzed patient. *Ann Intern Med* 1978;89(5 pt 1):644–5.
166. Leapman SB et al. *Strongyloides stercoralis* in chronic renal failure: safe therapy with thiabendazole. *South Med J* 1980;73:1400–2.
167. Lowenthal DT et al. Timolol kinetics in chronic renal insufficiency. *Clin Pharmacol Ther* 1978;23:606–15.
168. Raehl CL et al. Tocainide pharmacokinetics during continuous ambulatory peritoneal dialysis. *Am J Cardiol* 1987;60:747–50.
169. Kroboth PD et al. Effects of end stage renal disease and aluminum hydroxide on triazolam pharmacokinetics. *Br J Clin Pharmacol* 1985;19:839–42.
170. Glew RH et al. Vancomycin pharmacokinetics in patients undergoing chronic intermittent peritoneal dialysis. *Int J Clin Pharmacol Ther Toxicol* 1982;20:559–63.
171. Blevins RD et al. Pharmacokinetics of vancomycin in patients undergoing continuous ambulatory peritoneal dialysis. *Antimicrob Agents Chemother* 1984;25:603–6.
172. Rogge MC et al. Vancomycin disposition during continuous ambulatory peritoneal dialysis: a pharmacokinetic analysis of peritoneal drug transport. *Antimicrob Agents Chemother* 1985;27:578–82.
173. Harford AM et al. Vancomycin pharmacokinetics in continuous ambulatory peritoneal dialysis patients with peritonitis. *Nephron* 1986;43:217–22.
174. Whitby M et al. Pharmacokinetics of single dose intravenous vancomycin in CAPD peritonitis. *J Antimicrob Chemother* 1987;19:351–7.
175. Quale JM et al. Removal of vancomycin by high-flux hemodialysis membranes. *Antimicrob Agents Chemother* 1992;36:1424–6.
176. Torras J et al. Pharmacokinetics of vancomycin in patients undergoing hemodialysis with polyacrylonitrile. *Clin Nephrol* 1991;36:35–41.
177. Bohler J et al. Rebound of plasma vancomycin levels after haemodialysis with highly permeable membranes. *Eur J Clin Pharmacol* 1992;42:635–9.
178. Barth RH et al. Vancomycin pharmacokinetics in high-flux hemodialysis. *Clin Res* 1990;38:a339. Abstract.
179. Figg WD et al. The effect of hemodialysis using polysulfone dialyzers on vancomycin clearance and the significance of rebound post-dialysis. *Pharmacotherapy* 1991;11:34.
180. Tan CC et al. Pharmacokinetics of intravenous vancomycin in patients with end-stage renal failure. *Ther Drug Monit* 1990;12:29–34.
181. Bailie GR et al. Prediction of serum vancomycin concentrations following intraperitoneal loading doses in continuous ambulatory patients with peritonitis. *Clin Pharmacokinet* 1992;22:298–307.
182. Morse GD et al. Comparative study of intraperitoneal and intravenous vancomycin pharmacokinetics during continuous ambulatory peritoneal dialysis. *Antimicrob Agents Chemother* 1987;31:173–7.
183. Barth RH, DeVincenzo N. Use of vancomycin in high-flux hemodialysis: experience with 130 courses of therapy. *Kidney Int* 1996;50:929–36.
184. Scott MK et al. Effects of dialysis membrane on intradialytic vancomycin administration. *Pharmacotherapy* 1997;17:256–62.
185. Gonzalez-Martin G et al. Pharmacokinetics of vancomycin in patients with severely impaired renal function. *Int J Clin Pharmacol Ther* 1996;34:71–5.
186. Zoer J et al. Dosage recommendation of vancomycin during haemodialysis with highly permeable membranes. *Pharm World Sci* 1997;19:191–6.
187. Shah GM, Winer RL. Verapamil kinetics during maintenance hemodialysis. *Am J Nephrol* 1985;5:338–41.
188. Beyerlein C et al. Verapamil in antihypertensive treatment of patients on renal replacement therapy—clinical implications and pharmacokinetics. *Eur J Clin Pharmacol* 1990;39(suppl 1):S35–7.
189. Hanyok JJ et al. An evaluation of the pharmacokinetics, pharmacodynamics, and dialyzability of verapamil in chronic hemodialysis patients. *J Clin Pharmacol* 1988;28:S31–6.
190. Kremer D et al. Zidovudine pharmacokinetics in five HIV seronegative patients undergoing continuous ambulatory peritoneal dialysis. *Pharmacotherapy* 1992;12:56–60.

4 Immunization

■ GENERAL RECOMMENDATIONS ON IMMUNIZATION*

Recommendations for immunizing infants, children, and adults are based on characteristics of immunobiologics, principles of active and passive immunization, and judgments by public health officials and specialists in clinical and preventive medicine. Benefits and risks are associated with the use of all immunobiologics: No vaccine is completely safe or completely effective. Recommendations for immunization practices balance scientific evidence of benefits, costs, and risks to achieve optimal levels of protection against infectious diseases. The recommendations in this chapter describe this balance and attempt to minimize the risks by providing information regarding dose, route, and spacing of immunobiologics, and delineating situations that warrant precautions or contraindicate the use of these immunobiologics. These recommendations are for use only in the United States because vaccines and epidemiologic circumstances often differ in other countries. *Individual circumstances may warrant deviations from these recommendations.* Tables 4–1 and 4–2 list the immunobiologics available in the United States.

■ IMMUNOBIOLOGICS

The specific nature and content of immunobiologics can differ. When immunobiologics against the same infectious agent are produced by different manufacturers, active and inert ingredients in the various products are not always the same. Practitioners are urged to become familiar with the constituents of the various products.

Suspending Fluids.   These may be sterile water, saline, or complex fluids containing protein or other constituents derived from the medium or biologic system in which the vaccine is produced (eg, serum proteins, egg antigens, and cell culture–derived antigens).

Preservatives, Stabilizers, Antibiotics.   These components of vaccines, antitoxins, and globulins are used to inhibit or prevent bacterial growth in viral cultures

---

*Excerpted from reference 1.

TABLE 4–1. LICENSED VACCINES AND TOXOIDS AVAILABLE IN THE UNITED STATES, BY TYPE AND RECOMMENDED ROUTES OF ADMINISTRATION

VACCINE	TYPE	ROUTE
Adenovirus[a]	Live virus	Oral
Anthrax[b]	Inactivated bacteria	Subcutaneous
Bacillus of Calmette and Guérin (BCG)	Live bacteria	Intradermal/percutaneous
Cholera	Inactivated bacteria	Subcutaneous or intradermal[c]
Diphtheria-tetanus-pertussis (DTP)	Toxoids and inactivated whole bacteria	Intramuscular
DTP–*Haemophilus influenzae* type b conjugate (DTP-Hib)	Toxoids, inactivated whole bacteria, and bacterial polysaccharide conjugated to protein	Intramuscular
Diphtheria-tetanus-acellular pertussis (DTaP)	Toxoids and inactivated bacterial components	Intramuscular
Hepatitis A	Inactivated virus	Intramuscular
Hepatitis B	Inactive viral antigen	Intramuscular
Haemophilus influenzae type b conjugate (Hib)[d]	Bacterial polysaccharide conjugated to protein	Intramuscular
Influenza	Inactivated virus or viral components	Intramuscular
Japanese encephalitis	Inactivated virus	Subcutaneous
Measles	Live virus	Subcutaneous
Measles-mumps-rubella (MMR)	Live virus	Subcutaneous
Meningococcal	Bacterial polysaccharides of serotypes A/C/Y/W-135	Subcutaneous
Mumps	Live virus	Subcutaneous
Pertussis[b]	Inactivated whole bacteria	Intramuscular
Plague	Inactivated bacteria	Intramuscular
Pneumococcal	Bacterial polysaccharides of 23 pneumococcal types	Intramuscular or subcutaneous
Poliovirus vaccine, inactivated (IPV)	Inactivated viruses of all 3 serotypes	Subcutaneous
Poliovirus vaccine, oral (OPV)	Live viruses of all 3 serotypes	Oral
Rabies	Inactivated virus	Intramuscular or intradermal[f]
Rubella	Live virus	Subcutaneous
Tetanus	Inactivated toxin (toxoid)	Intramuscular[f]
Tetanus-diphtheria (Td or DT)[g]	Inactivated toxins (toxoids)	Intramuscular[f]

(*continued*)

TABLE 4–1. LICENSED VACCINES AND TOXOIDS AVAILABLE IN THE UNITED STATES, BY TYPE AND RECOMMENDED ROUTES OF ADMINISTRATION (continued)

VACCINE	TYPE	ROUTE
Typhoid (parenteral)	Inactivated bacteria	Subcutaneous[h]
(Ty21a oral)	Live bacteria	Oral
(Vi CPS)	Bacterial polysaccharide	Intramuscular
Varicella	Live virus	Subcutaneous
Yellow fever	Live virus	Subcutaneous

[a]Available only to the U.S. Armed Forces.

[b]Distributed by the Division of Biologic Products, Michigan Department of Public Health.

[c]The intradermal dose is lower than the subcutaneous dose.

[d]The recommended schedule for infants depends on the vaccine manufacturer; consult the package insert and ACIP recommendations for specific products.

[e]The intradermal dose of rabies vaccine, human diploid cell (HDCV), is lower than the intramuscular dose and is used only for pre-exposure vaccination. **Rabies vaccine, absorbed (RVA) should not be used intradermally.**

[f]Preparations with adjuvants should be administered intramuscularly.

[g]Td = tetanus and diphtheria toxoids for use among persons ≥7 years of age. Td contains the same amount of tetanus toxoid as DTP or DT, but contains a smaller dose of diphtheria toxoid. DT = tetanus and diphtheria toxoids for use among children <7 years of age.

[h]Booster doses may be administered intradermally unless vaccine that is acetone killed and dried is used.

TABLE 4–2. IMMUNE GLOBULINS AND ANTITOXINS[a] AVAILABLE IN THE UNITED STATES, BY TYPE OF ANTIBODIES AND INDICATIONS FOR USE

IMMUNOBIOLOGIC	TYPE	INDICATION(S)
Botulinum antitoxin	Specific equine antibodies	Treatment of botulism
Cytomegalovirus immune globulin, intravenous (CMV-IGIV)	Specific human antibodies	Prophylaxis for bone marrow and kidney transplant recipients
Diphtheria antitoxin	Specific equine antibodies	Treatment of respiratory diphtheria
Hepatitis B immune globulin (HBIG)	Specific human antibodies	Hepatitis B postexposure prophylaxis
Immune globulin (IG)	Pooled human antibodies	Hepatitis A pre- and post-exposure prophylaxis; measles postexposure prophylaxis
Immune globulin, intravenous (IGIV)	Pooled human antibodies	Replacement therapy for antibody deficiency disorders; immune thrombocytopenic purpura (ITP); hypogammaglobulinemia in chronic lymphocytic leukemia; Kawasaki disease
Rabies immune globulin[b] (HRIG)	Specific human antibodies	Rabies postexposure management of persons not previously immunized with rabies vaccine
Tetanus immune globulin (TIG)	Specific human antibodies	Tetanus treatment; postexposure prophylaxis of persons not adequately immunized with tetanus toxoid
Vaccinia immune globulin (VIG)	Specific human antibodies	Treatment of eczema vaccinatum, vaccinia necrosum, and ocular vaccinia
Varicella-zoster immune globulin (VZIG)	Specific human antibodies	Postexposure prophylaxis of susceptible immunocompromised persons, certain susceptible pregnant women, and perinatally exposed newborn infants

[a]Immune globulin preparations and antitoxins are administered intramuscularly unless otherwise indicated.
[b]HRIG is administered around the wounds in addition to the intramuscular injection.

or the final product or to stabilize the antigens or antibodies. Allergic reactions can occur if the recipient is sensitive to one of these additives (eg, mercurials [thimerosal], phenols, albumin, glycine, and neomycin).

Adjuvants.   Many antigens evoke suboptimal immunologic responses. Efforts to enhance immunogenicity include mixing antigens with a variety of substances or adjuvants (eg, aluminum adjuvants such as aluminum phosphate or aluminum hydroxide).

Storage and Handling of Immunobiologics.   Failure to adhere to recommended specifications for storage and handling of immunobiologics can make these products impotent. Recommendations included in a product's package insert should be followed closely to ensure maximum potency of vaccines. Vaccines should be stored at recommended temperatures immediately upon receipt. Certain vaccines, such as oral polio vaccine (OPV) and yellow fever vaccine, are very sensitive to increased temperature. Other vaccines are sensitive to freezing, including diphtheria and tetanus toxoids and pertussis vaccine, adsorbed (DTP); diphtheria and tetanus toxoids and acellular pertussis vaccine, adsorbed (DTaP); diphtheria and tetanus toxoids for pediatric use (DT); tetanus and diphtheria toxoids for adult use (Td); inactivated poliovirus vaccine (IPV); *Haemophilus influenzae* type b conjugate vaccine (Hib); hepatitis B vaccine; pneumococcal vaccine; and influenza vaccine. Mishandled vaccine may not be easily distinguished from potent vaccine, and, when in doubt, contact the manufacturer.

■ ADMINISTRATION OF VACCINES

General Instructions.   Persons administering vaccines should take precautions to minimize risk for spreading disease and be adequately immunized against hepatitis B, measles, mumps, rubella, and influenza. Tetanus and diphtheria toxoids are recommended for all persons. Hands should be washed between patients. Gloves are not required when administering vaccinations, unless the persons who administer the vaccine will come in contact with potentially infectious body fluids or have open lesions on their hands. Syringes and needles used for injections must be sterile and preferably disposable to minimize the risk of contamination. A separate needle and syringe should be used for each injection. Different vaccines should not be mixed in the same syringe unless specifically licensed for such use.* Disposable needles and syringes should be discarded in labeled, puncture-proof containers to prevent inadvertent reuse or needlestick injury.

Routes of administration are recommended for each immunobiologic (*see* Table 4–1). Injectable immunobiologics should be administered where there is little likelihood of local, neural, vascular, or tissue injury. In general, vaccines containing adjuvants should be injected into the muscle mass; when administered subcutaneously or intradermally, they can cause local irritation, induration, skin

---

*The only vaccines currently licensed to be mixed in the same syringe by the person administering the vaccine are PRP-T *Haemophilus influenzae* type b conjugate vaccine, lyophilized, which can be reconstituted with DTP vaccine produced by Connaught. PRP-T can be mixed with Connaught's DTaP for injection of booster doses for toddlers only.

discoloration, inflammation, and granuloma formation. Once the needle is inserted into the injection site, the syringe plunger should be pulled back. If blood appears in the needle hub, the needle should be withdrawn and a new site selected before the vaccine is expelled. The process should be repeated until no blood appears.

Subcutaneous Injections. SC injections are usually administered into the thigh of infants and into the deltoid area of older children and adults. A ⅝- to ¾-inch, 23- to 25-gauge needle should be inserted into the tissues below the dermal layer of the skin.

Intramuscular Injections. The preferred sites for IM injections are the anterolateral aspect of the upper thigh and the deltoid muscle of the upper arm. *The buttock should not be used routinely for active vaccination of infants, children, or adults because of the potential for injury to the sciatic nerve.* In addition, injection into the buttock has been associated with decreased immunogenicity of hepatitis B and rabies vaccines in adults. If the buttock is used for passive immunization when large volumes are to be injected or multiple doses are necessary (eg, large doses of immune globulin), the central region should be avoided; only the upper, outer quadrant should be used, and the needle should be directed anteriorly (ie, not inferiorly or perpendicular to the skin) to minimize the possibility of involvement with the sciatic nerve. For all IM injections, the needle should be long enough to reach the muscle mass and prevent vaccine from seeping into subcutaneous tissues, but not so long as to endanger the underlying neurovascular structures or bone.

Infants (<12 Months of Age). Among most infants, the anterolateral aspect of the thigh provides the largest muscle mass and is therefore the recommended site. However, the deltoid can also be used with the thigh, for example, when multiple vaccines must be administered on the same visit. In most cases, a ⅞- to 1-inch, 22- to 25-gauge needle is sufficient to penetrate muscle in the thigh of a 4-month-old infant. The free hand should bunch the muscle, and the needle should be directed inferiorly along the axis of the leg at an angle appropriate to reach the muscle while avoiding nearby neurovascular structures and bone.

Toddlers and Older Children. The deltoid may be used if the muscle mass is adequate. The needle size can range from 22 to 25 gauge and from ⅝ to 1¼ inches, based on the size of the muscle. As with infants, the anterolateral thigh may be used, but the needle should be longer—generally ranging from ⅞ to 1¼ inches.

Adults. The deltoid is recommended for routine intramuscular vaccination among adults, particularly for hepatitis B vaccine. The suggested needle size is 1 to 1½ inches and 20- to 25-gauge.

Intradermal Injections. Intradermal injections are generally administered on the volar surface of the forearm, except for human diploid cell rabies vaccine (HDCV), for which reactions are less severe when the vaccine is administered in the deltoid area. With the bevel facing upward, a ⅜ to ¾ inch, 25- or 27-gauge needle can be inserted into the epidermis at an angle parallel to the long axis of the forearm. The needle should be inserted so that the entire bevel penetrates the skin and the injected solution raises a small bleb. Because of the small amounts of antigen used in intradermal injections, care must be taken not to inject the vaccine subcutaneously, because it can result in a suboptimal immunologic response.

Multiple Vaccinations.   If more than one vaccine preparation is administered or if live vaccine and an immune globulin preparation are administered simultaneously, it is preferable to administer each at a different anatomic site. It is also preferable to avoid administering two IM injections in the same limb, especially if DTP is one of the products administered. However, if more than one injection must be administered in a single limb, the thigh is usually the preferred site because of the greater muscle mass; the injections should be sufficiently separated (ie, 1–2 inches apart) so that any local reactions are unlikely to overlap.

Regurgitated Oral Vaccines.   Infants may sometimes fail to swallow oral preparations (eg, OPV) after administration. If a substantial amount of the vaccine is spit out, regurgitated, or vomited shortly after administration (ie, within 5–10 min), another dose can be administered at the same visit. If this repeat dose is not retained, neither dose should be counted, and the vaccine should be readministered at the next visit.

■ AGE AT WHICH IMMUNOBIOLOGICS ARE ADMINISTERED

Recommendations for the age at which vaccines are administered are influenced by several factors: age-specific risks of disease, age-specific risks of complications, ability of persons of a given age to respond to the vaccine(s), and potential interference with the immune response by passively transferred by maternal antibody. In general, vaccines are recommended for the youngest age group at risk for developing disease whose members are known to develop an adequate antibody response to vaccination (*see* Tables 4–3, 4–4, and 4–5).

■ SPACING OF IMMUNOBIOLOGICS

Interval Between Multiple Doses of Same Antigen.   Some products require administration of more than one dose for development of an adequate antibody response. In addition, some products require periodic reinforcement or booster doses to maintain protection (*see* Tables 4–3, 4–4, and 4–5.) Longer-than-recommended intervals between doses do not reduce final antibody concentrations. Therefore, an interruption in the immunization schedule does not require reinstitution of the entire series of an immunobiologic or the addition of extra doses. However, administering doses of a vaccine or toxoid at less-than-recommended minimum intervals may decrease the antibody response and therefore should be avoided. Doses administered at less-than-recommended minimum intervals should not be counted as part of a primary series.

Some immunobiologics produce increased rates of local or systemic reactions in certain recipients when administered too frequently (eg, adult Td, pediatric DT, tetanus toxoid, and rabies vaccine). Such reactions are thought to result from the formation of antigen-antibody complexes.

TABLE 4-3. RECOMMENDED CHILDHOOD IMMUNIZATION SCHEDULE[a]
UNITED STATES JANUARY–DECEMBER 1998

VACCINE	Birth	1 Mo	2 Mo	4 Mo	6 Mo	12 Mo	15 Mo	18 Mo	4-6 Yr	11-12 Yr	14-16 Yr
Hepatitis B[b,c]	Hep B-1	Hep B-2			Hep B-3					Hep B[c]	
Diphtheria and tetanus toxoids and pertussis[d]			DTaP or DTP	DTaP or DTP	DTaP or DTP		DTaP or DTP[d]		DTaP or DTP	Td	Td
Haemophilus influenzae type b[e]			Hib	Hib	Hib	Hib					
Poliovirus[f]			Polio	Polio	Polio[f]				Polio		
Measles-mumps-rubella[g]						MMR			MMR	MMR	
Varicella virus[h]						Var				Var	

Range of acceptable ages for vaccination.

Vaccines to be assessed and administered if necessary.

(continued)

949

TABLE 4–3. RECOMMENDED CHILDHOOD IMMUNIZATION SCHEDULE[a] UNITED STATES, JANUARY–DECEMBER 1998 (continued)

[a]From reference 8. This schedule indicates the recommended age for routine administration of currently licensed childhood vaccines; vaccines are listed under the ages for which they are routinely recommended. Catch-up immunization should be done during any visit when feasible. Some combination vaccines are available and may be used whenever administration of all components of the vaccine is indicated. Providers should consult the manufacturers' package inserts for detailed recommendations.

[b]**Infants born to hepatitis B surface antigen (HBsAg)-negative mothers** should receive 2.5 µg of Merck vaccine (Recombivax HB®) or 10 µg of SmithKline Beecham (SB) vaccine (Engerix-B®). The second dose should be administered at least 1 month after the first dose. The third dose should be administered at least 2 months after the second, but not before 6 months of age. **Infants born to HBsAg-positive mothers** should receive 0.5 mL hepatitis B immune globulin (HBIG) within 12 hours of birth, and either 5 µg of Merck vaccine (Recombivax HB®) or 10 µg of SB vaccine (Engerix-B®) at a separate site. The second dose is recommended at age 1–2 months and the third dose at age 6 months. **Infants born to mothers whose HBsAg status is unknown** should receive either 5 µg of Merck vaccine (Recombivax HB®) or 10 µg of SB vaccine (Engerix-B®) within 12 hours of birth. The second dose of vaccine is recommended at age 1 month and the third dose at age 6 months. Blood should be drawn at the time of delivery to determine the mother's HBsAg status; if it is positive, the infant should receive HBIG as soon as possible (no later than age 1 week). The dosage and timing of subsequent vaccine doses should be based on the mother's HBsAg status.

[c]Children and adolescents who have not been vaccinated against hepatitis B in infancy may begin the series during any visit. Those who have not previously received three doses of hepatitis B vaccine should initiate or complete the series during the routine visit to a health-care provider at age 11–12 years, and unvaccinated older adolescents should be vaccinated whenever possible. The second dose should be administered at least 1 month after the first dose, and the third dose should be administered at least 4 months after the first dose and at least 2 months after the second dose.

[d]Diphtheria and tetanus toxoids and acellular pertussis vaccine (DTaP) is the preferred vaccine for all doses in the vaccination series, including completion of the series in children who have received one or more doses of whole-cell diphtheria and tetanus toxoids and pertussis vaccine (DTP). Whole-cell DTP is an acceptable alternative to DTaP. The fourth dose (DTP or DTaP) may be administered as early as age 12 months, provided 6 months have elapsed since the third dose and if the child is unlikely to return at age 15–18 months. Tetanus and diphtheria toxoids, absorbed, for adult use (Td), is recommended at age 11–12 years if at least 5 years have elapsed since the last dose of DTP, DTaP, or diphtheria and tetanus toxoids, absorbed, for pediatric use (DT). Subsequent routine Td boosters are recommended every 10 years.

(continued)

950

TABLE 4-3. RECOMMENDED CHILDHOOD IMMUNIZATION SCHEDULE[a] UNITED STATES, JANUARY–DECEMBER 1998 (continued)

[e]Three *Haemophilus influenzae* type b (Hib) conjugate vaccines are licensed for infant use. If *Haemophilus* b conjugate vaccine (meningococcal protein conjugate) (PRP-OMP) (PedvaxHIB® [Merck]) is administered at ages 2 and 4 months, a dose at age 6 months is not required.

[f]Two poliovirus vaccines are currently licensed and distributed in the United States: inactivated poliovirus vaccine (IPV) and oral poliovirus vaccine (OPV). The following schedules are all acceptable to the ACIP, AAP, and AAFP. Parents and providers may choose among these options: 1) two doses of IPV followed by two doses of OPV; 2) four doses of IPV; or 3) four doses of OPV. ACIP recommends two doses of IPV at ages 2 and 4 months followed by a dose of OPV at age 12–18 months and at age 4–6 years. IPV is the only poliovirus vaccine recommended for immunocompromised persons and their household contacts.

[g]The second dose of measles-mumps-rubella vaccine (MMR) is recommended routinely at age 4–6 years but may be administered during any visit, provided at least 1 month has elapsed since receipt of the first dose and that both doses are administered beginning at or after age 12 months. Those who have not previously received the second dose should complete the schedule no later than the routine visit to a health-care provider at age 11–12 years.

[h]Susceptible children may receive varicella vaccine (Var) at any visit after the first birthday, and those who lack a reliable history of chickenpox should be vaccinated during the routine visit to a health-care provider at age 11–12 years. Susceptible children aged ≥13 years should receive two doses at least 1 month apart.

Use of trade names and commercial sources is for identification only and does not imply endorsement by CDC or the U.S. Department of Health and Human Services.

Source: Advisory Committee on Immunization Practices (ACIP), American Academy of Pediatrics (AAP), and American Academy of Family Physicians (AAFP).

TABLE 4–4. RECOMMENDED ACCELERATED IMMUNIZATION SCHEDULE FOR INFANTS AND CHILDREN <7 YEARS OF AGE WHO START THE SERIES LATE[a] OR WHO ARE >1 MONTH BEHIND IN THE IMMUNIZATION SCHEDULE[b] (ie, children for whom compliance with scheduled return visits cannot be assured)

TIMING	VACCINE(S)	COMMENTS
First visit (≥4 mo of age)	DTP,[c] IPV[d] or OPV, Hib,[c,e] Hepatitis B, MMR (should be given as soon as child is age 12–15 mo)	All vaccines should be administered simultaneously at the appropriate visit.
Second visit (1 mo after first visit)	DTP,[c] Hib,[c,e] Hepatitis B	
Third visit (1 mo after second visit)	DTP,[c] OPV,[d] Hib,[c,e]	
Fourth visit (6 weeks after third visit)	OPV	
Fifth visit (≥6 mo after third visit)	DTaP[c] or DTP, Hib,[c,e] Hepatitis B	
Additional visits (Age 4–6 yr)	DTaP[c] or DTP, OPV, MMR	Preferably at or before school entry.
(Age 14–16 yr)	Td	Repeat every 10 yr throughout life.

DTP, diphtheria-tetanus-pertussis; DTaP, diphtheria-tetanus-acellular pertussis; Hib, *Haemophilus influenzae* type b conjugate; MMR, measles-mumps-rubella; OPV, poliovirus vaccine, live oral, trivalent; Td, tetanus and diphtheria toxoids (for use among persons ≥7 years of age).

[a]If initiated in the first year of life, administer DTP doses 1, 2, and 3 and OPV doses 1, 2, and 3 according to this schedule; administer MMR when the child reaches 12–15 mo of age.

[b]See individual ACIP recommendations for detailed information on specific vaccines.

[c]Two DTP and Hib combination vaccines are available (DTP/HbOC [TETRAMUNE]; and PRP-T [ActHIB, OmniHIB] which can be reconstituted with DTP vaccine produced by Connaught). DTaP preparations are currently recommended only for use as the fourth and/or fifth doses of the DTP series among children 15 mo–6 yr of age (before the seventh birthday). DTP and DTaP should not be used on or after the seventh birthday.

[d]The Advisory Committee on Immunization Practices (ACIP) of the Centers for Disease Control and Prevention (CDC) recommends the use of enhanced inactivated poliomyelitis vaccine (IPV) injection for the first 2 doses of the series to minimize OPV-related paralysis.[5]

[e]The recommended schedule varies by vaccine manufacturer. For information specific to the vaccine being used, consult the package insert and ACIP recommendations. Children beginning the Hib vaccine series at age 2–6 mo should receive a primary series of three doses of HbOC [HibTITER] (Lederle-Praxis), PRP-T [ActHIB, OmniHIB] (Pasteur Merieux; SmithKline Beecham; Connaught), or a licensed DTP-Hib combination vaccine;

(*continued*)

TABLE 4–4. RECOMMENDED ACCELERATED IMMUNIZATION SCHEDULE FOR INFANTS AND CHILDREN <7 YEARS OF AGE WHO START THE SERIES LATE[a] OR WHO ARE >1 MONTH BEHIND IN THE IMMUNIZATION SCHEDULE[b] (ie, children for whom compliance with scheduled return visits cannot be assured) (continued)

or two doses of PRP-OMP [PedvaxHIB] (Merck, Sharp, and Dohme). An additional booster dose of any licensed Hib conjugate vaccine should be administered at 12–15 mo of age *and* at least 2 mo after the previous dose. Children beginning the Hib vaccine series at 7–11 mo of age should receive a primary series of two doses of a vaccine containing HbOC, PRP-T, or PRP-OMP. An additional booster dose of any licensed Hib conjugate vaccine should be administered at 12–18 mo of age *and* at least 2 mo after the previous dose. Children beginning the Hib vaccine series at ages 12–14 mo should receive a primary series of one dose of a vaccine containing HbOC, PRP-T, or PRP-OMP. An additional booster dose of any licensed Hib conjugate vaccine should be administered 2 mo after the previous dose. Children beginning the Hib vaccine series at ages 15–59 mo should receive one dose of any licensed Hib vaccine. Hib vaccine should not be administered after the fifth birthday except for special circumstances as noted in the specific ACIP recommendations for the use of Hib vaccine.

TABLE 4–5. RECOMMENDED IMMUNIZATION SCHEDULE FOR PERSONS ≥7 YR OF AGE NOT VACCINATED AT THE RECOMMENDED TIME IN EARLY INFANCY[a]

TIMING	VACCINE(S)	COMMENTS
First visit	Td,[b] OPV,[c] MMR,[d] and Hepatitis B[e]	Primary poliovirus vaccination is not routinely recommended for persons ≥18 yr of age.
Second visit (6–8 weeks after first visit)	Td, OPV, MMR,[d,f] Hepatitis B[e]	
Third vist (6 mo after second visit)	Td, OPV, Hepatitis B[e]	
Additional visits	Td	Repeat every 10 yr throughout life.

MMR, measles-mumps-rubella; OPV, poliovirus vaccine, live oral, trivalent; Td, tetanus and diphtheria toxoids (for use among persons ≥7 yr of age).

[a]See individual ACIP recommendations for details.

[b]The DTP and DTaP doses administered to children <7 yr of age who remain incompletely vaccinated at age ≥7 yr should be counted as prior exposure to tetanus and diphtheria toxoids (eg, a child who previously received two doses of DTP needs only one dose of Td to complete a primary series for tetanus and diphtheria).

[c]When polio vaccine is administered to previously unvaccinated persons ≥18 yr of age, inactivated poliovirus vaccine (IPV) is preferred. For the immunization schedule for IPV, see specific ACIP statement on the use of polio vaccine.

[d]Persons born before 1957 can generally be considered immune to measles and mumps and need not be vaccinated. Rubella (or MMR) vaccine can be administered to persons of any age, particularly to nonpregnant women of childbearing age.

[e]Hepatitis B vaccine, recombinant. Selected high-risk groups for whom vaccination is recommended include persons with occupational risk, such as health care and public safety workers who have occupational exposure to blood, clients and staff of institutions for the developmentally disabled, hemodialysis patients, recipients of certain blood products (eg, clotting factor concentrates), household contacts and sex partners of hepatitis B virus carriers, injecting drug users, sexually active homosexual and bisexual men, certain sexually active heterosexual men and women, inmates of long-term correctional facilities, certain international travelers, and families of HBsAg-positive adoptees from countries where HBV infection is endemic. Because risk factors are often not identified directly among adolescents, universal hepatitis B vaccination of teenagers should be implemented in communities where injecting drug use, pregnancy among teenagers, and/or sexually transmitted diseases are common.

[f]The ACIP recommends a second dose of measles-containing vaccine (preferably MMR to ensure immunity to mumps and rubella) for certain groups. Children with no documentation of live measles vaccination after the first birthday should receive two doses of live measles-containing vaccine not less than 1 mo apart. In addition, the following persons born in 1957 or later should have documentation of measles immunity (ie, 2 doses of measles-containing vaccine [at least one of which being MMR], physician-diagnosed measles, or laboratory evidence of measles immunity): (a) those entering post-high school educational settings; (b) those beginning employment in health care settings who will have direct patient contact; and (c) travelers to areas with endemic measles.

Simultaneous Administration.   Many of the commonly used vaccines can safely and effectively be administered simultaneously (ie, on the same day, *not* at the same anatomic site). Simultaneous administration is important in certain situations, including imminent exposure to several infectious diseases, preparation for foreign travel, and uncertainty that the person will return for further doses of vaccine.

Killed Vaccines.   In general, inactivated vaccines can be administered simultaneously at separate sites. However, when vaccines commonly associated with local or systemic side effects (eg, cholera, parenteral typhoid, and plague) are administered simultaneously, the side effects might be accentuated. When feasible, it is preferable to administer these vaccines on separate occasions.

Live Vaccines.   The simultaneous administration of the most widely used live and inactivated vaccines has not resulted in impaired antibody responses or increased rates of adverse reactions. Administration of combined measles, mumps, and rubella (MMR) vaccine yields results similar to administration of the individual vaccines at different sites. Concern has been raised that oral live attenuated typhoid (Ty21a) vaccine theoretically might interfere with the immune response to OPV when OPV is administered simultaneously or soon after live oral typhoid vaccine, but no published data exist to support this theory.

Routine Childhood Vaccines.   The simultaneous administration of routine childhood vaccines does not interfere with the immune response to these vaccines. When administered at the same time and at separate sites, DTP, OPV, and MMR have produced seroconversion rates and rates of side effects similar to those observed when the vaccines are administered separately. Simultaneous vaccination of infants with DTP, OPV (or IPV), and either Hib vaccine or hepatitis B vaccine has resulted in acceptable response to all antigens. Routine simultaneous administration of DTP (or DTaP), OPV (or IPV), Hib vaccine, MMR, and hepatitis B vaccine is encouraged for children who are the recommended age to receive these vaccines and for whom no specific contraindications exist at the time of the visit. Individual vaccines should not be mixed in the same syringe unless they are licensed for mixing by the U.S. Food and Drug Administration (FDA).*

Other Vaccines.   The simultaneous administration of pneumococcal polysaccharide vaccine and whole-virus influenza vaccine elicits satisfactory antibody responses without increasing the frequency or severity of adverse reactions in adults. Simultaneous administration of the pneumococcal vaccine and split-virus influenza vaccine also yields satisfactory results in both children and adults.

Hepatitis B vaccine administered with yellow fever vaccine is as safe and efficacious as when these vaccines are administered separately. Measles and yellow fever vaccines have been administered together safely and with full efficacy.

---

*The only vaccines currently licensed to be mixed in the same syringe by the person administering the vaccine are PRP-T *Haemophilus influenzae* type b conjugate vaccine, lyophilized, which can be reconstituted with DTP vaccine produced by Connaught. PRP-T can be mixed with Connaught's DTaP for injection of booster doses for toddlers only.

The antibody response to yellow fever and cholera vaccines is decreased if administered simultaneously or within a short time of each other. If possible, separate yellow fever and cholera vaccinations by at least 3 weeks. If time constraints exist and both vaccines are necessary, the injections can be administered simultaneously or within a 3-week period with the understanding that antibody response may not be optimal. Yellow fever vaccine is required by many countries and is highly effective in protecting against a disease with substantial mortality and for which no therapy exists. The currently used cholera vaccine provides limited protection of brief duration; few indications exist for its use.

Antimalarials and Vaccination.   The antimalarial mefloquine (Lariam) could potentially affect the immune response to oral live attenuated typhoid (Ty21a) vaccine if both are taken simultaneously. To minimize this effect, it may be prudent to administer Ty21a typhoid vaccine at least 24 hours before or after a dose of mefloquine. Because chloroquine phosphate (and possibly other structurally related antimalarials, such as mefloquine) may interfere with the antibody response to human diploid cell rabies vaccine (HDCV) when HDCV is administered by the intradermal route, HDCV should be administered by the intramuscular route when chloroquine, mefloquine, or other structurally related antimalarials are used.

Nonsimultaneous Administration.   Inactivated vaccines generally do not interfere with the immune response to other inactivated vaccines or to live vaccines except in certain instances (eg, yellow fever and cholera vaccines). In general, an inactivated vaccine can be administered either simultaneously or at any time before or after a different inactivated vaccine or a live vaccine. However, limited data indicate that prior or concurrent administration of DTP vaccine may enhance anti-PRP antibody response following vaccination with certain *Haemophilus influenzae* type b conjugate vaccines (ie, PRP-T, PRP-D, and HbOC). For infants, the immunogenicity of PRP-OMP appears to be unaffected by the absence of prior or concurrent DTP vaccination.

Theoretically, the immune response to one live-virus vaccine might be impaired if administered within 30 days of another live-virus vaccine. Whenever possible, live-virus vaccines administered on different days should be administered at least 30 days apart. However, OPV and MMR vaccines can be administered at any time before, with, or after each other, if indicated. Live-virus vaccines can interfere with the response to a tuberculin test. Tuberculin testing, if otherwise indicated, can be done either on the same day the live-virus vaccines are administered or 4–6 weeks later.

IMMUNE GLOBULIN

Live Vaccines.   OPV and yellow fever vaccines can be administered at any time before, with, or after the administration of immune globulin or specific immune globulins (eg, hepatitis B immune globulin [HBIG], rabies immune globulin [RIG]). The concurrent administration of immune globulin should not interfere with the response to Ty21a typhoid vaccine. Recent evidence suggests that high doses of immune globulin can inhibit the immune response to measles vaccine for more than 3 months. Administration of immune globulin can also inhibit the response to rubella vaccine. The effect of immune globulin preparations on the response to mumps and varicella vaccines is unknown, but commercial immune globulin preparations contain antibodies to these viruses.

Blood (eg, whole blood, packed RBCs, and plasma) and other antibody-containing blood products (eg, immune globulin; specific immune globulins; and immune globulin, intravenous [IGIV]) can diminish the immune response to MMR or its individual component vaccines. Therefore, after an immune globulin preparation is received, these vaccines should not be administered before the recommended interval has passed. However, postpartum vaccination of rubella-susceptible women with rubella or MMR vaccine should not be delayed because anti-Rho(D) IG (human) or any other blood product was received during the last trimester of pregnancy or at delivery. These women should be vaccinated immediately after delivery and, if possible, tested at least 3 months later to ensure immunity to rubella and, if necessary, to measles.

If administration of an immune globulin preparation becomes necessary because of imminent exposure to disease, MMR or its component vaccines can be administered simultaneously with the immunoglobulin preparation, although vaccine-induced immunity might be compromised. The vaccine should be administered at a site remote from that chosen for the immune globulin inoculation. Unless serologic testing indicates that specific antibodies have been produced, vaccination should be repeated after the recommended interval.

If administration of an immune globulin preparation becomes necessary after MMR or its individual component vaccines have been administered, interference can occur. Usually vaccine virus replication and stimulation of immunity occurs 1–2 weeks after vaccination. Thus, if the interval between administration of any of these vaccines and subsequent administration of an immune globulin preparation is less than 14 days, vaccination should be repeated after the recommended interval unless serologic testing indicates that antibodies were produced.

Killed Vaccines. Immune globulin preparations interact less with inactivated vaccines and toxoids than with live vaccines. Therefore, administration of inactivated vaccines simultaneously with or at any interval before or after receipt of immune globulins should not substantially impair the development of a protective antibody response. The vaccine or toxoid and immune globulin preparation should be administered at different sites.

Interchangeability of Vaccines From Different Manufacturers. When at least one dose of a hepatitis B vaccine produced by one manufacturer is followed by subsequent doses from a different manufacturer, the immune response has been shown to be comparable with that resulting from a full course of vaccination with a single vaccine.

Both HDCV and rabies vaccine, adsorbed (RVA) are considered equally efficacious and safe. When used as licensed and recommended, they are considered interchangeable during the vaccine series. *RVA should not be used intradermally.* The full 1 mL dose of either product, administered by IM injection, can be used for both pre-exposure and postexposure prophylaxis.

When administered according to their licensed indications, different diphtheria and tetanus toxoids and pertussis vaccines as single antigens or various combinations, as well as the live and inactivated polio vaccines, also can be used inter-changeably.

Currently licensed *Haemophilus influenzae* type b conjugate vaccines (ie, PRP-OMP, PRP-T, HbOC, and combination DTP-Hib vaccines) have been shown to induce different temporal patterns of immunologic response in infants. Data suggest that infants who receive sequential doses of different vaccines produce a satisfactory antibody response after a complete series. The primary vaccine series should be completed with the same Hib vaccine, if feasible. However, if different vaccines are administered, a total of 3 doses of Hib vaccine is considered adequate for the primary series among infants, and any combination of Hib conjugate vaccines licensed for use among infants may be used. Any of the licensed conjugate vaccines can be used for the recommended booster dose at 12–18 months of age.

■ HYPERSENSITIVITY TO VACCINE COMPONENTS

Vaccine components can cause allergic reactions in some recipients. These reactions can be local or systemic, and can include mild to severe anaphylaxis or anaphylactoid responses (eg, generalized urticaria or hives, wheezing, swelling of the mouth and throat, difficulty breathing, hypotension, and shock). The responsible vaccine components can derive from vaccine antigen, animal protein, antibiotics, preservatives, and stabilizers.

Egg Allergy. The most common animal protein allergen is egg protein found in vaccines prepared using embryonated chicken eggs (eg, influenza and yellow fever vaccines) or chicken embryo cell cultures (eg, measles and mumps vaccines). Ordinarily, persons who are able to eat eggs or egg products safely can receive these vaccines; persons with histories of anaphylactic or anaphylactoid allergy to eggs or egg proteins should not. Asking persons whether they can eat eggs without adverse effects is a reasonable way to determine who might be at risk for allergic reactions. Protocols for testing and vaccinating those persons with anaphylactic reactions to egg ingestion or vaccinating children with egg hypersensitivity and severe asthma have been developed. Rubella vaccine is grown in human diploid cell cultures and can be safely administered to persons with histories of severe allergy to eggs or egg proteins.

Antibiotic Allergy. Some vaccines contain trace amounts of antibiotics to which patients may be hypersensitive. The information provided in the vaccine package insert should be carefully reviewed before deciding if the uncommon patient with such hypersensitivity should receive the vaccine(s). No currently recommended vaccine contains penicillin or penicillin derivatives. MMR and its individual component vaccines contain trace amounts of neomycin and, although the amount present is less than would usually be used for a skin test to determine hypersensitivity, persons who have experienced anaphylactic reactions to neomycin should not receive these vaccines. Most often, neomycin allergy is a contact dermatitis—a manifestation of a delayed-type (cell-mediated) immune response—rather than anaphylaxis. A history of delayed-type reactions to neomycin is not a contraindication for these vaccines.

Thimerosal Allergy.   Exposure to vaccines containing the preservative thimerosal (eg, DTP, DTaP, DT, Td, Hib, hepatitis B, influenza, and Japanese encephalitis) can lead to induction of hypersensitivity. However, most patients do not develop reactions to thimerosal given as a component of vaccines even when patch or intradermal tests for thimerosal indicate hypersensitivity, which usually consists of local delayed-type hypersensitivity reactions.

Vaccine Allergy.   Certain parenteral bacterial vaccines (ie, cholera, DTP, plague, and typhoid) are frequently associated with local or systemic adverse effects, such as redness, soreness, and fever. These reactions are difficult to link with a specific sensitivity to vaccine components and appear to be toxic rather than hypersensitive. Urticarial or anaphylactic reactions in DTP, DT, or Td or tetanus toxoid recipients have been reported rarely. When these reactions are reported, appropriate skin tests should be performed to determine sensitivity to tetanus toxoid before its use is discontinued. Alternatively, serologic testing to determine immunity to tetanus can be performed to evaluate the need for a booster dose of tetanus toxoid.

■ VACCINATION IN SPECIAL POPULATIONS

Preterm Infants.   Infants born prematurely, regardless of birth weight, should be vaccinated at the same chronologic age and according to the same schedule and precautions as full-term infants and children. Birthweight and size generally are not factors in deciding whether to postpone routine vaccination of a clinically stable premature infant. The full recommended dose of each vaccine should be used. To prevent the theoretical risk of poliovirus transmission in the hospital, the administration of OPV should be deferred until discharge.

Any premature infant born to a hepatitis B surface antigen (HBsAg)-positive mother should receive immunoprophylaxis with hepatitis B vaccine and HBIG beginning at or shortly after birth. For premature infants of HBsAg-negative mothers, the optimal timing of hepatitis B vaccination has not been determined. Some studies suggest that decreased conversion rates might occur in some premature infants with low birthweights (ie, <2000 g) following administration of hepatitis B vaccine at birth. Such low-birthweight premature infants of HBsAg-negative mothers should receive the hepatitis B vaccine series, which can be initiated at discharge from the nursery if the infant weighs at least 2000 g or at 2 months of age along with DTP, OPV, and Hib vaccine.

Breastfeeding and Vaccination.   Neither killed nor live vaccines affect the safety of breastfeeding for mothers of infants. Breastfeeding does not adversely affect immunization and is not a contraindication for any vaccine. Breast-fed infants should be vaccinated according to routine recommended schedules.

Inactivated or killed vaccines do not multiply within the body. Therefore, they should pose no special risk for mothers who are breastfeeding or for their infants. Although live vaccines do multiply within the mother's body, most are not excreted in breastmilk. Although rubella vaccine virus may be transmitted in breastmilk, the virus usually does not infect the infant, and, if it does, the infection is well tolerated. There is no contraindication for vaccinating breastfeeding mothers with yellow fever vaccine. Breastfeeding mothers can receive OPV without any interruption in feeding schedule.

Vaccination During Pregnancy. Risk from vaccination during pregnancy is largely theoretical. The benefit of vaccination among pregnant women usually outweighs the potential risk when the risk for disease is high, infection would pose a special risk to the mother or fetus, and the vaccine is unlikely to cause harm.

Combined tetanus and diphtheria toxoids are the only immunobiologic agents routinely indicated for susceptible pregnant women. Previously vaccinated pregnant women who have not received a Td vaccination within the past 10 years should receive a booster dose. Pregnant women who are unimmunized or only partially immunized against tetanus should complete the primary series. Depending on when a woman seeks prenatal care and the required interval between doses, one or two doses of Td can be administered before delivery. Women for whom the vaccine is indicated but who have not completed the required three-dose series during pregnancy should be followed up after delivery to ensure they receive the doses necessary for protection.

There is no convincing evidence of risk from immunizing pregnant women with other inactivated virus or bacteria vaccines or toxoids. Hepatitis B vaccine is recommended for women at risk for hepatitis B infection, and influenza and pneumococcal vaccines are recommended for women at risk for infection and for complications of influenza and pneumococcal disease.

OPV can be administered to pregnant women who are at substantial risk of exposure to natural infection. Although OPV is preferred, IPV may be considered if the complete vaccination series can be administered before the anticipated exposure. Pregnant women who must travel to areas where the risk of yellow fever is high should receive yellow fever vaccine. In these circumstances, the small theoretical risk from vaccination is far outweighed by the risk of yellow fever infection. Known pregnancy is a contraindication for rubella, measles, and mumps vaccines. Although a theoretical concern, no cases of congenital rubella syndrome or abnormalities attributable to rubella vaccine virus infection have been observed in infants born to susceptible mothers who received rubella vaccine during pregnancy.

Persons who receive measles, mumps, or rubella vaccines can shed these viruses, but generally do not transmit them. These vaccines can be administered safely to the children of pregnant women. Although live poliovirus is shed by persons recently immunized with OPV (particularly after the first dose), this vaccine can also be administered to the children of pregnant women because experience has not revealed any risk of polio vaccine virus to the fetus.

All pregnant women should be evaluated for immunity to rubella and tested for the presence of HBsAg. Women susceptible to rubella should be immunized immediately after delivery. A woman infected with hepatitis B virus should be followed carefully to ensure that the infant receives HBIG and begins the hepatitis B vaccine series shortly after delivery.

There is no known risk to the fetus from passive immunization of pregnant women with immune globulin. Further information regarding immunization of pregnant women is available in the American College of Obstetricians and Gynecologists Technical Bulletin Number 160, October 1991.[2]

Altered Immunocompetence.   This section is a summary of the more extensive recommendations on vaccines and immune globulin preparations for immunocompromised persons. Additional information can be found in references 3 and 6.

Severe immunosuppression can be the result of congenital immunodeficiency. HIV infection, leukemia, lymphoma, generalized malignancy, or therapy with alkylating agents, antimetabolites, radiation, or large amounts of corticosteroids. Severe complications have followed vaccination of immunocompromised patients with live, attenuated-virus vaccines and with live-bacteria vaccines. In general, these patients should not receive live vaccines except in certain circumstances that are noted below. In addition, OPV should *not* be administered to any household contact of a severely immunocompromised person. If polio immunization is indicated for immunosuppressed patients, their household members, or other close contacts, IPV should be administered. MMR is not contraindicated in close contacts of immunocompromised patients.

Killed or inactivated vaccines can be administered to all immunocompromised patients, although response to such vaccines may be suboptimal. All such childhood vaccines are recommended for immunocompromised persons in usual doses and schedules. Certain vaccines such as pneumococcal vaccine or Hib vaccine are recommended specifically for certain groups of immunocompromised patients, including those with functional or anatomic asplenia.

HIV Infection.   Limited studies of MMR vaccination in HIV-infected patients have not documented serious or unusual adverse events. Because measles may cause severe illness in persons with HIV infection, MMR vaccine is recommended for all asymptomatic HIV-infected persons and should be considered for all symptomatic HIV-infected persons. HIV-infected persons on regular IGIV therapy may not respond to MMR or its individual component vaccines because of the continued presence of passively acquired antibody. However, because of the potential benefit, measles vaccination should be considered approximately 2 weeks before the next monthly dose of IGIV (if not otherwise contraindicated), although an optimal immune response is unlikely to occur. Unless serologic testing indicates that specific antibodies have been produced, vaccination should be repeated (if not otherwise contraindicated) after the recommended interval. An additional dose of IGIV should be considered for persons on routine IGIV therapy who are exposed to measles 3 or more weeks after administration of a standard dose (100–400 mg/kg) of IGIV.

Chemotherapy or Radiation Therapy.   Vaccination during chemotherapy or radiation therapy should be avoided because antibody response is poor. Patients vaccinated while on immunosuppressive therapy or in the 2 weeks before starting therapy should be considered unimmunized and should be revaccinated at least 3 months after therapy is discontinued. Patients with leukemia in remission whose chemotherapy has been terminated for 3 months may receive live-virus vaccines.

Corticosteroid Therapy.   The exact amount of systemically absorbed corticosteroids and the duration of administration needed to suppress the immune system of an otherwise healthy child are not well defined. Most experts agree that corticosteroid therapy usually does not contraindicate administration of live-virus vaccine when it is short term (ie, <2 weeks); low to moderate dose; long-term, alternate-day treatment with short-acting preparations; maintenance physiologic doses (replacement therapy); or administered topically (skin or eyes), by aerosol, or by intra-articular, bursal, or tendon injection. Although of recent theoretical concern, no evidence of increased severe reactions to live vaccines has been reported among persons receiving corticosteroid therapy by aerosol, and such therapy is not in itself a reason to delay vaccination. The immunosuppressive effects of corticosteroid treatment vary, but many clinicians consider a dose equivalent to a total of 20 mg/day of prednisone in adults as sufficiently immunosuppressive to raise concern about the safety of vaccination with live-virus vaccines. Corticosteroids used in greater than physiologic doses can also reduce the immune response to vaccines. Physicians should wait at least 3 months after discontinuation of therapy before administering a live-virus vaccine to patients who have received high systemically absorbed doses of corticosteroids for 2 or more weeks.

Vaccination of Persons with Hemophilia. Persons with bleeding disorders such as hemophilia have an increased risk of acquiring hepatitis B and at least the same risk as the general population of acquiring vaccine-preventable diseases. However, because of the risk of hematomas, intramuscular injections are often avoided among persons with bleeding disorders by using the subcutaneous or intradermal routes for vaccines that are normally administered by the intramuscular route. Hepatitis B vaccine administered intramuscularly to hemophiliacs using a 23-gauge needle, followed by steady pressure at the site for 1 to 2 minutes has resulted in a 4% bruising rate with no patients requiring clotting factor supplementation. Whether an antigen that produces more local reactions, such as pertussis, would produce an equally low rate of bruising is unknown.

When hepatitis B or any other intramuscular vaccine is indicated for a patient with a bleeding disorder, it should be administered intramuscularly if, in the opinion of a physician familiar with the patient's bleeding risk, the vaccine can be administered with reasonable safety by this route. If the patient received antihemophilic or other similar therapy, intramuscular vaccination can be scheduled for shortly after such therapy is administered. A fine needle (≤23 gauge) can be used for the vaccination and firm pressure applied to the site (without rubbing) for at least 2 minutes. The patient or family should be instructed concerning the risk of hematoma from the injections.

■ REFERENCES

1. General recommendations on immunization. Recommendations of the Advisory Committee on Immunization Practices (ACIP). *MMWR* 1994;43(RR-1):1–38.
2. Immunization during pregnancy. ACOG technical bulletin number 160—October 1991. *Int J Gynaecol Obstet* 1993;40:69–79. Also available from the American College of Obstetricians and Gynecologists. Attention: Resource Center, 409 12th Street SW, Washington, DC 20024–2188.
3. Recommendations of the Advisory Committee on Immunization Practices (ACIP): use of vaccines and immune globulins for persons with altered immunocompetence. *MMWR* 1993;42(RR-4):1–18.
4. Recommended childhood immunization schedule—United States, January–June 1996. *MMWR* 1996;44:940–3.
5. Marwick C. Switch to inactivated polio vaccine recommended. *JAMA* 1996;276:89. News.
6. Gardner P et al. Update: adult immunizations. *Ann Intern Med* 1996;12(1 pt 1):35–40.
7. Update: vaccine side effects, adverse reactions, contraindications, and precautions. *MMWR* 1996;45(RR-12):1–35.
8. Recommended childhood immunization schedule—United States, January–June 1998. *MMWR* 1998;47:8–12.

Medical Emergencies: Anaphylaxis, Cardiac Arrest, Poisoning, Status Epilepticus

5

Outline of Drug Therapy

The clinical management of medical emergencies is an area in which there continues to be some variability in treatment philosophy. Thus, the therapeutic approaches, drugs, and adult dosages given here are based on somewhat divergent and conflicting sources of information. In addition, some recommendations have been made based on the authors' experience and suggestions from specialists and researchers in the field. As a result, the therapeutic concepts and dosages contained herein, although conforming to medical standards, may differ from those advocated by specific practitioners and institutions.

Anaphylaxis

Lawrence R. Borgsdorf

An anaphylactic reaction is an *urgent* medical problem that can be fatal. Although the onset of symptoms can vary from minutes to hours, most reactions occur within 5–30 min following ingestion or parenteral administration of an antigen. Symptoms may progress from extreme apprehension and cutaneous reactions to more severe systematic manifestations, such as severe respiratory distress and/or profound shock. Reactions include conjunctivitis, GI edema (nausea, vomiting, diarrhea), cutaneous reactions (urticaria, pruritus, angioedema), rhinitis, laryngeal edema, and bronchospasm (coughing, wheezing, dyspnea, cyanosis), vascular collapse, cardiac arrhythmias, and cardiac arrest. (*See* the following section on Cardiac Arrest.)

■ DEFINITIVE THERAPY

(*See also* Adjunctive Therapy.)
Adult dosages only are given in this section.

1a. Treatment of anaphylaxis is always initiated with *immediate* **epinephrine HCl (aqueous), SC or IM, 0.3–0.5 mg** (0.3–0.5 mL of 1:1000); may repeat q 10–15 minutes,
or, for nonresponding or severe reactions,
epinephrine HCl, IV slow push, 0.2–0.5 mg (0.2–0.5 mL of 1:1000 diluted to 10 mL with NS, or 2–5 mL of 1:10,000); may repeat q 5–20 minutes.

1b. Patient should be in a recumbent position with legs elevated, patent airway established, and oxygen given; if applicable, a tourniquet should be placed proximal to the antigen injection site (remove temporarily q 10–15 min), and give
epinephrine HCl, infiltrate 0.1–0.3 mg (0.1–0.3 mL of 1:1000) at antigen injection site.

2. *Bronchospasm* alone (no cutaneous or cardiovascular manifestations) may respond to **albuterol,** via nebulization (0.5 mL of 0.5% solution in 2.5 mL of NS); may repeat q 20 min.

3a. *Hypotension* not responding to epinephrine may be treated by the use of fluids (*see* 3b) and vasopressor agents; for example, **dopamine HCl, IV slow infusion,** adjust rate to response (400 mg in 500 mL NS or D5W = 800 mg/L),
or, if dopamine fails to maintain blood pressure,
norepinephrine bitartrate, IV infusion, adjust rate to maintain a systolic blood pressure of about 90–100 mm Hg (2 mL of 0.2% solution in 500 mL D5W = 4 mg base/L).

3b. *Hypovolemia* may be the underlying cause of hypotension and this requires rapid expansion of the intravascular fluid volume with **NS** or **lactated Ringer's injection,**
or, for failure to respond to above or in severe hypotension,
hetastarch or **albumin human.** Monitor cardiac filling pressures to avoid hemodynamic pulmonary edema (ie, keep pulmonary capillary wedge pressure between 15 and 20 mm Hg).

■ ADJUNCTIVE THERAPY

Adult dosages only are given in this section.
There is no clear evidence that the following measures are effective in the treatment of acute, life-threatening anaphylaxis; therefore, use only after life-threatening symptoms have been controlled.

1. To prevent prolonged antigen-antibody reactions, give **hydrocortisone phosphate or succinate, IV, 100 mg;** may repeat q 6 hours.
2. To prevent further cutaneous reactions, give **diphenhydramine HCl, PO, IM, or slow IV, 25–50 mg;** may repeat q 6 hours.

3. To manage urticarial manifestations, give **cimetidine, PO, IM, or slow IV, 300 mg;** may repeat q 6 hours (unlabeled indication).

4. To manage prolonged bronchospastic manifestations, give **aminophylline, IV slow infusion, 5 mg/kg** (0.2 mL/kg of 25 mg/mL solution in 250 mL fluid) over 20 min, followed by continuous infusion for maintenance. (*See* Theophylline monograph.)

■ REFERENCES

1. Carlson RW et al. Anaphylactic, anaphylactoid, and related forms of shock. *Crit Care Clin* 1986;2:347–72.
2. Kelly JS, Prielipp RC. Is cimetidine indicated in the treatment of acute anaphylactic shock? *Anesth Analg* 1990;71:104–5. Letter.
3. Bochner BS, Lichtenstein LM. Anaphylaxis. *N Engl J Med* 1991;324:1785–90.
4. Yunginger JW. Anaphylaxis. *Ann Allergy* 1992;69:87–96.

Cardiac Arrest

Amy J. Guenette

A cardiac arrest is a medical emergency requiring a systematic approach. Early recognition (unconsciousness, apnea, no pulse) must be followed by prompt, effective application of Basic Cardiac Life Support (BCLS) techniques to sustain the patient until Advanced Cardiac Life Support (ACLS) capabilities are available. With ACLS capabilities, a definitive treatment plan can then be attempted.

Thus, management of cardiac arrest is a four-step approach:

- **Diagnosis**
- **Emergency Treatment (BCLS)**
- **Definitive Therapy (ACLS)**
- **Postresuscitation Care**

■ DIAGNOSIS

Verify that respiration and perfusion have ceased:

1. Loss of consciousness.
2. Loss of functional ventilation (apnea).
3. Loss of functional perfusion (no pulse).

■ EMERGENCY TREATMENT (BCLS)

The findings listed above are sufficient to justify the immediate application of BCLS techniques listed below. The goal of BCLS is to rapidly and effectively reperfuse the CNS with oxygenated blood. It is well recognized that delays in initiating BCLS or in providing ineffective BCLS can result in irreversible hypoxic brain damage in an otherwise "successful" resuscitation.

1. Summon help and resuscitation equipment.
2. If this is a witnessed arrest and a defibrillator is readily available:
   - Defibrillate with 200 joules of direct current shock if ventricular tachycardia or ventricular fibrillation are documented.
   - If the first shock fails to terminate the dysrhythmia, a second shock with 200–300 joules should be attempted. If the first two shocks fail, a third shock of 360 joules should be attempted.
3. If this is a witnessed arrest and a defibrillator is *not* readily available:
   - Deliver a sharp precordial blow.
4. If no response to above, or if an unwitnessed arrest, start artificial ventilation:
   - Establish an adequate airway.
   - Ventilate by mouth-to-mask or bag-valve-mask technique.

- The first two ventilations should be slow and deep, then ventilate at approximately 12 per minute.
5. Begin artificial perfusion via external chest compressions:
   - Position patient supine on firm surface.
   - Ensure proper placement of hands on sternum.
   - Depress sternum at rate of 80–100 cycles per minute (50% of cycle should be compression).

■ DEFINITIVE THERAPY (ACLS)

Adult dosages only are given in this section.

Initiate attempts by trained personnel to maintain a patent airway, establish an intravenous route for administration of fluids and drugs, establish an electrocardiographic diagnosis, and apply specific treatments to correct a recognized electrical and/or mechanical abnormality.

Definitive therapy can be divided into **General Therapy**—modalities to be considered in all cases of cardiac arrest before a specific electrical abnormality has been identified, and **Specific Therapy**—modalities designed for specific electrocardiographic or mechanical abnormalities.

GENERAL THERAPY

Management of Acidosis. Severe acidosis can develop within 5 minutes after cardiac arrest and will continue unless BCLS is provided. Acidosis is due primarily to a respiratory component (hypoventilation) and to a lesser extent to a metabolic component (lactic acidosis), which occurs later.

1. *Respiratory acidosis:*
   - Etiology: Accumulation of CO_2 secondary to hypoventilation.
   - Treatment: Adequate ventilation, *no* role for sodium bicarbonate.
2. *Metabolic acidosis:*
   - Etiology: Slow accumulation of lactic acid secondary to anaerobic metabolism within hypoperfused (hypoxic) tissues.
   - Treatment: Adequate perfusion of oxygenated blood will delay development of clinically important lactic acidosis. Thus, early administration of sodium bicarbonate (buffer) is not indicated unless pre-existing acidosis, hyperkalemia, or tricyclic antidepressant (TCA) overdose is documented. There are no proven benefits of bicarbonate, and it can produce devastating complications, including shift of the oxyhemoglobin saturation curve to the left (decreasing release of oxygen), hyperosmolarity, hypernatremia, paradoxical intracellular acidosis (because of production of carbon dioxide, which diffuses readily into cells), exacerbation of central venous acidosis, and possible inactivation of simultaneously administered catecholamines.

   Therefore
   - Do *not* administer sodium bicarbonate until after specific therapy (eg, incubation, antidysrhythmics) has been employed and only at the discretion of the team leader after considering the possible complications noted above.

If the decision to use bicarbonate is made, then the following guidelines should be followed:

- *If arterial blood gases (ABGs) are not available,* then empiric administration of **sodium bicarbonate, IV slow push, 1 mEq/kg initially,** then not more than **0.5 mEq/kg** q 10 minutes (50 mL of 7.5% solution = 44.6 mEq [0.9 mEq/mL]; 50 mL of 8.4% solution = 50 mEq [1 mEq/mL]).
- *If ABGs are available,* then sodium bicarbonate doses can be calculated from the base deficit:

$$\text{NaHCO}_3 \text{ dose in mEq} =$$
$$\text{Base deficit in mEq/L} \times 0.2 \times \text{body weight in kg}$$

EPINEPHRINE—EMPIRIC USE

Epinephrine is often given empirically at the start of definitive therapy, even before an ECG diagnosis has been made. The basis for this empiric use is epinephrine's α-adrenergic receptor agonist activity, which increases systemic vascular resistance, enhancing perfusion of the myocardium and CNS during CPR. Thus, the following is appropriate:

- **epinephrine HCl, IV push, 1 mg** (10 mL of 1:10,000 solution, or 1 mL of 1:1000 diluted to 10 mL with NS); may repeat q 3–5 minutes. (*See* Special Considerations/Precautions: high-dose epinephrine.)

If IV access has not been established or has been lost, *then:*

- **epinephrine HCl, via endotracheal tube, 2–2.5 mg** (20–25 mL of 1:10,000 solution), followed by 3 or 4 rapid ventilations to disperse drug. If neither IV nor endotracheal access is available, consider intraosseous administration. (*See* Special Considerations/Precautions.)

SPECIFIC THERAPY

In order to simplify the pharmacologic management of cardiopulmonary arrest, disturbances of cardiac activity associated with cardiac arrest may be grouped into three major categories, each of which can be approached in a logical manner: ventricular tachydysrhythmias, bradydysrhythmias (including asystole), and pulseless electrical activity.

Ventricular Tachydysrhythmias.   Considered in this category, and treated in the same way, are ventricular fibrillation, ventricular flutter, and ventricular tachycardia when associated with ineffective cardiac output.

1. *Electrical defibrillation, 200 joules delivered.* If tachydysrhythmias persist, then subsequent defibrillation should deliver more energy (eg, 200–300 joules for second shock; 360 joules for third shock).
2. Epinephrine HCl, IV push, 1 mg (10 mL of 1:10,000 solution) is commonly stated to be an effective adjunct for successful defibrillation, especially

when ventricular fibrillation is monitored as "fine" fibrillatory waves. There are no scientific data to support this concept; *thus, epinephrine is not recommended as an aid to defibrillation specifically, but rather as an aid to myocardial perfusion.* (*See* Epinephrine—Empiric Use.)

3. In intractable ventricular tachydysrhythmias or when there is repeated reversion to tachydysrhythmias following electrical defibrillation, an irritable focus in the myocardium may be the source of persistent tachydysrhythmias and an antidysrhythmic drug is indicated (if digitalis toxicity is suspected, *see* item 7):
   - **lidocaine HCl, IV push, 50–100 mg (1–1.5 mg/kg)** (2.5–5 mL of 2% or 5–10 mL of 1% solution); may repeat q 3–5 min to a total of 3 mg/kg.

   If IV access has not been established or has been lost, *then:*
   - **lidocaine HCl via endotracheal tube, 150–300 mg (3 mg/kg)** (7.5–15 mL of 2% solution), followed by 3 or 4 rapid ventilations to disperse drug.

   If neither IV nor endotracheal access is available, consider intraosseous administration. (*See* Special Considerations/Precautions.)

   If response to loading dose occurs, *then maintenance:*
   - **lidocaine HCl, IV infusion, 2–4 mg/min (20–50 μg/kg/min)** (10 mL of 20% in 500 mL D5W = 4 mg/mL).

4. If lidocaine fails to maintain electrical stability, *then:*
   - **bretylium tosylate, IV push, 350–500 mg (5 mg/kg)** (50 mg/mL, 7–10 mL); may repeat with 10 mg/kg q 5 minutes to total of 30–35 mg/kg. Note that bretylium frequently has a slow onset of action (>10 min). While waiting for this effect, one could administer procainamide HCl (*see* item 5) in an attempt to gain control of the dysrhythmia rapidly. The important point to recognize is that once primary therapy fails, second-line agents are not predictably effective. Should procainamide fail to suppress tachydysrhythmias, the slower-acting bretylium will already have been administered. Should procainamide be effective, then subsequent doses of bretylium will not be necessary.

   If response to loading dose occurs, *then maintenance:*
   - **bretylium tosylate, IV infusion, 1–2 mg/minute**.

5. If lidocaine- and bretylium-resistant dysrhythmias persist, or if one elects to administer procainamide concurrently with bretylium, *then:*
   - **procainamide HCl, IV push, 500 mg** (5 mL of 100 mg/mL vial, or 1 mL of 500 mg/mL vial); may repeat in 5 min to a total of 1 g. Note that this rate is greater than the commonly reported 20–50 mg/min; however, this is a life-threatening dysrhythmia and a delay in drug administration may result in treatment failure.

   If response to loading dose occurs, *then maintenance:*
   - **procainamide HCl, IV infusion, 1–5 mg/min** (20–80 μg/kg/min).

6. If lidocaine-, bretylium- and procainamide-resistant dysrhythmias persist, *then:*
   - **propranolol HCl, IV push, 1 mg over 1 min** (1 mg/mL ampule); may repeat q 5 min to a total of 0.1 mg/kg.

7. If all of the above fail or if digitalis toxicity or hypomagnesemia is suspected, *consider:*
   - **magnesium sulfate, IV push, 1–2 g (8–16 mEq) over 1–2 minutes** (2–4 mL of 50% solution diluted in 10 mL D5W); may repeat after 5 minutes if no response.
8. IV amiodarone is approved for the treatment and prophylaxis of frequently recurring ventricular fibrillation and hemodynamically unstable ventricular tachycardia refractory to other therapy. Amiodarone may present an alternative to available therapies and has been effective in the cardiac arrest setting in small studies. However, its role in the arrest setting and in treatment algorithms remains to be defined.

Bradydysrhythmias.   Considered in this category, and treated in the same way, are asystole, complete heart block, slow ventricular focus, sinus bradycardia, and agonal rhythm. In dealing with any of these dysrhythmias (except asystole), transvenous pacing is probably the best long-term approach, but is usually not readily available. Thus, drugs are used to enhance or initiate cardiac activity, at least until transvenous or transthoracic pacing equipment becomes available.

It is important to note that true asystole, unless it is the result of excessive vagal tone (bradyasystole event), is frequently associated with irreversible cardiac damage.

1. Treatment of bradydysrhythmias should be initiated with:
   - **atropine sulfate, IV push, 0.5–1 mg** (5–10 mL of 0.1 mg/mL solution); may repeat with 0.5–1 mg q 3–5 minutes to a total of 3 mg.
   If IV access has not been established or has been lost, *then:*
   - **atropine sulfate, via endotracheal tube, 1–2.5 mg** (10–25 mL of 0.1 mg/mL solution), followed by 3 or 4 rapid ventilations to disperse drug.
   If neither IV nor endotracheal access is available, consider intraosseous administration. (*See* Special Considerations/Precautions.)
2. For bradydysrhythmias failing to respond to atropine, *then:*
   - **epinephrine HCl, IV push, 0.5–1 mg** (5–10 mL of 1:10,000); may repeat after 3–5 min. (*See* Special Considerations/Precautions: high-dose epinephrine.)
3. For bradydysrhythmias failing to respond to the above, some experts have recommended isoproterenol. The use of isoproterenol, although supported by AHA-ACLS guidelines, is probably inappropriate, because β-adrenergic agonist–mediated vasodilation may actually lower perfusion pressures during CPR. Thus, the use of isoproterenol cannot be justified.

Pulseless Electrical Activity (PEA).   PEA was previously known as electromechanical dissociation. Considered in this category are ineffective cardiac output (hypotension) in the face of ECG evidence of electrical myocardial activity, hypotension secondary to inadequate peripheral vasoconstriction, volume depletion, cardiac tamponade, tension pneumothorax, or massive pulmonary embolism. Hypoventilation and hypoxia, as well as a number of drug overdoses including tricyclic antidepressants, digoxin, and calcium-channel antagonists, can produce PEA. Many causes of PEA have specific interventions. Recognition and treatment of an underlying cause, whenever possible, is the hallmark of PEA management.

1. Nonspecific treatment measures include administration of epinephrine HCl (1 mg IV push every 3–5 min) and, if bradycardic, atropine (1 mg IV push every 3–5 min to a total of 3 mg).
2. Since hypovolemia is the most common underlying cause, rapidly assess volume status—if depleted, fluid challenge with crystalloid (NS or lactated Ringer's injection) or colloid (hetastarch or albumin human).
3. If volume is adequate and no evidence of tamponade, then consider cardiac sympathomimetics for vasoconstricting and inotropic/chronotropic effects. Begin with:
   - **dopamine HCl, IV infusion, 5 µg/kg/minute initially,** increasing prn to a maximum of 20 µg/kg/minute, adjusting rate to keep systolic blood pressure between 90 and 100 mm Hg (400 mg in 500 mL D5W = 800 µg/mL).
4. If dopamine fails, *then:*
   - **norepinephrine bitartrate, IV infusion, 8 µg/min initially,** adjusting, as needed, to keep systolic blood pressure between 90 and 100 mm Hg (8 mL of 0.1% solution [1 mg/mL] in 500 mL D5W = 16 µg/mL).
5. If norepinephrine fails, consider high-dose epinephrine. (*See* Special Considerations/Precautions.)
6. Calcium administration in the therapy of pulseless electrical activity has not been shown to be effective and, in fact, may be harmful. Therefore, its use should be confined to situations in which acceptable therapy has failed or in situations in which calcium therapy is antidotal (eg, hyperkalemia, hypocalcemia, calcium-channel blocker toxicity), in which case add:
   - **calcium chloride, IV slow push, 0.5–1 g** (5–10 mL of 10% solution = 6.8–13.6 mEq), *or*
   - **calcium gluconate, IV slow push, 1–2 g** (10–20 mL of 10% solution = 4.7–9.4 mEq), *or*
   - **calcium gluceptate, IV slow push, 1.1–2.2 g** (5–10 mL = 4.5–9 mEq).

■ POSTRESUSCITATION CARE

Patients who have been successfully resuscitated are at great risk of experiencing subsequent events. Thus, if the patient is not already in an intensive care setting with constant monitoring, readily available resuscitation equipment, and skilled nursing staff, transport the patient to such an area as soon as possible. The cause of the initial episode must be sought and corrected if possible.

■ SPECIAL CONSIDERATIONS/PRECAUTIONS

Because of concern regarding the possibility that dextrose-containing fluids administered during ACLS may worsen neurologic outcome. NS or lactated Ringer's injection should be considered the fluids of choice, with dextrose-containing solutions reserved for patients believed to be hypoglycemic.

Systemic circulation times are grossly prolonged during external chest compression. Remember to allow *at least* 2 minutes between the time of peripheral injection of pharmacologic agents and anticipated response. To enhance the onset and activity of peripherally administered medications, they should be administered by rapid bolus injection, followed by a 20 mL bolus of IV fluid and elevation of the extremity, if possible.

Initial studies of **high-dose epinephrine** (up to 0.2 mg/kg IV q 5 minutes) indicated that the higher doses may be more effective than standard ACLS doses. However, more recent studies have found no advantage of high-dose over standard-dose epinephrine. In any event, ACLS guidelines allow options for **intermediate** (2–5 mg IV push q 3–5 minutes); **escalating** (1 mg, then 3 mg, then 5 mg separated by 3 minutes); or **high-dose** (0.1 mg/kg IV push q 3–5 minutes) epinephrine.

Endotracheal administration of epinephrine, lidocaine, or atropine can be used in situations in which IV access has not been established or has been lost. Doses 2–3 times the IV dose and diluted in 10 mL NS or distilled water are advised. Endotracheal administration may not be as effective as IV administration.

Intraosseous administration of epinephrine, atropine, sodium bicarbonate, lidocaine, vasopressors, or calcium via the distal tibia can be used in situations in which IV access and endotracheal intubation have not been established.

Intracardiac injections of drugs play *no* role in modern management of cardiopulmonary arrest. Drugs do not work within the chambers of the heart, but rather at the cellular level after delivery via the coronary circulation. Stopping BCLS to attempt intracardiac injections only serves to interrupt vital CNS perfusion.

Be aware of the possible **physical incompatibilities** of sodium bicarbonate and catecholamines. In addition, sodium bicarbonate and calcium-containing solutions may form a precipitate if infused at the same time in the same IV line.

■ REFERENCES

1. Otto CW et al, eds. Wolf Creek III conference on cardiopulmonary resuscitation. *Crit Care Med* 1985;13: 881–951.
2. Raehl CL. Endotracheal drug therapy in cardiopulmonary resuscitation. *Clin Pharm* 1986;572–9.
3. Iserson KV. Intraosseous infusions in adults. *J Emerg Med* 1989;7:587–91.
4. Callaham ML. High-dose epinephrine therapy and other advances in treating cardiac arrest. *West J Med* 1990; 152:697–703.
5. Anon. Adult advanced cardiac life support. *JAMA* 1992;268:2199–41.
6. Niemann JT. Cardiopulmonary resuscitation. *N Engl J Med* 1992;327:1075–80.
7. Grillo JA, Gonzalez ER. Changes in the pharmacotherapy of CPR. *Heart Lung* 1993;22:548–53.
8. Chow MSS. Advanced cardiac life support controversy: where do antiarrhythmic agents fit in? *Pharmacotherapy* 1997;17(2 Pt 2):84S–8S.

Poisoning

William G. Troutman

Management of the poisoned patient involves procedures designed to prevent the absorption, minimize the toxicity, and hasten the elimination of the suspected toxin. The prompt employment of appropriate emergency management procedures can often prevent unnecessary morbidity and mortality.

A regional poison center is a practitioner's best source of definitive treatment information and should be consulted in all poisonings, regardless of the apparent simplicity of the case. Contact the regional poison center in your area to learn of its staffing, resources, and capabilities before a need for its services arises. Well-qualified regional centers are certified by the American Association of Poison Control Centers.

In all cases, every attempt should be made to accurately identify the toxin, estimate the quantity involved, and determine the time that has passed since the exposure. These data, plus patient-specific parameters such as age, weight, sex, and underlying medical conditions or drug use, will assist you and the regional poison center in designing an appropriate therapeutic plan for the patient.

The techniques described below are intended for the initial management of the poisoned patient using materials that should be readily available.

■ TOPICAL EXPOSURES

1. *Immediately* irrigate affected areas with a copious amount of water; use soap only if a stubborn, oily substance is the contaminant. Skin should be gently washed, not scrubbed, and special attention should be given to the hair, skin folds, umbilicus, and other areas where the contaminant might be trapped.
2. If the patient's clothes have been contaminated, remove them during the irrigation and either clean them before they are worn again or destroy them. Clothing can interfere with the irrigation process and can serve as a reservoir of toxic material.
3. Do not attempt to "neutralize" the contaminant with another chemical (eg, acids and alkalis). Attempts at neutralization waste valuable time, are of no benefit, and may be harmful.
4. Do not cover the affected area with emollients. These may trap unremoved contaminant against the skin. Severely damaged skin may be temporarily covered with a light, dry dressing.
5. Protect yourself from contamination. Gloves, aprons, or a change of clothes may be necessary.
6. After the irrigation is complete, contact a regional poison center for definitive treatment information.

■ EYE EXPOSURES

1. *Immediately* irrigate the eye; damage can occur within seconds. The stream of water from the tap or a pitcher should strike the patient on the forehead, temple, or bridge of the nose and then flow into the eye.
2. The eyelids should be open with frequent blinking during the irrigation.
3. The irrigation should continue for at least 15 minutes (by the clock) to ensure adequate removal of the contaminant and normalization of the conjunctival pH. Body temperature water or saline may be substituted for tap water as the irrigation proceeds, but only if they can be obtained without interrupting the irrigation.
4. After the irrigation is complete, contact a regional poison center for definitive treatment information.

■ INHALATION EXPOSURES

1. Remove the patient from the suspected contaminated area, regardless of its apparent safety. Carbon monoxide, a common inhaled toxin, cannot be detected by sight, smell, or taste.
2. Institute artificial ventilation, if necessary, and provide supplementary humidified oxygen if available and needed.
3. Protect yourself from contamination at all times.
4. Contact a regional poison center for definitive treatment information.

■ INGESTIONS

1. Remove any remaining contaminant from inside and around the mouth of the patient.
2. Give a small amount of water to clear the mouth and esophagus.
3. Contact a regional poison center for definitive treatment information.
4. In many cases, it will not be necessary to take further steps. The following information can be utilized if additional care is recommended by the regional poison center.

■ GASTROINTESTINAL DECONTAMINATION

Gastrointestinal (GI) decontamination may be accomplished by the administration of activated charcoal, gastric lavage, ipecac-induced emesis, and whole-bowel irrigation. Indications for GI decontamination are ingestion of a known toxic dose, ingestion of an unknown dose of a known toxic substance, and ingestion of a substance of unknown toxicity. For all methods of GI decontamination, the value of the procedure diminishes rapidly with time. Some authors now question the usefulness of gastric lavage or ipecac-induced emesis more than 1 hour after ingestion. None of these techniques should be presumed to provide complete removal or binding of the ingested toxin(s). Comparative experimental studies have shown only limited success with these techniques and there is considerable interpatient variability in the results. In general, activated charcoal is the most useful agent for preventing absorption of ingested toxic substances. Other methods of GI decontamination may be considered if the ingested contaminant is not adsorbed by activated charcoal or if circumstances do not permit its prompt administration.

ACTIVATED CHARCOAL

Activated charcoal is a nonspecific absorbent that binds unabsorbed toxins within the GI tract. There is limited experience using activated charcoal in the home setting. Activated charcoal is not effective for absorbing strong acids and alkalis, cyanide, ethanol, methanol, ethylene glycol, iron, or lithium.

1. Activated charcoal is administered orally or by gastric tube in doses that range from 30 to 120 g.
2. Activated charcoal is commercially supplied as a slurry in water or a concentrated solution of sorbitol. The water-based products are preferred because the large amount of sorbitol that accompanies a typical dose of activated charcoal may result in excessive sorbitol-induced catharsis, producing fluid and electrolyte imbalance. Gentle encouragement may be needed to make children swallow the charcoal. Having the child take the liquid through a drinking straw from an opaque container is sometimes helpful.
3. Activated charcoal administration is commonly followed by the administration of a cathartic (eg, sorbitol, magnesium citrate, or magnesium sulfate) to hasten the elimination of the activated charcoal-toxin complex. There is no evidence to support cathartic use.
4. Alert the patient that charcoal will cause the stools to turn black.
5. Repeated oral doses of activated charcoal (eg, 20–30 g q 4 hours) have been used to enhance the elimination of some drugs, most notably carbamazepine, phenobarbital, salicylate, or theophylline. Multiple-dose activated charcoal is only suitable for patients with active bowel sounds.

GASTRIC LAVAGE

Lavage may be more effective in recovering toxin than ipecac-induced emesis, and it has the advantage of being useful in patients with CNS depression.

1. If the patient's gag reflex is weak or absent, the airway must be protected by the use of a cuffed endotracheal tube.
2. The largest possible orogastric tube should be used (26–28 F for children and 34–42 F for adults): the larger the tube diameter, the more efficient the lavage. The tube should be introduced through the mouth with the aid of a water-soluble lubricant. Nasogastric passage is not recommended.
3. Gastric lavage may be done with water, but a solution like 0.45% NaCl may be used to minimize the risk of dilutional hyponatremia, especially in children. Aliquots of fluid up to 100 mL in children and 200 mL in adults are introduced through the tube and then removed by gravity or suction-assisted drainage. The lavage should be continued for several cycles after the returning fluid is clear. Warming the lavage fluid will reduce the risk of hypothermia.

INDUCTION OF EMESIS

Do not induce emesis if the patient is experiencing or is at risk for CNS depression, seizures, or loss of gag reflex, or if the patient has ingested a caustic substance.

1. Induce emesis only with syrup of ipecac. Salt water, mustard water, other "home remedies," or gagging have no place in the management of the poisoned patient. These techniques are ineffective and can be dangerous.
2. The usual initial dose of **syrup of ipecac** is 30 mL in persons over 5 years of age, 15 mL in children 1–5 years old, and 10 mL in children between 6 months and 1 year of age.
3. Give the patient additional water to drink: 125–250 mL (4–8 fl oz) in children, 250–500 mL (8–16 fl oz) in adults. Activated charcoal should not be given until after ipecac-induced emesis has occurred.
4. Emesis usually occurs within 15–20 minutes. If 30 minutes have passed without emesis, administer an additional dose of syrup of ipecac and more water.
5. Have the patient vomit into a bowl or other container so that the vomitus can be inspected for the presence of the ingested toxin. The endpoint is clearing of the rectal effluent.

WHOLE-BOWEL IRRIGATION

Whole-bowel irrigation with an orally administered **polyethylene glycol electrolyte solution** (eg, GoLYTELY or CoLyte) is commonly used prior to bowel procedures. It has drawn attention as an alternative to other methods of GI decontamination in the management of acute poisoning. Results of studies are promising and the technique may have value in cases of ingestion of iron, enteric-coated or sustained-release products, foreign bodies, and drug-smuggling packets. Instillation rates have ranged from 500 mL/hour in children to 2 L/hour in adults. Typically, 4–6 L of fluid are administered.

■ REFERENCES

1. Smilkstein MJ, Flomenbaum NE. Techniques used to prevent absorption of toxic compounds. In, Goldfrank LR, Flomenbaum NE, Lewin NA, et al., eds. *Goldfrank's toxicologic emergencies.* 5th ed. Norwalk, CT: Appleton & Lange; 1994;47–59.
2. Olson KR. Comprehensive evaluation and treatment of poisoning and drug overdose. In, Olson KR, ed. *Poisoning and drug overdose.* 2nd ed. Norwalk, CT: Appleton & Lange; 1994:1–58.
3. Shannon MW, Haddad LM. The emergency management of poisoning. In, Haddad LM et al, eds. *Clinical management of poisoning and drug overdose.* 3rd ed. Philadelphia: WB Saunders; 1998:2–31.
4. Gut decontamination. In, Ellenhorn MJ. *Ellenhorn's medical toxicology: diagnosis and treatment of human poisoning.* 2nd ed. Baltimore: Williams & Wilkins; 1997:66–78.
5. Herrington AM, Clifton GD. Toxicology and management of acute drug ingestions in adults. *Pharmacotherapy* 1995;15:182–200.
6. Oderda GM. Gastrointestinal decontamination. *J Pharm Pract* 1993;6:48–56.
7. Kulig K. Initial management of ingestions of toxic substances. *N Engl J Med* 1992;326:1677–81.
8. Manoguerra AS. Gastrointestinal decontamination after poisoning: where is the science? *Crit Care Clin* 1997;13:709–25.
9. Wheeler-Usher DH et al. Gastric emptying. Risk versus benefit in the treatment of acute poisoning. *Med Toxicol* 1986;1:142–53.

10. Palatnick W, Tenenbein M. Activated charcoal in the treatment of drug overdose. An update. *Drug Saf* 1992;7:3–7.

11. Merigian KS et al. Prospective evaluation of gastric emptying in the self-poisoned patient. *Am J Emerg Med* 1990;8:479–83.

12. Shannon M et al. Cathartics and laxatives. Do they still have a place in management of the poisoned patient? *Med Toxicol* 1986;1:247–52.

13. Tenenbein M et al. Efficacy of ipecac-induced emesis, orogastric lavage, and activated charcoal for acute drug overdose. *Ann Emerg Med* 1987;16:838–41.

14. Tandberg D, Troutman WG. Gastric lavage in the poisoned patient. In, Roberts JR, Hedges JR, eds. *Clinical procedures in emergency medicine.* 2nd ed. Philadelphia: WB Saunders; 1991;655–62.

15. Kirshenbaum LA et al. Whole-bowel irrigation versus activated charcoal in sorbitol for the ingestion of modified-release pharmaceuticals. *Clin Pharmacol Ther* 1989;46:264–71.

Status Epilepticus

Brian K. Alldredge

Status epilepticus is a medical emergency in which prompt recognition and effective medical intervention are required to reduce the risk of permanent sequelae and death. Status epilepticus is defined as either continuous seizures lasting at least 5 minutes, or two or more sequential seizures without full recovery of consciousness between seizures.

Status epilepticus can be divided into two major types: convulsive and nonconvulsive. Convulsive status epilepticus is associated with the highest risk of morbidity and mortality, so this section focuses on the clinical features and management of this form of status epilepticus.

In about one-half of patients, status epilepticus is the first manifestation of seizures. The causes of status epilepticus are similar to those for new-onset seizures and include CNS infection, cerebral tumor, trauma, stroke, metabolic disorders, cardiopulmonary arrest, and drug toxicity. In the remainder of patients, status occurs in the setting of a pre-existing seizure disorder. Among persons with a history of epilepsy, antiepileptic drug withdrawal (usually noncompliance with prescribed therapy) is the most common cause of status epilepticus.

The primary determinant of patient outcome after status epilepticus is the underlying cause of the episode. In general, patients with status caused by an acute or progressive neurologic insult (eg, cardiopulmonary arrest, stroke) have poorer outcomes than patients in whom status epilepticus occurs in the setting of a more chronic or stable underlying condition (eg, antiepileptic drug withdrawal or medically refractory epilepsy). Nonetheless, aggressive medical intervention and administration of effective antiepileptic drug therapy are important to reduce status-related morbidity and mortality, regardless of the etiology.

Status epilepticus should be managed in an emergency department or in an environment where continuous skilled medical and nursing support are available. The emergency management of status epilepticus should include the following:

- Ensure airway patency and adequate oxygenation.
- Obtain blood specimens for baseline laboratory measurements, including CBC, serum electrolytes (including calcium and magnesium), toxicologic screen, and anticonvulsant serum levels.
- Establish IV access.
- Administer IV glucose (100 mg thiamine followed by 50 mL of 50% glucose in adults).
- Administer IV antiepileptic drugs.
- Monitor blood pressure and temperature. Treat hyperthermia with passive cooling.
- Obtain other diagnostic studies as needed.
- Treat precipitating factors.

■ DRUG THERAPY OF STATUS EPILEPTICUS

Adult doses only are given in this section.

If a treatable cause of status epilepticus can be identified rapidly, then drug therapy to terminate seizures may be unnecessary. In these situations, treatment of the underlying cause may be sufficient to stop status. Examples include status caused by an acute metabolic derangement (where correction of the underlying abnormality often stops seizures) or status following isoniazid overdose (where IV pyridoxine is usually effective). However, when a treatable cause is not found, drug therapy should begin immediately. The goal of drug treatment is to terminate seizures as rapidly as possible. Evidence from animal and human studies indicate that 60–120 min of status epilepticus is associated with neurologic sequelae and that the risk increases as status continues. Thus, it is important to have a clear, stepwise plan for the administration of effective drug therapy. Figure 5–1 is an example of a status epilepticus treatment protocol. Additionally, adequate support should be available to manage cardiac and respiratory complications that may occur during drug administration.

1. For rapid termination of seizures:
   - **lorazepam, IV, 0.1 mg/kg (4–8 mg) at rate of 2 mg/minute;** may repeat in 10 min if seizures continue (to maximum of 0.2 mg/kg). Lorazepam

Figure 5–1. Timeline for administration of drug therapy for convulsive status epilepticus. Heavy bars (▬) indicate duration (in minutes) of intravenous drug administration. PE = phenytoin equivalents.

has a longer duration of anticonvulsant effect than diazepam and is often preferred for this reason.

or

- **diazepam, IV, 0.2 mg/kg (5–10 mg) at rate of 5 mg/minute;** may repeat in 10 minutes if seizures continue (to maximum of 20 mg). Diazepam has a short duration of anticonvulsant effect (15–60 minutes) and must be immediately followed by a long-acting agent (eg, phenytoin).

2a. Following benzodiazepine administration, give:
- **phenytoin, IV infusion, 20 mg/kg at rate of 50 mg/minute** or **fosphenytoin 20 mg/kg phenytoin equivalents IV at a rate of 150 mg/minute.** Monitor blood pressure and ECG during administration of phenytoin loading dose. Elderly and severely ill patients are predisposed to phenytoin-related hypotension.

2b. If status persists, *then:*
- **phenytoin** or **fosphenytoin, IV,** up to 2 additional doses of 5 mg/kg, to a total dosage of 30 mg/kg.

2c. If status is terminated, then begin maintenance phenytoin therapy.

3. If seizures are not terminated after administration of phenytoin or fosphenytoin 30 mg/kg,
   then:
- **phenobarbital, IV, 20 mg/kg at rate of 100 mg/minute.** The risk of hypoventilation is increased markedly when phenobarbital is administered after benzodiazepines; respiratory support is often required.

4. For patients who continue in status epilepticus despite the above recommendations, anesthetic doses of benzodiazepines, barbiturates, or propofol are often required to suppress seizure activity. Ventilatory assistance and vasopressor drug therapy are often required; therefore, the patient should be admitted to the ICU and the following therapies considered:

4a. **midazolam, IV slow push, 200 µg/kg,** *then maintenance:*
- **midazolam, IV infusion, 0.75–10 µg/kg/minute.** High-dose midazolam is probably associated with a lower risk of hypotension than high-dose pentobarbital; however, there is less experience with its use.

4b. **pentobarbital, IV infusion, 1–2 mg/kg/hour.** Hypotension is a frequent complication of high-dose pentobarbital therapy; vasopressor (eg, dopamine) may be required.
   or

4c. **propofol, IV slow push, 1 mg/kg,** *then maintenance:*
- **propofol, IV infusion 2–4 mg/kg/hour.** Reduce dosage by one-half in elderly or hemodynamically unstable patients.

The EEG should be monitored continuously during the first 1–2 hours of therapy, and infusion rates should be adjusted until suppression of electrographic seizures is evident. After seizures are terminated, the rate of the maintenance infusion can be slowed periodically to determine if status has remitted.

■ REFERENCES

1. Working Group on Status Epilepticus. Treatment of convulsive status epilepticus. Recommendations of the Epilepsy Foundation of America's working group on status epilepticus. *JAMA* 1993;270:854–9.
2. Lowenstein DH, Alldredge BK. Status epilepticus at an urban public hospital in the 1980s. *Neurology* 1993;43(3 pt 1):483–8.
3. Lowenstein DH et al. Barbiturate anesthesia in the treatment of status epilepticus: clinical experience with 14 patients. *Neurology* 1988;38:395–400.
4. Parent JM, Lowenstein DH. Treatment of refractory generalized status epilepticus with continuous infusion of midazolam. *Neurology* 1994;44:1837–40.
5. Shorvon SD. *Status epilepticus: its clinical features and treatment in children and adults.* New York, NY: Cambridge University Press; 1994.
6. Stecker MM et al. Treatment of refractory status epilepticus with propofol: clinical and pharmacokinetic findings. *Epilepsia* 1998;39:18–26.
7. Lowenstein DH, Alldredge BK. Current concepts: status epilepticus. *N Engl J Med* 1998;338:970–6.

6 Nutrition Support

Fred Shatsky

Nutrition status is a major determinant of patients' morbidity and mortality. Morbidity increases with malnutrition as is manifested by depressed immunocompetence and impaired wound healing.[1] Conditions that indicate a possible need for nutrition support include inadequate oral nutrition for longer than 7 days, recent body weight loss >10%, an illness lasting more than 3 weeks, recent major surgery, a lymphocyte count <1.2×10^3 μL, serum albumin <3 g/dL, serum transferrin <150 mg/dL, and serum prealbumin <15 mg/dL. Sepsis, trauma, and other factors that induce hypermetabolism may intensify the need.

The term "nutrition support" can be applied to any nutrition regimen that is provided for conditions that preclude the use of regular foods. There are two broad categories of nutrition support, enteral and parenteral, determined by their route of administration. Enteral nutrition applies to regimens provided via any portion of the gastrointestinal (GI) tract. Parenteral nutrition (PN), although implying all routes other than the GI tract, refers primarily to regimens that are provided directly by the intravenous route of administration. Less frequently used modes of PN such as intradialytic parenteral nutrition (IDPN) and intraperitoneal nutrition (IPN) are not discussed in this chapter.

Whenever possible, maintenance rather than repletion should be the primary objective of nutrition support. Early provision of nutrition requirements without exceeding energy balance promotes the synthesis of lean body mass rather than adipose tissue.[2]

■ NUTRITION ASSESSMENT

Nutrition assessment of the patient can aid in diagnosing malnutrition and determining its degree of severity, so that a proper nutrition support regimen can be formulated. The patient's physical and dietary history should be obtained to establish baseline data. Clinical parameters for assessing the patient's nutrition status can be evaluated through the use of an assessment form (Table 6–1). Because a patient's nutrition status is best reflected by body protein, nutrition assessment should focus on the protein compartments. Protein compartments are classified into two types: somatic (muscle protein) and visceral (all other protein).

TABLE 6–1. NUTRITION ASSESSMENT[a]

NAME: AGE: HT (CM): DATE: SEX: WT (KG):	STANDARD	Mild	Moderate	Severe
Triceps Skinfold (TSF), mm =	M 12.5	11.3	11.3–7.5	<7.5
Ideal Body Weight:	F 16.5	14.9	14.9–9.9	<9.9
$\frac{ABW}{IBW} \times 100 =$	100%	90%	90–60%	<60%
Mid–Upper Arm Circumference	M 29.3	26.4	26.4–17.6	<17.6
(MUAC), cm	F 28.5	25.7	25.7–17.1	<17.1
Mid–Upper Arm Muscle Circumference	M 25.3	22.8	22.8–15.2	<15.2
MUAC (cm) – [0.314 × TSF (mm)] =	F 23.2	21.0	21.0–13.9	<13.9
Creatinine/Height Index:				
$\frac{Cr_u}{ICr_u \text{ for height}} \times 100 =$	100%	90%	90–60%	<60%
Serum Albumin, g/dL =	3.5–5.0	3.5–3.0	3.0–2.1	<2.1
Serum Prealbumin, mg/dL =	>20	20–15	15–10	<10
Serum Transferrin, mg/dL =	200–400	200–150	150–100	<100
Total Lymphocyte/μL:	1800–3000	1800–1200	1200–800	<800
$\frac{WBC/\mu L \times \% \text{ Lymphocytes}}{100}$				

[a] The standards specified represent those of healthy persons. Measurements in patients may be additionally affected by nonnutritional as well as nutritional factors.
ABW, actual body weight; Cr_u, urinary creatinine; IBW, ideal body weight; ICr_u, ideal urinary creatinine; MUAC, mid–upper arm circumference; TSF, triceps skinfold.

SOMATIC PROTEIN ASSESSMENT PARAMETERS

Percentage Ideal Body Weight. A simple initial measurement of a patient's nutrition status is body weight expressed as a percentage of ideal body weight. (*See* Appendix 2, Anthropometrics.)

$$\text{Percentage Ideal Body Weight} = \frac{\text{Actual Body Weight}}{\text{Ideal Body Weight}} \times 100$$

Creatinine/Height Index. Creatinine/height index (CHI), when accurately obtained, is a more sensitive indicator of somatic protein and nutrition status than is percentage ideal body weight. Creatinine, a product of muscle metabolism, is normally excreted in urine at a constant rate proportional to the amount of skeletal muscle and lean body mass catabolized. CHI is calculated from a 24-hr urinary creatinine measurement and the ideal urinary creatinine value found in Table 6–2, using the following formula:

$$CHI = \frac{\text{Actual Urinary Creatinine}}{\text{Ideal Urinary Creatinine for Height}} \times 100$$

It is important that the urine sample be an aliquot drawn from a 24-hour collection of urine rather than a random sample.

TABLE 6–2. IDEAL URINARY CREATININE

MALES[a]		FEMALES[b]	
Height *(cm)*	*Ideal Creatinine* *(mg/24 hr)*	*Height* *(cm)*	*Ideal Creatinine* *(mg/24 hr)*
157.5	1288	147.3	830
160.0	1325	149.9	851
162.6	1359	152.4	875
165.1	1386	154.9	900
167.6	1426	157.5	925
170.2	1467	160.0	949
172.7	1513	162.6	977
175.3	1555	165.1	1006
177.8	1596	167.6	1044
180.3	1642	170.2	1076
182.9	1691	172.7	1109
185.4	1739	175.3	1141
188.0	1785	177.8	1174
190.5	1831	180.3	1206
193.0	1891	182.9	1240

[a]Creatinine coefficient (men) = 23 mg/kg of ideal body weight.
[b]Creatinine coefficient (women) = 18 mg/kg of ideal body weight.
From Blackburn GL et al, Nutritional and metabolic assessment of the hospitalized patient. JPEN 1977;1:11–22, reproduced with permission.

There are limitations in using CHI as an indicator of malnutrition. Patients sometimes excrete amounts of creatinine and nitrogen that vary with different diets, medications, degree of renal function, conditions of illness, or stress. Certain drugs interfere with urine creatinine determinations. (*See* Drug–Laboratory Test Interferences, page 1035.)

Anthropometric Measurements. Anthropometric measurements may be of questionable value because of slow change over time and interobserver variability. If used, the triceps skinfold (TSF) and mid–upper arm circumference (MUAC) should be taken on the mid–upper portion of the nondominant arm by trained personnel. Detailed procedures and methods of measurement are available.[3,4] TSF measurement with calipers is compared to the standards in Table 6–1 to give a reasonable estimate of subcutaneous fat reserves. Both TSF and MUAC, obtained with a tape measure, can be used to derive the mid–upper arm muscle circumference (MUAMC) by the formula:

$$MUAMC = MUAC \text{ (cm)} - (0.314 \times TSF \text{ [mm]})$$

VISCERAL PROTEIN ASSESSMENT PARAMETERS

The status of visceral protein reflects the patient's ability to respond to stress by means such as immunocompetence and wound healing. Visceral protein status can be determined by measurements of serum albumin, serum thyroxine–binding prealbumin (also referred to as transthyretin or prealbumin), and serum transferrin. These visceral protein indicators usually decrease after trauma or surgical procedures; however, consistently low levels for a period of at least 1 week may indicate a degree of malnutrition.[4] Serum albumin is unreliable as an assessment parameter in certain patients. Serum albumin may be elevated as a result of dehydration, shock, hemoconcentration, or administration of anabolic hormones or IV albumin. Decreased albumin levels can result from chronic illness, malabsorption, pregnancy, nephrotic syndrome, hepatic insufficiency, protein-losing enteropathy, overhydration, or severe burns.[5,6]

Prealbumin and transferrin are visceral proteins with a more rapid turnover than albumin; they are effective assessment parameters with half-lives of approximately 2 and 8 days, respectively.

Visceral protein levels and nitrogen balance are expected to decline postoperatively. In a comparison between postoperative prealbumin and transferrin serum levels, the decline in prealbumin was much greater, and changes in transferrin were more closely correlated with changes in nitrogen balance.[7] Transferrin levels may be elevated in patients who are iron deficient, pregnant, or taking estrogens or oral contraceptives. Serum albumin, prealbumin, and transferrin values indicative of varying degrees of depletion are given in Table 6–1.

■ PERIODIC REASSESSMENT

An initial assessment can be made prior to beginning a nutrition support regimen. Periodic reassessment of the patient, using some or all of the previously mentioned parameters, can provide a means of objectively evaluating the efficacy of nutrition support. Additional parameters to consider during this stage of assessment are nitrogen balance and body weight.

NITROGEN BALANCE

Nitrogen balance determinations indicate the extent to which exogenous protein is being used and can serve as a method for evaluating the efficacy of nutrition support. Because nitrogen balance data are subject to errors of collection and other variables, they should be used only as a relative index of daily change and not an absolute measure of depletion or improvement. Nitrogen balance is calculated for a 24-hr period using the following formula:[4]

$$\text{Nitrogen Balance} = \text{Total Nitrogen In} - \text{Total Nitrogen Out}$$

Urinary urea nitrogen (UUN), although a less sensitive indicator of nitrogen output than total urea nitrogen, is a more simplified laboratory procedure and is therefore a more frequently used measurement to estimate nitrogen balance. Nitrogen balance is calculated as follows:

$$\text{Nitrogen Balance} = \frac{\text{Protein Intake (in g)}}{6.25} - [\text{UUN (in g)} + 4]$$

Urinary urea nitrogen is usually reported in mg/dL; therefore, to derive the amount in grams for use in the above formula, the value must be multiplied by the total 24-hr volume of urine output. The urine sample sent to the laboratory should be an aliquot drawn from an accurate 24-hr urine collection. The factor 4 is added as an empirical number to account for nonurinary nitrogen such as that excreted in feces, sweat, and other normal losses. Excessive nitrogen losses that cannot be measured, such as nitrogen lost in exudates from severe burns or other fluid losses, render nitrogen balance data less reliable.

Positive nitrogen balance can indicate a retention of nitrogen, both as newly synthesized body protein tissue and as nitrogen retained in body fluids. A positive nitrogen balance of 4–6 g/day is the maximum that should be expected;[8] greater amounts are not considered efficient. Because only synthesized protein is of therapeutic interest, increments in BUN above baseline (in grams) should be subtracted from total nitrogen balance. This calculation is summarized as follows:

$$\text{Corrected Nitrogen Balance} = \text{Nitrogen Balance} - \text{BUN Increment (g)}$$

To derive the BUN increment above baseline in grams, the total body water volume of the patient must be considered. Body water can be estimated to be 55% of total body weight (0.55 L/kg).[8] A BUN of 10 mg/dL above baseline in a 70-kg patient represents a BUN increment of 3.85 g (70 kg × 0.55 L/kg × 100 mg/L = 3850 mg).

BODY WEIGHT

The weight difference between body water and tissue is indistinguishable unless water balance is measured. Body weight gain alone is therefore not a reliable maintenance assessment parameter. It is known, however, that weight gain in excess of 200 g/day is undesirable because patients cannot synthesize lean body tissue at a greater rate.[8] Despite its shortcomings as a monitoring parameter, body weight should nevertheless be measured throughout the support regimen at the same time each day, and intake and output should be considered in the interpretation of body weight changes.

■ NUTRIENT REQUIREMENTS

The nutrients required for enteral and parenteral nutrition are virtually the same. Either mode of nutrition support must consist of the basic components of a normal diet: water, carbohydrate, fat, protein, electrolytes, vitamins, and trace elements.

CALORIC REQUIREMENTS

Accurate estimation of caloric requirements is essential, particularly for the severely stressed or depleted patient, to avoid problems associated with overfeeding as well as underfeeding.[9] Requirements can be calculated accurately by indirect calorimetry using instruments that measure respiratory gas exchange. When this is not possible, requirements can be estimated as a multiple of the patient's basal energy expenditure (BEE). BEE is the amount of energy required to maintain basic metabolic functions in the resting state and can be derived from the Harris-Benedict equations:[9]

$$\text{BEE (Men): } 66 + (13.8 \times \text{wt in kg}) + (5 \times \text{ht in cm}) - (6.8 \times \text{age in yr})$$

$$\text{BEE (Women): } 655 + (9.6 \times \text{wt in kg}) + (1.8 \times \text{ht in cm}) - (4.7 \times \text{age in yr})$$

Mechanically ventilated nonsurgical patients without stress or sepsis should receive a total caloric intake no greater than the calculated BEE.[9] Trauma and sepsis increase energy and protein requirements, and the nutrition support regimen should be adjusted accordingly. One means of determining the severity of catabolism in stress conditions is by measurement of UUN excreted per 24 hr. Caloric requirements can then be estimated as a multiple of BEE as shown in Table 6–3.[10]

TABLE 6–3. CALORIC REQUIREMENTS DURING CATABOLISM

24-HR UUN	DEGREE OF NET CATABOLISM	CALORIC REQUIREMENTS
0–5 g	1° (normal)	1 × BEE
5–10 g	2° (mild)	1.5 × BEE
10–15 g	3° (moderate)	1.75 × BEE
>15 g	4° (severe)	2 × BEE

In estimating the calories to be provided by each substrate, yields may be considered as follows: dextrose, 3.4 kcal/g; fat, 9 kcal/g; and protein, 4 kcal/g. Although protein is considered a calorigenic substrate, it is not usually included in estimating caloric goals because the main role of protein is for preservation or synthesis of lean body mass.

PROTEIN REQUIREMENTS

The minimum requirement for protein is about 0.8 g/kg/day of a balanced mixture of amino acids (AAs), and can be as high as 2.5 g/kg/day in severely stressed or traumatized patients. For optimal synthesis of protein, concurrent provision of nonprotein calories must be sufficient. To calculate the nonprotein calorie–to–nitrogen ratio, it may be assumed that the nitrogen content is 1 g/6.25 g of AAs. The optimal ratio of nonprotein calories to nitrogen for efficient nitrogen retention and nitrogen balance is not definite, but varies with the metabolic state of the patient,

Nonprotein calorie–to-nitrogen ratios of standard enteral nutrition and PN formulas are typically about 150:1. Lower ratios are indicated for stress or trauma, and higher ratios for nonstressed patients and those with impaired protein metabolism.

■ ENTERAL NUTRITION

For physiologic and economic reasons, the enteral route should be used whenever possible, but adequacy of the GI tract must be established before enteral nutrition is provided. The IV route should be strictly reserved for patients who cannot be adequately nourished by the enteral route.

Formulas for enteral nutrition are available for supplemental oral feeding or enteral feeding through various types of tubes. When the oral route is not feasible, transnasal passage of a feeding tube into the stomach (nasogastric) or intestine (nasoduodenal or nasojejunal) are generally the feeding routes employed. Feeding ostomies, most commonly the gastrostomy, jejunostomy, or combination gastrostomy-jejunostomy, are generally indicated when insertion through the nares is not feasible or when long-term feeding is anticipated.

FORMULA SELECTION

The abundance of products and lack of an ideal system of categorization may present confusion in selecting the most appropriate enteral formula for a patient. It is not within the scope of this chapter to fully describe criteria for formula selection or to provide a complete list of formulas.

Some nutritionally complete, ready-to-use liquid enteral formulas that are suitable for a variety of patients are presented in Table 6–4. Carbohydrate, fat, and protein sources differ with products and may be important criteria for selecting a product. Because patients with abnormal intestinal function are usually lactose intolerant, only lactose-free products are included. Disease-specific formulas, such as those with high content of branched-chain amino acids for liver disease or essential amino acids for renal disease, may be nutritionally incomplete and are not included because of inadequate evidence of their superiority.

ADMINISTRATION

Either of two types of feeding schedules may be employed, continuous or intermittent. Continuous drip infusion is the preferred method of administration, particularly for patients who have not eaten for a long time. Large 24-hr volumes may be given by infusion without challenging the GI tract, thereby allowing readaptation of the starved gut. Although gravity may be used, an infusion pump is recommended when initiating therapy. For most patients, it is recommended that the first day's feeding be infused at a rate of 50 mL/hr using a lactose-free, nutrient-intact, isotonic formula of 1 kcal/mL. Many protocols recommend diluting the initial formula to one-half strength; however, this practice has been questioned.[11]

Incremental advances in rate and strength can be attempted daily until the desired rate of a full-strength formula is achieved. To minimize the risk of aspira-

TABLE 6–4. REPRESENTATIVE ENTERAL FORMULAS

PRODUCT	CALORIES (per mL)	PROTEIN (g/L)	FAT (g/L)	CARBOHYDRATE (g/L)	NONPROTEIN CALORIES:N (cal/g nitrogen)	SODIUM (mEq/L)	POTASSIUM (mEq/L)	CALCIUM (mg/L)	PHOSPHORUS (mg/L)	OSMOLARITY (mOsm/L)
Compleat Modified	1.07	43	37	140	131	29	36	670	930	300
Criticare HN	1.06	38	5	220	149	28	34	530	530	650
Ensure Plus	1.5	55	53	200	146	50	54	705	705	690
Ensure Plus HN	1.5	63	50	200	125	51	47	1057	1057	650
Impact	1.0	56	28	132	71	48	33	800	800	375
Isocal	1.06	34	44	133	167	23	34	630	530	300
Isocal HCN	2.0	75	91	225	145	35	43	1000	1000	690
Isosource HN	1.2	53	41	157	115	31	43	670	670	390
Jevity	1.06	44	37	152	126	40	40	910	760	310
Magnacal	2.0	70	80	250	154	43	32	1000	1000	590
Nitrolan	1.24	60	40	160	104	30	30	800	800	310
Osmolite	1.06	37	38	145	153	28	26	528	528	300
Osmolite HN	1.06	44	37	141	125	41	40	758	758	300
Pulmocare	1.5	63	92	106	125	57	49	1060	1060	490
Reabilan	1.0	31	39	131	174	30	32	500	500	350
Suplena	2.0	30	96	225	342	34	29	1386	728	600
Sustacal	1.3	61	23	140	78	40	54	1010	930	620
Sustacal HC	1.5	61	58	190	134	37	38	850	850	650
TraumaCal	1.5	83	68	142	91	52	36	750	750	490
Ultracal	1.06	44	45	123	126	40	41	850	850	310

tion, proper placement of the tube must be confirmed, and the patient's head and shoulders must be kept at a 30–45° angle during and for 1 hr after feeding. The stomach should be checked periodically for residual volumes during gastric feedings.

Once a patient has been stabilized on maintenance therapy, intermittent infusions may be used, allowing the patient to rest from feedings at selected hours. A volume of 250–400 mL may be administered 5–8 times/day. This method is preferred for ambulatory patients, because it permits more freedom of movement than does continuous feeding.

Formulas should be given at room temperature and should be kept no longer than 12 hr after the time of preparation and 6 hr from the start of administration to avoid excessive bacterial growth. The delivery system, including bag and tubing, should be changed q 24 hr.

COMPLICATIONS

Mechanical and GI complications known to occur with tube feedings are summarized in Table 6–5. Metabolic complications that occur with enteral nutrition are similar to those of parenteral nutrition and are included in Table 6–12.

TABLE 6–5. TUBE FEEDING COMPLICATIONS AND MANAGEMENT

COMPLICATION	PREVENTION OR MANAGEMENT
Mechanical	
Clogged Tube	Flush with water, replace tube if necessary. Avoid passing crushed tablets through small-bore feeding tubes.
Nasal, Pharyngeal, Esophageal Irritation	Use small-lumen flexible tube. Provide daily care of nose and mouth.
Aspiration	Ensure proper tube placement and verify location. Maintain patient's head and shoulders at 30–45° upright position during and for 1 hr after feeding. Monitor for gastric reflux and abdominal distention. Stop infusion if vomiting occurs. Check residual gastric volume prior to and q 2–4 hr during infusion. Hold if the residual exceeds the hourly volume or 150 mL.
Dislocated Tube	Verify tube location and mark tube at insertion site.
Gastrointestinal	
Diarrhea and Cramps	Reduce flow rate, dilute formula, or consider alternative formula. Rule out alternative causes. If persistent, add anti-diarrheal agent.
Vomiting or Bloating	Check stool output and measure residual formula in gut q 2–4 hr if necessary, stop or reduce flow.
Constipation	Consider different formula or a laxative.

To prevent metabolic complications, monitoring of the patient as suggested in Table 6–13 is recommended.

■ PARENTERAL NUTRITION

Parenteral nutrition (PN) may be administered by either of two routes of access: peripheral veins or larger central veins. The peripheral route is indicated for those patients who require only short-term supplementation or supplementation in addition to enteral support, or for those in whom the risks of central venous administration are too great. Peripheral veins are susceptible to thrombophlebitis, particularly when the osmolarity of the solution exceeds 600 mOsm/L. Therefore, it is recommended that formulas for peripheral administration not exceed final concentrations of 10% dextrose and 4.5% amino acids plus electrolyte and vitamin additives. A number of techniques to prevent or delay onset of peripheral vein thrombophlebitis have been reported.[12] Addition of small amounts of hydrocortisone (5 mg/L) and heparin (1000 units/L) to PN formulas, as well as the topical use of agents such as nitroglycerin, have demonstrated success. Concurrent administration of IV fat emulsion, which is a concentrated, iso-osmotic calorie source, is vital, because it increases the caloric content of a peripheral regimen while minimizing the risk of thrombophlebitis.

The complete nutrition needs of the malnourished or hypermetabolic patient are difficult to provide via peripheral vein for long periods of time. The concentrated, hyperosmolar solutions required by such patients for PN *must* be administered into a large central vein, such as the superior vena cava, where rapid dilution occurs.

ADMINISTRATION

Initiation of PN should be gradual, particularly in the malnourished patient, to avoid glucose intolerance and the dangers of refeeding syndrome.[13] With high concentrations of dextrose and amino acids intended for central vein administration, an initial rate of 40 mL/hr for the first 24 hr is suggested. Infusion rates may then be increased daily in accordance with assessment goals. Less concentrated formulas that are suited for peripheral vein administration do not warrant such slow initial rates of infusion.

A variety of catheters exist for infusion of PN formulas by central or peripheral vein. Use of an in-line filter is recommended to minimize adverse consequences in case precipitation occurs in the PN solution.[14]

PARENTERAL NUTRIENTS

Each of the following nutrient substrate groups are required in formulas for effective PN.

Water. The average healthy adult can tolerate a fluid infusion volume of about 5 L/day. The patient who is fluid restricted might be limited to an intake of 2 L/day or less. This may be the deciding factor in selecting a hypertonic concentrated solution for infusion through a large central vein rather than a more dilute solution for peripheral administration.

Carbohydrate. Presently, the preferred carbohydrate substrate for PN is dextrose. The concentration of dextrose should be determined by the osmotic limitation of the administration route and the nonprotein calorie requirement of the patient. The concentrations of available dextrose solutions with their corresponding caloric concentrations and osmolarities are as shown in Table 6–6.

Dextrose remains the primary source of calories for PN via central vein, and the rate of infusion should be limited to its maximum rate of oxidation, which is 5 mg/kg/min or 7.2 g/kg/day.[15] On a calorie-for-calorie basis, carbohydrate is more efficient than fat in sparing body protein during hypocaloric feedings.[16] The inclusion of both dextrose and fat is recommended in PN regimens, but the optimal proportion of each has not been established.

Fat. Fat is an important parenteral substrate for three major reasons: (1) it is a concentrated source of calories in an isotonic medium, which makes it useful for peripheral administration; (2) it is a source of essential fatty acids (EFAs) required

TABLE 6–6. IV DEXTROSE SOLUTIONS

CONCENTRATION	kcal/L	mOsm/L
5%	170	252
10%	340	505
20%	680	1010
40%	1360	2020
50%	1700	2520
60%	2040	3030
70%	2380	3530

for prevention or treatment of EFA deficiency, which may develop during prolonged fat-free PN;[17] and (3) it is a useful substitute for carbohydrate when dextrose calories must be limited because of glucose intolerance or diminished ventilatory capacity. When a patient's ventilatory effort is hampered, it is important to avoid excessive calories of any type. In comparison to dextrose, the metabolism of fat results in an increase in heat production, a decrease in respiratory quotient (RQ), and an increase in oxygen consumption. Having a lower RQ, fat produces less CO_2 for a given number of calories, thereby minimizing the ventilatory effort required to eliminate CO_2. The RQ of fat is 0.7 compared to 1 for carbohydrate. An RQ in excess of 1 indicates net lipogenesis and is undesirable.[18]

Fat is available as emulsions of 10, 20, or 30% soybean oil, or 10 or 20% soybean–safflower oil mixtures. Clinical studies have not shown any major advantages of one lipid source over the other. The major differences between these products are their fatty acid contents, which are summarized in Table 6–7. The 20 and 30% emulsions are more readily cleared than the 10% because of the lower proportion of phospholipid to triglyceride.[19]

Fat emulsions that are currently marketed in the United States contain only long-chain triglycerides (LCTs); however, the use of fat emulsions that contain both LCTs and medium-chain triglycerides (MCTs) is being investigated. MCTs are reported to be more rapidly cleared from the blood and more ketogenic than LCTs, and emulsions containing both MCTs and LCTs have greater protein-conserving properties than pure LCT emulsions.[20] LCTs are required for their essential fatty acid content, however.

TABLE 6–7. IV FAT EMULSIONS

FATTY ACID	SOYBEAN OIL	SOYBEAN OIL/ SAFFLOWER OIL
Linoleic Acid	54%	65.8%
Linolenic Acid	8%	4.2%
Oleic Acid	26%	17.7%
Palmitic Acid	9%	8.8%
Stearic Acid	2.5%	3.4%

The caloric density of 10% fat emulsions is 1.1 kcal/mL, of which 1 kcal is supplied by lipid and 0.1 kcal by glycerol (carbohydrate); the 20 and 30% emulsions have caloric densities of 2 and 3 kcal/mL, respectively, of which 0.1 kcal/mL is glycerol. The average particle size (0.5 micron) is the same in all concentrations, and all are nearly iso-osmotic.

Fat emulsion may be infused concurrently with amino acid/dextrose solution through peripheral or central veins. The 10 or 20% emulsion may be infused separately or combined with amino acids and dextrose in a single container to form a total nutrient ("3-in-1") admixture (TNA).[21] The 30% concentration is intended only for compounding TNA. Because lipid emulsion is iso-osmolar, it reduces the thrombophlebitic effect of hyperosmolar amino acid/dextrose solutions on the endothelium of peripheral veins when they are infused concurrently.[22] For this reason as well as its potential adverse effect on the immune system, fat emulsion should be infused as slowly as possible.[23] The use of IV fat emulsion in patients with pancreatitis is often questionable because it is harmful if lipid is not adequately cleared from the blood. IV fat emulsion can be used safely if serum triglyceride levels are monitored and remain below 400 mg/dL (4.5 mmol/L).[24] Product literature suggests that fat be provided in quantities no greater than 3 g/kg or 60% of total calories. For further information on dosage, administration, and precautions of fat emulsion, the product literature should be consulted.

Protein. Various brands and concentrations of amino acid solutions are available as sources of protein for parenteral use. The AA profile differs in each, and therefore their nitrogen contents are not equivalent. A comparison of formulations is summarized in Table 6–8. Amino acid solutions >3.5% concentration should be diluted to a lower final concentration with dextrose and other additives.

TABLE 6-8. AMINO ACID SOLUTIONS COMPARISON CHART

AA SOLUTION AND OSMOLARITY CONCENTRATION	TOTAL BCAAs (g/dL)	TOTAL ESSENTIAL AAs (g/dL)	TOTAL N (g/dL)	ELECTROLYTES (mEq/L)					PO₄ (mmol/L)	Osmolarity (mOsm/L)
				Na^+	K^+	Mg^{++}	Cl^-	Ac^-	PO_4 (mmol/L)	Osmolarity (mOsm/L)
FOR GENERAL PURPOSE										
Aminosyn 3.5%[a]	0.86	1.65	0.55	7	—	—	—	46	—	357
Aminosyn 5%[a]	1.23	2.35	0.79	—	5.4	—	—	86	—	500
Travasol 5.5%	0.86	2.15	0.95	—	—	—	22	48	—	575
(with electrolytes)				70	60	10	70	102	30	850
Aminosyn 7%[a]	1.73	3.32	1.1	—	5.4	—	—	105	—	700
(with electrolytes)				70	66	10	96	124	30	1013
Aminosyn 8.5%[a]	2.11	4.06	1.34	—	2.7	—	11.7	90	—	856
(with electrolytes)				70	66	10	98	142	30	1160
Travasol 8.5%	1.32	3.34	1.43	—	—	—	34	73	—	890
(with electrolytes)				70	60	10	70	141	30	1160
FreAmine III 8.5%	1.92	3.94	1.43	10	—	—	<3	73	10	810
(with electrolytes)				60	60	10	60	125	20	1045
Aminosyn 10%	2.46	4.7	1.57	—	5.4	—	—	148	—	1000
Aminosyn II 10% (with electrolytes)	2.16	4.3	1.53	87	66	10	86	72	30	1130
FreAmine III 10%	2.26	4.63	1.53	10	—	—	<3	89	10	950
Travasol 10%	1.91	4.05	1.65	—	—	—	40	87	—	1000
Novamine	2.09	5.11	1.8	—	—	—	—	114	—	1057

(continued)

TABLE 6-8. AMINO ACID SOLUTIONS COMPARISON CHART (continued)

AA SOLUTION AND OSMOLARITY CONCENTRATION	TOTAL BCAAs (g/dL)	TOTAL ESSENTIAL AAs (g/dL)	TOTAL N (g/dL)	ELECTROLYTES (mEq/L)						Osmolarity (mOsm/L)
				Na^+	K^+	Mg^{++}	Cl^-	Ac^-	PO_4 (mmol/L)	
Aminosyn II 15%	3.24	6.42	2.3	63	—	—	—	107	—	1300
Novamine 15%	2.75	6.72	2.37	—	—	—	—	151	—	1388
FOR PROTEIN SPARING										
ProcalAmine 3%[b]	0.68	1.4	0.46	35	24	5	41	47	3.5	735
FreAmine III 3% (with electrolytes)	0.68	1.4	0.46	35	24	5	41	44	3.5	405
Aminosyn 3.5% M[a]	0.86	1.65	0.55	47	13	3	40	58	3.5	477
3.5% Travasol (with electrolytes)	0.55	1.38	0.59	25	15	5	25	52	7.5	450
FOR RENAL FAILURE										
Aminess 5.2%	1.95	5.18	0.66	—	—	—	—	50	—	416
Aminosyn RF 5.2%	1.72	4.83	0.79	—	5.4	—	—	105	—	475
NephrAmine 5.4%	2.08	5.33	0.65	5	—	—	<3	44	—	435
RenAmin 6.5%	1.92	4.32	1.0	—	—	—	31	60	—	600
FOR TRAUMA										
BranchAmin 4%[c,d]	4.0	4.0[d]	0.44	—	—	—	—	—	—	316
FreAmine HBC 6.9%[c]	3.01	4.28	0.97	10	—	—	<3	57	—	620
Aminosyn HBC 7%[c]	3.15	4.21	1.12	7	40	—	—	72	—	665

(continued)

TABLE 6–8. AMINO ACID SOLUTIONS COMPARISON CHART (continued)

AA SOLUTION AND OSMOLARITY CONCENTRATION	TOTAL BCAAs (g/dL)	TOTAL ESSENTIAL AAs (g/dL)	TOTAL N (g/dL)	ELECTROLYTES (mEq/L)					
				Na^+	K^+	Mg^{++}	Cl^-	Ac^-	PO_4 (mmol/L)	Osmolarity (mOsm/L)
FOR LIVER DISEASE										
HepatAmine 8%[c]	2.84	4.17	1.2	10	—	—	<3	62	10	785
FOR PEDIATRICS										
Aminosyn PF 7%	1.82	3.2	1.07	3.4	—	—	—	33	—	586
Aminosyn PF 10%	2.63	4.61	1.52	3.4	—	—	—	46	—	834
TrophAmine 6%	1.8	4.28	0.93	5	—	—	<3	56	—	525
TrophAmine 10%	3.0	7.2	1.55	5	—	—	<3	97	—	875

[a]Also available as Aminosyn II which contains glutamic and aspartic acids, and differs slightly in content of other amino acids, acetate, and chloride.
[b]Contains glycerol as a nonprotein calorie source.
[c]Branched-chain amino acid–enriched products. Each of these products has distinct indications for use and should not be interchanged.
[d]Contains only the branched-chain amino acids. Other essential amino acids are not included.
BCAAs, branched-chain amino acids.

SPECIAL AMINO ACID SOLUTIONS

Special amino acid solutions are available for specific metabolic or disease states. Discretion is recommended in the use of these solutions, because they are expensive and clinical benefit is not proved.

Protein Sparing.   A low concentration of amino acids infused with or without concurrent nonprotein calories conserves endogenous nitrogen more efficiently than the traditional 5% dextrose infusion alone.[25] For a limited infusion of no more than 1 week's duration in patients who are not severely catabolic, low-concentration AA formulas merit consideration. Low-concentration AA formulas are available with or without electrolytes and with or without a nonprotein calorie source (*see* Table 6–8).

Renal Failure.   The objective of PN in patients with renal failure is to provide sufficient amino acids and calories for protein synthesis without exceeding the renal capacity for excretion of fluid and metabolic wastes. Four parenteral products that contain primarily essential amino acids have been developed for this purpose (*see* Table 6–8), but controversy exists regarding their use. Patients who undergo renal replacement therapy such as peritoneal or hemodialysis require both essential and nonessential amino acids and should receive standard amino acid solutions.

Hepatic Failure.   Patients with hepatic failure, in whom muscle breakdown and an altered serum and CNS amino acid profile may contribute to hepatic encephalopathy, may benefit from a special AA formula. This formula has relatively greater amounts of branched-chain amino acids (BCAAs—leucine, isoleucine, and valine) and smaller amounts of the aromatic acids (ie, phenylalanine, tyrosine, tryptophan), and methionine.[26] One parenteral formula, HepatAmine, is currently available specifically for therapeutic and nutrition support of patients with liver disease (*see* Table 6–8).

Stress and Trauma.   The hypermetabolism that occurs in response to stress and trauma presents difficulty in providing nutrition support. BCAAs, in addition to their useful effect in metabolic support of the patient with liver disease, are reported to be useful for patients with stress and trauma.[27,28] Three BCAA-enriched products are available (*see* Table 6–8). FreAmine HBC and Aminosyn HBC are solutions of nonessential and essential AAs enriched with BCAAs. BranchAmin 4% is a solution of only BCAAs intended for use as a supplement to be admixed with a complete amino acid and a nonprotein caloric source. These products are indicated only for stress and trauma, and should not be confused with the BCAA-enriched product that is indicated for hepatic encephalopathy.

Pediatrics.   It is beyond the scope of this chapter to describe procedures for nutrition support of pediatric patients except in this brief mention of parenteral amino acid products. Crystalline AA solutions marketed for infants are based on the essentiality of certain AAs in these patients (*see* Table 6–8).[29] Compared to adult AA formulations, these products contain taurine and glutamic and aspartic acids. Increased amounts of tyrosine and histidine, and lower amounts of phenylalanine, methionine, and glycine are included. Although cysteine is also assumed to be essential for infants, adequate amounts cannot be included in AA formulas, because of its limited solubility. A cysteine solution (50 mg/mL) is available separately for admixture to the formula prior to administration.

ELECTROLYTES

Formulas are also available with standard electrolyte compositions that may be suitable for most patients, after the addition of certain additives. Electrolyte provision, however, should be based on close monitoring of patients' laboratory values. Average daily requirements are summarized in Table 6–9.

TABLE 6-9. ELECTROLYTES AND REQUIREMENTS

ELECTROLYTES	AVERAGE DAILY REQUIREMENT	DOSAGE FORMS	COMMENTS
CATIONS			
Sodium	60–150 mEq	Sodium chloride concentrate (4 mEq/mL) Sodium acetate (2 mEq/mL) Sodium phosphate (4 mEq Na^+/mL)	Requirements during parenteral nutrition should not differ from normal fluid therapy requirements unless there is excessive sodium loss. Lactate and bicarbonate salts of sodium should not be used.
Potassium	40–240 mEq	Potassium chloride (2 mEq/mL) Potassium acetate (2 mEq/mL) Potassium phosphate (4.4 mEq K^+/mL)	Requirements are related to glucose metabolism and therefore increase with higher concentrations of dextrose infused.
Magnesium	10–45 mEq	Magnesium sulfate (4 mEq/mL)	Requirements increase with anabolism, however, with less variation than does potassium.
Calcium	5–30 mEq	Calcium gluconate 10% (4.5 mEq/10 mL) Calcium chloride 10% (13 mEq/10 mL)	Requirements increase only slightly during parenteral nutrition. Limited amounts of calcium and phosphate, as determined by compatibility references, may be combined in solutions that contain AAs.
ANIONS			
Phosphate	10 mmol/1000 kcal	Potassium phosphate (3 mmol P/mL, Abbott) Sodium phosphate (3 mmol P/mL, Abbott) (other concentrations may vary according to manufacturer)	Requirements increase with anabolism. Safe empirical dosage guidelines should be developed, taking into account the sodium or potassium content of the phosphate solution.
Acetate and Chloride	The amounts of acetate and chloride contained in each amino acid solution vary (*see* Table 6–8). Acetate is metabolized to bicarbonate. Bicarbonate salts should not be added to PN solutions because of incompatibility.		

VITAMINS

Vitamin requirements for PN have been suggested in a report by an advisory group to the American Medical Association (AMA).[30] Multiple vitamins are available in adult and pediatric formulations for once-daily IV administration (*see* Table 6–10). The usual daily dosage of the adult formulation is 10 mL to provide the amounts of vitamins specified in Table 6–10. The daily dosage of the pediatric formulation for infants who weigh <1 kg is 1.5 mL. For infants weighing 1–3 kg, the daily dosage is 3 mL. For infants and children weighing ≥3 kg up to 11 yr of age, the daily dosage is 5 mL. Vitamin K is included in the pediatric product only. Phytonadione 5 mg may be given to adults weekly in the PN formula, or by IM or SC administration, if needed.[30]

Fat emulsion contains vitamin K. Intralipid 10% contains about 0.31 mg/L and Liposyn II contains 0.13 mg/L; 20% products contain twice as much. Intralipid 20% 500 mL provides about 300 μg of vitamin K, an amount that exceeds maintenance recommendations and interferes with oral anticoagulant therapy.[30]

TABLE 6–10. IV MULTIVITAMINS

	AMOUNT	
TYPICAL FORMULA	*Adult (per vial)*	*Pediatric (per 5 mL)*
Ascorbic Acid (C)	100 mg	80 mg
Vitamin A	3300 IU	2300 IU
Vitamin D	200 IU	400 IU
Vitamin E	10 IU	7 IU
Thiamine (B_1)	3 mg	1.2 mg
Riboflavin (B_2)	3.6 mg	1.4 mg
Niacinamide (B_3)	40 mg	17 mg
Pantothenic Acid (B_5)	15 mg	5 mg
Pyridoxine (B_6)	4 mg	1 mg
Biotin	60 μg	20 μg
Folic Acid	400 μg	140 μg
Cyanocobalamin (B_{12})	5 μg	1 μg
Phytonadione (K)	0	200 μg

TRACE ELEMENTS

Solutions of individual trace elements are available in several concentrations from various manufacturers. Solutions of multiple trace elements are also commercially available in products containing 4, 5, 6, or 7 elements and in concentrations suitable for adult or pediatric use. Guidelines for the use of trace elements in PN have been reported in an AMA statement[31] and the recommended daily dosages appear in Table 6–11. Although a need for molybdenum and iodine in long-term PN has been described, there are no officially recommended requirements for these elements.[32–34]

TABLE 6–11. SUGGESTED DAILY IV DOSAGE OF TRACE ELEMENTS

TRACE ELEMENT	PEDIATRIC PATIENTS (μg/kg)[a]	STABLE ADULT	ADULT IN ACUTE CATABOLIC STATE[b]	STABLE ADULT WITH INTESTINAL LOSSES[b]
Zinc	400 (preterm)[c] 250 (<3 mo)[d] 100 (>3 mo–1 yr)[d] 50 (>1 yr)[d]	2.5–4 mg	Additional 2 mg	Add 12.2 mg per liter small-bowel fluid lost; 17.1 mg per kg of stool or ileostomy output.[e]
Copper	20	0.5–1.5 mg	—	—
Chromium	0.14–0.2	10–15 μg	—	20 μg[f]
Manganese	1	0.15–0.8 mg	—	—
Selenium	2	20–60 μg	—	—

[a]Limited data are available for infants weighing <1500 g. Their requirements may be more than the recommendations because of their low body reserves and increased requirements for growth.
[b]Frequent monitoring of plasma levels in these patients is essential to provide proper dosage.
[c]Premature infants (weight <1500 g) up to 3 kg of body weight. Thereafter, the recommendations for full-term infants apply.
[d]Full-term infants and children ≤5 years old. Thereafter, the recommendations for adults apply, up to a maximum dosage of 4 mg/day.
[e]Values derived by mathematical fitting of balance data from a 71-patient-week study in 24 patients.
[f]Mean from balance study.
Modified from references 31 and 35.

IRON

Iron deficiency can occur in patients deprived of iron during long-term PN. Although other parenteral sources of iron have been tested, the only commercially available iron product for IV use in the United States at this time is iron dextran. Iron dextran can be added to PN solutions, but the advisability of its routine use as well as its compatibility with fat emulsion is questionable. Dosage recommendations by this route range from 1–12.5 mg/day of iron.[36]

INSULIN

Many patients who receive PN become hyperglycemic. When feasible, the cause should be investigated and controlled by means other than insulin before insulin is employed (*see* Table 6–12). Although the efficacy of PN is reportedly enhanced by insulin,[37] it should be used cautiously to avoid hypoglycemia, and also because it promotes deposition of fatty acids in body fat stores, making them less available for important biochemical pathways.[38] When it is required, insulin may be provided separately by SC or IV administration, or added to the PN formula. Until a patient is stabilized on a consistent dosage of insulin, it is more cost effective to provide insulin separately to avoid wasting of PN formulations that may be discarded if the insulin dosage needs to be changed.[39] Human insulin is the least immunogenic and is therefore the insulin of choice. Guidelines for dosage are empirical; one-half to two-thirds of the previous day's sliding scale requirements may be added as regular human insulin to the daily PN formula. Standardized admixture procedures should be used to minimize variations of insulin activity caused by absorption loss.

ALBUMIN

Albumin is compatible when admixed with PN formulas; however, its supply is too limited and its cost is too prohibitive for casual use. Although inclusion of albumin in PN is reported to rapidly increase serum albumin levels[40] and enhance tolerance of enteral feedings,[41] the clinical benefits of such treatment are not proved. For synthesis of endogenous protein, albumin is inferior to crystalline amino acids as a parenteral source of nitrogen. If administration of albumin is necessary, it should not be included in the PN formula.

CARNITINE

Carnitine is an amino acid that is vital to energy metabolism because of its role in transporting long-chain fatty acids across the mitochondrial membrane. Certain patients, such as those with chronic renal failure on dialysis and premature neonates, are at increased risk of developing carnitine deficiency, especially if they are receiving long-term PN.[42,43] L-carnitine, the physiologically active form, is available for IV administration as a 1 g/5 mL solution that is stable when added to PN formulas.[44] Consult the carnitine product information for detailed usage information.

MEDICATIONS

There may be advantages to the admixture of certain medications such as antibiotics, chemotherapeutic agents, and H_2-receptor antagonists to PN, if there is compatibility reported with all components of the formula. Consult other sources for information regarding the stability and compatibility of medication/PN admixtures.

■ MONITORING THE PATIENT

Metabolic complications known to occur with enteral or parenteral nutrition are summarized in Table 6–12. Most of these can be avoided by proper precautions and close monitoring of the patient. Laboratory parameters for patient monitoring are summarized in Table 6–13.

TABLE 6–12. NUTRITION SUPPORT: METABOLIC COMPLICATIONS AND MANAGEMENT

COMPLICATION	FREQUENT CAUSES	MANAGEMENT
Hyponatremia	Excessive GI or urinary sodium losses, or inadequate sodium intake.	Increase sodium provision.
	Excessive water intake.	Limit free water.
Hypokalemia	Excessive GI or urinary potassium losses; deficit of potassium; or large glucose infusion.	Increase potassium provision.
Hypocalcemia	Insufficient calcium.	Increase calcium provision.
	Magnesium deficit.	Increase magnesium provision.
Hypomagnesemia	Insufficient magnesium; or excessive GI or urinary losses.	Increase magnesium provision.
Hypophosphatemia	Inadequate phosphate.	Increase phosphate provision.
	Refeeding syndrome.	Refeed gradually.
Hypoglycemia	Abrupt interruption of formula infusion.	Begin dextrose infusion and monitor blood glucose and potassium.
	Excessive insulin.	Decrease insulin.
Hyperglycemia	Deficit of potassium or phosphorus.	Increase potassium or phosphate provision.
	Insufficient insulin.	Give insulin.
	Corticosteriod use.	Reduce rate of glucose infusion.
	Sepsis.	Sepsis workup and treatment.
Hypertriglyceridemia	Impaired clearance.	Hold IV lipid if serum triglycerides >400 mg/dL (4.5 mmol/L).
Elevated BUN	Dehydration.	Correct dehydration.
	Renal dysfunction; or calorie:nitrogen ratio imbalance.	Increase nonprotein calorie:nitrogen ratio.
Elevated Liver Function Tests	Underlying disease; lack of GI use; or GI bacterial overgrowth.	Attempt enteral feeding.
	Essential fatty acid deficiency.	Provide lipid.
	Excessive nutrients.	Decrease PN.
Metabolic Acidosis	Excessive GI or urinary losses of base.	Increase acetate provision.
	Inadequate amount of base-producing substance in formula.	Decrease chloride in formula or increase acetate provision.

(*continued*)

TABLE 6–12. NUTRITION SUPPORT: METABOLIC COMPLICATIONS AND MANAGEMENT (continued)

COMPLICATION	FREQUENT CAUSES	MANAGEMENT
Osmotic Diuresis	Failure to recognize initial hyperglycemia and increased glucose in urine.	Reduce infusion rate. Give insulin to correct hyperglycemia. Give 5% dextrose and 0.2% or 0.45% NaCl, rather than PN solution to correct dehydration. Continue to monitor blood glucose, sodium, and potassium.
Essential Fatty Acid Deficiency	Insufficient provision of fat during PN.	Provide lipid.

■ FUTURE DEVELOPMENTS

Technological advancements in nutrition formulas and the means of preparing, providing, and monitoring their effects on patients continue to be made. These modifications enable safer and more cost-effective nutrition support of patients in the hospital or at home.

Body composition research is presenting innovative approaches to metabolic and nutrition assessment.[45] Formulas with specialized amino acid mixtures continue to be investigated. The benefits of using branched-chain amino acid–enriched formulas are reported for patients with hepatic encephalopathy[46] or hypermetabolism,[47] but remain unproved in terms of morbidity and mortality. Recombinant human growth factors,[48] arginine,[49] and glutamine[50] offer promise

TABLE 6–13. ROUTINE PATIENT MONITORING PARAMETERS

PARAMETER	FREQUENCY[a]
Urinary glucose and specific gravity.	Every voided specimen until stable, then daily.
Finger stick glucose.	Every 6 hr until stable.
Vital signs, weight, intake, and output.	Daily.
Serum glucose, electrolytes, creatinine, and BUN.	Daily until stable, then twice weekly.
Magnesium, calcium, and phosphorus.	Daily until stable, then once weekly.
CBC, hemoglobin, WBC, platelets, and prothrombin time.	Baseline, then weekly.
Serum protein, albumin, prealbumin, and liver function tests.	Baseline, then weekly.
Serum cholesterol and triglycerides.	Baseline, then weekly.
Blood ammonia.	Baseline, then weekly in renal and hepatic patients.

[a]Frequency should be increased in critically ill patients.

for their beneficial influences on protein synthesis rates, immunocompetence, and intestinal mucosal barrier protection, respectively.

In vitro and animal studies report an improvement in tissue protein synthesis and reduction in hypermetabolic response with the enteral use of structured lipids containing medium-chain triglycerides and omega-3 fish oil.[51,52] Because of difficulties reported with the IV use of currently available long-chain triglyceride emulsions, such as hepatic and pulmonary complications and immunosuppression, alternate shorter-chain lipid preparations have been investigated.[53] MCTs continue to be explored for IV use as an obligate fuel and as an important component of PN.[54] Animal studies with short-chain triglycerides such as triacetin show potential for better protein-sparing properties than MCTs, with less toxicity.[53] Short-chain fatty acids have also been shown to be beneficial in inhibiting small-bowel mucosal atrophy when infused IV or intracolonically.[55]

New insights into the relationship between nutrition and immune function are emerging through advances with recombinant monokines and new discoveries concerning the involvement of interleukin-1 and tumor necrosis factor in energy metabolism.[52,56] Although all of these are promising areas of research, they are not yet considered to be standard therapy in nutrition support.

■ REFERENCES

1. Albina JE. Nutrition and wound healing. *JPEN* 1994;18:367–76.
2. Elwyn DH. Nutritional requirements of adult surgical patients. *Crit Care Med* 1980;8:9–19.
3. Grant JP et al. Current techniques of nutritional assessment. *Surg Clin North Am* 1981;61:437–63.
4. Blackburn GL et al. Nutritional and metabolic assessment of the hospitalized patient. *JPEN* 1977;1:11–22.
5. Traub SL, ed. *Basic skills in interpreting laboratory data.* Bethesda, MD: American Society of Hospital Pharmacists; 1992.
6. Vanlandingham S et al. Prealbumin: a parameter of visceral protein levels during albumin infusion. *JPEN* 1982; 6:230–1.
7. Fletcher JP et al. A comparison of serum transferrin and serum prealbumin as nutritional parameters. *JPEN* 1987;11:144–7.
8. Bistrian BR. Recent advances in parenteral and enteral nutrition: a personal perspective. *JPEN* 1990;14:329–34.
9. Liggett SB, Renfro AD. Energy expenditures of mechanically ventilated nonsurgical patients. *Chest* 1990;98: 682–6.
10. Rutten P et al. Determination of optimal hyperalimentation infusion rate. *J Surg Res* 1975;18:477–83.
11. Rees RGP et al. Elemental diet administered nasogastrically without starter regimens to patients with inflammatory bowel disease. *JPEN* 1986;10:258–62.
12. Payne-James JJ, Khawaja HT. First choice for total parenteral nutrition: the peripheral route. *JPEN* 1993;17: 468–78.
13. Solomon SM, Kirby DF. The refeeding syndrome: a review. *JPEN* 1990;14:90–7.
14. Food and Drug Administration. Safety alert: hazards of precipitation associated with parenteral nutrition. *Am J Hosp Pharm* 1994;51:1427–8.
15. Barton RG. Nutrition support in critical illness. *Nutr Clin Pract* 1994;9:127–39.
16. Shizgal HM, Forse RA. Protein and calorie requirements with total parenteral nutrition. *Ann Surg* 1980; 192:562–9.
17. Barr LH et al. Essential fatty acid deficiency during total parenteral nutrition. *Ann Surg* 1981;193:304–11.
18. Mattox TW, Teasley-Strausberg KM. Overview of biochemical markers used for nutrition support. *DICP* 1991; 25:265–71.
19. Roulet M et al. Effects of intravenously infused egg phospholipids on lipid and lipoprotein metabolism in postoperative trauma. *JPEN* 1993;17:107–12.
20. Crowe PJ et al. A new intravenous emulsion containing medium-chain triglyceride: studies of its metabolic effects in the perioperative period compared with a conventional long-chain triglyceride emulsion. *JPEN* 1985;9:720–4.
21. Driscoll DF et al. Practical considerations regarding the use of total nutrient admixtures. *Am J Hosp Pharm* 1986;43:416–9.

22. Pineault M et al. Beneficial effect of coinfusing a lipid emulsion on venous patency. *JPEN* 1989;13:637–40.

23. Hardin TC. Intravenous lipids—depression of the immune function: fact or fantasy? *Hosp Pharm* 1994;29: 182,185–6.

24. Guidelines for the use of parenteral and enteral nutrition in adult and pediatric patients. American Society for Parenteral and Enteral Nutrition. *JPEN* 1993;17(4 suppl);1SA–52SA.

25. Humbestone DA et al. Relative importance of amino acid infusion as a means of sparing protein in surgical patients. *JPEN* 1989;13:223–7.

26. Freund H et al. Infusion of branched-chain enriched amino acid solution in patients with hepatic encephalopathy. *Ann Surg* 1982;196:209–20.

27. Freund H et al. Infusion of the branched-chain amino acids in postoperative patients: anticatabolic properties. *Ann Surg* 1979;190:18–23.

28. Cerra FB et al. Branched-chains support postoperative protein synthesis. *Surgery* 1982;92:192–9.

29. Heird WC et al. Pediatric parenteral amino acid mixture in low birth weight infants. *Pediatrics* 1988;81:41–50.

30. Baumgartner T, ed. *Clinical guide to parenteral nutrition,* 3rd ed. Deerfield, IL: Fujisawa, Inc; 1997.

31. American Medical Association Department of Foods and Nutrition. Guidelines for essential trace element preparations for parenteral use: a statement by an expert panel. *JAMA* 1979;241:2051–4.

32. Lane HW et al. The effect of selenium supplementation on selenium status of patients receiving chronic total parenteral nutrition. *JPEN* 1987;11:177–82.

33. Abumrad NN et al. Amino acid intolerance during prolonged total parenteral nutrition reversed by molybdate therapy. *Am J Clin Nutr* 1981;34:2551–9.

34. Shils ME, Jacobs DH. Plasma iodide levels and thyroid function studies in long term home TPN patients. *Am J Clin Nutr* 1983;37:731. Abstract.

35. Greene HL et al. Guidelines for the use of vitamins, trace elements, calcium, magnesium, and phosphorus in infants and children receiving total parenteral nutrition: report of the Subcommittee on Pediatric Parenteral Nutrient Requirements from the Committee on Clinical Practice Issues of the American Society for Clinical Nutrition. *Am J Clin Nutr* 1988;48:1324–42.

36. Norton JA et al. Iron supplementation of total parenteral nutrition: a prospective study. *JPEN* 1983;7:457–61.

37. Shizgal HM, Posner B. Insulin and the efficacy of total parenteral nutrition. *Am J Clin Nutr* 1989;50:1355–63.

38. Rothkopf MM et al. Nutritional support in respiratory failure. *Nutr Clin Pract* 1989;4:166–72.

39. Sajbel TA et al. Use of separate insulin infusions with total parenteral nutrition. *JPEN* 1987;11:97–9.

40. Brown RO et al. Response of serum albumin concentrations to albumin supplementation during central total parenteral nutrition. *Clin Pharm* 1987;6:222–6.

41. Andrassy RJ, Durr ED. Albumin: use in nutrition and support. *Nutr Clin Pract* 1988;3:226–9.

42. Wolk R. Micronutrition in dialysis. *Nutr Clin Pract* 1993;8:267–76.

43. Bonner CM et al. Effects of parenteral L-carnitine supplementation on fat metabolism and nutrition in premature neonates. *J Pediatr* 1995;126:287–92.

44. Borum PR. Is L-carnitine stable in parenteral nutrition solutions prepared for preterm neonates? *Neonatal Intensive Care* 1993;Sept/Oct:30–2.

45. Heymsfield SB, Matthews D. Body composition: research and clinical advances—1993 ASPEN research workshop. *JPEN* 1994;18:91–103.

46. Alexander WF et al. The usefulness of branched chain amino acids in patients with acute or chronic hepatic encephalopathy. *Am J Gastroenterol* 1989;84:91–6.

47. Teasley KM, Buss RL. Do parenteral nutrition solutions with high concentrations of branched-chain amino acids offer significant benefits to stressed patients? *DICP* 1989;23:411–6.

48. Hatton J et al. Growth factors in nutritional support. *Pharmacotherapy* 1993;13:17–27.

49. Daly JM et al. Immune and metabolic effects of arginine in the surgical patient. *Ann Surg* 1998;208:512–23.

50. Li J et al. Glycyl-L-glutamine-enriched total parenteral nutrition maintains small intestine gut-associated lymphoid tissue and upper respiratory tract immunity. *JPEN* 1998;22:31–6.

51. Teo TC et al. Administration of structured lipid composed of MCT and fish oil reduces net protein catabolism in enterally fed burned rats. *Ann Surg* 1989;210:100–6.

52. Endres S. The effect of dietary supplementation with n-3 polyunsaturated fatty acids on the synthesis of interleukin-1 and tumor necrosis factor by mononuclear cells. *N Engl J Med* 1989;320:265–71.

53. Bailey JW et al. Triacetin: a potential parenteral nutrient. *JPEN* 1991;15:32–6.

54. Mascioli EA et al. Thermogenesis from intravenous medium-chain triglycerides. *JPEN* 1991;15:27–31.

55. Koruda MJ et al. Parenteral nutrition supplemented with short-chain fatty acids: effect on the small-bowel mucosa in normal rats. *Am J Clin Nutr* 1990;51:685–9.

56. Pomposelli JJ et al. Role of biochemical mediators in clinical nutrition and surgical metabolism. *JPEN* 1988;12: 212–8.

Part III

APPENDICES

- CONVERSION FACTORS
- ANTHROPOMETRICS
- PHARMACOKINETIC EQUATIONS
- LABORATORY INDICES
- DRUG–LABORATORY TEST INTERFERENCES

Conversion Factors

■ MICROMOLECULES

SI units (*le Système International d'Unités*) are being introduced in the United States to express clinical laboratory and serum drug concentration data. Instead of employing units of mass (such as micrograms), the SI system uses moles (mol) to represent the amount of a substance. A molar solution contains one mole (the molecular weight of the substance in grams) of the solute in 1 L of solution. The following formula is used to convert units of mass to moles (μg/mL to μmol/L or, by substitution of terms, mg/mL to mmol/L, or ng/mL to nmol/L).

Micromoles per Liter (μmol/L)

$$\mu mol/L = \frac{\text{Drug concentration } (\mu g/mL) \times 1000}{\text{Molecular weight of drug } (g/mol)}$$

■ MILLIEQUIVALENTS

An equivalent weight of a substance is that weight which will combine with or replace 1 g of hydrogen; a milliequivalent is 1/1000 of an equivalent weight.

Milliequivalents per Liter (mEq/L)

$$mEq/L = \frac{\text{Weight of salt } (g) \times \text{Valence of ion} \times 1000}{\text{Molecular weight of salt}}$$

$$\text{Weight of salt } (g) = \frac{mEq/L \times \text{Molecular weight of salt}}{\text{Valence of ion} \times 1000}$$

APPROXIMATE MILLIEQUIVALENTS— WEIGHTS OF SELECTED IONS

SALT	mEq/g SALT	mg SALT/mEq
Calcium Carbonate [$CaCO_3$]	20.0	50.0
Calcium Chloride [$CaCl_2 \cdot 2H_2O$]	13.6	73.5
Calcium Gluceptate [$Ca(C_7H_{13}O_8)_2$]	4.1	245.2
Calcium Gluconate [$Ca(C_6H_{11}O_7)_2 \cdot H_2O$]	4.5	224.1
Calcium Lactate [$Ca(C_3H_5O_3)_2 \cdot 5H_2O$]	6.5	154.1
Magnesium Gluconate [$Mg(C_6H_{11}O_7)_2 \cdot H_2O$]	4.6	216.3
Magnesium Oxide [MgO]	49.6	20.2

(*continued*)

APPROXIMATE MILLIEQUIVALENTS— WEIGHTS OF SELECTED IONS (continued)

SALT	mEq/g SALT	mg SALT/mEq
Magnesium Sulfate [MgSO₄]	16.6	60.2
Magnesium Sulfate [MgSO₄ · 7H₂O]	8.1	123.2
Potassium Acetate [K(C₂H₃O₂)]	10.2	98.1
Potassium Chloride [KCl]	13.4	74.6
Potassium Citrate [K₃(C₆H₅O₇) · H₂O]	9.2	108.1
Potassium Iodide [KI]	6.0	166.0
Sodium Acetate [Na(C₂H₃O₂)]	12.2	82.0
Sodium Acetate [Na(C₂H₃O₂) · 3H₂O]	7.3	136.1
Sodium Bicarbonate [NaHCO₃]	11.9	84.0
Sodium Chloride [NaCl]	17.1	58.4
Sodium Citrate [Na₃(C₆H₅O₇) · 2H₂O]	10.2	98.0
Sodium Iodide [NaI]	6.7	149.9
Sodium Lactate [Na(C₃H₅O₃)]	8.9	112.1
Zinc Sulfate [ZnSO₄ · 7H₂O]	7.0	143.8

VALENCES AND ATOMIC WEIGHTS OF SELECTED IONS

SUBSTANCE	ELECTROLYTE	VALENCE	MOLECULAR WEIGHT
Calcium	Ca^{++}	2	40.1
Chloride	Cl^-	1	35.5
Magnesium	Mg^{++}	2	24.3
Phosphate (pH = 7.4)	$HPO_4^=$ (80%) $H_2PO_4^-$ (20%)	1.8	96.0*
Potassium	K^+	1	39.1
Sodium	Na^+	1	23.0
Sulfate	$SO_4^=$	2	96.0*

*The molecular weight of phosphorus only is 31; that of sulfur only is 32.1.

■ ANION GAP

The anion gap is the concentration of plasma anions not routinely measured by laboratory screening. It is useful in the evaluation of acid-base disorders. The anion gap is greater with increased plasma concentrations of endogenous (eg, phosphate, sulfate, lactate, ketoacids) or exogenous (eg, salicylate, penicillin, ethylene glycol, ethanol, methanol) species. The formulas for calculating the anion gap follow:

$$(A) \qquad \text{Anion Gap} = (Na^+ + K^+) - (Cl^- + HCO_3^-)$$

or

$$(B) \qquad \text{Anion Gap} = Na^+ - (Cl^- + HCO_3^-)$$

where

the expected normal value for A is 11–20 mmol/L;
the expected normal value for B is 7–16 mmol/L.*

*Note that there is variation at the upper and lower limits of the normal range.

■ TEMPERATURE

Fahrenheit to Centigrade: $(°F - 32) \times 5/9 = °C$
Centigrade to Fahrenheit: $(°C \times 9/5) + 32 = °F$
Centigrade to Kelvin: $°C + 273 = °K$

■ WEIGHTS AND MEASURES

Metric Weight Equivalents

1 kilogram (kg)	=	1000 grams
1 gram (g)	=	1000 milligrams
1 milligram (mg)	=	0.001 gram
1 microgram (mcg, μg)	=	0.001 milligram
1 nanogram (ng)	=	0.001 microgram
1 picogram (pg)	=	0.001 nanogram
1 femtogram (fg)	=	0.001 picogram

Metric Volume Equivalents

1 liter (L)	=	1000 milliliters
1 deciliter (dL)	=	100 milliliters
1 milliliter (mL)	=	0.001 liter
1 microliter (μL)	=	0.001 milliliter
1 nanoliter (nL)	=	0.001 microliter
1 picoliter (pL)	=	0.001 nanoliter
1 femtoliter	=	0.001 picoliter

Apothecary Weight Equivalents

1 scruple (ℨ)	=	20 grains (gr)
60 grains (gr)	=	1 dram (ℨ)
8 drams (ℨ)	=	1 ounce (ℨ)
1 ounce (ℨ)	=	480 grains
12 ounces (ℨ)	=	1 pound (lb)

Apothecary Volume Equivalents

60 minims (m)	=	1 fluidram (fl ʒ)
8 fluidrams (fl ʒ)	=	1 fluid ounce (fl ʒ)
1 fluid ounce (fl ʒ)	=	480 minims
16 fluid ounces (fl ʒ)	=	1 pint (pt)

Avoirdupois Equivalents

1 ounce (oz)	=	437.5 grains
16 ounces (oz)	=	1 pound (lb)

Weight/Volume Equivalents

1 mg/dL	=	10 µg/mL
1 mg/dL	=	1 mg%
1 ppm	=	1 mg/L

Conversion Equivalents

1 gram (g)	=	15.43 grains
1 grain (gr)	=	64.8 milligrams
1 ounce (ʒ)	=	31.1 grams
1 ounce (oz)	=	28.35 grams
1 pound (lb)	=	453.6 grams
1 kilogram (kg)	=	2.2 pounds
1 milliliter (mL)	=	16.23 minims
1 minim (m)	=	0.06 milliliter
1 fluid ounce (fl oz)	=	29.57 mL
1 pint (pt)	=	473.2 mL
0.1 mg	=	1/600 gr
0.12 mg	=	1/500 gr
0.15 mg	=	1/400 gr
0.2 mg	=	1/300 gr
0.3 mg	=	1/200 gr
0.4 mg	=	1/150 gr
0.5 mg	=	1/120 gr
0.6 mg	=	1/100 gr
0.8 mg	=	1/80 gr
1 mg	=	1/65 gr

Anthropometrics 2

■ CREATININE CLEARANCE FORMULAS

FORMULAS FOR ESTIMATING CREATININE CLEARANCE IN PATIENTS WITH STABLE RENAL FUNCTION

Adults [Age 18 Years and Older][1]

$$Cl_{cr} (Males) = \frac{(140 - Age) \times (Weight)}{Cr_s \times 72}$$

$$Cl_{cr} (Females) = 0.85 \times Above\ value*$$

where

Cl_{cr} = creatinine clearance in mL/min
Cl_s = serum creatinine in mg/dL
Age is in years
Weight is in kg.

*Some studies suggest that the predictive accuracy of this formula for women is better *without* the correction factor of 0.85.

Children [Age 1–18 Years][2]

$$Cl_{cr} = \frac{0.48 \times (Height) \times (BSA)}{Cr_s \times 1.73}$$

where

BSA = body surface area in m^2
Cl_{cr} = creatinine clearance in mL/min
Cr_s = serum creatinine in mg/dL
Height is in cm.

FORMULA FOR ESTIMATING CREATININE CLEARANCE FROM A MEASURED URINE COLLECTION

$$Cl_{cr} (mL/min) = \frac{U \times V*}{P \times t}$$

where

U = concentraton of creatinine in a urine specimen (in same units as P)
V = volume of urine in mL

P = concentration of creatinine in serum at the midpoint of the urine collection period (in same units as U)

t = time of the urine collection period in minutes (eg, 6 hr = 360 min; 24 hr = 1440 min).

*The product of U × V equals the production of creatinine during the collection period and, at steady state, should equal 20–25 mg/kg/day ideal body weight (IBW) in males and 15–20 mg/kg/day IBW in females. If it is less than this, inadequate urine collection may have occurred and Cl_{cr} will be underestimated.

■ IDEAL BODY WEIGHT

Ideal body weight (IBW) is the weight expected for a nonobese person of a given height. The IBW formulas below, as well as various life insurance tables, can be used to estimate IBW. Most dosing methods described in the literature utilize IBW as a method in dosing obese patients.

Adults [Age 18 Years and Older][3]

IBW (Males) = 50 + (2.3 × Height in inches over 5 feet)

IBW (Females) = 45.5 + (2.3 × Height in inches over 5 feet)

where IBW is in kg.

Children [Age 1–18 Years][2]
Children Under 5 Feet Tall:

$$IBW = \frac{(Height^2 \times 1.65)}{1000}$$

where

IBW is in kg;
Height is in cm.

Children 5 Feet or Taller:

IBW (Males) = 39 + (2.27 × Height in inches over 5 feet)

IBW (Females) = 42.2 + (2.27 × Height in inches over 5 feet)

where IBW is in kg.

■ SURFACE AREA NOMOGRAMS

Nomograms represent the relationship between height, weight, and surface area in infants and adults. To use a nomogram, a ruler is aligned with the height and weight on the two lateral axes. The point at which the center line is intersected gives the corresponding value for surface area.

NOMOGRAM FOR DETERMINATION OF BODY SURFACE AREA
FROM HEIGHT AND WEIGHT (INFANTS)[4]

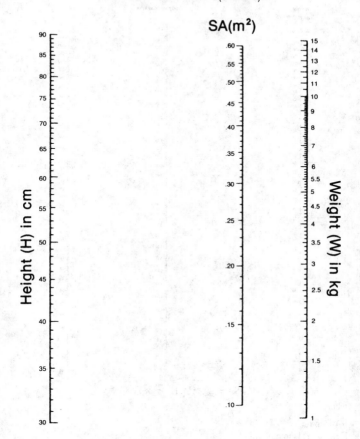

$$SA = W^{0.5378} \times H^{0.3964} \times 0.024265$$

where

SA is in m^2
Height (H) is in cm
Weight (W) is in kg.

Reproduced from reference 4, with permission.

NOMOGRAM FOR DETERMINATION OF BODY SURFACE AREA FROM HEIGHT AND WEIGHT (ADULTS)[5]

$$SA = W^{0.425} \times H^{0.725} \times 71.84$$

where

SA is in m^2
Height (H) is in cm
Weight (W) is in kg.

Reproduced from reference 5, with permission.

REFERENCE

1. Cockcroft DW, Gault MH. Prediction of creatinine clearance from serum creatinine. *Nephron* 1976;16:31–41.
2. Traub SL, Johnson CE. Comparison of methods of estimating creatinine clearance in children. *Am J Hosp Pharm* 1980;37:195–201.
3. Devine BJ. Gentamicin therapy. *Drug Intell Clin Pharm* 1974;8:650–5.
4. Haycock GB et al. Geometric method for measuring body surface area: a height-weight formula validated in infants, children, and adults. *J Pediatr* 1978;93:62–6.
5. DuBois and DuBois. *Arch Intern Med* 1916;17:863.

Pharmacokinetic Equations **3**

James R. Lane, Jr.

Abbreviations used in this appendix:

Alb_{meas} = measured serum albumin
Alb_{nl} = normal serum albumin
α = fraction of drug unbound to albumin
C_{adj} = adjusted serum concentration
C_{des} = desired serum concentration
Cl = serum drug clearance
C_{meas} = measured serum concentration
ΔCp = desired increase in serum concentration
Cp_t = serum concentration at time t
C_{ss} = steady-state serum concentration
$C_{ss\ ave}$ = average steady-state serum concentration
$C_{ss\ max}$ = maximum (peak) steady-state serum concentration
$C_{ss\ min}$ = minimum (trough) steady-state serum concentration
C_{ti} = initial serum concentration
D = dose
F = fraction of dose absorbed
k_0 = infusion rate (dose/t_{inf})
ka = absorption rate constant
kd = elimination rate constant
km = Michaelis–Menten constant in mg/L
S = salt fraction
τ = dosage interval in hours
$t_{1/2}$ = elimination half-life
t_{inf} = duration of infusion
t_{max} = time of peak serum concentration
$t_{max\ ss}$ = time of peak serum concentration at steady state
V_d = apparent volume of distribution
V_m = maximum rate of metabolism in mg/day

■ ONE COMPARTMENT EQUATIONS

$$kd = \frac{Cl}{Vd}$$

$$t_{1/2} = \frac{0.693 \times Vd}{Cl}$$

$$kd = \frac{0.693}{t_{1/2}}$$

$$kd = \frac{\ln (Cp_1 / Cp_2)}{t}$$

Where t = time between serum concentrations Cp_1 and Cp_2.

SINGLE-DOSE EQUATIONS

Concentration at time t (IV bolus):

$$Cp_t = \frac{S \times D}{Vd} \times e^{-kd \times t}$$

Concentration at time t (during IV infusion):

$$Cp_t = \frac{S \times k_0}{Cl} \times (1 - e^{-kd \times t_{inf}})$$

Concentration at time t (after the end of an IV infusion):

$$Cp_t = \frac{S \times k_0}{Cl} \times (1 - e^{-kd \times t_{inf}}) \times e^{(-kd \times [t - t_{inf}])}$$

Concentration at time t (PO or IM):

$$Cp_t = \frac{S \times F \times D \times ka}{Vd \times (ka - kd)} \times (e^{-kd \times t} - e^{-ka \times t})$$

Time to Peak (PO or IM):

$$t_{max} = \frac{\ln (ka/kd)}{ka - kd}$$

Loading Dose (negligible drug loss during administration):

$$LD = \frac{\Delta Cp \times Vd}{S \times F}$$

Loading Dose (IV loading dose when drug is lost during administration):

$$LD = \frac{Cl \times t_{inf} \times (C_{des} - [C_{ti} \times e^{-kd \times t_{inf}}])}{S \times (1 - e^{-kd \times t_{inf}})}$$

Loading Dose (IM or PO):

$$LD = \frac{Vd \times (C_{des} - [C_{ti} \times e^{-kd \times t_{max}}])}{S \times F \times (1 - e^{-kd \times t_{max}})}$$

STEADY-STATE EQUATIONS

Peak Concentration (IV):

$$C_{ss\,max} = S \times k_0 \times \frac{1 - e^{-kd \times t_{inf}}}{Cl \times (1 - e^{-kd \times \tau})}$$

Peak Concentration (PO or IM):

$$C_{ss\,max} = \frac{S \times F \times D \times e^{-kd \times t_{max\,ss}}}{Vd \times (1 - e^{-kd \times \tau})}$$

Trough Concentration (IV):

$$C_{ss\,min} = C_{ss\,max} \times e^{-kd \times (\tau - t_{inf})}$$

Trough Concentration (PO or IM):

$$C_{ss\,min} = \frac{S \times F \times D \times ka}{Vd \times (ka - kd)} \times \left[\frac{e^{-kd \times \tau}}{1 - e^{-kd \times \tau}} - \frac{e^{-ka \times \tau}}{1 - e^{-ka \times \tau}} \right]$$

Average Concentration (IV, PO, or IM):

$$C_{ss\,ave} = \frac{S \times F \times D}{Cl \times \tau}$$

Time to Peak (PO or IM):

$$t_{max\,ss} = \frac{\ln (ka \times [1 - e^{-kd \times \tau}])/[kd \times \{1 - e^{-ka \times \tau}\}]}{ka - kd}$$

Dosage Interval:

$$Interval = T + \frac{[\ln (C_{max}/C_{min})]}{kd}$$

where T = infusion time for IV doses and t_{max} for PO and IM doses.

■ MICHAELIS–MENTEN EQUATIONS

$$\text{Daily Dosage (phenytoin)} = \frac{Vm \times C_{ss\,ave}}{S \times F \times (km + C_{ss\,ave})}$$

$$C_{adj} = \frac{C_{meas}}{\left([1-\alpha] \times \dfrac{Alb_{meas}}{Alb_{nl}}\right) + \alpha}$$

$$C_{ss\,ave} = \frac{S \times F \times Dosage/day \times km}{Vm - (S \times F \times daily\,dosage)}$$

Laboratory Indices 4

Blood, Serum, Plasma Chemistry; Urine, Renal Function Tests; Hematology

William G. Troutman

The following table includes typical reference ranges for clinical laboratory tests in common use. Reference ranges for laboratory tests may vary widely among testing facilities, often as a result of methodologic differences. It is therefore always advisable to obtain reference ranges from the laboratory performing the analyses. Laboratory test results should never be accepted without correct identification of the units of measurement, because most tests can be reported in several systems of measurement. The table presents both conventional and international (usually the same as *Système International,* or SI) units.

The following abbreviations are used to identify the specimen:

(P)	– Plasma
(S)	– Serum
(U)	– Urine
(WB)	– Whole Blood
(WB, art)	– Whole Blood, Arterial

The table begins on page 1022.

BLOOD, SERUM, PLASMA CHEMISTRY

TEST/SPECIMEN	AGE GROUP OR OTHER FACTOR	REFERENCE RANGE	
		Conventional	*International Units*
Acid Phosphatase (S)		0.11–0.60 unit/L	0.11–0.60 unit/L
Alanine Aminotransferase (S)		*units/L*	*units/L*
(ALT, SGPT)	Adult	8–20	8–20
	>60 yr, M	7–24	7–24
	>60 yr, F	7–16	7–16
Alkaline Phosphatase (S)		*units/L*	*units/L*
	Child	20–150	20–150
	Adult	20–70	20–70
	>60 yr	30–75	30–75
Ammonia Nitrogen (S,P)	Adult	15–45 µg/dL	11–32 µmol/L
Amylase (S)		*units/L*	*units/L*
	Adult	25–125	25–125
	>70 yr	20–160	20–160
Anion Gap ($Na^+ - [Cl^- + HCO_3^-]$) (P)		7–16 mEq/L	7–16 mmol/L
Aspartate Aminotransferase (S)		*units/L*	*units/L*
(AST, SGOT)	Adult	8–20	8–20
	>60 yr, M	11–26	11–26
	>60 yr, F	10–20	10–20
Bicarbonate (S)		*mEq/L*	*mmol/L*
	Arterial	21–28	21–28
	Venous	22–29	22–29
(WB, art)	Adult	18–23	18–23
Bilirubin (S)		*mg/dL*	*mmol/L*
Total	Child, Adult	0.2–1.0	3.4–17.1
Conjugated (direct)	Child, Adult	0–0.2	0–3.4
Calcium (S)		*mg/dL*	*µmol/L*
Ionized	Adult	4.48–4.92	1.12–1.23
Total	Child	8.8–10.8	2.20–2.70
	Adult	8.4–10.2	2.10–2.55
Carbon Dioxide, Partial Pressure (WB, art)		*mm Hg*	*kPa*
(pCO_2)	Adult, M	35–48	4.66–6.38
	Adult, F	32–45	4.26–5.99
Chloride (S,P)		98–107 mEq/L	98–107 mmol/L
Cholesterol, Total (S,P)		*mg/dL*	*mmol/L*
	Child	120–200	3.11–5.18
	Adolescent	120–210	3.11–5.44
	Adult	140–310	3.63–8.03
	Desired, Adult	140–220	3.63–5.70
Cortisol (S,P)		*µg/dL*	*nmol/L*
	08:00 hr	5–23	138–635
	16:00 hr	3–15	83–414
	20:00 hr	≤50% of 08:00 hr	≤50% of 08:00 hr

(*continued*)

BLOOD, SERUM, PLASMA CHEMISTRY (continued)

TEST/SPECIMEN	AGE GROUP OR OTHER FACTOR	REFERENCE RANGE	
		Conventional	*International Units*
Creatine Kinase (CK) (S)		*units/L*	*units/L*
	Adult, M	38–174	38–174
	Adult, F	26–140	26–140
Creatinine (S,P)		*mg/dL*	*μmol/L*
	Child	0.3–0.7	27–62
	Adolescent	0.5–1.0	44–88
	Adult, M	0.7–1.3	62–115
	Adult, F	0.6–1.1	53–97
(γ)-Glutamyltransferase (S) (GGT)		*units/L*	*units/L*
	Adult, M	9–50	9–50
	Adult, F	8–40	8–40
Glucose, 2-hr Postprandial (S)		<120 mg/dL	<6.7 mmol/L

Glucose Tolerance Test (S) (Oral)		*mg/dL*		*mmol/L*	
		Normal	Diabetic	Normal	Diabetic
	Fasting	70–105	>140	3.9–5.8	>7.8
	60 min	120–170	≥200	6.7–9.4	≥11.1
	90 min	100–140	≥200	5.6–7.8	≥11.1
	120 min	70–120	≥140	3.9–6.7	≥7.8

TEST/SPECIMEN	AGE GROUP OR OTHER FACTOR	Conventional	International Units
HDL-Cholesterol (S,P)		*mg/dL*	*mmol/L*
	15–19 yr, M	30–65	0.78–1.68
	15–19 yr, F	30–70	0.78–1.81
	20–29 yr, M	30–70	0.78–1.81
	20–29 yr, F	30–75	0.78–1.94
	30–39 yr, M	30–70	0.78–1.81
	30–39 yr, F	30–80	0.78–2.07
	>40 yr, M	30–70	0.78–1.81
	>40 yr, F	30–85	0.78–2.20
	Values for blacks 10 mg/dL higher.		
Iron (S)		*μg/dL*	*mmol/L*
	Child	50–120	8.95–21.48
	Adult, M	65–170	11.64–30.43
	Adult, F	50–170	8.95–30.43
Iron-Binding Capacity, Total (S) (TIBC)		250–450 μg/dL	44.75–80.55 μmol/L
Isocitrate Dehydrogenase (S)		1.2–7.0 units/L	1.2–7.0 units/L
Lactate Dehydrogenase (S)		*units/L*	*units/L*
	Child	60–170	60–170
	Adult	100–190	100–190
	>60 yr	110–210	110–210
Isozymes (S)		*% of Total*	*Fraction of Total*
	Fraction 1	14–26	0.14–0.26
	Fraction 2	29–39	0.29–0.39
	Fraction 3	20–26	0.20–0.26
	Fraction 4	8–16	0.08–0.16
	Fraction 5	6–16	0.06–0.16

(*continued*)

BLOOD, SERUM, PLASMA CHEMISTRY (continued)

TEST/SPECIMEN	AGE GROUP OR OTHER FACTOR	REFERENCE RANGE	
		Conventional	*International Units*
Lead (WB)		*μg/dL*	*μmol/L*
	Child	<15	<0.72
	Adult	<30	<1.45
Lipase (S)		*units/L*	*units/L*
	Adult	10–150	10–150
	>60 yr	18–180	18–180
β-Lipoprotein (LDL) (S)	28–53% of total lipoproteins.		0.28–0.53
Magnesium (S)		*mEq/L*	*mmol/L*
	6–12 yr	1.7–2.1	0.70–0.86
	12–20 yr	1.7–2.2	0.70–0.91
	Adult	1.6–2.6	0.66–1.07
Osmolality (S)		*mOsmol/kg*	*mOsmol/kg*
	Child, Adult	275–295	275–295
	>60 yr	280–301	280–301
Osmolal Gap		≤10	≤10
Measured Osmolality − Calculated Osmolality			
Calculated Osmolality = 2(Na$^+$) + (Glucose/18) + (BUN/2.8)			
Oxygen, Partial Pressure (WB, art)		83–108 mm Hg	11.04–14.36 kPa
(pO$_2$) (Decreases with age and altitude)			
pH (WB, art)		7.35–7.45	7.35–7.45
Phosphorus, Inorganic (S)		*mg/dL*	*mmol/L*
	Child	4.5–5.5	1.45–1.78
	Adult	2.7–4.5	0.87–1.45
	>60 yr, M	2.3–3.7	0.74–1.20
	>60 yr, F	2.8–4.1	0.90–1.32
Potassium (S,P)		*mEq/L*	*mmol/L*
	Child	3.4–4.7	3.4–4.7
	Adult	3.5–5.1	3.5–5.1
Protein, Total (S)		*g/dL*	*g/L*
	Adult		
	Ambulatory	6.4–8.3	64–83
	Recumbent	6.0–7.8	60–78
	>60 yr	lower by 0.2	lower by 2
Albumin	Adult	3.5–5.0	35–50
	>60 yr	3.7–4.7	37–47
Globulins	Adult	2.3–3.5	23–35
Prealbumin	Adult	10–40 mg/dL	100–400 mg/L
Sodium (S,P)		*mEq/L*	*mmol/L*
	Child	138–145	138–145
	Adult	136–146	136–146
Thyroid-Stimulating Hormone (S,P)		*μunits/mL*	*munits/L*
(TSH)	Child	4.5 ± 3.6	4.5 ± 3.6
	Adult	<10	<10
	>60 yr, M	2–7.3	2–7.3
	>60 yr, F	2–16.8	2–16.8

(continued)

BLOOD, SERUM, PLASMA CHEMISTRY (continued)

TEST/SPECIMEN	AGE GROUP OR OTHER FACTOR	REFERENCE RANGE			
		Conventional		International Units	
Thyroxine, Total (S)		*µg/dL*		*nmol/L*	
(T$_4$)	5–10 yr	6.4–13.3		83–172	
	Adult	5–12		65–155	
	>60 yr, M	5–10		65–129	
	>60 yr, F	5.5–10.5		71–135	
	4–9 mo pregnant	6.1–17.6		79–227	
Transferrin (S)		*mg/dL*		*g/L*	
	Adult	220–400		2.20–4.00	
	>60 yr	180–380		1.80–3.80	
Triglycerides (S)		*mg/dL*		*mmol/L*	
		M	F	M	F
	12–15 yr	36–138	41–138	0.41–1.56	0.46–1.56
	16–19 yr	40–163	40–128	0.45–1.84	0.45–1.45
	20–29 yr	44–185	40–128	0.50–2.09	0.45–1.45
	30–39 yr	49–284	38–160	0.55–3.21	0.43–1.81
	40–49 yr	56–298	44–186	0.63–3.37	0.50–2.10
	50–59 yr	62–288	55–247	0.70–3.25	0.62–2.79
	Desired, Adult	40–160	35–135	0.45–1.81	0.40–1.53
Triiodothyronine Resin Uptake (S)		*% of Total*		*Fraction of Total*	
(T$_3$RU)	Adult	24–34		0.24–0.34	
	>60 yr, M	24–32		0.24–0.32	
	>60 yr, F	22–32		0.22–0.32	
Triiodothyronine, Total (S)		*ng/dL*		*nmol/L*	
(T$_3$)	10–15 yr	80–210		1.23–3.23	
	Adult	120–195		1.85–3.00	
	>60 yr, M	105–175		1.62–2.69	
	>60 yr, F	108–205		1.66–3.16	
Urea Nitrogen (S)		*mg/dL*		*mmol/L urea*	
(BUN)	Child	5–18		0.8–3.0	
	Adult	7–18		1.2–3.0	
	>60 yr	8–21		1.3–3.5	
Uric Acid (S)		*mg/dL*		*mmol/L*	
(Uricase Method)	Child	2.0–5.5		0.12–0.32	
	Adult, M	3.5–7.2		0.21–0.42	
	Adult, F	2.6–6.0		0.15–0.35	

URINE, RENAL FUNCTION TESTS

TEST/SPECIMEN	AGE GROUP OR OTHER FACTOR	REFERENCE RANGE	
		Conventional	International Units
Catecholamines, 24-hr (U)		<110 µg	<650 nmol
Creatinine, 24-hr (U)		mg/kg	µmol/kg
	Child	8–22	71–195
	Adolescent	8–30	71–265
	Adult, M	14–26	124–230
	Adult, F	11–20	97–177
	Decreases with age to 10 mg/kg/day at age 90.		
Creatinine Clearance (S, P, and U)		mL/min/1.73 m^2	mL/sec/m^2
	<40 yr, M	97–137	0.93–1.32
	<40 yr, F	88–128	0.85–1.23
	Decreases with age <40 yr.		

Inulin Clearance (S and U)		mL/min/1.73 m^2		mL/sec/m^2	
		M	F	M	F
	20–29 yr	90–174	84–156	0.87–1.68	0.81–1.50
	30–39 yr	88–168	82–150	0.85–1.62	0.79–1.44
	40–49 yr	78–162	82–146	0.75–1.56	0.79–1.41
	50–59 yr	68–152	66–142	0.65–1.46	0.63–1.37
	60–69 yr	57–137	58–130	0.55–1.32	0.56–1.25
	70–79 yr	42–122	45–121	0.40–1.17	0.43–1.17
	80–89 yr	39–105	39–105	0.38–1.01	0.38–1.01

TEST/SPECIMEN	FACTOR	Conventional	International Units
pH (U)		4.5–8	4.5–8
Protein, Total (U)		1–14 mg/dL	10–140 mg/L
	At Rest	50–80 mg/day	50–80 mg/day
Specific Gravity, Random (U)		1.002–1.030	1.002–1.030
Uric Acid, 24-hr (U)		250–750 mg	1.48–4.43 mmol

HEMATOLOGY

TEST/SPECIMEN	AGE GROUP OR OTHER FACTOR	REFERENCE RANGE	
		Conventional	*International Units*
Bleeding time		3–9 min	180–540 sec
Erythrocyte Count (WB)		$\times 10^6/\mu L$	$\times 10^{12}/L$
	M	4.6–6.2	4.6–6.2
	F	4.2–5.4	4.2–5.4
Erythrocyte Indices (WB)			
Mean Corpuscular Volume		80–96 μm^3	80–96 fL
Mean Corpuscular Hemoglobin		27–31 pg	27–31 pg
Erythrocyte Sedimentation Rate (WB)		*mm/hr*	*mm/hr*
	M	1–13	1–13
	F	1–20	1–20
Fibrinogen (P)		200–400 mg/dL	2.00–4.00 g/L
Hematocrit (WB)		*% Packed RBC Volume*	*Volume Fraction*
	6–12 yr	35–45	0.35–0.45
	12–18 yr, M	37–49	0.37–0.49
	12–18 yr, F	36–46	0.36–0.46
	18–49 yr, M	41–53	0.41–0.53
	18–49 yr, F	36–46	0.36–0.46
Hemoglobin (WB)		*g/dL*	*mmol/L*
	6–12 yr	11.5–15.5	1.78–2.40
	12–18 yr, M	13.0–16.0	2.02–2.48
	12–18 yr, F	12.0–16.0	1.86–2.48
	18–49 yr, M	13.5–17.5	2.09–2.71
	18–49 yr, F	12.0–16.0	1.86–2.48
Hemoglobin A$_{1c}$ (WB)		5.3–7.5% of total Hb	0.053–0.075
Leukocyte Count (WB)		$4.5–11 \times 10^3/\mu L$	$4.5–11 \times 10^9/L$
	Segs	31–71%	31–71%
	Bands	0–12%	0–12%
	Lymphocytes	15–50%	15–50%
	Monocytes	0–12%	0–12%
	Eosinophils	0–5%	0–5%
	Basophils	0–2%	0–2%
Absolute Neutrophil Count (ANC)			
ANC = (% Segs + % Bands) × Leukocyte Count			
Partial Thromboplastin Time,			
Activated (WB) (aPTT)		25–37 sec	25–37 sec
Platelets (WB)		$150–440 \times 10^3/\mu L$	$0.15–0.44 \times 10^{12}/L$
Prothrombin Time (WB)		Less than 2-sec deviation from control.	
Reticulocytes (WB)		0.5–1.5% of erythrocytes	0.005–0.015

■ REFERENCES

1. Burtis CA, Ashwood ER, eds. *Tietz textbook of clinical chemistry,* 2nd ed. Philadelphia: WB Saunders; 1994.
2. Henry JB, ed. *Clinical diagnosis and management by laboratory methods,* 18th ed. Philadelphia: WB Saunders; 1991.
3. Preventing lead poisoning in young clildren: a statement by the Centers for Disease Control. 4th Rev. ed. Atlanta: Centers for Disease Control; 1991.
4. Système International (SI) units conversion table for common laboratory tests. *Ann Pharmacother* 1995;29:100–7.
5. Tietz NW, ed. *Clinical guide to laboratory tests,* 2nd ed. Philadelphia: WB Saunders; 1990.
6. Wallach J. *Interpretation of diagnostic tests: a synopsis of laboratory medicine,* 6th ed. Boston: Little, Brown; 1996.

Drug—Laboratory Test Interferences: Blood, Serum, Plasma Chemistry; Urine Tests; Hematology

David G. Dunlop

The following table lists common clinical laboratory tests and drugs that may interfere with those tests. Drugs may interfere with laboratory tests through a pharmaologic or toxic effect, or through actual chemical interference with the testing process. Either effect may lead to an altered value of the laboratory test, resulting in an inappropriate diagnosis or treatment. It is essential that the clinician recognize possible drug–laboratory test interferences and use this information in the overall assessment of a patient's clinical status.

For the purpose of this section, a pharmacologic or toxic effect refers to change in a laboratory test that occurs because of the action of the drug in vivo. The alteration in laboratory value is often expected and reflects a true measure of what is taking place in the body. With a change of this type, the test is interpreted as being accurate even if it falls outside the normal range. Examples are hyperglycemia following corticosteroid administration or electrolyte disturbances after diuretic use. An illustration of a toxic effect is elevated transaminase levels subsequent to an acetaminophen overdose.

An analytical interference differs from a pharmacologic effect, in that the true laboratory value is not measured accurately. The result is inaccurate because of a problem with in vitro laboratory test procedures. The chemical and physical characteristics of a drug may account for the interference. Examples of an analytical interference include cefoxitin mimicking creatinine in a colorimetric assay or fluoride being misread as chloride due to chemical similarities.

This table lists drug interferences with the most common laboratory tests. For detailed information on laboratory tests not covered here, refer to references 1–3 at the end of this section. A drug may interfere with various laboratory tests by different mechanisms. Also, a drug may cause more than one type of interference (eg, a physiologic increase and an analytical decrease). New laboratory procedures and improved assays are being developed at a rapid pace and this information is constantly changing. Therefore, it may be necessary to compare the original citation against the procedures carried out at your laboratory. Refer to the references cited in the table, as well as other relevant sources, to obtain further information about a specific test.

The following abbreviations are used in the table:

(B)   = Blood
(CSF) = Cerebrospinal Fluid
(S)   = Serum
(I)   = Analytical Interference of Drug
(P)   = Pharmacologic/Toxic Effect of Drug

DRUG–LABORATORY TEST INTERFERENCES

TEST	DRUGS THAT MAY AFFECT RESULTS AND CAUSE OF INTERFERENCE
BLOOD, SERUM, PLASMA CHEMISTRY	
Alkaline Phosphatase (S)	*Elevated* by albumin (I), anticonvulsants (P), hepatotoxins (P), ticlopidine (P).[1,3,4]
	Decreased by citrate salts (I), diphosphonates (eg, etidronate) (P), EDTA (I), estrogens (P), fluoride salts (I), vitamin D (P), zinc salts (I). [1,3]
Aminotransferases (ALT [SGPT]/AST [SGOT]) (S)	*Elevated* by acarbose (P), acetaminophen (I,P), ascorbic acid (I), cholinergic drugs (P), danazol (P), dexrazoxane (P), erythromycin (I,P), hepatotoxins (P), HMG-CoA reductase inhibitors (P), IM injections (P), isotretinoin (P), methyldopa (I), narcotics (P), parenteral nutrition (P), salicylate (P), tacrine (P), ticlopidine (P).[1–5]
	Decreased by interferon alfa (P), interferon beta (P), naltrexone (P).[1]
Ammonia (B)	*Elevated* by acetazolamide (P), alcohol (P), ammonium chloride (P), asparaginase (P), barbiturates (P), carbamazepine (P), diuretics (loop, thiazide) (P), divalproex (P), isoniazid (P), parenteral nutrition (P), valproic acid (P).[1,3,6]
	Decreased by cefotaxime (I), kanamycin (oral) (P), lactulose (P), neomycin (oral) (P), potassium salts (P), tetracyclines (P).[1,2,4]
Amylase (S)	*Elevated* by asparaginase (P), chloride salts (I), cholinergic drugs (P), contraceptives (oral, combination) (P), dexrazoxane (P), fluoride salts (I), narcotics (P), pancreatotoxins (P), potassium iodide (P).[1,3,6]
	Decreased by somatostatin (P).[1]
Bilirubin, Total (S)	*Elevated* by ascorbic acid (I), dexrazoxane (P), dextran (I), epinephrine (I), hemolytic agents (P), hepatotoxins (P), isoproterenol (I), levodopa (I), methyldopa (I,P), narcotics (I), nitrofurantoin (I,P), phenazopyridine (diazo reaction) (I), phenelzine (I), propranolol (I), rifampin (I,P), sulfonamides (I), theophylline (I).[1–3,6]

(*continued*)

DRUG–LABORATORY TEST INTERFERENCES (continued)

TEST	DRUGS THAT MAY AFFECT RESULTS AND CAUSE OF INTERFERENCE

BLOOD, SERUM, PLASMA CHEMISTRY

Decreased by barbiturates (especially in newborns) (P), corticosteroids (P), phenazopyridine (colorimetric) (I), pindolol (I), sulfonamides (P).[3,4]

Calcium (S)

Elevated by anabolic steroids (P), androgens (P), calcium salts (P), cefotaxime (I), chlorpropamide (I), contraceptives (oral, combination) (P), diuretics (thiazide) (P), estrogens (P), ferrous salts (I), hydralazine (I), interferons (I), lithium salts (P), magnesium salts (I), progestins (P), tamoxifen (P), thyroid (P), vitamin A (P), vitamin D (P).[1–4,6]

Decreased by acetazolamide (P), albuterol (P), alcohol (P), aldesleukin (P), amifostine (P), asparaginase (P), aspirin (I), calcitonin (P), carbamazepine (P), cisplatin (P), corticosteroids (P), diphosphonates (eg, etidronate) (P), diuretics (loop) (P), EDTA (I), fluoride salts (I,P), foscarnet (P), heparin (I), laxatives (P), magnesium salts (P), phenobarbital (P), phenytoin (P), phosphate salts (P), plicamycin (P), saquinavir (P), sulfisoxazole (I), zalcitabine (P).[1–4,6]

Carbon Dioxide (B)

Elevated by bicarbonate salts (P), diuretics (loop, thiazide) (P), respiratory depressants (P).[1,3]

Decreased by aldesleukin (P), aspirin overdose (P), nephrotoxins (P), theophylline (P).[1,3]

Chloride (S)

Elevated by androgens (P), carbamazepine (P), cefotaxime (I), cholestyramine (P), corticosteroids (by salt retention) (P), cyclosporine (P), diuretics (carbonic anhydrase inhibitor, thiazide—chronically by alkalosis) (P), estrogens (P), guanethidine (P), halides (eg, fluoride salts) (I), lithium salts (P), methyldopa (P), NSAIDs (P), propantheline (I), pyridostigmine (I).[1,3]

Decreased by bicarbonate salts (P), cefotaxime (metabolite) (I), chlorpropamide (P), corticosteroids (by alkalosis) (P), diuretics (loop, thiazide—by acute diuresis) (P), fludrocortisone (by alkalosis) (P), laxatives (long-term use) (P).[1,3]

Cholesterol (S)

[Does not include antilipemics]. *Elevated* by alcohol (P), anabolic steroids (by cholestasis) (P), ascorbic acid (I), aspirin (I), β-adrenergic blockers (P), cefotaxime (I), contraceptives (oral, combination) (P), corticosteroids (I,P), cyclosporine (P), diuretics (thiazide) (P), hepatotoxins (cholestatic effect) (P), isotretinoin (P), mycophenolate (P), phenothiazines (I,P), smoking (P), ticlopidine (P), vitamin A (I), vitamin D (I).[1–4,6]

Decreased by aldesleukin (P), anabolic steroids (by inhibiting synthesis) (P), ascorbic acid (I,P), chlorpropamide (P), estrogens (P), haloperidol (P), heparin (I), hepatotoxins (decreased synthesis) (P), kanamycin (oral) (P),

(continued)

DRUG–LABORATORY TEST INTERFERENCES (continued)

TEST	DRUGS THAT MAY AFFECT RESULTS AND CAUSE OF INTERFERENCE

BLOOD, SERUM, PLASMA CHEMISTRY

	metformin (P), metronidazole (P), neomycin (oral) (P), niacin (P), nitrates (I), penicillamine (I).[1–4,6]
Coombs' [Direct]	*Positive* by cephalosporins (P), chlorpromazine (P), chlorpropamide (P), ethosuximide (P), hemolytic agents (P), hydralazine (P), indomethacin (P), isoniazid (P), levodopa (P), mefenamic acid (P), methyldopa (P), penicillins (P), rifampin (P), quinidine (P), quinine (P), sulfonamides (P), tetracyclines (P).[1,3–5]
Creatine Kinase (S)	*Elevated* by alcohol (chronic) (P), aminocaproic acid (P), cefotaxime (I), clofibrate (P), danazol (P), gemfibrozil (P), HMG-CoA reductase inhibitors (P), IM injections (P), niacin (P), probucol (P), succimer (I).[1,2,4]
Creatinine (S)	*Elevated* by acetohexamide (I), aldesleukin (P), ascorbic acid (I), cephalosporins (Jaffe method) (I,P), cimetidine (P), cyclosporine (P), flucytosine (I), furosemide (I), lactulose (I), levodopa (I), lidocaine (I), lithium salts (P), methyldopa (I), nephrotoxins (P), nitrofurantoin (I), penicillin (I), pentamidine (P), salicylates (P), trimethoprim/sulfamethoxazole (P).[1–4,7]
Glucose (S)	*Elevated* by acetaminophen (SMA 12/60 method) (I), albuterol (P), antidepressants (heterocyclic) (P), ascorbic acid (neocuproin method) (I), asparaginase (P), β-adrenergic blockers (type 1 diabetes) (P), cefotaxime (I), clonidine (P), corticosteroids (P), cyclosporine (P), dextran (I), dextrothyroxine (P), diazoxide (P), diuretics (loop, thiazide) (P), epinephrine (I,P), estrogens (P), glucagon (P), isoniazid (P), levodopa (SMA 12/60 method) (I), lithium salts (P), methyldopa (I), metronidazole (I), mycophenolate (P), niacin (I,P), pentamidine (IV) (P), phenothiazines (P), phenytoin (P), progestins (P), salicylates (acute toxicity) (I,P), somatostatin (P), tacrolimus (P), thiabendazole (P), thyroid (P), zalcitabine (P).[1–4,6]
	Decreased by acetaminophen (GOD-Perid method) (I,P), alcohol (P), anabolic steroids (P), ascorbic acid (GOD-Perid method) (I), β-adrenergic blockers (in type 2 diabetes) (P), clofibrate (P), disopyramide (P), gemfibrozil (P), isoniazid (I), levodopa (glucose oxidase) (I), MAOIs (P), metformin (P), pentamidine (IV) (P), salicylates (acute and long-term toxicity) (P), sulfonamides (P).[1–3,5]
Iron (S)	*Elevated* by cefotaxime (I), chloramphenicol (P), cisplatin (P), citrate salts (I), contraceptives (oral, combination) (P), dexrazoxane (P), estrogens (P), ferrous salts (I), iron dextran (I,P), methyldopa (P), rifampin (I).[1,3,6]
	Decreased by acarbose (P), cholestyramine (P), colchicine (P), deferoxamine (I), heparin (I).[1,3,6]

(continued)

DRUG–LABORATORY TEST INTERFERENCES (continued)

TEST	DRUGS THAT MAY AFFECT RESULTS AND CAUSE OF INTERFERENCE

BLOOD, SERUM, PLASMA CHEMISTRY

Iron-Binding Capacity, Total (S)

Elevated by estrogen (P).[1,3,6]
Decreased by chloramphenicol (P), corticotropin (P).[1,3,6]

Magnesium (S)

Elevated by amiloride (P), calcium salts (I), cefotaxime (I), lithium salts (P), magnesium salts (P).[1,3–5]
Decreased by albuterol (P), alcohol (P), aldesleukin (P), amifostine (P), aminoglycosides (P), amphotericin B (P), calcium salts (I), cefotaxime (I), cisplatin (P), cyclosporine (P), digitalis glycosides (toxic concentrations) (P), diphosphonates (eg, etidronate) (P), diuretics (loop, thiazide) (P), foscarnet (P), insulin (P), phosphate salts (I), tacrolimus (P).[1,3–5]

Osmolality (S)

Elevated by alcohol (ADH suppression) (P), corticosteroids (P), demeclocycline (ADH inhibition) (P), glucose (I), lithium salts (ADH inhibition) (P), mannitol (I,P).[1,4]
Decreased by carbamazepine (P), chlorpropamide (P), vasopressin (P).[1,4]

Phosphorus, Inorganic (S)

Elevated by foscarnet (P), vitamin D (excessive) (P).[1,4]
Decreased by aldesleukin (P), anabolic steroids (P), androgens (P), antacids (phosphate binders) (P), anticonvulsants (P), diphosphonates (eg, etidronate) (P), foscarnet (P), lithium salts (P), mycophenolate (P), parenteral nutrition (P), sucralfate (P).[1,4–6]

Potassium (S)

Elevated by aminocaproic acid (P), ACE inhibitors (P), antineoplastics (cytotoxic effect) (P), β-adrenergic blockers (P), cyclosporine (P), diuretics (potassium-sparing) (P), iodine salts (I), isoniazid (P), lithium salts (P), mannitol (P), mycophenolate (P), nephrotoxins (P), NSAIDs (especially indomethacin) (P), pentamidine (P), potassium penicillin (P), propranolol (P), salt substitutes (P), succinylcholine (P), tacrolimus (P).[1–6]
Decreased by acetazolamide (P), aminoglycosides (P), ammonium chloride (P), amphotericin B (P), bicarbonate salts (P), β-adrenergic agonists (P), corticosteroids (P), diphosphonates (eg, etidronate) (P), diuretics (loop, thiazide) (P), fludrocortisone (P), foscarnet (P), glucose (P), insulin (P), laxatives (P), mycophenolate (P), ondansetron (P), penicillins (extended-spectrum) (P), salicylates (P), saquinavir (P).[1–6]

Protein, Total (S)

Elevated by anabolic steroids (P), corticosteroids (P), heparin (I), phenazopyridine (I).[1–3]
Decreased by estrogens (P), hepatotoxins (P).[1–3]

Protein, Total (CSF)

Elevated by methotrexate (I), penicillins (I), phenothiazines (I), sulfonamides (I), tetracyclines (I).[1–3]
Decreased by cytarabine (I).[1–3]

Sodium (S)

Elevated by anabolic steroids (P), carbamazepine (P), clonidine (P), contraceptives (oral, combination) (P), corticosteroids (P), diazoxide (P), estrogens (P), fludrocortisone (P), methyldopa (P), NSAIDs (P), tetracycline (P).[1,3,6]

(continued)

DRUG–LABORATORY TEST INTERFERENCES (continued)

TEST	DRUGS THAT MAY AFFECT RESULTS AND CAUSE OF INTERFERENCE

BLOOD, SERUM, PLASMA CHEMISTRY

Thyroxine (S)

Decreased by ammonium chloride (P), amphotericin B (P), carbamazepine (P), chlorpropamide (P), diuretics (P), interferons (P), lithium salts (P), sulfonylureas (P), vasopressin and analogues (P), vincristine (P).[1,3,4,6]

Elevated by amiodarone (P), clofibrate (P), contraceptives (oral, combination) (P), estrogens (P), heparin (I), insulin (P), levodopa (P), propranolol (P), radiographic agents (I,P), tamoxifen (P).[1–6]

Decreased by anabolic steroids (P), androgens (P), asparaginase (P), carbamazepine (P), cholestyramine (P), clofibrate (P), corticosteroids (P), danazol (I), heparin (I), iodide (P), lithium salts (P), phenytoin (P), salicylates (P), sulfonamides (P), sulfonylureas (P).[1–4,6]

Triglycerides (S)

Elevated by alcohol (P), β-adrenergic blockers (P), cholestyramine (P), colestipol (P), contraceptives (oral, combination) (P), dexrazoxane (P), diuretics (loop, thiazide) (P), estrogens (P), isotretinoin (P).[2–4,6]

Decreased by ascorbic acid (I,P), asparaginase (P), clofibrate (P), danazol (P), gemfibrozil (P), metformin (P), niacin (P), sulfonylureas (P).[1–4]

Urea Nitrogen (S)

Elevated by acetohexamide (I), aldesleukin (P), anabolic steroids (P), chloral hydrate (I), chloramphenicol (Nesslerization method) (I), dextran (I), diuretics (loop, thiazide) (P), nephrotoxins (P), pentamidine (P), sulfonamides (I), tetracyclines (P).[1,3,4,6]

Decreased by ascorbic acid (I), chloramphenicol (Berthelot method) (I), fluoride salts (I), streptomycin (I).[1,3,4,6]

Uric Acid (S)

Elevated by acetaminophen (I), acetazolamide (P), anabolic steroids (P), androgens (P), antineoplastics (P), ascorbic acid (Bittner method) (I), caffeine (Bittner method) (I), cyclosporine (P), diazoxide (P), diuretics (carbonic anhydrase inhibitor, loop, thiazide) (P), epinephrine (I), ethambutol (P), hydralazine (I), isoniazid (I), levodopa (I,P), methyldopa (I), niacin (P), phenytoin (P), propranolol (P), pyrazinamide (P), rifampin (I), salicylates (low doses) (I,P), spironolactone (P), tacrolimus (P), theophylline (I,P).[2–4,6]

Decreased by acetohexamide (P), allopurinol (P), ascorbic acid (by seralyzer) (I), clofibrate (P), contrast media (iodinated) (P), corticosteroids (P), diflunisal (P), glucose infusions (P), guaifenesin (P), indomethacin (P), levodopa (I), lithium salts (P), methyldopa (I), phenothiazines (P), probenecid (P), salicylates (large doses) (P), sulfinpyrazone (P).[2–4,6]

(continued)

DRUG–LABORATORY TEST INTERFERENCES (continued)

TEST	DRUGS THAT MAY AFFECT RESULTS AND CAUSE OF INTERFERENCE

URINE TESTS

Bilirubin

Elevated by hepatotoxins (P), mefenamic acid (I), phenazopyridine (I), phenothiazines (I,P).[1,6]

Catecholamines

Elevated by acetaminophen (I), alcohol (P), α_1-adrenergic blockers (P), aspirin (I), caffeine (P), chloral hydrate (I), chlorpromazine (I), epinephrine (I), erythromycin (I), hydralazine (I), insulin (P), labetalol (I), levodopa (I), methenamine (I), methyldopa (I), niacin (I), nitroglycerin (P), quinidine (I), reserpine (P), tetracyclines (I,P).[1,2,4,6]

Decreased by α_2-adrenergic blockers (P), bromocriptine (P), clonidine (P), contrast media (iodinated) (I), disulfiram (P), guanethidine (P), methenamine (destroys catecholamines in bladder urine) (P), reserpine (P).[1,2,4]

Creatinine

Elevated by ascorbic acid (I), cephalosporins (except cefotaxime, ceftazidime; Jaffe method) (I), corticosteroids (P), levodopa (I), methyldopa (I), nephrotoxins (P), nitrofurantoin (I).[1,4,6]

Decreased by anabolic steroids (P), androgens (P), cimetidine (P), diuretics (thiazide) (P).[1,4,6]

Glucose

False positive by aminosalicylic acid (copper reduction) (I), ascorbic acid (copper reduction) (I), aspirin (copper reduction) (I,P), cephalosporins (except cefotaxime; copper reduction) (I), chloral hydrate (copper reduction) (I), corticosteroids (P), diuretics (loop, thiazide) (P), ifosfamide (P), levodopa (copper reduction) (I), niacin (P), penicillins (I), phenazopyridine (Tes-Tape) (I), phenothiazines (P).[1–6]

False negative by ascorbic acid (glucose oxidase) (I), bisacodyl (I), chloral hydrate (glucose oxidase) (I), diazepam (I), digoxin (I), ferrous salts (I), levodopa (glucose oxidase) (I), phenazopyridine (glucose oxidase) (I), tetracyclines (I).[1–6]

Gonadotropins (Pregnancy Test)

False positive by phenothiazines (I).[1,6]

Ketones

Elevated by albuterol (P), ifosfamide (I), isoniazid (P), levodopa (Labstix) (I), mesna (P), phenazopyridine (I), phenothiazines (I), salicylates (I), succimer (I).[1,2,4,6]

Protein

Elevated by acetazolamide (I), bicarbonate salts (I), captopril (P), cephalosporins (I), chlorpromazine (I), contrast media (iodinated) (I), diuretics (carbonic anhydrase inhibitor) (I or P), ifosfamide (P), nephrotoxins (P), phenazopyridine (I), salicylates (I), sulfonamides (I), tolbutamide (I).[1,6]

Specific Gravity

Elevated by contrast media (iodinated) (P), dextran (P), sucrose (P).[1,4,6]

Decreased by lithium salts. (P).[1]

(*continued*)

DRUG–LABORATORY TEST INTERFERENCES (continued)

TEST	DRUGS THAT MAY AFFECT RESULTS AND CAUSE OF INTERFERENCE
HEMATOLOGY	
Erythrocyte Sedimentation Rate (B)	*Elevated* by dextran (P), methyldopa (P), methysergide (P), penicillamine (P), theophylline (P), vitamin A (P).[1,6]
	Decreased by corticosteroids (P), gold salts (P), penicillamine (P), quinine (P), salicylates (P), drugs that cause hyperglycemia (P).[1,6]
Prothrombin Time (B)	[Does not include anticoagulants or drugs that potentiate or antagonize them]. *Elevated* by antibiotics (gut steriliz- ing) (P), aspirin (P), cephalosporins (P), chloral hydrate (P), chloramphenicol (P), cholestyramine (P), colestipol (P), cyclophosphamide (P), dexrazoxane (P), hepatotox- ins (P), laxatives (P), mercaptopurine (P), propyl- thiouracil (P), quinidine (P), quinine (P), sulfonamides (P).[1,4,6]
	Decreased by anabolic steroids (P), azathioprine (P), con- traceptives (oral, combination) (P), estrogens (P), vita- min K (P).[1,3,6]

■ REFERENCES

1. Young DS. *Effects of drugs on clinical laboratory tests.* 3rd ed. Washington, DC: AACC Press; 1990, and Sup- plement, 1991.
2. Salway JG ed. *Drug-test interaction handbook.* 1st ed. New York: Raven Press; 1990.
3. Sher PP. Drug interferences with clinical laboratory tests. *Drugs* 1982;24:24–63.
4. McEvoy GK, ed. *AHFS drug information 98.* Bethesda, MD: American Society of Health-System Pharmacists; 1998.
5. Dukes MNG, ed. *Meyler's side effects of drugs,* 13th ed. Amsterdam: Elsevier; 1996.
6. Wallach J. *Interpretation of diagnostic tests: a synopsis of laboratory medicine.* 6th ed. Boston: Little, Brown; 1996.
7. Ducharme MP et al. Drug-induced alterations in serum creatinine concentrations. *Ann Pharmacother* 1993;27:622–33.

Index